New
Medical
Dictionary

Fifth Edition

Compilation edited by

PS Shankar

MD, FRCP (Lond), FAMS, DSc(h.c.Gul), DSc(h.c. NTR)
DSc (h.s RGUHS), DSc(h.c.TU), DLitt(Hampi)

Emeritus Professor of Medicine
Rajiv Gandhi University of Health Sciences
Bengaluru

Oxford & IBH Publishing Co. Pvt. Ltd.

New Delhi

(A Unit of CBS Publishers & Distributors Pvt Ltd **)**

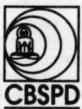

CBSPD

CBS Publishers & Distributors Pvt Ltd

New Delhi • Bengaluru • Chennai • Kochi • Kolkata • Lucknow • Mumbai

Hyderabad • Jharkhand • Nagpur • Patna • Pune • Uttarakhand

New Medical Dictionary

Fifth Edition

ISBN-13: 978-81-204-1788-5
ISBN-10: 81-204-1788-7

© 2016 Copyright Reserved
Previous editions: 2012, 2008, 2004, 2000
Reprint: 2017, 2018, 2019, 2020, 2021, 2022, **2024**

OXFORD & IBH
New Delhi
(A Unit of CBS Publishers & Distributors Pvt Ltd)

Published by **Satish Kumar Jain** and produced by **Varun Jain** for

CBS Publishers & Distributors Pvt Ltd
4819/XI Prahlad Street, 24 Ansari Road, Daryaganj, New Delhi 110 002, India.
Ph: 011-23289259, 23266861   Website: www.cbspd.com
                                e-mail: delhi@cbspd.com

Corporate Office: 204 FIE, Industrial Area, Patparganj, Delhi 110 092
Ph: 011-4934 4934   Fax: 011-4934 4935
                           e-mail: publishing@cbspd.com; publicity@cbspd.com

Branches
- **Bengaluru:** Seema House 2975, 17th Cross, KR Road, Banasankari 2nd Stage, Bengaluru 560 070, Karnataka, India
  Ph: +91-80-26771678/79   Fax: +91-80-26771680   e-mail: bangalore@cbspd.com
- **Chennai:** 7, Subbaraya Street, Shenoy Nagar, Chennai 600 030, Tamil Nadu, India
  Ph: +91-44-26680620, 26681266   Fax: +91-44-42032115   e-mail: chennai@cbspd.com
- **Kochi:** 42/1325, 1326, Power House Road, Opp KSEB, Power House, Ernakulum Kochi 682 018, Kerala, India
  Ph: +91-484-4059061-65,67   Fax: +91-484-4059065   e-mail: kochi@cbspd.com
- **Kolkata:** 147, Hind Ceramics Compound, 1st Floor, Nilgunj Road, Belghoria, Kolkata-700056, West Bengal, India
  Ph: +033-25633055, 033-25633056   e-mail: kolkata@cbspd.com
- **Lucknow:** Basement, Khushnuma Complex, 7 Meerabai Marg (Behind Jawahar Bhawan), Lucknow-226001, UP, India
  Ph: +0522-4000032   e-mail: tiwari.lucknow@cbspd.com
- **Mumbai:** PWD Shed, Gala no 25/26, Ramchandra Bhatt Marg, Next to JJ Hospital Gate no. 2, Opp. Union Bank of India, Noorbaug, Mumbai-400009, Maharashtra, India
  Ph: 022-66661880/89   e-mail: mumbai@cbspd.com

Representatives
Hyderabad	0-9885175004	Jharkhand	0-9811541605	Nagpur	0-8692091830
Patna	0-9334159340	Pune	0-9664372571	Uttarakhand	0-9716462459

Printed at Chaman Enterprises, Daryaganj, New Delhi, India

Preface to the Fifth Edition

The history of medicine is as old as the history of mankind. The practice of medicine has evolved from the days of witchcraft to empirical symptomatic treatment to recent times where we are talking of basics such as life style to evidence-based medicine. The health care system is in a constant state of flux and Medicine is an ever changing field.

There is a continuous quality improvement with new information, new techniques and new technology. The growth and development of the medical science is phenomenal and it has made enormous accomplishments that have bewildered even the most futuristic person. It has brought a sea of changes in understanding of disease, its diagnosis and management. New words are added to the vocabulary. The advances in nano-technology, genetics, oncology, cardiology, computer science and imageology have added many new words in recent years.

New words have been added and the tables have been revised. These additions have been given at the end. Simplicity and preciseness have been maintained while describing the meaning of the words. As in earlier editions, earnest attempt has been made to keep the dictionary concise and complete to provide details of various terms.

I acknowledge the support and help given by my wife Ambikashankar.

September 2015
Kalaburagi

P.S. Shankar

Preface to the Fifth Edition

January, 2015
Allahabad

Preface to the First Edition

There is a tremendous growth in the knowledge of science in general and medical science in particular, in the recent years. This dictionary has been produced to provide a concise and compact guide to medical science terminology.

An attempt has been made to include as many new words as possible in different specialities of medical science. Tables, line diagrams, spelling and pronunciation have been provided. Care has been taken to provided accurate information.

Medical terms are included as main entries or sub-entries. Most of the terms consisting of two (essential tremor), three (transcutaneous oxygen monitor) or four (transcutaneous electrical nerve stimulation) words appear as subentries under the main entry. However there are some exceptions (traveller's diarrhoea tea pot stomach) which appear as main entries because of their importance. The main entry is repeated in the subentries in abbreviated form (e.g. alveolar sac under sac.) The plural form of subentry is indicated by the addition of an 's to the abbreviation of main entry (Curschmann's s's). Adjectives are given at the end of the entry (e.g., sporicide . . . . sporicidal, adj). The plural forms are mentioned against the singular forms (e.g., staphylococcus . . . . pl staphylococci). The pronunciation of words is mentioned in parenthesis immediately after each main entry. e.g., serendipity (ser'endip'i-te).

If the main entry is in the form of abbreviation (UTI) it is expanded immediately after the entry (urinary tract infection).

There are many Western dictionaries available in the country. This work provides a Medical Dictionary which incorporates terms pertinent to India and to the medicine practised. Hence it excludes terms which do not have an occurrence in India. My thanks are to Dr. M. Gopalan for illustrations, Prof. Lalit Mehta for tables and to Mrs. Geeta Kumar, Mrs. Geeta Balvalli and Mrs. Shailaja Dalvi for their secretarial assistance. A large number of medical experts advised on the terms entered in this dictionary. I am grateful to my wife Ambika whose help and support this work could never have been done.

April 2000   **P.S. Shankar**
Mumbai   Editor

Abbreviations

a	artery
adj	adjective
Ayu	Ayurveda
Chi	Chinese
Dent	Dental
ECG	electrocardiogram
Ger	German
Hom	Homoeopathy
Jap	Japanese
n	nerve
pl	plural
pres	Prescription
Psy	Psychiatry
Radiol	Radiology
s	Sanskrit
stat	statistics
	vein

A

α alpha the first letter of Greek alphabet

A symbol for Angstrom unit, alveolar gas, adenosine, the floppy disk drive on a PC

A₂ aortic second sound

a anterior, area, aqua, ampere, accommodation, arterial blood gas

AA abbreviation for amino acids

ab abbreviation for antibody

A band a dark staining area in the middle of a sarcomere in skeletal or cardiac muscle

abarognosis (ab'ar-og-no'sis) loss of ability to appreciate sense of weight

abarthrosis (ab-ar-thro'sis) a moveable joint

abasia (a-ba'ze-a) inability to walk due to impaired co-ordination

abate (a-bat) to lessen or to cease

abatement (a-bat'ment) decrease in severity

ABC sequence the first level of life support measures used in cardiopulmonary resuscitation consisting of airway, breathing and circulation

abdomen (ab-do'men) belly; the portion of the trunk between the pelvis and thorax. It contains lower part of the oesophagus, stomach, small and large intestines, liver, gall bladder, pancreas, spleen and kidney. acute a sudden onset of severe pain in the abdomen requiring surgical intervention pendulous a markedly relaxed anterior wall of the abdomen hanging over the lower part of abdomen scaphoid a hollowed anterior wall of abdomen, making abdomen boat shaped. surgical a acute abdomen. a angina intermittent severe ischaemia resulting in colicky abdominal pain within half an hour after taking food and lasting for an hour or two. Noted when superior and inferior mesenteric and coeliac arteries have atherosclerosis. a apoplexy acute haemoperitoneum.

abdominal (ab-dom'i-nal) pertaining to the abdomen a apron abdominal wall hanging down in front of genitalia in extreme obesity a bath a treatment field in radiotherapy extending from the diaphragm to pelvis , used in treatment of abdominal lymphomas or ovarian carcinoma a cavity the cavity of the abdomen whose interior is lined by peritoneum. It contains most of the organs of the digestive system and the urinary system, and also internal reproductive system a muscle four muscles that make up the abdominal wall such as external oblique, internal oblique, rectus abdominis and transverse abdominis a reflex contraction of the muscles of the abdominal wall on stimulation of the overlying skin a quadrant division of abdomen into nine regions by two horizontal lines one at the level of the ninth costal cartilage and another at the level of the highest point on the iliac crest, and two vertical lines through the centre of the inguinal ligaments on either side. The quadrants so formed are right and left hypochondrium (lateral) and epigastrium (middle); right and left lumbar (lateral) and umbilical (middle) and right and left iliac (lateral) and hypogastrium (middle) a rings the apertures in the abdominal wall, present in the aponeurosis of the external oblique

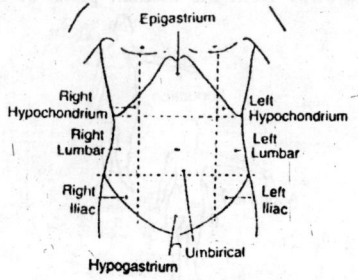

Abdominal quadrants

muscle just above and to the lateral side of the crest of the pubic bone (external), and in the transverse fossa midway between the anterior superior iliac spine and the pubic symphysis 1.3 cm above the inguinal ligament (internal)

abdominocentesis (ab-dom'i-no-sen-te'sis) abdominal paracentesis, puncture of the abdomen with a trocar to remove fluid from the abdominal cavity through the cannula

abdominocyesis (ab-dom'in-o-si-es'is) abdominal pregnancy

abdominohysterectomy (-his'ter-ek'ta-me) removal of the uterus through abdominal incision

abdominoperineal pertaining to the abdomen and perineal region

abdominoscopy (ab-dom'i-nos'ko-pe) examination of the abdominal cavity and its contents by the use of an endoscope; peritoneoscopy

abdominothoracic (ab-dom'i-no-tho-ra'sik) pertaining to the abdomen and thorax **a arch** the costal arch

abducens (ab-du'sens) drawing away from the midline of the body **a muscle** lateral rectus muscle of the eye that moves the eye ball outwards **a nerve** the sixth cranial nerve supplying lateral rectus muscle

abducent (ab-du'sent) drawing away

abduct (ab-dukt) to draw away from the median plane of the body

abduction (ab-duk'shun) lateral movement away from the median plane of the

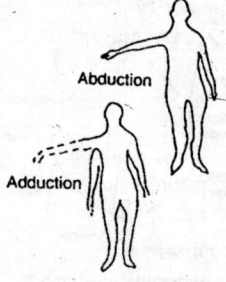

Abduction and Adduction

body or the axial line of an extremity.

abductor (ab-duk'tor) a muscle that on contraction draws the part away from the median plane of the body or the axial line of an extremity

aberrant (ab-er'ant) 1. deviating from the normal 2. wandering off. Certain ducts, vessels or nerves taking an unusual course

aberration (ab-er-a'shun) 1. deviation from the normal 2. imperfect refraction of light rays 3. deviant development

abeyance (a-be'ans) a temporary suspension of activity

ABG abbreviation for arterial blood gases

abhraka (s) mica

ability capability to undertake a given task

abiosis (ab-e-o'sis) absence of life

abiotrophy (ab-e-ot'ro-fe) premature degeneration of tissues and cells

ablate (ab-lat) 1. to remove 2. to destroy the function

ablation (ab-la'shun) removal or destruction of a part

ablepsia (a-blep'se-a) blindness

ablution (ab-lu'shun) a cleansing or washing

abnormal (ab-nor'mal) deviating from the normal

abnormality (ab'nor-mal'i-te) deviation from the normal

ABO blood groups the major classification of human blood into 4 groups - A, B, AB and O - based on the presence or absence of specific proteins on red blood cells

abocclusion (ab'o-kloo'zhun) teeth of upper and lower jaw not in contact

aboral (ab-o-ral) away from the mouth

abort (a-bort) 1. to expel an embryo or foetus prior to viability 2. to arrest the progress of disease 3. to arrest in growth or development

abortifacient (a-bor-ti-fa'shent) any drug or measure used to induce abortion

abortion (a-bor'shun) termination of pregnancy before the foetus is capable of maintaining an independent existence. The foetus is not viable until the seventh calendar month. **complete a** an abortion in which all products of conception are expelled **criminal a** induction of abortion without any clear medical indications **habitual a** three or more consecutive spontaneous abortions **imminent a** impending abortion characterised by bleeding and pain, with effaced and patulous cervix **incomplete a** an abortion in which some portion of the placenta or of the embryo has been retained in the uterus **induced a** termination of pregnancy before the foetus is viable **inevitable a** an abortion in which the ovum has been detached and felt in the cervix or there is escape of amniotic fluid and the process of abortion cannot be arrested **missed a** death of foetus before completion of 20 weeks of gestation and retention of the products of conception for a variable time **saline a** termination of pregnancy during the second trimester by replacing 200 ml amniotic fluid with 200 ml of 20% saline solution stimulating uterine contractions. **septic a** abortion in which there is an infection of uterine contents **spontaneous a** abortion without any apparent cause **therapeutic a** performance of abortion when the continuance of pregnancy would involve risk to the life or to the physical and mental health of pregnant woman or when the foetus has a known condition incompatible with life **threatened a** haemorrhage during early pregnancy unaccompanied by pain or dilatation of the cervix **tubal a** detachment of the ovum from its base and expulsion through the abdominal ostium

abortive (a-bor'tiv) 1. preventing the completion of some thing 2. that which prevents continuation of pregnancy

ABPA abbreviation for allergic bronchopulmonary aspergillosis

abrachia (a-bra'kia) congenital absence of arms

abrade (a-brad) to roughen or remove by friction

Abrams box a diagnostic instrument to determine a patient's electromagnetic radiation or biocurrents, named after Albert Abrams, the American neurologist

abrasion (a-bra'zhun) scraping away of skin or mucosa

abrasive producing abrasion

abreaction (ab're-ac-shun) recollection of repressed memories and the release of and from the emotions that are associated with experiences buried in the unconscious

abruptio (a-brup'she-o) tearing away **a placentae** premature detachment of a normally situated placenta after 20th week of gestation

abscess (ab-ses) a localised collection of pus in any part of the body as a result of infection by pyogenic organisms **alveolar a** abscess in dentoalveolar process **amoebic a** liquefactive necrosis of liver or organs containing amoebae **appendicular a** an intraperitoneal abscess resulting from extension of infection in appendicitis, especially with perforation of the appendix. **Brodie's a** deep seated bony swelling from chronic osteomyelitis situated near a joint named after Sir Benjamin-Brodie, London surgeon. **cold a** an abscess without usual signs of inflammation **collarstud a** a cystic swelling in the neck that has connection with tuberculous lymphadenitis. The diseased node(s) beneath the cervical fascia being connected by a small opening in the fascia to a more superficially placed 'cold' abscess. Similar abscess may be seen in localised cellulitis of the fingers or hand **cryptic a** abscess in crypts of Lieberkuhn of large intestinal mucosa as in ulcerative colitis **dental a** abscess with foetor, local tenderness and some degree of trismus **diffuse a** a collection of pus not circumscribed by a well defined capsule **ischiorectal a** a redness and swelling between the anal verge and the ischiorectal tuberosity **lung a** a localised collection of pus in the parenchyma of the lung as a result of tissue necrosis and suppuration from a pyogenic infection **perforating a** an abscess that breaks down tissue barriers to enter adjacent areas **peritonsillar a** extension of tonsillar infection beyond the capsule with abscess formation; quinsy **popleteal a** abscess in popleteal space which is often deep seated, giving slight fullness of the space. The patient inclines to keep the knee joint somewhat flexed and full extension causes pain **Potts' a** tuberculous abscess of the spine **psoas a** an abscess usually tuberculous originating in tuberculous spondylitis and extending through iliopsoas muscle to the inguinal region. **pyaemic a** abscess resulting from pyaemia, septicaemia or bacteraemia **ring a** an acute purulent corneal inflammation wherein a central necrotic area is surrounded by an annular girdle of leucocytic infiltration **satellite a** an abscess having relation to a parent abscess. **stellate a** a starshaped necrotic area surrounded by epitheloid cells in the enlarged glands in lymphogranuloma venereum. **stitch a** an abscess around a stitch or suture **tropical a** amoebic abscess **tuberculous a** an abscess caused by tubercle bacilli. **wandering a** an abscess occurring at a distance from the primary focus of a disease, and pus burrows along fascial planes

abscissa (ab-sis'a) the horizontal line or axis in a graph of a two-dimensional coordinate system

abscission (ab-si'shun) removal by excision

absence (ab'senz) brief temporary loss of consciousness **a seizure** seizure in which there is loss of consciousness over a brief period characterised by blank facial expression; petit mal seizures

absolute complete **a alcohol** ethyl alcohol with not more than 1% of water by weight **a scale** temperature scale in which zero is at the point of absolute zero, that is the lowest possible temperature **a temperature** temperature measured on the absolute scale

absorb (ab-sorb) 1. to take in by absorption 2. to reduce the intensity of light

absorbance (ab-sor'bans) the ability of a tissue to absorb radiation

absorbefacient (ab-sor'be-fa'shent) an agent that causes absorption

absorbent (ab-sor'bent) a substance that absorbs

absorption (ab-sorp'shun) 1. taking up of liquids by solids or of gases by solids or liquids 2. removal of antibody from serum by addition of an antigen or removal of an antigen by addition of an antibody

abstinence (ab'sti-nens) going without something voluntarily such as refraining from alcoholic beverages or sexual intercourse

abstract (ab'strakt) 1. summary of an article 2. a concentrated drug mixed with lactose

abstraction (ab-strak-shun) 1.distillation of a volatile constituent from a mixture 2. exclusive mental concentration 3. malocclusion of teeth. 4. the process of selection of a certain aspect of a concept from the whole

abulia (a-bu'li-a) loss or impaired ability to perform voluntary actions or to make decisions

abuse (a-bus) 1. misuse, excessive use 2. injurious, harmful

abutment (a-but'ment) the tooth to which a partial denture is anchored.

abhakta (s) on empty stomach

a.c. antecibum, before food

acacia (a-ka'she-a) a dried gummy exudate from *Acacia calculare* that is used as a suspending agent in pharmaceutical products.

acalculia (a-kal-ku'li-a) a form of aphasia with an inability to do mathematical calculations.

acantha (a-kan'tha) spine or spinous process

acanthesthesia (a-kan'thes-the-ze-a) a form of parasthesia, in which there is a sensation of a pin prick.

acanthion the tip of the anterior nasal spine

acanthocyte (a-kan'tho-sit) protoplasmic projections on an abnormal red blood cell which gives an impression of being covered with thorns.

acanthocytosis (a-kan'tho-si-to'sis) presence of acanthocytes in the blood, a feature of a betalipoproteinaemia

acanthokeratodermia (a-kan'tho-ker'a-to-der'me-a) hypertrophy of the horny portion of the skin of the palms of the hands and soles of the feet

acantholysis (a-kan-thol'i-sis) any disease of skin exhibiting degeneration of the horny layers of the skin

acanthoma (ak'an-tho'ma) a benign tumour of the skin with hypertrophy of epidermal squamous cells

acanthosis (ak'an-tho'sis) increased thickness of the prickle cell layer of the skin **a nigricans** hyperpigmented, hyperkeratotic growth on the skin flexures as a skin manifestation of internal malignancy

acapnia (a-kap'ne-a) absence of carbon dioxide in the blood

acarbia (a-kar'be-a) decreased level of bicarbonate in the blood

acardia (a-kar'de-a) congenital absence of the heart

acariasis (ak'a-ria-sis) any disease caused by an infestation with a burrowing mite, *Sarcoptes scabei*

acaricide (a-kar'i-sid) an agent that destroys acarids

acaridae (ak'a-ri'de) a family of mites that irritate the skin

acarina (ak'a-ri'na) ectoparasites such as mites or ticks, which act as vectors of diseases

acarodermatitis (ak'a-ro-der'ma-ti'tis) inflammation of the skin caused by a mite

acarophobia (ak'a-ro-fo'be-a) morbid fear of small parasites, small particles or of itching

acarus (ak'ar-us) a genus of mites

acaryote (a-kar-e-ot) without a nucleus

acatalasia (a'kat-a-la'ze-a) a rare inherited disorder marked by the absence of enzyme, catalase. It makes the gingival and oral tissues to be susceptible to bacterial infection leading to gangrene and destruction of alveolar bone

acatamathesia (a-kat-a-ma-the'zea) loss of faculty of understanding

acataphasia (a-kat'a-fa'ze-a) loss of power to correctly formulate a statement

acathesia (a'ka-thiz'e-a) an inability to sit down with restlessness and muscular quivering , may occur as a complication of treatment with phenothiazine group of drugs

acathexia (a-ka-theks'ia) abnormal body secretions

acathexis (a-ka-theks'is) a mental disorder where certain objects or ideals fail to arouse an emotional response

acceleration (ak-sel'er-a'shun) 1. an increase in the speed of action or function. 2. the rate of change in velocity for a given unit of time. **a deceleration injury** any injury caused when the body abruptly comes to a halt and the internal organs collide with each other inside the body **a injury** head injury that occurs when a moving object hits the head remaining stationary

accelerator (ak-sel'er-a'tor) anything that increases action or function. **linear a** a device which produces high energy photons for use in radiation therapy

acceptor (ak-sep'tor) a compound that will take up a chemical group from another compound

accessory (ak-ses'o-re) supplementary, auxiliary **a cell** a macrophage that aids in immune recognition by binding circulating antigens **a nerve** eleventh cranial nerve **a nipple** supernumerary nipple

accident (ak'si-dent) 1. a mishap 2. an unexpected complicating event **cerebrovascular a** cerebral arterial disease may present as an acute focal stroke by sudden appearance of a focal deficit of brain function. Other presentations are due to cerebral infarction from thromboembolic disease secondary to atherosclerosis in carotid artery and aortic arch or intracerebral or subarachnoid haemorrhage

acclimatization (ak-li-ma-ti-za'shun) the act of getting to a different environment or altitude

acclimatize (ak-kli-ma-tiz) to become accustomed to a different environment

accommodation (a-kom'o-da'shun) adaptation or adjustment **a reflex** constriction of the ciliary muscles causing contraction of the pupil and convergence of eyes in accommodation to a near vision.

accoucheur (a-koo-shur) an obstetrician

accreditation a process of recognition of an institute or a hospital. facility

accretion (a-kre'shun) 1. accumulation 2. the growing together of similar parts 3. accumulation of foreign material on the surface of tooth or in a cavity

ACE abbreviation for angiotensin converting enzyme. **ACE inhibitors** agents that inhibit the conversion of angiotensin I to angiotensin II, used in the treatment of moderate-to-severe hypertension, diabetic nephropathy and heart failure

acedia (a-se'de-a) a state of indifference, lack of energy or emotion

acellular not containing cells

acenaesthesia (a-sen-es-the'zi-a) 1. absence of normal sensation of physical existence 2. absence of consciousness of visceral activity

acentric (a-sen'trik) 1. not central 2. a chromosome without a centromere

acephalia (a-se-fa'le-a) congenital absence of the head

acetabular (as'e-tab'ular) pertaining to the acetabulum

acetabulum (as'e-tab'u-lum) a cup-shaped depression on the lateral surface of the innominate bone (hip bone) that provides the socket into which the head of the femur rotates

acetaldehyde (as'et-al'de-hid) an interme-

diate in yeast fermentation and alcohol metabolism

acetaminophen (a-set'a-min'o-fen) a sy..thetic preparation having antipyretic and analgesic properties.

acetazolamide (as'et-a-zol'a-mid) a drug that inhibits the enzyme carbonic anhydrase, used as a diuretic and to reduce raised intraocular tension

acetic (a-se'tik) acid characteristic compound of vinegar. **diluted aa** contains 6% W/V of acetic acid. **glacial aa** contains 99% absolute acetic acid

acetoacetic acid a ketone body formed in excess and appearing in urine in starvation or diabetic ketoacidosis

acetoacetyl coenzyme an intermediate in the oxidation of fatty acids

acetobactor (a-se'to-bak-ter) a genus of nonpathogenic bacteria of the family of pseudomonadaceae

acetohexamide (as'e-to-heks'a-mid) an oral hypoglycaemic agent that stimulates pancreatic insulin secretion useful in the treatment of type 2 diabetes

acetone (as'e-ton) dimethyl ketone having a sweet fruity odour. It is produced when fats are not properly oxidised as in diabetes and after prolonged fasting. **a body** ketone body

acetonaemia (as'e-to-ne'me-a) presence of excess amounts of acetone in the blood.

acetonuria (as'e-to-nu're-a) presence of acetone bodies in the urine

acetowhite lesions white condylomatous lesions of the uterine cervix exhibiting hyperkeratosis

acetylation (a-set'i-la-shun) the introduction of one or more acetyl groups into an organic compound

acetylcholine (as'e-til-ko'len) ACh a choline ester that acts as a neurotransmitter at neuromuscular junction in the parasympathetic nervous system and sympathetic paraganglionic fibres (cholinergic fibres) It is inactivated by the enzyme cholinesterase

acetylcholinesterase (as'e-til-ko

AChE an enzyme that inactivates the action of acetylcholine

acetylcysteine (as'e-til-sis'te-in) a mucolytic agent

acetylsalicylic (a-se'til-sal'i-sil'ik) **acid** aspirin

acetyltransferase (as'e-til-trans'fer-as) enzyme capable of transferring an acetyl group from one compound to another

ACh abbreviation for acetyl choline

achalasia (ak'a-la'ze-a) failure to relax. **a of the cardia** failure of the cardia (lower oesophageal) sphincter to relax restricting the passage of food to the stomach

achara (s) regimen

AChE abbreaviation for acetylcholinesterase

ache (ak) a persistent fixed pain

achetana (s) inert

achilles (a-kil'ez) the strong tendon connecting gastrocnemius and soleus muscles to the heel named after Achilles, hero of Iliad whose vulnerable spot was his heel.

achlorhydria (a'kolr-hi'dre-a) absence of free hydrochloric acid in the stomach

achloropsia (a-klo-rop'se-a) colour blindness with an inability to recognise green colour

acholuria (a-ko-lu're-a) absence of bile pigments in the urine

achondrogenesis (a-kon'dro-jen'e-sis) failure of bone to grow especially those of the extremities

achondroplasia (a-kon'dro-pla'se-a) a genetic disorder characterised by short stature and disproportionately short limbs but normal trunk

achoo (a-koo) **syndrome** sneezing upon passing from dark to bright light; photic sneeze

achroma (a-kro'ma) absence of colour or pigmentation as in leucoderma, vitiligo and albinism.

achromasia (ak'ro-me'ze-a) 1. absence of normal pigmentation of the skin 2. inability of tissues or cells to be stained

achromate (a-kro'mat) colour blind

achromatic (ak'ro-mat'ik) 1. colourless 2. not containing chromatin 3. difficult to stain 4 non dispersion of light into

constituent components

achromatin (a-kro'ma-tin) the weakly staining substance of a cell nucleus

achromatism (a-kro'ma-tizm) colourlessness

achromia (a-kro'me-a) 1. absence of colour or pallor 2. lack of capacity to accept stains in cells or tissues

achylia (a-ki'le-a) absence of chyle **a gastrica** absence or decrease in secretion of gastric juice **a pancreatica** absence or decrease in pancreatic secretion

achylous (a-ki'lus) lacking digestive secretion

acicular (a-sik'u-lar) needle-shaped **acid a** substance that liberates hydrogen ions (protons) in solution

acid-base balance the pH of the extracellular fluid is maintained at about 7.4 despite production of upto 100mmol of hydrogen ions each day by the average adult. Homeostasis is maintained by short-term mechanisms in the form of buffers involving bicarbonate and phosphate system and haemoglobin and long term compensation involving the kidney and normal lung function

acidaemia (as-i-de'me-a) an increase in the hydrogen ion concentration or a fall in pH below normal

acid-fast not decolourised easily by acid-alcohol after staining as acid-fast bacteria, classic example being *Mycobacterium tuberculosis.*

acidification (a-sidi-fi-ka'shun) conversion into an acid

acidifier (a-sid'i-fi'er) a substance that causes acidity

acidity (a-sid'i-te) 1. possession of hydrogen ions (protons) 2. sourness

acid mucosubstrate a polymer of glucose and amino groups such as mucopolysaccharides, glycosaminoglycans that takes a stain in acid medium

acidophil (a-sid'o-fil) 1. acidophilic 2. an acid-staining cell of the anterior pituitary 3. a bacteria growing well in an acid medium

acidophilic (a-sid'o-fil'ik) 1. having affinity to acid 2. pertaining to a cell capable of being stained by acid dyes.

acidosis (as'i-do'sis) a state of increased acid content of the blood

acid phosphatase an enzyme that liberates inorganic phosphate from phosphoric esters with an optimum pH of 5.4 and is present in the prostate gland

acid poisoning ingestion of a toxic acid

acid reflux disorder a condition produced by entry of acid contents of the stomach to the oesophagus

aciduria (as-id-u're-a) passage of excess amount of acid in the urine

aciduric (as'i-du'rik) capable of growth in an acid medium

acinar (as'i-nar) pertaining to an acinus

acinetobacter (as'i-net'o-bak'ter) a gram-negative coccobacillus found in fresh water and soil, and is a skin and throat commensal in humans, can cause noscomial infection in intensive care setting

acini (as-i-ni) pl. of acinus

acinitis (as'i-ni-tis) inflammation of glandular acini

acinous (as'i-nus) pertaining to glanas resembling a bunch of grapes

acinus (as'i-nus) 1. the smallest division of a gland 2. the basic respiratory unit of pulmonary tissue taking part in gas exchange. It is the portion of the lung distal to and supplied by a single terminal bronchiole. It includes several generations of respiratory bronchioles, alveolar ducts and alveolar sacs. Alveoli project from them

ACLS abbreviation for advanced cardiac life support

acme (ak'me) 1. peak 2. the time of maximum intensity of a symptom 3. greatest muscle tension noted in a segment of uterine labour contraction

acne (ak'ne) an inflammatory follicular, papular and pustular eruption involving the sebaceous apparatus **a conglobata** a chronic disease characterised by presence of comedones, papules, nodules, cysts and severe scarring on chest, shoulders, back and nape of the neck, found in men during late puberty. **a excoriae** acne associated with extensive excoriations, seen in young females **a neonatorum** acne on the nose and cheek in newborns around 3 months, mostly males. **a vulgaris** common during adolescence, characterised by comedones, papules, pustules, nodules and cysts on face. There is increase in size of sebaceous glands and increased secretion of sebum with inflammatory changes. **drug a** acneiform lesions from drugs such as corticosteroids, phenytoin. **occupational a** exposure to oils and tars among workers producing acne at site of contact with the skin. **tropical a** variant of acne with large painful cysts, nodules and pustules leading to scarring and seen on the back, nape of neck, buttocks, thighs and arms

acnegenic (ak'ne-jen'ik) causing acne

acneiform (ak-ne'i-form) resembling acne

aconite (ak'o-nit) a powerful alkaloid from the root of Aconitum

acorea (a-ko-re'a) absence of the pupil of the eye

acousia (a-koo'ze-a) the hearing faculty

acoustic (a-koos'tik) pertaining to sound or to sense of hearing **a meatus** the opening of the auditory canal **a nerve** *see* vestibulocochlear nerve **a reflexometry** a procedure to measure the level of sound transmitted and reflected from the middle ear **a reflex threshold** a test for measurement of the intensity of a sound at which stapedius muscle contracts **a trauma** injury to hearing by loud noise

acoustics (a-koos'tiks) the science of sound, its production, transmission and effects.

acquired (a-kwird) developed as a result of factors acting from outside. **a immunodeficiency syndrome** AIDS an infection with the human immunodeficiency virus (HIV-1 and HIV 2) resulting in the development of AIDS. The infection is transmitted by sexual, perinatal and parenteral route. HIV in-

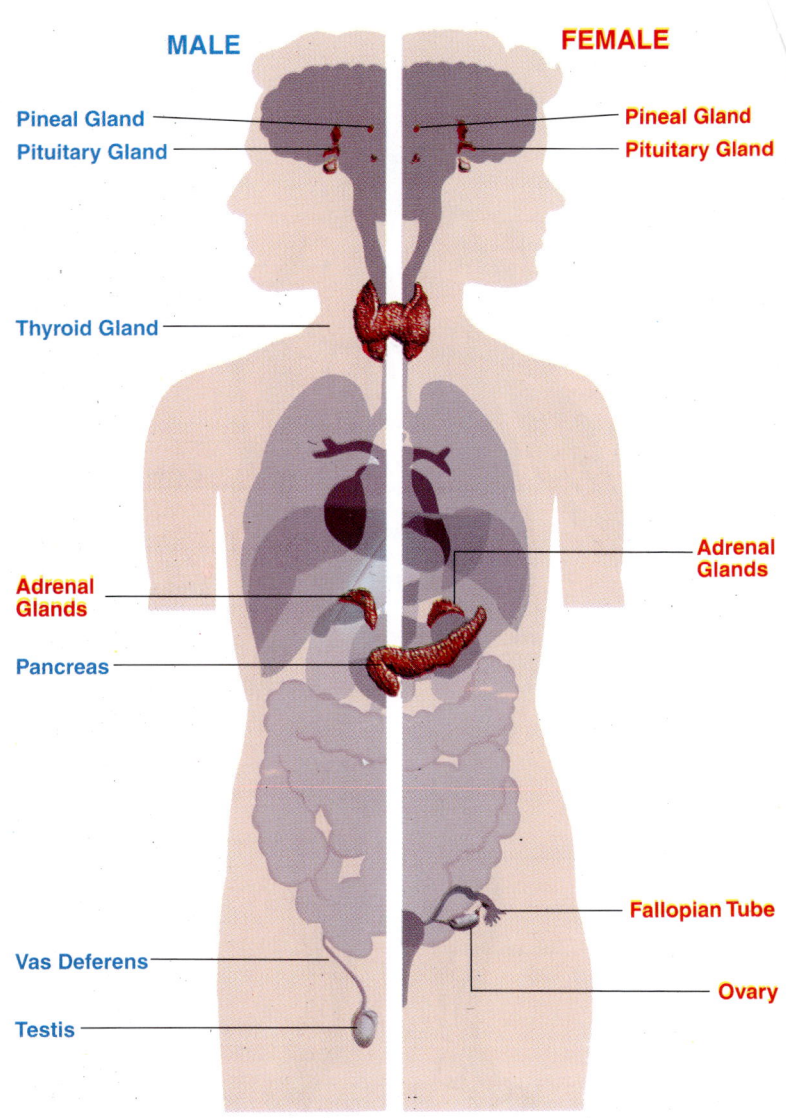

MALE

FEMALE

Pineal Gland

Pituitary Gland

Pineal Gland

Pituitary Gland

Thyroid Gland

Adrenal
Glands

Adrenal
Glands

Pancreas

Fallopian Tube

Vas Deferens

Ovary

Testis

Endocrine System

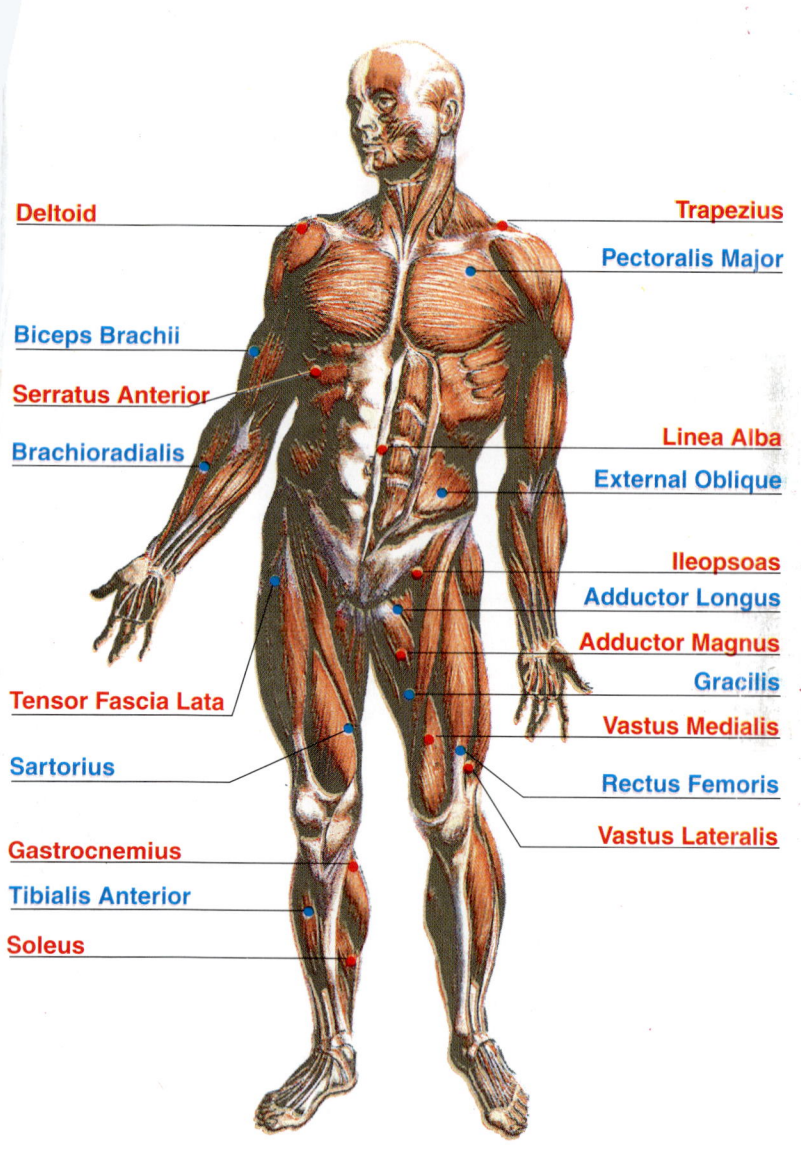

Deltoid

Trapezius

Pectoralis Major

Biceps Brachii

Serratus Anterior

Brachioradialis

Linea Alba

External Oblique

Ileopsoas

Adductor Longus

Adductor Magnus

Gracilis

Tensor Fascia Lata

Vastus Medialis

Sartorius

Rectus Femoris

Vastus Lateralis

Gastrocnemius

Tibialis Anterior

Soleus

Muscular System

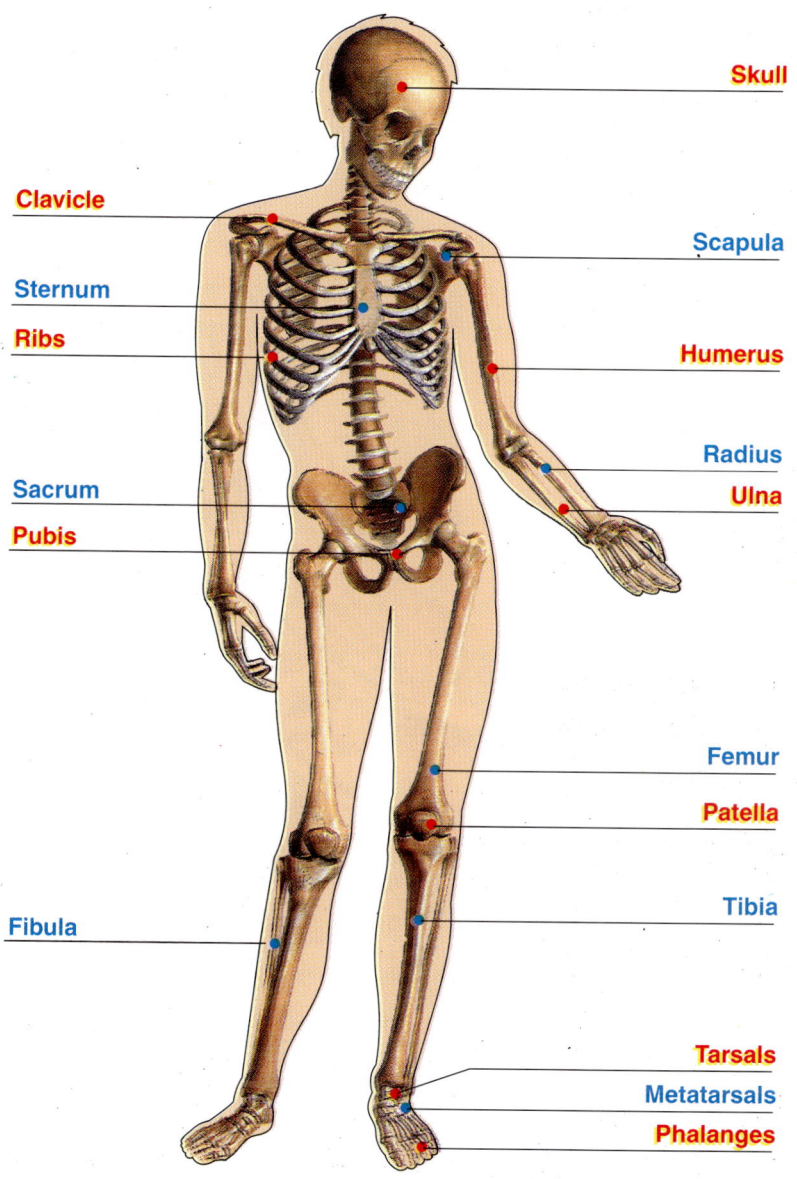

Skull

Clavicle

Scapula

Sternum

Ribs

Humerus

Radius

Sacrum

Ulna

Pubis

Femur

Patella

Tibia

Fibula

Tarsals

Metatarsals

Phalanges

Skeletal System

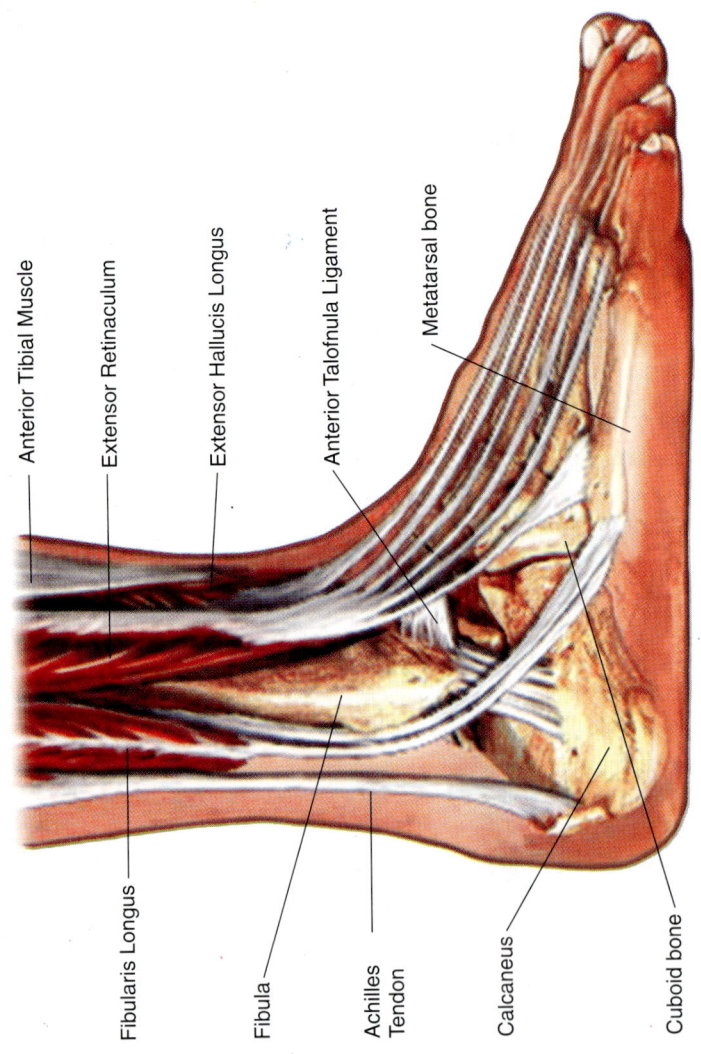

Anterior Tibial Muscle

Extensor Retinaculum

Extensor Hallucis Longus

Anterior Talofnula Ligament

Metatarsal bone

Fibularis Longus

Fibula

Achilles Tendon

Calcaneus

Cuboid bone

Foot

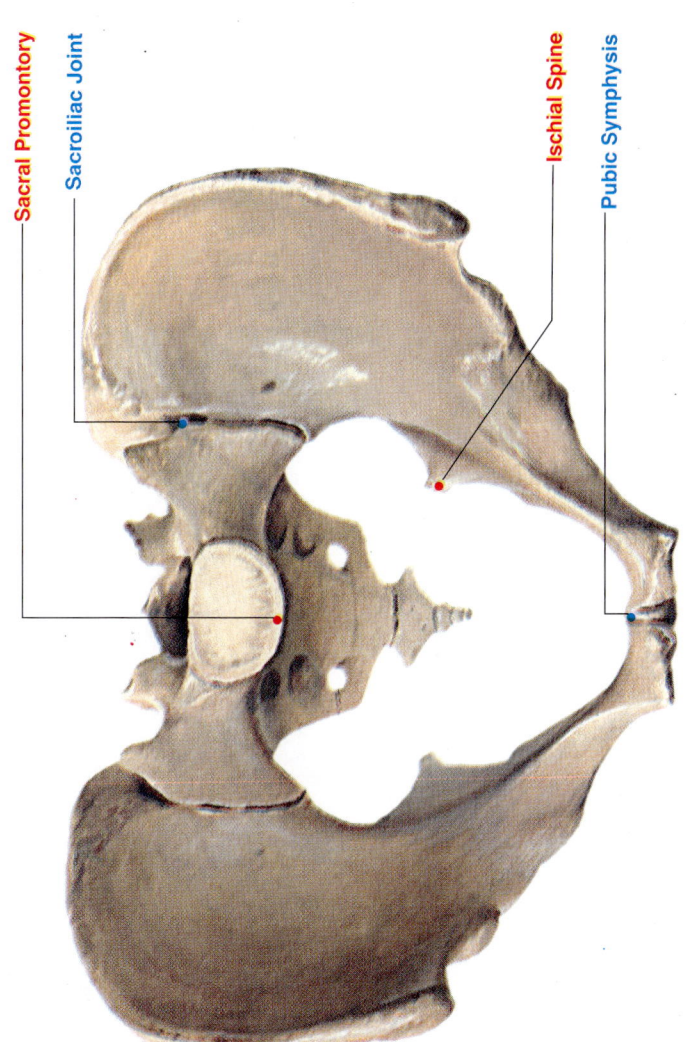

Sacral Promontory

Sacroiliac Joint

Ischial Spine

Pubic Symphysis

Pelvic Inlet-Anterior View

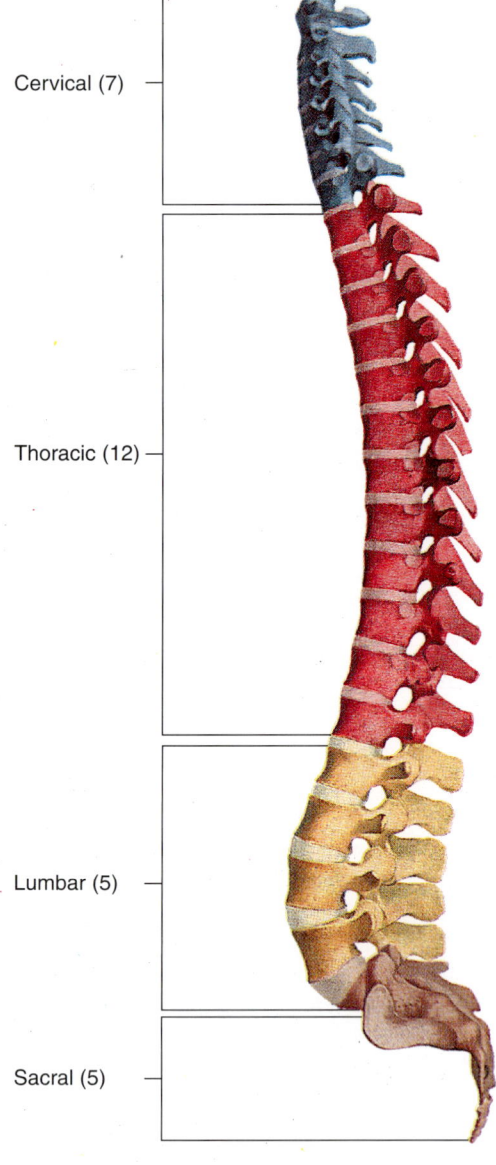

Cervical (7)

Thoracic (12)

Lumbar (5)

Sacral (5)

Vertebral Column

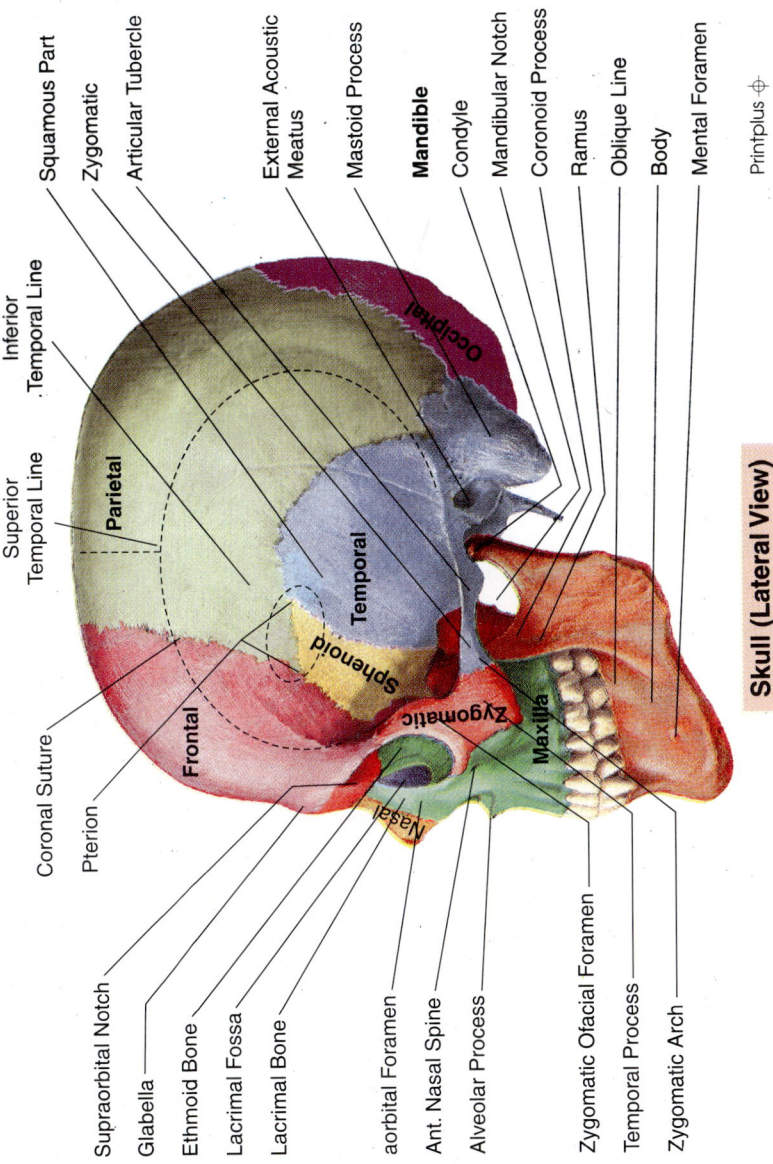

Skull (Lateral View)

Superior Temporal Line
Inferior Temporal Line
Squamous Part
Zygomatic
Articular Tubercle
External Acoustic Meatus
Mastoid Process
Mandible
Condyle
Mandibular Notch
Coronoid Process
Ramus
Oblique Line
Body
Mental Foramen

Printplus

Parietal
Occipital
Temporal
Sphenoid
Zygomatic
Maxilla
Frontal
Nasal

Coronal Suture
Pterion

Supraorbital Notch
Glabella
Ethmoid Bone
Lacrimal Fossa
Lacrimal Bone
aorbital Foramen
Ant. Nasal Spine
Alveolar Process
Zygomatic Ofacial Foramen
Temporal Process
Zygomatic Arch

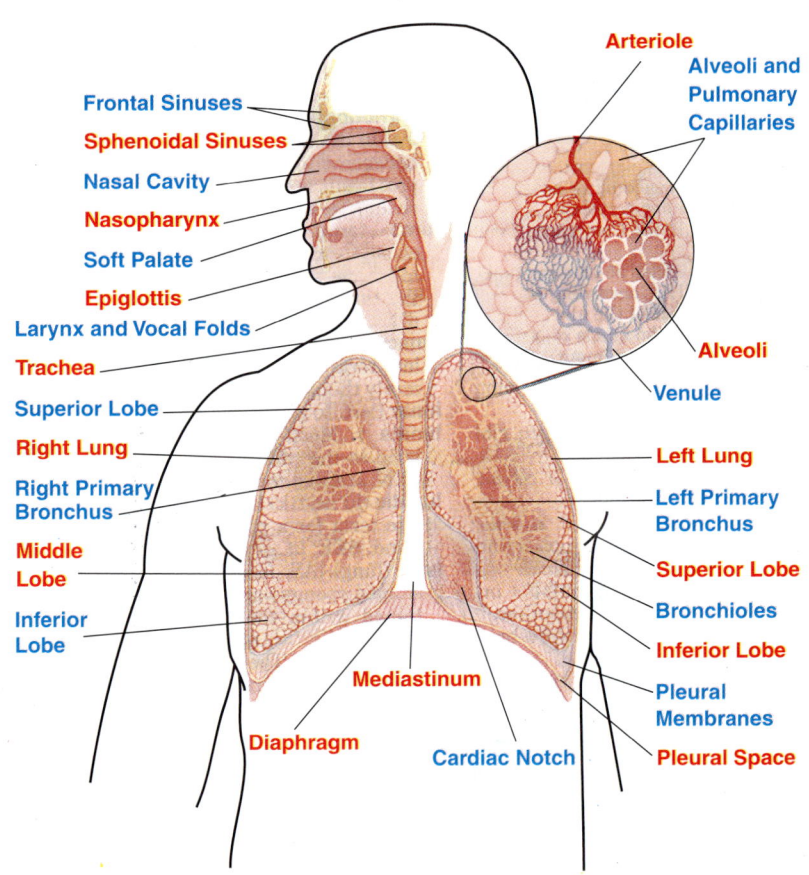

Arteriole

Alveoli and Pulmonary Capillaries

Frontal Sinuses

Sphenoidal Sinuses

Nasal Cavity

Nasopharynx

Soft Palate

Epiglottis

Larynx and Vocal Folds

Trachea

Superior Lobe

Right Lung

Right Primary Bronchus

Middle Lobe

Inferior Lobe

Alveoli

Venule

Left Lung

Left Primary Bronchus

Superior Lobe

Bronchioles

Inferior Lobe

Pleural Membranes

Pleural Space

Mediastinum

Diaphragm

Cardiac Notch

Anterior view of upper and lower Respiratory tracts

Respiratory System

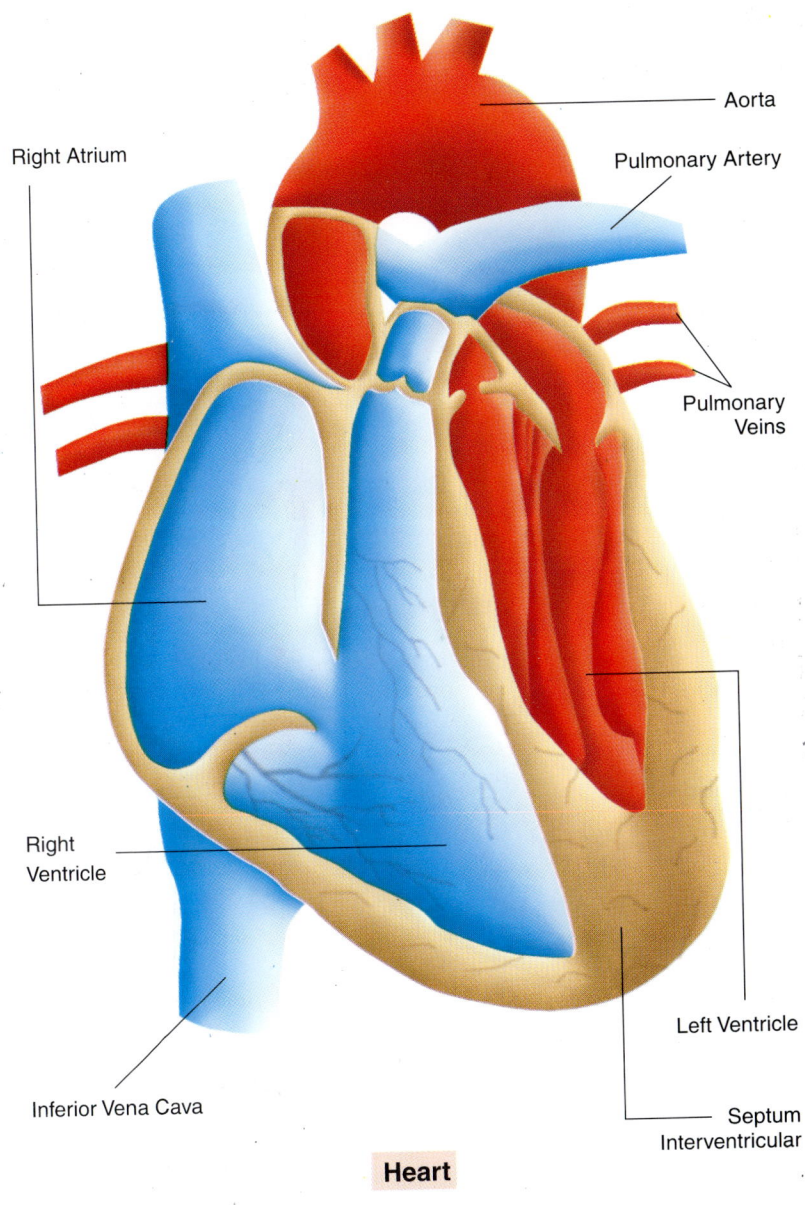

Right Atrium

Aorta

Pulmonary Artery

Pulmonary Veins

Right Ventricle

Inferior Vena Cava

Left Ventricle

Septum Interventricular

Heart

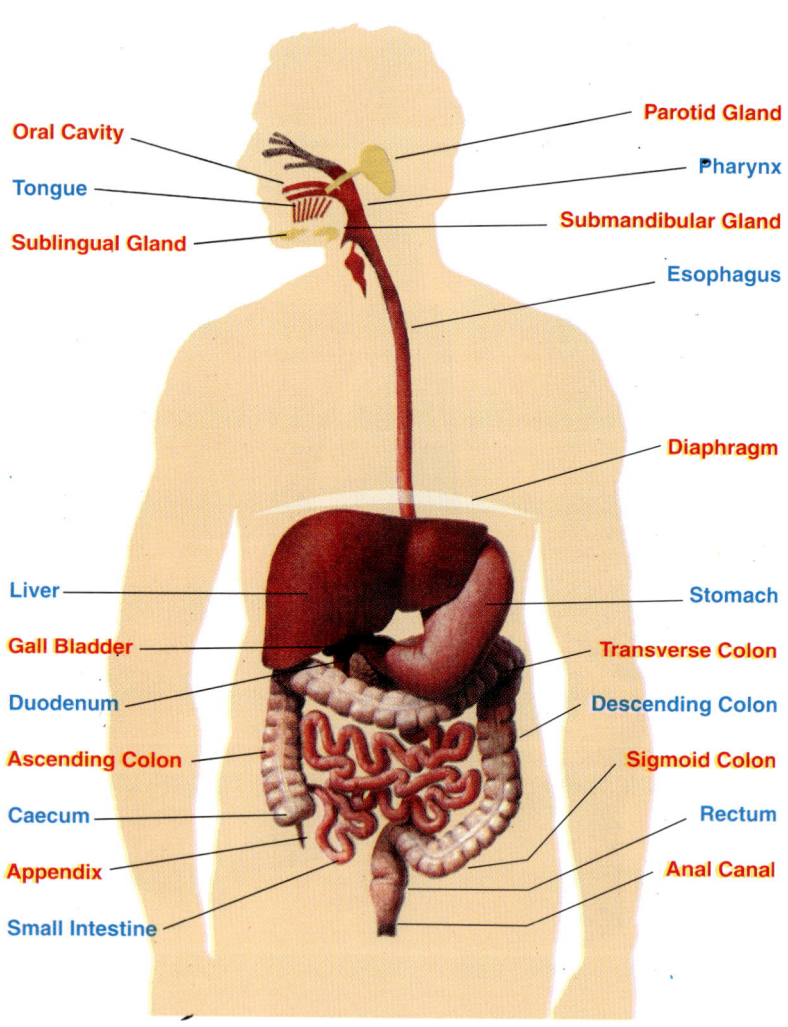

Oral Cavity

Tongue

Sublingual Gland

Parotid Gland

Pharynx

Submandibular Gland

Esophagus

Diaphragm

Liver

Gall Bladder

Duodenum

Ascending Colon

Caecum

Appendix

Small Intestine

Stomach

Transverse Colon

Descending Colon

Sigmoid Colon

Rectum

Anal Canal

Digestive System

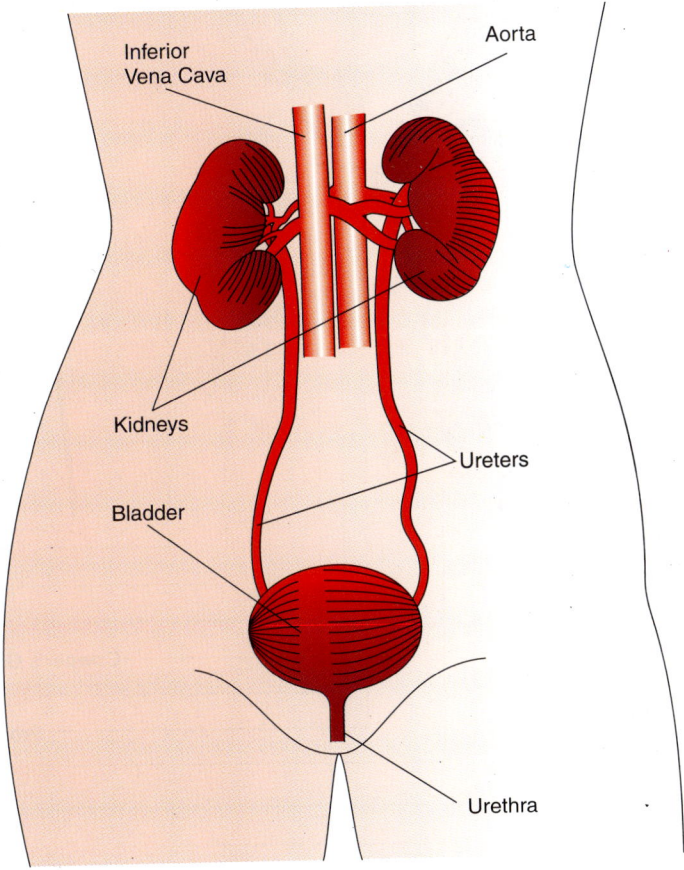

Inferior
Vena Cava

Aorta

Kidneys

Ureters

Bladder

Urethra

Urinary System

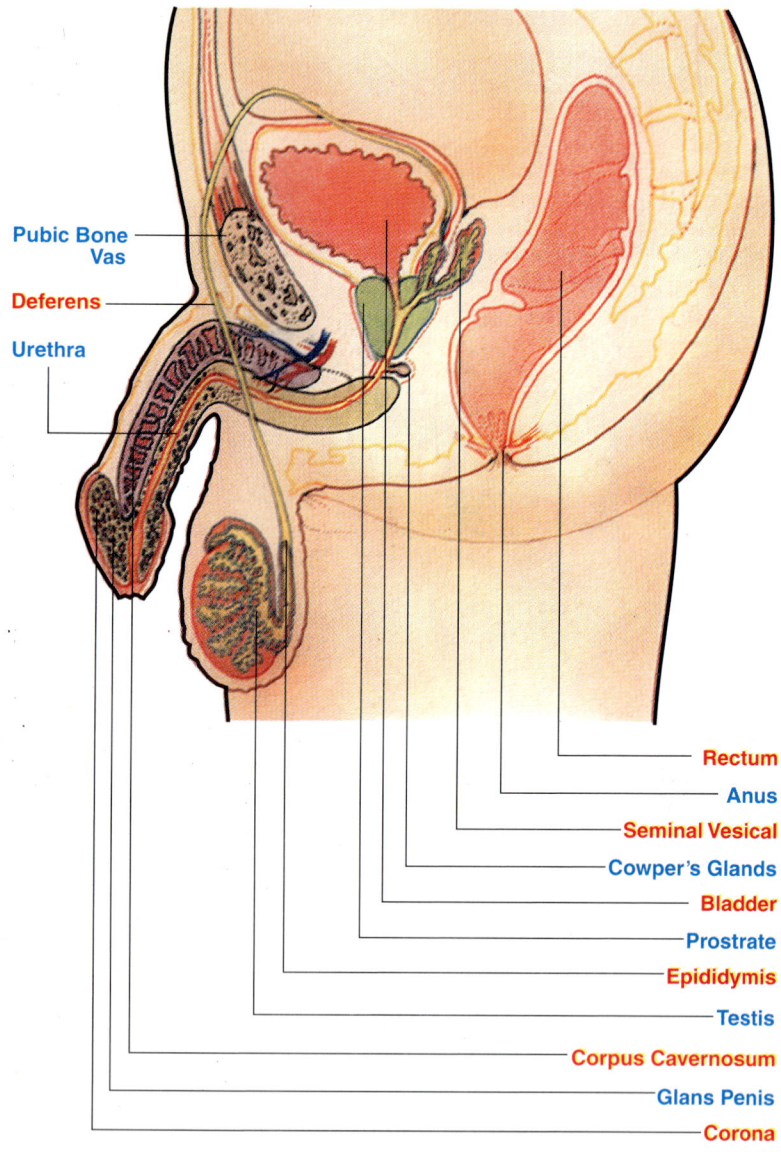

Pubic Bone

Vas

Deferens

Urethra

Rectum

Anus

Seminal Vesical

Cowper's Glands

Bladder

Prostrate

Epididymis

Testis

Corpus Cavernosum

Glans Penis

Corona

Male Reproductive System

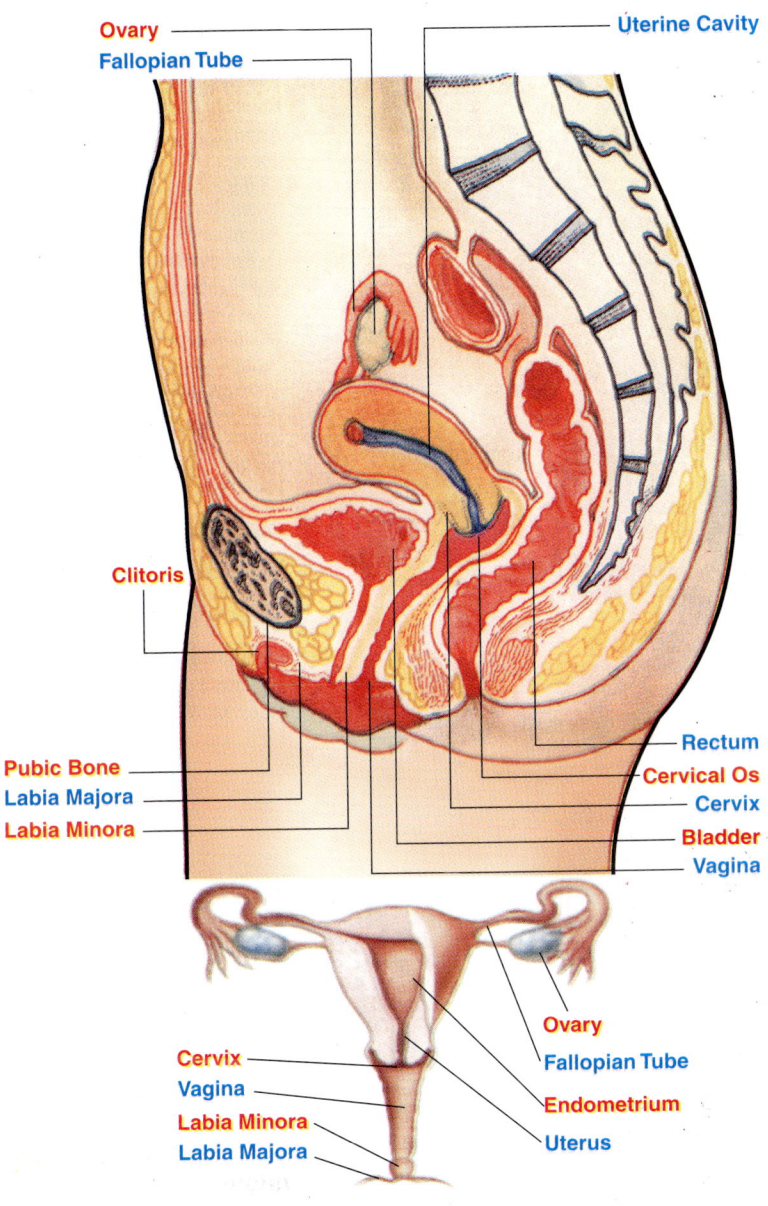

Ovary
Fallopian Tube
Uterine Cavity

Clitoris

Pubic Bone
Labia Majora
Labia Minora

Rectum
Cervical Os
Cervix
Bladder
Vagina

Cervix
Vagina
Labia Minora
Labia Majora

Ovary
Fallopian Tube
Endometrium
Uterus

Female Reproductive System

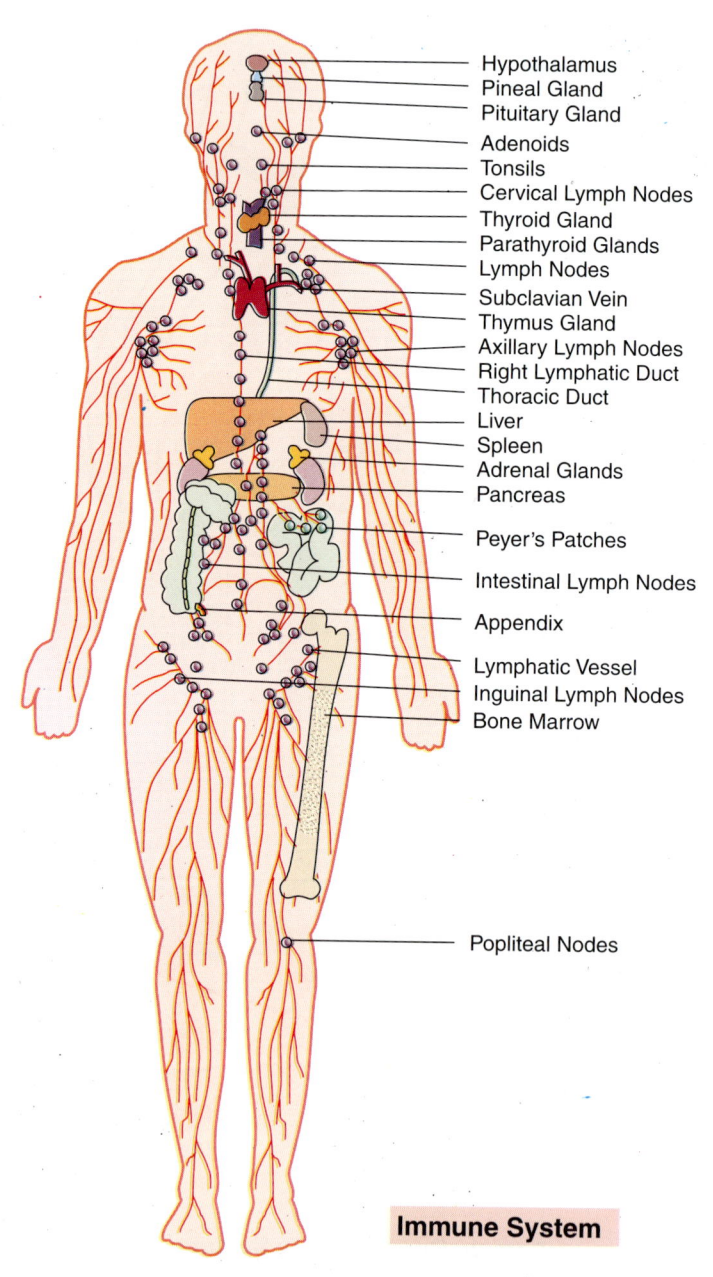

Hypothalamus
Pineal Gland
Pituitary Gland

Adenoids
Tonsils
Cervical Lymph Nodes
Thyroid Gland
Parathyroid Glands
Lymph Nodes
Subclavian Vein
Thymus Gland
Axillary Lymph Nodes
Right Lymphatic Duct
Thoracic Duct
Liver
Spleen
Adrenal Glands
Pancreas

Peyer's Patches

Intestinal Lymph Nodes

Appendix

Lymphatic Vessel
Inguinal Lymph Nodes
Bone Marrow

Popliteal Nodes

Immune System

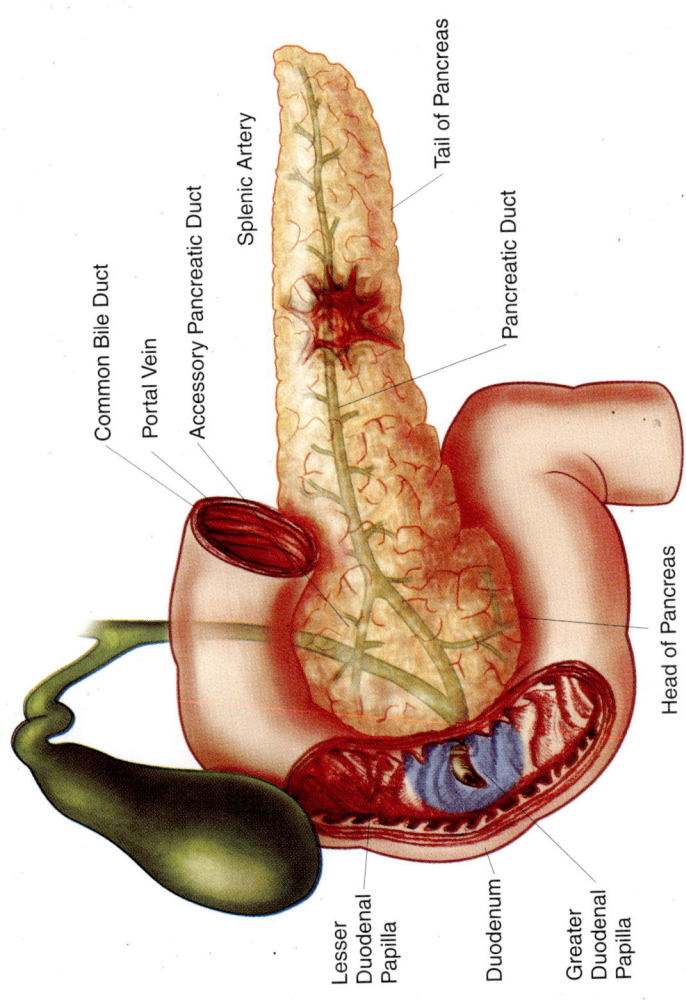

Common Bile Duct

Portal Vein

Accessory Pancreatic Duct

Splenic Artery

Tail of Pancreas

Pancreatic Duct

Head of Pancreas

Lesser Duodenal Papilla

Duodenum

Greater Duodenal Papilla

Pancreas

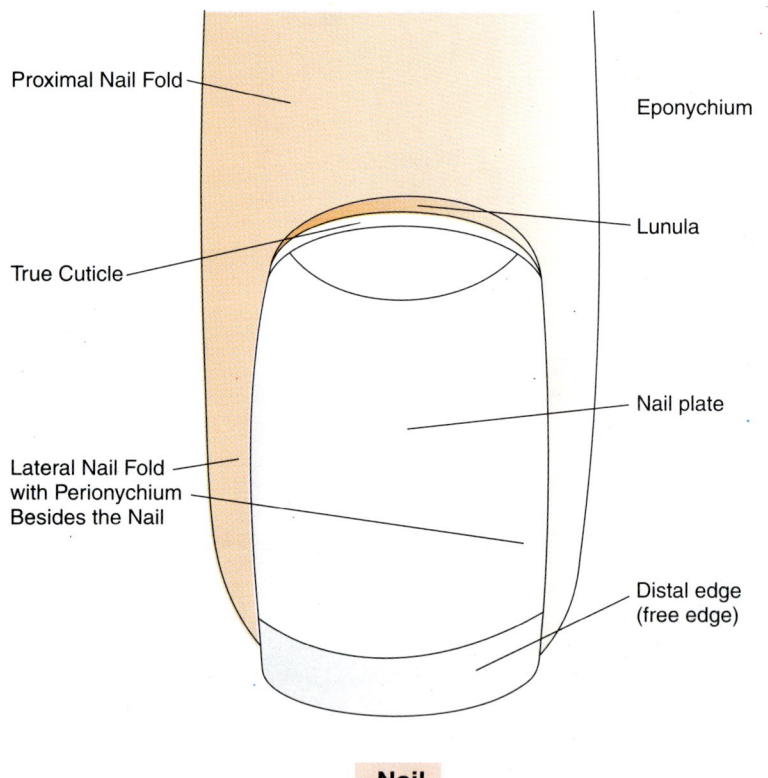

Proximal Nail Fold

Eponychium

True Cuticle

Lunula

Nail plate

Lateral Nail Fold
with Perionychium
Besides the Nail

Distal edge
(free edge)

Nail

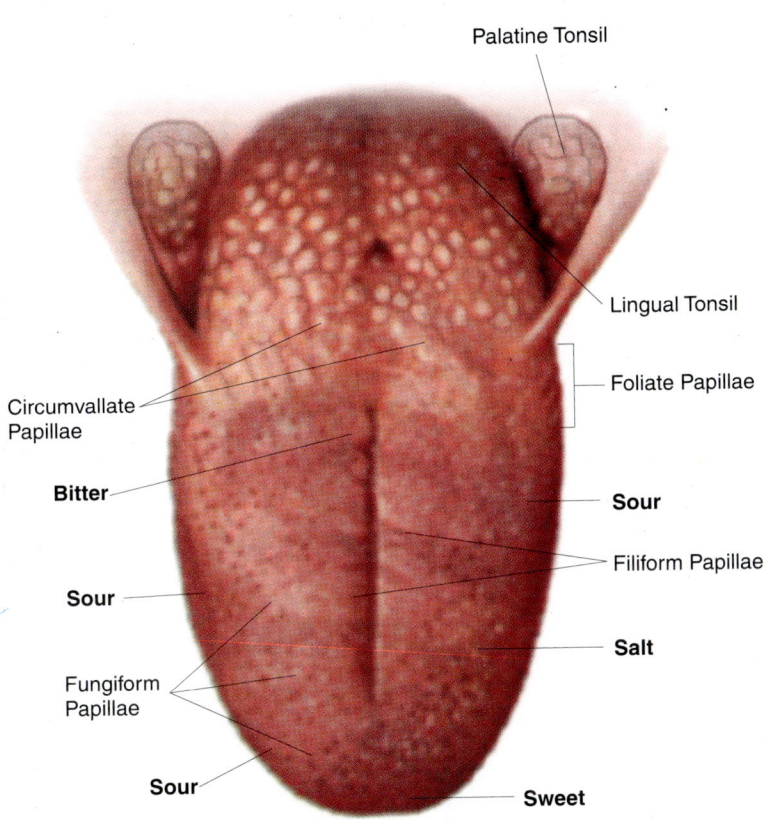

Palatine Tonsil

Lingual Tonsil

Foliate Papillae

Circumvallate
Papillae

Bitter

Sour

Filiform Papillae

Sour

Salt

Fungiform
Papillae

Sour

Sweet

Bold entry denotes teste sensation

Tongue

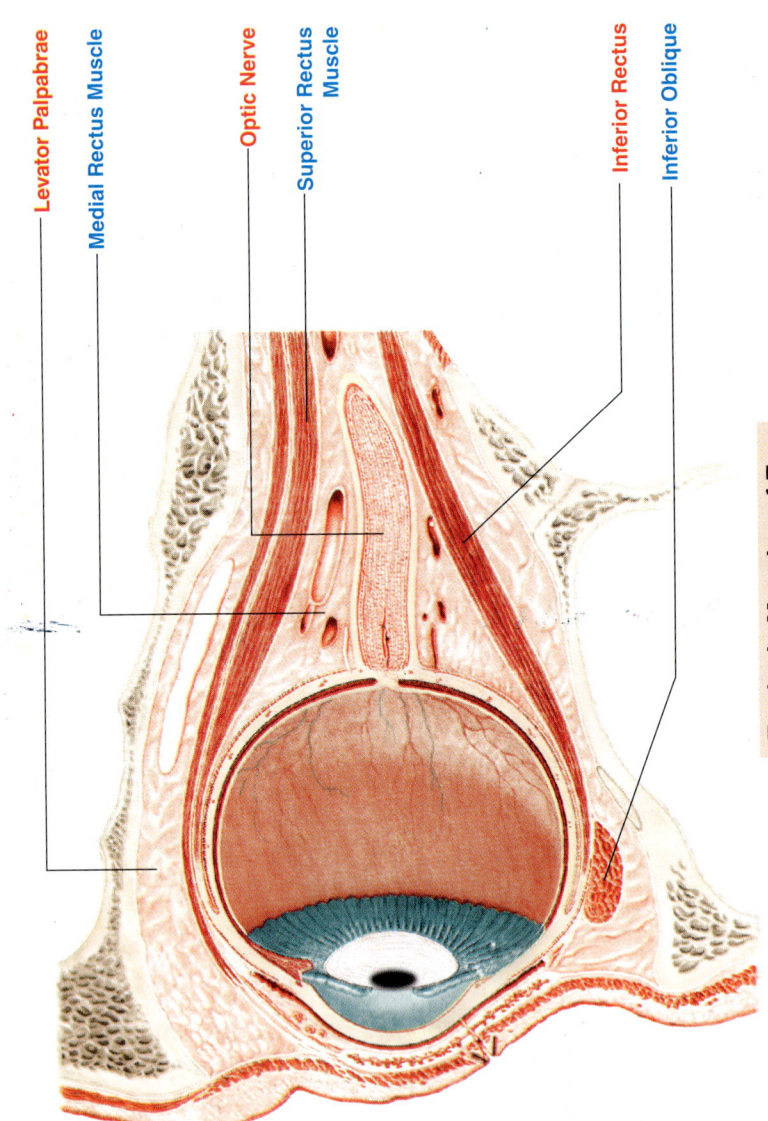

Levator Palpabrae

Medial Rectus Muscle

Optic Nerve

Superior Rectus Muscle

Inferior Rectus

Inferior Oblique

Extrinsic Muscles of Eye

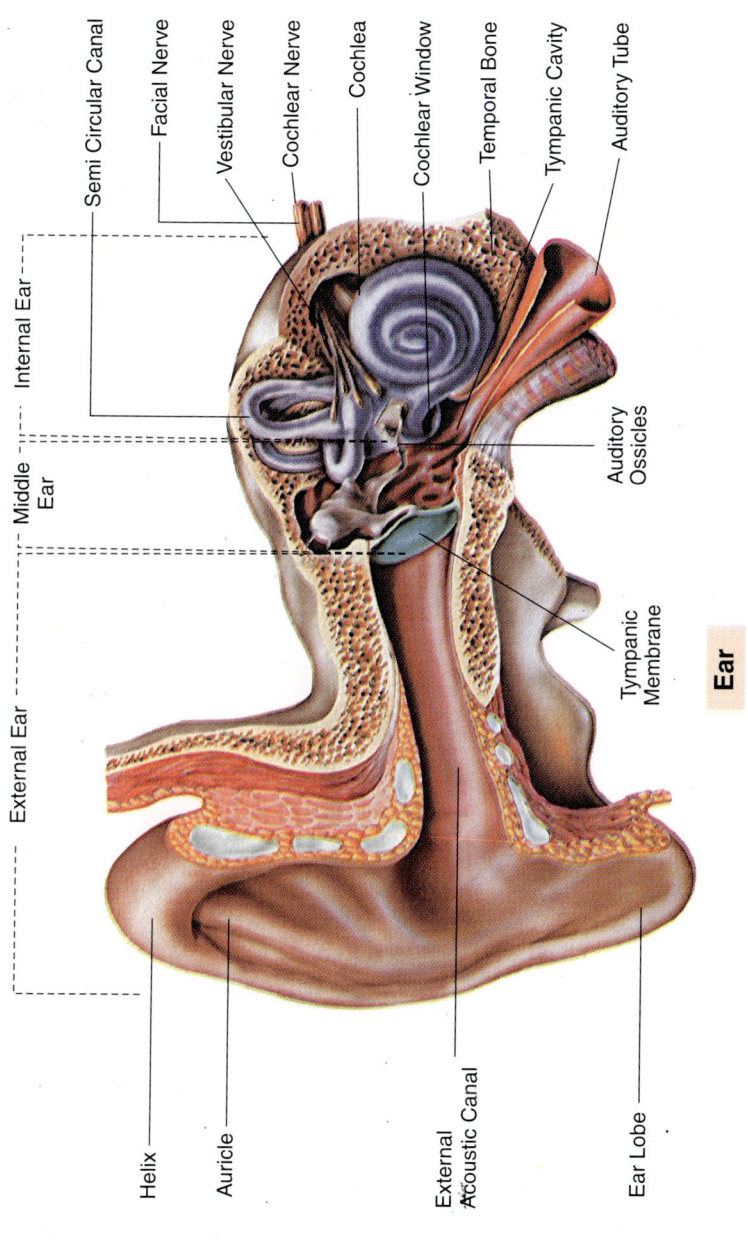

Semi Circular Canal

Facial Nerve

Vestibular Nerve

Cochlear Nerve

Cochlea

Cochlear Window

Temporal Bone

Tympanic Cavity

Auditory Tube

Internal Ear

Middle Ear

External Ear

Auditory Ossicles

Tympanic Membrane

Ear

Helix

Auricle

External Acoustic Canal

Ear Lobe

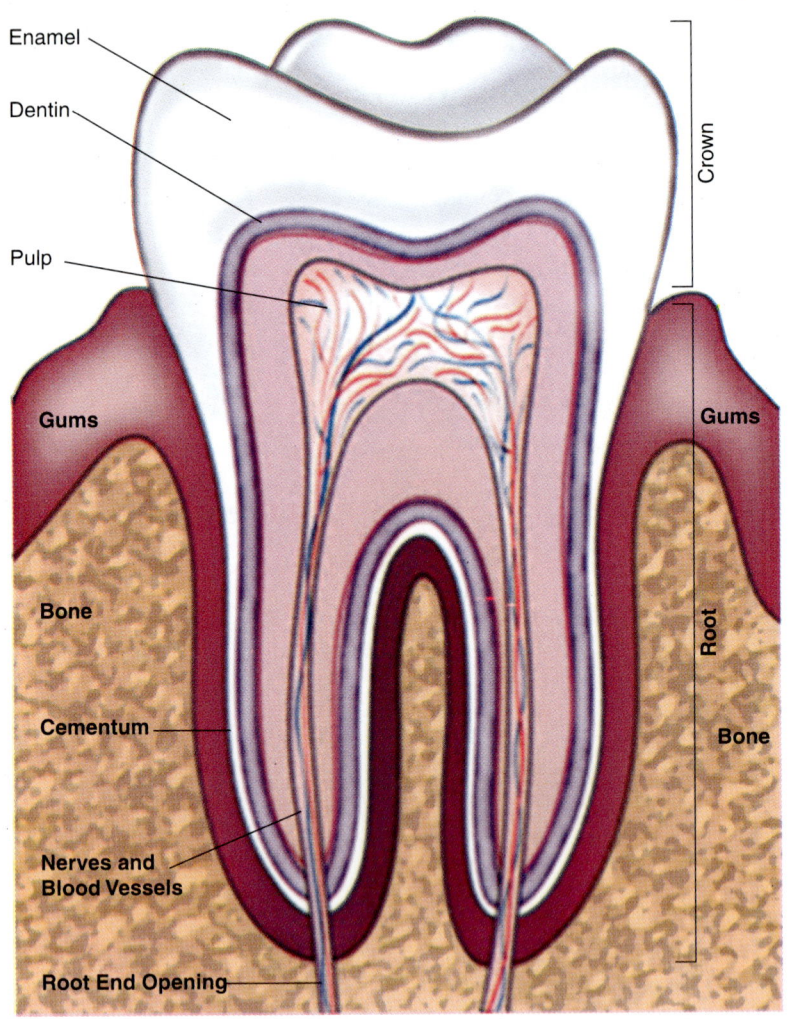

Enamel

Dentin

Pulp

Gums

Bone

Cementum

Nerves and
Blood Vessels

Root End Opening

Crown

Gums

Root

Bone

Tooth

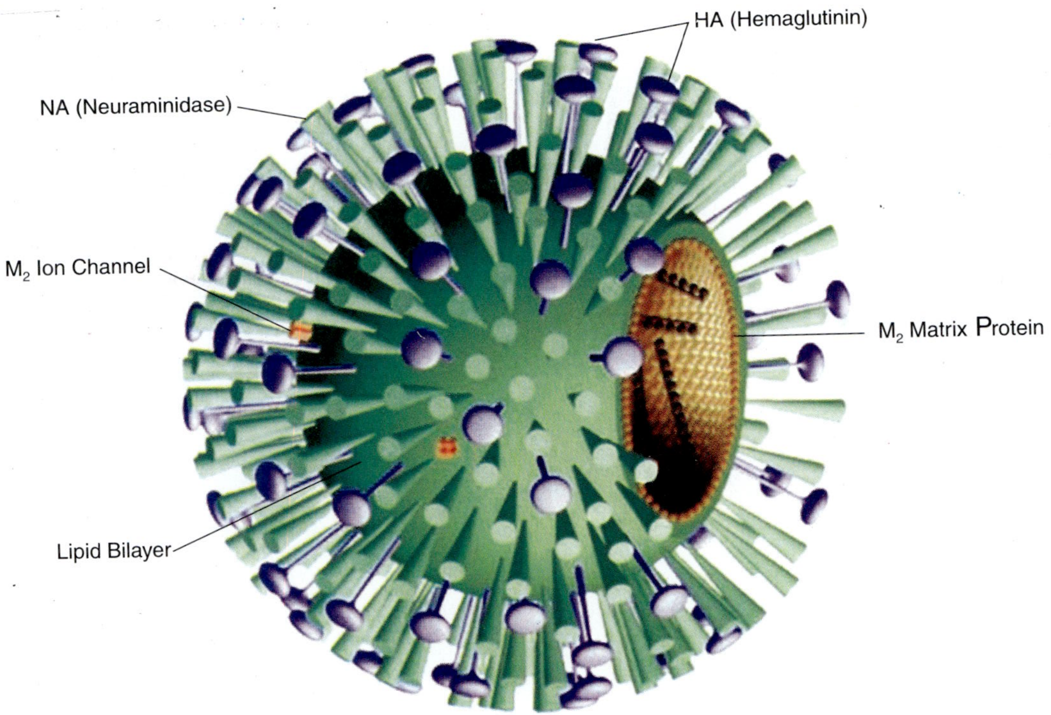

Influenza Virus

M₂ Matrix Protein

HA (Hemaglutinin)

NA (Neuraminidase)

M₂ Ion Channel

Lipid Bilayer

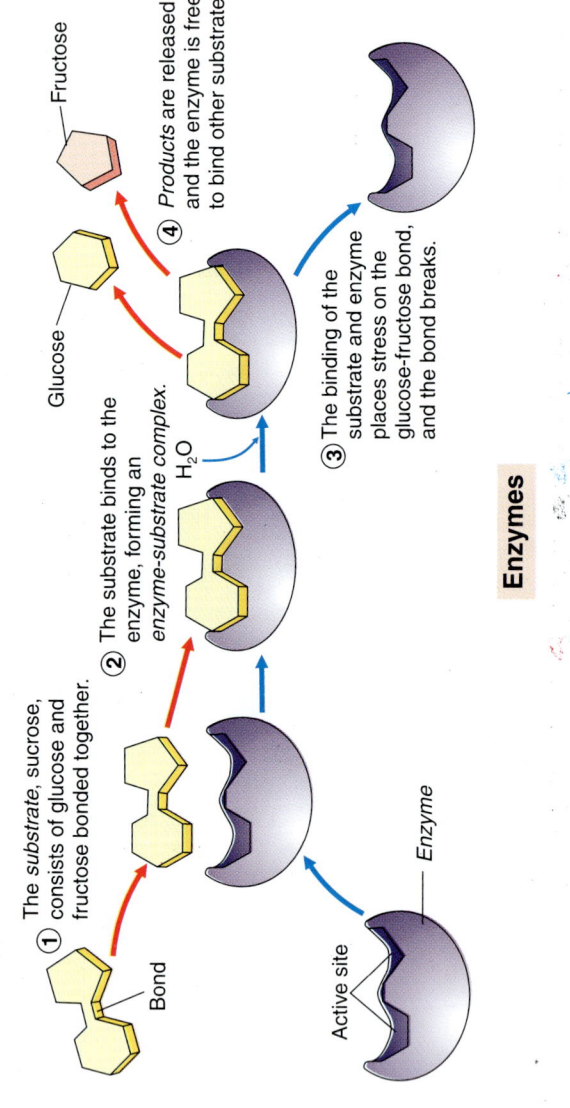

Enzymes

① The *substrate*, sucrose, consists of glucose and fructose bonded together.

Bond

② The substrate binds to the enzyme, forming an *enzyme-substrate complex*.

H_2O

Glucose

Fructose

④ *Products* are released, and the enzyme is free to bind other substrates.

③ The binding of the substrate and enzyme places stress on the glucose-fructose bond, and the bond breaks.

Active site

Enzyme

Skin Structure

Labels (top, left to right): Epidermis, Dermis, Sebaceous Gland, Arrector Pili Muscle, Subcutaneous Layer, Sweat Gland

Labels (left): Pore, Hair

Labels (bottom, left to right): Dermal Papillea, Receptors, Blood Vessel, Connective Tissue, Fat Lobule

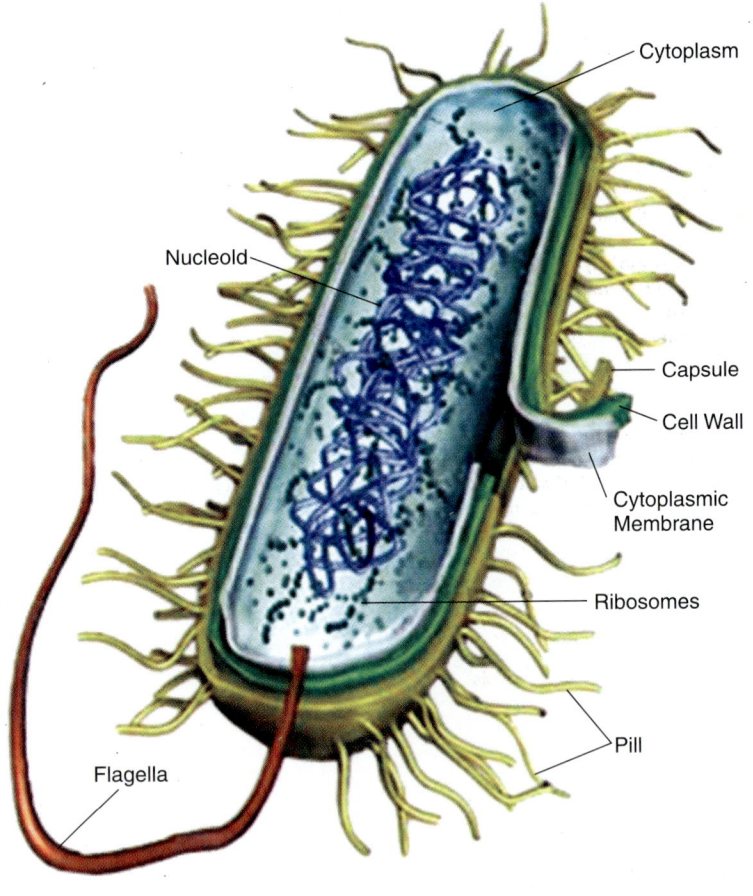

Cytoplasm

Nucleoid

Capsule

Cell Wall

Cytoplasmic
Membrane

Ribosomes

Pill

Flagella

Bacteria

fects CD4 + helper lymphocytes resulting in a decrease in their numbers and there is failure of most aspects of immune function, particularly cell mediated immunity. There is defect and reduced responses by B lymphocytes, monocytes and macrophages. It presents with fatigue, fever, malaise, weight loss, diarrhoea, lymphadenopathy, opportunistic infections and Kaposi's sarcoma. The condition is diagnosed by demonstration of the presence of antibodies to HIV in serum (ELISA test) and confirmed by immunoblot (westernblot) test which also detects the presence of anti-HIV antibodies

acral (ak'ral) pertaining to extremities

acrid (ak'rid) bitter, burning, irritating

acrimony (ak'ri-mo'ne) quality of being acrid, pungent or imitating

acritical (a-krit'i-kal) not marked by crisis

acro - combining word for extremity; top

acroagnosis (ak'ro-ag-no'sis) absence of feeling of one's limb

acroanaesthesia (ak'ro-an-es-the'ze-a) lack of sensation of one or more limbs

acrocentric (ak'ro-sen'trik) location of a centromere at one end of a chromosome

acrocephaly (ak-ro-sef'a-le) a malformed skull with a peaked appearance

acrocyanosis (ak'ro-si-a-no'sis) cyanosis of the hands and feet due to spasm of the arterioles

acrodermatitis (ak'ro-der-ma-ti'tis) dermatitis of the extremities.

acrodermatosis (ak'ro-der'ma-to'sis) any disease of the skin of the hand and feet.

acrodolichomelia (ak-ro-dol'i-ko-me'le-a) a condition associated with abnormally long hands and feet

acrodynia (ak'ro-din'e-a) a toxic neuropathy following exposure to mercury in infants and young children characterised by pain and swelling, and pink colouration of the fingers and toes, listlessness, irritability, profuse sweating and failure to thrive

acroesthesia (ak'ro-es-the'ze-a) 1. pain in the extremities 2. abnormal sensitiveness of the extremities

acrohyperhidrosis (ak'ro-hi'per-hi-dro'sis) excessive perspiration of the hands and feet

acrohypothermy (ak'ro-hi'po-ther'me) abnormal coldness of the hands and feet

acrokeratosis (ak'ro-ker'a-to'sis) horny growths on the skin of the extremities

acrokinesia (ak'ro-kin-e'se-a) abnormal movement of the extremities

acromegaly (ak'ro-meg'a-le) a condition caused by the growth hormone (GH), secretion from a pituitary tumour in adult. GH acts by stimulation of secretion of insulin-like growth factor 1 and its binding proteins from liver. It is characterised by large hands and feet, growth of lower jaw, and skull, skin thickening, increased sweating, enlargement of lips, nose and tongue and visceromegaly

acromelic (ak'ro-mel'ik) pertaining to the end of the extremities

acrometagenesis (ak'ro-met'a-jen'i-sis) abnormal growth of the extremities

acromial (ak-ro'me-al) relating to the acromion **a process** acromion

acromioclavicular (a-kro'me-o-kla-vik'u-lar) pertaining to the acromion and clavicle

acromion (a-kro'me-on) the lateral projection of the spine of the scapula that articulates with the clavicle and forms the highest point of the shoulder

acromionectomy (a-kro'me-on-ek'ta-me) surgical resection of the acromion

acromioplasty (a-kro'me-o-plas'te) surgical removal of distal portion of acromion to relieve mechanical compression of the rotator cuff during movement of the glenohumeral joint

acromioscapular (a-kro'me-o-skap'u-lar) pertaining to the acromion and scapula

acromphalus (ak'rom'fal-us) 1. the centre of the umbilicus 2. bulging of the umbilicus

acromyotonia (ak'ro-mi'o-to're-a) spasmodic deformity from contraction of the extremities acroneurosis (ak'ro-nu-ro'sis) nervous disorder in the hands and feet

acronym (ak'ro-nim) a word coined by the initial letters of the main components of a compound term

acroosteolysis (ak'ro-os'te-ol'i-sis) 1. dissolution of distal portion of distal phalanges of the fingers and toes 2. bone destruction of the distal phalanges in persons engaged in vinyl chloride polymerisation process

acropachy (ak'ro-pak'e) clubbing of the fingers and toes

acropachyderma (ak'ro-pak'e-der'ma) thickening of the skin over the face, scalp and extermities, clubbed digits and deformities of long bones

acroparalysis (ak'ro-pa-ral'i-sis) paralysis of one or more extremities

acroparesthesia (ak'ro-par'es-the'ze-a) tingling and numbness in the extremities

acropathology (ak'ro-pa-thol'a-je) pathology of diseases of the extremities

acropathy (a-krop'a-the) any disease of the extremities

acrophobia (ak'ro-fo'be-a) morbid fear of heights

acroposthitis (ak'ro-pos-thi'tis) inflammation of the prepuce of the penis.

acroscleroderma (ak'ro-skler'o-der'ma) hard and thickened skin of the extremities

acrosclerosis (ak'ro-skl'er'o-sis) a combination of Raynaud's disease and scleroderma affecting distal parts of the extremities, and of the neck and face

acrosome (ak'ro-som) a caplike-lysosomal structure on the head of a spermatozoa that contains enzymes to digest the membrane of the ovum

acrotism (ak'ro-tizm) absence or imperceptible pulse

acrotrophoneurosis (ak'ro-trof'o-nu-ro'sis) trophic, neuritis and vascular disturbances of the extremities

acrylate (ak'ri-lat) a salt or ester of acrylic acid

act (akt) 1. to perform a function 2. the accomplishment of a function.

ACTH adrenocorticotropic hormone of anterior pituitary that stimulates the adrenal cortex to produce adrenal cortical hormones

actin (ak'tin) a muscle protein found in the myofibrils. Along with myosin it causes contraction and relaxation of muscle. It occurs in globular (G-actin) and fibrous (F-actin) forms.

acting out (ak'ting-out) a behaviour abnormality when one expresses hidden emotional conflicts through actions rather than speech

actinic (ak-tin'ik) radiant energy causing photochemical effects **a burns** burns caused by ultraviolet or sun rays. **a cancer** any cutaneous malignancy that is ascribed to excess exposure to solar radiation, most commonly noted in head and neck. **a dermatitis** inflammation and erythema of the skin following exposure to radiation

actino - combining word for a ray or radiation

actinobacillus (ak'ti-no-bas'i-lus) small gram-negative coccobacillus of genus schizomycetes capable of infecting domestic animals, rarely man

actinodermatitis (ak'tin-o-der'ma-ti'tis) dermatitis caused by exposure to radiation

actinomadura (-ma-ju'ra) a genus of schizomycetes including *A. madurae* the cause of maduromycosis. The discharged pus contains white granules. The granules are red in discharged pus in infection by *A. pelletierii*

actinomyces (-mi'sez) a genus of bacteria containing gram-positive filaments belonging to the genus of schizomycetes. They cause various diseases in humans and animals. *A. antibioticus* a species of Actinomyces from which the antibiotic actinomycin is produced. *A. bovis* a species of actiomyces responsible for actinomycosis in cattle. *A. israelii* a species of Actinomyces that causes human actinomycosis. It is gram-positive, anaerobic branching, filamentous bacterium that exists as a normal flora in the oral cavity. *A. naeslundii* and aerobic form of actinomyces are found in the oral cavity and may produce human actinomycosis and periodontal disease

actinomycetaceae (-misa-ta'se-e) an order of bacteria consisting of the families of actinomycetales, mycobacteriaceae, nocardiaceae, dermatophilaceae and streptomycetaceae

actinomycete (-mi-set) any bacterium belonging to the order actinomycetales

actinomycin (-mi'sin) a highly toxic antibiotic produced from *A. antibioticus* effective against bacteria and certain neoplastic conditions

actinomycosis (-mi-ko'sis) a chronic suppurative and granulomatous infection by *A. israelii*. It involves face, and neck commonly. The organisms invade lungs, pleura, iliocaecal and pelvic regions. The abscesses discharge pus containing sulphur granules. It is treated with penicillin

actinotherapy (-ther'a-pe) phototherapy

action (ak'shun) 1. performance of a function. 2. accomplishment of an effect **active** adj. **a potential** *see* potential **antagonistic a** ability to oppose or result of the action, as in a drug or muscle. **bactericidal a** ability to kill the bacteria. **bacteriostatic a** ability to stop the multiplication of the bacteria without killing them **ball-valve a** intermittent obstruction of a passage in the normal direction. **cumulative a** cumulative effect by a drug after administration of several doses. **reflex a** an involuntary movement produced by a sensory stimulus **sparing a** the way in which a nonessential nutrient substance, by its presence in the diet decreases the requirement of an essential substance. **specific a** a drug having direct action upon a causative agent. **specific dynamic a** increase of heat production by ingestion of certain foods especially proteins. **synergistic a** an ability of a drug or muscle to help or enhance the effect of another drug or muscle. **trigger a** the

initiation of physiologic or pathologic activity

activate (ak'ti-vat) to make active

activated charcoal an adsorbent agent produced by subjecting carbonaceous materials to steam and acid. It is capable of binding to a toxic substance in the gastrointestinal tract due to the presence of innumerable interstices capable of trapping organic chemicals

activated macrophage a mononuclear phagocyte stimulated by lymphokines. They are twice the size of resting macrophages and play a major role in defending against micro-organisms

activated partial thromboplastin time APTT the time taken for the formation of a fibrin clot after addition of activating factors, which varies from 16 to 40 seconds

activation (ak'ti-va'shun) 1. the process of making active 2. the process of transformation of an inactive or proenzyme into an active enzyme 3. the process of stimulation of CNS by the reticular activating system

activator (ak'ti-va'ter) 1. a substance which renders another substance active or accelerate a process or reaction 2. a substance that stimulates the development of a specific structure in the embryo 3. a fragment produced during chemical proactivator inducing enzymatic activity of another substance **active plate a** a recoverable orthodontic appliance capable of providing force for movement of teeth. **plasminogen a** any of a group of substances that are capable of cleaving plasminogen and converting it into the active form, plasmin. **prothrombin a** any one of the substances activating coagulation

active principle the chemical substance found in a pharmaceutical preparation that is responsible for its therapeutic action.

active range of motion the range of movement of a joint performed by a patient without any assistance

active transport the process of movement of molecules against a concentration or electrochemical gradient.

activity (ak-tiv'i-te) 1. the quality of accomplishing an effect 2. presence of neurogenic electrical activity. **blocking a** a phenomenon of repression of electrical activity in the brain following arrival of a sensory stimulus. **endplate a** spontaneous activity at the motor end plates that can be recorded. **enzyme a** the catalytic effect exerted by an enzyme. **graded a** presentation of tasks gradually in occupational therapy. **intrinsic sympathomimetic a** ISA the ability of beta blocker to stimulate beta-adrenergic receptors during beta-blockade. **optical a** the ability of a chemical compound to rotate the plane of polarized light either clockwise or counter-clockwise **pulseless electrical a** pulse may not be palpable even though the heart is beating as shown on ECG

actomyosin (ak'to-mi'o-sin) a protein complex of actin and myosin in the muscle fibres

actual (ak'chu-al) real. **a cautery** cautery acting by heat

actuate (ak'chu-at) to put into action or motion

acumentin (ak'u-men'tin) a motility protein found in neutrophils and macrophages that regulate the length of actin

acuity (a-ku'i-te) sharpness, clearness **a of vision** sharpness of vision, determined by asking the patient to read the letters of a Snellen's chart at a distance of six metres and each eye is tested separately. It is expressed as a fraction (d/D), the numerator indicates the distance at which the patient is standing from the chart (d), and the denominator indicates the distance at which a normal person is able to read the same (D). The individual having normal vision is able to read all letters and the acuity is described as 6/6 vision. The acuity of vision is determined by finger counting at bed side

acuminate (a-ku'mi-nat) pointed

acupoint (a'ku-poin-t) a point on the body used in acupuncture and acupressure

acupressure (ak'u-presh'ur) compression of blood vessels by application of needles in surrounding tissue

acupuncture (ak'u-punk'chur) a Chinese procedure in which specific areas of the body along the peripheral nerves are pierced with fine needles to relieve pain, to produce surgical anaesthesia and to promote treatment

acus (a'kus) needle

acusis (a'ku-sis) ability to hear

acute (a-kut) 1. rapid onset with severe symptoms and sharp course. **ac abdomen** *see* abdomen. **ac confusional state** a global impairment in mental function with varying degrees of impaired level of consciousness and memory defect especially for recent events leading to disorientation in time and place. **ac congestive glaucoma** a condition noted in middle aged persons, commonly women having hypermetropia with small eyeballs and presents with severe headache, neuralgic pains and vomiting. The eyes are red and lids oedematous. The anterior chamber is shallow and pupils dilated and vertically oval. The eye ball is stony hard. **ac disseminated encephalitis** an acute complication of viral infection or vaccination affecting entire brain and spinal cord or focally affecting a nerve or cord root. **ac mountain sickness** a symptom complex of less than a week duration associated with rapid ascent to greater than 2500-4500 metres, characterised by marked frontal throbbing headache, nausea, vomiting and insomnia. There may be retinal haemorrhage and sometimes life-threatening high altitude pulmonary oedema or cerebral oedema. The person has to be descended immediately and treated with dexamethasone **ac necrotising ulcerative gingivitis** a condition characterised by progressive necrosis of oral tissues seen in individuals with poor oral hygiene **ac phase protein** a group of proteins which show characteristic change in response to inflammation and tissue injury. **ac radiation injury syndrome** a disorder noted in nuclear reactor accidents which may be asymptomatic with chromosomal aberrations, asymptomatic with mild decrease of leucocytes and platelets, or nausea, anorexia and vomiting, or bone marrow depression **ac renal failure** a sudden failure of the kidney to maintain normal biochemical homeostasis in the body. It is characterised by a failure to excrete waste products of metabolism leading to an increase in the levels of blood urea and serum creatinine. The condition may be prerenal, renal or postrenal **ac respiratory distress syndrome** a severe, life threatening catastrophe occurring suddenly in patients without any evidence of previous lung diseases following a variety of unrelated pulmonary injuries. There is outpouring of protein-rich fluid into the alveolar spaces from damaged alveolar-capillary membrane, collapse of peripheral gas exchanging units and deficiency of surfactant. The condition is characterised by marked dyspnoea, progressive hypoxaemia, reduced pulmonary compliance, marked impairment in oxygen transportation despite ventilatory assistance and roentgenographic evidence of bilateral pulmonary infiltrates. The condition may be followed by systemic manifestations in the form of multiple organ system failure (MOSF) notably liver, kidneys, gastrointestinal tract, CNS and haematologic system **ac respiratory failure** an inability to keep the arterial blood gases at normal level while breathing ambient air at sea level and the individual exhibits the partial pressure of oxygen below 60 mmHg with or without an elevation of carbon dioxide tension above 49 mmHg in the arterial blood. Acute respiratory failure

may develop from inadequate gas exchange (type I) and/or inadequate ventilation (type II). The former is associated with hypoxaemia, seen in diseases affecting the peripheral gas exchanging parts of the lungs, and the latter with hypoxaemia and hypercarbia, seen in obstructive pulmonary diseases, neuromuscular diseases and disorders of chest bellows.

acyanotic (a-si'-a-not'ik) characterised by absence of cyanosis

acyclovir (a-si'klo-vir) an antiviral agent used in the treatment of herpes simplex infections of genitals and herpes infections of the skin

Acyl-CoA-acyl coenzyme A. a metabolic intermediate especially in the oxidation of fat **a-dehydrogenase** any of the several enzymes that catalyse the oxidation of acyl co-enzyme A thioesters as a step in the degradation of fatty acids.

acylation (as'i-la'shun) incorporation of an acid radical into a chemical

acyltransferase (a'sil-trans'-fer-as) any of a group of enzymes that catalyse the transfer of acyl group from one substance to another

ad- prefix indicating adherence, increase, or movement toward.

-ad suffix denoting toward or in the direction of

ADA adenosine de-aminase an enzyme catalysing simple hydrolysis of C-NH$_2$ bonds.

ADA deficiency a condition resulting from inheritance of mutation in both copies of the gene and associated with severe combined immunodeficiency. First condition for which gene therapy was attempted.

adactyly (a-dak'ti-le) congenital absence of fingers or toes **adactylous** adj.

adamantine (ad'a-man'tin) very hard, pertaining to enamel of the teeth.

adamantinoma (ad'a-man'ti-no'ma) ameloblastoma a benign tumour of the jaw especially mandible arising from enamel forming cells.

adamantoblast (ad'a-man'to-blast) a enamel forming cell found during the formation of tooth; ameloblast

adamantoma (ad'a-man-to'ma) adamantinoma

Adam complex a guilt, complex that a person who breaks a 'parental' law that the person was not aware it was forbidden.

ADAM Complex development of amniotic deformity, adhesions and mutilations in utero

Adam's apple laryngeal prominence formed by the two laminae of the thyroid cartilage named after Adam who took a piece of the forbidden fruit for Eve, which stuck in his throat

Adams-Stokes syndrome *see* Stokes-Adams syndrome

adaptation (ad'ap-ta'shun) 1. adjustment of an organism to its environment 2. ability of the eyes to adjust to variations in the intensity of light 3. property of certain receptors becoming less responsive or cease to show any response to constant intensity of stimulation 4. proper fitting of dentures or restorative material to the teeth 5. adjustment of the microorganism to a new environment **colour a** prolonged visual stimulation lessening the intensity of colour perception **dark a** the adaptation of the vision in dark or in reduced illumination **genetic a** the progeny of a mutant organism better adapted to a new environment, especially seen in drug resistant organisms **light a** adjustment of the eye to vision in bright light **phenotypic a** alteration in the properties of an organism in response to genetic mutation or to a change in the environment. **photopic a** light adaptation **retinal a** adjustment of the eye to the degree of illumination **scotopic a** dark adaptation

adapter (a-dap-ter) a device to join one part of an instrument or apparatus to another part

adaptive design a type of clinical trial design in which the probability that a patient receives a given treatment is at least partly, determined by the results obtained with patients so far

adaptive thermogenesis physiological response of the body to adjust its metabolic rate to the presence or absence of calories

adaptometer (ad-ap-tom'e-ter) an instrument for measuring the time required for ocular dark adaptation and for measurement of the minimum light threshold

adaxial (ad-ak'se-al) towards main axis

add an abbreviation used in prescriptions meaning let there be added

addict (ad'ikt) a person who is physically or psychologically or both dependent on a substance especially alcohol or drug

addiction (a-dik'shun) psychological or physical dependence on a substance (alcohol, drug) or practice (eating, gambling) which is beyond voluntary control

Addisonian crisis a state of acute adrenal insufficiency induced by stress of infections, trauma or surgery characterised by hypotension, shock, fever, dehydration, anorexia and weakness

Addisonian pernicious anaemia megaloblastic anaemia due to a failure of secretion of intrinsic factor by the stomach other than from total gastrectomy. An autoimmune disorder exhibiting very low serum vitamin B_{12} and anti-intrinsic factor antibodies in 50%

Addison's disease a disease resulting from deficiency in the secretion of either glucocorticoids or mineralocorticoids initially and later of any class of adrenocortical hormones. It may present with an acute adrenal crisis (circulatory shock with severe hypotension, hyponatraemia and hyperkalaemia) or chronic features (weight loss, malaise, weakness, anorexia, nausea, pigmentation and decrease in body hair) . The condition is treated by glucocorticoid replacement therapy and mineralocorticoid named after Thomas Addison who described the disease when he was a medical student in Edinburgh.

addisonism (ad'i-son-izm) symptoms simulating Addison's disease, debility and pigmentation in pulmonary tuberculosis

additive (ad'i-tiv) a substance deliberately added to fulfil certain purpose **food a** substance added to food to improve its nutritive value, to enhance palatability or to improve its consistency or texture.

adducent (a-du'sent) causing adduction

adduct (a-dukt) 1. to draw towards the median line or the main axis of the body or limb 2. an inclusion product.

adduction (a-duk'shun) movement of a limb or eye towards the median line or beyond it

adductor (a-duk'tor) a muscle that draws a part toward the midline

adelomorphous (a-del'o-mor'fus) of not having a clearly defined form

adenalgia (ad'en-al'jah) pain in a gland

adenase (ad'en-nas) an enzyme that converts adenine into hypoxanthine

adendritic (a'den-drit'-ik) without dendrites

adenectomy (ad'e-nek'to-me) surgical removal of a gland

adenectopia (ad'e-nek-to'pe-a) presence of a gland elsewhere than in its normal anatomic position

adenemphraxis (ad'e-nem-frak'sis) obstruction to the discharge of a glandular secretion

adenia (a-de'ne-a) chronic enlargement of a lymph gland

adenine (ad'e-nin) a major purine found in RNA and DNA

adenitis (ad'e-ni'tis) inflammation of a lymph node or a gland

adenisation (ad'e-ni-za'shun) conversion into a gland-like structure.

aden (o) combining word for gland.

adenoacanthoma (ad'e-no-ak'an-tho'-ma) a well-differentiated adenocarcinoma with foci of metaplasia to squamous neoplastic cells.

adenoameloblastoma (-a-mel'o-blast-to-ma) a benign tumour developing in the maxilla and it consists of ducts lined by cuboidal cells.

adenoblast (ad'e-no-blast) an embryonic cell with the potential to form gland tissue.

adenocarcinoma (ad'e-no-kar'si-no'ma) a malignant condition of the epithelial cells in glandular tissue or glandular pattern.

adenocoele (ad'e-no-sel) a cystic tumour from a gland

adenocellulitis (ad'e-no-sel'u-li'tis) inflammation of a gland and its surrounding tissues

adenocystoma (-sis-to-ma) cystadenoma

adenocyte (ad'e-no-sit) a gland cell

adenoepithelioma (ad'e-no-epi-the'-leo'ma) a tumour composed of glandular and epithelial elements

adenofibroma (-fi-bro'ma) a benign tumour composed of glandular and fibrous tissues

adenogenous (ad'e-noj'e-nus) developing from glandular tissue

adenography (-nog'ra-fi) radiography of the glands

adenohypophysectomy (ad'e-no-hi-pof'i-sek'ta-me) anterior lobe of the pituitary gland

adenoid (ad'e-noid) hypertrophied lymphoid tissue situated at the roof of the nasopharynx, present at birth and gradually undergoes atrophy; nasopharyngeal tonsil.

adenoiditis (ad'e-noid'i-tis) inflammation of the adenoids.

adenolipoma (ad'e-no-li-po'ma) a tumour composed of glandular and fatty elements.

adenolymphitis (-lim-fi'tis) lymphadenitis

adenolymphoma (-lim-fo'ma) a benign tumour of parotid gland containing both epithelial and lymphoid tissues. Epithelial cells proliferate to form multiple acini within the lymphatic tissue. It presents as a slow growing painless swelling on the side of the face

adenoma (ad'e-no'ma) a benign epithelial tumour in which the tumour cells form glands or gland-like structures in the stroma **acidophilic a** a tumour of eosinophilic chromophil cells of the anterior pituitary associated with gigantism and acromegaly. **basal cell a** a benign, encapsulated slow growing painless salivary gland tumour especially in the parotid gland **basophilic a** a tumour of basophilic cells of the anterior pituitary associated with Cushing's syndrome. **bronchial a** a tumour arising either in the main or lobar bronchus from the duct epithelium of bronchial mucous glands and includes three histologically distinct types of tumours: carcinoid, cylindroma and mucoepidermoid tumours. The tumour may obstruct bronchial passage or grow out as a dumb-bell tumour or bleed. **chromophil a** a pituitary basophilic or an eosinophilic adenoma **chromophobe a** a tumour of chromophobe cells of the anterior pituitary **Hurthle cell a** a tumour of thyroid gland containing eosinophil-staining cells **islet a** a tumour of pancreas that may contain beta cells and lead to hypoglycaemia **a sebaceum** benign growth from the epithelium of sebaceous glands **villous a** large polyp arising from mucosa of large intestine

adenomalacia (ad'e-no-ma-la'shah) marked softness of a gland

adenomatoid (ad'e-no'ma-toid) resembling adenoma

adenomatosis (ad'e-no-ma-to'sis) development of multiple glandular overgrowths

adenomere (ad'e-no-mer) a blind terminal end of a glandular cavity of a developing gland which develops into a functional part

adenomyofibroma (ad'e-no-mi'o-fi-bro-ma) a tumour composed of glandular and muscular tissues

adenomyoma (-mi-o'ma) a benign tumour of muscle with glandular elements, occurs in the uterus and uterine ligaments

adenomyomatosis (-mi'o-ma-to'sis) development of multiple adenomyomatous nodules in the uterus

adenomyometritis (-mi'o-me-tri'tis) a hyperplastic condition of uterus developing from pelvic inflammation

adenomyosarcoma (-mi'o-sar-ko'ma) an adenosarcoma containing muscle tissue

adenomyosis (-mi-o'sis) a benign ingrowth of the endometrium into the uterine muscles

adenoncus (ad'e-nong'kus) enlargement of a gland

adenopathy (ad'e-nop'a-the) enlargement of glands , especially of the lymph nodes

adenopharyngitis (ad'e-no-far'in-ji'tis) inflammation of the adenoids and pharynx

adenosarcoma (-sar-ko'ma) a mixed tumour arising in the mesodermal tissue and glandular epithelium of the same part

adenosclerosis (-skle-ro'sis) hardening of the gland

adenosine (a-din'o-sen) 1. purine nucleotide consisting of adenine and ribose and is a component of RNA. 2. a cardiac depressant

adenosis (ad'e-no'sis) proliferation of the acini of the glands

adenotome (ad'e-no-tom) an instrument for excision of a gland, especialy adenoid glands

adenoviridae (ad'e-no-vir'i-de) a family of double-stranded DNA viruses. It develops in the nuclei of infected cells and is responsible for infection of respiratory tract and conjunctiva

adenovirus (ad'e-no-vi'rus) any virus belonging to the family of adenoviridae. Adeno-pharyngo-conjunctival (APC) virus is an example

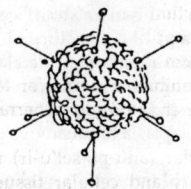

Adeno virus

adenyl (ad'e-nil) the radical of adenine cyclase an enzyme linked to the G-proteins on the cell membrane which generates second messenger cyclic adenosine monophosphate (cAMP) on stimulation

adenylate (a-den'i-lat) salt or ester of adenylic acid **a cylase** adenyl cyclase **a kinase** an enzyme that catalyses the phosphorylation of one molecule of ADP by another to yield ATP and AMP

adenylic (ad'e-nil'ik) **acid** a condensation product of adenosine and phosphoric acid

adequacy (ad'i-kwa-se) the state of being adequate; sufficiency

adermogenesis (a-der'mo-jen'i-sis) imperfection in the regeneration

ADH abbreviation for antidiuretic hormone

adherence (ad-her'ins) ability to adhere, as of bacteria adhering to specific receptors found on some cells or antibody-coated bacteria adhering to red blood cells in presence of complement component C_3

adhesin a molecule on the surface of bacteria involved in specific binding to receptor

adhesion (ad-he'shun) 1. a property of uniting two surfaces or parts as in wound healing 2. a fibrous band holding parts together 3. substances adhering to each other

adhesiotomy (ad-he'ze-ot'a-me) surgical division of adhesions

adhobhakta (s) after meals

adhyayana (s) study

adiadochokinesia (a-di'a-do'ko-ki-ne'zhah) inability to perform rapid alternating movements

adiaphoria (a'di-a-for'e-a) nonresponsiveness to stimulation after a series of previously applied stimuli

ad infinitum L endlessly, to infinity

adip (o) combining word for fat

adipocoele (ad'i-po-sel) a hernia containing fat

adipocellular (ad'i-po-sel'u-lr) relating to both fatty and cellular tissues.

adipocyte (-sit) fat cell

adipogenic (ad'i-po-jen'ik) inducing the formation of fat

adipokinesis (-ki-ne'sis) mobilisation of body fat

adipokinin (-ki'nin) a hormone from anterior pituitary that brings about mobilisation of fat from adipose tissues

adipolysis (ad'i-pol'i-sis) lipolysis **adipolytic** adj

adiponecrosis (ad'-po-na-kro'sis) necrosis of fatty tissue

adipopexis (-pek'sis) storage of fat

adiposis (ad'i-po'sis) excessive accumulation of fat in the body

adiposity (ad'ipos'i-te) obesity

adiposuria (ad'i-po-su're-a) presence of fat in the urine

adipsia (a-dip'se-a) lack of thirst

aditus (ad'i-tus) an entrance to a cavity or channel

adjuvant (aj'oo-vant) 1. a non-specific immune enhancer 2. the agent added to a drug affects the action of the active ingredient in a predictable manner. **Freund's complete a** a water in oil emulsion with inclusion of killed mycobacteria to further enhance antigenicity. **Freund's incomplete a** a water in oil emulsion in which the antigen solution is emulsified in mineral oil

adjunct something joined or added to another, as in the treatment modality

adjunctive therapy a treatment modality used with conventional modality of treatment such as radiotherapy or immunotherapy

adjuvanticity (aj'oo-van-tis'i-te) the ability to modify the immune response.

ad lib L as desired

adnerval (ad-ner'vil) 1. situated near a nerve 2. in the direction of a nerve

adneural (ad-noor'al) adnerval

adnexa (ad-nek'sa) things connected, appendages.

adolescence (ad'o-les'ins) the period between puberty and attainment of complete growth and maturity, **second a** a period of life roughly between the ages of 35 and 50 when the orientation of our lives is more with the growth of the self and less with the opinions of others

adoral (ad-o'ral) towards or near the mouth

adoption assumption of full parental rights over a child

ADP abbreviation for adenosine diphosphate

ADR abbreviation for adverse drug reaction

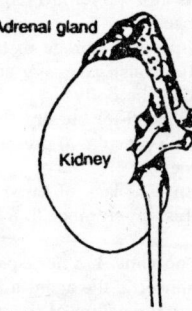

Adrenal gland

adrenal (a-dre'nil) 1. near the kidney 2. an adrenal gland **a cortex** the outer portion of adrenal gland fused with medulla. It is concerned with the production of mineralocorticoids, glucocorticoids and androgens **a crisis** sudden development of adrenal cortical failure. It may complicate chronic adrenal insufficiency or may develop acutely in patients who develop fulminant infections **a gland** a triangular secretory organ on the superior surface of the kidneys. Each consists of an outer cortex and inner medulla, each having different functions. The cortex in response to ACTH of anterior pituitary secretes cortisol and androgens **a medulla** inner part of adrenal gland concerned with secretion of adrenaline and nor adrenaline **a reserve** a test to determine the responsiveness of the adrenal cortex to ACTH by estimating plasma and/or urinary steroids before and during ACTH administration

adrenalectomy (a-dre-nal-ek'to-mi) removal of one or both adrenal glands.

adrenaline (a-dren'a-lin) an endogenous adrenal hormone and a synthetic vasoconstrictor

adrenalinuria (a-dren'a-lin-u're-a) presence of adenaline in the urine

adrenalism (a-dren'al-izm) adrenal dysfunction

adrenalitis (a-dre'nal-i'tis) inflammation of adrenal gland

adrenarche (a-dre'n-ar'ke) stimulation of growth of axillary and pubic hairs by adrenal androgens during puberty

adrenergic (ad'ren-er'jik) acting through the agency of adrenaline or non-adrenaline, **a bronchodilator** a drug that acts on the sympathetic receptors to relax bronchial smooth muscle **a drug** a sympathomimetic agent **a fibres** autonomic nerve fibres that release the neurotransmitter nor adrenaline and in some regions, dopamine **a nerve** a nerve controlling the release of nor adrenaline at its synapses **a receptor** a site in a sympathetic effector cell that reacts to adrenergic stimulation. They are alpha-adrenergic responding to sympathomimetic stimuli and beta-adrenergic inhibiting the sympathomimetic activity.

adren(o) combining word for adrenal gland

adrenoceptor (a-dre'no-sep'ter) adrenergic receptor **adrenoceptive** adj

adrenocortical (-kor'ti-kal) pertaining to adrenal cortex. **a insufficiency** hypofunction of the adrenal cortex due to a primary disorder of the adrenal gland or secondary to hyposecretion of ACTH

adrenocorticohyperplasia (a-dre'no-kor'ti-ko-hy-per-plas'zhah) adrenal cortical hyperplasia

ad-enocorticoid (-kor'ti-koid) any of the steroid hormones synthesised in the adrenal cortex

adrenocorticotrophic (-trof'ik) corticotropic

adrenocorticotropin (-trop'in) corticotropin

adrenogenital sydrome congenital adrenal hyperplasia characterised by virilisation in female and precocious puberty in male children. There is a congenital deficiency of enzymes leading to a metabolic block in hormone synthesis

adrenoleukodystrophy (-loo'ko-dis'tro-fe) an x-linked recessive disorder causing diffuse abnormality of white matter of the brain and atrophy of the adrenal glands. It is characterised by adrenocortical insufficiency, skin hyperpigmentation, intellectual and neurologic disturbances

adrenolytic (-lit'ik) inhibiting the activity of adrenergic nerves or interfering with the response of adrenaline

adrenomegaly (-meg'a-le) enlargement of one or both adrenal glands

adrenomimetic (-mi-met'ik) sympathomimetic

adrenomyeloneuropathy (-mi'e-lo-noorop'a-the) a hereditary disorder with diffuse abnormality of white matter of brain, degeneration of spinal cord, peripheral neuropathy and atrophy of adrenal gland

adrenoreceptor (-re'sep'ter) adrenergic receptor

adrenotoxin (-tok'sin) a substance toxic to adrenal glands

adriamycin (a'dre-a-mi'sin) an antineoplastic antibiotic; doxorubicin

Adson's test forced inspiration with hyperextended neck turned to the side of lesion such as cervical rib causes loss of pulse and pain in the hand

adsorb (ad-sorb) to take up by absorption

adsorbent (ad-sor'bent) 1. a substance that absorbs. 2. a substance capable of attaching other substances to its surface without any chemical action, such as activated charcoal or magnesia

adsorption (ad-sorp'shun) the property of a substance to attract and hold to its surface other substances, gas or liquid.

adult (a-dult) fully grown and mature individual or organism

adulteration (a-dul'ter-a'shun) addition of impure, cheap or even toxic substances in a formation, preparation or food material

advancement (ad-vans'ment) a surgical procedure in which a tendon or a skin flap is detached from its attachment and sutured to a point further forward

adventitia (ad'ven-tish'e-a) outermost connective tissue coat of a blood vessel

adventitious (ad'ven-tish'is) 1. acquired ; not natural 2. coming from without **a breath sounds** sounds audible in disease but not present in normal persons. They may arise in the lungs (wheeze, crackles) or in the pleura (pleural rub).

adverse event any untoward occurrence in any subject given a pharmaceutical product,

adverse reaction an undesired side-effect or toxic manifestation following administration of drugs

adynamia (a'di-na'me-a) loss of normal power

Aedes (a-e'dez) a genus of mosquitoes, some of them are vectors of diseases. *A. aegypti* a vector of dengue fever and yellow fever

aegophony (eg'o-pho-ny) nasal quality of vocal resonance, may be elicited above the level of pleural effusion

aeration (ar-a'shun) 1. exchange of carbon dioxide for oxygen by the blood in the lungs 2. airing 3. saturating a liquid with air or gas

aero- combining form for the word air, gas

aerobacter (ar'o-bak'ter) family of enterobacteriaceae consisting genera of enterobacter and klebsiella

aerobe (ar'ob) micro-organism that can live and grow in presence of free oxygen. **aerobic** adj **fecultative a's** micro-organisms that can live in presence or absence of oxygen **obligate a's** microorganisms that require oxygen for growth

aerobic using oxygen; surviving in presence of oxygen **a exercise** intense excercise facilitating re-synthesis of high energy compounds in presence of oxygen

aerobiology (ar'o-bi-ol'o-je) study of distribution of micro-organisms by air

aerobiosis (-bi-o'sis) existence in an atmosphere containing oxygen

aerocoele (ar'o-sel) air containing cyst

aerodermectasia (ar'o-der'mek-ta'zhah) subcutaneous emphysema

aerodontalgia (-don-tal'je-a) pain in the teeth due to an alteration of atmospheric pressure

aeroembolism (-em'bo-lizm) obstruction of a blood vessel by air or gas

aeroemphysema (-em'fi-ze'ma) decompression sickness

aerogen (ar'o-jen) a gas producing bacteria

aeromonas (ar'o-mo'nas) a genus of schizomycetes, found in water and soil, and rarely may cause opportunistic infection in man

aerootitis (-o-ti'tis) barotitis due to pressure changes

aeropathy (ar-op'a-the) any disorder induced by alteration in the atmospheric pressure

aeroperitonia (ar'o-par'i-to'ne-a) pneumoperitoneum

aerophagy (-pha-ge) excessive swallowing of air.

aerophilic (-fil'ik) aerobic

aeroplethysmograph (-ple-thiz'mo-graf) an instrument to measure respiratory volumes by recording the changes in the body volume

aerosinusitis (-si'nus-i-tis) barosinusitis

aerosol (ar'o-sol) a suspension of fine liquid or solid particles in air which gets dispersed over a wide surface on inhalation into the lungs. Beta-adrenergic bronchodilators, anticholinergic bronchodilators and corticosteroids can be administrated in the form of an aerosol

aerotitis (-ti'tis) barotitis

aesculapius (es'ku-la'pe-us) God of healing in Roman mythology **staff of A** a rod with a snake wound around it signifies the art of healing, and it is used as an emblem of some medical organisations

AFB abbreviation for acid fast bacillus often *Mycobacterium tuberculosis*

afebrile (a-feb'ril) without fever

affect (af'ekt) the experience of emotion expressed by the patient. It is variable over time in response to changing emotional states and is observed by others. **appropriate a** existence of harmony between the emotional tone and the accompanying idea, thought or speech. **inappropriate a** disharmony between emotional tone with the idea, thought or speech accompanying it

affection (a-fek'shun) 1. a state of emotion or feeling 2. a disease state affecting the body or mind

affective (a-fek'tiv) pertaining to affect **a disorder** a maniac-depressive psychosis where the affect varies between the poles of depression and elation **a personality** persistent excessive cheerfulness or depression or alternation of each

afferent (af'er-ent) directed from periphery towards centre such as nerves or signals

affiliate (a-fil'i-ate) to join, to associate

affinity (a-fin'i-te) 1. a natural liking for or attraction to a person or thing. 2. close resemblance or connection 3. a phylogenetic relationship between two organisms or groups of organisms 4. the force by which atoms are held together in chemical compounds

afibrinogenemia (a-fi'brin-o-ji-no'me-a) absence or deficiency of fibrinogen in the blood, leading to its incoagulability

aflotoxicosis acute toxicity noted on consumption of mouldy cereals, pulses or nuts particularly during drought and famine. Aflatoxin produces a picture of acute hepatitis, cirrhosis of the liver or hepatoma depending on dose and duration of exposure

aflatoxin (af'la-tok'sin) toxic products of fungi, particularly *Aspergillus flavus* and *A. parasiticus* which contaminate groundnuts, cereals or pulses stored in damp environment

afterbirth (af'ter-birth) the placenta and membranes that are expelled from the uterus after childbirth

aftercataract residual opacity following lens extraction, usually in posterior capsule

afterdepolarisation (af'ter-de-po'lar-i-za'shun) a depolarising after potential

AFMC The Armed Forces Medical College, Pune, established in 1948

after image (-im'ij) image that remains after cessation of the stimulus.

afterload (af'ter-lod) the force against which cardiac muscle shortens, and it refers to the tension that develops in the ventricular wall during systole

afterpains (-panz) cramplike pain noted after childbirth due to contractions of the uterus

afterpotential (-po-ten'shul) a small alteration in electrical potential in a stimulated nerve following the main potential

aftertaste (-tast) a taste persisting after contact of the tongue with the substance caused

Ag chemical symbol for silver (argentum); antigen

agada(**s**) vegetable or animal poison. *a* A *tantra* toxicology

agalactia (a'ga-lak'she-a) absence of milk in the breasts after childbirth

agammaglobulinaemia (a-gam-a-glob'u-li-ne'me-a) absence of or markedly diminished levels of gamma globulin in the blood, due to an abnormal B lymphocyte function

aganglionosis (a-gang'gle-on-o'sis) absence of ganglion cells as from the myenteric plexus, seen in congenital megacolon.

agantu (s) exogenous

agar (ag'ar) polysaccharide forming stable gel, used in solid culture media in bacteriology

agastric (a-gas'trik) without stomach or alimentary canal

age (aj) 1. the time that has elapsed since the birth of a living individual 2. a particular period of life 3. to grow old. **achievement a** the age of a person expressed as chronologic age of an average person showing the same level of

attainment **chronological a** a record of time elapsed since birth **mental a** the age of a child's relative intelligence as determined by standard intelligence tests

agenesia (a'je-ne'zhah) 1. failure of an organ to develop 2. impotence

agenesis (a-jen'i-sis) absence of an organ, failure to form or imperfect development of an organ

agenitalism (a-jen'i-til-izm) congenital absence of genitals

agenosomia (a-jen'a-so-me-a) absence or defective formation of genitals and eventration of the lower abdominal parts

agent (a'jint) 1. a substance capable of producing an effect 2. cause of disease **disease a** a substance, living or non-living, or a force, tangible or intangible, the excessive presence or relative lack of which may initiate or perpetuate a disease process

ageusia (a-gu'si-a) lack of sense of taste

agger (aj'er) mound; an eminence

agglutinant (a-gloo'ti-nant) 1. a substance that holds parts together, as in wound healing 2. a substance causing adhesion 3. an antibody produced in response to stimulation by an antigen

agglutination (a-gloo'ti-na'shun) adhesion together of small particles to form visible clumps by antibodies

agglutinator (a-agloo'ti-na'tar) an agglutinin.

agglutinin (a-gloo'ti-nin) 1. an antibody found in the blood that attaches to an antigen found on red blood causing them to clump together 2. a substance capable of agglutinating organic particles **anti Rh a** an agglutinin produced in plasma by Rh-negative mothers carrying an Rh positive foetus or following transfusion of Rh-positive blood into an Rh-negative person **cold a** a red blood cell agglutinin that acts only at low temperatures

agglutinogen (ag'loo-tin'o-jen) any substance that stimulates the production of agglutinin

agglutinophilic (a-gloo'ti-no-fil'ik) readily undergoing agglutination.

aggregation (ag're-ga'shun) 1. a mass of materials together 2. a cluster of similar units

aggression (a'gresh'in) exaggeration of drive toward a personal goal

aging (ag'ing) 1. the process of growing old 2. the gradual structural changes that occur with passage cf time

agitation (aj'i-ta'shun) anxiety associated with severe motor restlessness

aglutition (a'gloo'tish'un) dysphagia

aglycaemia (a'gli-se'me-a) absence of sugar in the blood

aglycon (a-gli'kon) the non-carbohydrate moiety of a glycoside molecule

agni(s) fire *a karman* cautery

agnogenic (ag-no-jen'ik) of unknown origin; idiopathic

agnosia (ag-no'zhah) inability to recognise despite an intact sensory apparatus.

agogue combining form for something which leads or induces

agonadism (a-go'na-dism) absence of sex glands

agonist (ag'o-nist) 1. a muscle in a state of contraction 2. a drug capable of combining with receptors and stimulate physiologic activity

agony (ag'o-ne)1. mental or physical suffering 2. death struggle

agoraphobia (ag'o-ra-fob'e-a) fear of open spaces

agranulocyte (a-gran'u-lo-sit) a non-granular leucocyte

agranulocytosis (a-gran'u-lo-si-to'sis) a symptom complex of severe depression of neutrophils often associated with infection. It is characterised by severe prostration, fever, necrotic lesions in the mouth and throat and almost complete absence of neutrophils in peripheral blood

agraphia (a-graf'e-a) loss of power of writing inspite of normal muscles of writing

ague (a'gu) 1. malaria 2. a chill

agyria (a-ji're-a) an improper development of the gyri of the cerebral cortex

ahankara (s) ego

ahara(s) food

ahitara (s) unfavourable

aid (ad) help or assistance to a person **hearing a** sound amplifying instrument used by persons with impaired hearing **first a** an emergency assistance given to the injured or diseased before arrival of a physician or transportation to the hospital **robotic a** a mechanical device operated by a person

AIDS acquired immunodeficiency syndrome

AIIMS All India Institute of Medical Sciences, New Delhi

ailurophobia (i-loor'o-fo'bi-a) morbid fear of cats

ainhum (i'num) linear groove at the root of toe with swelling of distal part as if tied by a ligature and severe pain. The groove invades circumferentially to cause auto amputation, noted in bare footed males, in Africa

air (ar) the invisible, colourless mixture of gases that make up the atmosphere. The approximate per cent of the gas after removal of water vapour is oxygen 20.94, nitrogen 78.03, argon and other rare gases 0.99, and carbon dioxide 0.04 **a bags** protective devices in automobiles that are designed to expand upon impact to protect the driver and passengers from injury **alveolar a** air in the alveoli that is involved in the pulmonary exchange of gases **complemental a** inspiratory reserve volume **functional residual a** the volume of air that remains in the lungs at the end of a normal expiration **reserve a** expiratory reserve volume **residual a** air remaining in the lung without being expelled even after forceful expiration **supplement a** expiratory reserve volume **tidal a** amount of air breathed in and out of the lungs during a normal quiet breathing and it is about 500 ml in adults

air borne (ar'born) an agent suspended in, and spread by air

airway (ar'wa) 1. air passage 2. a device to keep the main airway patent

ajmaline rauwolfia alkaloid

akaryocyte (a-kar'e-o-sit) a non-nucleated cell such as a red blood cell

akaryote (a-kar'e-ot) akaryocyte

akathisia (ak'a-thi'zhah) inability to sit still with motor restlessness

akin (a-kin) of similar nature

akinesia (a'ki-ne'zhah) absence or poverty of movements **akinetic** adj

akinetic epilepsy a mild form of epilepsy with brief loss of muscle tone causing fall to the ground

akinetic deaf mutism minimal recovery from major brain damage with awareness but without speech or spontaneous movement

akinesthesia (a-kin'es-the'zhah) absence of sense of perception of movement

akriti (s) appearance

akshi(s) eye

Al chemical symbol, aluminium

ala (a'la) pl **alae** a winglike structure **a nasi** the broad and lateral flaring wall of each nostril

alacrima (a-lak'ri-ma) a deficiency or absence of lacrimal secretion

alactasia (a'lak-ta'zhah) inability to absorb lactose due to an abnormality of brushborder of small intestine leading to an osmotic diarrhoea

Alagille syndrome a rare inherited liver disorder in infants and young children due to a builtup of bile in the liver due to deformity or absence of normal bile ducts, and presents with jaundice, stunted growth, fatty deposits in the skin and facial deformities

alalia (a-la'le-a) inability to speak due to paralysis of vocal organs

alanine (al'a-nen) one of the amino acids found widely in proteins

alanine transaminase (-trans-am'i-nas) ALT. glutamic-pyruvic transaminase. An

aminoenzyme transferring amino groups from L-alanine to 2 ketoglutarate or the reverse, and is found in high concentrations in muscle, liver and brain.

alar (a'lar) 1. pertaining to an ala or wing 2. axillary

alba (al'ba) white

albedo (al-be'do) whiteness

Albers-Schonberg (al'bars-skon'barg) **disease** a hereditary condition characterised by increased bone density secondary to defective resorption named after Albers-Schonberg, German radiologist

albicans (al'bi-kans) white

albiduria (al'bi-du're-a) passage of pale or white urine

albinism (al'bi-nizm) congenital absence of pigment in the skin, hair and eyes due to tyrosine abnormality in production of melanin **oculocutaneous a** a condition without melanin, inherited as an autosomal recessive trait, characterised by white skin, deficient pigment in the hair, iris and retina, poor vision, photophobia, and rotary nystagmus.

albino (al-bi'no) an individual with albinism

albinoidism (al-bi'noid'izm) deficiency of pigmentation in hair, skin and eyes and it is less than that seen in albinism

albinuria (al'bi-nu're-a) albiduria

Albright's syndrome a condition characterised by precocious puberty, irregular pigmentation and dysplasia of several bones named after Fuller Albright, US physician

Albuginea (al'bu-jin'e-a) 1. a white fibrous tissue covering a part or organ 2. the tunica albuginea

albumin (ab-bu'min) a simple protein distributed widely in tissues and fluids of plants and animals **blood a** a serum albumin **egg a** albumin of egg whites. **human a** sterile preparation of serum albumin obtained by fractionating blood plasma proteins from healthy blood donors **serum a** The principal protein found in the blood plasma

albuminoid (al-bu'mi-noid) 1. resembling albumin 2. any protein 3. scleroprotein found in horny and cartilaginous tissues and in the lens of the eye

albuminuretic (al-bu'mi-nu-re-tik) relating to, characterised by or suffering from albuminuria

albuminuria (al-bu'mi-nu're-a) presence of protein, chiefly albumin in the urine

alcaligenes (al-ka-lij i-nes) a genus of rod-shaped, gram-negative bacteria of the family achromobacteraceae found in the intestinal tract in the dairy products and in soil

alcohol (al'ka-hol) derived from arabic word al-koh'l. One of a series of organic chemical compounds containing hydroxyl (-OH) functional group. **absolute a** a solution containing 99% alcohol **benzyl a** a colourless liquid used as a bacteriostatic and as a local anaesthetic **cetyl a** a solid alcohol used as an emulsifying agent **dehydrated a** a volatile liquid used as a solvent and injected into nerves and ganglia for relief of pain **denatured a** ethyl alcohol rendered unfit for consumption **ethyl a** ethanol, ordinary grain alcohol **isopropyl a** a volatile liquid used as a solvent and disinfectant **ethyl a** methanol, liquid obtained by distillation of wood **wood a** methanol.

alcoholics anonymous AA. A self-help programme for fighting addition to alcohol

alcoholism (-izm) a disorder characterised by alcohol abuse, dependence or addiction

aldehyde (al'de-hid) a compound containing CH=O that can be reduced to an alcohol or oxidised to an acid, which includes acetaldehyde

aldehyde reductase (re-duk'tas) an enzyme that catalyses the reduction of aldoses.

aldolase (al'do-las) an enzyme participating in the conversion of glycogen into lactic acid, found in the skeletal and cardiac muscle and liver

aldose (al'dos) a monosaccharide containing aldehyde (-CHO) group

aldosterone (al-dos'ter-on) a mineralocorticoid hormone secreted by adrenal cortex. Its major action is in the regulation of electrolyte and water balance by promoting the retention of sodium and excretion of potassium in the distal convoluted renal tubules

aldosteronism (al-dos'te-ro-nizm) hyperaldosteronism, a disorder caused by excessive secretion of aldosterone **primary a** see Conn's syndrome **secondary a** extraadrenal stimulation of aldosterone secretion as in nephrotic syndrome, cardiac failure, cirrhosis and hypoproteinaemia.

alecithal (a-les'i- thal) without yolk

alendronate (a-en'dro-nate) drug used in osteoporosis

alepa(s) plaster

aleucocytosis (a-loo'ko-si-to'sis) absence or marked reduction in the number of circulating white blood cells.

aleukaemia (a'loo-ke'me-a) 1. a decrease in the number of leucocytes in the blood.2. leukaemic changes in the bone marrow with a decrease in number of leucocytes in the peripheral blood

aleukia (a-loo'ke-a) absence or markedly decreased number of leucocytes in the peripheral blood

alexia (a-lek'se-a) loss of ability to understand the meaning of written or printed words or sentences

alexic (-sik) pertaining to alexia

alexithymia inability or difficulty to describe one's emotions or moods

aleydigism (a-li'dig-izm) absence of secretion of interstitial cells of Leydig

alga (al'ga) individual organism of algae.

algae (al'je) chlorophyll containing water plants, living in both sea and fresh water, varying in size

algefacient (ál'je-fa'shint) cooling or refregerant

algesia (al-je'ze-a) 1. appreciation of pain sense 2. excessive sensitivity to pain

algesimeter (al'je-sim'e-ter) an instrument for measuring the degree of sensitivity to a painful stimulus.

algesinogenic (al-je'ze-no-jen'ik) producing pain

algesthesis (al'jes-the'sis) algesia

-algia combining word for pain

algicide (al'ji-sid) 1. destructive to algae 2. an agent which destroys algae

algid (al'jid) chilly; cold

algophobia fear of pain

algorithm (al'go-rith'm) step by step set of instructions on hand to accomplish a task. They provide a useful skeleton to illustrate the major factors of decision

Alice in wonderland syndrome bizarre perceptional distortions of the body image, space and size

alienia (a'li-e'ne-a) absence of the spleen

aliform (al'i-form) wing-shaped

alimentary (al'i-men'ta-ri) relating to food or to organs of digestion **a system** digestive system from mouth to anus consisting of oesophagus, stomach, small and large intestines and rectum

alimentation (al'i-men-ta'shun) providing nourishment

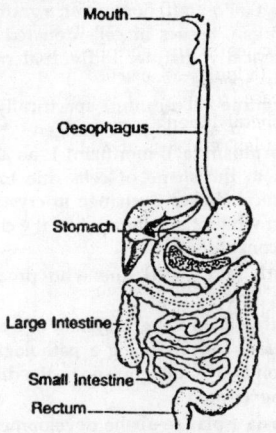

Alimentary system

alinasal (al'i-na'zl) pertaining to ala nasi

aliphatic (al-i-fat'ik) 1. fatty or oily 2. pertaining to acyclic carbon compounds **a acids** acids of nonaromatic hydrocarbons such as acetic, propionic and butyric acids

aliquot (al'i-kwot) pertaining to a portion of the whole

alisphenoid (al-i-sfe'noid) pertaining to the greater wing of the sphenoid bone

alkalaemia (al'ka-le'me-a) a fall in H^+ ion concentration of the blood or a rise in pH

alkali (al'ka-li) a strong basic substance yielding hydroxide (OH-) ions in solution, such as sodium hydroxide

alkaline (al'ka-lin) relating to or having the reaction of an alkali

alkalinuria (al'ka-li-nu're-a) the passage of alkaline urine

alkalizer (al'ka-lizer) an agent that causes alkalisation

alkaloid (al'ka-loid) heterocyclic nitrogen-containing plant product having pharmacologic activity and the examples are atropine, nicotine, caffeine, cocaine, strychnine, morphine and quinine. **Vinca a's** alkaloids produced by *Vinca rosea;* vincristine and vinblastine are used in treatment of malignancy

alkalosis (al'ka-lo'sis) an increase in base or decrease in acid. **compensated a** alkalosis in which there is rise in bicarbonate but the pH of the body fluids is near normal due to compensatory mechanisms of the body **metabolic a** an increase in plasma bicarbonate concentration. There is marked loss of acid other than H_2CO_3 from the stomach and kidney and a fall in plasma chloride **respiratory a** a condition where CO_2 in the arterial blood is below normal range. There is hyperventilation and pH is raised **uncompensated a** rise in bicarbonate concentration and pH of body fluids is raised due to lack of compensatory mechanisms

alkyl (al'kl) a monovalent hydrocarbon radical

alkylation (al'ki-la'shun) substitution of an alkyl radical for a hydrogen atom

ALL abbreviation for acute lymphoblastic leukaemia

all (o) combining form for the word other; deviating from normal

allantochorion (a-lan'to-kor'e-on) an extraembryonic membrane formed by fusion of allantois and chorion

allantoid (a-lan'toid) 1. sausage-shaped 2. resembling the allantois

allantoin (a-lan'to-in) a substance found in the allantoic fluid, and urine of the foetus

allantois (a-lan'to-is) a vestigeal foetal membrane developing from the yolk sac

allele (a'lel) one of two or more variations of a gene located at a particular site of chromosome

allelochemics (al-le'lo-kem'iks) chemical interaction between species and it is associated with release of active chemical substances

allelotaxis (-tak'sis) development of an organ from a number of embryonic structures or tissues

allergen (al'er-jen) an antigenic substance capable of producing hypersensitivity (immediate and late) reaction.

allergic relating to any response stimulated by an allergen. **a shiners** dark, discoloured circles under the eyes in children with allergic rhinitis

allergist (al'er-jist) a person specialised in the treatment of allergic disorders

allergy (al'er-je) 1. an immunologic response in a susceptible person to exposure to an allergen. The exposure to antigen in atopic individuals stimulates peripheral lymphoid tissues to synthesise IgE antibodies. They possess 2 Fab and Fc pieces. They get fixed by Fc piece to the mast cells. The cytoplasmic matrix of the mast cells is filled with granules. Any further exposure to the same antigen leads to the union of antigen with the antigen receptors on Fab portion of two molecules of IgE antibody. There is degranulation of the cells following entry of calcium and release of mediators of anaphylaxis 2. an acquired hypersensitivity to certain drugs and biologic products

allesthesia (al'es-the'zhah) experiencing a sensation remote from the place where stimulus is applied, stimulus in one limb being referred to opposite limb

alleviate (a'liv'i-at) relieve

Allgrove syndrome a syndrome of primary adrenocortical insufficiency with achalasia of cardia and deficient tear production *see* triple A syndrome

alloantibody (al'o-anti-bod-e) an antibody occurring in some members of a species

alloantigen (-an'ti-gen) an antigen occurring in some members of a species

allobarbital (-bar'bi-tal) a barbituric acid preparation acting as a sedative and hypnotic

allochromasia (-okro-ma-zhah) change of colour of the skin or hair

allodynia (din'e-a) pain from non-noxious stimulus

alloerotism (-er'o-tizm) sexual attraction towards another person

allogeneic (-je-ne'ik) pertaining to different gene constitutions within the same species

allogenic (-jen'ik) allogeneic

allograft (al'o-graft) homograft; a graft such as organ, tissues or cells donated from genetically distinct individual of the same species

alloimmune (al'o-i-mun) specifically immune to an allogenic antigen

allomorphism (al'o-mor'fizm) 1. an alteration in the shape of cells due to mechanical causes 2. change in crystalline form without an alteration in the chemical constitution

allopath (al'o-path) one who practices allopathy

allopathy (al'op'a-the) a system of treating diseases by producing a pathologic reaction that is antagonistic to the disease being treated

alloplasia (-plas'ze-a) the development of tissues at a site where such tissue does not occur

alloplast (al'o-plast) a graft of an inert or plastic material

alloplasty (al'o-plas'te) 1. repair of defects by alloplast 2. adaptation by altering the external environment

allopsychic (-si'kik) pertaining to the mental processes in their relation to the external world

allopurinol (-pur'i-nol) a drug capable of inhibiting xanthine oxidase and bring down the serum and urinary level of uric acid. Used in the treatment of gout

allorhythmia (-rith'me-a) irregularity of the heart recurring regularly

all or none (awl or non) any stimulus, however weak exciting a cardiac contraction will produce as powerful contraction as the strong stimulus

allosensitization (al'o-sen'si-ti-za'shun) sensitisation to alloantigens as to Rh antigens during pregnancy

allosome (al'o-som) one of the chromosomes differing in appearance or behaviour from an ordinary chromosome

allostasis (al'o-sta-sis) ability to achieve stability of body systems through change

allotherm (al'o-therm) an animal where body temperature exhibits variation according to the temperature of the environment

allotope (-top) a site on the constant region of an antibody that can be recognised by a combining site of other antibodies

allotropic (al'o-trop'ik) 1. allotropism 2. *psy* a type of personality preoccupied with the reactions of other

allotropism (a-lot'ro-pizm) existence of certain elements in several forms

allotype (al'o-tip) any one of the genetically determined antigenic differences within a given class of immunoglobulins

alloxan (a-lok'san) an oxidation product of uric acid capable of destroying islets of Langerhans in experimental animals and produce diabetes

alloy (al'oi) a metallic substance resulting from a mixture of two or more metals.

Alma-Ata Declaration a declaration made at a conference on primary health care held at Alma-Ata, Kazakhistan (1978), that primary health care is the key to attain health for all by 2000 A.D.

aloe (al'o) dried juice from the leaves of *Aloe*

alopaecia (al'o-pa'she-a) absence or loss to hair from skin areas where it is normally found **a aerata** circumscribed loss of hair on the scalp and beard **a capitis totalis** total loss of hair on the scalp **cicatricial a** loss of hair associated with scarring **male pattern a** hair loss in males, which begins in the frontal region and progresses to leave behind a horse shoe area of hair remains in the back and temples due to the influence of androgenic hormone **a medicamentosa** diffuse hair loss of the scalp due to administration of cytotoxic agents **a totalis** total loss of hair of the scalp **a universalis** total loss of hair from all parts of the body

alpha (al'fa) the first letter of Greek alphabet; α

alpha fetoprotein (alfa-fe'to-pro'ten) AFP a plasma protein formed in foetal liver, yolk sac, and gastrointestinal tract and by hepatocellular carcinoma

alpha antitrypsin (an'ti-trip'sin) an alpha 2 globulin produced by the liver which inhibits the activity of trypsin and other proteolytic enzymes

alphalytic (-lit'ik) an alpha-adrenergic receptor blocking agent

alphamimetic (-mi-met'ik) simulating the stimulation of alpha adrenergic receptors of the sympathetic nervous system

alphavirus (al'fa-vi'rus) a genus of viruses belonging to the family togaviridae

ALT alanine aminotransferase

Alport's syndrome an inherited cause of renal failure due to progressive degeneration of glomerular basement membrane with deafness, named after Arthur Alport, South African physician

Alstrom (al-strom) syndrome a rare hereditary recessive condition with progressive pigmentary retinopathy, childhood truncal obesity, hearing loss, type 2 diabetes mellitus, hypogonadism, and normal intelligence, named after C.H. Alstrom, Swedish physician

alteplase (al'te-plas) a tissue plasminogen activator produced by recombinant DNA technology

alternans (awl-ter'nanz) alternating, often applied to alternation of the heart **electrical a** a disorder showing ventricular complexes regular but alternating in pattern **mechanical a** the contractions of heart are regular in time but are alternatively stronger and weaker **pulsus a** regular heart rhythm in which strong beats alternate weak ones

alternation (all'ter-na'shun) the occurrence of two opposing or different events in succession

alternative medicine the approach to the diagnosis and treatment by other modalities which do not fall in the generally accepted scientific methods which include acupressure, acupuncture, ayurveda, faith healing, herbal medicine, homoeopathy, hypnosis, electrotherapy, naturotherapy, *siddha*, unani, and yoga

altruism (al'trui-zam) unselfishly giving help when it is needed

alum (al'um) an astringent and styptic, a double-sulphate of aluminium and ammonium compound

alumina (a-loo'mi-na) aluminium oxide

aluminosis (a-loo'mi-no'sis) a pneumoconiosis developing from inhalation of aluminium particles

aluminium (a-loo'mi-num) a metallic element, symbol Al atomic number 13, used as an astringent, antiseptic and antipyretic.

alveolar relating to an alveolus

alveolectomy surgical excision of a portion of dentoalveolar process

alveoli (al-ve'o-li) pl of alveolus

alveolitis (al-ve'o-li'tis) 1. inflammation of alveoli 2. inflammation of a tooth socket. **Cryptogenic fibrosing a** a fibrosing lesion from the beginning **extrinsic allergic a** a hypersensitivity reaction occurring at the peripheral gas exchanging parts of the lungs in response to repeated inhalation of antigens contained

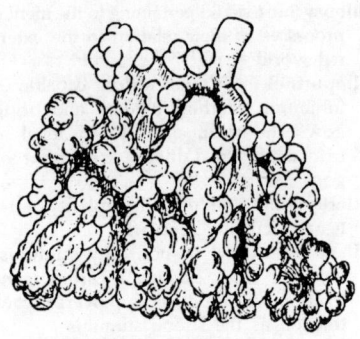

Pulmonary alveoli

in finely particulate organic dusts of wide variety and other agents by a susceptible individual. External agents like spores of thermophilic actinomycetes and other fungi, moulding stored vegetable matters (hay, bagasse) and animal protein (avian, bovine, porcine or insect material) act as antigens **fibrosing a** an inflammatory process of the lung with predominant involvement of alveolar walls. It is characterised by inflammatory cellular thickening of the alveolar walls with marked tendency to fibrosis (mural) or the presence of a large number of large mononuclear cells (desquamative)

alveoloclasia (al-ve'o-lo-kla'se-a) destruction of the inner wall of tooth alveolus.

alveoloplasty (al-ve'o-lo-plas'te) surgical preparation of the alveolar ridges for the reception of dentures

alveolus (al-ve'o-lus) pl **alveoli** 1. a small cavity 2. a sac-like dilatation **a dentalis** tooth socket. **pulmonary a** terminal blind ending structures of the respiratory bronchioles where gas exchange takes place

alveus (al've-us) a channel or groove

alymphocytosis (a-lim'fo-si-to'sis) absence or marked reduction in the number of lymphocytes

alymphoplasia (-pla'zhah) failure of development of lymphoid tissue

Alzheimer's (alts'hi-merz) **disease** a condition with atrophy of brain particularly the cerebral cortex and hippocampus, characterised by gradual impairment of memory and dementia, named after Alois Alzheimer, German neurologist

ama(s) products of digestion *a dosa* indigestion a sakti   digestive power a vata rheumatoid arthritis

amacrine (am'a-kren) a cell or structure with long fibrous process

amalgum (a-mal'gum) an alloy of a metal with mercury, such as a mixture of silver and mercury is used to fill teeth

amanita (am'a-ni'ta) a genus of fungi, many members of which are poisonous

amantadine (a-man'ta-den) an antiviral agent used in prophylaxis against influenza A virus and in the treatment of Parkinsonism

amapitta (s) acidity

amasaya (s) stomach

amastia (a-mas'te-a) congenital absence of breast

amaurosis (am'aw-ro'sis) blindness occurring without any apparent cause. **amaurotic** adj **a fugax** a temporary loss of vision from a transient ischemia due to carotid artery insufficiency

ambidextrous (am'bi-dek-strus) having ability to use either hand effectively.

ambilateral (-lat'er-il) relating to both sides

ambilevous (-le'vus) inability to use either hand efficiently

ambiopia (am'be-o'pe-a) diplopia

ambisexual (am'bi-sek'shoo-al) bisexual

ambivalence (am-biv'a-lens) coexistence of two opposing impulses towards the same thing in the same person at the same time

amblyomma (am'ble-om'a) a genus of hard-bodied ticks

amblyopia (-o'pe-a) reduction or dimness of vision without any detectable organic lesion

amblyoscope (am'ble-o-skop) an instrument to measure binocular vision and for stimulation of vision in the amblyopic eye

amboceptor (am'bo-sep'ter) a haemolysis having double receptors, to combine with the red blood cell and with complement

ambon (am'bon) the raised ring of fibrocartilage around the edge of a bone socket

ambu bag a self-refilling bag-valve mask unit of 1 to 1.5 litre capacity, used for artificial respiration

ambulance a vehicle for transporting the sick and injured persons. It is equipped and staffed to give medical aid during shifting, **air a** helicopters used to bring injured people to hospitals

ambulatory (am'bu-la-tor'e) able to walk; not confined to bed

amelia (a-me'le-a) congenital absence of a limb or limbs

amelification (a-mel'i-fi-ka'shun) development of enamel cells into enamel

amelioration (a-mel'yo-ra'shun) improvement, as of patient's condition

ameloblast (a-mel'o-blast) a cylindrical epithelial cell found in the innermost layer of the enamel

ameloblastoma (a-mel'o-blas'to'ma) a benign but locally invasive tumour of enamel organ

amelogenesis (am'e-lo-jen'i-sis) the formation of enamel

amelogenin (-jen'in) any of several proteins secreted by ameloblasts and forming the organic matrix of enamel

amenorrhoea (a-men'o-re'a) absence or abnormal cessation of the menstruation **lactation a** absence of menstruation incidental to lactation **physiologic a** absence of menstruation during pregnancy **primary a** failure of menstruation to occur at puberty **secondary a** cessation of menstruation in a woman who was menstruating earlier

amentia (a-men'shah) 1. mental retardation 2. mental disorder characterised by confusion, disorientation and sometimes stupor

ametria (a-me'tre-a) congenital absence of the uterus

ametropia (am'i-tro'pe-a) a refractory error with failure of parallel rays to get focussed on retina

AMI abbreviation for acute myocardial infarction

amidase (am'i-das) an enzyme that catalyses the hydrolysis of amide

amide (am'id) substance derived from ammonia through substitution of an acid radical for hydrogen or from an acid through replacing-OH group by - NH$_2$

amikacin (am'ika'sin) aminoglycoside-antibiotic, active against many gentamicin resistant organisms

amimia (a-mim'e-a) loss of power to expression by gestures or signs

amine (a-men) a substance derived from ammonia by replacement of one or more hydrogen atoms by hydrocarbon or other radicals **sympathomimetic a** a substance that evokes responses similar to those produced by adrenergic nerve activity

amino (a-me'no) combining word for a compound containing the radical group- NH$_2$

amino acid organic compounds containing both amino (NH$_2$) and a carboxyl (COOH) group. Amino acids are essential building blocks for proteins and poly-peptides **branched chain a** a essential amino acids leucine, isoleucine and valine. They bypass liver and are available for the cells from the circulation. **dispensable a** a amino acids that can be synthesised in the body by transamination if there is sufficient supply of amino group **essential a** a amino acids that cannot be synthesised by the organism and are to be supplied in the diet. They are histidine, isoleucine, leucine, lysine, methionine, cysteine, phenylalanine, tyrosine, threonine, tryptophan and valine. Arginine is also needed in infants **indispensable a** a amino acids required in the diet **non-essential a** a amino acid that may be synthesized by ¡e organism

aminoacidaemia (a-me'no-as'i-de'me-a) an excess amount of amino acids in the blood

aminoaciduria (-as'i-du're-a) excretion of amino acids in urine, in excessive amounts

aminobenzoate (-ben'zo-at) any salt or ester of p-aminobenzoic acid

p-aminobenzoic acid (-ben-zo'-ik) PABA a substance required for synthesis of folic acid. It is capable of absorption of ultraviolet light.

γ aminobutyric acid (-bu-ter'ik) GABA an inhibitory neurotransmitter substance found in CNS

ε aminocaproic acid (-ka-pro'ik) a nonessential amino acid that acts as an inhibitor of plasmin and of plasminogen activators.

aminoglutethimide (-gloo-teth'i-mid) a substance that inhibits cholesterol metabolism, thus of production of adrenocortical hormone

aminoglycoside (-gli'ko-sid) any of a group of antibiotics derived from *Streptomyces* or produced synthetically. Streptomycin, gentamicin, tobramycin, netilmycin, amikacin and neomycin possess similiar structure and adverse effects

p-aminohippurate (-hip'urat) any salt of aminohippuric acid.

p-aminohippuric acid (-hi-pur'ik) PAHA glycine amide of p-aminobenzoic acid used intravenously to determine renal blood flow and excretory capacity of the renal tubules

δ-aminolevulinic acid (-lev'u-lin'ik) ALA an intermediate in the biosynthesis of haem

6-aminopenicillanic acid (a-me'no-pen'isil-an'ik) the active nucleus common to all penicillins. Semisynthetic penicillins are prepared by substitution at the 6-amino position

aminophylline (am'i-nof'i-lin) a mixture of theophylline and ethylenediamine used as a bronchodilator

aminopterin (am'i-nop'ter-in) a folic acid antagonist

aminoquinoline (a-me′no-kwin′o-len) a compound derived from quinoline by addition of an amino group. It comprises 4 aminoquinolines and 8 aminoquinolines used as antimalarial agents

aminosalicylate (-sa-lis′i-lat) any salt of p-aminosalicylic acid

p-aminosalicylic (-sal′i-sil′ik) **acid** PAS a bacteriostatic substance used in treatment of tuberculosis. It is less effective, possesses antipyretic action. It has to be administered in large doses, and deteriorates on storage for long time

aminotransferase (-trans′fer-as) transaminase enzyme transferring amino groups from α-amino acid to a 2-keto acid

aminuria (am′i-nu′re-a) presence of excess amounts of amines in the urine

amiodarone (a-me′o-da-ron) antiarrhythmic agent whose main effect is to prolong action potential in the heart and is effective for controlling paroxysmal atrial fibrillation and recurrent ventricular tachycardia. It has a very long tissue half life

amitosis (am′i-to′sis) a direct cell division by simple cleavage of the nucleus

amitriptyline (am′i-trip′ti-len) a tricyclic anti-depressant

AML abbreviation for acute myelogenous leukaemia

amla (s) acid, sour

amlodipine (am-lo′di-pen) an ultra long acting calcium channel blocker used in the management of angina pectoris and hypertension

amnioaciduria (am′o-as′i-du′re-a) presence of an excess amount of ammonia and amino acids in the urine

ammonia (a-mon′ya) a volatile gas NH_3, soluble in water forming a base NH_4OH

ammonium (a-mo′ne-um) the radical, NH_4^+ formed by combination of NH_3 and $H+$

ammoniuria (a-mo′ne-u′re-a) presence of an excess amount of ammonia in the urine

amnesia (am-ne′zhah) partial or total inability to recall past experiences. It may be organic or emotional in origin **anterograde a** amnesia in reference to the events following injury or disease **dissociative a** patchy and inconsistent memory loss and is a characteristic feature of a loss of personal identity. **retrograde a** amnesia in reference to the events that occurred before the injury or disease **transient a** loss of memory for a period of time due to a toxic confusional state, psychological fugue state or postictal period after a seizure **transient global a** an abrupt discrete and reversible loss of short-term memory function

amniocele (am′ne-o-sel) omphalocele

amniocentesis (am′ne-o-sen-te′sis) aspiration of fluid from the amniotic sac by transabdominal or trans-cervical approach guided by ultra sound scanning. It is a prenatal diagnostic procedure performed to study for genetic and biochemical disorders, and to determine foetal maturity

amniogenesis (-jen′i-sis) the development of amnion

amnion (am′ne-on) the innermost of the membranes that envelop the embryo in uterus and filled with amniotic fluid

amniorhexis (am′ne-o-rek′sis) rupture of the amnion

amnioscope (am-ne-o-skop) an endoscope to visualise the foetus and amniotic fluid

amniotic cavity the fluid filled cavity of the amnion

amniotic fluid liquor amni. The albuminous, transparent fluid in the amnion protects the foetus from injury, helps in maintenance of an even temperature and prevent development of any adhesions between the amnion and the foetus **a embolism** a syndrome resulting from traumatic delivery and injection of amniotic fluid into the maternal circulation

amniotic sac a thin-walled bag containing the foetus and amniotic fluid during pregnancy

amniotomy (am'ne-ot'a-me) artificial rupture of the foetal membranes to induce labour

amobarbital (am'o-bar'bi-tal) an intermediate acting sedative

amodiaquine (-di-a-kwin) an antimalarial and anti-inflammatory agent

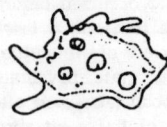

Amoeba

amoeba (a-me'ba) a pseudopod forming protozoa of the class sarcodina found in water. It constantly changes its shape by sending out finger-like processes of protoplasm for mobility and to obtain food. Some species of the genus amoeba such as entamoeba, iodamoeba and acanthamoeba are parasites of man

amoebiasis (am'e-bi-a-sis) a disease caused by *Entamoeba histolytica*, a pathogenic intestinal amoeba. It spreads between humans by its cysts. It gives rise to amoebic dysentery or extra intestinal amoebiasis such as amoebic liver abscess. The amoebic cysts gain entry into the body by faecal oral route. The vegetative trophozoites emerge from the cysts in the colon, and invade the mucous membrane and produce flask-shaped ulcers. Amoebae reach the liver through portal venous system and cause destruction of parenchyma of the liver to produce an amoebic abscess. The liquid contents are chocolate brown in colour **hepatic a** *see* hepatic amoebiasis **intestinal a** presents with a chronic course with mucous diarrhoea, sometimes with streaks of blood, abdominal pain, tenderness along the line of colon; or with acute symptoms of dysen-

tery. Metronidazole, tinidazole are useful

amoebicide (a-me'bi-sid) an agent that kills amoeba

amoebocyte (a-me'bo-sit) a cell showing amoeboid movement

amoeboid (a-me'boid) resembling amoeba

amoeboma(am'e-bo'ma) a localised granuloma due to *E. histolytica* causing a palpable mass in the rectum

amok a psychotic reaction in which the person goes on a homicidal rampage.

amorph (a'morf) a silent mutated allele that has no effect on the phenotypic expression of a trait

amorphia (a-mor'fi-a) quality of being amorphous

amorphous (a-mor'fus) 1. without definite shape 2. not crystallised

amosite (a-mo'sit) brown asbestos

amotio (a-mo'she-o) removal or detachment

amotivation (a-moti'va-shun) **syndrome** behavioural pattern characterised by widespread apathy toward productive activities

amoxycillin (a-mok'si-sil'in) an analogue of ampicillin with a similar antibacterial spectrum. It is reliably absorbed from the gastroinstestinal tract

AMP adenosine monophosphate

amp ampere

ampere (am'per) a unit of electric current produced by one volt acting through a resistance of one ohm, named after Andre Ampere

amphetamine (am-fet'a-men) a sympathomimetic amine having CNS stimulating effects

amph(i) combining word for both; on both sides

amphiarthrosis (am-fe-ar-thro-sis) an articulation permitting little motion as the opposing surfaces of bone are connected by fibrocartilage, such as articulations of the bodies of the vertebrae

amphibia (am-fib'e-a) a cold blooded vertebrate that breaths by gills in larval state and by lungs on metamorphosis.

It includes frogs and toads. They live on land and in water

amphibolic (am'fi-bol'ik) 1. uncertain 2. possessing both anabolic and catabolic functions

amphidiarthrosis (-di'ar-thro'sis) a joint articulation with amphiarthrosis and diathrosis, such as lower jaw

amphigonadism (-geon'a-dizm) having both ovarian and testicular tissue; true hermaphroditism

amphitrichous (am-fit'ri-kus) having a single flagellum

amphocyte (am'fo-sit) a cell that stains readily with acid or basic dyes

amphophilic (am'fo-fil'ik) stainable with either acidic or basic dyes

amphoric (am-for'ik) resembling the sound made by blowing across the mouth of a bottle, **a breath sound** a variant of bronchial breathing having a hollow reverboratory quality, audible over an open pneumothorax and over a thin walled cavity communicating with a bronchus.

amphoteric (am'fo-ter'ik) capable of acting either as an acid or base

amphotericin B (-ter'i-sin) an antibiotic preparation used in the treatment of systemic fungal infections. It is administered by intravenous infusion in increasing daily doses

ampicillin (amp'i-sil'in) a semi-synthetic penicillin having a bactericidal action against both Gram-positive and some Gram-negative organisms. It is susceptible to degradation by beta-lactamases

amplification (am-pli-fi-ka'shun) 1. a process of making bigger such as an increase of an auditory stimulus 2. multiple copies of a DNA sequence

amplify (am'pli-fi) to elaborate, to enlarge

amplitude (am'pli-tood) width or breadth of range or extent

ampule (am'pul) a small sealed glass container that preserves its contents sterile, such as medication for parenteral administration

ampulla (am-pul'ah) a flask-like dilatation of a tubular structure pl **ampullae a ductus differentis** dilatation of vas deferens where it approaches its fellow prior to it is joined by the duct of seminal vesicle **hepato pancreatic a** the dilatation formed by junction of the common bile duct and main pancreatic duct proximal to their opening into the duodenum; a of Vater **membranous a** the dilatations at one end of each of the three semicircular ducts (anterior, posterior and lateral) where they connect with the utricle **osseous a** the dilatation of one end of each of the three bony semicircular canals (anterior, posterior and lateral), each contains a membranous ampulla **rectal a** dilated portion of the rectum just above the anal canal **a of Thoma** one of the small terminal expansion of an interlobar arteries in the splenic pulp **a of uterine tube** the wide portion of fallopian tube near the fimbriated end

amputation (am'pu-ta'shun) the surgical removal of limb/or part of a limb or an outgrowth **above knee (AK) a** division of femur in the supra-condylar region at mid-thigh **below knee (BK) a** division of tibia and fibula distal to tibial tuberosity **Chopart's a** amputation of the foot through mid-tarsal joint **congenital a** amputation of foetal parts as a developmental defeat **double-flap a** amputation in which a flap is cut from the soft parts on either side of the limb. **Dupuytren's a** amputation of arm or shoulder joint **flap a** an amputation in which flaps of muscle and skin are made to cover the end of the bone **guillotine a** amputation performed by a circular incision through the skin, and the muscles and bone are kept and left open for dressing **primary a** amputation performed before inflammation sets in **secondary a** amputation performed during suppuration **spontaneous a** amputation as a result of disease process rather than external trauma as in leprosy or diabetes mellitus **Syme's a** amputation of the foot at the ankle joint with removal of the malleoli **traumatic a** amputation resulting from accident

amputation sign sharp cut-off on air bronchograms in pulmonary thromboembolism

amputee a person with an amputated limb

amusia (a-mu'ze-a) a form of aphasia with loss of ability to appreciate simple musical tones.

amyelinic (a-mi'e-lin'ik) 1. without myelin 2. without medullary sheath

amygdala (a-mig'da-la) 1. an almond-shaped structure 2. corpus amygdaloideum 3. tonsilla cerebelli 4. lymphatic tonsils.

amygdaline (-len) 1. like an almond 2. pertaining to tonsil or to an amygdala

amyl (am'il) the radical formed from a pentane **a nitrate** a vasodilator, used in angina by inhalation

amylaceous (am'i-la'she-us) starchy

amylase (am'i-las) an enzyme that catalyses the hydrolysis of starch into smaller molecules

amyl (o) combining word for starch

amylin (a'my-lin) islet amyloid polypeptide found in beta cells found in all persons and is cosecreted with insulin

amyloid (am'i-loid) any of a group of chemically diverse proteins that appear microscopically homogeneous, that get deposited in the walls of blood vessels especially in association with reticuloendothelial tissue. **a AA** secondary amyloid derived from serum protein **a AL** amyloid made up of light chain immunoglobulin

amyloidosis (am'i-loi-do'sis) a disease associated with amyloid deposition. **primary a** monoclonal over production of a normal immunoglobulin light chain often presents with nephrotic syndrome, renal impairment, restrictive cardiomyopathy, malabsorption, macroglossia, and peripheral neuropathy **reactive a** deposition of normal protein, amyloid A component. It is produced in the liver in response to long-standing inflammation. It is associated with nephrotic syndrome, progressive renal impairment and hepatosplenomegaly

amylopectin (am'i-lo-pek'tin) insoluble branched chain starch, found in cereals.

amylopectinosis (-pek'ti-no'sis) glycogen storage disease, type IV

amylorrhoea (-re'a) presence of abnormal amount of strach in the stools

amyluria (am'il-u're-a) presence of starch in the urine

amyloplasia (-pla'zhah) absence of muscle formation.

amylostasia (-sta'shah) muscular tremor seen in motor ataxia.

amyotonia (a'mi-o-to'ne-a) lack of muscle tone **a congenita** congenital disease of children exhibiting general hypotonia of the muscles.

amyotrophic lateral sclerosis a motor neuron disease characterised by distal and proximal muscle wasting, fasciculations, spasticity, exaggerated reflexes and extensor plantars.

amyotrophy (a'mi-ot'ra-fe) atrophy of muscle **diabetic a** severe and progressive weakness and wasting of the proximal muscles of lower limbs accompanied by pain.

amyxia (a-mik'se-a) absence of mucus

amyxorrhoea (a'mik'sa-re'ah) absence of mucous secretion

ANA abbreviation for anti-nuclear antibodies

ana (an'ah) of each

ana-combining word for upward; again; backward; excessively

anabiosis (an'a-bi-o'sis) restoration of vital processes.

anabolism (a-nab'o-lizm) a metabolic activity in which the simple substances are converted into complex compounds by the cells.

anabolite (a-nabo-lit) any product of anabolism

ANCA abbreviation for antineutrophil cytoplasmic antibodies

anacidity (an'a-sid'i-te) lack of normal acidity

anaclisis (an'a-kli'sis) depending on something

anacrotism (a-nak'ro-tizm) an abnormal type of pulse exhibiting a prominent notch on its ascending limb.

anadipsia (an'a-dip'se-a) intense thirst

anadrenalism (an'a-dre'nil'izm) complete lack of adrenal function.

anaerobe (an'e-rob) microorganism that grow optionally without oxygen **fecultative a's** microorganisms that can grow under either anaerobic or aerobic condition **obligate a's** micro-organisms that can grow only in complete absence of oxygen.

anaerobic (an'er-o-bic) **energy production** body's production of energy when needed amounts of oxygen are not readily available

anaerobiosis (an-ar'o-bi-o'sis) life in total absence of molecular oxygen

anaerogenic (-jen'ik) 1. producing little or no gas 2. suppressing the production of gas

anagen (an'a-jen) phase of active growth of hair

anaha (s) constipation

anakùsis (an'a-koo'sis) deafness

anal (a'n-l) relating to the anus **a canal** the terminal portion of the large intestine that opens out in anus. It remains closed except during defecation or passage of flatus **a fissure** traumatic and ischaemic damage to anal mucosa resulting in a mucosal tear in the midline posteriorly. There is severe pain on defecation, bleeding, mucus discharge and pruritus. **a fistula** fistula- in-ano an indurated track with external opening and internal orifice in the anal canal **a reflex** an immediate contraction of the anal sphincter on scratching the skin around the anus **a tag** swollen skin at the distal end of an anal fissure. It is often accompanied by pain on defecation and fresh bleeding.

analeptic (an'a-lep'tik) 1. restorative 2. a central nervous stimulant

analgesia (an'al-je'ze-a) absence of pain sensibility

analgesic (-je'sik) 1. substance relieving pain¯ 2. insensitive to pain **a nephropathy** tubulointerstitial inflammation associated with papillary necrosis caused by ingestion of analgesics such as acetaminophen, aspirin and phenacetin and manifest in haematuria, renal colic and pyelonephritis

analgia (an-al'ja) absence of pain.

analogous (a-nal'a-gus) resembling in appearance or function

analogue (an'a-log) 1. a drug whose effect mimics that of another, having a dissimilar chemical structure. 2. A part or organ possessing similar function as another, but of different origin

analogy (a-nal'o-je) the quality of being analogous, resemblance or similarity in appearance or function

analysis (a-nal'i-sis) 1. separating complex material into constituent parts and identifying them 2. determination of concentration of one arterial constituent in a mixture **blood gas a** the determination of oxygen and carbon dioxide concentrations and pH, using O_2, CO_2 and pH electrodes. HCO_3 is determined by a nomogram

analysis of variance ANOVA *stat* a technique to define and segregate the causes of variability affecting a set of observations

analyser (an'a-li'zer) any instrument that performs an analysis

anamnesis (an'am-ne'sis) 1. history taking from a patient 2. faculty of memory

anaphase (an'a-faz) stage of mitosis or meiosis with division of centromere in which daughter chromosomes move toward the poles of the cell

anaphia (an-a'fe-a) loss of sense of touch

anaphoria (an'a-for'e-a) a tendency of the visual axes of both eyes to divert above the horizontal plane

anaphrodisiac (an'af-ro-diz'e-ak) 1. a drug that causes subsidence of sexual desire 2. repressing sexual desire

anaphylactic shock severe reaction occurring suddenly following injection of a drug or serum. There is bronchospasm, hypotension, and laryngeal oedema

anaphylactogenesis (an'a-fi-lak'to-gen'e-sis) the production of anaphylaxis

anaphylactoid reaction an anaphylaxis-like reaction occurring as a non-immune reaction

anaphylaxis (-fi-lak'sis) a hypersensitivity reaction that occurs upon exposure to an antigen to which the body has previously formed on IgE antibody

anaplasia (-pla'z-e-a) a loss of differentiation of cells and their orientation to one another as in tumour tissue

anapophysis (-pof'i-sis) an accessory vertebral process may be found in thoracic or lumbar vertebrae

anarthria (an-ar'thre-a) a severe dysarthria with speechlessness

anasarca (an'a-sar-ka) oedema involving the whole body; dropsy

anastomosis (a-nas'ta-mo'sis) 1. a communication between two vessels by collaterals 2. an opening between two organs or spaces, which can be natural or resulting from injury, surgery or disease

anatomical deadspace the air remaining in the conducting system, from nose to the beginning of respiratory bronchioles does not participate in the gas exchange and that part of the ventilation is considered wasted. However it helps in saturation of the inspired air with moisture brings it to the level of body temperature, and enables the removal of particulate matter.

anatomist (a-nat'o-mist) a specialist in the field of anatomy

anatomy (a-nat'a-me) 1. the structure of an organism 2. the branch of science dealing with morphology or structure of organisms **applied a** application of anatomical knowledge in diagnosis and treatment **comparative a** comparison of homologous structures of different animals **descriptive a** a description of individual parts of the body **developmental a** embryology **gross a** study of structures by naked eye **microscopic a** histology **pathologic a** study of diseased or abnormal tissues **physiologic a** anatomy studied in relation to function **radiological a** study of body through X-ray imaging **surface a** study of the configuration of the surface of the body in its relation to deeper structures **surgical a** applied anatomy in relation to surgical diagnosis and treatment **topographic a** the study of parts in their relation to surrounding parts.

anatropia (an'atro'pe-a) an upward deviation of visual axis of one eye when the other eye is fixing

ANC abbreviation for antenatal clinic

anchorage (ang'ker-ij) fixation especially of the displaced viscera by operative procedure 2. fixation of fillings or of artificial crowns or bridges in operative dentistry

ancillary (an'sil-lar'e) secondary, supplementary

ancipital (an-sip'i-t'l) two-edged or two-headed

anconad (ang'ko-nad) toward the elbow

anconagra (ang'kon-ag'ra) gout of the elbow

anconeal (ang-ko'ne-il) pertaining to the elbow

anconeus (ang-ko'ne-us) short extensor of elbow *see* table of muscles.

anconitis (ang'ko-ni'tis) inflammation of the elbow joint

ancrod (an'krod) an enzyme purified by the venom of Malaysian pit viper, used as an anticoagulant.

ancylostomiasis (an-si-los-to-mi'a-sis) ankylostomiasis

ancyroid (an'si-roid) anchor-shaped

and(o) combining word for male; masculine

androblastoma (an'dro-blas-to'ma) a benign tumour of testis, which histologically resembles foetal testis. Sertoli cells may produce oestrogens to cause feminisation

androgen (an'dro-jen) masculinising hormone

androsterone metabolite of testosterone.

anecdotal (an'ek-do'tl) unsubstantiated, as a response to unproven therapy or a cause-and-effect relationship

anechoic (an-e-ko'ik) without echoes

anectasis (an-ek'ta-sis) congenital atelectasis

anaemia (a-ne'me-a) a state in which haemoglobin of blood is below the normal range for the patient's age and sex and the clinical features of anaemia reflect the diminished oxygen carrying capacity of the blood. **Addisonian pernicious a** megaloblastic anaemia due to a failure of secretion of intrinsic factor by the stomach other than total gastrectomy **a of chronic disease** anaemia developing in presence of chronic infections, chronic inflammation or malignancy. Anaemia is mild, normocytic and normochromic. It occurs due to abnormality of iron metabolism and erythropoiesis **aplastic a** hypoplastic or aplastic bone marrow resulting in decreased formation of erythrocytes and haemoglobin. There is associated granulocytopaenia and thrombocytopaenia **congenital haemolytic a** disorders such as hereditary spherocytosis, glucose-6-phosphate dehydrogenase deficiency and haemoglobinopathies (sickle-cell disease, thalassaemia) are associated with anaemia **hyperchromic a** anaemia with mean corpuscular haemoglobin concentration (MCHC) greater than normal **hypochromic a** anaemia with deficient haemoglobin and MCHC being less than normal **immune-autoimmune haemolytic a** the condition is associated with the formation of antibodies against red cell antigens and cause inappropriate destruction of red cells. Based on thermal characteristic of the antibodies, they are categorised as warm (IgG with a thermal optimum of 37°C) or cold (IgM with a thermal optimum of 4°C, that bind complement) **iron deficiency a** develops from loss of iron from bleeding, inadequate diet or malabsorption. There is reduced haemoglobin, low mean cell volume, hypochromia and microcytosis **macrocytic a** anaemia in which the average size of circulating erythrocytes are greater than normal **mediterranean a** thalassemia major **megaloblastic a** vitamin B_{12} and folic acid are necessary for DNA synthesis and deficiency of either or both causes a failure in DNA synthesis and disordered cell proliferation. The cells are abnormally large (megaloblastic). Haemoglobin is reduced, mean cell volume is raised with low erythrocyte count, oval macrocytosis and red cell fragmentation **non-immune haemolytic a** shearing of red cells from mechanical trauma, *Plasmodium falciparum* infection, *Clostrium perfringens* septicaemia, administration of dapsone or salazopyrin are associated with haemolysis **microcytic a** anaemia in which the average size of circulating erythrocytes is smaller than normal **normochromic a** anaemia in which the concentrations of haemoglobin in the erythrocytes is within the normal range **normocytic a** anaemia in which the erythrocytes are normal in size **refractory a** any of a group of anaemic conditions exhibiting persistent anaemia despite treatment with a variety of haematenics. **sickle-cell a** presence of haemoglobin S on deoxygenation, the molecules of haemoglobin polymerise to form pseudocrystalline structure (tactoids) which distort the red cell membrane and produce sickle-shaped cells. Though polymerisation is reversible, the distortion of the red cell membrane may become permanent and the red cells become irreversibly sickled. These cells increase blood viscosity, traverse capillaries poorly, tend to obstruct the blood flow, and cause thrombosis, and infarction of the part. **sideroblastic a** refractory anaemia exhibiting presence of sideroblasts in the bone marrow **spherocytic a** hereditary spherocytosis

anaesthesia (an'es-the'zhah) loss of sensation due to a neurologic disease or as a result of pharmacologic depression of nerve function **basal a** parenteral administration of sedatives as premedication to produce a state of depressed consciousness short of general anaesthesia **block a** injection of local anaesthetic agent in close proximity of a nerve supplying the area (nerve block) or encircling the operative field (field block) to inhibit nerve transmission **caudal a** regional anaesthesia produced by injection of a local anaesthetic agent into the epidural space via sacrococcygeal notch **closed circuit a** inhalation anaesthesia in which there is continuous rebreathing of an anaesthetic in a closed system with removal of CO_2 **conduction a** block anaesthesia **dissociated a** loss of sensation of pain and temperature with preservation of touch sensation as in syringomyelia **dissociative a** a form of anaesthesia without complete unconsciousness, characterised by cataplexy, amnesia, and analgesia, and patient feels a dissociation from the environment **endotracheal a** anaesthesia produced by introduction of gaseous mixture through a tube inserted into the trachea **epidural a** regional anaesthesia produced by injection of a local anaesthetic between the vertebral spines and beneath ligamentum flavum into the extradural space **general a** a state of unconsciousness and loss of ability to perceive pain produced by administration of anaesthetic agents by intravenous or inhalation route **girdle a** anaesthesia distributed in the form of a band around the abdomen **glove and stocking a** loss of sensation in the area that would be covered by a glove and stocking as in peripheral neuropathy **infiltration a** local anaesthesia produced by injection of anaesthetic directly into the tissues **inhalation a** general anaesthesia produced by inhalation of vapour or gaseous anaesthetic agents such as ether, nitrous oxide and methoxyflurane **insufflation a** maintenance of inhalation anaesthesia by blowing a mixture

of gases or vapours into the airway **local a** regional anaesthesia produced by direct infiltration of an anaesthetic into the operative field **open a** application usually by dropping of volatile anaesthetic agent onto gauge held over the nose and mouth and there is no significant rebreathing **primary a** the first stage of anaesthesia before loss of consciousness **pudendal a** a type of local anaesthesia produced by blocking the pudendal nerve on either side near the ischial spine **rectal a** general anaesthesia produced by instillation into the rectum of liquid inhalation anaesthetics **refrigeration a** local anaesthesia induced by lowering temperature of a part of body to near freezing either by spraying it with ethyl chloride or by immersion in ice **regional a** nerve or field block by anaesthetic agent to produce a circumscribed area of anaesthesia **retrobulbar a** injection of a local anaesthetic behind the eyeball **saddle block a** a type of spinal anaesthesia limited to buttocks, perineum and inner surfaces of thigh produced by injection of anaesthetic agent into fourth lumbar space **segmental a** anaesthsia limited to an area supplied by one or more spinal nerve roots, due to neurologic lesion **spinal a** 1. loss of sensation produced by disease of spinal cord 2. anaesthetic into the subarachnoid space of the spinal canal **splanchnic a** anaesthesia produced by injection into splanchnic ganglia **surgical a** loss of sensation and muscle relaxation enabling safe performance of surgery **tactile a** loss of sense of touch **thermal a** loss of heat sense **topical a** local anaesthesia induced by direct application of local anaesthetic solutions, ointments or jellies **traumatic a** loss of sensation from a nerve injury **twilight a** a state of light anaesthesia **anaesthesiologist** (an'es-the'ze-ol'o-jist) a medical specialist trained in anaesthesiology

anaesthesiology (an'es-the'ze-ol'aje) the medical speciality concerned with the study of anaesthesia and anaesthetic agents

anaesthetic (an'es-thet'ik) 1. pertaining to, characterised by or producing anaesthesia 2. a medication used to induce anaesthesia

anaesthetist (a-nes'the-tist) a person trained in the administration of anaesthesia

anencephaly (an'en-sef'a-le) the congenital absence of a major portion of the brain, skull and scalp

anergy (an'er-je) a condition in which T cells have decreased or absence of lymphokine secretion when the T cell receptor is engaged by an antigen.

anerythroplasia (an'e-rith'ro-pla'zhah) absence of red cell formation.

anerythropoiesis (-poi-e'sis) decreased production of red blood cells.

aneuploidy (an'u-ploi'de) a congenital or acquired alteration in the number of chromosomes that deviates from multiple of a haploid of chromosomes.

aneurine thiamine

aneurysm (an'u-rizm) localised rounded distension of a vessel in continuity of its lumen **abdominal aortic a** localised dilatation of the wall of abdominal aorta **aortic a** an abnormal dilatation of the aortic wall due to atheroma, Marfan's syndrome, or aortitis **arteriovenous a** a dilated arteriovenous shunt **berry a** aneurysmal bulging from the bifurcation of cerebral arteries particularly in the region of circle of Willis, and they develop from defects in the media of the arterial wall **cirsoid a** a dilatation of a group of vessels due to congenital malformations **dissecting a** splitting of an arterial wall with entry of blood through an intimal tear **mycotic a** aneurysm due to impaction of a septic embolus **popliteal a** a cystic swelling of the popliteal space exhibiting an expansile impulse **Rasmussen's a** dilated artery traversing a pulmonary

tuberculous cavity causing massive haemoptysis **ventricular a** persistent occlusion of the infarct-related artery causes thinning and stretching of the infarcted segment of the ventricle

aneurysmoplasty (an'u-riz'mo-plas'te) plastic restoration of an artery in aneurysm

aneurysmorrhaphy (an'u-riz-mor'a-fe) the operative removal of aneurysm with suturing of neck

ANF abbreviation for antinuclear factor

anga (s) organ *a mardana* massaging

angi(o) combining word for vessel

angiasthenia (an'je-as-the'ne-a) loss of tone in the vascular system

angiectasis (-ek'ta-sis) marked dilatation and often lengthening of a blood vessel.

angiectomy (-ek'ta-me) excision of a vessel

angiectopia (-ek-to'pe-a) abnormal position or course of a vessel.

angiitis (-i'tis) inflammation of a vessel, refers to a blood or lymph vessel; vasculitis.

angina (an-ji-na) 1. a severe constricting pain referring to angina pectoris 2. sore throat **abdominal a** intermittent cramping abdominal pain, frequently occurring after food, caused by inadequacy of mesenteric circulation **a pectoris** discomfort due to transient myocardial ischaemia and occurs when there is an imbalance between myocardial oxygen supply and demand. Coronary atheroma is the most common cause **crescendo a** unstable angina showing rapidily worsening angina at rest or prolonged and severe chest pain without ECG or enzyme abnormalities. **Ludwig's a** cellulitis under deep cervical fascia **noctural a** angina developing either soon after patient lies down due to an increase in venous return that increases myocardial oxygen demand beyond the capacity of supply or several hours later due to an increase in myocardial oxygen demand or vasospasm **postprandial a** angina developing during or soon after meals due to an increased oxygen demand in splanchnic vascular bed **Prinzmetal's a** a variant of angina pectoris in which pain occurs during rest, severe and of longer duration associated with ECG abnormalities with elevation of ST segment **stable a** characterised by central chest pain that is precipitated by exertion and promptly relieved by rest. The pain may radiate to the neck , and often accompanied by discomfort in the arms, wrists and sometimes hand **unstable a** acute coronary insufficiency in which the symptoms are intermediate in severity between stable angina pectoris and myocardial infarction **variant a** a form of angina attributed to a local magnesium deficiency **Vincent's angina** an ulcerative infection of tonsils and pharynx **walk-through a** angina occurring during exercise, but disappearing with continued exercise.

anginose (an'je-nos) characterised by an angina

angioblast (an'je-o-blast) a cell concerned with the formation of blood vessels

angioblastoma (an'je-o-blas-to'ma) haemangloblastoma

angiocardiogram (an'je-o-kar'de-og'ram) radiographic image produced by angiocardiography

angiocardiography (-kar'de-og'ra-fe) radiographic imaging of the heart and blood vessels following injection of radioopaque solution

angiocarditis (-kar-di'tis) inflammation of heart and blood vessels

angiocentric (-sen'trik) pertaining to the lesions taking origin in blood vessels

angiodysplasia (-dis-pla'zhah) development of vascular malformations in the proximal colon and it is associated with aortic valve disease. There is acute and profuse bleeding that stops spontaneously

angioedema (-e-de'ma) development of urticaria and oedematous areas of skin, mucous membrane or viscera. It is caused by dilatation and increased permeability of the capillaries.

angioendothelioma (-en'do-the'le-o'ma) a vascular tumour containing endothelial cells

angioendotheliomatosis (-en'do-the'le-o-ma-to'sis) a B-cell or less commonly T cell lymphoma with a predilection for intravascular spaces . It is characterised by multiple indurated and erythematous plaques, fever and neurologic signs

angiofibroma (-fi-bro'ma) a tumour consisting of fibrous tissue and vascular proliferation

angiofollicular (-fo-lik'u-ler) pertaining to a lymphoid follicle and its blood vessels

angiogenesis (-jen'i-sis) development of blood vessels in the embryo

angiogenic (-jen'ik) 1. pertaining to angiogenesis 2. vascular in origin

angiography (an'je-og'ra-fe) a radiologic procedure used to visualise the interior of blood vessels following injection of a contrast medium **coronary a** performed to detect stenoses and guide revascularisation procedures in patients with coronary artery disease **digital subtraction a** (DSA) a technique whereby images obtained before contrast injection are digitised and subtracted from post-contrast images **pulmonary a** to diagnose pulmonary emboli, contrast medium is passed down a catheter inserted via the femoral vein into the main pulmonary artery **renal a** performed to investigate renal artery stenosis, following injection of contrast material into the aorta

angiohaemophilia (an'je-o-he'mo-fil'e-a) *see* Von Willebrand's disease

angiohyalinosis (-hi'a-li-no'sis) hyaline degeneration of the walls of the blood vessels

angioid (an'je-oid) resembling blood vessels.

angiokeratoma (an'je-o-ker'a-to'ma) telangiectatic wart

angiokinetic (-ki-net'ik) vasomotor

angioleiomyoma (-li'o-mi-'oma) vascular leiomyoma

angiolipoleiomyoma (-lip'o-li'o-mi-o'ma) a benign tumour consisting of blood vessels, adipose tissue, and smooth muscle, may develop in kidney

angiolipoma (-li-po'ma) a lipoma containing large number of vascular channels.

angiology (an'je-ol'a-je) the study of vessels of the blood, as related to blood vessels and lymphatics.

angiolysis (an'je-ol'i-sis) obliteration of a blood vessel, noted in new born infant after tying the umbilical cord.

angioma (an'je-o'ma) vascular tumour of blood vessels **cavernous a** cavernous haemangioma **telangiectatic a** angioma with dilated vessels

angiomatosis (an'je-o-ma-to'sis) a condition associated with multiple angiomas

angiomyolipoma (-mi'o-lip'o-ma) a benign tumour consisting of vascular, fatty and muscular tissue

angiomyoma (-mi-o'ma) a tumour consisting of blood vessels and muscle tissue

angiomyosarcoma (-mi'o-sar-ko'ma) a tumour composed of blood vessels, muscle tissue and connective tissue

angioneuropathy (-nu-rop'a-the) any neuropathy affecting the blood vessels.

angionoma (-no'ma) ulceration of a blood vessel

angioparalysis (pa-ral'i-sis) vasoparalysis

angioparesis (-pa-re'sis) vasoparesis

angiopathy (-p'a-the) any disease of the vessels. **percutaneous transluminal coronary a** (PTCA) , performed by passing a fine guidewire across a coronary stenosis under radiographic control and using it to position a balloon which is then inflated to dilate the stenosis.

angiopoiesis (an'je-o-poi-e'sis) the formation of blood vessels

angiopressure (an'je-o-presh'er) application of pressure to control bleeding

angiorrhaphy (an'je-or'a-fe) suture of a vessel(s)

angiosarcoma (an'je-o-sar-ko'ma) malignant neoplasm arising from blood vessels

angiosclerosis (-skl-ro'sis) hardening of the walls of blood vessels.

angioscope (an'je-o-skop) a microscope for observation of capillaries

angioscopy (an'je-os'ka-pe) visualisation of capillary blood vessels by an angioscope

angioscotoma (an'je-o-sko-to'ma) a defect in the visual blood vessels

angiospasm (an'je-o-spazm) vasospasm

angiostenosis (an'je-o-ste-no'sis) narrowing of vessels

angiosteosis (an'je-os'te-o'sis) calcification of a blood vessel

angiostrophe (an'je-os'tra-fe) twisting of a cut end of a blood vessel to arrest bleeding

angiotelectasis (an'je-o-te-lek'ta-sis) dilatation of arterioles.

angiotensin (-ten'sin) decapeptide with vasoconstrictive activity produced by enzymatic action of renin upon angiotensinogen **a I** a decapeptide produced by the action of renin on angiotensinogen, a mild vasopressor and promotes release of aldosterone **a II** an octapeptide produced from angiotensin I by angiotensin converting enzyme, a powerful vasopressor and promotes release of aldosterone **a II receptor antagonists** drugs act by blocking the action of angiotensin II on heart, peripheral vasculature and kidney

angiotensinase (-ten'sin-as) the enzyme that degrades angiotensin II

angiotensin converting enzyme (ACE) cleaves the angiotensin I and converts to angiotensin II which stimulates synthesis of aldosterone **ACE inhibitors** act to prevent conversion of angiotensin I to angiotensin II , thereby counteract salt and water retention, peripheral arterial and venous vasoconstriction and activation of sympathetic nervous system. It causes reduction in after load in heart failure and effective in moderate to severe hypertension

angiotensinᴄgen (an'je-o-ten'sin-o-jen) α_2 globulin, an inactive precursor of angiotensin produced in the liver

angiotome (an'je-o-tem) one of the segments of vascular system of the embryo

angiotonic (an'je-o-ton'ik) increasing arterial tension

angiotrophic (an'je-o-trof'ik) relating to nutrition of blood vessels or lymphatics

angle (ang'gl) a figure or space formed by the junction of two lines or planes **acromial a** the bony point at which the lateral border becomes continuous with the spine of the scapula **cardiophrenic a** the medial inferior corner of thoracic cavity bordered by the heart and diaphragm **carrying a** the angle made at the elbow by extending the long axis of the forearm and the upper arm **cerebellopontine a** the angle formed by the junction of the cerebellum and the pons **costal a** the meeting point of lower border of the false ribs with the axis of sterum **costovertebral a** the angle formed on either side of vertebral column between the last rib and lumbar vertebrae **iridocorneal a** the acute angle between iris and cornea at the periphery of the anterior chamber of the eye **mandibular a** the angle formed by the lower margin of the body and the posterior margin of the ramus of the mandible **sternal a** junction of the manubrium with the body of the sternum and it corresponds with the attachment of the second costal cartilage on either side of the sternum; Louis angle **a of Treitz** sharp curve at the duodenojejunal junction . **visual a** angle formed by lines drawn from the nodal point of the eye to the edges of the object viewed

angstrom (ang'strom) Å a unit of length used for atomic dimensions and light

wave, named after A. Angstrom, Swedish physicist

angulation (ang'gu-la'shun) formation of an angle

angular stomatitis inflammation of the angles of the mouth.

angulus (ang'gu-lus) pl **anguli**, angle

anhedonia (an'he-do'ne-a) absence of pleasure from activities which are normally pleasurable

anhidrotic (an'hi-drot'ik) 1. an agent which suppresses sweating 2. reduction or absence of sweat glands

anhidrosis (an'hi-dros'is) failure to sweat

anhydrase (an'hidr'ase) an enzyme that catalyses the removal of water from a compound

anhydremia (an'hi-dre'me-a) deficiency of water in the blood

anhydride (an'hi-drid) an oxide that can combine with water to form an acid or that is derived from an acid by abstraction of water

aniline (an'i-len) aminobenzene, parent substance of many dyes derived from coal tar

anilism (an'i-lism) methaemoglobinaemia following exposure to aniline and its derivatives

anima (an'i-ma) the soul

animal (an'i-m'l) a living organism requiring oxygen and organic foods for existence and having sensation and power of voluntary movement

animation (an'i-ma'shun) the state of being alive **suspended a** a temporary state resembling death with absence of breathing

anion (an'i-on) an ion carrying negative charge **a gap** represents those negative ions not normally measured and it includes phosphate, sulphate , lactate, keto acids and albumin = plasma $Na^+ -$ (plasma $Cl^- +$ plasma HCO_3). In health it ranges from 8 to 14 mmol/L

aniridia (an'i-rid'e-a) congenital absence of iris.

aniseikonia (an'i-si-ko'ne-a) inequality of retinal images of both eyes

anis (o) combining word for unequal

anismus (a-nis'mus) inappropriate contraction of external anal sphincter and puborectalis resulting in obstructed defecation.

anisochromatic (an-i'so-kro-mat'ik) not of same colour throughout.

anisocoria (-kor'e-a) inequality in the size of pupils

anisocytosis (-si-to'sis) inequality in the size of red cells, which is prominently seen in megaloblastic anaemia

anisogamete (-gam'et) a gamete differing in size and structure from the one with which it unites

anisokaryosis (-kar'e-o'sis) inequality in the nuclei of cells

anisomelia (an-i-so-me'li-a) inequality of two paired limbs.

anisometropia (-ma-tro'pe-a) inequality in the refractive power of both eyes.

anisopiesis (-pi-e'sis) inequality in the blood pressure as registered in different limbs

anisopoikilocytosis (-poi'ki-lo-si-to'sis) erythrocytes of varying sizes and shapes

anisosphygmia (an-i-so-sfig'mi-a) inequality of pulses.

anisosthenic (an-i'sos-then'ik) unequal power, as of muscles

anisotonic (an-i'so-ton'ik) 1. differing in tonicity or tension 2. having different osmotic pressure

anisuria (an'i-su're-a) alternating, decrease and increase in the amount of urine passed

anjana (s) eye ointment; sulphide of lead

ankle (ang'k'l) tarsus; the region of joint between leg and foot

ankyl (o) combining word for bent; in the form of a loop

ankyloblepharm (ang'ki-lo-blef'a-rm) adhesion of ciliary edges of the eyelids

ankyloglossia (-glos'e-a) tongue tie due to short wide frenum

ankylosed (ang'ki-lozd) fused; obliterated

ankylosing stiffening **a hyperostosis** diffuse idiopathic skeletal hyperostosis, a chronic age related disorder exhibiting new bone formation which radiologically shows by the presence of flowing ossification along the anterolateral aspect of four contiguous vertebral bodies **a spondylitis** chronic inflammatory arthritis with a predilection for sacroiliac joints and spine. There is progressive stiffening and fusion of axial skeleton

ankylosis (ang'ki-lo'sis) immobilisation of joint by fibrous or bony union **artificial a** arthrodesis **bony a** union of bony surfaces resulting in complete immobility. **extracapsular a** stiffness of a joint due to rigidity of the surrounding tissues **false a** fibrous ankylosis **fibrous a** decreased mobility of the joint due to proliferation of the surrounding fibrous tissues **intracapsular a** stiffness of the joint due to adhesions between the articular surfaces of the joint

ankylostoma (an'kil-os'to-ma) a genus of nematodes of the family Ankylostomatidae, whose members are intestinal parasites. Of them *Ankylostoma duodenale Necator americanus* belonging to the suborder Strongylata causes ankylostomiasis

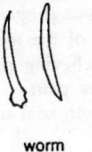 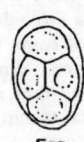

worm   Egg

Ankylostoma

ankylostomiasis (an'kil-os'to-mi'a-sis) hook worm disease caused by infestation of *A. duodenale* or *N. americanus*. They are greyish white, of 1 cm length, found in duodenum and upper jejunum. The eggs passed in the faeces develop in warm, moist soil and penetrate human skin as filariform larvae and develop as adult worms. The disease is common in insanitary conditions. The worms attach to the intestinal mucosa and suck the blood, and result in iron deficiency anaemia

ankyroid (ang'ki-roid) hook-shaped

anlage (an-lah'ge) primordium

Ann arbor (an'ar-bar) **classification** a system for staging Hodjkin's tumours to guide therapy

annapaka (s) digestion of food

annectent (an-nek'tint) connecting; joining together

annelid (an'e-lid) any member of Annelida

Annelida (a-nel'i-da) segmented worms, includes leeches.

annihilate (an'in'le-t) to destroy completely, to reduce to nothing

annular (an'u-ler) ring-shaped

annuloplasty (an'u-lo-plas'te) reconstruction of an incompetent cardiac valve

annulorrhaphy (an'u-lor'a-fe) closure of a hernia by sutures.

annulus (an'u-lus) pl **annuli** a small ring or an encircling structure **a fibrosus** 1. major outer part of intervertebral disc made of cartilage 2. ring of attachment of cardiac valve

anode (an'od) an electrode at which oxidation takes place

anoderm (an'o-derm) lining of anal canal

anodontia (an'o-don'she-a) congenital absence of some or all of the teeth

anodyne (an'o-din) 1. relieving pain 2. a medicine that relieves pain

anogenital relating to both anal and genital regions.

anomalad (a-nom'a-lad) sequence

anomalous (a-nom'a-lus) deviating from normal

anomaly (a-nom'a-le) deviation from normal especially as a result of congenital or hereditary defects.

anomia (a-nom'e-a) inability to produce correct word

anonychia (an'o-nik'e-a) congenital absence of nail(s)

anopheles (a-nof'e-lez) a genus of mosquitoes belonging to anophilinae subfamily, many of which are vectors of malaria

anophthalmia (an'-of-thal'me-a) complete absence of the eyes

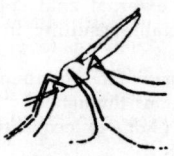

Anopheles Mosquito

anopia (an'o-pe-a) absence or major defect of vision

anoplasty (a'no-plas'te) reconstructive surgery of the anus

anorchism (an-or'kizm) absence of testes

anorectal (a'no-rek'tal) relating to both anus and rectum

anorectic (an'o-rek'tik) 1. causing or characterised by anorexia 2. an agent producing anorexia

anorexia (-rek'se-a) **a nervosa** a psychoneurotic condition which develops during adolescence and affects predominantly girls who want to maintain a slim figure. It is characterised by weight loss, avoidance of high-calorie diet, distortion of body image and amenorrhoea

anorexigenic (-rek-si-jen'ik) causing anorexia

anorgasmic (an'or-gas'mic) one who does not experience orgasm

anorthopia (an'or-tho'pe-a) asymmetrical or distorted vision

anoscopy (an-us-ku-pee) examination of the anal canal and rectum using a short speculum

anosigmoidoscopy (a'no-sig'moi-dos'ka-pe) endoscopy of the anus, rectum and sigmoid colon

anosmia (an-oz'me-a) loss of sense of smell

anosognosia (an-o-sog-no'ze-a) non-recognition by patient of existence of manifest disability, specially of paralysis

anostosis (an'os-to'sis) failure of ossification

anotia (an-o'shah) absence of ears

anovarism (an'o'var-izm) absence of ovaries

anovesical relating to both anus and urinary bladder

anovular (an-ov'u-ler) without ovulation

anovulatory (an-ov'u-la-tor'e) not accompanied by ovulation

anoxaemia (an'ok-se'me-a) a state of insufficient oxygen in the blood. It develops from one or more mechanisms such as alveolar hypoventilation, ventilation perfusion imbalance, right-to-left shunt and diffusion abnormalities

anoxia (a-nok'se-a) a deficiency of oxygen in a body tissue **anaemic a** due to decrease in haemoglobin in the blood **anoxic a** due to reduced oxygen pressure in high altitudes **histotoxic a** an inability of tissue cells to utilise oxygen **stagnant a** ischaemic hypoxia.

ansa (an'sa) pl **ansae** any structure in the form of a loop or an arc

anserine bursitis inflammation of sartorius bursa. Persons with valgus deformities of knee present with pain and tenderness on the medial side of lower femur

ansiform in the form of a loop or an arc

antacid (an'ta-sid) substance neutralising acid in the stomach and duodenum and are combinations of calcium, aluminium and magnesium salts

antagonism (an-tag'o-nism) mutual opposition in action between muscles, drugs, organisms, disease or physiologic processes

antagonist (an-tag'o-nist) something opposing the action of another, such as muscle or drug. α-**adrenergic a** α-blocker, β-**adrenergic a** β blocker. **folic acid a** an antimetabolite H_1 **receptor a** any agent blocking the action of histamine by competitive binding to H_1 receptors H_2 **receptor a** an agent that blocks the action of histamine by competitive binding to H_2 receptor.

antarbhakta (s) between meals

ante- combining word for before

antebrachium (an'to-bra'ke-um) forearm

antecedent (-se'dent) a precursor; something coming before

antecibum (an'te-se'bum) before food

antecubital in front of the elbow

antegrade (an'te-grad) moving forward a **pyelography** injection into renal pelvis

antereflexion (-flek'shun) a bending forward

ante-mortem (an'temor'tem) before death

antenatal (an'te-na'tal) before birth

antenna (an-ten'a) either of two lateral appendages on anterior segment of the head of arthropods

antepartal (an'te-par-t'l) occurring before labour or childbirth

antepartum (an'te-par'tum) before delivery

antepyretic (-pi-ret'ik) before the occurrence of fever

anterior (an-ter'e-or) 1. before in relation to time or space 2. ventral 3. front surface of the body **a chamber** in front of aqueous cavity of the eye, between the cornea and iris **a horn cell** motor neuron cell in the anterior horn of the gray matter of the spinal cord, whose axon innervates skeletal muscle

antero- combining word for anterior; in front of

anterograde (an'ter-o-grad) moving forward

anteroinferior (an'ter-o-in'feri-er) in front and below

anterolateral (an'ter-o-lat'er-al) in front and away from the midline

anteroposterior (-pos-ter'eo-er) relating both front and back

anterosuperior (-sup-eri'er) in front and above

anteversion (an'te-ver'zhun) turning or tilting forwards

anthelix (ant'he-liks) an elevated ridge of cartilage anterior to the posterior part of the auricle helix

anthelmintic (ant'hel-min'tik) an agent that destroys or expels intestinal worms

anthracene (an'thra-sen) a hydrocarbon obtained from coal tar, used in manufacture of dyes.

anthracoid (an'thra-koid) 1. resembling a carbuncle 2. resembling anthrax

anthracosilicosis (-sil'i-ko'sis) pneumoconiosis due to accumulation of carbon and

46

silica in the lungs from inhaled coal
dust
anthracosis (an'thra-ko'sis) a blackening of lungs by carbon dust in city
dwellers
anthracycline (an'thra-si'klen) antineoplastic antibiotics that includes
daunomycin and doxorubicin
anthraquinone (an'thra-kwin'on) a quinone
derivative of anthracene used in the
manufacture of dyes
anthrax (an'thrax) an occupational disease
of farmers, butchers and dealers in
hides, hair, wool and bonemeal, and a
disorder of domestic animals infected
by inhalation or ingestion of spores of
Bacillus anthracis. Initially there is an
itchy papule on the skin which becomes a vesicle containing
serosanguinous fluid. It dries to form a
thick black eschar . It can give rise to
pharyngitis, laryngitis or
bronchopneumonia
anthrop (o) combining word for man
anthropoid (an'thro-poid) resembling
man such as higher apes **a pelvis**
long, narrow and oval, ape-like female pelvis
anthropology (an'thro-pol'o-je) the branch
of science concerned with the man's
origin and development.
anthropometry (an'thro-pom'i-tre) measurements of human body and parts,
such as skull, bone, height and
weight
anthropophilic (-fil'ik) human-seeking,
with reference to parasite
anti- combining word for counteractive,
against
antiabortifacient (an'te-a-bor'ti-fa'shint)
agent preventing abortion
antiadrenergic (-ad're-ner'jik) an agent antagonising the effects of the sympathetic
nervous system
antiagglutinin (-a-gloo'ti-nin) a specific antibody that inhibits the action of an
agglutinin
antiamoebic (-a-me'bik) an agent destroying or suppressing growth of
amoebae

antianaemic (-a-ne'mik) factors that prevent or correct anaemia
antiandrogen (-an'dro-jen) drugs that act
as androgen receptor antagonists, or prevent conversion of testosterone to active
dihydrotestosterone or suppress ovarian steroid production or suppress adrenal androgen production
antianginal (-an-ji'nal) drugs that relieve
the symptoms of angina pectoris by
increasing the blood flow to the cardiac
muscle and by decreasing the work
load on the cardia
antianxiety (-ang-zi'it-e) drugs relieving
anxiety or useful in anxiety-related disorders such as benzodiazepines, beta-
adrenoceptor blockers (propranolol) and
azapirons.
antiarrhythmic (-a-rith'mik) drugs used to
prevent or correct an abnormal cardiac
rhythm. They act by suppressing excitability and slowing conduction in atrial
and ventricular muscle (quinidine,
disopyramide, lignocaine, mexiletine,
flecainide, propafenons), or as
adrenoceptor antagonists (propranolol,
metoprolol, atenolol, sotalol) or by prolonging the plateau phase of the action
potential (amiodarone), or by blocking
slow calcium channel affecting impulse
generation and conduction in atrial and
nodal tissue (verapamil). Other agents
are adenosine and digoxin
antibacterial (anti'bak-ter'e-al) preventing
the growth of or destructive to bacteria
antibiogram (-bi'o-gram) tabulation of antibiotic resistances of organism
antibiosis (-bi-o'sis) suppression of growth
of one microorganism by another
antibiotic (-bi-ot'ik) a chemical substance
derived from mold or bacteria that kills
or inhibits the growth of microorganisms **aminoglycoside a** bactericidal
agents that have been administered
parenterally for systemic treatment
betalactam a penicillins and cephalosporins containing a four-membered
betalactam ring. They are bactericidal
killing bacteria by interfering with their
cell wall synthesis **broad spectrum a**

effective against a wide range of bacteria **macrolide a** used to treat infections caused by gram-positive organisms. Erythromycin, clarithromycin, azithromycin and spiramycin are examples. **tetracycline a** bacteriostatic agent inhibiting the growth of gram-positive and gram-negative bacteria **a resistance** ability of micro-organisms to resist the action of antibiotic **a sensitivity test** response of the culture of bacteria to the antibiotic

antibody (an'ti-bod-e) (Ab) immunoglobulin with ability to react with specific antigen and are classified as agglutinin, bacteriolysin, haemolysin, opsonin or precipitin on the mode of their action. Antibodies are synthesised by B-lymphocytes that have been stimulated by the antigen bound to a cell surface receptor **anticardiolipin a** anti-phosphatid antibodies **antimitochondrial a** antibodies directed against mitochondrial antigens **antineutrophil cytoplasmic a's** (ANCA's) antibodies to proteinase 3 resulting in granular staining of neutrophil cytoplasm, found in vasculitis, Wegener's granulomatosis and rapidly progressive idiopathic glomerulonephritis **antinuclear a's** (ANA) autoantibodies directed against nuclear components such as DNA, RNA and histones **antiphospholipid a's** a group of heteregeneous autoantibodies that are primarily directed against a complex antigen of which B2-glycoprotein-1 is an essential component, found in SLE, primary antiphospholipid syndrome and recurrent cerebral ischaemia **blocking a** IgG reacting with an antigen, preventing it from reacting with IgE and prevent hypersensitivity reaction **complement-fixing a** activation of complement by IgM and IgG in the classic pathway and by IgA by alternate pathway **heterophile a** antibody directed against heterophile antigens **immune a** induced by immunisation **incomplete a** 1. an antibody that binds to bacteria or erythrocytes, but does not result in agglutination. 2. an univalent antibody fragment, such as Fab fragment **monoclonal a's** a highly specific antibody formed by fusing a myeloma cell to a cell producing an antibody against a desired antigen **natural a's** antibodies that react with antigens to which the individual had no exposure **neutralizing a** antibody on mixing with homologous infectious agent reduces the infectious titre **protective a** antibody responsible for immunity to an infectious agent as seen in passive immunity

anticancer drugs drugs acting as antineoplastic agents and they are antimetabolites, alkylating agents, plant alkaloids (inhibit cell division), antibiotics and taxanes (stabilise the mitotic spindle)

anticholesteraemic (an'ti-ka-les'ter-e'mik) agent promoting reduction of cholesterol levels in the blood

anticholinergic (-ko'lin-er'jik) antagonist to the action of parasympathetic or other cholinergic nerve fibres

anticholinesterase (-ko'lin-es'ter-as) inhibitor of breakdown of acetylcholine by inhibiting the enzyme acetylcholinesterase

anticipation (-si-pa'shun) increasing severity or early age at onset of a genetic disease in successive generation

anticoagulant (-ko-ag'u-lant) 1. prevent clotting of blood 2. any substance which prevents blood coagulation

anticoagulation (-ko-ng'u-la-shun) prevention of coagulation

anticodon (-ko'don) a triplet of nucleotides in the transfer RNA that is complementary to messenger RNA which determines the amino acid

anticomplement (-kom'pli-ment) a substance that combines with a complement and neutralises its action

anticonvulsant (-kon-vul'sant) agent preventing or arresting convulsions

anticus (an-ti'kus) anterior

anti D antibody against D antigen (Rh antigen)

antidepressant (an'ti-de-pres'ant) drugs used in the treatment of depressive illness and they include tricyclic compounds (amitriptyline, imipramine), 5HT reuptake inhibitors (fluoxetine) monoamine oxidase inhibitors (phenelzine) and nor adrenergic and 5HT reuptake inhibitors (venlafaxine)

antidiarrhoeal (-dia-r'e-al) drugs used to relieve the symptoms of diarrhoea

antidiuretic (-di'u-rat'ik) an agent that reduces the output of urine; a hormone, vasopressin

antidote (an'ti-dot) an agent that neutralises a toxin or poison **chemical a** a substance that unites with a poison to form a harmless chemical compound **mechanical a** a substance that prevents the absorption of a poison **physiologic a** substance counteracting the effects of poison by production of opposing physiologic effects **universal a** a substance that is effective against many poisons, such as activated charcoal

antidyskinetic (-dis'ki-net'ik) 1. relieving dyskinesia 2. an agent relieving or preventing dyskinesia

antiemetic (an'te-e-met'ik) 1. preventing or relieving nausea and vomiting 2. an agent that prevents or relieves nausea and vomiting

antifibrinolysin (-fi'bri-nol'i-sin) inhibitor of fibrinolysin

antifibrinolytic (-fi'bri-no-lit'ik) inhibiting fibrinolysis

antifibrotic (-fi-brot'ik) causing regression of fibrosis

antiflatulent (-fla'tu-lent) 1. relieving or preventing flatulence 2. an agent relieving or preventing flatulence

antifungal (-fung'g'l) agents that suppress the growth or reproduction of fungi which may be used topically in superficial infections (nystatin, clotrimazole) or orally (miconazole, ketoconazole) or intravenously (amphotericin B) in systemic fungal infections

antigen (an'ti-jen) (Ag) substance that is able to produce specific detectable immune reaction **antigenic** adj. **Australia a** hepatitis B surface antigen **blood group a's** antigen found on the surface of erythrocytes that determine a blood grouping reaction with specific antiserum **capsular a** antigen found in the capsule of certain microorganisms **carcinoembryonic a** (CEA) a glycoprotein of embryonic endodermal origin found in certain carcinomas **complete a** antigen capable of stimulating the formation of antibody with which it reacts **flagellar a** the heat labile antigen associated with bacterial flagella **hepatitis-associated a** (HAA) surface antigen of hepatitis B virus; Australia antigen **hepatitis B core a** (HBc Ag) antigen found in the core of hepatitis B virus (Dane particle) **hepatitis Be a** (HBe Ag) an antigen of DNA core of hepatitis B virus **hepatitis B surface a** (HBs Ag) a surface coat antigen of the hepatitis B virus **heterophile a** an antigen common to more than one species **histocompatibility a's** genetically determined isoantigens found on the surface of nucleated cells of most tissues **human lymphocyte a's** (HLA) histocompatibility antigens on the surface of nucleated cells determined by a region on chromosome 6 having several genetic loci (A,B,C,DP,DQ,DR,MB,MT, and Te) that have a strong influence on human allotransplantation **incomplete a** haptene **O a** a somatic antigen of nonmotile bacteria **oncofetal a** carcinoembryonic antigen **organ-specific a** tissue specific antigen with a specificity to a particular organ **partial a** a haptene **prostate specific a** (PSA) an endopeptidase secreted by the epithelial cells of prostate **sensitised a** a complex formed when antigen combines with specific antibody **somatic a** antigen in the body of a bacteria **species-specific a** antigenic components in the tissues and fluids that distinguish the species **tissue-specific a** organ specific antigens **tumour-specific a** an antigen produced by certain tumours. **V a** viral antigen that is intimately associated with virus

antigenaemia (an'ti-je-ne'mi-a) persistence of antigen in the blood

antigen-antibody reaction the combination of an antigen with its specific antibody

antigenic (an-ti-jen'ik) capable of eliciting the production of an antibody **a determinant** the specific area of an antigen that binds with an antibody combining site and determines the specificity of antigen-antibody reaction **a variation** circumvention of immune mechanism by organisms which vary in surface antigens

antigenicity the capacity to stimulate the production of antibodies or the capacity to react with an antibody

antigen presenting cell (APC) macrophages, dendritic and B-cells activate and provide signals to cells required for activation of T lymphocytes, to produce immunity and expand clonal expansion

antigen-specific receptor cell B and T cells express a vast array of antigen-specific receptors that are clonally distributed, to recognise a variety of potentially pathogenic microbes

antiglobulin (an'ti-glob'u-lin) an antibody directed against gamma globulin, as in Coomb's reagent

antihaemolysin (an'ti-he-mo'li-sin) a substance that inhibits or prevents the effect of haemolysin

antihaemophilic globulin clotting factor VIII involved in activation of factor X whose defect produces haemophilia

antihaemorrhagic (-hem'o-raj'ik) haemostatic; arresting haemorrhage

antihistamine (-his'ta-min) drug that blocks the effects of histamine

antihypercholesterolaemic (-hi-per-ko-ter-ol-e'mik) preventing or controlling rise in the level of serum cholesterol

antihyperlipoproteinaemic (-lip'o-pro'ten-e'mik) promoting a reduction of lipoprotein levels in the blood

antihypertensive (-hi-per'ten-siv) drug to reduce high blood pressure such as thiazide diuretics, Beta adrenoceptor antagonists, calcium channel blockers, ACE inhibitors and vasodilators

antiinfective (ante-in-fek'tiv) drugs active against infection

antiinflammatory (-in-flam'a-tor'e) drugs to reduce inflammation without directly antagonising the causative agent.

antilipaemic (-li-pe'mik) preventing the accumulation of fatty substances in the blood

antilymphocyte serum serum containing antibodies directed against lymphocytes that promote some degree of immunosuppression, used to reduce the occurrence of rejection of transplanted organs

antilysis (-li'sis) prevention or inhibition of lysis

antimetabolite (an'ti-me-tab'o-lit) a substance that competes with or antagonises a particular metabolite

antimethaemoglobinaemic (-met-he'mo-glo'bi-ne'mik) promoting the reduction of methaemoglobin levels in the blood

antimalarial (-mal'a-re'al) drugs used to prevent or treat malaria

antimicrobial (-mi-kro'be-il) antibiotics and chemotherapeutic agents active against microorganisms. Those that kill microorganisms are bactericidal and those that inhibit their growth are bacteriostatic

antimony (an'ti-mo'ne) metallic element Sb (stibium) at no. 51. Antimony preparations are used in the treatment of leishmaniasis

antimycotic (an'ti-mi-kot'ik) antagonistic to fungi

antineoplastic (-ne'o-plas'tik) preventing the development and spread of neoplastic tissue

antinociceptive (an'ti-no'si-sep'tiv) reducing the sensitivity to painful stimuli

antinuclear factor (ANF) anti-DNA antibody found in SLE, connective tissue diseases and chronic hepatitis

antioxidant (an'te-ok'si-dant) agents that protect against cell damage caused by oxygen free radicals

antiparkinsonian (-par′kin-so′ne-an) pertaining to the therapy for Parkinsonism

antiperistalsis (-per′i-stal′sis) reversed peristalsis

antiplasmin (-plaz′min) a substance that prevents or inhibits the effects of plasmin

antiplastic (-plas′tik) preventing or inhibiting the wound healing

antiprotease (-pro′te-as) a substance that interferes with proteoloysis α_1 **a inhibitor** agent that binds with a proteolytic enzyme, human neutrophil elastase released by polymorphs to form an inactivated complex

antiprothrombin (an′ti-pro-throm′bin) an anticoagulant that inhibits or prevents the conversion of prothrombin into thrombin

antipruritic (-proo-rit′ik) preventing or relieving itching

antipsychotic (-si-kot′ik) an agent effective in the management of psychotic disorders.

antipyretic (-pi-ret′ik) 1. reducing fever 2. antifebrile

antiretroviral (-ret′ro-vi′ral) agents against retroviruses such as HIV. They are reverse transcriptase inhibitors that prevent spread of infectious virus into unaffected cells (zidovudine), protease inhibitors and non-nucleoside reverse transcriptase inhibitors

antiscorbutic (-skor-bu′tik) preventing or relieving scurvy

antisecretory (-se-kre′ta-re) inhibitory to secretion

antisense (anti-sens) the non-coding strand in double-stranded DNA, that serves as the template to mRNA synthesis

antiseptic (-sep′tik) an agent capable of preventing infection by inhibiting growth of infectious agents

antiserum (an′ti-se-rum) serum containing one or more specific antibodies

antisialic (-si-al′ik) reducing the flow of saliva

antisocial (-so′sh′l) behaving in violation of social norms of the society

antispasmodic (-spaz-mod′ik) preventing or relieving spasm

antisudorific (-su-dor-ifik) anhidrotic

antithrombin (-thrombin) any substance capable of inhibiting the effects of thrombin so that blood does not clot

antithromboplastin (-throm′bo-plas′tin) any agent that interferes with the interaction of blood coagulation factors as they generate thromboplastin

antithyroid (-thi-roid) drugs to treat a hyperactive thyroid gland

antitoxin (-tok′sin) antibody formed in response to poisonous substances of biologic origin such as diphtheria, gas gangrene, botulism or tetanus

antitragus (-tra-gus) a projection of the auricle posterior to the tragus

antitrypsin (-trip′sin) a glycoprotein acting as a major protease inhibitor in the serum α_1 **a α_1** - protease inhibitor α_1 **a deficiency** familial absence is associated with panacinar emphysema

antituberculosis drugs the drugs capable of killing actively multiplying large bacterial population in a cavity, slow and intermittently multiplying small population in a solid caseous lesion and a slow occasionally multiplying population inside macrophages, of *Mycobacterium tuberculosis*

antitussive (-tus′iv) drugs that suppress or relieve coughing

antivenin (-ven′in) an antitoxin specific for an animal or insect venom

antiviral drugs used to treat an infection caused by a virus. They arrest viral replication (Aciclovir, amantadine, ribovirin, ganciclovir)

antixerotic (-ze-rot′ik) preventing dryness of the skin

antr (o) combining word for chamber; cavity, especially maxillary sinus

antritis (an-tri′tis) inflammation of an antrum, mainly of maxillary antrum

antrochoanal emerging from maxillary sinus and blocking posterior nares, as of nasal polyp

antrocoele (an'tro-sel) accumulation of fluid in a cyst in the maxillary antrum

antroscope (an'tro-skop) an instrument for visualisation of maxillary antrum

antrostomy (an'tros'to-me) creation of a permanent opening for drainage from maxillary sinus into inferior meatus

antrotomy (an-tro'ta-me) incision through the wall of an antrum

antrum (an'trum) 1. any nearly closed cavity having bony walls 2. pyloric end of the stomach **a of Highmore** maxillary sinus **a of stomach** an upward sloping segment beyond angular notch on lesser curvature, and the mucosa does not secrete acid **mastoid a** a cavity in the petrous portion of the temporal bone, communicating posteriorly with the mastoid cells and anteriorly with the middle ear **puncture of a** puncture of maxillary sinus by inserting a trochar near the floor of the nose through the sinus wall to drain fluid

ANUG acute necrotising ulcerative gingitivitis, Vincent's disease

anulomana (s) carminative

anulus (an'u-lus) a circular or ring-shaped structure **a conjunctivae** a narrow ring at the junction of the cornea with the conjunctiva **a femoralis** femoral ring; the abdominal opening of femoral canal **a fibrosus** concentric rings of collagen fibres at the outer portion of intervertebral discs **a inguinalis profundus** deep inguinal ring found in the transversalis fascia through which the ductus deferens in male or round ligament in female, enter the inguinal canal **a inguinalis superficialis** superficial inguinal ring found in the aponeurosis of the external oblique muscle through which ductus deferens in male or round ligament in female emerge from the inguinal canal **a umibicalis** an opening in the linea alba, through which umbilical vessels pass in the foetus. It is represented by naval in adult **a**

urethralis a muscular ring surrounding the opening of bladder into the urethra.

anumana (s) logical inference

anupana (s) medication; prescription

anuresis (an'u-re'sis) inability to pass urine.

anuria (an-u're-a)absence of urinary secretion; secretion less than 50ml per day

anus (a'nus) the opening of the rectum through which faecal material is excreted. It is the lower opening of the alimentary tract found in the fold between the buttocks **artificial a** an opening into the bowel formed by colostomy **imperforate a** anal atresia

anvil (an'vil) incus, the second of the three small bones found in the middle ear

anxiety (ang-zi'te) feeling of apprehension from the anticipation of danger, which may be internal or external **a neurosis** a predominant causeless fear and uncertainty **free floating a** pervasive unfocussed fear not attached to any idea

anxiolytic (ang'zi-o-lit'ik) 1. relieving anxiety 2. drugs so acting

aorta (a-or'ta) the main trunk of the systemic arterial system. It arises from the base of the left ventricle and passes upward as the ascending aorta, then takes a turn backward and left as the arch of the aorta, and passes down as descending aorta. It has thoracic and abdominal portions and terminates at the left side of the body of the fourth vertebra by dividing into right and left common iliac arteries **abdominal a** gives branches to the abdominal organs and pelvic organs **ascending a** gives right and left coronary arteries to supply the myocardium **thoracic a** gives branches such as bronchial, oesophageal, pericardial and nine pairs of intercostal arteries

aortic pertaining to aorta **a arch** gives three branches as innominate artery, left common carotid artery and left subclavian artery **a area** right of the sternum in the second intercostal space **a bodies** chemoreceptors located in the wall of aortic arch **a aneurysm** *see* aneurysm **a arch syndrome** pulseless disease a chronic inflammatory granulomatous panarteritis of the aorta and its major branches, associated with loss of pulses, bruits, hypertension and aortic incompetence; Takayashu's disease **a dissection** develops by a tear in the intima of the aorta exposing the diseased media to blood at intra-aortic pressure. It presents with very sudden onset of extremely severe pain in the chest and back **a insufficiency** a condition developing from congenitally abnormal cusps (bicuspid valves) or from valve damage due to rheumatic heart disease or infective endocarditis. Other causes are trauma and aortic dilatation. There is leakage of blood from the aorta through the aortic valve back into the left ventricle following left ventricular contraction. It is associated with collapsing pulse and early diastolic murmur **a regurgitation** aortic insufficiency **a sinuses** shallow ballooning of aortic valve corresponding to each cusp of aortic valve **a stenosis** narrowing of the aortic valve. It may be congenital, rheumatic or due to calcification of the aortic valve. The condition develops slowly and leads to hypertrophy of the left ventricle. There is fixed outflow obstruction and is associated with an ejection systolic murmur. **a valve** the semilunar valve between the left ventricle and the ascending aorta and it closes at the end of systole

aortitis (a'or-ti'tis) inflammation of the aorta **aorto a** condition affecting the aortic arch or thoracoabdominal aorta and its branches or both and exhibit features of cough, breathlessness, haemoptysis and pain

aortography (a-or-tog'ra-fe) radiographic visualisation of aorta and its branches after injection of a contrast medium

aorto-combining word for aorta; aortic wall

aortoplasty (a-or'to-plas'te) surgical repair or reconstruction of the aorta

aortorrhaphy (a'or-tor'a-fe) suture of the aorta

aortosclerosis (a-or'to-skle'ro'sis) arteriosclerosis of the aorta

aortotomy (a'or-tot'a-me) incision of the aorta

APACHE II an acronym for acute physiology and chronic health evaluation, second generation evaluation, to predict the outcome of critically ill patients in an I.C.U.

apasmrti (s) memory disorder

apathy (ap'a-the) lack of emotion; indifference

apatite (a p'a-tit) phosphate of calcium, a major constituent of bone and teeth

APC gene a gene located on chromosome 5q. probably encodes a protein with tumour suppressor activity

apellous (a-pel'us) 1.absence of skin 2.lacking in foreskin as in circumcision

apana (s) downward moving

aparient (a-per'e-ent) mild purgative

apasmara (s) epilepsy

aperistalsis (a-per-i-stal'sis) absence of peristalsis

ape thumb paralysis of the opponens pollicis muscle due to the lesion of the median nerve

Apert's syndrome a familial disorder with peaked skull due to suture closure and marked syndactyly named after Eugene Apert, French paediatrician

aperture (ap'er-cher) 1. an opening; 2. the diameter of the objective of a microsocope allowing entry of light rays

apex (a'peks) pl **apices** the pointed extremity of a conical or pyramidal structure **a beat** apical impulse **a of lung** apical segment of the lung rising 2-3 cm above the clavicle **a of heart** lowermost and outermost part of the heart formed by the left ventricle

apexcardiogram (a'peks-kar'de-o-gram) a tracing of the chest wall movement obtained by an apexcardiography

apexcardiography (-kar'de-og'ra-fe) a technique of recording low frequency precardial pulsations of a circumscribed area relative to its motion of the surrounding chest wall

Apgar score a simple test to evaluate neonate's post-partum status and potential for survival in the neonatal period by giving 0-2 marks to each of five parameters: appearance, pulse, grimace-reflex, activity or muscle tone and respiratory effort. Higher score is better. It is acronym of Virginia Apgar, US anaesthetist

aphagia (a-fa'jah) inability to swallow

aphakia (a-fa'ke-a) absence of lens of eye.

aphalangia (a'fa-lan'jah) absence of one or more digits

aphasia (a-fa'zhah) total loss of the spoken speech due to dysfunction of the central mechanism in the brain **amnestic a** inability to remember words **auditory a** inability to understand spoken words in presence of normal hearing **Broca's a** expressive aphasia with impaired speech production with lesion in posterior end of left inferior frontal gyrus **conduction a** a lesion in the association tracts between motor and speech centres result in skipping or repeating words on substitution of one word to another **expressive a** motor aphasia or Broca's aphasia **fluent a** inability to understand the spoken word, but able to produce an incoherent speech. **global a** a combination of a grossly nonfluent aphasia and fluent aphasia **jargon a** aphasia in which nonsense words are repeated **motor a** Broca's aphasia **nominal a** difficulty in finding correct name for an object **sensory a** loss of ability to comprehend the meaning of written or spoken words **syntactical a** inability to arrange words in proper sequence **Wernicke's a** sensory aphasia due to an injury to Wernicke's area in the temporal lobe of dominant hemisphere

apheresis (af'e-re-sis) a process of separation of unwanted components from the patient's blood by use of a continuous-flow separator

aphonia (a-fo'ne-a) loss of voice.

aphotic (a-fot'ik) dark; absence of light

aphrasia (a-fa'zhe-a) inability to speak

aphrodisiac (af'ro-dis'e-ak) an agent that is alleged to increase libido or the duration of sexual activity

aphtha (af'thah) pl **aphthae** small ulcers on the mucous membrane of the mouth.

aphthosis (af-tho'sis) any condition characterised by the presence of aphthae

aphthous stomatitis recurrent shallow painful ulcers in the mouth

aphthovirus (af'tho-vi'rus) viruses of foot and mouth disease, belonging to any genus of *Picorna viridae*

aphylaxis (a'fi-lak'sis) absence of protection against disease

API Association of Physicians of India

apical (ap'i-k'l) pertaining to an apex **a impulse** lowest and outermost point of pulsation of the cardia. It is visible and distinctly palpable 9 cm from the midsternal line or 1.25 cm medial to mid-clavicular line in the left fifth intercostal space

apicectomy (a'pi-sek'to-me) excision of air cells in the apex of the petrous part of the temporal bone

apicitis (a'pi-si'tis) inflammation of the apex as of a lung or the root of a tooth.

apicoectomy (a'pi-ko-ek'to-me) resection of the apex of the root of a tooth

apicolysis (a'p-i-kol'i-sis) surgical collapse of the upper part of the lung

aplasia (a-pl'zhah) 1. lack of development of an organ or tissue 2. improper or defective regeneration

aplastic anaemia *see* anaemia

apnoea (ap'ne'-a) temporary cessation of breathing **sleep a** absence of airflow at the nose and mouth for at least 10 seconds during sleep and they are repetitive. It may be central due to cessation of respiratory efforts of the chest due to failure of rhythm genesis or obstructive due to obstruction to extrathoracic airway at the level of oropharynx or mixed

apneusis (ap-noo'sis) a sustained inspiratory effort leading to an abnormal respiration

apo-combining word for away from; separated; derived from; the component of a protein molecule

apochromat (ap'o-kro-mat) an apochromatic objective

apochromatic (-kro-mat'ik) absence of any chromatic and spherical aberrations.

apocope (a-pok'a-pe) cutting of

apocrine (ap'o-krin) coiled tubular glands, such as sweat glands

apoenzyme (ap'o-en'zim) a protein portion of an enzyme

apoferritin (-fer'i-tin) a protein found in the intestinal wall that combines with iron to form ferritin

apolar (a-po'ler) without poles or processes

apolipoproteins (apo-lipo-pro'tens) molecules comprising the protein moiety of lipoproteins and given an ABC designation. Coronary artery disease is associated with decreased Apo A-I, Apo A-II or increased Apo B **Apo A** major protein component of HDL. Both Apo A subtypes are synthesised in the liver and intestine **Apo B** major protein component of LDL.

apomorphine (-mor'fen) a morphine derivative that acts as an emetic and expectorant.

aponeurorrhaphy (-nor-ror'a-fe) suture of an aponeurosis

aponeurosis (-noo-ro'sis) an expanded fibrous sheet that attaches muscle to a bone or other tissue.

apophysis (a-pof'i-sis) pl. **apophyses** a projection from a bone; bony outgrowth without an independent centre of ossification.

apophysitis (a-pof'i-zi'tis) inflammation of an apophysis.

apoplexy (ap'o-plex'se) 1. sudden stroke 2. an effusion of blood into a tissue or organ.

apoprotein (ap'o-pro'ten) a protein moiety of a molecule, as of a lipoprotein.

apoptosis (a-pop-to'sis) an intrinsic program of cell death. It is characterised by chromatin condensation and DNA degradation.

apothecary (a-poth'e-kar'e) a druggist or pharmacist.

apparatus (ap'a-ra'tus) 1. an instrument made of several parts 2. a collection of instruments used for a special purpose 3. a group of structures or organs that participate in the performance of some function **juxtaglomerular a** close to glomerulus containing cells of the afferent arteriole and the macula densa of the distal tubule. It is concerned with activation of the renin-angiotensin mechanism

apparent (ap'a-rent) obvious

appendage (a-pen'dj) a subordinate structure - in size and function - attached to a main structure

appendectomy (ap'en-dek'ta-me) surgical removal of vermiform appendix

appendicitis (a-pen'di-si'tis) an inflammation of the mucous membrane or lymph follicles of the vermiform appendix. It may be obstructive (colicky abdominal pain later shifting to the right iliac fossa, nausea, vomiting, fever) or non-obstructive (continuous dull aching pain in the abdomen, aggravated by movement)

appendicostomy (a-pen'di-kos'ta-me) surgical opening into the intestine through the tip of appendix

appendicular mass comonest swelling of right iliac fossa consisting of inflamed and turgid appendix surrounded by thickened and oedematous omentum and matted coils of intestine

appendix (a-pen'diks) pl **appendices** 1. various appendages to organs 2. When unqualified refers to vermiform appendix **a epiploica** a number of small sacs of the peritoneum distended with fat projecting from serous coat of the large intestine along taeniae coli **a of the eye** eyelid, eyelashes, eyebrow, lacrimal apparatus and conjunctiva **a of skin** the nails, hair, sebaecous and sweat gland' **vermiform a** a short blind ended, worm-like intestinal diverticulum extending from the blind end of the caecum

apperception (ap'er-sep'shun) comprehension modified by one's own emotions

appestat (ap'i-stat) brain centre concerned in controlling appetite

appetite (ap'e-tit) a natural desire for food

applenometer (ap'la-nom'e-te) a tonometer to determine the intraocular pressure

apple (ap'l) the edible fruit of rosaceous tree **a core appearance** circumferential narrowing of the femoral neck caused by erosion **Adam's a** prominence in the midline of the neck by the thyroid cartilage **a jelly nodule** small, soft yellow brown cutaneous papule which oozes on application of pressure, seen in lupus vulgaris.

apple core lesion a focal stricture of the bowel in annular carcinoma of the colon, at contrast material enema examination, where the shouldered margins of stricture resemble the core of an apple that has been partially eaten

appliance (a-pli'ans) a device used to provide function to a part such as artificial dentures, cane, crutch or walker.

apply (ap-pli) to administer a remedy; to lay or put to

apposition (ap'o-zish'in) 1. positioning of things in proximity 2. the condition of being placed together 3. the relationship of fracture fragments to one another.

apprehension (ap're-hen'shun) to be conscious by means of the senses; conscious perception; anticipatory fear

approved name name of drugs found in official pharmacopoeia.

apractagnosia (a-prak'tag-no'zhah) a lesion in the parietal cortex giving rise to an inability to use common tools or to perform skilled motor activities.

APPT activated partial thromboplastin

apraxia (a-prak'se-a) 1. an inability to execute purposeful movements without impairment of muscle power, sensation or coordination

apron (a'pron) outer dress protecting the front of the body during surgery or any diagnostic or therapeutic procedure **lead a** an apron containing lead worn as a protection from ionising radiation.

aprosexia (ap'ro-seksia) inability to concentrate.

aprotes elementary ions that are either positively-charged cations (sodium, potassium, calcium and magnesium) or negatively-charged anions (chloride and sulphate)

apt ('apt) fitting, suitable

aptitude (ap'ti-tude) skill, potential ability

aptyalism (ap-ti-a-lizm) absence or deficiency of secretion of saliva.

APUD amine precursor uptake and decarboxylation, concerns to a group of cells in different organs secreting polypeptide hormones. These cells contain amines, take up precursors of these amines and contain amino-acid decarboxylase.

apudoma (a'pud'o-ma) a gut-related neuroendocrine tumour producing small peptide hormones from the APUD system

apyogenic (a'pi-o-jen'ik) not caused by pus

apyretic (a'pi-ret'ik) afebrile; without fever

apyrexia (a'pi-rek-se'a) absence of fever

aqua (ah'kwah) 1. water 2. different dilute solutions of essential oils. 3. watery fluid.

aquaphobia (ak'wa-fo'be-a) morbid fear of water

aqueduct (ak'we-dukt) a conduit or canal **cerebral a** a canal lined by ependymal cells in the mid-brain connecting the third and fourth ventricles; aqueduct of Sylvius **a cochleae** ductus perilymphaticus

aqueous (a'kwe-us) watery; of the nature of water **a chambers** anterior and posterior chambers of the eye and they contain aqueous humour **a humour** transparent fluid found in the aqueous chambers of the eye and it is produced by the ciliary processes **a pores** channels found in intestinal cell membranes allowing passage of water soluble molecules of monosaccharide level **a veins** small subconjunctival veins carrying aqueous of eye

Ar symbol for argon

arabinose pentose of gum arabica

arachidic (ar-a-kid'ik) **acid** straight-chain saturated 20-carbon fatty acid

arachidonic (a-rak'i-don'ik) **acid** a 20-carbon polyunsaturated fatty acid with 4 double bonds, found in the phospholipid component of cell membranes, precursor of prostaglandins and leukotrienes

arachnide (a-rak'ni-de) a class of arthropodes, including spiders, scorpions, ticks and mites

arachnodactyly (a-rak'no-dak'ti-le) abnormally long and slender toes

arachnoid (a-rak'noid) 1. resembling a cobweb 2. arachnoid membrane **a mater** a delicate fibrous membrane interposed between the duramater and the pia mater, which cover the brain **(a encephali)** and spinal cord **(a spinalis)**. It is closely applied to dura, but there is a subarachnoid space between arachnoid and pia mater

ARA American Rheumatism Association

arachnoiditis (a-rak'noi-di'tis) inflammation of arachnoid membrane **chronic a** may be a complication of meningitis or spinal surgery or myelography with oil-based contrast agents

araphia (a-ra'fe-a) defective closure of a raphe, specially of the neural tube

arbor (ar'bor) 1. a tree-like 2. arthropod-borne

arborization (ar'bo-ri-za'shun) ramification; terminal branching of nerve fibres or arterioles

arborvirus (ar'bor-vi'rus) RNA viruses which multiply in both vertebrate host and insect vector; arthropod-borne viruses **a group A** genus of Alphavirus of togavirus family (eastern and western equine encephalitis) **a group B** flavovirus of togavirus family (dengue, Kyasanur forest, Japanese B) **a group C** non-togavirus

arbuda (s) cancer; malignant growth

ARC AIDS – related complex

arc (ark) a curved line; part of a circle **a eye** conjunctivitis and keratitis from exposure to welding arc **reflex a** a neural arc where the impulse travels from the periphery through the afferent nerve to the nerve centre and response passes through the efferent nerve to the effector organ

arcanobacterium (ar-ka'no-bak-ter'e-um) an irregular, rod-shaped, gram-positive bacteria, *A. haemolyticus* causes pharyngitis and rash in adolescents

arch any anatomical structure having a curved outline. **abdominothoracic a** boundary between the abdomen and thorax formed by the line of the false ribs on either side with the lower end of the sternum **aortic a** the curved part between the ascending aorta and descending aorta **aortic a's** a series of arterial channels encircling the embryonic pharynx of potentially six pairs 1 and 2 disappear; pair 3 takes part in the formation of carotids, 4th becomes the arch of the aorta, 5th disappears and 6th forms the proximal part of the pulmonary arteries, and until birth, the ductus arteriosus **costal a** abdominothoracic arch **crural a** the inguinal ligament extending from the anterior superior iliac spine to the pubic tubercle **deep palmar a** the arch in the palm formed by the communicating branch of ulnar and radial artery **dental a** the curved structure formed by the teeth in each jaw **glossopalatine a** the anterior piller of the fauces **longitudinal a** the anteroposterior arch of the foot. The medial longitudinal arch consists of the calcaneus, talus, navicular, three cuneiform bones and the three medial metatarsals. The lateral longitudinal arch is formed by calcaneus, cuboid and two lateral metatarsals **mandibular a** mandibular process **neural a** a vertebral arch, the posterior projection from the body of a vertebra that encloses the vertebral foramen **palatal a** the roof of the mouth **plantar a** the arterial arch formed by the external plantar artery running across the bases of metatarsal bones and the deep branch of dorsalis pedis artery **pubic a** arch formed by inferior rami of the pubic bone **pulmonary a** the fifth aortic arch on left side becoming pulmonary artery **superciliary a** a curved process of the frontal bone lying just above the orbit, below the eye brow **superficial palmar a** arterial arch in the hand formed by the ulnar artery and a communication with superficial palmar branch of the radial artery **supraorbital a** bony arch formed by the upper margin of the orbit **vertebral a** neural arch **zygomatic a** arch formed by temporal process of the zygomatic bone and zygomatic process of the temporal bone.

archenteron (ark-en'ter-on) gastrocoele; primitive digestive cavity of embryo

archetype (ar'ke-tip) a primitive form from which different modifications have evolved

archiform (ar'chi-form) arcuate; having a shape of a bow

arcuation (ar'ku-a'shun) a bending; curvature

arcus (ar'kus) an arch **a alveolaris** the arch formed by the alveolar process of the mandible or maxilla **a dentalis** dental arch **a juvenilis** an opaque greyish ring at the periphery of the cornea in young individuals **a plantaris** plantar arch **a senilis** an opaque, greyish ring at the periphery of the cornea within the sclerocorneal junction frequently occurring in elderly persons

ardita (s) facial paralysis

ARDS adult respiratory distress syndrome *see* acute respiratory distress syndrome

area (ar'e-a) 1. a circumscribed surface or space 2. part of an organ performing a special function 3. the part supplied by a specific artery or nerve **association a** association cortex **auditory a** auditory cortex **Broca's a** an area comprising inferior frontal gyrus **a of cardiac dullness** area corresponding to the heart in front of the chest **catchment a** geographical region served by a health centre **macular a** portion of the retina giving central vision **mitral a** area over the apex of the heart **motor a** motor cortex **sensorimotor a** the precentral and post-

central gyri of the cerebral cortex **silent a** any cortical area of the brain which on stimulation does not produce any detectable motor or sensory phenomenon **trigger a** a point or circumscribed area, which on irritation gives rise to disturbances at other areas

arenaviridae (a-ren'a-vir'i-de) arenaviruses, a family of RNA virus

arenavirus (a-re'na-vi'rus) any virus of arenaviridae which includes choriomeningitic virus and Lassa virus

areola (a-re'o-la) 1. any small area 2. a circular area of diffuse pigmentation, as around the nipple of the breast or around a wheal or the part of iris around the pupil

argentaffin (ar-jen'ta-fin) refers to cells that reacts with silver and get stained brown or black **a reaction** a staining that involves reduction of ammoniacal silver to metallic iron, used to identify APUD system

argentaffinoma (ar'jen-taf'i-no-ma) carcinoid tumour

argentum (ar-jen'tum) silver sym. Ag.

arginase (ar'ji-nas) an enzyme found in the liver that hydrolyses arginine to produce urea and ornithine in urea cycle

arginine (ar'ji-nen) an amino acid found in proteins. It participates, in urea cycle to produce urea, and in the synthesis of creatine

argininosuccinate synthase (ar'ji-ne-no-suk'si-nat-sin'thas) an enzyme that catalyses condensation of citrulline and aspartate, in the hepatic urea cycle

argininosuccinic (-suk-sin'ik) **acid** an amino acid formed in the urea cycle as an intermediate in the conversion of citrulline to arginine

argininosuccininaciduria (-asid-ur'e-a) excessive excretion of argininosuccinic acid, with epilepsy, mental retardation, ataxia, liver disease and friable hair

argon (ar'gon) chemical element at no. 18.

Argyll Robertson's pupil unequal, irregular, miotic pupils having presence of accommodation reflex but absence of light and ciliospinal reflexes, noted in neurosyphilis named after Douglas Moray Cooper Lamb Argyll Robertson, Scottish physician

argyria (ar-ji're-a) silver poisoning with slate-grey discolouration of skin and deeper tissues

argyrophil (ar-ji-ro-fil) ability to bind silver salts

ariboflavinosis (a-ri'bo-fla'vi-no'sis) a condition caused by deficiency of riboflavin in the diet presenting with cheilitis, angular stomatitis and magenta tongue

arishta (s) unfavourable symptoms

arm 1. brachium; the part between shoulder and elbow 2. an arm-like structure such as the portion of the chromatid extending in either direction from the centromere of a mitotic chromosome

armamentarium (ar'ma-men-ta're-um) the therapeutic means such as drugs and instruments available to the medical practitioner.

armouring (ar'mo-ring) a physical condition resulting from mental and emotional factors

arocakahara (s) that which cures anorexia

arochaka (s) loss of appetite

arogya (s) health

aromatic (ar'o-mat'ik) having an agreeable somewhat spicy odour

arrector (a-rek'tor) 1. raising 2. that which rises

arrest (ah-rest) 1. to stop; restrain 2. a stoppage **cardiac a** stoppage of heart beat resulting in cessation of circulation **epiphyseal a** early and premature fusion between the epiphysis and diaphysis **maturation a** stoppage of complete differentiation of a cell at an immature stage **pelvic a** presentation part of the foetus getting fixed in the maternal pelvis **respiratory a** stoppage of spontaneous respiration **sinus a** cessation of cardiac sinus activity, necessitating implantation of a pace maker

arrestin (ah-rest'in) a vision-related protein-maximally activated in bright sunlight affecting the activity of rods

arrheno- combining word for male; masculine

arrhenoblastoma (a-re'no-blas-to'ma) a rare tumour of ovary that secretes male sex hormone to cause virilization

arrhythmia (a-rith'me-a) loss or an irregularity of rhythm **cardiac a** a disturbance in the electrical activity of the heart. It may be paroxysmal or continuous. It may cause bradycardia or tachycardia. Arrhythmia may be supraventri_ular (sinus, atrial or junctional) or ventricular **reperfusion a** arrhythmia occurring in the damaged heart following thrombolysis or angioplasty due to reperfusion **respiratory a** disturbance in normal quiet rhythm of inspiration and expiration becoming abnormal as in Cheyne-Stokes breathing, and Biot's breathing **sinus a** a phasic alteration of the heart rate during respiration. There is an increase in sinus rate during inspiration and decrease during expiration

arrhythmogenesis (a-rith'mo-gen'e-sis) the development of arrhythmia

arrhythmogenic (-jen'ik) producing arrhythmia

arseniasis (ar'se-ni-a-sis) chronic arsenic poisoning

arsenic (ar'se-nik) a highly poisonous, steel-grey metal, symbol As at no. 33. Acute poisoning results in shock and death. Chronic poisoning is associated with skin pigmentation, hyperkeratosis of palms and soles, transverse lines on the finger nails and peripheral neuropathy.

artefact (ar'te-fakt) artifact

arteralgia (ar'ter-al-jah) pain arising from an artery, as of headache

arteria (ar'ter'e-a) artery, a blood vessel carrying blood away from the heart. **a lusoria** an abnormally placed artery in the retrooesophageal region causing dysphagia

arterial (ar-te're-al) pertaining to one or more arteries **a bleeding** bleeding from an artery. It is bright red and comes in spurts. **a blood gases** (ABG) estimation of PaO_2 and $PaCO_2$ using arterial blood to determine the alveolar ventilation

• and acid-base status **a circulation** movement of blood through arteries **a line** introduction of a catheter and connecting it to a transducer and monitor

arteriectasis(ar-te-re-ek'ta-sis) dilatation and stretching of an artery

arter(o) combining word for artery

arteriogram (ar'te-re-o-gram) a radiogram of an artery taken after injection of radio-opaque substance into an artery.

arteriography (ar-ter'e-og'ra-fe) radiographic visualisation of artery

arteriola (ar-ter'e-o-la) pl **arteriolae,** arteriole

arteriole (ar-ter'e-ol) a minute branch of an artery with muscular wall; a terminal artery continuous with the capillary network

arteriol(o) combining word for arteriole

arteriolonecrosis (ar-ter'e-o'lo-ne-kro'sis) necrosis in the media of arterioles

arteriolopathy (ar-ter'e-o-lop'a-the) any disease of arterioles

arteriolosclerosis (ar-ter'e-olo-skle-ro-sis) thickening and sclerosis affecting the walls of arterioles

arteriomotor (ar-ter'e-o-mo'ter) causing an alteration in the calibre of an artery

arteriomyomatosis (-mi'o-ma-to'sis) thickening of the wall of an artery by an overgrowth of muscle fibres.

arteriopathy (ar-ter'e-op'a-the) any disease of the arteries.

arterioplasty (ar-ter'e-o-plas'te) surgical reconstruction of the wall of an artery.

arteriorrhaphy (ar-ter'e-or'a-fe) suture of an artery

arteriorrhexis (ar-ter'e-o-rek'sis) rupture of an artery

arteriosclerosis (-skle-ro'sis) arterial hardening.

arteriostenosis (ar-ter'o-ste-no'sis) narrowing of an artery

arteriotony (ar-ter'e-ot'a-ne) blood pressure

arteriovenous (ar-ter'i-o-ve'nus) pertaining to both artery and a vein; both arterial and venous.

arteritis (ar'te-ri'tis) inflammation of an artery. **giant cell a** temporal arteritis condition found in elderly people predominantly females involving temporal artery, causing severe headaches and scalp tenderness. Arterial wall is infiltrated by an inflammatory infiltrate of lymphocytes, plasma cells, giant cells, macrophages and eosinophils, with marked necrosis of media and fragmentation of internal elastic lamina **Takayashu's a** pulseless disease; aortic arch syndrome

artery (ar'ter-e) pl **arteries** a vessel carrying blood away from the heart. There are two divisions: pulmonary and systemic. Pulmonary and umbilical arteries convey deoxygenated blood. Systemic arteries carry oxygenated blood to the different parts of the body (table 1)

Table 1: Arteries

acromiothoracic: branch of axillary artery distributing blood to thoracic, deltoid and clavicular regions through its four branches.

alveolar anterior: superior-branch of infraorbital artery supplying blood to upper incisors, canine teeth and maxillary sinus.

alveolar inferior: branch of maxillary artery for lower jaw and lower lip regions

alveolar posterior: superior-branch of maxillary artery to supply blood to

premolar, molar region of upper jaw and also maxillary sinus.

angular branch of facial artery for lower eye-lid, nose and lacrimal sac.

aorta: largest artery, arising from left ventricle of the heart having different parts-ascending, arch, thoracic and abdominal aorta.

ascending: proximal part of aorta arising from left ventricle, gives right and left coronary arteries and continues as arch of aorta

arch: continuation of ascending aorta gives 3 large branches-brachiocephalic, left common corotid and left subclavian, and continues as thoracic aorta.

thoracic: extends from distal part of arch to opening in diaphragm, gives bronchial, oesophageal, pericardial, mediastinal and posterior intercostal arteries, continues as abdominal aorta.

abdominal: continuation of thoracic aorta, extends from opening in diaphragm to bifurcation into common iliac arteries, gives branches-inferior phrenic, lumbar, median sacral, superior and inferior mesenteric, renal, middle suprarenal, coeliac and gonadal arteries.

appendicular: branch of iliocolic artery to supply appendix

auricular deep: branch of maxillary artery, distributes blood to tympanic membrane, auditory canal and temporomandibular joint.

axillary: continuation of subclavian artery, main artery of the upper limb gives superior thoracic, acromiothoracic, lateral thoracic , subscapular and anterior posterior cicumflex and humeral branches

basilar : formed by union of right and left vertebral arteries at the lower border of pons, supplies brain stem, internal ear, cerebellum and part of cerebrum by its pontine, labyrnthine, anterior inferior cerebellar and superior cerebellar branches, bifurcates into posterior cerebral arteries at the upper border of pons.

brachial: continuation of axillary artery, supplies shoulder, arm, forearm and hand by its branches.

brachiocephalic: origin from arch of aorta, supplies right side of head and neck and right arm, gives right common carotid and right arm.

buccal: branch of maxillary artery, supplies buccinator muscle and oral mucous membrane.

caecal anterior: branch of iliocolic supplies caecum **Inferior**-branch of iliocolic supplies caecum

caroticotympanic: branch of internal carotid artery, supplies middle ear cavity.

carotid common: branch of brachiocephalic on the right side and from arch of aorta on the left side, divides into external and internal carotid branches.

carotid external: origin from common carotid artery supplies neck, face and skull by its branches - superior thyroid, ascending pharyngeal, lingual, facial, sternomastoid, occipital, posterior auricular, terminates into superficial temporal and maxillary arteries.

carotid internal: origin from common carotid, supplies brain, orbit and middle ear, gives ophthalmic, caroticotympanic, posterior communicating, anterior choroid, anterior cerebral and middle cerebral

central artery of retina: branch of ophthalmic artery supplies retina

cerebellar anterior inferior: branch of basilar artery, supplies cerebellum, pons and medulla oblongata.

cerebellar posterior inferior: branch of vertebral artery supplies cerebellum and medulla oblongata.

cerebellar superior: branch of basilar artery supplies cerebellum, midbrain and pineal gland.

cerebral anterior: branch of internal carotid supplies orbital, frontal, parieta cortex, corpus collosum, diencephalon corpus striatum, internal capsule and choroid plexus of lateral ventricle.

cerebral middle: branch of internal carotid supplies orbital, frontal, parietal, temporal cortex, corpus striatum and internal capsule.

cerebral posterior: origin as terminal bifurcation of basilar supplies occipital temporal cortex, basal ganglia, thalamus, and midbrain.

cervical ascending: branch of inferior thyroid artery supplying muscles of neck and vertebrae.

cervical deep: branch of costocervical trunk, supplies deep muscles of neck.

cervical transverse: branch of subclavian artery, gives deep and superficial branches to muscles of scapular region

ciliary anterior and posterior: branches of ophthalmic artery, supplies iris, ciliary process and choroid.

circumflex: branch of left coronary artery, supplies left ventricle and left atrium by its atrial, marginal and posterior ventricular branches

circumflex femoral: origin from femoral artery supplies hip joint and muscles of thigh by its ascending, descending and transverse branches.

circumflex humeral posterior: branch of axillary artery, supplies shoulder joint, deltoid, teres minor and triceps muscles.

circumflex humeral anterior: branch of axillary artery, supplies shoulder joint, head of biceps and pectoralis major near their insertions.

circumflex iliac deep: branch of external iliac, supplies iliac fossa, groin and abdominal muscles.

circumflex iliac superficial: branch of femoral artery supplies groin and abdominal wall.

circumflex scapular: branch of subscapular artery, supplies muscles of scapula.

coliac: branch of abdominal aorta supplies oesophagus, stomach, duodenum, spleen, pancreas, liver and gall bladder, by its branches left gastric, common hepatic, and splenic artery

colic left: branch of inferior mesenteric artery for descending colon.

colic middle and right: branches of superior mesenteric artery supplying transverse colon and ascending colon.

coronary left: origin from left aortic sinus, supplies left atrium and left ventricle by its anterior interventricular and circumflex branches.

coronary right: origin from right aortic sinus supplies right ventricle, right atrium, atrioventricular node and sinoatrial node by its atrial, right mar-

ginal and posterior interventricular branches.

cremasteric: branch of inferior epigastric supplies cremaster muscle and coverings of spermatic cord.

cystic: branch of hepatic artery, supplies gall bladder.

digital in foot: dorsal-branch of dorsal metatarsal artery, supplies dorsum of toes.

digital in hand: dorsal branch of dorsal metacarpal artery, supplies dorsum of fingers.

digital palmar: origin from superficial palmar arch, gives digital proper branches to supply fingers.

digital plantar: origin from plantar metatarsal arteries gives digital proper branches to supply toes.

dorsal artery of clitoris: branch of internal pudendal artery, supplies clitoris.

dorsal artery of penis: branch of internal pudendal , supplies glans and prepuce of penis.

dorsalis pedis: continuation of anterior tibial, supplies foot and toes, tarsal joint by its lateral and medial tarsal branches.

epigastric inferior: branch of external iliac artery supplies anterior abdominal wall.

epigastric superior: terminal branch of internal thoracic artery, supplies abdominal wall and diaphragm.

epigastric superficial: branch of femoral artery, supplies abdominal wall and groin.

ethmoidal: anterior and posterior-branches of ophthalmic artery, supplies ethmoidal air sinuses, duramater, frontal air sinuses and nose.

facial: branch of external carotid artery, supplies face, tonsils, palate and submandibular gland by its various branches.

facial transverse: branch of superficial temporal artery, supplies parotid region

femoral: continuation of external iliac artery in the front of thigh, main artery of the lower limb, also supplies lower abdominal wall and external genitalia.

femoral deep: also called as profunda femoris, branch of femoral artery, supplies thigh muscles and hip joint.

gastric left: branch of coeliac artery, supplies lower end of oesophagus and lesser curvature of stomach.

gastric posterior: branch of splenic artery, supplies posterior surface of stomach

gastric right: branch of common hepatic artery supplying lesser curvature of stomach

gastric short: branches from splenic artery, supplying upper part of stomach

gastroduodenal: origin from common hepatic artery, supplies stomach, duodenum, pancreas and greater omentum by its superior pancreatic duodenal and gastroepiploic branches.

genicular descending: branch of femoral artery, supplies knee joint and upper part of leg.

genicular lateral inferior: branch of popliteal artery for knee joint.

genicular lateral superior: branch of popliteal artery, supplies knee joint, and lower end of femur.

genicular medial inferior: branch of popliteal artery for knee joint.

genicular medial superior: branch of popliteal artery, supplies knee joint and lower end of femur.

genicular middle: branch of popliteal artery, supplies knee joint and cruciate ligaments.

gluteal inferior: branch of internal iliac artery, supplies muscles of gluteal region and back of thigh

gluteal superior: branch of internal iliac artery, supplies muscles of gluteal region.

helicine: branch of deep and dorsal artery of penis, supplies erectile tissue of penis by its superficial and deep branches.

hepatic common: originates from coeliac trunk. Supplies stomach, pancreas, duodenum liver, gall bladder and greater omentum.

hepatic proper: branch of common hepatic artery, supplies liver and gall bladder by its right and left branches.

hyaloid: branch of ophthalmic artery in foetus, atrophies after birth.

hypophyseal inferior and superior: branches of internal carotid artery to supply pituitary gland.

iliac common: originates from abdominal aorta, supplies pelvic viscera, abdominal wall and lower limb by its internal and external iliac branches.

iliac external: originates from common iliac artery, supplies abdominal wall, external genitalia and lower limb, continues as femoral artery.

iliac internal: continuation of common iliac artery, supplies pelvic viscera and wall, buttock and medial side of thigh by its various branches.

iliolumbar: branch of internal iliac artery, supplies pelvic wall, lumbar and sacral vertebrae.

ileal: branch of superior mesenteric artery, supplies ileum.

ileocolic: branch of superior mesenteric, supplies ileum, caecum, appendix and ascending colon.

infraorbital: terminal branch of maxillary artery supplies maxillary sinus, bone, upper jaw, lower eyelid, nose and cheek.

intercostal: highest-branch of costocervical trunk, supplies upper part of thoracic wall by its Ist and IInd intercostal branches.

intercostal: posterior nine pair of arteries arising from thoracic aorta to supply thoracic wall by its dorsal and lateral branches.

interosseous anterior: branch of posterior or common interosseous artery to supply deep muscles on the front of forearm.

interosseous common: branch of ulnar artery in the elbow region, supplies cubital region and gives anterior and posterior interosseus branches.

interosseous recurrent: branch of ulnar artery in the elbow region, supplies cubital region and gives anterior and posterior interosseus branches.

interosseous recurrent: branch of posterior or common interosseus, supplies back of elbow joint.

interosseous posterior: originates from common interosseus artery, supplies deep parts at the back of the fore arm.

labial superior and inferior: branches of facial artery, supplies upper and lower lip.

labyrinthine: branch of basilar artery , supplies internal ear by its cochlear and vestibular branches.

lacrimal: branch of ophthalmic artery, supplies lacrimal gland, eyelids and conjunctiva

laryngeal inferior: branch of inferior thyroid artery, supplies larynx trachea and oesophagus

laryngeal superior: branch of superior thyroid artery, supplies larynx.

lingual: branch of external carotid artery supplies tongue, sublingual gland, tonsil and epiglottis by its suprahyoid sublingual, dorsal lingual, and *profunda linguae* branches

lumbar: branches of abdominal aorta. Supplies posterior abdominal wall by its dorsal and spinal branches.

lumbar: lowest branch of median sacral artery supplies sacrum and gluteus maximus muscle

masseteric: branch of maxillary artery, supplies masseter muscle

maxillary: branch of external carotid artery supplies teeth, muscles of mastication, ear, nose, paranasal sinuses, palate and meninges.

median: branch of anterior interosseous artery, supplies muscles on the front of forearm and median nerve.

meningeal middle: branch of maxillary artery, supplies cranium and dura-mater

meningeal posterior: arising from ascending pharyngeal artery supplies occipital bone and dura mater

mesenteric inferior: originates from abdominal aorta, supplies descending colon and rectum by its left colic, sigmoid and superior rectal branches.

mesenteric superior: originates from abdominal aorta, supplies small intestine pancreaticoduodenal, jejunal, ileal, iliocolic, right colic and middle colic branches.

musculophrenic: branch of internal thoracic, supplies diaphragm and part of thoracic and abdominal wall.

nasal posterior lateral: branch of sphenopalatine, supplies paranasal sinuses.

nutrient: arteries supplying to the bone, usually a branch of large artery in that region.

obturator: originates from internal iliac artery, supplies pelvic muscles and hip joint.

obturator accessory: branch of inferior epigastric, supplies pelvic muscles and hip joint.

occipital: branch of external carotid artery, supplies back of the neck and scalp muscles.

occipital lateral: branch of posterior cerebral artery, supplies temporal lobe by its anterior, middle and posterior temporal branches.

occipital middle: branch of posterior cerebral, supplies corpus callosum , cuneus and posterior part of lateral surface of occipital lobe.

ophthalmic: origin from internal carotid artery, supplies eye, orbit and lacrimal gland.

ovarian: branch of abdominal aorta, supplies ovary, uterine tube and ureter.

palatine ascending: branch of facial artery, supplies soft palate, pharynx, tonsil and pharyngotympanic tube.

palatine descending: branch of maxillary artery, supplies hard and soft palate by its greater palatine and lesser palatine branches palpebral lateral: branch of lacrimal artery, supplies eye lids and conjunctiva

palpebral medial: branch of ophthalmic artery, supplies eye lids

pancreaticoduodenal anterosuperior: branch of gastroduodenal artery, supplies pancreas and duodenum

pancreaticoduodenal inferior: branch of superior mesenteric supplies pancreas and duodenum

paracentral: branch of anterior cerebral artery supplies cerebral cortex and medial central sulcus

parietal: branch of middle cerebral artery, supplying parietal lobe and temporal lobe

parietooccipital: branch of anterior cerebral artery, supplying parietal and occipital lobe

perforating: branches from deep femoral, supplies muscles at the back of the thigh and gluteal region

pericardiophrenic: branch of internal thoracic artery supplying pericardium, pleura and diaphragm

perineal: branch of internal pudendal artery supplying perineum and external genitalia

peroneal: branch of posterior tibial artery supplying muscles of lateral compartment of leg and ankle region

pharyngeal ascending: branch of external carotid artery supplying soft palate , ear and meninges

phrenic inferior: branch of abdominal aorta, supplies diaphragm and suprarenal gland

phrenic superior: branch of thoracic aorta, supplies diaphragm

plantar lateral: branch of posterior tibial, forms plantar arch, gives metatarsal branches to supply sole, toes and joints

plantar medial: branch of posterior tibial supplies sole and toes by its superficial and deep branches

pontine: branch from basilar artery, supplies pons

popliteal: continuation of femoral artery, supplies knee joint and calf muscles by its genicular and muscular branches

posterior: branch of external carotid artery supplying parotid gland, pinna, middle ear and muscles.

princeps pollices: branch of radial artery supplying thumb

profunda linguae: branch of lingual artery supplying tongue

pudendal external: branch of femoral artery, supplies external genitalia and adjacent part of the thigh

pudendal internal: branch of internal iliac artery, supplies genitalia , anal canal and perineum

pulmonary: left and right originate from pulmonary trunk, distributes blood to the left and right lung by its various segmental branches for oxygenation

pulmonary trunk: originates from right ventricle, divides into left and right pulmonary arteries to convey deoxygenated blood to lungs

radial: one of the terminal branches of brachial artery, supplies forearm, wrist and hand

radialis indices: branch of princeps pollices artery supplying index finger

rectal inferior: branch of internal pudendal artery, supplies rectum and anal canal

rectal middle: branch of internal iliac artery, supplies rectum, prostate and seminal vesicles

rectal superior: branch of inferior mesenteric artery supplies rectum

recurrent: branches given by arteries in different regions which course in opposite direction to the parent artery. These can be seen as branches of radial, ulnar and tibial arteries

renal: branch of abdominal aorta, supplies kidney, suprarenal gland and ureter, gives arcuate, interlobar and intralobular branches inside kidney

sacral lateral: branch of iliolumbar artery supplies sacrum and coccyx

sacral median: lowest branch of abdominal aorta, supplies sacrum, coccyx and rectum.

scapular dorsal: branch of transverse cervical artery, supplies trapezius, rhomboids and latissimus dorsi muscles

sciatic: branch of inferior gluteal artery, seen along with sciatic nerve and supplies it.

septal anterior and posterior: branches of left and right coronary arteries supplying anterior and posterior part of interventricular septum

sigmoid: branch of inferior mesenteric artery, supplies sigmoid colon

sphenopalatine: branch of maxillary artery, supplies nasal cavity and nasopharynx by its posterior lateral nasal and posterior septal branches

spinal anterior and posterior: branches of vertebral artery, supplies spinal cord

splenic: branch of coeliac trunk, supplies spleen, pancreas stomach and greater omentum

stylomastoid: branch of posterior auricular artery supplies middle ear and mastoid cells by its mastoid and stapedial branches

subclavian: branch of brachiocephalic trunk on the right side and directly from arch of aorta for left side, supplies neck, thoracic wall, spinal cord, brain and upper limb

subcostal: origin from thoracic aorta, supplies posterior abdominal wall

submental: branch of facial artery in submental region

subscapular: branch of axillary artery supplies scapular muscles by its thoracodorsal and circumflex scapular branches

supraduodenal: branch of gastroduodenal artery, supplies first part of duodenum

supraorbital: branch of ophthalmic artery, supplies scalp, orbital muscles, upper eye lid and frontal sinus

suprarenal inferior: branch of renal artery for suprarenal gland.

suprarenal middle: branch of abdominal aorta, supplies suprarenal gland

suprarenal superior: branch of inferior phrenic, supplies suprarenal gland.

suprascapular: originates from thyrocervical trunk, supplies deltoid, scapular and clavicular regions.

supratrochlear: terminal branch of ophthalmic artery, supplies forehead

tarsal lateral and medial: branches of dorsalis pedis artery, supplies tarsal bones and joints

temporal anterior: branch of middle cerebral artery supplying cortex of the temporal lobe anteriorly

temporal deep: branch of maxillary artery, supplies temporalis muscles and fossa

temporal middle: branch of middle cerebral artery, supplies cortex of temporal lobe

temporal superficial: terminal branch of external carotid artery, supplies temporal and parotid region

testicular: originates from abdominal aorta, supplies testes, ureter and epididymis

thoracic superior: branch of axillary artery supplying anterior chest wall and mammary gland

thoracic internal: branch of subclavian, supplies anterior thoracic wall, mammary gland and diaphragm

thoracic lateral: branch of axillary artery, supplies pectoral region and mammary gland

thoracoacromial: branch of axillary artery, gives acromial, deltoid, clavicular and pectoral branches to supply deltoid, clavicular and pectoral region.

thoracodorsal: branch of subscapular artery, supplies subscapularis and teres muscles.

thyrocervical trunk: branch of subclavian artery, supplies neck, thyroid gland and scapular regions.

thyroid superior: branch of external carotid supplies thyroid gland and adjacent structures.

thyroid inferior: branch of thyrocervical trunk, supplies thyroid gland and adjacent structures.

thyroidima: originates from arch of aorta or brachiocephalic trunk, supplies isthmus of thyroid gland.

tibial anterior: branch of popliteal artery supplies ankle and foot

tibial posterior: branch of popliteal artery, supplies leg and foot.

tympanic anterior: branch of maxillary artery supplying tympanic cavity.

tympanic inferior: branch of ascending pharyngeal artery supplying tympanic cavity.

tympanic posterior: branch of stylomastoid artery supplying tympanic cavity.

tympanic superior: branch of middle meningeal artery supplying tympanic cavity

ulnar: branch of brachial artery supplying forearm, wrist and hand.

umbilical: branch of internal iliac artery supplies vas deferens, seminal vesicles, testes, ureter and urinary bladder in male, and atrophies in female.

urethral: branch of internal pudendal, supplies urethra

uterine : branch of internal iliac artery, supplies uterus, fallopian tubes, ovary and vagina.

vaginal: branch of uterine artery, supplies vagina and urinary bladder.

vertebral: branch of subclavian artery supplies muscles of neck, vertebrae, spinal cord, cerebellum and cerebrum.

vesical inferior: branch of internal iliac, supplies urinary bladder, prostate and seminal vesicles.

vesical superior: branch of umbilical artery, supplies urinary bladder, ureter and urachus.

zygomatico orbital: branch of superficial temporal, supplies lateral wall of orbit.

---

arthralgia (ar-thral'jea) pain in the joint

arthritide (ar'thri-tid) a skin eruption of gouty or rheumatic origin

arthritis (ar-thri'tis) pl **arthritides**, adj **arthritic.** inflammation of a joint **acute septic a** bacterial infection of the joint presenting with hot, painful, tender, swollen joint **degenerative a** osteoarthritis **gouty a** an inflammatory arthritis from crystals of monosodium urate monohydrate derived from hyperuricaemic body fluids **gonococcal a** arthritis usually of knee joint produced by gonococcal infection **infective a** septic arthritis and arthritis associated with specific infections such as gonorrhoea, brucellosis, tuberculosis, leprosy, and syphilis **juvenile idiopathic a** inflammatory arthritis of children **juvenile rheumatoid a** arthritis with an age of onset less than 16 years that may present as oligoarthritis, polyarthritis with systemic manifestations such as hepatosplenomegaly and lymphadenopathy **Lyme a** large joint arthritis from *Borrelia burgdorferi* **polindromic a** transient recurrent arthritis of large joints, of undetermined aetiology **psoriatic a** a seronegative inflammatory arthritis found in patients with psoriasis **reactive a** arthritis following an enteric infection Reiter's disease is characterised by reactive arthritis **rheumatoid a** chronic inflammatory polyarthritis. There is symmetrical, deforming polyarthritis affecting small and large synovial joints, with associated systemic disturbances. There is presence of circulating antiglobulin antibodies (rheumatoid factor). The course of the disease is prolonged with exacerbations and remissions **syphilitic a** painful para articular swelling or painless effusion (congenital syphilis) joint involvement (acquired syphilis) **tuberculous a** joint involvement in tuberculosis

arth(o) combining word for joint; articulation

arthrocentesis (ar'thro-sen-te'sis) needle aspiration of fluid from a joint cavity

arthrochalasis (-kal'a-sis) lax joint

arthrochondritis (-kon-dri'tis) inflammation of the cartilage of a joint

arthrodia (ar-thro'de-a) a synovial joint permitting only simple gliding movement

arthrodysplasia (ar'thro-dis-pla'ze-a) a hereditary disorder characterised by deformity of various joints

arthroempyesis (-em'pi-e'sis) pus formation within a joint

arthrography (ar-throg'ra-fe) 1. radiography of a joint 2. radiography of a synovial joint after injection of a contrast medium

arthrogryposis (ar'thro-gri-po-sis) a fixation of joint by contractures and fusion

artholith (ar'thro-lith) calculus in a joint

arthroneuralgia (ar'thro-noo-ral'je-a) pain in or around a joint

arthro-ophthalmopathy (-of'thal-mop'a-the) disease affecting the joint and eye.

arthropathy (ar-throp'a-the) any joint disease

arthroplasty (ar'thro-plas'te) 1. creation of an artificial joint 2. plastic repair of a joint to restore its integrity and function

arthropoda (ar-throp'o-da) a phylum of metazoa having a bilateral symmetry, a hard exoskeleton, segmented body and jointed paired appendages. housefly, tsetsefly, mosquito, sandfly and louse are examples. It includes crustacea (crabs, cray fish), arachnida (spiders, scorpions, ticks, mites). They may act as vectors of infectious agents or envenomate through stings and bites or cause infestation or cause allergic dermatitis

arthropyosis (ar'thro-pi-o'sis) formation of pus in a joint cavity

arthroscope (ar'thro-skop) an endoscopy for examining the interior of a joint

arthroscopy (ar-thros'ko-pe) examination of the interior of a joint with an arthroscope

arthrosis (ar-thro'sis) atrophic degenerative disorder of a joint

arthrostomy (ar-thros'to-me) surgical creation of a temporary opening into a joint cavity to facilitate drainage

arthrosynovitis (ar-thro-sin'o-vi'tis) inflammation of the synovial membrane of a joint

articular (ar-tik'u-lar) pertaining to a joint

articulare (ar-tik'u-lar'e) a point of insertion of the articular process of mandible and temporal bone

articulate (ar-tik'u-lat) 1. to join together allowing movement between joints 2. to speak distinctly and clearly 3. to arrange teeth in proper relation to each other while making an artificial denture

articulation (-la'shun) 1. the place of union between two or more bones as in joint. It may be immovable (synarthrosis), slightly movable (amphiarthrosis) or freely movable (diarthrosis) 2. pronunciation of words and sentences

articulo (ar-tik'u-lo) at the moment **a mortis** at the moment of death

artifact (ar'ti-fakt) 1. a substance or signal that interferes with or obscures the interpretation of a study 2. any abnormality in histology and radiography produced by the technique used 3. anything produced artificially

artificial not natural **a blood** artificial oxygen carrier such as perfluorochemicals. **a heart** ventricular assist device **a insemination** depositing of sperm-of the partner or of a donor- in the female reproductive tract in an attempt to impregnate **a pancreas** a selectively permeable tubular membrane containing xenotic pancreatic islets **a reproduction** artificial insemination, ovum donation, *in vitro* fertilisation, surrogate motherhood, and cryopreserved embryo transplantation **a skin** a porous mat of collagen chondroitin 6 sulphate strands covered by a thin skin of silastic **a sweeteners** substances having a taste similar to dietary sugar, which do not supply calories (saccharine, cyclamates, aspartame) **a tears** a solution containing 0.5% carboxymethyl cellulose or 5%

polyvinyl alcohol for treatment of xerophthalmia

arytenoid (ar'i-te'noid) 1. one of a pair of small pyramidal cartilage of the larynx 2. arytenoideus muscle of the larynx

arytenoidopexy (ar'i-te-noi'do-pek'se) surgical fixation of arytenoid cartilage

asadhya (s) impossible, refers to cure

asanas (s) body posture used in yoga

asankhya (s) innumerable

asava (s) drugs mixed with water and allowed to ferment

asbestos (as-bes'tos) an indestructible, fibrous mineral with great tensile strength, flexibility and heat resistance. It is a family of crystalline hydrated silicates. It consists of a mixture of silicates of iron, magnesium, chromium, calcium and aluminium which break into fibres when crushed. The mineral existing as amphibole with straight thin fibres (crocidolite, amosite, anthrophillite and tremolite) or as serpentine form with curly long fibres (chrysotile) **a body** ferruginous body. It has a beaded necklace of dumb-bell appearance and its presence is an index of asbestos exposure.

asbestosis (as-bes-to'sis) a diffuse interstitial fibrosis of lung parenchyma caused by exposure to asbestos. The fibrosis is diffuse with airspace enlargement or honeycombing

ascariasis (as'kar-ri'a-sis) round worm infestation. The nematode *Ascaris lumbricoides* is a pale yellow worm of 20 cm and gains entry by eating food contaminated with mature ova. They hatch in the duodenum and larva migrate through the lungs ultimately reach small intestine and mature. The presentation may be abdominal discomfort, passage of worms in stools or vomiting of worms, intestinal obstruction, blockage of bile or pancreatic duct and obstruction of appendix

ascaricide (as-kar'i-sid) an agent that kills the ascarids **ascaricidal** adj

ascarid (as'ka-rid) any nematode belonging to the family of Ascarididae

ascaris (-ris) a genus of round worm that is parasitic in small intestine of man

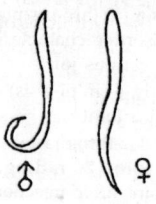

Ascaris

ascites (a-si'tez) accumulation of free fluid in the peritoneal cavity. It causes abdominal distension with fullness of flanks. Its presence is demonstrable by shifting dullness on percussion and a fluid thrill when the amount of fluid is large. Cirrhosis of liver, nephrotic syndrome, congestive heart failure, hypoproteinaemia, tuberculosis, malignancy form the common causes for ascites. Ascites is a physical sign

ascomycetes (as'ko-mi-se'tez) a class of fungi exhibiting a sexual and asexual reproductive phases

ascorbic (a-skor'bik) **acid** vitamin C, antiscorbutic vitamin preventing scurvy.

-ase termination denoting an enzyme

asemia (a-se'me-a) inability to appreciate by touch the form and nature of an object

asepsis (a-sep'sis) a condition without any living pathogenic microorganisms.

ASI Association of Surgeons of India

Asian paralysis syndrome acute flaccid para¹ sis bilaterally symmetrical, without sensory loss in children, due to motor axonal neuropathy and recovery is partial

asialia (a'si-a'le-a) absence of saliva

asiderosis (a-sid-er'o-sis) deficiency of iron reserve in the body

-asis combining word for state; condition

asmari (s) urinary calculi

ASO anti-streptolysin O a serologic test for group A-β haemolytic streptococcal infection. Test is based on haemolysis inhibition and it is raised in acute rheumatic fever, expressed as Todd units.

asparaginase (as-par'a-jin-as) 1. an enzyme catalysing the hydrolysis of asparagine to aspartic acid and ammonia 2. an enzyme from *Escherichia coli* used in the treatment of acute leukaemia

asparagine (as-par'a-jen) a non-essential amino acid occurring in proteins.

aspartate (a-spar-tat) a salt or ester of aspartic acid **a aminotransferase** (AST) glutamic-oxaloacetic transferase catalysing the transfer of an amine group from glutamic acid to oxaloacetic acid

aspartic (a-spar'tik) **acid** aminosuccinic acid, amino acid found in the protein

aspect (as'pekt) 1. appearance; looks 2. the side of an object directed to any direction

aspergilloma (as'per-jil'o-ma) *A. fumigatus* or *A. niger* can develop in the form of a fungus ball by having a saprophytic growth in a nidus provided by damaged lung tissue

aspergillosis (-o'sis) a disorder initiated by inhalation of the spores liberated by the fungi of Aspergillus, mainly *A. fumigatus* the clinical manifestations depend on the immunological reactivity of the individual and present as hypersensitivity reaction of aspergillus (allergic bronchopulmonary aspergillosis, bronchocentric granulomatosis, and mucoid impaction of bronchus, extrinsic allergic alveolitis, and asthma) saprophytic colonisation (aspergilloma) or tissue invasive aspergillosis

aspergillus (as'per-jil'is) a mould-like fungus with a worldwide distribution in the soil and decaying vegetation. The spores of size of two to three microns in diameter are arranged like a holy water sprinkler at the end of a filament. The spores get separated readily and present in air in large numbers especially during winter months and can be readily inhaled. *Aspergillus fumigatus* is the common example. Other species are *A. niger*, *A. terreus* and *A. nidulans*

aspermia (a-sper'me-a) lack of expulsion of semen following ejaculation

asphyxia (as-fik'se-a) condition produced by lack of oxygen in air and it results in hypoxaemia and hypercapnia

aspiration (as'pi-ra'shun) 1. the act of inhaling 2. removal of fluid or gas by suction from body cavity. **a pneumonia** inhalation of acidic gastric contents in comatose patients, leading to acute inflammation of lung parenchyma **vacuum a** removal of uterine contents by application of vacuum.

aspirin (as'pi-rin) acetylsalicylic acid, widely used analgesic and antipyretic. It inhibits platelet aggregation, used prophylactically in small doses in coronary artery disease, transient ischaemic disease and thromboembolic condition of the brain.

asplenia (a-sple'ne-a) absence of spleen

asrapitta (s)   haemorrhagic disease

asrk (s) blood

assay (as'a) 1. analysis 2. to examine; to subject to analysis

assimilation (a-sim'i-la'shun) 1. conversion of nutrient substances into living tissue 2. *psy* absorption of new experience

assistant (a-sis'tent) one who helps or supports in carrying out activities of patient care; an auxiliary

association (a-so'sea-a'shun) 1. the act of joining; co-ordination with another structure or idea

assortment (a-sort'ment) random distribution of non-homologous chromosomes to daughter cells in metaphase

AST aspartate transaminase, a cytoplasmic and mitochondrial transaminase enzyme, earlier called glutamic oxaloacetic transaminase.

astasia (as-ta'zhah) inability to stand due to muscular incoordination

asteatosis (as'te-a-to'sis) a scaly skin condition due to diminished secretion of sebaceous glands

astemizole (a-stem'i-zol) a H_1-receptor antagonist used in treatment of urticaria and allergic rhinitis

asterion (as-ter'e-on) the point on the skull at the junction of occipital, parietal and temporal bones

asterixis (as'ter-ik'sis) flapping tremor with involuntary jerking movements especially of hand, often encountered in hepatic precoma or encephalopathy

asteroid (as'ter-oid) star-shaped **a bodies** acidophilic, stellate inclusions in giant cells, seen in sarcoidosis, berylliosis

asthenia (as-the'ne-a) loss of strength; disability

asthenocoria (as-the'no-kor'e-a) sluggish pupillary light reflex

asthenopia (as'thi-no'pe-a) weakness of eyes accompanied by pain, headache and dimness of vision

asthi (s) bone *a bhanga* fracture

asthma (az'mah) bronchial asthma a complex and heterogeneous syndrome characterised by episodic intrathoracic airways obstruction, airways hyper-responsiveness and airways inflammation resulting in occurrence of dyspnoea and wheezing which varies widely over time either spontaneously or in response to treatment **aspirin-sensitive a** asthma following aspirin or NSAIDs. It develops without any previous history of asthma or atopy **exercise induced a** initiation or exacerbation of bronchospasm by exercise. Dyspnoea may be a relatively occult manifestation of hypersensitive airways **extrinsic atopic a** exposure to antigen in atopic individuals stimulates peripheral lymphoid tissues to synthesise IgE, and initiate asthma **extrinsic non-atopic a** constant exposure to a large amount of antigen may stimulate appearance of antibodies, which combine with allergens to form immune complexes and initiate asthma **intrinsic a** asthma in middle aged in whom an extrinsic allergen can't be identified **nocturnal a** asthma associaed with deep, nocturnal worsening **occupational a** asthma

due to inhalation of airborne dusts, vapours and fumes encountered in work place

astigmatism (a-stig'ma-tizm) 1. a lens having different curvatures in different meridians 2. a condition of unequal curvatures in the refractive surfaces of eye and prevent the focussing of rays at a single point in retina

astrogalus (as-trag'a-lus) - talus *see* table of bones

astringent (a-strin'joint) 1. drawing together; constricting; binding 2. an agent that has power to do so

astroblast (as'tro-blast) an embryonic cell that develops into an astrocyte

astroblastoma (as'tro-blas-toma) a relatively poorly differentiated glioma composed of immature neoplastic cells of the astrocytic series

astrocyte (as'tro-sit) spider cell, form the structural framework for the neurons. Their foot processes are closely associated with blood vessels to form the blood-brain barrier.

astrocytoma (as'tro-si-to'ma) a diffuse and infiltrating tumour which may be solid or partly cystic occurs at any age. In children it occurs in the cerebellum **malignant a** glioblastoma multiforme, which undergoes degenerative changes, and occurs in cerebrum of adults. It contains all types of glial cells.

astroglia (as-trog'le-a) astrocyte that makes neuroglial tissue

astrovirus (as'tro-vi'rus) a small non-enveloped RNA virus, infects children and causes gastroenteritis

asukari (s) quick acting

asymmetry (a'sim-i-tre) absence of symmetry; presence of dissimilarity in corresponding parts or organs on opposite sides of the body

asynchronism (a-sing'kro-nizm) lack of co-ordination

asynclitism (a-sing'kli'tizm) 1. oblique presentations of the foetal head during labour 2. maturation of the nucleus and cytoplasm of blood cells at different times.

asyndesis (a-sin'de-sis) a disorder of language wherein the related elements of a sentence can't be brought together

asynechia (a'sin-ek'e-a) absence of continuity of structure

asynergy (a-sin'er-je) lack of coordination between different parts or organs.

asystole (a-sis'to-le) cardiac arrest, absence of heart beat

atactiform (a-tak'ti-form) resembling ataxia

atanka (s) anxiety.

ataractic (at'a-rak'tik) 1. pertaining to ataxia 2. a tranquilliser

atavism (a'ta-vi-zm) recurrence of a trait found in a remote ancestor but not in near generations

ataxia (a-tak'se-a) imperfect control over voluntary actions **cerebellar a** ataxia due to cerebellar disease, with ataxic gait **Friedrich's a** *see* Friedrich's ataxia **frontal a** inability to walk normally due to frontal lobe lesions, walks with slow, short shuffling steps, dragging feet on the ground **kinetic a** a motor ataxia **motor a** incoordination occurs only during movement **sensory a** loss of proprioception, ataxia is apparent in the affected limb on closure of eyes **static a** limb outstretched horizontally sways up and down **a-telangiectasia** an autosomal recessive condition characterised by sinopulmonary infections, choreoathetosis, slurring speech and muscle atrophy and oculocutaneous telangiectasia

atel(o) combining word for incomplete, imperfectly developed

atelectasis (at'a-lek'ta-sis) 1. collapse, referring to lung 2. failure of expansion of lung in neonate

atelia (a-te'le-a) imperfect or incomplete development **ateliotic** adj

atelocardia (at'e-lo-kar'de-a) imperfect development of the heart

athelia (a-the'le-a) congenital absence of nipples.

atherectomy (ath'er-ek'ta-me) removal of an atherosclerotic plaque from an artery

athermic (a-ther'mik) without rise of temperature; afebrile.

atheroembolus (ath'er-o-em'bo-lus) an embolus of fragments of atheromatous plaques

atherogenesis (-jen'i-sis) formation of atheromatous lesions in the arterial walls

atheroma (ath'er-o'ma) atherosclerosis, a patchy focal disease of the arterial wall. Coronary arteries are at high risk.

atheromatosis (ath'er-o-ma-to'sis) diffuse atheromatous lesion of the arteries

atherosclerosis (-skle-ro'sis) a condition caused by intramural deposition of LDL, secondary to exposure of smooth muscle to lipid, resulting in platelet induced smooth muscle proliferation, formation of fibrotic plaques and calcification.

athetosis (ath'i-to'sis) slower writhing movements at the limbs

athlet's foot dermatomycosis of the toe webs and soles of the feet of athletes resulting in maceration, erosion and pruritus. *Trichophyton rubrum* is the common causative agent.

athletic heart highly trained athletes exhibiting an increased left ventricular diastolic volume and increased thickness of the left ventricular wall.

athrepsia (a-threp'se-a) marasmus

athymia (a-thim'e-a) 1. dementia 2. absence of thymus

athyreosis (a-th're-o'sis) hypothyroidism

athyria (a-thi're-a) hypothyroid state *atisara* (s) diarrhoea

atlantoaxial (at-lan'to-ak'se-al) pertaining to the atlas and the axis

atlas (at'las) the first cervical vertebra; *see* table of bones

atman (s) soul

atmosphere (at-mos-fer) the gaseous envelope surrounding the earth ; the air

atmospheric (-fer'ik) pertaining to, existing in or consisting of the atmosphere

atocia (a-to'shah) sterility in the female

atom (at'om) the smallest particle of an element and it comprises protons, neutrons and electrons atomisation (at'om-i-za'shun) the process of breaking up of a liquid into a fine spray

atony (at'a-ne) lack of tone or strength

atopic (a-top'ik) relating to or marked by atopy

atopognosia (a-top'og-no'zhzh) inability to locate a sensation properly

atopy (at'a-pe) a genetic predisposition to develop an immediate hypersensitivity against substances of day-to-day exposure from the environment and there is an incrased production of IgE. Common examples of diseases of atopy are bronchial asthma, allergic rhinitis, and atopic dermatitis

atoxic (a-tok'sik) non-toxic

ATP adenosine triphosphate

ATPase adenosine triphosphatase

atraumatic (a'traw-mati'ik) not producing injury or damage

atresia (a-tre-zhah) congenital absence of a normal opening or normally patent lumen

atreomegaly (a'tre-o-meg'a-lę) enlargement of the atrium.

atrial pertaining to atrium a ectopic beat atrial extrasystole. Often asymptomatic, or produce a sensation of a missed beat or an abnormal strong beat. ECG shows a premature beat otherwise normal QRS complex a fibrillation atria beating rapidly and chaotically and ineffectively. Ventricle responds at irregular intervals. Pulse is irregularly irregular. Noted in rheumatic heart disease, coronary artery disease, thyrotoxicosis. It presents with palpitation and may precipitate cardiac failure. ECG shows irregular QRS complexes with no P waves. Digoxin, β- blockers and verapamil reduce the ventricular rate a flutter there is rapid atrial rate of around 300 per minute and is associated with AV block. ECG shows 'saw tooth' pattern waves a myxoma single or multiple gelatinous polypoid mass arising in the left ventricle that is attached by a pedicle to interatrial septum. It may present with pyrexia, syncope, and arrhythmia. There is a 'diastolic plop' due to prolapse of the mass through mitral valve a septal defect (ASD) a common congenital heart disease. Common presentation is as 'ostium secondum' defect from a defect involving the fossa ovalis. 'ostium primum' defect occurs from a defect in the atrioventricular septum and is associated with a cleft mitral valve. In ASD, there is shunt of a large volume of blood through the defect in interatrial septum from left to right atrium and then to the right ventricle and pulmonary arteries. The presentation is with dyspnoea, chest infections and cardiac failure a tachyarrhythmias atrial ectopic beats, atrial tachycardia, atrial fibrillation and atrial flutter a tachycardia an ectopic tachycardia due to an increased automaticity. ECG shows an atrial rate of 140-220 per minute with abnormal P waves

atrionatriuretic peptide a peptide hormone derived from atriopeptigen, released from cardiac myosite storage granules. It suppresses ion flow at sodium channel and increases calcium channel permeability and causes inhibition of sodium absorption in the collecting tubules of the kidney

atrioseptopexy (-sep'to-pek'se) a closed surgical correction of atrial septal defect

atrioventricularis communis (-ven-trik'u-la'ris'ko-mu'nis) a congenital cardiac abnormality due to failure of fusion of the endocardial cushions, resulting in persistence of ostium primum, and atrioventricular canal remains single and undivided

atrium (a'tre-um) pl. atria 1. a chamber, or cavity to which several chambers are connected 2. upper smaller chamber of the heart on either side which receive blood from vena cavae (right) and from pulmonary veins (left) and convey it to the ventricles of the same side 3. tympanic cavity that lies deep to the tympanic membrane 4. a part of gas exchanging portion of the lung, the alveolar duct from which alveolar sacs open.

atrophy (at'ro-fe) wasting wherein there is diminution in the size of a cell, tissue, organ or part

atropine (at'ro-pen) an anticholinergic alkaloid obtained from *Atropa belladonna* used as a smooth muscle relaxant. It is antisecretory, mydriatic and anticholinergic

attack (ah-tak) occurrence of some disease or episode, often it has a dramatic onset. **Adam-Stokes a** episodes of ventricular asystole causing recurrent syncope which occurs without warning. **transient ischaemic a** a brief attack of cerebral ischaemia which recovers within 24 hours **vasovagal a** a transient vascular and neurogenic condition characterised by pallor, bradycardia, sweating and rapid fall in blood pressure. It is due to sudden stimulation of vagus nerve mediated through the receptors in the carotid sinus, aortic arch or heart

attending physician physician who is legally responsible for the care given to a patient while in the hospital or outside.

attention deficit hyperactive disorder ADHD a neurobehavioural disorder in child characterised by impulsiveness, distractibility, hyperreactivity and emotional lability

attenuate (a'ten-uat) to make a culture of genus harmless without actually killing them

attenuation (a-ten'u-a'shun) diminution of an effect; reduction of virulence

attic (at'ik) upper recess of middle ear containing malleus and incus

attitude (at'i-tood) 1. position of the body; posture 2. reaction in a certain way 3. the relation of various parts of foetal body

attraction (a-trak'shun) 1. tendency of two bodies to approach each other. 2. the force causing the fluids to rise up

attribute (a'tri-but) characteristic quality

atypia (a-tip'e-a) deviation from normal

atypical (-i-k'l) not typical; unusual type. **a mycobacteria** mycobacteria other than *M. tuberculosis*, weak pathogens ubiquitously distributed in the environment. Pulmonary infection causes disease similar to tuberculosis

Au chemical symbol of gold (aurum)

audi(o) combining word for hearing

audiogenic (aw'de-o-jen'ik) produced by sound

audiologist (-ol'o-jist) a person trained in audiology

audiology (aw'de-ol'a-je) the science of hearing

audiometer (aw'de-om'e-ter) an instrument to test the power of hearing

audiometry (aw'de-om'i-tre) measurement of efficiency of hearing, expressed in dB as a ratio of person's hearing threshold to reference normal threshold of different frequencies

audiovisual (aw'de-o-viz'u-al) pertaining to simultaneous stimulation of the sense of both hearing and sight

audition (aw'dish'un) 1. act of hearing 2. ability to hear

auditory (aw'de-ta'ri) acuity and clarity at which a particular sound can be heard

Auerbach's (ow'er-baks) **plexus** autonomic plexus found between the layers of gut muscle from midoesophagus downwards that exhibits a motor control of peristalsis, named after Leopold Auerbach, German anatomist

augmentin a combination of amoxycillin and clavulanic acid

augmentation therapy therapy with prolastin to improve the antiprotease activity in patients with a documented deficiency of alpha$_1$ antitrypsin

aura (aw'rah) a subjective (illusionary or hallucinatory) or objective (mator) event marking the onset of epileptic attack or migraine

aural (aw'r'l) 1. pertaining to or perceived by ear 2. pertaining to aura

auric (aw'rik) pertaining to or containing gold

auricle (aw'ri-k'l) part of the external ear not contained within the head; the pinna, or flap of the ear

auricula (aw-rik'u-la) auricle

auriculare (aw-rik'u-lar'e) a point at the top of the opening of the external auditory meatus

auricularis (aw'rik'u-lar'is) auricular; pertaining to the ear

auriculotermporal syndrome flushing and sweating of the skin innervated by the auriculotemporal nerve at the time of meals, occurs, following injury to the auriculotemporal nerve

auris (aw'ris) ear; the organ of hearing **a externa** external ear comprising the auricle and the external acoustic meatus **a interna** internal ear comprising the vestibule, cochlea and semicircular canals **a media** middle ear, containing auditory ossicles .

auriscope (aw'ri-skop) otoscope

aurothioglucose (aw'ro-thi'o-glo'okos) a monovalent preparation of gold salt.

aurum (aw'rum) gold

auscultation (aws'kul-ta'shun) listening for sounds made by different structures of the body directly (by applying ear) or indirectly (through stethoscope).

aushadhalaya(s) dispensary

aushadhi(s) medicine

Austin Flint (aws'tin-flint) **murmur** a diastolic murmur at the apex in severe aortic regurgitation, named after Austin Flint, US physiologist

Australia antigen hepatitis B virus antigen first isolated from an Australian aborgine. It is found in hepatocyte cytoplasm

aut(o) combining word for self

autism (aw'tizm) a condition wherein the subjective, self-centred trends of thought dominate the person

autistic think. 1g thinking that gratifies unfulfilled desires. It has no regard for reality

autoagglutination (aw'to-a-gloo'ti-na'shun) clumping of an individual's cells by his own serum, as in auto-haemagglutination.

autoagglutinin (-a-gloo'ti-nin) an agglutinating autoantibody

autoamputation (-am'pu-ta'shun) the spontaneous separation from the body of an appendage or of an abnormal growth

autoantibody (-an'ti-bod'e) an antibody produced in response to and reacting against an endogenous body constituent

autoantigen (-an'ti-jen) a normal tissue constituent acting as an antigen, as in autoimmune disease

autoclasis (aw-tok'la-sis) destruction of a part from internal causes, as by autoimmune process

autoclave (aw'to-klav) an apparatus for effective sterilisation by steam under pressure

autocrine (-krin) a secretion of a cell which binds to the receptors and influence the function of cell type that produced it

autodigestion (aw'to-di-jes'chun) self-digestion; autolysis

autoeczematization (aw'to-ek-zem'a-ti-za'shun) spread of lesions from an initial focus of eczema

autoeponym a term applied for a condition affecting the author who described it and/or who died of the disease such as Carrion's disease, Jones fracture (a diaphyseal fracture of fifth metatarsal), Rickettsia (after Howard Ricketts), Thomsen's disease (after Julius Thomsen with an autosomal dominant myopathy)

autoerotism (-er'o-tizm) erotic behaviour directed toward oneself

autograft (aw'to-graft) a graft of tissue obtained from another site in or on the body of an individual receiving it; autologous graft

autohaemolysin (-he-mol'i-sin) an autoantibody that causes lysis of the erythrocytes in the same person

autohaemolysis (-he-mol'i-sis) haemolysis of blood cells of a person by his own serum

autohaemotherapy (-he'mo-ther'a-pe) reinjection of the individual's own blood.

autoimmune (-i-mun) directed against the body's own tissue

autoimmune lymphoproliferative syndrome a disorder due to a failure of lymphocytes to die once they have completed their activity. It results in splenomegaly and lymphadenopathy. The immune cells may attack the body's own tissues

autoimmunity (-i-mun'i-te) reaction of an organism's immune system to self-antigens and there is production of autoantibody. It is closely linked to connective tissue disease

autoimmunization (-im'u-ni-za'shun) induction of an immune response to its own tissue constituents

autoinoculation (-in-ok'u-la'shun) inoculation with micro-organisms from one's own body

autokeratoplasty (-ker'a-to-plas'te) corneal grafting with tissue from patient's other eye

autolesion (-le'shun) a self-inflicted injury

autologous (aw-tol'a-gus) related to self **a blood transfusion** collection and reinfusion of the patient's own blood **a bone marrow transfusion** a treatment modality for leukaemia patients, a cytopreserved bone marrow taken from the patient during remission is reinfused during relapse

autolysin (aw-tol'i-sin) an antibody that causes lysis of cells and tissues in the body of the person in whom it was formed

autolysis (aw-tol'i-sis) 1. destruction of cells as a result of the action of autolysin 2. enzymatic digestion of cells

automaticity (aw'to-ma-tisite) 1. the state of being spontaneous or involuntary 2. the capacity of a cell to initiate an impulse without an external stimulus

automatism (aw-tom'a-tizm) automatic performance of acts representative of unconscious symbolic activity

autonomic (aw'to-nom'ik) 1. functioning independently 2. referring to autonomic nervous system **a nervous system** the part of nervous system that controls involuntary body functions. It has two divisions as sympathetic or

thoracolumbar division and the parasympathetic or craniosacral division **a triad** dilated pupils, moist palms and tachycardia, noted in schizophrenics

autophagosome (-fag'o-sum) an intracytoplasmic vacuole with elements of a cell's own cytoplasm. It has capability to fuse with a lysosome

autophagy (aw-tof-a-je) lysosomal digestion of a cell's own cytoplasmic contents

autoplasty (aw'to-plas'te) repair of defects with tissues taken from another region of patient's body

autopsy (aw'top-se) the postmortem examination of a body; necropsy

autorad (aw'to-rad) autoradiograph similar to an X-ray picture. It is the final step in making a genetic fingerprint visible.

autoregulation (-reg'u-la'shun) 1. any biologic system equipped with inhibitory feedback system. 2. an intrinsic tendency of an organ or tissue to maintain a constant blood flow despite changes in the pressure in the artery

autosensitization (-sen'si-ti-za'shun) autoimmunisation

autosome (-som) non-sex chromosome

autosplenectomy (a.vt'o-sple-nek'to-me) disappearance of spleen by progressive fibrosis and shrinkage

autosuggestion (-sug-jes'chin) suggestion arising in one's self by constant dwelling of an idea or concept, a form of self hypnosis

autotransfusion (-trans-fu'zhun) transfusion back into the body of blood removed

autovaccine (aw'to-vak'sen) a vaccine prepared from cultures of organisms isolated from the patient's own tissues or secretions

auxocyte (awk'so-sit) an oocyte, spermatocyte in the early stage of development

AV atrioventricular; arteriovenous

avascular (a-vas'ku-ler) not vascular; without blood

AV bundle atrioventricular bundle

AV block atrioventricular block. Any delay in conduction or failure of an electrical impulse to reach the ventricular conduction system **first-degree AV b** a delay in conduction with prolonged PR interval and all the P waves are conducted to the ventricle **second-degree AV b** there are dropped beats as some impulses from atria fail to reach ventricle **third-degree AV b** no atrial beats are conducted to the ventricle

AV dissociation atrioventricular dissociation wherein there is independent depolarisation of the atria and ventricles. The rate of ventricular pacemaker is faster than that of the atrial pacemaker

Avellis' (av-el'ez) **syndrome** ipsilateral paralysis of vocal cord and soft palate, and loss of pain and temperature sense contralaterally due to lesion of nucleus ambiguus and spinothalamic tract, named after George Avellis, German laryngologist

aversion (a'vur-shun) a strong or intense dislike

avian (a've-in) pertaining to birds

avidity (a-vid'i-te) 1. a strong attachment to something 2. ability of antibodies to bind to antigen

avirulent (a-vir'u-lant) not virulent

AV node atrioventricular node

avoidance (a-void'ins) a conscious or unconscious defensive reaction to escape anxiety, danger, or conflict

avolition (a'voli-shun) an inability to initiate and persist in goal-directed activities

avulsion (a-vul'shun) a tearing away of a part of structure

avyakta(s) not manifest; hidden

a wave a positive 'a' wave in normal jugular venous pulse. It corresponds to presystole and is due to the right atrial contraction and precedes the carotid pulsation. The 'a' wave begins before the first heart sound. The wave is prominent in tricuspid stenosis, severe pulmonary stenosis, pulmonary hypertension and disappears in atrial fibrillation

axenic (a-zen'ik) sterile referring to pure culture

axialis (ak'se-a'lis) 1. axial, relating to an axis 2. relating to or situated in the central part of the body 3. relating to or parallel with the long axis of a tooth

axiation (ak'se-a'shun) the establishment of an axis or development of polarity in an ovum, embryo or organ

axilla (ak-sil'a) pl **axillae** the armpit

axillary: continuation of subclavian artery, main artery of the upper limb gives superior thoracic, acromiothoracic, lateral thoracic , subscapular and anterior posterior cicumflex and humeral branches

axiomatic (a'ksi-o-met'rik) self evident, needing no proof

axipetal (ak-sip'i-t'l) directed towards an axon or axis

axis (ak'sis) pl **axes** 1. the line passing through the centre of a body or about which a structure revolves 2. central line of the body 3. second cervical vertebra 4. an artery that divides immediately upon its origin

axo-axonic (ak'so-ak-son'ik) referring to the synaptic connection between the axon of one neuron and that of another

axodendritic (-den'drit'ik) referring to the synaptic relationship between an axon and a dendrite

axolemma (ak'so-lem'a) the surface membrane of an axon

axolysis (ak-sol'i-sis) degeneration and destruction of an axon of a nerve cell.

axon (ak'son) 1. the axis of the body 2. long outgoing process of nerve cell by which impulses travel away from a neuron 3. vertebral column

axoneme (ak'so-nem) central structure of the cilia and the sperm tails with a ring of 9 peripheral doublets around a pair of central microtubules (9 plus 2 pattern)

axonopathy (ak-so-nop'a-the) a disorder causing disruption of the normal function of axons

axonotmesis (ak'son-ot-me'sis) an incomplete division where the axons are divided and the nerve sheath is intact. It may occur from compression or traction injuries as in closed fractures and dislocations

axoplasm (-plasm) the cytoplasm of an axon

axotomy (ak-sot'a-me) transection of an axon

Ayerza's (a-yer'zhaz) **disease** pulmonary hypertension associated with sclerosis of pulmonary artery and polycythaemia vera and chronic cyanosis named after Abel Ayerza, Argentinian physician

ayu (s) life

Ayurveda the oldest existing medical system practised in India. It considers that disease is caused by an imbalance of homeostatic mechanisms related to three physiologic principles known as 'doshas' – *vata, pitta* and *kapha*. The therapeutic modalities consist of transcendental meditation, a healthy life style, herbal preparations and behaviour modification

ayushya (s) longevity

azathioprine (az'ah-thi'o-prin) a cytotoxic and immunosuppressive agent used in the treatment of leukaemia, auto immune diseases and organ transplantation

azidothymidine (az'i-do-thi'mi-den) AZT

azithromycin a macrolide antibiotic active against certain gram-negative organisms, including *H. influenzae*. Its serum half life is prolonged allowing once – daily administration

azlocillin (az'lo-sil'in) an acylureidopenicillin active against Pseudomonas infections

azo dyes a group of dyes produced from amino compounds by diazotization and coupling the reactants

azoospermia (a-zo'o-sper'me-a) 1. absence of spermatozoa in the semen. 2. failure of spermatogenesis

azotaemia high blood urea

azoto (az'ot) nitrogen

azoturia (az'o-tu're-a) an increased excretion of urea in the urine

AZT *see* zidovudine (azidothymidine)

aztreonam (az'tre-o-nam) a monocylic β-lactam antibiotic acting on gramnegative-aerobes such as *Ps. aeruginosa* and *Haemophilus influenzae*

azure (azh'er) basic blue methionine or phenothiazine dye used to stain blood cells and nuclei

azurophil (azh-u'ro-fil) red blood cells containing granules that stain readily with an azure dye **a granules** primary lysosomes appear as large, coarse non-specific blue-purple granules within myelocytes and neutrophils containing myeloperoxidase

azurophilia (azh'u-ro-fil'e-a) a condition in which blood contains cells having azurophilic granules

azygography (az'i-gog'ra-fe) radiography of the azgygos venous system following injection of contrast media

azygos (az'i-gos) an unpaired (single) anatomical structure

B

β beta, second letter of the Greek alphabet

B symbol for blood, bacillus, base

b symbol for base

Ba chemical symbol of barium

babbling quasi random vocalisations in infants that precede language acquisition.

Babcock's (bab'koks) operation extirpation of the saphanous vein to treat varicose veins, devised by William Babcock, US surgeon.

Babes-Ernst (ba'baz-ernst) granules metachromatic granules, named after Victor Babes, Rumanian bacteriologist and Paul Ernst, German pathologist

Babesia (ba-be'ze-a) a plasmodium-like organism, that infests red blood cells in animals, named after Victor Babes

babesiosis (ba-be-ze-o'sis) a tick-borne malaria-like disease caused by *Babesia microti*

Babinski's (ba-bin-skez) reflex dorsiflexion of the big toe at the metacarpophalangeal joint on stimulation of the sole of the foot due to the contraction of the extensor hallucis longus. It is accompanied by the extension and spread of the other toes like a fan indicating a lesion of the pyramidal tract, described by Joseph Babinski, French neurologist

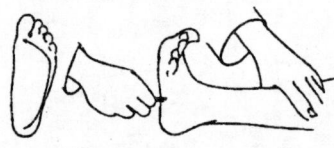

Babinski's reflex

baby an infant or young child battered b evidence of physical abuse of a baby in the form of bruises, scars, cuts, fractures or abdominal visceral injuries

blue b newborn child with cyanosis, due to a congenital anomaly that allows entry of blood from the right-to-the left side of the heart giving the infant a bluish complexion collodion b an infant born completely covered by a parchment like membrane

bacciform (bak'si-form) berry-shaped; coccal

Bachelor of Science in Nursing an academic degree awarded on completion of a 4-year course of study in a college of Nursing

Bachmann's bundle a branch of the anterior tract from SA node conducting impulses to the left atrium

Bacillaceae (bas'-i-la'se-e) a family of rod-shaped organisms that can produce endospores. They are gram-positive, commonly found in soil such as bacillus and clostridia

bacillary (bas'il-ar-e) pertaining to or caused by bacilli b dysentery *see* dysentery

bacillaemia (bas-i-leme-a) the presence of bacilli in the circulating blood

bacille (ba-sel) calmette-guerin attenuated strain of *Mycobacterium bovis* used in the preparation of BCG vaccine named after Albert Calmette and Camille Guerin, French bacteriologists

bacillin an antibiotic isolated from strains of *Bacillus subtilis*

bacillosis (bas'i-lo'sis) bacillary infection

bacilluria (bas-i-lu're-a) the presence of bacilli in the urine

bacillus (ba-sil'us) rod-shaped bacteria belonging to the family of Bacillaceae. They are aerobic, and gram-positive pl. bacilli acid fast b not readily discoloured by acids when stained B. *anthracis* a bacillus pathogenic to man causing anthrax B. *cereus* an aerobic spore-forming bacillus that may cause opportunistic infection in an immuno-compromised host. *B. subtilis* a laboratory contaminant, generally non-pathogenic, **Ducrey's b** *Haemophilus ducreyi* responsible for soft chancre or chancroid infection **Friedlander's b** *Klebsiella pneumoniae* causing necrotising pneumonia. **Hansen's b** *Mycobacterium leprae*, causative agent of leprosy **Koch-Weeks b** *Haemophilus aegyptius*, causative agent of infectious conjunctivitis. *B. melaninogenicus* a gram-negative non-spore forming organism responsible for lung abscess and Vincent's angina **tubercle b** *Mycobacterium tuberculosis*, causative agent of tuberculosis **typhoid b** *Salmonella typhi*, causative agent of typhoid fever

bacitracin (bas-i-tra'sin) an antibiotic produced by *Bacillus subtilis* and it is applied locally in infections from haemolytic streptococci and staphylococci

back 1. dorsum 2. posterior region of the trunk from neck to pelvis **b ache** pain in the back **b board** a stiff board placed on the stretcher or cot so that the patient's back is kept flat in spinal injuries **b bone** the vertebral column **b pain** any pain in the back **b rest** an adjustable device that gives support to the back in bed **b up** anything that served to replace a function or system that fails

back flow an abnormal backward flow of fluids; regurgitation

back-up (bak'up) a duplicate copy of a file, made in case of accidental loss or damage to the original document

backward failure cardiac failure from elevated filling pressure of the ventricles. It is seen in mitral or tricuspid stenosis which causes increased venous pressure with congestion

bacteraemia (bak-ter-e'me-a) the presence of bacteria in the blood

bacteria (bak-te're-a) any microorganism of the class schizomycetes

bacterial (bak-te're-al) pertaining to bacteria **b endocarditis** an acute or subacute bacterial infection of the endocardium or the heart valves or both **b inflammation** any inflammation occurring in response to a bacterial infection **b resistance** development of resistance to a drug by an organism previously susceptible to it **b toxin** any poisonous substance produced by a bacterium **b vaginosis** a chronic inflammation of vagina by *Gardnerella vaginalis*

bacterial artificial chromosome BAC a cloning vector used to propagate DNA in bacteria grown in culture

bactericidal (bak-ter-i-si'dal) destructive to or destroying bacteria

bactericide (bak-ter'i-sid) an agent destroying the bacteria

bacterid (bak'ter-id) a skin eruption caused by a bacteria or its toxin. The infection is at a remote place in the body

bacterio- (bak-te're-o) pertaining to bacteria

bacteriological index smears obtained from 4 skin lesions, from both ear lobes and from nose are stained for presence of acid fast bacilli. It is estimated as 0 (no bacilli in any field) 1+ (few bacilli in few fields), 2+ (few bacilli in all 100 fields), and 3+ (many bacilli found in all fields). For the scores of 7 sites are added and divided by 7. The score if less then 2 the case is paucibacillary leprosy and if 2 or more, it is multibacillary leprosy

bacteriologist (bak-te're-ol'o-jist) person concerned with the study of bacteria

bacteriology (bak-te're-o' lo-ge) the branch of science concerned with the study of bacteria

bacteriolysin (bak-te're-ol'i-sin) an antibacterial antibody, causing lysis of bacteria

bacteriolysis (bak-te're-ol'i-sis) the destruction or dissolution of bacteria

bacteriophage (bak-te're-o'fag) a virus with specific affinity for bacteria. Bacteriophages are widely distributed in nature

bacteriosis (bak-te're-o'-sis) any bacterial disease

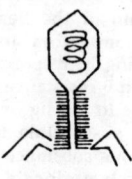

Bacteriophage

bacteriostasis (bak-te're-os'ta-sis) inhibition of growth or multiplication of bacteria

bacteriostatic (bak-te-re-o-stat'ik) an agent inhibiting the growth or multiplication of bacteria

bacteriotoxaemia (bak-te-re-o-tok'se-me-a) the presence of bacterial toxins in the blood

bacterium (bak-te're-um) pl. **bacteria** non-spore forming single-celled organisms that multiply by simple cell division. They may be spherical, rod-shaped or spirilliform. The spherical cocci and other bacilli are non-motile and spiral forms are motile

bacteriuria (bak-te're-u're-a) the presence of bacteria in the urine, which often indicates a urinary tract infection

bacteroid (bak'ter-oyd) resembling a bacterium

bacteroides (bak-ter-oyd'ez) anaerobic filamentous non-sporulating gram-negative bacteria found as normal flora in the oral cavity and colon, and as secondary invader in the necrotic tissue. *B. fragilis* is an important example of the genus

badge (baj) a distinguishing sign or mark **film b** a radiographic film worn on the body during potential exposure to radioactivity. It helps in quantifying the dosage of exposure

baffle a component of a nebuliser that helps in removal of large airborne particles

bag a sack or pouch **colostomy b** a water tight container that holds the discharge from a colostomy site **Douglas' b** the peritoneal space that lies behind uterus and in front of rectum, named after James Douglas, Scottish anatomist **b of waters** amnion.

bagasse (be-gas) the crushed fibres or the residue of sugarcane, a source of the thermophilic actinomycetes antigen.

bagassosis (bag-a-so'sis) occupational respiratory disorder caused by inhalation of sugarcane dust containing *Thermoactinomyces sacchari*, a fungus. It is characterised by fever, dyspnoea and malaise

bagging the artificial respiration performed with a respirator bag such as an Ambu bag. The bag is squeezed to deliver air to the patient's lungs as the mask is held over the mouth

bags loose infraorbital skin caused by inflammation and oedema, often associated with vasodilation, noted in lack of sleep and smoking

Baghdad sore oriental sore due to *Leishmania tropica*

Bainbridge's reflex a cardiac reflex consisting of an increased pulse rate that results from stimulation of stretch receptors in the wall of left atrium, described by Francis Bainbridge, English physiologist

Baker's cyst a cystic swelling arising from the synovial lining of the knee in the popliteal space and is associated with osteoarthritis of the knee, described by William Baker, British surgeon

BAL British anti-lewisite, dimercaprol, used as an antidote in poisoning from heavy metals.

Bala strength

Bal ahar a mixture of groundnuts, wheat, Bengal gram and jaggery

balance (bal'ans) 1. an instrument to measure weight, scale 2. a state of equilibrium 3. ability to maintain the centre of gravity **acid-base b** mechanism of maintenance of equilibrium so as to keep pH of arterial blood at 7.4 **fluid b** the balance between intake and output of fluids in the body **metabolic**

b intake and output of a specific nutrient. It may be negative when an excess of nutrient is excreted and positive when taken in an excess amount **nitrogen b** a state in which intake of nitrogen in protein foods is equal to loss of nitrogenous substances **water b** fluid balance

balanced diet a diet that contains carbohydrates, proteins, fats, minerals, vitamins and water in proper proportions and in quantity that is adequate for current needs as well as for the needs in future. It provides requisite energy, maintains health and vitality and provides roughage. It is palatable, pleasing in appearance and varied from day to day. It conforms to the local customs and habits

balanic (ba-lan'ik) pertaining to glans penis or glans clitoris

balanitis (bal-a-ni'tis) inflammation of the glans penis or glans clitoridis, associated with a purulent discharge

balano (bal'a-no) combining form pertaining to the glans penis or the glans clitoris

balanoblennorrhoea (bal'a-no-blen'o-re'a) an inflammation of the glans penis from gonococcal infection

balanochlamyditis (bal'a-no-klam'e-di'tis) an inflammation of glans clitoridis.

balanoplasty (bal'a-no-plas'te) plastic surgery of the glans penis

balanoposthitis (bal'a-no-pos-thi'tis) inflammation of the glans penis and overlying prepuce

balantidiasis (bal'an-ti-di'a-sis) infection of large intestine by protozoan parasites of the genus balantidium. It presents with abdominal pain, diarrhoea, vomiting and loss of weight and is treated with tetracyclines or metronidazole

balantidium (bal-an-tid'e-um) a ciliated protozoan parasite found in the large intestine. *B. coli* a species of balantidium, is the largest protozoan parasite causing balantidiasis

balanus (bal'a-nus) the glans penis or glans clitoridis

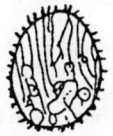

Balantidium coli

bala roga disease of children.

baldness (bawld'ness) lack of or loss of hair on head.

bald tongue complete atrophy of lingual papillae seen in anaemias and pellegra

Balkan frame strong, horizontal support that fits over a bed. The weights suspended from the frame through ropes and pulleys produce desired continuous traction while permitting freedom of motion. It helps in maintaining desired immobilisation of the part being treated.

ball (bawl) a spherical-shaped object **b of hair** mass of hair that has accumulated in the stomach or intestine; trichobezoar, **b of foot** the padded portion of the anterior region of the sole of the foot **b of thumb** thenar eminence of the thumb **b thrombus** a rounded blood clot **fungus b** a granulomatous mass due to colonisation of fungus such as Aspergillus in a body cavity; aspergilloma.

ball and socket joint a synovial joint in which one rounded bone head moves within the concavity of another bone, such as in hip and shoulder joints.

ballismus (ba-liz'mus) violent flinging movements of the proximal limb muscles seen in chorea

ballistic (ba'lis-tik) **stretching** a bouncing form of stretching in which a muscle group is lengthened repetitively to produce multiple quick, forceful stretches **trauma** injury secondary to bullets and blast

ballistocardiogram (ba-lis'to-kar'de-o-gram) the tracing from a ballistocardiograph.

ballistocardiograph (ba-lis'to-kar'de-o-gra-f) an instrument used to take ballistocardiogram.

ballistocardiography (ba-lis'to-kar'de-o-gra-fe) the graphic recording by ballistocardiograph of the bodily movements occurring due to cardiac contraction and ejection of the blood.

ball of the foot the part of the foot composed of the distal heads of the metatarsals and their surrounding fatty fibrous tissue pad.

balloon angioplasty a technique to reopen arteries narrowed by atheromatous plaques by inserting and inflating a balloon catheter inside the blood vessels.

balloon catheter a catheter with a balloon near its tip used to open a narrowed artery or instestine or to drain an obstructed organ such as urinary bladder

balloon cell any cell with abundant clear cytoplasm which includes carcinoid cells, ependymal cells and hepatocytes

ballooning biconcave compression of the end plate of the vertebral body by pressure arising in the intervertebral discs as in osteoporosis

balloon tamponade a haemostatic procedure for upper gastrointestinal bleeding using a Sengstaken-Blackemore tube

balloon valvuloplasty a method of using a balloon catheter to widen the stenotic cardiac valves

ballotment (bal-ot-mon') a palpatory method to toss an organ and feel, especially a floating organ such as kidney, or foetus.

ball thrombus a round coagulated mass of blood that may cause obstruction of a blood vessel or an orifice

ball-valve action action of a mass moving to open and close the passage of a tube or chamber. It causes intermittent obstruction

balm (bahm) a healing or soothing ointment

balsam (bawl'sam) a fragrant oily exu-date from herbs used in topical preparations

baltarism stuttering

Bamberger-Marie disease hypertrophic pulmonary osteoarthropathy, described by Eugene Bamberger, Austrian physician and Pierre Marie, French physician

bamboo spine roentgenogram of the spine exhibiting syndesmophytosis in ankylosing spondylitis that resembles the stalk of a bamboo

banana sign an ultrasonographic image where cerebellum gives a banana-like appearance as it is wrapped around the posterior brain stem, seen in foetal cranial abnormality from a neural tube defect

Bancroftiosis infection with *Wuchereria bancrofti*, named after Joseph Bancroft, British physician

band 1. a tape-like tissue that connects or holds structures together 2. an appliance that encircles the body or a limb **b keratopathy** a broad deposit of opaque calcium phosphate in vertical lines on Bowman's membrane, recognised by slit lamp examination noted in hyperparathyroidism

bandage a roll of gauze used to wrap any part of the body as a dressing **b lens** contact lens used as corneal dressing

band cell an immature neutrophil with nucleus lacking the segmentation.

band form a mature intraerythrocytic form of trophozoite of *Plasmodium malariae.*

bandicoot (ban'de-koot) an Indian rodent

Bang's bacillus *Brucella abortus*, isolated by a Danish physician, Bernhard Bang

bank a stored supply of body tissues or tissues for use of another person such as blood bank, eye bank, or tissue bank.

Bannister's (ban'eis-terz) **disease** angioneurotic oedema described by a Chicago physician, Henry Bannister

Banti's (ban'tez) **disease** congestive

splenomegaly with cirrhosis, described by Italian pathologist, Guido Banti

bar 1. a metal piece attaching two or more units of a removable dental prosthesis 2. a rigid component of a splint 3. a section of tissue connecting two similar structures 4. an unit of pressure, 10^5 pascal

baragnosis (bar-ag-no'sis) impaired ability to differentiate weights, and is indicative of parietal lobe lesion

Barany's (bah'ra-nez) **pointing test** making a patient to point at a fixed object with the eyes open and closed; in brain lesion the patient fails to point at the object with the eyes closed, described by an Austrian otologist, Robert Barany

barba beard

barber's chair sign electric-shock like radiation into arms on flexing neck seen in cervical cord lesions

barber's itch 1. an infection of hair follicles in the face by staphylococci, presenting with papules and pustules; folliculitis barbae 2. a dermatomycosis caused by a fungus - trichophyton, *Tinea barbae*

barbiturate (bar-bit'u-rat) a salt of barbituric acid that is depressant of the central nervous system. It is used as a sedative or hypnotic, named after Saint Barbara

barbotage (bar-bo-tozh) repeated injection and withdrawal of fluid, as in gastric lavage, or of CSF in spinal anaesthesia

bar diagram a diagramatic representation in which frequencies are represented by bars extending from the ordinate. It allows visualisation of the distribution of the entire sample at once

bare foot doctors countryside health aides

baresthesia (bar-es-the'ze-a) perception of weight or pressure

Bariatrician (bari-a'tri-shun) physician who specialises in the study and treatment of obesity

bariatrics (bar'e-a'triks) scientific study of obesity and its related disorders.

baritosis pneumoconiosis due to inhalation of barium dust

barium (ba're-um) a metallic alkaline earth element atomic No. 56 **b sulphate** a radiopaque barium compound used in roentgenography of the gastrointestinal tract **b enema** use of barium sulphate as an enema to enable x-ray and fluoroscopic examination of the colon **b meal** ingestion of barium sulphate to visualise the outline of the oesophagus, stomach and small intestine during roentgenologic examination of the upper gastrointestinal tract **b sandwich** a mixture of solid food and barium contrast used for evaluation of oesophageal deglutition by fluoroscopy **b swallow** roentgenologic examination of the oesophagus during and after ingestion of barium sulphate **double contrast b enema** a technique of barium enema x-ray study of the large bowel in which air is insufflated into the rectum and colon. It helps in demonstrating pathologic lesions of the large intestine better than an ordinary barium enema.

barium X-ray examination any of a group of imaging procedures that are used to diagnose diseases of gastrointestinal tract using barium sulphate as a contrast medium

barley a cereal

Barlow's (bar'loz) **disease** infantile scurvy, described by a British physician, Sir Thomas Barlow. The condition is noted in both breast-fed and bottle-fed babies who do not receive adequate supplement of vitamin C

Barlow's syndrome floppy (prolapsing, billowing) mitral valve

barognosis (bar-og-no'sis) perception of weight

baroreceptor (bar'o-re-sep'tor) a sensory nerve ending in the wall of the auricle of the heart, aortic arch, carotid sinus and vena cava sensitive to stretching of the wall from an increased pressure within

baroreflexes (bar'o-re'flek-ses) reflexes mediated or activated through barore-ceptors

barotitis (bar'o-ti'tis) acute vertigo due to otitis media or the passage of water into the middle ear at depths of from 5 to 20 m; inflammation of the middle ear due to sudden changes in baro-metric pressure as may occur while flying or diving

barosinusitis (bar'o-sinu-si'tis) sinus pain and later damage to the walls of paranasal sinuses that occur due to having ascended or descended to a different altitude

barotrauma (bar'o-traw'ma) injury to the eustachian tube and the tympanic membrane due to an imbalance be-tween ambient pressure and intratympanic pressures

Barr body sex chromatin mass found in the nuclei of the somatic cells of nor-mal females, described by Murray Barr, a Canadian anatomist. It repre-sents an inactivated X-chromosome.

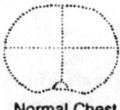

Normal Chest

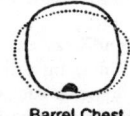

Barrel Chest

barrel chest overinflated chest. The anteroposterior diameter of the chest is increased. The ribs are horizontal. The sternum is prominently arched. The chest appears circular on cross section, noted in chronic airflow obstruction and in thoracic kyphosis

barren sterile; incapable of producing off-spring

Barrett's oesophague occurrence of co-lumnar epithelium lining of a segment of oesophagus occasionally accompa-nied by peptic ulceration. The patient has an increased risk of development of adenocarcinoma, named after Nor-man Barrett, British surgeon

barrier an impediment **b cream** applica-tion of cream to prevent the chemical coming into direct skin contact **b method** contraceptives such as condom or diaphragm that prevent meeting of sperm and ova **b precautions** any method or device used to reduce the contact with potentialty infectious body fluids such as face masks, gloves or gowns

Bar's (bahrz) **incision** an incision for caesarian section made in the middle of the abdomen, described by a French obstetrician, Paul Bar

Bartholin's (bar'to-linz) **duct** duct drain-ing the sublingual gland, described by Casper Bartholin, a Danish anato-mist

Bartholin's glands a pair of pea-sized vulvovaginal glands that secrete a fluid that lubricates the vagina during sexual arousal. These glands are felt on pal-pating the posterior part of the labia majora between the finger and thumbs

Bartholinitis (bar'to-lin-i'tis) inflammation of Bartholin's glands

bartonella (bar'to-nel'a) a rickettsia found in man and in arthropod vectors, described by a Peruvian physician, Alberto Borton

bartonellosis (bar'to-nel-o'sis) a disease caused by bartonella and transmitted by the bite of sandfly. It presents with fever, haemolytic anaemia and multi-ple eruptions on the skin and mucous membranes and responds to antibiot-ics such as chloramphenicol.

Bartter's syndrome hyperplasia of juxtaglomerular cells of the kidney as-sociated with hypokalaemic alkalosis and hyperaldosteronism without hy-pertension, named after Frederic Bartter, US physician.

baruria (ba-roo're-a) the passage of urine of a high specific gravity.

baryglossia (bar-i-glos'e-a) thick slow speech

barylalia (bar-i-la'le-a) thick indistinct speech, due to imperfect articulation.

basal (ba'sal) 1. pertaining to the base 2. of primary importance **b acid output** production of gastric H+ under baseline conditions **b body temperature** temperature of the body at absolute rest **b cell** deepest layer of epidermis, stratum germinativum. **b deficit** measure of acidosis, base needed to bring blood pH to 7.4 **b excess** measure of alkalosis, acid needed to bring blood pH to 7.4 **b energy expenditure** the amount of oxygen consumed while resting and fasting, which equals to 25 Kcal/kg **b ganglia** part of extrapyramidal system containing corpus striatum (caudate and lentiform nuclei) amygdaloid nuclei and the putamen **b lamina** a thin non-cellular layer of ground substance lying just under epithelial surfaces **b metabolic rate** (BMR) the metabolic rate as measured under basal conditions, expressed as kilocalories per square metre of body surface per hour **b metabolism** the amount of energy required when the person is at rest to maintain vital body functions.

base 1. the supporting structure 2. the principal substance in a mixture 3. any substance that combines with hydrogen ions 4. one component of nucleic acids. **denture b** artificial teeth, which rest on abutment teeth of the residual alveolar ridge **b pair** a pair of linked nucleotide bases that forms a single 'rung' in the ladder-like structure of DNA **b triplet** a group of three nucleotide bases found in DNA and RNA and it codes specific amino acid production.

baseball finger *see* mallet finger

Basedow's (baz'e-doz) **disease** exophthalmic goitre, described by Karl von Basedow, German physician

baseline (bas'lin) an initial value with which the subsequent measurement can be compared

Basel Nomina Anatomica BNA an international system of anatomic terminology adopted at Basel, Switzerland

basement membrane a structure involved in cell growth, adhesion and differentiation, consists of a multi-molecular layer composed of collagen glycoprotein, fibronectin and proteoglycans and is subjacent to epithelium and endothelium

Base pair two bases which form a 'rung of the DNA ladder'. A DNA nucleotide is made of a molecule of sugar, a molecule of phosphoric acid and a molecule of base. The bases are the 'letters' that spell out the genetic code. In base pairing, adenine always pairs with thymine, and guanine with cytosine

baseplate (bas'plat) a temporary preformed shape made of wax, acrylic resin or metal that makes the base of a denture.

basic life support cardiopulmonary resuscitation.

basilar (bas'i-lar) pertaining to a basal part **b artery** the single posterior arterial trunk formed by union of two vertebral arteries at the base of the skull **b impression** upward displacement of the basal part of the occipital bone constricting posterior fossa structures **b membrane** cellular structure giving a base for spiral organ of Corti

basilic (ba-sil'ik) important; prominent **b vein** *see* table of veins

basiloma (bas-i-lo'ma) basal cell carcinoma.

basin an open, bowl-like container for holding liquids

basion (ba'se-on) mid-point of the anterior border of the foramen magnum

basket cell a cell of the cerebellar cortex whose axons enclose the Purkinje cells in a basket-like fashion

basophil (ba'so-fil) 1. a granular leucocyte that stains with basic dyes that may have a role in some allergic reaction, and constitutes 0.5% to 1%

of leucocytes 2. a type of cell found in the anterior lobe of the pituitary that produces corticotropin

basophilia (ba-so-fil'e-a) an abnormal increase in the number of basophils in the blood or in an organ

basophilic (ba-so-fil'ik) pertaining to the staining characteristics of various cells **b adenoma** pituitary tumour composed of cells that can be stained with basic dyes **b stippling** punctate stippling of erythrocytes which appear as 'blue' dots in Wright-Giemsa stain as in lead poisoning

Bateman's (bat'manz) **disease** molluscum contagiosa, described by an English physician, Thomas Bateman

Bateman's purpura capillary fragility in Cushing's syndrome or after prolonged corticosteroid therapy

bath the medium and method of cleansing the body or any part of it, or treating it with air, light, vapour or water

bathyanaesthesia (bath-e-an'es-the'ze-a) loss of deep sensibility

bathyesthesia (bath'e-es-the'ze-a) deep sensibility

bathypnoea (bath'e-p-nea) deep breathing

bat wing distribution shaggy, bilateral perihilar lung opacity on a PA view chest film seen in pulmonary oedema and pulmonary alveolar proteinosis

battered woman syndrome repeated episodes of physical assault of a woman by husband or partner

battery 1. a device to generate electricity 2. a series of tests performed on a patient, to determine the cause of a particular illness

Battle's sign in fracture of the posterior cranial fossa, blood accumulates beneath the deep fascia, producing discolouration near the tip of the mastoid process, named after William Battle, British surgeon

Battey (bat'e) **bacillus** a mycobacteria recognised at Battey, tuberculosis hospital in Rome, Georgia, US.

Baudelocque's (bod-loks) **method** manipulation to convert a foetal face presentation into a vertex presentation, named after Jean Baudelocque, French obstetrician

Bayes' theorem a formula for the probability of disease in the presence of a positive test result, named after Thomas Bayes, an English clergyman

Bazette's formula ECG QT interval denotes the total electromechanical systole. It varies inversely with the heart rate, and it is of use if expressed in relation to the heart rate and is expressed as QTc (corrected QT interval), which is obtained by the formula

$$\frac{QT \text{ (milliseconds)}}{R - R \text{ interval (milliseconds)}}$$

Bazin's (ba-zaz') **disease** erythema induratum described by a French dermatologist, Antoine Bazin

BBB abbreviation for bundle branch block; blood brain barrier.

B-cell bursa associated lymphocyte present in the blood, lymph and connective tissue that produces antibodies to fight infection

BCG Bacille Calmette Guerin **BCG vaccine** a freeze-dried vaccine of a live, attenuated strain of Mycobacterium bovis used in children for immunisation against tuberculosis.

BCNU Carmustine

beaked pelvis forward projection of symphysis due to inward pressure of femoral heads in osteomalacia

beam alignment alignment of radiographic tube head properly with X-ray film.

beam collimation restriction of X-radiation only to the area being examined

beam quality energy of the X-ray beam.

bearing down the explusive effort of parturient woman in second stage of labour

beat a pulsation as in contraction of the heart or the passage of blood through an artery **apex b** the lowest and outermost point of pulsation of cardia. It is produced by the contraction of left ventricle, and left ventricular and septal forces. It is well circumscribed, visible and palpable 9 cm from mid-sternal line in the left fifth intercostal space **dropped b** absence of a ventricular contraction of the heart **ectopic b** a heart beat beginning at a place other than SA node **premature b** a heart beat that arises from a site other than SA node and occurs early in the cardiac cycle before the expected sinus beat

beaten silver appearance radiologic appearance of the skull in raised intracranial tension with premature closure of the cranial sutures. There is variably sized rounded zones of bony attenuation of the skull bones caused by pressure from cerebral cortical gyri

Beau's (boz) **lines** transverse ridging noted on the finger nails as a sign of systemic disease, described by a French physician, Joseph Beau

Becker's muscular dystrophy a genetic disorder with muscular dystrophy starting later in childhood and progressing more slowly

Beck's (beks) **triad** a symptom complex of cardiac tamponade consisting of high venous pressure, low arterial pressure and a small quiet heart, described by Claude Beck, US physician

beclomethasone dipropionate a glucocorticoid used in an inhaler in the treatment of bronchial asthma.

bed 1. a couch that supports during sleep 2. a supporting structure or tissue

bed bug a blood sucking arthropod and it elicits pruritus

bed occupancy a 24-hour patient occupancy in a hospital inpatient services

bedpan a pan-shaped container placed under a bedridden patient for collecting faecal material and urine

bedrest confining a patient to bed for rest

bedsore decubitus ulcer, pressure sore; ischaemic necrosis and ulceration of tissue especially over a bony prominence

bed wetting enuresis

bee a inset of the order Hymenoptera, such as honey bee **b sting** injury caused by bee venom. It is associated with pain, redness and swelling

beef tape worm *Taenia saginata*

beeturia purplish hue of urine following eating beetroot

Beevor's (be'vorz) **sign** paralysis of lower part of rectus abdominis muscle. There is upward movement of the umbilicus, named after Charles Beevor, British neurologist

behaviour 1. the manner in which one acts 2. any response elicited from an organism **b disorder** any antisocial behaviour patterns occurring in children and adolescents **b modification** behavioural therapy designed to change the learned behaviour of an individual **b therapy** treatment of psychoneurosis by attempts to modify behaviour.

Behcet's (be'sets) **disease** diffuse vasculitis causing orogenital lesions and uveitis in young males, described by a Turkish dermatologist, Hulusi Behcet

bejel (bej'l) a non-venereal form of syphilis affecting children, caused by a strain of *Treponema pallidum*

Bel a unit of measurement of the intensity of sound and is expressed as a logarithm of the ratio of two sounds of acoustic intensity and is expressed in decibels

belching eructation

Bell's nerve nerve to serratus anterior, named after Sir Charles Bell, Scottish surgeon

Bells' palsy lower motor neuron facial paralysis which is associated with immobility of one half of the face

Bell's phenomenon palpebro-oculogyric reflex. Normally the eyeballs roll up reflexly while attempting to close the eyes. This is exaggerated in lower motor neuron facial palsy. The whole cornea goes under the upper eyelid

belladonna (bel'a-don'a) deadly nightshade, a herb *Atropa balladonna,* whose leaves and root contain atropine and related alkaloids (stramonium, hyoscyamus and scopalamine). Anticholinergic used as a sedative and spasmolytic.

Bellini's (be-le'nez) **tubule** the terminal excretory ducts of the kidney, formed by fusion of numerous collecting tubules, named after Lorenzo Bellini, Italian anatomist

belly 1. the abdomen or abdominal cavity 2. the fleshy central part of a muscle **b button** umbilicus **b tap** abdominal tap

belt any broad geographical region with an increased incidence of a particular disease process

Bence Jones protein thermosensitive urinary protein in multiple myeloma, described by an English physician, Henry Bence Jones. A precipitate forms when urine is heated to $50°$ to $60°C$ and it disappears on further heating. It reappears on cooling

bench a long worktable.

bend a flexure or curve

bendroflumethiazide (ben'dro-floo'meti'azid) a thiazide diuretic

bends pain in the limbs and abdomen noted following rapid reduction of air pressure. It is caused by bubbles of nitrogen in blood and tissues

Benedict's test a test to demonstrate presence of sugar in the urine, described by American chemist, Stanley Benedict. 5 ml of fresh Benedict's copper sulphate- based reagent is taken in a test tube and boiled. 8 drops of urine added to it by a dropper. Then it is heated to vigorous boiling and allowed to cool. The presence of reducing substance is revealed by the appearance of a precipitate varying from light green turbidity to a red precipitate. If the reduction is due to glucose the amount

is assessed as 0.5, 1.0, 1.5 and 2% when it shows light green turbidity, green, yellow and red precipitate respectively

Benedikt's syndrome a syndrome of ipsilateral hemiplegia with oculomotor palsy and contralateral tremors due to involvement of the third nerve and red nucleus, described by Moritz Benedikt, an Austrian physician

benign (be-nin) non-malignant, mild **b lymphadenopathy** any non-malignant regional or generalised enlargement of lymph nodes **b prostatic hypertrophy** a non-malignant enlargement of the prostate due to excessive growth of prostate tissue, presents in elderly males as nocturia, difficulty in initiating urination and diminished force of urinary stream **b tumour** a growth that does not spread to other parts of the body. However it can grow to a large size

Bennett's fracture a fracture through the base of the first metacarpal bone and into the carpometacarpal joint, named after Edward Bennett, Irish surgeon

bent inclination, tendency, propensity

bentonite (ben'ton-it) a hydrated aluminium silicate

benzene (ben'zen) an aromatic hydrocarbon. It is a volatile liquid that is immiscible with water and it dissolves fats. It is used as a solvent

benzathine penicillin long acting penicillin.

benzidine (ben'zi-din) a substance used in detecting presence of blood in faeces.

benzocaine (ben'zo-kan) a local anaesthetic derived from aminobenzoic acid

benzodiazepine (ben'zo-di-az'e-pen) a psychotropic drug possessing hypnotic and sedative action

benzoic acid a white crystalline material used in keratolytic ointments and in food preservation

benzoin (ben'zoyn) a resin from trees *Syrax benzoin* used as a stimulant expectorant and as a protective coating for ulcers

benzpyrene a carcinogenic polycyclic hydrocarbon

benzyl benzoate a colourless liquid used as a topical scabicide

bephenium anthelminthic, especially active against hookworms.

benzyl penicillin penicillin G. bactericidal antibiotic that is rapidly absorbed following intramuscular injection

bereavement reaction of grief and sadness upon learning of the death of loved one

Berger's disease idiopathic, focal glomerulonephritis with mesangial deposits of IgA

Beri-beri (ber'e-ber'e) a disease caused by a deficiency of thiamine in diet, derived from a sinhalese word. There is failure of metabolism of glucose aerobically and there is accumulation of pyruvic and lactic acid **dry b** a peripheral polyneuropathy presenting with parasthesia, cramps and impaired sensation **wet b** a high output cardiac failure

Berkefeld (ber'ke-feld) **filter** a filter that allows passage of virus-sized particles, named after Wilhelm Berkefeld, German manufacturer

Bernard-Souller Syndrome an autosomal recessive disease with decreased number of platelets, prolonged bleeding time and qualitatively large platelets in circulation

Bernoulli effect the sum of the velocity and the kinetic energy of a fluid flowing through a tube, is constant. The greater the velocity, the lesser the lateral pressure on the wall of the tube, named after Daniel Bernoulli, Swiss mathematician

berry small sack-like swelling **b aneurysm** a small saccular dilatation of arteries at the base of the brain at or adjacent to circle of Willis or rarely at the vertebrobasilar arteries. They rupture when their diameter exceeds 1 cm and cause subarachnoid haemorrhage

Berry's sign enlarged thyroid gland displaces the carotid artery backwards and outwards. In large goitre the pulsation of carotid artery is felt behind the posterior edge of the swelling and displaced artery is much less in evidence in thyroid malignancy as it tends to be surrounded by the tumour, described by Sir James Berry, British surgeon

berylliosis (ber'il-le-o'sis) beryllium poisoning. Acute inhalation causes a generalised acute inflammatory reaction in the respiratory tract and alveoli. Chronic disease, following inhalation in a low dose over a long time causes progressively increasing dyspnoea and fatigue

beryllium (be-ril'e-um) a metallic element used in aircraft industries, atomic reactors, manufacture of X-ray tubes and heat resistant ceramics

bestiality (bes-te-al'i-te) 1. sexual relation with an animal 2. a brutal character

beta (be'ta) second letter of Greek alphabet: β-**adrenergic agent** a drug that stimulates β (sympathetic) receptors β-**adrenergic blocking agent** an agent that blocks sympathetic inhibitory stimuli, and useful in treatment of hypertension, angina and cardiac arrhythmis β-**adrenergic receptors** adenergic receptors present in various organs responsible for a variety of physiologic responses that may be stimulatory or inhibitory. β_1 receptors exhibit an equal affinity to catecholamines β_2 receptors exhibit greater affinity to epinephrine. They are present in smooth muscle of bronchi and their stimulation results in bronchodilatation. Similar receptors are found in the blood vessels, skeletal muscle and liver and their stimulation results in relaxation of vascular smooth muscle, tremors of skeletal muscle and stimulation of glycolysis respectively β **carotene** a carotenoid precursor of vitamin A, found in fresh vegetables and fruits β **cells** 1. basophilic cells in the anterior lobe of pituitary 2. insulin secreting cells of the islets of Langerhans of pancreas. β **haemolysis**

development of a clear zone around a bacterial colony growing on a blood agar medium. β **haemolytic streptococci** the pyogenic streptococci that cause haemolysis of red blood cells in blood agar β-**lactamase resistance** the ability of certain microorganisms that produce the enzyme β-lactamase (penicillinase) resisting the action of certain types of antibiotics including some forms of penicillin. β **wave** one of the four types of brain waves and it is characterised by relatively low voltage. These waves are recorded by EEG from the frontal and the central area of cerebrum when the patient is awake and alert with eyes open

betamethasone (be'ta-meth'a-son) a synthetic glucocorticoid used as a topical anti-inflammatory agent

betelnut chewing 'chew' composed of ground areca nut, lime, ground spices wrapped in a betel leaf. Tobacco may also be added to the chew, associated with high incidence of oral cancer

Betz's (bet'zes) **cells** large pyramidal cells in the motor area of the cerebral cortex described by Vladimir Betz, a Russian anatomist

bevel (bev'el) 1. a slanting edge 2. dent to produce a slanting surface in the margin of enamel of a cavity preparation.

bezoar (be'zor) a ball of entangled material formed in the stomach and intestine, such as a hair ball (trichobezoar), ball of hair and vegetable fibre (trichophytobezoar) or food ball (phytobezoar)

Bezold's mastoiditis mastoid process grows slowly after birth until puberty. If it is infected at that time the pus penetrating the bone forms an abscess in the neck beneath the mastoid process, named after Friederich Bezold, otologist in Munich

bhang less active form of marihuana

bhaya(s) fear

Bl:edana (s)cathartic

Bhishak(s) physician

Bhopal gas tragedy acute air pollution on 3rd December 1984 by methyl isocyanate (MIC), an intermediate chemical in the manufacture of pesticides at Bhopal, Madhya Pradesh, India killing 2,500 people

Bhutgragha (s) mental illness

bias (bi'us) 1. any systemic error in the determination of the association between the exposure and disease. Some of the important bias in epidemiologic studies are due to confounding, recall, selection, or may be ascribed to interviewer or due to different rates of admission to hospital for people with different diseases. 2. the systematic deviation of an estimate from the true value

bibasic (bi-ba'sik) pertaining to an acid with two hydrogen atoms that can be replaced by bases to form salts

bibliomania (bib'le-o-ma'ne-a) an intense desire to collect books

bibliotherapy (bib'le-o-ther'a-pe) inducing a patient with mental illness to read books

bicameral (bi-kam'er-al) having two chambers

bicarbonate (bi-kar'bo-nat) any salt containing the HCO_3^- (bicarbonate) anion

biceps (bi'seps) a muscle having two heads **b brachii** muscle of the upper arm with two heads. It flexes the arm and forearm and supinates hand **b femoris** one of the hamstring muscles lying posterolaterally in the thigh. It flexes knee and rotates it outwards **b reflex** contraction of biceps muscles on percussing its tendon.

bicipital (bi-sip'a-tal) 1. having two heads 2. pertains to a biceps muscle **b groove** a groove between the greater and lesser tubercles of the humerus for the passage of biceps tendon.

biconcave (bi 'kon' kav) concave on each side

bicornuate (bi-kor'nu-at) having two horns, especially of uterus with body partly divided into two.

biconvex (bi kon'veks) convex on each side.

bicuspid (bi-cus'pid) having two cusps **b tooth** a premolar tooth having two cusps on the grinding surface and a flattened root. There are two premolars on either side of jaw between the canines and molars **b valve** mitral valve between the left atrium and left ventricle of the heart

b.i.d. *bis in die* twice a day

bidet (be-da) a basin used for cleaning perineum

biennial (bai'en-ial) occurring every two years

bifid (bifid) divide into two parts **b spine** congenital fissure of vertebral column **b tongue** tongue divided by a longitudinal furrow

bifocal (bi-fo'kal) lens having two parts with different focusing powers

bifurcation (bi-fur-ka'shun) the site at which a single structure separates into two branches

bigeminal (bi-jem'-nal) occurring in twos, double **b pulse** two coming in couples where second beat is weaker. It is due to premature contraction and is followed by a pause. It is noted in partial heart block and digitalis toxicity

bigeminy (bi-jem'i-ne) occurring in pairs. adj. **bigeminal atrial b** an arrhythmia consisting of repetitive sequence of one atrial premature complex followed by a narrow sinus impulse **ventricular b** an arrhythmia consisting of repeated sequence of one ventricular premature complex followed by a normal beat.

biguanides hypoglycaemic agent

bijou bottle small, capacity screw-top culture bottle

bilateral (bi-lat'er-al) 1. having two sides 2. appearing on two sides

bilayer a two-component layer

bile (bil) gall, secretion of the liver consisting bile salts, bilirubin, cholesterol, phospholipid and electrolytes, which aid in the emulsification of fats **b acids** acids such as cholic, glycocholic and taurocholic acids which occur as salts in bile. They help in digestion of fats **cystic b** bile stored in gall bladder **b ducts** intercellular passages that convey bile from the liver to the hepatic duct which joins the duct from gall bladder (cystic duct) to form common bile duct that opens into the duodenum **hepatic b** bile secreted by the liver cells **b pigments** highly coloured substances such as bilirubin and biliverdin found in bile that are derived from haemoglobin. They impart brown colour to the stools **b salts** alkali salts of bile such as sodium glycocholate and sodium taurocholate **lithogenic b** bile supersaturated with cholesterol

Bilharzia (bil-har'ze-a) blood fluke, Schistosoma, described by Theodor Bilharz, a German physician

Bilharziasis (bil'har-zi'a-sis) schistosomiasis

biliary (bil'e-ar-e) relating to the bile, or bile duct or gall bladder **b atresia** a birth defect in which the bile ducts fail to develop or under-developed. **b calculus** gall stone **b cirrhosis** a form of cirrhosis of the liver resulting from destruction of intrahepatic bile ducts (primary) or secondary to prolonged obstruction **b colic** severe pain in upper right abdomen caused by passing of gall stones by gall bladder's attempt to expel gall stones **b sludge** bile in a gel form that contains numerous crystals of calcium bilirubinate granules, cholesterol crystals and glycoproteins and essential precursor to the formation of gall stones **b tract** the organs and ducts in which the bile is formed, concentrated and carried from the liver to the duodenum

bilin (bil'i-n) yellow bile pigment.

bilious (bil'yus) 1. relating to bile 2. a disorder affecting the bile

biliousness (bil'yus-nes) a disorder of the liver characterised by nausea, abdominal discomfort and constipation

bilirubin (bil-l-roo'bin) an orange-yellow

bile pigment formed as a degradation product of haemoglobin **conjugated b** bilirubin that has been taken up by the liver cells and conjugated to form the water-soluble form of bilirubin **unconjugated b** the lipid soluble form of bilirubin that is circulated in loose combination with plasma proteins

bilirubinaemia (bil'i-roo-bin-e'me-a) the presence of bilirubin in excess amounts in the blood

bilirubinuria (bil'i-roo-bin-u're-a) presence of bilirubin in excess amounts in the urine

biliverdin (bil-i-ver'din) a green pigment produced by catabolism of haemoglobin which later gets reduced to bilirubin

billiard ball testis in tertiary interstitial orchitis due to syphilis the testicle is round, densely hard, completely insensitive and freely moveable in its scrotal coverings

Billroth's operation partial gastrectomy for peptic ulcer initiated by Theodore Billroth, an Austrian surgeon **Billroth I** excision of pylorus of the stomach with anastomosis of the upper part of the stomach to the duodenum **Billroth II** subtotal excision of the stomach with closure of the proximal end of the duodenum and side-to-side anastomosis of the jejunum to the remaining part of the stomach

bimanual (bi-man'u-al) performed by both hands **b compression** a technique used to make uterus to contract after childbirth to control bleeding **b palpation** a technique to palpate kidney mass that is sandwiched between two hands

bimodal (bi-mo'dal) having two peaks, of frequency distribution

binary (bi-nar-e) two equal parts or branches **b fission** direct division of a cell or nucleus into two equal parts

binasal hemianopia loss of vision from the nasal half of each visual field

binaural (bin-aw'ral) pertaining to both ears

bind to fasten, wrap or encircle with a bandage

binder (bind'er) 1. a broad bandage 2. an inert substance that holds a mixture of solid particles together

bindu(s) drop

binge - purge syndrome bouts of over eating followed by self induced vomiting or purging with laxatives

Binet age determination of the mental age of a child by Binet-Simon tests, named after Alfred Binet, and Theodore Simon French psychologists

binocular (bin-ok'u-lar) pertaining to both eyes

binomial (bi-no'me-al) 1. an equation containing two variables 2. composed of two terms such as a combination of genus and species name

binovular developing from two distinct ova.

Binswanger's disease rare cause of vascular dementia from diffuse or multifocal white matter degeneration

bio-combining word for, relating to life

bioassay (bi'o-as'a) determination of the effectiveness of a specific sample of a drug on a live animal or an isolated organ preparation

bioavailability (bi'o-a-val'a-bil'i-te) the degree to which a drug is available to act on the target organ. It is affected by the route of administration, rate of metabolism, lipid solubility and binding proteins

biochemical (bi-o-kem'i-kal) relating to biochemistry **b marker** any biochemical substance such as antigen, antibody, enzyme or hormone that is altered by disease process acting as an aid to diagnose a disease

biochemistry the science dealing with living organisms and of chemical changes occurring in them

biochips (bi-o'chips) computer-chip-like devices that contain miniature DNA sequencing and analysis components, making it possible to run several genetic tests at one time in a very small space and to provide genetic analysis quickly and cheaply

biocompatibility (bi'o-kom-pat'i-bil'it-e) the quality of not exhibiting any toxic effects on biologic systems adj. **biocompatible**

biodegradable susceptible to degradation by biologic processes.

bioequivalence (bi'o-i-kwiv'a-lens) the property of possessing the same biologic effects of that to which a medicine is compared adj **bioequivalent**

biofeedback a learning technique wherein a desired response is learnt on the basis of the information received from the eyes or ears on the status of an autonomic body function

biogenesis (bi'o-jen'e-sis) origin of life from a pre-existing life

biogenic (bi-o-jen'ik) produced by living organisms

biohazard anything that is harmful to humans and environment

biokinesthesiology (bi'o-kinis-thio'loji) a system of body energetics which uses muscle testing as a means of understanding an individual's inner state

biological 1. pertaining to biology 2. a medical compound such as serum, vaccine, antitoxin prepared from living organisms and their products **b clock** circadian rhythm. **b response modifiers** molecules that modulate the immune response **b warfare** use of infectious agents as a weapon of war **b toxin** poison produced by microorganisms during the course of an infectious disease

biologist a specialist in biology

biology (bi-ol'o-je) the science of life and living things **molecular b** branch of biology dealing with analysis of the structure and development of biological systems

biomass (bi'o-mas) the total body weight of all living things in a given area

biomechanics (bi'o-me-kan'iks) the action of forces on the living body

biomicroscopy (bi'o-mi'kro-sko-pe) microscopic examination of living tissue in the body.

biomedical application of the natural sciences to the study of medical science

biometrics (bi'o-met'riks) a statistical science applied to the study of biological phenomenon

biometry (bi-om'e-tre) application of statistical methods to biologic facts

bionics (bi-on'iks) bioelectronics

biopharmaceutics the study of the physical and chemical properties of a drug and its dose

biophilia (b'o-fili'a) passionate love of life

biophysics (bi'o-fiz'iks) the study of physical processes occurring in organisms

biopsy (bi-op-se) removal of a piece of tissue from the body and examining it microscopically after staining, for purpose of diagnosis **aspiration b** removal of tissue by a needle and syringe **brush b** removal of a tissue by brushing **needle b** removal of tissues by a needle attached to a syringe **percutaneous transthoracic needle aspiration b** using a fluoroscopically guided aspiration needle to obtain a sample of a tissue from a pulmonary lesion. **punch b** removal of a small bit of tissue by a hollow punch. **sternal b** biopsy of bone marrow of the sternum either by puncture or trephine

biorhythm (bi'o-rith'um) a biologically inherent cyclic variation of an event or state

bioscience (bi'o-si'ens) life science

biosis (bi'os-is) combining form indicating mode of life

biosphere (bi'o-sfer) part of the universe wherein the living organisms are known to exist

biostatistics (bi'o-sta-'tis'tiks) vital statistics; application of statistical methods to analyse biologic data

biosynthesis (bi'o-sin'the-sis) formation of a chemical compound by living organisms

biosystem a living organism that interacts with others

biotechnology genetic engineering

biotelemetry (bi'o-tel-em'e-tre) monitoring of vital processes of a person and transmission of the data to a remote place without wires

biotics (bi-ot'iks) the science pertaining to life

biotin (bi'o-tin) a member of B complex involved in carboxylase reactions and is essential for the metabolism of fat and carbohydrates. Liver, kidney, milk, egg yolk and yeast are rich in biotin. Biotin deficiency causes scaly dermatitis, muscle pain and anorexia

biotoxin (bi-o-tok'sin) any toxic substance formed in a living body

biotransformation conversion of a substance within an organism

Biot's (be-oz) **breathing** an irregular respiration that can become slow or rapid, shallow or deep with irregular pauses, found in meningitis, named after Camille Biot, French physician

biotype (bi'o-tip) a group of persons with same genotype

bipartite (bi-par'tit) having two parts

biped (bi'ped) an animal with feet

biphasic (bi-faz'ik) consisting of two phases

bipolar (bi-po'lar) having two poles **b affective disorder** a disorder wherein the patient exhibits both maniac and depressive episodes **b cells** primitive cells found in the bone marrow that are yet to terminally differentiate and are capable of giving rise to erythroid and megakaryotic daughter cells **b traits** personality traits that represent extreme opposites of expression

bird handler's disease a hypersensitivity pneumoritis caused by an allergic reaction to a protein in bird droppings

birefringence (bi're-frin'jens) the splitting of a ray of light into two

birth the act of being born; passage of a child from uterus **b canal** the canal through which foetus passes in birth and it comprises the cervix, vagina and vulva **b certificate** a legal record of the birth of a child **b control** prevention of conception or implantation of fertilised ovum or termination of

pregnancy **b control pill** oral contraceptive containing synthetic oestrogen and progesterone or synthetic progesterone alone **b defect** a congenital anomaly **b injury** an injury sustained by the neonate during the birth process **b mark** naevus, mole **b rate** the number of live births per 1000 estimated mid-year population in a given year **b weight** weight recorded within the first hour of life, and is considered as the single most important determinant of its chances of survival, healthy growth and development. It should be at least 2.5 kg **high b weight** birth weight over 4 kg **low b weight** birth weight less than 2.5 kg. Such babies are those born prematurely and those with foetal growth retardation **multiple b** the birth of two or more offsprings produced in the same gestation period **premature b** birth of a premature baby

birthing rooms hospital facilities that serve as both a labour and a delivery room

bisacodyl (bis-ak'o-dil) a cathartic having direct effect on the colon

bisection (bi-sek'shun) cutting into two equal parts

bisexual (bi-seks'u-al) 1. having gonads of both sexes, in one person; hermaphrodite 2. a person who is sexually attracted to others of either sex

bisexuality (bi-seks'u-al-i-te) sexual attraction to persons of both sexes

bisferiens (bis-fer'e-un-s) widely notched **pulsus b** a slow upstroke and a collapsing pulse giving a feel of double humps

bis in die twice in a day *abbr* b.d; bid

bismuth (biz'muth) a silvery metallic element used as a protective for inflammed surfaces. Bismuth salts such as bismuth subcarbonate, bismuth subgallate and bismuth subnitrate are astringents, and used to treat diarrhoea

bistoury (bis'too-re) a long narrow straight or curved surgical knife

bit a contraction of binary digit, the smallest unit of computer memory that is used to process the data and the value can only 0 or 1

bite 1. to cut with teeth 2. an injury wherein the body surface is torn by an animal or insect **b lock** (bit'lok) a dental device to retain bite rims

bitemporal (bi-tem'po-ral) pertaining to both temples or temporal bone **b hemianopia** lesions at the level of the optic chiasma interrupting the impulses from the nasal halves of both retina thus resulting in loss of vision from the temporal side

bitolterol a long acting inhaled beta agonist bronchodilator

Bitot's (be'toz) **spots** triangular, shiny gray spots on the conjunctiva seen in vitamin A deficiency, described by Pierre Bitot, French physician

bitter (bit'er) having a disagreeable taste.

bituminous (bi'tu-mi-nus) soft coal

biuret (bi'u-ret) a crystalline decomposition derivative of urea **b test** a method for detecting urea and other soluble proteins in serum

biventer (bi-ven'ter) a muscle with two bellies

biventricular (bi'ven-trik'u-ler) pertaining to or affecting both ventricles of the heart

Bjerrum's (byer'oomz) **screen** target screen, prepared by a Danish ophthalmologist, Jannik Bjerrum. It is useful to plot the physiological blind spot

black (blak) reflecting no light or true colour.

black death plague

black eye beefy red eye from extravasated blood which extends beyond the oribital margins. There may be haemorrhage in the conjunctiva

black fever *see* kala azar

black head a black tipped semisolid sebum that obstructs the opening of a hair follicle

black lung coal workers' pneumoconiosis; anthracosis with deposits of carbon dust in the lungs of urban dwellers

Blackfan-Diamond syndrome inherited disorder with erythroid hypoplasia and anaemia

blackout transitory loss of consciousness.

black tongue dorsal surface of the tongue covered with black or brown fur. The filiform papillae are much lengthened; hairy tongue

blackwater fever production of dark brown-black urine due to intravascular haemolysis seen in falciparum malaria

bladder (blad'der) a hollow muscular organ commonly refered to urinary bladder **atonic b** loss of bladder control with loss of bladder sensation. There is overflow incontinence with dribbling. It develops in spinal cord lesion above S_2 in acute stage **automatic b** sudden complete reflex evacuation of bladder. There is absence of bladder distension and its capacity is small. It develops in spinal cord lesion above S_2 in chronic stage **autonomous b** overflow incontinence with absence of bladder sensation. There is loss of bladder control noted in spinal cord or cauda equina $S_{2,3,4}$ lesions **b cancer** most common site of urinary tract for malignancy. It is a transitional cell carcinoma which spreads locally by direct invasion. Painless haematuria is the presenting symptom **b irrigation** the washing out of the bladder by water or medicated solution **b stone** large round stone in the bladder **neurogenic b** any dysfunction of the urinary bladder due to lesions of CNS or nerve supply to bladder **pear-shaped b** extensive compression of the urinary bladder from an excess tissue in the pelvis giving a pear-shape to the bladder following intravenous pyelogram **urinary b** a musculo-membranous distensible reservoir situated in the pelvic cavity. It receives urine from kidneys through ureters and stores it for some time and then discharges out through urethra

Blalock-Taussig shunt an anastomosis of a subclavian artery to the pulmonary artery on the same side in cyanotic heart disease characterised by reduced pulmonary flow such as tetrology of Fallot and pulmonary atresia, named after Alfred Blalock, US surgeon and Halen Taussig, US paediatrician

blanch to lose colour especially of the face **b test** application of pressure on a finger nail or toe nail and then quickly releasing it to determine circulation. In presence of normal circulation the nail bed loses its colour and returns back to normal within 2 sec or less

bland mild or having a soothing effect. **bland diet** *see* diet

blast an immature stage in the development of a cell **b cell** early precursor cells, especially large undifferentiated cells with basophilic cytoplasm as seen in acute leukaemia **b crisis** shift especially of chronic myeloid leukaemia to acute form with appearance of many myeloblasts in peripheral blood

blastocoele (blas'to-sel) the fluid-filled cavity of the mass of cells produced by cleavage of a fertilised ovum

blastocyst (blas'to-sist) an early stage of embryo wherein there is a two-layer sphere of cells surrounding a fluid-filled cavity

Blastocystis hominis an intestinal protozoan causing diarrhoea in immunocompromised patients

blastoma (blas-to'ma) tumour, arising from embryonic layers

blastomyces (blast-o-mi'sez) biphasic fungi growing as mycelia at room temperature and as yeast-like forms at body temperature

blastomycosis (blas'to-mi-ko'sis) systemic infection cause ' by blastomyces. It may present like a pneumonitis or as a long term illness affecting the lungs, skin and bones

blastula (blas'tu-la) an early stage of development through which a zygote develops into an embryo. It is a fluid-

filled sphere formed by a single layer of cells. It is the form in which embryo gets implanted in the wall of the uterus

BLB mask mask for administration of oxygen at high altitudes, named after inventors, Boothby, Lovelace and Bulbulion

bleaching use of an oxidising chemical to remove stain **b powder** calcium hypochlorite

bleb 1. an irregular elevation of the epidermis 2. a thin-walled lucent area contiguous with pleura

bleeding 1. flow of blood from an injured vessel; haemorrhage **arterial b** bleeding in spurts of bright red blood **b time** time required for blood to stop flowing from the site of pin prick or a small wound. **breakthrough b** intermenstrual bleeding **dysfunctional uterine b** abnormal bleeding from the uterus from undertermined cause **internal b** haemorrhage from an internal organ **menstrual b** *see* menstruation **occult b** inapparent bleeding especially that occurring in the intestine **venous b** a continuous flow of dark red blood

blennorrhagia (blen'o-ra'je-a) excess discharge of mucus

blennorrhoea (blen'o-re'a) discharge from the urethra or vagina due to gonorrhoea

bleomycin an anti-tumour drug

blepharism continuous blinking.

blepharitis (blef'ar-i'tis) inflammation of the hair follicles and glands along the border of the eyelids. The eyelids become red, tender and sore with sticky exudate

blepheroplasty (blef'a-ro-plas'te) surgical removal of wrinkled skin on the eyelid.

blepharospasm (blef'a-ro-spa-sm) spasm of the orbicularis oculi causing closure of the eyelids

blepharotomy (blet-a-rot'o-me) surgical incision of an eyelid

blighted (bli'tid) **ovum** a fertilised ovum that fails to develop

blind 1. without sight 2. in clinical trials the treating physician being unaware of the content of the drug **b fistula** sinus **b loop syndrome** bacterial overgrowth in duodenum and jejunum from achlorhydria, or impaired intestinal motility or structural abnormality causing watery diarrhoea, steatorrhoea with anaemia due to B_{12} deficiency. Tetracyclines are useful **b spot** optic disc devoid of rods and cones.

blindness inability to see from injuries to the eye, corneal opacity, cataract, glaucoma and muscular degeneration

blink involuntary opening and closing of the eye **b reflex** the automatic closure of the eyelid when an object is approaching the eye rapidly

blister an elevation of the epidermis containing fluid

bloated swollen

bloating abdominal distress from distension and abnormal intestinal motility

block 1. obstruction 2. a method of regional anaesthesia to stop passage of sensory impulses 3. to obstruct any passage or opening **b dissection** removal of local lymphatic drainage area with tumour as a single block of tissue **caudal b** extradural injection of anaesthetic agent **epidural b** single injection in lumbar spaces **spinal b** subarachnoid block causing rapid anaesthesia

blockade (block-ad) prevention of action of a drug or body function.

blocker a drug that prevents the normal action of a system or cell receptor

blocking *psy* abrupt interruption in train of thinking before a thought or idea is finished, after a brief pause, person indicates no recall of what was being said or was going to be said **b antibody** antibody (lgG) that combines with antigen preventing access of other antibodies

blood (blud) the liquid pumped by the heart through the circulatory system consisting of arteries, veins and capillaries. It consists of a clear yellow fluid (plasma) and formed elements (red blood cells, white blood cells and platelets). The major functions of the blood is to transport oxygen and nutrient substances to the cells and remove from the cells carbon dioxide and other waste products for elimination **arterial b** oxygenated blood found in the pulmonary veins, the left chambers of the heart and the systemic arteries **b agar** a culture medium consisting of blood and nutrient agar used for cultivation of microorganisms **b bank** an unit concerned with collecting, processing and storing blood for transfusion **b borne pathogens** pathogenic microorganisms found in the blood that can cause disease in humans **b brain barrier** the phenomenon by which several substances found in the blood including drugs fail to reach neurons and cerebrospinal fluid **b capillaries** hairlike vessels that convey blood from the arterioles to the venules **b cell** any of the formed elements of blood **b circulation** the circuit of blood in the body through which blood circulates **b clot** the end result of blood clotting consisting of a semisolid mass of erythrocytes, leucocytes and platelets that are enmeshed in an insoluble fibrin network **b clotting** the conversion of blood from a free flowing liquid to a semisolid gel **b corpuscle** a blood cell, either red or white blood cell **b count** determination of the number of red and white blood cells per cubic millimetre of blood **b donor** a person donating blood **b dyscrasia** a condition wherein the constituents of blood are abnormal in structure and function **b fluke** flatworm of genus schistosoma **b gas** gas dissolved in liquid part of the blood. It includes oxygen, carbon dioxide and nitrogen **b gas analysis** determination of the concentration and pressure of oxygen and carbon dioxide and bicarbonate levels in the arterial blood **b gas tension** partial pressure of a gas in the blood **b group** the classification of blood based on the presence or absence of genetically determined antigens located on the surface of the erythrocyte. There are a number of human blood group systems, each system is determined by a series of two or more genes that are closely linked on a single autosomal chromosome. ABO blood group discovered by Karl Landsteiner is of great significance in blood transfusion. The population is divided into four blood groups as A, B, AB and O. The Rhesus (Rh) system is of value in obstetrics **b level** the concentration of a drug or other substance in the plasma, serum or whole blood **b osmolality** the osmatic pressure of blood. The normal values in serum are 280 to 295 mOsm/L **b pH** the hydrogen ion concentration of the blood and the normal values are 7.38 to 7.44 **b smear** a drop of blood spread on a slide for examination **b transfusion** the replacement of blood or one of its components **b urea nitrogen** (BUN) the level of nitrogen in the blood in the form of urea **b vessel** any one of the network of muscular tubes that carry blood such as arteries, arterioles, veins, venules and capillaries **cord b** blood in the umbilical vessels at the time of delivery of the infant **occult b** blood found in minute quantity that is detectable only by chemical tests **venous b** blood that has given up its oxygen to the cells and is carrying carbon dioxide **whole b** blood from which none of the elements has been removed.

blood pressure the pressure exerted by the flow of blood as it is pumped by the heart through the main arteries **basal bp** blood pressure obtained after making the patient to rest for about an hour in bed or after a sedative to allay anxiety **bp estimation** gives an indication of the overall cardiovascular status as it depends upon cardiac output and peripheral resistance **casual bp** the values of blood pressure obtained when the patient is examined in a clinic without any prior preparation

Bloom syndrome immunodeficiency disease with reduction in immunoglobulin levels

blowing test lump in the lateral regions of the abdomen are made visible by asking the patient to shut his mouth, hold his nose and then blow. It raises the intraabdominal pressure and makes the abdominal musculature tense

blue asbestos crocidolite

blue baby a neonate with cyanosis of any aetiology

blue belly periumbilical bluish discolouration due to intraperitoneal haemorrhage

blue bloater chronic bronchitis with CO_2 retention, cyanosis and heart failure

blue bodies laminated PAS-positive iron containing bodies in alveolar macrophages of desquamative interstitial pneumonia

blue line grey black dots situated about 1 mm from the free margin of the gum, seen best with the aid of magnifying glass. They are to be looked for in patients who work with lead

blue sclera sclera that retains the normal foetal transparency so that blue uvea is visible. It may occur alone or in association with brittle bones and deafness

B lymphocyte an immune cell derived from bursa. They comprise 30% of circulating lymphocytes and are concentrated in the follicular zones of the lymphoid tissue. They are responsible for antibody production.

board-like rigidity the abdominal wall becoming rigid and immobile in generalised peritonitis

Boas's sign in cholecystitis there may be an area of hyperaesthesia posteriorly. The tenderness extends from about 2.5 cm lateral to the spines of the vertebrae to the posterior axillary line, and vertically from the level of the 11th thoracic to the 1st lumbar spine.

Bodansky unit the quantity of phosphatase in 100 ml of serum required to liberate 1 mg of phosphorous, named after Aaron Bodansky, US biochemist

body 1. the whole physical structure of an individual with all organs 2. a cadaver or a corpse 3. the largest or main part of any organ **b cavity** any of the spaces in the chest and abdomen that contain body organs **b composition** quantitation of the various components of the body **b fluid** a fluid contained in the three compartments of the body such as plasma, interstitial fluid between the cells and intracellular fluid within the cells **b image** a person's subjective concept of his or her physical appearance **b language** a set of non-verbal signals such as postures, gestures and facial expression that give expression of the individual **b mass index** an index for estimating obesity. It is weight (kg)/ height (m2) **b mechanics** study of muscular actions and functions of muscles in maintaining the posture of the body **b odour** an unpleasant smell emanating from the human body **b piercing** a penetration of jewellary into openings made in such regions of the body such as helix of the ears, and nose **b plethysmograph** a device permitting rapid estimation of the volume of air in the thorax **b temperature** the level of heat produced and sustained by body processes **b type** classification of the human body according to the distribution of muscles and fat **Donovan's b** intracellular bacillus *(Calymmato-bacterium donovani)* seein in histiocyte in the genital skin of patients affected with granuloma inguinale

Boerhaave (boor'ha-ve) **syndrome** spontaneous rupture of the oesophagus leading to mediastinitis and pleural effusion. Usually associated with violent retching and vomiting, named after Hermann Boerhaave, Danish physician

Bohr effect the effect of acid environment on haemoglobin. Increasing levels of PCO2 and H + decrease oxyhaemoglobin saturation, whereas decreasing concentration have opposite effect, described by Christian Bohr, Danish physiologist

boil furuncle, infection of a hair follicle by staphylococci. It is characterised by redness, swelling, heat and tenderness.

bolus (bo'lus) 1. a rounded mass of food material 2. material injected intravenously and rapidly at one time for a quick response 3. a rounded soft mass of pharmaceutical preparation ready to swallow

Bombay phenotype The O_h phenotype, a variant of the ABO antigens on red cells. These red cells do not agglutinate with antisera containing anti-A, anti-B or anti-'H' type antibody. These red cells lack the H antigen and H substance. The condition was described in Mumbai.

bombesin a neuropeptide produced in the gastrointestinal tract, stimulating gastrointestinal smooth muscle contraction, release of gastric acid and most gastrointestinal hormones except secretin

bonding the emotional ties formed between the infant and mother that occur in early postpartum period

bone 1. the dense, hard tissue forming the skeleton 2. any distinct piece of the skeleton of the body (see table 2). **b age** radiologic study of estimation of biologic age based on the stage of development of ossification centres of the wrist bones and long bones of extremities **b cancer** a skeletal malignancy occurring primarily as a sarcoma or as metastasis from cancer elsewhere in the body **b cell** osteocyte, a nucleated cell with spidery processes in the septate lacuna of bone **b cyst** a cystic structure replacing the bone **b density** the concentration of protein and mineral salts in bone; their concentra-

Table 2. Bones

Name	Region	Character	Articulations
Atlas	neck	ring-shaped first cervical vertebra under skull, having no body	occipital bone above and axis vertebra below
Axis	neck	second cervical vertebra with fused body of atlas as odontoid process	with atlas above and 3rd cervical vertebra below
Calcea-neus	foot (heel)	largest of the tarsal bones, irregular in shape	with talus and cuboid bone
Capitate	wrist	central carpal bone with rounded head	with metacarpals distally and other carpal bones proximally
Carpals	wrist	8 in number, small irregular bones scaphoid, lunate, triquetral, pisiform trapezoid, capitate, trapezium and hamate arranged in two rows of 4 each	with radius proximally and metacarpals distally
Clavicle	front of shoulder	horizontally placed long bone, with concavo-convex curve, in the upper part of a thorax	with sternum, scapula and first rib
Coccyx	tip of the vertebral column at lower end	triangular in shape, formed by fusion of last 4 vertebrae	with sacrum
Concha inferior	lateral wall of nasal cavity	thin curved piece of bone attached on the lateral wall of nasal cavity	with ethmoid, lacrimal and palatine processes of maxilla
Cuboid	foot	irregular cubical bone placed laterally	with calcaneus, cuneiform and 4th and 5th metatarsal bones
Cuneiform	foot	three in number, medial, intermediate and lateral, wedge-shaped bones	with bases of 1st to 4th metatarsal bones and other tarsal bones
Ethmoid	skull	single bone below frontal bone extending into nasal cavity contributing to nasal septum and forming superior and middle nasal conchae	with sphenoid, frontal, vomer, maxilla, lacrimal and nasal bones
Fabella	knee	a small rounded sesamoid bone, present in the lateral head of gastrocnemius near its origin	with femur, reduces friction of tendon with bone

Femur	thigh	longest bone of the skeleton	forms hip joint with *os-inno-minatum* and knee joint with tibia and patella distally
Fibula	leg	thin long bone placed laterally in leg	with tibia at both ends and also with talus distally
Frontal	skull	single bone on the anterior part of skull, having frontal air sinus in it	with parietal, sphenoid, maxilla, ethmoid, zygomatic, lacrimal and nasal bones
Hamate	wrist	carpal bone, hammer-shaped, placed medially in distal row of carpal bones	with bases of 4th and 5th meta-carpal bones and other carpal bones
Hip bone	pelvis	irregular bone formed by fusion of 3 bones ischium, ilium and pubis. Bones of two sides together with sacrum form bony pelvis	hip joint, with head of femur, sacro-iliac joint with sacrum and symphysis pubis with pubic bone of other side.
Humerus	arm	long bone with head, greater and lesser trichanter at upper end and trochlea and capitulum at lower end	forms shoulder joint with glenoid cavity of scapula and elbow joint with radius and ulna distally
Hyoid	front of neck	U-shaped small bone to which muscles of the tongue and ribbon muscles of neck are attached	suspended by ligament and muscles having no articulation with any bone
Ilium	pelvis	flat bony part of hip bone having crest and spines	with sacrum behind contributes to upper part of acetabulum which articulates with head of the femur
Incus	small bone in the middle ear cavity	anvil-shaped	with malleus and stapes
Ischium	pelvis	part of hip bone below and behind acetabulum	contributes to lower part of acetabulum which articulates with head of the femur
Lacrimal	skull	thin small flat bone contributes to medial wall of orbit near its margin	with ethmoid, frontal and maxilla
Lunate	wrist	half moon-shaped carpal bone in the proximal row of carpals	with radius and triquetral to form wrist joint and with other carpal bones forms intercarpal joints
Malleus	small bone in the middle ear cavity	hammer-shaped, placed laterally in contact with tympanic membrane	with incus

Mandible	lower jaw	horse shoe-shaped, having body, ramus and condyloid-coronoid processes. Body has sockets for teeth	with temporal bone forming temporo-mandibular joint, also with 16 teeth in adult
Maxilla	upper jaw	irregular paired bone below orbit and on lateral side of nasal cavity having maxillary air sinus in it, carries upper teeth	with ethmoid, frontal, vomer, lacrimal, nasal, palatine, zygomatic, maxilla of opposite side and inferior concha
Metacarpal	hand	five short-long bones, heads of which form knuckles	distally articulates with bases of proximal phalanges, proximally articulates with distal row of carpal bones
Metatarsal	foot	five short-long bones of foot with concavity on plantar surface	distally articulates with bases of proximal phalanges, proximally articulates with tarsal bones
Nasal	skull	small paired bone, together forming bridge of the nose	with frontal, ethmoid and maxilla
Navicular	foot	boat-shaped tarsal bone with a tuberosity on medial side	with talus proximally and 3 cuneiform bones distally
Occipital	skull	single bone at the back of skull, and at the base of skull having large foramen-foramen magnum-in it.	with sphenoid, both parietals and temporal bones
Palatine	skull	paired bone forming posterior part of hard palate	with ethmoid, sphenoid, vomer, maxilla and palatine of opposite side
Patella	knee	largest sesamoid bone, irregularly rectangular, placed in the tendon of quadriceps femoris, forms knee cap	with femur
Phalanges	fingers and toes	short-long bones, 3 in each fingers and toes, 2 in thumb and big toe arranged as proximal, middle and distal	with heads of metacarpal and metatarsal, with other phalanges proximal and distal to them
Pisiform	wrist	smallest sesamoid bone placed medially in proximal row of carpal bone	with triquetral bone
Pubic	pelvis	lower anterior part of hip bone, having body and 2 rami enclosing obturator foramen	with pubic bone of opposite side forming symphysis pubis bone
Radius	forearm	long bone placed laterally in forearm	proximally with ulna and humerus distally with ulna and carpal bones - scaphoid and lunate

Ribs	chest wall	12 pairs of thin ribbon-shaped bones forming posterolateral wall of chest	posteriorly all ribs articulate with corresponding vertebrae, anteriorly upper 7 ribs with sternum through costal cartilages, lower 3 ribs with costal cartilages of rib above and last 2 ribs are floating
Sacrum	lower back	wedge-shaped triangular bone formed by fusion of 5 vertebrae below lumbar vertebrae	with 5th lumbar vertebra above, coccyx below and ilium on the two sides
Scaphoid	wrist	boat shaped carpal bone placed laterally in proximal row of carpal bones	with radius proximally and with other carpal bones
Sesamoid	in the tendons of muscles of extremities	small, rounded or flat bones developing in the long tendons near the joints	
Sphenoid	base of skull	single, irregular bone having body and wing-shaped extensions forming part of lateral wall of orbit	with frontal, occipital, ethmoid, vomer, palatine, parietal, temporal and zygomatic bones
Stapes	middle ear	smallest bone, stirrup shaped, placed medially in middle ear cavity	with incus laterally, covers oval window of vestibule of internal ear medially.
Sternum	chest	flat bone placed in mid-line of anterior wall of chest, comprising 3 parts – manubrium, body and xiphoid process	with clavicle and upper 7 pairs of ribs on each side
Talus	ankle	large tarsal bone having no muscular attachment	with tibia, fibula, calcaneus and navicular
Tarsal bones	ankle-foot	irregular bones of foot, arranged in rows - talus, calcaneus, navicular, cuboid and 3 cuneiforms	forms ankle joint with tibia-fibula, intertarsal joints with each other and tarso-metatarsal joints with bases of metatarsal bones
Temporal	lateral side of skull	paired irregular bone having mastoid, squamous, petrous, tympanic and zygomatic parts, contains middle and internal ear.	with occipital, sphenoid, mandible, parietal and zygomatic bones
Tibia	leg	larger long bone in leg placed medially	with femur and fibula proximally and talus and fibula distally

Trapezium	wrist	carpal bone of the distal row placed laterally	with trapezoid and scaphoid and with bases of 1st and 2nd metacarpals
Trapezoid	wrist	carpal bone of distal row, trapezoid shape	with capitate, scaphoid, trapezium and bases of 2nd metacarpal bone
Triquetral	wrist	small 3 facet triangular carpal bone of proximal row of carpal bones	with hamate, lunate, pisiform and articular disc of wrist joint
Ulna	forearm	long bone placed medially in forearm	proximally with radius forming superior radio-ulnar joint and with humerus forming elbow joint distally with radius and articular disc
Vertebrae	vertebral column	irregular bones having body, neural arches, transverse processes, spine and vertebral canal. 7 cervical, 12 thoracic, 5 lumbar, 5 sacral fused to form sacrum and lower 3-5 coccygeal fused as coccyx.	1st cervical with occipital, 5th lumbar with sacrum, all vertebrae with adjacent vertebrae above and below. Thoracic also articulates with ribs
Vomer	skull	thin sheet-like bone forming postero-inferior part of nasal septum	with sphenoid and ethmoid
Zygomatic	skull	irregular bone forming bony prominence of cheek and lower margin of orbit	with frontal, sphenoid, maxilla and temporal bone

tion is lowered in osteoporosis **b densitometry** the measurement of bone mass or density **b graft** a surgical procedure in which a piece of bone is removed from one part of the body to repair the bone damaged in another part **b marrow** soft tissue found within bone cavities and it is the site of blood cell production **b marrow transplant** transplantation of bone marrow from healthy donors to stimulate production of blood cells **b spur** an abnormal bony excrescence often found in heel

bony landmark a prominence on a bone that serves as a guide to the location of other body structures

BOOP bronchiolitis obliterans organizing pneumonia

booster a follow-up dose of a vaccine administered to reinforce the effect of the first

borborygmus (bor'bo-rig'mus) rumbling noise or gurgling sound produced by the movement of fluid and gas through the intestines. pl. **borborygmi**

borderline any condition that cannot be placed in one of usually two categories **b hypertension** that range of systolic and diastolic blood pressures which are not benefited by therapy **b leprosy** dimorphous leprosy borderline lesions between two extremes of leprosy such as tuberculoid and lepromatous leprosy **b personality** a personality disturbance in which one lies between a neurotic, capable of coping with his environment and a psychotic who has lost contact with reality and there is persistent instability in emotions, relationships and behaviour **b tumour** a growth with low malignant potential

Bordetella (bor'de-te'la) gram-negative cocco-bacillus, named after a French bacteriologist, Jules Bordet **b pertusis** causative agent of whooping cough

Bornholm (born'hom) **disease** pleurodynia with involvement of intercostal muscles first noted in Danish island, Bornholm

Borrelia (bor-rel'e-a) a spirochaete causing relapsing fever, described by a French bacteriologist, Amedee Borrel *B burgedorferi* causative agent of lyme disease *B. duttonii* causative agent of tick-borne relapsing fever *B. recurrentis* causative agent of louse-borne relapsing fever *B. vincenti* causative agent of cancrum oris

bosselated (bo-sel'lat-ed) an intact surface that has numerous round emineneces

bossing rounded prominence of the frontal and parietal bones in an infant's cranial vault

Botallo's (bo-tal'oz) **duct** ductus arteriosus, described by an Italian surgeon, Leonardo Botallo

bothrium (both're-um) sucker in the form of a groove.

bottle feeding feeding an infant from a bottle with a rubber nipple on the end as a substitute for or supplement to breast-feeding.

botulin (boch 'u-lin) a powerful neurotoxin

botulism (bot'u-lizm) food poisoning due to botulin produced by the growth of *Clostridium botulinum* in improperly preserved or canned foods. The manifestations consist chiefly of vomiting and paresis of skeletal, ocular, pharyngeal and respiratory muscles

bougie (boo'zhe) a slender flexible cylindrical instrument introduced to dilate the constricted region such as urethra, or oesophagus

bouginage passage of bougie

Bourneville's (boor'ne-vez) **disease** tuberous sclerosis, described by a French neurologist, Desire-Magloire Bourneville

Boutonniere (boo-ton-yar') **deformity** deformity in rheumatoid arthritis with flexion at proximal interphalangeal joint and hyperextension at distal interphalangeal joint

bovine (bo'vin) pertaining to cattle **b cough** non-explosive cough as in laryngeal paralysis

bowel (bo'wel) the intestine **b movement** evacuation of faeces **b sounds** the normal sounds associated with movement of intestinal contents

Bowen's (bau'nz) **disease** a persistent progressive but potentially malignant intra-epidermal carcinoma

bow legs genu varum; outward curvature of the legs near the knee

Bowman's (bo'manz) **capsule** glomerular capsule described by an English physician, Sir William Bowman

Bowman's membrane the thin homogeneous membrane separating the corneal epithelium from the corneal substance

Boyle's apparatus continuous flow gasoxygen anaesthetic machine, designed by H. Boyle, British anaesthesiologist

Boyle's (boilz) **law** volume of gas varies inversely with pressure, after Robert Boyle, British physicist

BP abbreviation for blood pressure.

Brace mechanical support for damaged bones and ligaments

brachial (bra'ke-al) pertaining to the arm **b artery** the principal artery of upper arm **b plexus** a network of lower four cervical and the first thoracic spinal nerves that control the muscles of the upper limb

brachialgia (bra'ke-al'je-a) pain in the arm

brachialis (bra'ke-al'is) a muscle of the arm lying beneath biceps brachii

brachiocephalic (bra'ke-o-se-fal'ik) pertaining to the arm and head

brachioradialis (bra'ke-o-ra'de-a-lis) a muscle lying on the lateral side of the forearm

brachium (bra-ke-um) the arm or anatomical structure resembling an arm

brachy a combining word for short

brachycephalic (brak'e-se-fal'ik) having a short wide head

brachycephaly (brak'e-se-fal-i) short head

brachydactyly (brak'e-dak-til'i) short fingers and toes

brachygnathia (brak-ig-na'the-a) abnormally short lower jaw

branchytherapy (brak'e-ther'a-pe) treatment with ionising radiation whose source is near or on the surface of the body at a close distance

bracket a support of wood or metal, used as orthodontic appliances

Bradford frame an oblong frame which enables patients with fractures or diseases of the hip or spine to urinate or defecate without moving the spine or changing the positions, named after Edward Bradford, US orthopaedic surgeon

brady-a combining form of word meaning slow

bradyarrhythmia (brad'e-a-rith'me-a) a slow and irregular heart

bradycardia (brad'e-kar'de-a) slow heart beat exhibiting slow pulse rate, less than 60 per minute. Noted in myxoedema, obstructive jaundice, raised intracranial tension, digoxin toxicity, and complete heart block **relative b** normal relation of increase in pulse rate of 10 beats for each half degree centigrade rise of temperature is not maintained and pulse rate is relatively slow compared to the temperature. It is seen in typhoid, meningitis, dengue fever, cerebral abscess and in viral infections **b-tachycardia syndrome** heart rate alternating between abnormally slow and abnormally rapid rhythm

bradykinesia (brad'e-kin-ne'se-a) marked slowness of movement.

bradykinin (brad'e-ki'nin) a plasma kinin

bradypnoea (brad'ip-ne'a) decreased rate of breathing.

braille (bral) a system of reading and writing that enables the blind to see by using the sense of touch, named after Louis Braille, blind French educator

brain (bran) highest controlling centre of nervous system. It is a large soft mass of nerve tissue contained within the cranium. It consists of cerebrum, cerebellum, midbrain, pons and medulla. It is composed of neurons and neuroglia. Gray matter is composed of neuron cells and is concentrated in the cerebral cortex and nuclei and basal ganglia. White matter is composed of neuron processes which form tracts connecting parts of the brain with each

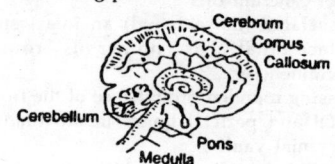

Brain section

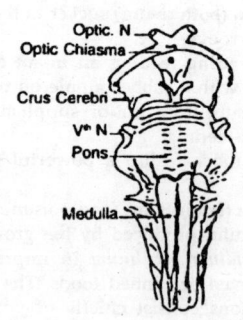

Brain stem

Brain stem

other and with the spinal card **b abscess** a pocket of infection in a part of the brain **b damage** degeneration or death of nerve cells in the brain **b death** the irreversible cessation of all brain functions while heart continues beating. There is lack of response to stimuli, lack of all reflexes, absent respirations and an isoelectric electroencephalogram **b oedema** swelling of the brain due to an increase in its water content **b fever** meningitis **b scan** the use of radioisotopes injected into circulation to detect abnormalities in the brain **b shift** displacement of parts of brain by expanding lesion **b stem** the stem-like part of midbrain comprising pons and medulla oblongata that connects cerebral hemispheres with the spinal cord **b tumour** any intracranial space occupying lesion such as neoplasm, cyst, or abscess **b washing** intense psychological indoctorination

bran the husk or outer envelope of cereal grains

brand name specific name assigned to a drug by the manufacturer

Branhamella catarrhalis organism associated with exacerbations of chronic bronchitis

brash a burning sensation in the stomach

brassy cough non-productive metallic cough heard in children with laryngotracheitis

brawny induration pathological hardening and thickening of tissues

Braxton Hicks contractions painless uterine contractions without cervical dilatation in latter half of pregnancy, named after Braxton Hicks, UK obstetrician.

bread and butter lesion diffuse fibrinous and serofibrinous adhesions on inflamed pericardium of rheumatic heart disease

breakbone fever Dengue fever

breakthrough bleeding midcycle bleeding in oral contraceptive users.

breast anterior aspect of the chest; mammary gland **b augmentation** enlarging breasts for cosmetic purposes **b cancer** a malignant neoplasm of breast tissue in women between the age of 30 and 50 may present as a small painless lump, thick or dimpled skin or nipple retraction, nipple discharge, ulceration and enlarged axillary lymph nodes, metastases through the lymphatics to axillary lymph nodes and to bone, lung, liver and brain. The extent of disease determines therapy. Surgery may be radical or simple mastectomy. Radiation or chemotherapy are adjuvant therapy **b examination** a process in which the breasts and their accessory structures are observed and palpated to find out any change or abnormality that could indicate malignant condition **b feeding** the act of providing milk to a new born or infant from mother's breasts **b implant** an inert sac filled with silicone covered by polyurethane foam used to augment cosmetically the female contour **b milk** contains 88% water, 3.5% fat, lactose, protein 1.0-1.5%, sterile, provides IgA and is more easily digestible **b mouse** fibroadenoma of the breast, an extremely mobile swelling of rubbery hard consistency **b pump** a device for withdrawing milk from the breast **b shadows** artifacts on chest radiography of women caused by breast tissue

breathanalyzer (breth'a-ny'li-zer) an apparatus used to test for blood alcohol levels in the expired air.

breathing the act of respiration - inhalation and exhalation **abdominal b** seen in men. There is downward excursion of the diaphragm with inspiration and free movement of the abdominal wall. It is more evident in paralysis of intercostal muscles, ankylosing spondylitis, pleurisy and fibrosis of the lung **Biot's b** an irregular respiration which may become slow or rapid, shallow or deep with irregular pauses, seen in meningitis, named after Camille Biot, French physician **bronchial b** sounds heard when the normal dampening effect of the air-containing alveoli is lost. The expiratory phase is longer as long as, or longer than inspiration. There is a pause between inspiration and expiration. The quality of the sound may be hollow or tubular. The breathing may be high pitched or low pitched **bronchovesicular b** an intermediate type of breathing exhibiting features of both vesicular and bronchial breathing **cavernous b** low pitched bronchial breathing heard over cavities **Cheyne-Stokes** (chan'stoks) **b** a periodic form of respiration wherein the successive respirations gradually become deeper and deeper and then diminish until there is temporary cessation of the respiration. It is noted in raised intracranial tension, narcotic poisoning of the respiratory centres, severe pneumonia, cardiac and renal failure, also when patient is asleep or comatose, named after John Cheyne, Scottish physician and William Stokes, Irish physician **cog-wheel b** breathing instead of being steady, appear jerky and inspiratory phase appears broken in nervous individual and in conditions of pleural adhesions **costal b** participation of intercostal muscles in the respiration, seen in women. It is encountered in paralysis of the diaphragm, peritonitis, ascites and diaphragmatic

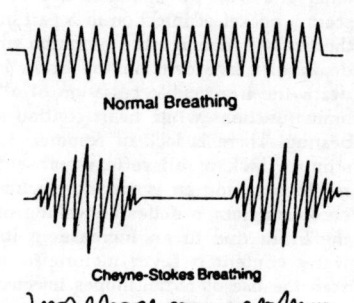

Normal Breathing

Cheyne-Stokes Breathing

Biot's Breathing

Breathing rhythm

paralysis; Thoracic respiration **Kussmaul's b** increased rate and depth of breathing in diabetic ketoacidosis and renal failure **puerile b** in children, the breath sounds are harsher than in adults **pursed lip b** slow exhalation promoting emptying of the lungs and retarding collapse of conducting airways **tubular b** a high pitched bronchial breathing heard over an area of consolidation **vesicular b** heard over the chest as a breezy rustling sound, inspiratory phase is fairly intense, longer and of low pitch. The expiratory phase is shorter with its length being equal to a third of the length of inspiration. The inspiration is harsher than expiration and its intensity is greater than that of expiration. There is no gap between inspiration and expiration. These sounds are heard on the greater part of the normal lungs except over trachea and the region where major bronchi are situated near the surface of the chest wall

breech buttocks **b birth** birth of a child with the buttocks, feet or knees first rather than head **b presentation** position of the foetus presenting with buttocks

bregma (breg'ma) the junction of the

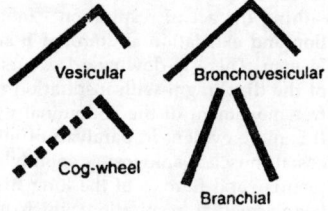

Vesicular

Bronchovesicular

Cog-wheel

Branchial

Breathing

coronal and sagittal sutures on the skull; anterior fontanella

Brenner's (bren'erz) **tumour** a benign fibroepithelioma of the ovary named after Fritz Brenner, German pathologist

bridge 1. a narrow band of tissue 2. a dental appliance that replaces a missing tooth and it is attached to adjacent teeth for support **b of nose** the upper part of nose formed by the junction of nasal bones

bridgework a partial denture held in place by attachments other than clasps

Bright's disease acute glomerulonephritis, described by an English physician, Richard Bright

brim an edge or margin **b of pelvis** the inlet of the lesser or true pelvis. It is formed by the iliopectineal line of the innominate bone and the sacral premontory. It is oval-shaped in female and heart-shaped in male

brittle bone syndrome bones with increased osseous fragility seen in osteogenesis imperfecta

brittle diabetes insulin-dependent diabetes mellitus in which blood glucose fluctuates widely despite frequent titration of the insulin dose

broach fine piercing instrument used in root canal surgery

broad ligament peritoneal fold from uterus to side of pelvis **b l of liver** a cresent- shaped fold of peritoneum attached to the diaphragm connecting with the liver and anterior abdominal wall

broad-spectrum antibiotic an antibiotic that is effective against a wide variety of bacteria

Broca's (bro'kas) **area** speech centre in the brain, described by a French anatomist, Pierre Broca

Broca index if a person has weight 20% more than his ideal weight, it is determined by height in cm–100

Brock's syndrome obstructive pneumonia of middle lobe due to enlarged hilar tuberculous lymph nodes, described by Russell Brock, UK surgeon

Brodie's abscess a deep-seated bony swelling situated near a joint in chronic osteomyelitis, named after Sir Benjamin Brodie, English surgeon

Brodmann's (brod'manz) **areas** division of cerebral cortex into 47 different areas that are associated with specific neurologic functions, named after Korbinian Brodmann, German anatomist

bromhexine mucolytic agent

bromhidrosis (bro'mi-dro'sis) sweat having an unpleasant odour due to bacterial decomposition

bromism (bro'mizm) poisoning by bromine or a bromine compound.

bromocriptin dopamine receptor stimulant used in hyperprolactinaemia and parkinsonism

bronchial (brong'ke-al) pertaining to bronchi or bronchioles **b adenoma** a benign tumour of the lung situated near the hilum. It arises either in the main or lobar branchus from the duct epithelium of bronchial mucous glands. It appears as a polypoid mass causing dry irritant cough and haemoptysis **b artery** one of the two bronchial arteries for each lung arising from the aorta or from the intercostal arteries or both **b asthma** see asthma **b breath sound** see breathing **b hyperactivity** airway hyperactivity manifested by the propensity for widespread but reversible narrowing of the airways in response to diverse stimuli and there is smooth muscle inflammation and mucosal oedema, accumulation of mucus and an influx of inflammatory cells including eosinophils **b isomerism** a congenital bronchial anomaly in which patient has bilateral right or left lungs **b secretion** mucus which is mostly secreted by goblet cells of the respiratory epithelium is composed of 95% water, the mucus glycoproteins and a variety of other proteins containing surfactant proteins, immunoglobulins, complement, bactericidal proteins and proteinase inhibitors **b tree** the branching, tree-like structure of airways in the lungs **b washing** irrigation of the bronchi and bronchioles to collect cells for cytologic study and to cleanse the region

bronchiectasis (brong'ke-ek'ta-sis) abnormal and permanent distortion and dilatation of the subsegmental airways. There is destruction of the components of bronchial wall. The condition develops insidiously and the manifestations depend on the degree of dilatation, infective episodes and secretion. There is profuse purulent expectoration and it has a postural relationship **dry b** bronchiectasis without infection presents with haemoptysis

bronchiole (brong'ke-ol) pl. **bronchioles** finer division of a bronchus. They are membranous and branch more frequently at a few millimetre distance. Smooth muscle forms its wall. There are no mucous glands **respiratory b** last division of bronchial tree. It contains both bronchiolar epithelium and alveoli in their walls. It ends by dividing into two or more air sacs **terminal b** the airway immediately proximal to the respiratory bronchiole. This last purely conducting structure supplies an acinus

bronchiolectasis (brong'ke-o-lek'ta-sis) dilatation of the bronchioles.

bronchiolitis (brong'ke-o-li'tis) inflammation of the bronchioles **b obliterans organising pneumonia** (BOOP) an infiltrative lung disease with a subacute clinical course where the granulation tissue plugs within the lumens of small airways

bronchioloalveolar carcinoma a subgroup of primary adenocarcinoma of the lung and it is a peripheral, well-differentiated neoplasm arising beyond a grossly recognisable bronchus with a tendency

to spread locally in the peripheral airspaces. It may present with dry cough, progressively increasing dyspnoea and haemoptysis

bronchitic (brong-ki'tic) pertaining to bronchitis.

bronchitis (brong-ki'tis) inflammation of the bronchi **acute b** bronchitis having a short clinical course with cough, expectoration and fever. Often caused by the spread of upper respiratory viral infections to the bronchi **chronic b** chronic or recurrent excess mucus secretion into the bronchial tree without a demonstrable cause either local or general occurring on most of the days during at least three months of the year for at least two successive years. It is caused by protracted bronchial irritation by cigarette smoke and airborne particulate and gaseous pollutants. There is bronchial mucous gland hyperplasia with chronic productive cough

bronchoalveolar (bron'ko-al-ve'o-lar) pertaining to the bronchus and alveoli **b lavage** removal of secretions and cells from lower respiratory passages by introduction of sterile saline solution through a fiberoptic bronchoscope.

bronchocoele (brong'ko-sel) a localised dilatation of a bronchus.

bronchoconstrictor a substance that causes the airways to narrow.

bronchoconstriction (brong'ko-kon-strik'shun) decrease in the calibre of the bronchial airways.

bronchodilator a drug that widens the constricted bronchial passages by relaxing the smooth muscles, Beta adrenergic receptor agonists, methylxanthines and anticholinergics are examples

bronchodilatation (brong'ko-dil-a-ta'shun) increase in the calibre of the bronchial airways

bronchogenic (brong-ko-jen'ik) originating in a bronchus **b carcinoma** lung cancer arising from the surface epithelium of the bronchial tree usually from either basal or mucosal cells. The incompletely differentiated cells in the basement membrane of the mucosa proliferate following a carcinogenic stimulus. The tumours are categorised as small cell lung cancer and nonsmall cell lung cancer comprising squamous cell carcinoma, adenocarcinoma and large cell carcinoma

bronchogram (brong-ko-gram) the roentgenogram obtained by bronchgraphy

bronchography (brong-kog'ra-fe) roentgenography of the bronchial tree after instilling a radioopaque medium into a bronchus

broncholith (brong'ko-lith) calcified material in the tracheobronchial tree

broncholithiasis (brong'ko-lith-i-a-sis) presence of calcified material within the tracheobronchial tree, or external compression of a bronchus by calcified peribronchial lymph nodes

bronchology (brong-kol'o-je) the study and treatment of the disorders of the tracheobronchial tree

bronchomalacia (brong'ko-ma-la'she-a) a deficiency in the cartilaginous wall of the trachea or a bronchus

bronchophony (brong-kof'o-ne) voice sounds heard through the stethoscope on a large bronchus and it can be heard in other regions of the chest in consolidation of the lung.

bronchopleural (brong'ko-ploor'al) pertaining to a bronchus and the pleura

bronchopneumonia (brong'ko-nu-mo'ne-a) a combination of bronchiolitis and pneumonia

bronchopulmonary (brong'ko-pul'mo-na-re) pertaining to the lungs and their air passages **b segment** a wedge-shaped lung supplied by a segmental bronchus

bronchorrhaphy (brong-kar'a-fe) the rapair of a bronchus

bronchorrhoea (brong'ko-re'a) excessive

secretion of the mucus from the airways

bronchoscope (brong'ko-skop) an instrument to visualise the interior of the airways, to aspirate secretions, to remove foreign body and to perform brush or biopsy

bronchoscopy (brong-kos'ke-pe) visual examination of the bronchi through a flexible or rigid bronchoscope

bronchosinusitis (brong'ko-si-nus-i'tis) inflammation of the paranasal sinuses and the lower respiratory passages

bronchospasm (brong'ko-spazm) spasmodic contraction of the bronchial smooth muscle of the airways causing the airways to narrow

bronchospirometry (brong'ko-spi-rom'e-tre) determination of the ventilatory function tests by a spirometer

bronchostaxis (brong'ko-stak'sis) bleeding from the bronchial wall

bronchostenosis (brong'ko-sten-o'sis) stricture of the bronchial passage

bronchotomy (brong-kot'o-me) surgical incision of a bronchus

bronchovesicular (brong'ko-ve-sik'u-lar) bronchoalveolar **b breath sound** see breathing

bronchus (brong' kus) air passage arising from the trachea which divides into lobar bronchi and in turn into segmental and subsegmental bronchi pl. **bronchi intermediate b** descending right main bronchus after giving upper lobe bronchus **large b** proximal five generations of bronchial division, contain abundant cartilage forming a complete ring in their walls and contain a large number of mucous glands **segmental b** bronchi leading to the segments of the lobes of the lung **small b** next 10 generations of bronchial division after large bronchi, contain sparse amount of cartilage in their walls and collapse easily. Number of mucous glands are less

bronze baby syndrome a complication of phototherapy characterised by dark gray-brown skin discolouration, marked elevation of direct bilirubin, and evidence of obstructive liver disease

bronze diabetes haemochromatosis

broth a liquid culture medium **enrichment b** broth designed to encourage the growth of small numbers of particular organism while suppressing other flora present

brown asbestos amosite

Brown-Sequard's (brown'sa-karz) **syndrome** hemisection of spinal cord causing ipsilateral spastic paralysis with loss of vibration and position sense and contralateral loss of pain and temperature, named after Charles Brown-Sequard, French physiologist

browse to navigate the Internet or the contents of the computer

brucella (bro-sel'a) non-motile gram-negative genus of micro-organisms belonging to the family of Brucellaceae, described by David Bruce, British army surgeon

brucellosis (broo'sel-o'sis) an infection caused by *Brucella abortus* which is usually spread to humans by ingestion of raw milk from infected cattle and cause both a blood stream infection and an intracellular infection. It presents with fever, sweating, weakness, headache, anorexia, pain in the limbs and back and splenomegaly. Tetracycline, streptomycin and rifampicin are useful in the treatment

Bruce protocol exercise electrocardiography while the individual is subjected to the stress of graded exercises. The subject is made to exercise in stages of increasing workloads until the end points are achieved. It is undertaken using the treadmill or bicycle ergometer

Brudzinski's (brood-zin'skez) **sign** Passive flexion of the neck causing flexion of limbs in meningitis, named after Jozef Brudzinski, Polish physician

brugia a genus of filarial worms *B malayi* nematode of filariasis that infects man

and other animals, and microfilaria are not confined to night

bruise (brooz) a superficial injury

bruit (broot) an abnormal sound or a murmur heard on auscultation **arterial b** systolic bruit audible over normal arteries with increased blood flow as in thyrotoxicosis or over the site where the lumen is narrowed as in renal artery stenosis or carotid stenosis **systolic b** arterial bruit **bruit de diable** *see* venous hum

Brunner's (brun'erz) **glands** submucosal glands in the first part of duodenum secreting alkaline fluid on stimulus of acid in the lumen, named after Johann Brunner, Swiss anatomist

brush border layer of absorbing surfaces of small intestine and first convoluted tubules of the kidney, consists of tightly packed microvilli

brush cells cells found in tracheal epithelium

bruxism (bruk'sizm) rhythmic or spasmodic grinding of the teeth especially during sleep

Bryant's triangle when the patient lies in the the the dorsal position, a plumb line is drawn towards the floor from the anterior superior iliac spine (base line), and another line to the tip of greater trochanter from the anterior superior iliac spine. Then a line is drawn by shortest route from the tip of greater trochanter to the base line (horizontal line). A difference in the horizontal line on both sides is useful to note shortening in femoral head or neck, named after Sir Thomas Bryant, British surgeon

BTPS abbreviation for body temperature, pressure, saturated

buba mucocutaneous leishmaniasis

bubo (boo'bo) an enlarged and inflamed lymph node in the axilla or groin **tropical b** inflamed lymph nodes along the iliac vessels in LGV

bubonic characterised by bubo **b plague** common type of plague characterised by painful, swollen lymph nodes (buboes) in the axilla, groin or neck

bubonocoele hernia limited to the inguinal canal

bucca (buk'a) the cheek

buccal (buk'al) pertaining to the cheek **b administration** drugs administered by tablet held in the mouth **b smear** scraping of epithelium of oral mucosa for sex chromatin.

buccinator (buk'sina'ter) the main muscle of the cheek

bucket handle fracture a fracture that produces a tear in a semilunar cartilage along the medial side of the knee joint

bucky very soft roentgen rays described by Gustav Bucky, German-born US roentgenologist **b diaphragm** a device consisting of a moving grid that limits the amount of scattered radiation reaching the film. The radiogram gives a better contrast and detail

Budd-Chiari (bud'ke-ar'e) **syndrome** obstruction to the venous outflow of the liver owing to occlusion of the hepatic vein described by Austrian pathologists, George Budd and Hans Chiari

budding an asexual reproduction in which the cell produces a bud-like projection containing chromatin. Later it gets separated and makes an independent existence.

budesonide corticosteroid used by inhalation in asthma

budgerigar a species of parakeet

Buerger's (bur'gerz) **disease** thromboangiitis obliterans, named after Leo Buerger, US urologist. It is a combination of thrombosis, inflammation and obliteration of small and medium sized arteries. The disease begins in distal small arteries and spreads upwards. Lower limbs are commonly affected and occurs in young smokers

Buerger's test a practical test to determine the arterial supply of a limb. It is performed in broad day light. The patient lying on his back, lifts both legs high keeping the knees straight. While legs are supported by the ex-

aminer the patient flexes and extends his ankles and toes to the point of mild fatigue. If the arterial blood supply to the limb is impaired the sole of the foot assumes a cadaveric pallor, the patient is then made to sit and feet lowered. In two or three minutes the affected foot shows a ruddy, cyanotic hue

buffalo hump a deposit of fat in the lower mid-cervical and upper thoracic area of the back characteristically seen in long-standing Cushing's disease

buffer (buf'er) a substance maintaining original hydrogen-ion concentration of its solution upon adding an acid or base

buffy coat a light coloured layer containing white cells appearing in the blood on centrifugation allowing to stand in a test tube. It is found between the red cells settled at the bottom and the plasma forming the top layer

bug an accidental error or fault in a computer programme

build general configuration of the individual **asthenic b** individual giving an exaggerated feature of hyposthenic build **hypersthenic b** short stocky build with a tendency towards obesity. The neck is short and thick, the chest broad and short and a thick abdominal wall **hyposthenic b** tall and thin build, normal shoulders, flat chest, poor development of musculature, underweight, abdominal wall is thin **sthenic b** athletic constitution with good musculature, broad shoulders, flat abdomen and average height

bulb a rounded mass

bulbar pertaining to medulla oblongata **b palsy** motor neuron disease affecting medulla and lower four cranial nerves

bulbourethral glands *see* Cowper glands

bulbitis (bul-bi'tis) inflammation of the bulbous portion of the urethra

bulbus cordis distal end of primitive heart from which outflow tracts of left and right ventricles are formed

bulimarexia (bul'i-marek-sia) binge eating followed by purging the body of the food

bulimia (bu-lim'e-a) episodes of uncontrolled excessive hunger **b nervosa** a psychologic abnormality with bouts of overeating which may or may not be followed by spontaneous or induced vomiting

bulk a substance that absorbs water in the intestinal tract making it into a mass that stimulates peristalsis

bulla (bul'ah) 1. a large vesicle 2. sharply demarcated avascular area in the lung with a wall thickness less than 1 mm and an internal diameter more than 1 cm

bull neck soft tissue oedema of the neck seen in presence of large nodes in the upper part of the neck as in faucial diphtheria

Bull's eye lamp equipment used to illuminate the area in ENT examination along with a head mirror.

bumetanide a potent diuretic

BUN abbreviation for blood urea nitrogen

bundle a collection of fibres **b branch block** a type of heart block in which interruption to the flow of electrical impulses through the right or left bundle of His delays activation of the appropriate ventricle that widens QRS complex and makes alteration in QRS morphology. Right bundle branch block is a common normal variant but,left bundle branch block signifies an underlying heart disease **b of His** a band of atypical cardiac muscle fibres arising from AV node extending along the AV groove to the top of,interventricular septum where it divides into right and left bundle branches, named after Wilhelm His, German physician

bunion (bun'yun) abnormal prominence of the inner aspect of the first metatarsal head

bunionelle prominent head of the fifth metatarsal due to an inflamed bursa

Bunsen burner a gas burner in which air

holes at the bottom of the tube can be closed or opened to adjust the heat produced, designed by Robert Bunsen, German chemist

bunyavirus single strand segmented RNA virus and all of them being arboviruses

buphthalmos (buf-thol'mos) enlargement of whole eye, seen in infantile glaucoma; oxy eye

burette (bu'ret) a special hollow glass tube usually with a stop cock at the lower end

Burgundy red urine a deep red urine produced in porphyria caused by uroporphyrin in the urine

burking murder by compression of chest combined with covering, mouth and nostrils, named after Burke and Hare

Burkitt's lymphoma massive jaw lesions and extranodal abdominal involvement, caused by Epstein-Barr virus. It is characterised by sheets of monotonous small round cells punctuated by a 'stary sky' pattern

burn tissue injury caused by heat, electricity, chemicals, radiation or gases. The effect depends on the type, duration, and intensity of the agent and the part of the body involved. The effect may be local or local and systemic. Superficial burns cause damage to the outer layers of the epidermis (first degree). The damage in second degree burns extends through the epidermis into the dermis. However, it does not interfere with regeneration of the epidermis. Full thickness of the skin including the tissue beneath it is affected in third degree burn. There is destruction of epidermis, dermis and underlying tissues

Burns' (bernz) **space** suprasternal area low in the neck in the middle line, named after Allan Burns, Scottish surgeon

burr (burr) a devise that rotates at high speed, used to cut tooth or bone **b cells** erythrocytes with scalloped margins, may appear in renal failure **b hole** a hole made to relieve pressure inside the skull or to gain access to brain

bursa (bur'sa) a sac filled with a viscid fluid located at the sites of friction and prevents friction between tissues around a moving joint pl. **bursae Anserine b** bursa related to the insertion of the tendons of the gracilis, sartorius and semitendinosus muscles, likened to a goose's foot **psoas b** bursa in the groin beneath inguinal ligament **semimembranosus b** swelling in the medial side of the popliteal space.

bursitis inflammation of a bursa **Achillis b** painful swelling nearer to *os calcis* **infrapatellar b** clergyman's knee. Tenderness and swelling below the patella at the insertion of quadriceps tendon **ischiogluteal b** swelling and tenderness over ischiogluteal bursa, and is detected when the hip is flexed **metatarsal b** pain and swelling situated more anteriorly over the metatarsal heads **olecranon b** a localised swelling over the olecranon **prepatellar b** housemaid's knee; localised pain and swelling in the antero- inferior part of the patella **sub-achilles b** painful swelling bulging out on either side of the Achilles tendon

burst 1. an abrupt onset of a reaction 2. rupture of cell filled with viral progeny **b therapy** administration of a relatively high dose of a drug such as corticosteroids

bursting fracture a fracture in which there is dispersal of bone fragments

Buruli ulcer a deeply penetrating mycobacterial ulcer seen in Buruli region in Uganda, caused by *Mycobacterium ulcerans*

busulphan alkylating cytotoxic agent, used in chronic myeloid leukaemia

butterfly bandage a small piece of adhesive tape with broad wing-shaped ends to hold the edges of a superficial wound together

butterfly fragment a wedge-shaped fragment of a long bone which is split off the main fragments encountered in a comminuted fracture

butterfly needle a short needle with flexible plastic handles that fold for insertion and lay flat for stabilisation with tape; scalp vein needle

butterfly pattern fine diffuse infiltrates that radiate bilaterally from the hilum to the lung periphery in chest radiographs of pulmonary alveolar microlithiasis

butterfly rash a photosensitive facial rash seen in SLE. It consists of an erythematous blush or scaly reddish patches on the malar region extending over nasal bridge

button (but'n) **hole** narrow slit-like orifice **b stenosis** fishmouth stenosis seen in mitral valve stenosis

Butyrophenones group of antipsychotic dopamine antagonists, such as haloperidol

bypass a shunt **b surgery** coronary artery bypass graft

byssinosis (bis'i-no'sis) an occupational lung disease in textile workers exposed to dust of cotton, flax, hemp or jute

byte a unit of computer memory, made up of eight bits. One byte of memory stores a single character

C

C symbol for carbon, centrigrade, Celsius, cervical vertebra, (C1 to C7) kilocalorie, and complement (C1 to C9), the hard drive of a PC on which all programmes and documents are stored

CA - 19-9 a tumour associated antigen, present in tissue associated with mucin and in certain blood groups

CA 125 a cell surface glycoprotein produced by tissues derived from coelomic epithelium and is associated with epithelial cancers such as ovarian cancer, adenocarcinoma of the uterine cervix, gastrointestinal tract and breast

Ca symbol for the element calcium; carcinoma

CABG abbreviation for coronary artery bypass graft

Cabot's (kab'ots) rings blue staining thread like inclusions seen in severe anaemia named after Richard Cabot, U.S. physician

cachectin (ka-kek'tin) tumour necrotic factor alpha released from endotoxin affected macrophages

cachexia (ka-keks'e-a) severe wasting and weakness

cachinnation (kak-i-na'shun) inappropriate loud laughter, may be associated with schizophrenia

CaCl$_2$ caicium chloride

cacogeusia (kak'o-gu'se-a) an unpleasant taste in the mouth

cacosmia (ka-koz'me-a) an unpleasant smell

cacumen (kak-u-men) the anterior part of superior vermis of the cerebellum

CAD abbreviation for coronary artery disease

cadaver (ka-dav'er) a dead body, a corpse, term applied to a body used for dissection

cadaveric spasm persistence of muscle contraction in some cases of sudden death

cadherin membrane glycoprotein specific for Ca++ dependent cell-cell adhesion molecules needed for tissue differentiation

cadherin (kad-herin) gene on chromosome 16 necessary for cell-cell attachment. Dysfunction of cell-cell adhesion system is involved in cancer invasion and metastasis

cadmium metallic element used in many alloys and plating, inhalation of the fumes may lead to fever, albuminuria and fibrosis of the lung

cadeceus (ka-du'se-us) a staff belonging to Apollo according to Greek mythology. It consists of two serpents entwined around a staff, surmounted by two wings

caecal (se'kal) pertaining to the caceum

c cell calcitonin-secreting cell of thyroid

c tumour calcitonin secreting tumour of thyroid

caecotomy (se-kot'o-me) an incision into caecum

caecum (se'kum) a blind pouch forming the first part of the large intestine, located below the entrance of ileum at the ileocaecal valve. Vermiform appendix is at its lower end

ceruloplasmin copper carrying alpha-2 globulin of blood

caesarian (se-sar'e-an) birth caesarian section

caesarian hysterectomy caesarian section immediately followed by hysterectomy

caesarian section removal of foetus from the gravid uterus by the abdominal route after 28th week of gestation. Julius Caeser was born so, hence the name

cafe'au lait macules pale brown areas of increased epidermal melanocytes and melanin in the skin. Often seen in neurofibromatosis

cafe coronary complete upper airway obstruction by a bolus of food with occlusion of both the oesophagus and larynx. The symptoms simulate a myocardial infarction

caffeine (kaf'en) an alkaloid present in coffee, chocolate, tea and cola drinks. It stimulates central nervous system, gastric secretion and raises free fatty acids in plasma. It acts by increasing the activity of beta-2 adrenoreceptors

Cain complex *psy* a destructive sibling rivalry in which one of the sibs resents the other for perceived favouritism from a parent, named after biblical Cain son of Adam and Eve, who killed his brother Abel

Cairn's syndrome hydrocephalus following tuberculous meningitis, named after H. Cairn, British neurologist

Caisson's disease a clinical complex caused by rapid body decompression with intravascular boiling of 'nitrogen' noted in Scuba divers, workers in high pressure environment and high-altitude pilots. It is characterised by headache, nausea, vomiting, vertigo, tinnitus, dyspnoea, convulsions and shock; decompression sickness

calabar swellings transient subcutaneous swellings of *Loa loa*

calamine (kal'a-min) a pink powder containing zinc oxide used externally in various skin conditions as a soothening agent. It is protective and astringent

calamus scriptorius the inferior portion of the floor of the fourth ventricle of the brain which is shaped like a pen. It is present between the restiform bodies

calcaneal spur a sharp spur projecting forwards from tuberosity of the calcaneum

calcaneoapophysitis (kal-ka'ne-o-a-pof'e-zi-tis) pain and inflammation of the posterior portion of the calcaneus at

the place of insertion of the Achilles tendon

calcaneocuboid (kal-ka'ne-o-ku'boyd) pertaining to the calcaneus and cuboid bone

calcaneodynia (kal-ka'ne-o-din'e-a) pain in the heel

calcaneofibular (kal-ka'ne-o-fib'u-lar) pertaining to the calcaneus and fibula

calcaneonavicular (kal-ka'ne-o-na-vik'u-lar) pertaining to the calcaneus and navicular bone

calcaneoscaphoid (kal-ka'ne-o-ska'foyd) pertaining to the calcaneus and scaphoid bone

calcaneotibial (kal-ka'ne-o-tib'e-al) pertaining to the calcaneus and tibia

calcaneum (kal-ka'ne-um) calcaneus

calcaneus (kal-ka-ne-us) the heel bone that articulates with cuboid bone and with the talus

calcaneodynia (kal-ka-ne-o-din'e-a) pain in the heel when standing or walking

calcar (kal'kar) a spur-like process

calcareous (kal-ka're-us) chalky

calcarine (kal-kar-in) spur-shaped

calcariuria (kal- kar'e-u're-a) the presence of calcium salts in the urine

calcicosis (kal'si-ko'sis) pneumoconiosis produced by inhalation of dust from limestone

calciferol (kal-sif'er-ol) vitamin D2 a synthetic preparation used in the treatment of vitamin D deficiency and hypocalcaemic tetany

calcification (kal'si-fi-ka'shun) deposition of calcium salts in body tissues and making them hard **arterial c** deposition of calcium in the arterial walls **dystrophic c** process of deposition of calcium and other minerals in the cellular debris **eggshell c** presence of shell-like calcification in the periphery of the lymph nodes, seen in hilar lymph nodes in silicosis **metastatic c** calcification of soft tissue with transference of calcium from bone **Monckeberg's c** deposition of calcium in the media of arteries **rice grain c**

multiple, small, ovoid calcifications resembling grains of rice in the soft tissues, may be seen in cysticercosis

calcific tendinitis deposition of calcium in a chronically inflamed tendon

calcination (kal'si-na'shun) drying by roasting to produce a powder

calcineurin a protein found in CNS which binds both Ca++ and calmodulin, inhibiting the latter's activity.

calcinosis (kal'si-no'sis) a condition characterised by abnormal deposition of calcium salts in tissues **c circumscripta** subcutaneous calcification **tumoral c** soft tissue calcification that usually involves the periarticular tissues

calcipaenia (kal'si-pe'ne-a) calcium deficiency in body tissues and fluids

calciphylaxis (kal-si-fil'ax-is) vascular calcification in the tunica media inducing painful violaceous skin lesions

calciprivia (kal'si-priv'e-a) deficiency of calcium

calcitonin (kal'si-to'nin) a thyroid hormone necessary to maintain a dense, strong bone matrix and to regulate the level of calcium in the blood **C-gene related peptide** CGRP, a regulatory peptide of CNS and lung

calcitriol a vitamin D metabolite promoting absorption of calcium and phosphate in the intestine and their deposition in the bone tissues

calcium (kal'se-um) lime, Ca. a metallic element atomic number 20, atomic weight 20, a major component of limestone. Calcium phosphate forms 75% of body ash and 85% of mineral matter in bones. Calcium gives firmness and rigidity to bones and teeth, and is necessary for blood coagulation, enzyme activation and acid-base balance. It is necessary for lactation, neuromuscular functions, and membrane permeability. Milk and milk products, and fish are good dietary sources of calcium **c carbonate** tasteless, odourless powder of precipitated chalk used as antacid and as an anti-

dote to corrosive acid poisoning **c chloride** solution of calcium salt, used to raise calcium level of the blood. It is administered intravenously in conditions like hypocalcaemic tetany **c cyclamate** an artificial sweetening agent **c gluconate** odourless and tasteless calcium powder **c glycerophosphate** calcium salt of glycerophosphoric acid used as a dietary supplement and in drug formulations **c hydroxide** white powder used as an astringent, and cavity liner **c lactate** a white odourless and tasteless powder **c oxalate** crystalline calcium **c oxide** a corrosive mineral **c phosphate** a white amorphous powder used as an antacid in gastric hyperacidity **c saccharin** an artificial sweetener

calcium channel blocker any of a group of drugs that slow the influx of calcium ions into muscle cells resulting in diminution of arterial resistance and myocardial oxygen demand. The preparations are used to treat angina, hypertension and supraventricular tachycardia

calciuria (kal'se-u're-a) calcium in the urine

calcospherite (kal'ko-sfe'rit) one of many small calcareous bodies found in tumours, nervous tissue, thyroid and prostate

calculogenesis (kal'ku-lo-jen'e-sis) formation of calculi

calculus (kal'ku-lus) pl **calculi**. any abnormal concretion, commonly referred to as a stone found within the body. It is composed of mineral salts and may occur in urinary and biliary systems and as a hard deposit on the teeth **biliary c** gall stone, cholelith. Composed of cholesterol. Bilirubin or calcium may be deposited in such stones **dental c** calcium deposits on teeth **haemic c** a stone formed from coagulated blood **pancreatic c** a stone in the pancreas, formed of calcium carbonate **renal c** a renal stone found in the kidney that may block urinary flow **salivary c** a calculus in the salivary duct especially that of the submandibular gland noted while eating **urinary c** a stone in any part of the urinary system **vesical c** a stone in the bladder

calefacient (kal'e-fe'shent) conveying a sense of warmth when applied to a part of the body

calender method a form of periodic abstinence in which the variable lengths of a woman's menstrual cycle are used to calculate her fertile period

calf (kaf) the fleshy muscular part of the back of the leg formed by the gastrocnemius and soleus muscles

caliber (kal'i-ber) the diameter of any orifice, tube or canal

calibration (kal-i-bra'shun) 1. determination of accuracy of an instrument by comparison with a known standard or an instrument known to be accurate

calibrator (kal'i-bra'tor) an instrument for measuring the inside diameter of tubes or orifices

caliceal (kal'i-se'al) pertaining to a calix

calicectasis (kal'i-sek'ta-sis) dilatation of the renal calyx

calicivirus (kal-is'i-virus) virus causing epidemic viral gastroenteritis

caliculus (ka-lik'u-lus) a cup-shaped structure **c gustatorius** a taste bud **c ophthalmicus** the optic cup

caliectasis (kal'e-ek'ta-sis) dilatation of the renal calyx

caligo (ka-li'go) dimness of vision

caliper (kal'i-per) 1. an instrument to measure the diameters of solids, such as those of arm or pelvis 2. weight bearing splints that permit walking

calisthenics (kal'is-then'iks) an exercise programme to develop a range of motion and strength needed for such movement

caliomania (kal'o-ma'ne-a) 1. belief in one's own beauty 2. an unrealistic attraction to something only because of beauty

CALLA common acute lymphocytic leukaemia antigen, a marker of childhood acute lymphocyte leukaemia and B cell lymphoma

callosal (ka-lo'sal) pertaining to corpus callosum

callosity (ka-los'i-te) a circumscribed thickened and hypertrophied horny layer of the skin. It occurs on the flexor surfaces of hands and feet and is caused by friction or pressure

callosum (ka-lo'sum) the great commissure between the cerebral hemispheres

callus (kal'us) 1. callosity 2. the osseous material woven across and around the ends of a fractured bone that is ultimately replaced by true bone in the healing process. 2. keratotic thickening of skin

calmative (kal'ma-tiv) sedative or soothing

Calmette-Guerin bacillus BCG attenuated bovine tubercle bacilli which have lost their virulence after repeated subcultures and are used for vaccination to protect against tuberculosis named after Albert Calmette and Camille Guerin, French bacteriologists

calomel (kal'o-mel) mercurous chloride

calmodulins intracellular proteins that combine with calcium and activate a variety of cellular processes

calor (ka'lor) heat

caloris (kal-o'rez) **bursa**. The bursa found between the arch of the aorta and trachea, named after Luigi Calori, Italian anatomist

caloric (ka-lor'ik) relating to heat or to a calorie **c test** a procedure to evaluate vestibular function in patients complaining of dizziness or imbalance while standing or loss of hearing using thermic stimuli to induce endolymphatic flow in the horizontal semicircular canal. Each ear is irrigated with warm water for 30 seconds followed by irrigation with cold water while the patient is supine. There is nystagmus to the side of irrigation with warm water and to the opposite side with cold water

calorie 120

calorie (kal'o-re) a unit of energy content of foods or the amount of energy expended by an organism. **large c** Kcl. The amount of heat required to change the temperature of 1 Kg of water from 14.5°C to 15.5°C. **small c** cal. The amount of heat required to change the temperature of 1 gram of water

calorifacient (ka-lor'i-fa'shent) producing heat

calorific (kal'o-rif'ik) producing heat

calorigenic (ka-lor'i-jen'ik) pertaining to the production of heat or energy

calorimeter (kal'o-rim'e-ter) an instrument to determine the amount of heat exchanged in a chemical reaction or by the animal body in specific conditions

calorimetry (kal'o-rim'e-tre) the determination of heat loss or gain

Calot's (kal-oz) triangle a triangle formed by the cystic artery superiorly, the cystic duct inferiorly and the hepatic duct medially, a dangerous area in cholecystectomy named after Jean-Francois Calot, French surgeon

calvaria (kal'va're-a) the dome-like superior portion of the cranium composed of the superior portions of the frontal, parietal and occipital bones, and covered by the scalp

Calve-Perthes (kal-va'per'taz) disease aseptic necrosis of the epiphysis of the head of the femur, named after Jacques Calve, French orthopaedic surgeon and Georg Perthes, German surgeon

calx (kal'ks) 1. lime 2. the heel

calyciform (ka-lis'i-form) cup-shaped

calymmatobacterium granulomatis (kalim'ma-to-bak-te're-um) a Gram-negative bacillus that causes granuloma inguinale

calyx (ka'lix) pl. calyces 1. any cup-like organ or cavity 2. a cup-like extension of the renal pelvis that encloses the papilla of a renal pyramid

CAM abbreviation for complementary and alternative medicine

camel back curve double quotidian febrile spikes seen in gonococcal endocarditis, measles and visceral leishmaniasis

camera (kam'er-a) a chamber or cavity

cAMP abbreviation for cyclic adenosine monophosphate

Campbell de Morgan spots raspberry red spots that do not blanch on stretching the skin, named after Campbell de Morgan, English surgeon

camphor (kam'for) an antipruritic agent

campimeter (kamp-im'e-ter) a device measuring the field of vision

campimetry (kamp-im'e-tre) perimetry

campodactylia (kamp'to-dak-til'e-a) flexion deformity of the fingers or toes

Campylobacter (kam'pi-lo-bak'ter) a gram-negative, motile, spirally curved, rod-shaped bacteria of the family Spirillaceae, reclassified as helicobacter

canal (ka-nal) a narrow tubular passage or channel **adductor c** a triangular space between the adductor longus and vastas medialis muscles. It extends from the apex of the femoral triangle to the popliteal space. It transmits femoral vessels and the saphenous nerve **alimentary c** the digestive tract from the mouth to the anus **alveolar c** one of the several canals in the maxilla that transmit the posterior superior alveolar blood vessels and nerves to the upper teeth **anal c** the terminal portion of the rectum opening at the anus **birth c** the passage way consisting of the cervix, vagina and vulva through which the foetus passes during delivery. **bony semicircular c** one of the several canals located in the bony labyrinth of the internal ear. It encloses the semicircular ducts that open into the vestibule. They are enclosed within the petrous portion of temporal bone **carotid c** a canal in the petrous portion of the temporal bone that transmits the internal carotid artery to the cranial cavity **central c** a small canal in the middle of the spinal cord **cervical c** a canal in the cervix of the uterus extending from the internal os to the external os **condylar c** a canal in the occipital bone for passage of emissary vein from transverse sinus and it opens anterior to the occipital condyle **c of Lambert** one of several bronchioalveolar communications in the lung **craniopharyngeal c** a canal in the foetal sphenoid bone that contains the stalk of Rathke's pouch **ethmoidal c** one of two grooves lying between the ethmoid and frontal bones. The anterior ethmoidal canal transmits the anterior ethmoidal vessels and nasociliary nerve and posterior ethmoidal vessels and nasociliary nerve are transmitted through posterior ethmoidal canal **external auditory c** external auditory meatus transmitting the sound waves **facial c** canal in the internal acoustic meatus of temporal bone transmitting the facial nerve **femoral c** *see* femoral **gastric c** a longitudinal groove on the lesser curvature of the stomach **haversian c** 1. one of the many minute canals found in compact bone each surrounded by lamellae of bone. Contains blood vessels, lymphatics, nerves and sometimes marrow, constitutes haversian system 2. a canal in the mandible that carries a neurovascular bundle to the teeth **hyaloid c** a canal in the vitreous body of the eye which serves as a lymph channel in foetus **hypoglossal c** a canal in the occipital bone transmitting hypoglossal nerve and a branch of the posterior meningeal artery **incisive c** a short canal in the maxillary bone transmitting nasopalatine nerve and the branches of great palatine arteries to the nasal fossa **infraorbital c** a canal in the maxilla lying in the floor of the orbit transmitting the infraorbital nerve and artery **internal auditory c** a canal in the petrous portion of the temporal bone that transmits the acoustic and facial nerves and the acoustic artery **intestinal c** the alimentary canal from pyloric opening to the anus **lacrimal c**

lacrimal duct **mandibular c** a canal in the mandible that transmits the inferior alveolar blood vessels and nerve to the teeth **maxillary c** alveolar canal **nasolacrimal c** canal lying between the lacrimal bone and inferior nasal conchae containing the nasolacrimal duct **nutrient c** opening on the surface of compact bone through which blood vessels reach medullary cavity of long bones **obturator c** an opening in the obturator membrane of the hip bone that transmits the obturator vessels and nerve **pharyngeal c** canal between the sphenoid and palatine bones that transmits branches of the sphenopalatine vessels **portal c** area between adjoining liver lobules consisting of connective tissue and interlobular branches of the hepatic artery, portal vein and bile duct **pterygoid c** a canal of the sphenoid bone transmitting the pterygoid vessels and nerve **pterygopalatine c** a canal between the maxillary and palatine bones that transmit the descending palatine nerve and artery **pudendal c** a canal on the pelvic surface of the obturator internus muscle that transmits pudendal vessels, named after Alcock Pudend **root c** passage in the root of a tooth through which nerve and blood vessels pass **sacral c** a cavity within the sacrum **semicircular c** one of several canals located in the bony labyrinth of the internal ear. It encloses superior, posterior and lateral semicircular ducts that open into the vestibule. They are found within the petrous portion of the temporal bone **spinal c** vertebral canal **spiral c of cochlea** bony labyrinth of the inner ear containing a spiral tube of 30mm long that makes a two and three quarters turn about a central bony axis. It contains the scala tympani, scala vestibuli and cochlear duct **uterine c** the cavity of uterus **vaginal c** the cavity of the vagina **vertebral c** the cavity formed by the foramina of the vertebral column that contains the spinal cord and its meninges **Volkmann's c** small canal found in bone through which blood vessels pass from periosteum

canaliculus (kan'a-lik'u-lus) pl **canaliculi** a small channel or canal

canalis (ka-na'lis) pl **canales** canal

canalisation (kan'al-i-za-shun) formation of channels in tissue

cancellous (kan'sol-us) having a reticular or latticework structure as the spongy tissue of bone

cancellous (kan-cel'us) a bony plate composed of cancellous bone

cancer (kan'ser) any of a group of diseases caused by unrestricted multiplication of cells in an organ or tissue that can spread throughout the body **c grading** degree of cancer cell differentiation **c screening** a program to detect cancer in its asymptomatic stage **c staging** extent of dissemination of cancer. T (tumour), N (regional extension to nodes), M (metastases) classification is used in staging of cancer according to size, and spread.

cancerous (kan'ser-us) pertaining to malignant growth

cancroid (kang' kroyd) 1. like a cancer 2. a type of keloid 3. epithelioma

cancrum (kang' krum) a rapidly spreading ulcer **c oris** gangrene-like lesions in the mouth in malnourished children caused by *Borrelia vincenti*

CANDA abbreviation used for computer-associated new drug application

Candida (kan'di-da) a genus of yeasts that develops a pseudomycelium and reproduces by budding. They form part of normal flora of the mouth formerly called monilia. *C. albicans* a small oral budding fungus, causative agent of candidiasis.

candidemia presence of Candida in the blood

candidiasis (kan'di-di'a-sn) thrush. any organ of the body can be invaded by candida, but vaginal and oral thrush are the common forms **cutaneous c**

occurs in intertriginous areas **chronic mucocutaneous c** occurs in children with T cell defect characterised by hyperkeratotic plaque-like lesions on the skin and endocrinopathies **oropharyngeal c** white plaques of fungus on the pharynx and palate. Rare in healthy, complicates treatment with broad-spectrum antibiotics, oral and inhaled corticosteroids and is found when immunity is defective. It may spread to the oesophagus and lung **vaginal c** dysuria, white, thick, ' cheesy' odourless discharge and irritation with inflammation of vulva and cervix

candle (kan'dl) a solid mass of combustible material **c fiame sign** Doppler colour flow imaging in mitral stenosis. There is a central blue colour corresponding to a zone of high velocity surrounded by a yellow-orange blush corresponding to turbulent zone of lower blood flow **c jar** simple device to produce an anaerobic environment

C and S culture and sensitivity. Isolation of potentially pathogenic bacteria, followed by antibiotic susceptibility testing

canine (ka'nin) pertaining to a dog **c tooth** any of the four teeth found between incisors and molars in upper and lower jaw

canities (kan-ish'e-ez) whiteness of hair

canker sore a small painful sore that occurs in the mouth; aphthous ulcer

cannabis (kan'a-bis) Marijuana

cannibalism the human consumption of human flesh

cannon 'a' wave an abnormal jugular venous pressure curve with an accentuated 'a' wave of sufficient intensity due to reduced right ventricular compliance, tricuspid stenosis or arrhythmia in which the atrium contracts against a closed or stenosed tricuspid valve

cannon ball metastases, one or many large, well-circumscribed metastatic nodules within the lungs seen in renal cell carcinoma

cannon sound the intensity of the first heart sound varies from beat to beat in complete heart block. The explosive sound is not synchronous with cannon waves

cannula (kan'u-la) a tube or sheath enclosing a trocar; a thin, flexible tube inserted into the body to withdraw or introduce fluids

cannulate (kan'u-lat) to introduce a cannula through a passage way

cantharides (kan-thar'i-dez) dried insects of species *Cantharis vesicatoria*, counter-irritant and vesicant

canthus (kan':hus) pl **canthi**. The angle at either end of the slit between the eyelids

CaO₂ the content of oxygen in arterial blood

cap (kap) a covering **knee c** patella

capacitance (ka-pas'i-tens) the ability to store an electrical charge

capacitation (ka-pasii-ta'shun) the process occurring in the female reproductive tract that enables the sperm to fertilise the ova

capacity 1. an ability to contain 2. an ability to perform mentally **closing c** cc. Lung volumes at which the closing of airways is detected during a slow expiration **forced vital c** FVC. The maximal volume of air expelled with force and speed following a maximal inspiration **functional residual c** FRC, gas volume in the lungs after a normal expiration. It is measured by a gas dilution method or body plethysmography. **maximum breathing c** MBC, the maximum volume of airflow can be breathed in and out of the lung in one minute **total lung c** TLC, the gas volume of the lung at the end of full inspiration. It is the sum of the residual volume and the vital capacity measured by gas dilution method **vital c** VC, the maximal volume of air which can be inspired after a complete expiration

CAPD abbreviation for continuous ambulatory peritoneal dialysis

capeline (kap'e-lin) a bandage used for the head or for the stump of an amputated limb

capillarectasia (kap'i-lar'ek-ta'se-a) distension of the capillary vessel.

capillary (kap'i-lar'e) pl **capillaries** any of the tiny blood vessels that connect the ends of the arterioles with the beginnings of the venules **c permeability** the ability of a substance to diffuse through capillary walls into tissue spaces

capital (cap'i-tal) pertaining to the head

capitate (kap'i-tat) head-shaped

capitatum (kap'i-ta-tum) the head bone in the distal row of the carpus

capitellum (kap'i-tel'um) the round eminence at the lower end of the humerus articulating with the radius

capitulum (ka-pit'u-lum) pl **capitula** a small rounded articular end of a bone.

Caplan's syndrome miners with rheumatoid arthritis are especially prone to rheumatoid nodules within the lung, named after Anthony Caplan, British physician, who worked in Kolar Gold Field Hospital, India

Capnocytophage a genus of gram-negative facultative, anaerobic bacteria found in oral cavity which may cause systemic infection in asplenic patients

capnography continuous recording of the carbon dioxide level in exhaled air in mechanically ventilated patients.

capnophilic (kap-no-fil'ik) referring to bacteria that grow best in an atmosphere containing carbon dioxide

capotement (ka-pot-ment) a splashing sound that may be heard when the dilated stomach contains air and fluid

capping (kap'ing) 1. placing a protective substance over the exposed pulp of a teeth 2. placing an artificial crown on a tooth for cosmetic purpose. 3. induction of a person into nursing profession

capreomycin a weak antituberculosis drug administered parenterally in drug resistant cases of tuberculosis. It has cross resistance with kanamycin and viomycin

capsicum (kap'si-kum) the fruit of pepper plant.

capsid (kap'sid) the protein covering of a virus that is composed of protein subunits known as capsomers

capsomer (kap'so-mer) short ribbons of protein that make up a portion of the capsid of a virus

capsula pl. capsulae a covering around an organ or structure; a sheath

capsular pertaining to a capsule

capsule 1. a sheath 2. a special container made of gelatin, to dispense a single dose of a drug glomerular c the glomerular capsule of the kidneys, named after Bowman joint c the sleeve-like membrane that encloses the bony ends in a diarthrodial joint. It consists of an outer fibrous layer and an inner synovial layer and contains synovial fluid lens c a transparent, structureless membrane that surrounds and encloses the lens of the eye

capsulectomy (kap'su-lek'to-me) surgical removal of capsule

capsulitis (kap'su-li'tis) inflammation of a capsule

capsuloplasty (kap'su-lo-pas'te) plastic surgery of a capsule, espcially a joint capsule

capsulorrhaphy (kap'su-lor'a-fe) suture of a joint capsule

capsulotome (kap'su-lo-tom) an instrument for incising the capsule of crystalline lens

capsulotomy (kap'su-ot'o-me) cutting of a capsule of the lens or a joint

captopril an antihypertensive agent that blocks the conversion of angiotensin I to angiotensin II.

caput (ka'put) the head c madusae a plexus of dilated veins radiating from the umbilicus as an evidence of obstruction to the portal venous system c succedaneum oedematous s velling of the foetal scalp that crosses the suture lines

carbamazepine (kar-ba-maz'e-pen) a drug used in the treatment of trigeminal neuralgia and temporal lobe epilepsy

carbenicillin (kar'ben-i-sil'in) a semi-synthetic penicillin

carbidopa (kar'bi-do'pa) decarboxylase inhibitor with levodopa in the treatment of Parkinsonism

carbimazole an imidazole derivative, antithyroid used in the treatment of thyrotoxicosis

carbohydrate (kar'bo-hi'drat) one of a group of chemical substances, including glucose, glycogen, starches, dextrines and celluloses, that contain only carbon, oxygen and hydrogen. Proximate principle needed by the body and is the main source of energy

carbolise (kar'bol-iz) to add carbolic acid

carbon non-metallic element, an important constituent of organic compounds

carbonate (kar'bon-at) any salt of carbonic acid.

carbon dioxide CO_2 final metabolic product of carbon as a colourless and odourless gas compound present in food. It is eliminated through the lungs mostly and a small amount in the urine and sweat c.d. combining power the amount of CO_2 that the blood serum can hold in chemical combination CO_2 in aqueous solution forms carbonic acid c.d. solid therapy snow used for therapeutic refrigeration

carbonaemia (kar'bo-ne'mea) an excess accumulation of carbonic acid in the blood

carbonic pertaining to carbon c acid H_2CO_3, an acid resulting from a mixture of CO_2 and water c anhydrase an enzyme that catalyses union of CO_2 with water to form carbonic acid

carbon monoxide CO, a poisonous gas resulting from the inefficient and incomplete combustion of coal. It is colourless, odourless and tasteless making it difficult to detect by senses. c.m. poisoning causes impairment of consciousness, hypertonia and hyper reflexia, coma, focal neurologic damage, myocardial ischaemia, and cardiac arrhythmias, treated with 100%

oxygen with mechanical ventilation

carbon tetrachloride CCl_4, a clear colourless liquid having an etheral odour. It is toxic causing acute atrophy of the liver and kidney

carbonyl (kar'bon-il) the divalent radical of carbon monoxide.

carboplatin a platinum containing cytotoxic agent used in treatment of ovarian cancer

carboxyhaemoglobin (kar-bok'si-he'moglo'bin) a compound formed by union of carbon monoxide and haemoglobin

carboxyhaemoglobulinaemia the presence of carboxyhaemoglobin in the blood

carboxyl (kar-bok'sil) COOH group of organic carboxylic acids

carboxylase (kar-bok'si-las) an enzyme that catalyses the removal of carboxyl group from amino acids

carboxylation replacement of hydrogen by a carboxyl molecule.

carbuncle (kar'bung'kl) large multilocular boil of the skin and deeper tissues. It terminates in a slough and suppuration. It is associated with systemic manifestations

carbutamide (kar-bu'ta-mid) an oral hypoglycaemic agent

carcass (kar'kas) a dead body, term applied to that of animals and insects

carcinoembryonic antigen CEA a glycoprotein of foetal endoderm, may be found elevated, may indicate recurrence of certain type of cancers

carcinogen (kar-sin'o-jen) any substance or agent that produces cancer or increases the risk of development of cancer

carcinogenesis (kar-cin'o-jen'e-sis) the production of cancer

carcinogenic (kar-cin'o-jen'ik) producing cancer

carcinoid (kar'si-noid) a tumour arising from argentaffin cells found in the intestine, and branchus. It is associated with secretion of serotonin **c syndrome** a symptom complex caused by carcinoids arising from the enterochromaffin system, most common in the ileum whose metastases to the liver release vasoactive substances such as serotonin, bradykinin, histamine, and prostaglandin. It presents with cutaneous flushing, diarrhoea, small bowel obstruction, bronchospasm, endocardial fibrosis involving the right sided cardiac valves and right ventricular wall leading to heart failure

carcinoma (kar'si-no'ma) a malignant tumour arising from cells in the surface layer or lining membrane of an organ. They tend to infiltrate and metastasise to distant organs or parts of the body **alveolar cell c** a variety of lung cancer **basal cell c** skin malignancy that rarely metasises **bronchogenic c** a malignant tumour orginating in the branchus. The examples are squamous cell carcinoma, adenocarcinoma, small cell carcinoma and large cell carcinoma **c in situ** malignant cell changes noted in the epithelial tissue that do not extend beyond the basement membrane **c encuirasse** a markedly indurated carcinoma involving a broad expanse of skin and subcutaneous breast tissue that is covered by papules and nodules progressing into morphea-like plaques **chorionic c** choriocarcinoma **epidermoid c** a tumour on surface, such as the skin or bronchus. **giant cell c** a tumour characterised by presence of unusually large cells **glandular c** adenocarcinoma **medullary c** a soft tumour composed of cells with little fibrous tissue **mucinous c** malignant tumour in which the glandular tissue secretes mucin **oat cell c** a variety of poorly differentiated small cell carcinoma that contains small oat-shaped cells **scirrhous c** hard carcinoma **squamous cell c** an epidermoid carcinoma developing from squamous cells

carcinomatosis (kar'si-no'ma-to'sis) a preterminal condition characterised by widespread dissemination of carcinoma in the body

carcinosarcoma (kar'si-no-sar-ko'ma) a malignant tumour containing elements of both carcinoma and sarcoma. These highly aggressive tumours are carcinomas and the cells display sarcoma-like spindling

cardamom dried ripe fruit of *Eleltaria cardamomum* used as a carminative and aromatic

cardia (kar'de-a) 1. junction of upper part of the stomach and oesophagus 2. heart

cardiac (kar'de-ak) 1. pertaining to the heart 2. pertaining to the cardia. **c ablation** a technique for correcting abnormal heart rhythms by destroying the tissue within the heart responsible for setting the faulty pace **c arrhythmia** an abnormality of cardiac rhythm. It may be in the form of bradycardia or tachycardia **c aneurysm** stretching of fibrotic area due to earlier myocardial infarction **c arrest** sudden stoppage of pumping action of the heart requiring institution of basic life support followed by advanced life support measures: sudden death due to cardiac causes **c asthma** dyspnoea and wheeze from bronchial endothelial oedema in left ventricular failure **c cachexia** loss of lean body mass that occurs in some patients with moderate to severe heart failure **c catheterisation** percutaneous intravascular insertion of a catheter into any chamber of the heart to monitor its function and to inject a contrast medium for imaging **c compensation** the ability of the heart to compensate for impaired function of the valves through the reserve power **c cirrhosis** hepatocellular atrophy, centrilobular necrosis and extensive fibrosis caused by repeated and/ or prolonged congestive heart failure **c enzymes** a group of three enzymes CPK (its isoenzyme CK-MB), AST and LDH which rise and fall in the same order over a period of weeks following myocardial infarction **c glycoside** a drug used in the treatment of rhythm disorders or heart failure **c failure** a condition resulting from the inability of the heart to pump sufficient amount of blood to meet the demands of the tissues. It may be high output failure when the demands are excessive as in thyrotoxicosis and anaemia or low output failure when the heart itself is defective, following myocardial infarction **c hormones** *see* atrial natriuretic peptides **c hypertrophy** enlargement of the heart **c index** cardiac output in litres per minute body surface area in sq. metres. **c insufficiency** inadequate cardiac output due to failure of the heart to function properly as in valvular abnormalities **c massage** rhythmic strong pressure on the lower end of sternum in cardiac arrest **c output** the amount of blood discharged from the left or right ventricles per minute **c plexus** the nerve plexus at the base of the heart with the branches of the vagus nerves and sympathetic trunks. It provides nerve supply to the heart **c reflex** an involuntary response of alteration in heart rate following stimulation of sensory nerve endings in the wall of the carotid sinus which slows the heart rate, and stimulation of vagus fibres by increased venous return resulting in increased heart rate **c reserve** the capacity of the heart to increase its output to meet the body requirement **c siphon** the intracavernous and supraclinoid segments of the internal carotoid artery **transplantation** transplantation of the heart in younger patients with severe intractable heart failure whose life expectancy is less than six months **troponin** a protein that is highly sensitive and specific indicator of myocardial infarction **c troponin T** a muscle protein whose presence can be detected in the blood following myocardial infarction. It is a rapid test to indicate myocardial damage at a very early stage

cardiectasis (kar'de-ek-ta'sis) dilatation of the heart

cardiectomy (kar'de-ek'to-me) excision of the cardiac end of the stomach

cardinal of primary importance.

cardio- combining form meaning heart

cardioactive (kar'de-o-ak'tiv) acting on the heart

cardioangiology (kar'de-o-an'je-ol'o-je) the science of the heart and blood vessels

cardiochalasia (kar'de-o-ka-la'ze-a) relaxation of the mucles of the cardiac sphincter of the stomach

cardiodilator (kar'de-o-di'la-tor) a device used in dilatation of the gastrooesophageal junction

cardio oesophageal pertaining to the junction of oesophagus and the stomach. **c reflux** regurgitation of contents of the stomach into the oesophagus

cardiogenic (kar'de-o-jen'ik) originating in the heart **c shock** a life threatening reduction of blood flow that results from a heart attack or pulmonary embolism

cardiogram (kar'de-o-gram) a graph of the electrical activity of the heart muscle obtained from an electrocardiograph machine

cardiograph (kar'de-o-graf) a device for registering the electrical activity of the heart muscle

cardioinhibitory (kar'de-o-in-hib'i-to-re) inhibiting the action of the heart

cardiolipin a phospholipid of mammalian heart with antigenic determinants similiar to *Treponema pallidum*, used in serologic tests. for syphilis

cardiologist (kar-de-ol'o-jist) a physician specialised in the treatment of heart diseases

cardiology (kar-de-ol'o-je) the study of pathophysiology, diagnosis and treatment of heart diseases

cardiolysis (kar-de-ol'i-sis) an operative procedure to seperate adhesions constricting the heart

cardiomalacia (kar-de-o-ma-la'she-a) softening of the heart muscle

cardiomegaly (kar-de-o-meg'a-le) enlargement of the heart which occurs in disorders that cause the heart to work harder than normal

cardiomyopathy (kar'de-o-mi-op'a-the) any disease that affects the heart muscle **alcoholic c** development of cardiomyopathy in the alcoholics who consume large quantites of alcholic beverages **dilated c** an impaired ventricular contraction leading to progressive left sided, and later right sided heart failure. Arrhythmia, thromboembolism and sudden death are common **hypertrophic c** a familial disorder characterised by inappropriate and elaborate ventricular hypertrophy with malalignment of the myocardial fibres. The hypertrophy may be generalised or confined to interventricular septum or apex **obliterative c** impaired ventricular filling as the ventricles are 'stiff'. The atrial pressure rises and there is atrial hypertrophy, dilatation and later atrial fibrillation **puerperal c** deterioration of cardiac status with successive pregnancies and development of cardiomyopathy during later stages of pregnancy or during puerperium **restrictive c** obliterative cardiomyopathy

cardiomyopexy (kar'de-o-mi'o-pek'se) surgical fixation of a vascular structure such as pectoral muscle to the cardiac muscle or pericardium to improve the blood supply to the myocardium

cardiomyotomy surgical treatment for achalasia cardia wherein the muscles surrounding the cardioesophageal junction are cut

cardioplegia (kar'de-o-ple'je-a) temporary arrest of cardiac function by hypothermia, medication or electrical stimuli to reduce the need of oxygen by heart muscle during surgery requiring cardio- pulmonary bypass

cardiopulmonary (kar'de-o-pul'mo-ner-e) pertaining to the heart and lungs

arrest sudden stoppage of ventilation and circulation **c bypass** provision of an extracorporeal device like a heart-lung machine to pump blood while a surgical procedure being carried on the heart **c endurance** ability of the heart, lungs and blood vessels to process and transport oxygen required by the muscle cells so that they can sustain aerobic energy production **c resuscitation** CPR. The process of ventilating and maintaining the circulation for a patient in cardiopulmonary arrest by combining mouth-to-mouth breathing with external chest compressions

cardiopyloric (kar′de-o-i-lor′ik) pertaining to the cardiac and pyloric ends of the stomach

cardiorrhexis (kar′de-o-rek′sis) rupture of the heart

cardiospasm (kar′de-o-spasm) disordered motor function of the distal end of the oesophagus and failure of the oesophageal orifice of the stomach to relax

cardiothoracic ratio width of heart as a percentage of width of chest inside the ribs. The transverse diameter of the heart should be less than 50% of the width of bony thorax. The ratio is higher in cardiomegaly

cardiotomy (kar′de-ot′o-me) incision of the heart

cardiovalvulitis (kar′de-o-val′vu-li-tis) inflammation of the cardiac valves

cardiovalvulotome (kar′de-o-val′vu-lo-tom) an instrument used in excision of a part of the cardiac valve

cardiovascular (kar′de-o-vas′ku-lar) pertaining to the heart and blood vessels **c collapse** sudden loss of effective blood flow to the tissues as in vasovagal attack or postural hypotension **c fitness** the capacity of the heart to pump blood and of the blo1d vessels to carry blood throughout the body **c system** the network of structures consisting of the heart and blood vessels, that pumps blood and transports it throughout the body

cardioversion (kar′de-o-ver′zhun) synchronised electric shock applied to ter-

minate cardiac arrhythmias; defibrillation

cardioverter (kar′de-o-ver′ter) a device used to administer electric shocks to the heart through electrodes placed on the heart.

cardiovocal syndrome hoarseness due to compression of the left laryngeal nerve between the aorta and dilated pulmonary artery; Ortner′s syndrome

Carey-Coombs murmur a transient soft low pitched mid diastolic murmur audible during mitral valvulitis due to acute rheumatic fever, described by Coombs, English physician

carditis (kar-di′tis) inflammation of the layers of the wall of the heart such as ′pericardium, myocardium and endocardium **rheumatic c** carditis occurring in rheumatic fever

Card test integrity of interossei muscles are tested by asking the patient to hold out his hand keeping the fingers absolutely straight. A pile of stiff paper is insinuated into the interdigital cleft and is asked to grip the paper between the fingers. Normally the clasping fingers offer resistance. The grip is feeble in interosseus weakness and the paper slides out of the cleft

care look after the needs **intensive c** care of critically ill patients **primary c** medical care of a person at the first contact **secondary c** medical care of a patient by a specialist **tertiary c** medical care of a patient in a large hospital that is staffed and equipped to provide comprehensive care

caries (kar′i-ez) gradual decay and disintegration of a tooth **d caries** see dental caries **c spine** see Pott′s spine

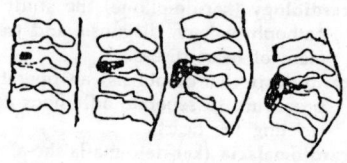

Caries spine

carina (ka-ri'na) a structure with a projecting central ridge **c tracheae** a ridge at the lower end of the trachea at its bifurcation as major bronchi

carious (ka're-us) 1. pertaining to caries 2. having pits

Carlen's tube double-lumen endotracheal catheter used for bronchospirometry of lungs separately named after E. Carlen, Scandinavian laryngologist

carminative (kar-min'ativ) a pleasant tasting agent preventing gas formation in the gastrointestinal tract

carmustine an anti-neoplastic nitrosurea compound; BCNU

L-carnitine an amino acid required for transport of long chain fatty acids across the mitochondrial membrane

carnal (kar'nal) sensual; pertaining to desires of the flesh

carneous (kar'ne-us) fleshy

carnitine (kar'ni-tin) a chemical metabolising palmitic and stearic acids

carnivore (kar'ni-vor) an animal that eats meat

carnivorous (kar-niv'o-rus) flesh eating

Caroli's (kar'o-liz) **disease** congenital intrahepatic cystic dilatation of bile ducts

Caroli's syndrome autosomal recessive disorder presenting Caroli's disease in association with congenital hepatic fibrosis

carotenaemia (kar'o-te-ne'me-a) presence of carotene in the blood leading to yellowish discolouration of the skin, and not of conjunctiva

carotenase (kar-ot'e-nas) an enzyme that converts carotene to vitamin A

carotene (kar'o-ten) an yellow crystalline pigment found in yellow vegetables such as carrots, corn and squash. It is converted in the liver to vitamin A

carotenoid (ka-rot'e-noyd) 1. resembling carotene 2 pigment varying from light yellow to red colour found in plants and animals. The examples are beta carotene in carrots, lycopene in tomatoes and lutein in spinach and are anti-oxidants

carotid (ka-rot'id) head and neck **c artery** pertains to the right and left common carotid arteries that supply to the head and neck **c artery syndrome** ipsilateral blindness and contralateral hemiplegia **c body** a collection of cells at the bifurcation of the common carotid artery that respond to the changes in oxygen concentration in the blood and to changes in blood pressure **c bruit** a continuous murmur audible over the neck particularly at the carotid bifurcation **c endartectomy** a surgical procedure to remove intra-arterial obstruction of the lower cervical portion of the internal carotid artery and restore normal blood flow **c sinus** slight dilatation at carotid bifurcation **c sinus massage** firm stroking of carotid artery at the sinus area slows SA node rhythm and may stop supraventricular tachycardia

carotidynia (kar-ot'i-din'e-a) spontaneous episodes of dull ache originating in the middle of the neck on one side and radiating to ipsilateral face, ear, jaw, tooth or down the neck. It is accompanied by tenderness on palpation over the carotid artery and induration of the overlying tissues

carpal (kar-pal) pertaining to the wrist **c bone** one of the eight bones that make up the wrist **c boss** a bony growth on the dorsal surface of the third metacarpocarpal joint **c tunnel** a canal in the wrist where the carpal bones form a concavity bridged by flexor retinaculum through which the flexor tendons and the median nerve pass **c tunnel syndrome** occurrence of tingling, pain and numbness in the region of the median nerve distribution of the hand. It is caused by compression of the median nerve as it passes between the bones and ligament at the front of the wrist

carpale (kar-pa'le) any wrist bone

carpometacarpal pertaining to the carpus and the metacarpus

carpopedal (kar'po-ped'al) pertaining to

both the wrist and the foot **c spasm** spasm of hands and feet as in tetany

carpoptosis (kar'pop-to'sis) wrist drop

carpus (kar'pus) the eight bones of the wrist.

carrier 1. an individual who harbours a specific microorganism without exhibiting any clinical features of the disease and is potentially capable of spreading the organisms to others; **convalescent c** a person harbouring an infective agent during recovery from the disease caused by the organism **genetic c** one whose chromosomes contain a pathologic mutant gene that may be transmitted to child **healthy c** a person harbouring an infectious agent without suffering from the disease **incubatory c** a person who harbours and spreads an infective agent during the incubation period of a disease 2. an insect passively carrying an infectious agent 3. a substance that when combined with another transport substance can pass through the cell membrane 4. a heterozygote carrying a recessive gene together with its normal allele 5. an apparatus or instrument used for transportation of some material such as an amalgam

Carrion's (kar-e-onz) **disease** Bartonellosis named after Danial Carrion, a Peruvian student who died following voluntarily injecting himself with a disease

cartilage (kar'ti-lij) a specialised type of dense connective tissue consisting of cells embedded in a firm and compact matrix or ground substance. It can withstand considerable pressure or tension. It forms part of the skeleton and is seen in the costal cartilages of the ribs, in the nasal septum, in the external ear, larynx, trachea, bronchi, between the vertebral bodies and covering of the articular surfaces of bones **articular c** the thin layer of smooth, elastic cartilage on the joint surfaces of a bone as in a synovial joint **costal c** a cartilage that connects the ends of a true rib

with the sternum or the end of a false rib with costal cartilage above **cricoid c** a signet ring-shaped lowermost cartilage of the larynx **cuneiform c** one of the small pieces of cartilage lying in the aryepiglottic fold of the larynx **fibrous c** fibrocartilage **hyaline c** a bluish white, flexible, glossy, transparent cartilage **semilunar c** medial or lateral crescentic cartilage of the knee joint between the femur and tibia **thyroid c** a shield-shaped large cartilage of the larynx found in front of the middle of the neck known as Adam's apple **yellow c** a network of yellow elastic fibres that holds cartilage cells

cartilaginous (kar'ti-laj'i-nus) pertaining to or consisting of cartilage

caruncle (kar'ung-k'l) a small fleshy growth **lacrimal c** a small reddish elevation on the conjunctiva near the inner canthus, at the medial angle of the eye **sublingual c** a protuberance on either side of the frenum of the tongue containing the openings of the ducts from submandibular and sublingual salivary glands **urethral c a** highly vascular, small papillary growth that may sometimes develop in the urinary meatus in female

caruncula (kar-ung'ku-la) pl. **carunculae** caruncle **c hymenales** small irregular nodules representing the remains of the hymen

Carvallo's (car-ve'loz) **sign** an increase in intensity of presystolic murmur during inspiration in patients with tricuspid stenosis. It is better audible in sitting posture, named after Rivero-Carvallo, Mexican physician

carver a knife or an instrument used to shape an object as in dentistry to carve amalgam or wax pattern

Casal's necklace *see* necklace

cascade (kas-kad) a continuous process of self-propagation or amplification through a series of steps, each step initiating the next, until the final is reached

case 1. occurrence of disease 2. a patient 3. an enclosing structure. **c control** a study in which the index cases are matched with comparison cases to discover risk factors or exposure **c finding** an active search to identify persons who have disease **c history** a detailed history of present, past, personal, and family of a patient at the time of admission for the present illness **c management** an individualised approach to the patient care

caseate (ka'se-at) to undergo cheesy degeneration

caseation (ka'se-a'shun) 1. the process of conversion of a necrotic tissue into a granular amorphous cheesy mass associated with a tuberculous lesion also seen in histoplasmosis 2. the precipitation of casein during coagulation of milk

casein (ka'-se-in) the principal milk protein that supplies all the amino acids necessary for growth and development.

caseinogen (ka-se-in'o-jen) the principal protein from which casein is derived in milk

caseous (ka'se-us) 1. resembling cheese 2. transformation of tissues into a cheesy mass

Casoni's (ka-so'nez) **test** intradermal injection of hydatid fluid followed by production of a wheal and flare reaction indicative of hydatid disease, named after Tommaso Casoni, Italian physician

caspase (kas'pe-s) protein that causes cell death on activation

cassava root of *Manihot esculenta* providing an excellent source of starch; tapioca

cassette (ka-set) a flat , light proof box with an intensifying screen for holding x-ray film; a case for film or magnetic tape; a segment of eukaryotic DNA that can be substitued by another sequence by transposition

cast 1. a positive copy of teeth and jaw over which denture bases are made 2. making an accurate metallic reproduction of a wax pattern of a dental appliance, tooth 3. material moulded to the shape of the part in which it has accumulated 4. a rigid casing applied to a part of the body to immobilise a fracture or dislocation. **epithelial c** an aggregation of renal epithelium filled with granules or fat droplets seen in acute nephritis **granular c** substance following degeneration of a hyaline cast **hyaline c** a urinary cast that is pale, transparent and having homogeneous rounded ends. **red blood cell c** a urinary cast composed mainly of red blood cells **urinary c** a cast found in the urine, formed from precipitation of proteins in the renal tubules **white blood cell c** a leucocyte cast found in urine in pyogenic infections of the kidney

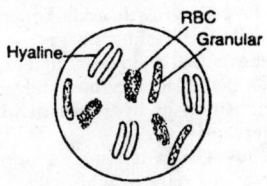

Urinary casts

casting forming of an object in a mould

Castle's intrinsic factor a substance secreted by the stomach essential for the absorption of vitamin B12, whose absence leads to pernicious anaemia, named after William Castle, US physician

castor oil oil from the plant *Ricinus communis* used internally as a laxative and externally as an emollient

castrate (kas'trat) to remove the testicles or ovaries

castrated rendered incapable of reproduction by removal of testicl⟨ ⟩ or ovaries

castration (kas-tra'shun) excision of one or both testicles or ovaries

casualty (kaz'u-al-te) 1. an accident causing injury or death 2. a person injured or killed in accident 3. an area in the hospital equipped to manage patients requiring emergency treatment

casuistics (kaz-u-is'tiks) analysis of clinical case records to establish the general characteristics of a disease

catabolism (ka-tab'o-lizm) a process of metabolism wherein the complex chemicals are broken down into simpler forms usually with the release of energy, and byproducts such as water and carbon dioxide

catabolite (ka-tab'o-lit) any product of catabolism

cataclysm (kata'k-lizm) disaster, sudden tragedy

catacrotic (kat'a-krot'ik) the downstroke of pulse tracing interrupted by an upstroke

catagen (kat'a-jen) the intermediate phase of the hair growth cycle between the growth and resting phase

catagenesis (kat'a-jen'e-sis) involution

catalase (kat'a-las) enzyme catalysing decomposition of hydrogen peroxide to water and oxygen

catalepsy (kat'a-lep'se) an abnormal trance-like state in which the muscles of the face, body, and limbs remain in a rigid position

catalysis (ka'tal'i-sis) hastening of a chemical reaction by a catalyst

catalyst (kat'a-list) a substance that hastens the rate of a chemical reaction without getting altered in the reaction. These are effective in small amounts and are not used up in the reaction

catalytic antibody a biologically selective enzyme wherein catalytic activity is introduced into the highly selective binding site of a monoclonal antibody

catamenia (kat-a-me'ne-a) menstruation

catamnesis (kat-am-ne'sis) the follow-up history of patient after treatment

cataplexy (kat'a-pleks-e) temporary loss of muscle tone and weakness following a strong emotional response

cataract (kat'a-rakt) opacity of the lens of the eye, its capsule or both **capsular c** cataract occurring in the capsule **hypermature c** overripe cataract **immature c** an early cataract which is not fully matured to require treatment **mature c** opaque lens with dense changes in anterior cortex of the lens preventing visualisation of the posterior portion of the lens and posterior portion of eye **nuclear c** a cataract in which the anterior portion of the lens is opacified **overripe c** stage following mature cataract where the lens is solidified and shrunken **radiation c** a cataract caused by exposure to radiation **ripe c** mature cataract **senile c** a cataract developing in an elderly person

cataractogenic (kat'a-rak'to-jen'ik) causing cataract

catarrh (ka-tar) inflammation of the mucous membrane of the nasopharyngeal mucosa

catatonia (kat-a-to'ne-a) motor anomalies in non-organic disorders, wherein there is increased tone and fixed postures

catatropia (kat'-tro'pe-a) a condition in which both eyes are directed downwards

cat bite fever an infection by *Pasteurella multocida* acquired by cat bite, is characterised by an abscess at the site of inoculation and focal arthralgia

catecholamine (kat'e-kol'a-men) one of two biologically active amines, epinephrine (adrenaline) nor epinephrine (nor adrenaline) and dopamine, which have important effect on nervous system

catgut sheep intestine twisted for use as an absorbable ligature

catharsis (ka-thar'sis) 1. purgative action of the bowel 2. emotion release

cathartic (ka-thar'tik) a purgative-producing-bowel movements **c colon** a colon affected by long-term abuse of cathartics and laxatives characterised by intractable diarrhoea, hypokalaemia, protein-losing enteropathy, cachexia and potentially increased constipation

cathepsin - D (ka'thep'sin) an oestrogen-induced lysosomal proteinase whose level may be raised in recurrence of breast carcinoma

catheter (kath'e-ter) a hollow, flexible tube passed through the body for evacuating fluids or injecting them into body cavities or vessels. It is made up of rubber, plastic, metal or elastic web **arterial c** a catheter inserted into an artery to inject medication or radioactive contrast material, to remove blood or to measure pressure **balloon c** a double-lumened catheter surrounded by a balloon **cardiac c** a long time catheter for passage through the lumen of a blood vessel into the chambers of the heart **central c** a catheter inserted into a central vein or artery **central venous c** a catheter inserted into the superior vena cava to permit intermittent or continuous monitoring of central venous pressure **condom c** a specially designed condom that includes a catheter bag **double channel c** a catheter providing for inflow and outflow **eustachian c** a cathetar passed into the eustachian tube through the nasal passage **female c** a catheter of 12.7 cm long used to pass into a women's bladder **Foley c** a urinary tract catheter with a balloon at one end. After insertion of the catheter, the balloon is filled with sterile water to prevent it leaving the bladder, named after Frederic Foley, US urologist **indwelling c** any catheter allowed to remain inside a vein, artery or body cavity **intravenous c** a catheter inserted into a vein to administer fluids or medications **male c** a catheter of 30.5 to 33 cm length used to pass into a man's bladder **pacing c** a catheter inserted into a vein or pulmonary artery that contains wires or leads for providing electrical stimuli from an external cardiac pacemaker **self-retaining c** a bladder catheter designed to remain in place **Swan-Ganz c** a thin, flexible, flow-directed catheter using a balloon to carry it through the heart to pulmonary artery and is positioned in a small arterial branch. Pulmonary wedge pressure is measured in front of inflated and wedged balloon

catheterisation (kath'e-ter-i-za'shun) insertion of a catheter into the body to drain, or inject fluids or to perform certain procedures such as widening of narrowed arteries **cardiac c** *see* cardiac catheterisation **urinary bladder c** introduction of a catheter through urethra into the bladder for removal of urine

catheterise (kath'e-ter-iz) to pass a catheter into a part, commonly it refers to bladder catheterisation

cathexis (ka-thek'sis) psychological attachment to an idea or object

cathode (kath'od) 1. negative electrode from which electrons are emitted. 2. source of the electron stream in a vacuum tube

cation (kat'i-on) an ion with a positive electric charge that moves to a negative pole.

cat-scratch disease. illness caused by the scratches or bite of cats, there is occurrence of a papule, and regional lymphadenopathy. It is thought to be caused by a bacterium and is a self-limiting illness

caucasian pertaining to the white race

cauda (kaw'da) a tail or tail-like structure. **c equina** the terminal portion of the spinal cord and the roots of the spinal nerves below L_1 nerve

caudad (kw'dad) in a posterior direction

caudal (kwad'al) 1. pertaining to any tail-like structure 2. inferior in position.

caudate (kwa'dat) possessing a tail **c lobe** lobe of liver on its inferior surface **c nucleus** an elongated curved mass of gray matter divided into head, body and tail which protrudes into the anterior horn of lateral ventricle

cauliflower ear recurrent auricular haematoma noted in boxers

cauliflower lesion pedunculated polypoid mass that grows into a lumen or hollow viscus

causalgia (kaw-sal'je-a) severe burning pain and trophic skin changes from injury to nerve fibres

cause something that brings about a particular condition or abnormality **antecedent c** a condition that predisposes to a disease or condition **predisposing c** a condition favouring the development of a disease **proximate c** a condition that immediately precedes and causes the disease **remote c** a condition that is not an immediate cause, but predisposes to the development of the disease **ultimate c** a remote event which initiates a train of events that culminate in the development of the disease

caustic (kaw'stik) corrosive agent particularly alkali that destroys the living tissue

cauterisation (kaw'ter-i-za'shun) application to the tissues a caustic chemical, an electric current, a hot iron or freezing in order to destroy them, to stop them from bleeding or to promote their healing

cauterise (kaw'ter-is) to burn with a cautery

cautery (kaw'ter-e) a device used to cause destruction of tissues by electricity, heat, freezing or caustic substances such as silver nitrate, potassium hydroxide or nitric acid

cava (ka'va) 1. a hollow area or body cavity 2. vena cava.

caval (ka'vaı) pertaining to vena cava

caveola (kav-e-o'la) a small pit

cavernositis (kav'er-no-si'tis) inflammation of corpus cavernosum

cavernosography radiography of penis following injection of a contrast material into the corpus cavernosa

cavernous (kav'er-nus) containing hollow spaces **c sinus** on either side of pituitary traversed by internal carotid artery and 3rd to 6th cranial nerves

cavitary (kar'i-ta're) pertaining to a cavity

cavitation formation of a cavity

cavity (kav'i-ti) a hollow space **abdominal c** the ventral cavity in the abdomen containing all abdominal organs **alveolar c** a tooth socket **amniotic c** the fluid- filled cavity around the developing embryo **articular c** the synovial cavity of the skull **dental c** a hole in the tooth caused by caries **oral c** the cavity of the mouth **pelvic c** the cavity of the pelvis. It consists of major pelvic cavity lying between the iliac fossa above iliopectineal line and minor pelvic cavity lying below the ileopectineal line or the inlet of the pelvis **pericardial c** the potential space between the visceral pericardium and parietal pericardium **peritoneal c** the potential space between the parietal peritoneum lining the inner aspect of abdominal wall and the visceral peritoneum covering the visceral organs **pleural c** the potential space between the parietal pleura lining the inner surface of the thoracic cavity and the visceral pleura covering the lungs **pulmonary c** irregular air-filled structures with a wall thickness greater than 1mm **serous c** the space between the two layers of serous membranes such as pleura, pericardium or peritoneum **spinal c** the cavity containing important organs such as cranial, thoracic or abdominal cavities **thoracic c** the space enclosed within the walls of thorax above the diaphragm **tympanic c** middle ear cavity **uterine c** the cavity of the body of the uterus

cavum (ka'vum) a cavity or space

CBC abbreviation for complete blood count

CCNU cyclonexyl-chloroethyl nitrosurea, highly toxic chemotherapeutic agent used in treatment of malignancy such as high grade astrocytoma

CD abbreviation for cluster of differentiation, name of surface antigens of human leucocytes characterised by monoclonal antibodies enabling leucocytes and other haemopoietic cells to be categorised by the expression on the cell surface.

CD 4 a surface glycoprotein that participates in adhesion of T cells to target cells and is involved in thymic maturation

CD 4/CD8 ratio of circulating T lymphocytes with 'helper cell' determinants (CD4 antigen) on the cell surface to T lymphocytes with 'suppressor cell' determinants (CD8 antigen)

CD4 cells circulating T lymphocytes with a 'helper' phenotype. The levels of CD4 + cells is a crude indicator of immune status and susceptibility to certain infections and new growths, in AIDS patients

CD8 cells T lymphocytes with a CD 8 antigen on the cell surface, which are suppressive. They are responsible for suppressing mitogen-induced and antigen-specific antibody production.

CDCP abbreviation for centres for disease control and prevention, located at Atlanta Georgia, US

cDNA DNA that is complementary to a messenger RNA actively translating various proteins

CD receptor one of the receptors specific to mature T lymphocytes that are responsible for the recognition of antigens

CD4 receptor receptors on T4 lymphocytes to which the human immunodeficiency virus binds producing an infection

CD-ROM compact disc read-only memory. A high-capacity form of storage-compact disc or CD. It contains up to 650 Mb of data. CD-ROM drive is necessary to use these discs.

CEA carcinoembryonic antigen. A glycoprotein present in circulation. It is found in nanogram amounts. It is used to monitor recurrent colon cancer

cecal (se'kal) *see* caecal

cecum (se'kum) *see* caecum

celerity (sel'e-riti) speed, quickness of motion

celibacy (sel'i-bas'i) the practice of being sexually abstinent

cell 1. basic structural unit of all cell animals/body containing a mass of protoplasm containing a nucleus or nuclear material 2. a small enclosed cavity like an air cell **acantholytic c** an epithelial cell that has separated from another epithelial cell and consequently has become round **acidophil c** a cell with affinity for staining with acid dyes **acinar c** a cell found in the acinus of an acinous gland, such as pancreas **adipose c** fat cell **adria c** cardiac myocyte that has lost its cross-striations and myofilaments seconday to adriomycin toxicity **alpha c** a cell present in the anterior lobe of the pituitary and pancreas. In the latter it is concerned with the secretion of glucagon **alveolar c** pneumocyte **ameloblast c** cell concerned with production of enamel of tooth crown **argentaffin c** *see* Kulchitsky cell **B c** B lymphocyte, a lymphoid stem cell from the bone marrow that migrates to, and becomes a mature antigen specific cell in the lymph nodes and spleen **band c** developing leucocyte at a stage when the nucleus is not segmented **basal c** a cell found in deepest layer of the epidermis **basaloid c** cell of the basal layer of the epidermis **basket c** a branching basal cell of salivary glands, and of cerebellum germinative cell **basophil c** a cell having an affinity for staining with basic dyes **beta c** 1. a cell found in the islets of Langerhans concerned with secretion of insulin 2. a cell found in anterior lobe of pituitary **Betz c** giant pyramidal cells in the motor area of the cerebral cortex whose axons form the corticospinal tract, named after Vladimir Betz, Russian anatomist **bipolar c** a neuron having two processes, an axon and a dendrite, found in the retina of the eye and in the cochlear and vestibular ganglia of the acoustic nerve **blast c** a newly formed cell of any type such as lymphoblast or myeloblast **blood c** any type of nucleated or non-nucleated cell found in the blood or blood forming tissues **burr c** an erythrocyte having spicules over its surface **caterpillar c** large multinucleated giant cell with lengthwise chromatin clumping in nucleus seen in heart in acute rheumatic fever **cementoblast c** one of the cells concerned with secretion of parathyroid hormone 2. one of the secretory cells found in gastric glands and secrete pepsin 3. a chromophobe cell of pituitary **chromaffin c** a cell found in adrenal medulla where granules stain brown with potassium bichromate **cleavage c** a cell following mitosis; blastomere **clue c** an epithelial cell of the vagina coated with coccobacillary organisms **columnar c** an epithelial cell with height greater than width **cone c** a light receptor cell in the retina **cornified c** corneocyte, the end product of the process of cornification **cuboid c** an epithelial cell with height about equal to width and depth **cytotoxic T c** a CD4 + T lymphocyte that can destroy microorganisms directly **daughter c** cell formed from the division of a mother cell **delta c** somatostatin secreting cell found in islets of Langerhans **endothelial c** one of the flat cells that line the blood and lymph vessels **ependymal c** one of the cells of the developing neural tube that gives rise to the ependyma **epithelial c** one of the cells forming the epithelial surfaces of skin and membranes **ethmoidal c** ethmoidal sinus cell **faggot c** malignant promyelocyte containing numerous Auer rods seen in acute myelogenous leukaemia **fat c** a cell that stores fat **foam c** a cell that contains vacuoles and lipid substance

ganglion c a neuronal cell found in ganglion **germ c** a cell concerned with reproduction of the organism. They possess a single set of chromosomes (haploid) and are called ova in females and spermatozoa in males **giant c** a large cell containing one or more nuclei **goblet c** an epithelial cell with a large globule of mucin giving it an appearance of goblet **golgi c** *see* Golgi cell **gustatory c** a taste cell in a taste bud **hair c** an epithelial cell having fine non-motile cilia found in the maculae and the organ of Corti of the membranous labyrinth of the inner ear. They act as receptors for the senses of position and hearing **hairy c** leucocytes possessing multiple cytoplasmic projections on the cell surface, found in hairy cell leukaemia **HeLa c** a cell from a strain continuously cultured from a patient's carcinoma of the cervix. The name has come from the first two letters of the patient's first and last names, Henrietta Lacks **helper Tc** a type of T lymphocytes required for the production of antibodies against certain antigens **horizontal c** a retinal cell where axons run horizontally connecting different parts of the retina **hyperchromatic c** densely staining cell which contains more than the normal number of chromosomes **interstitial c** one of the many cells found in the connective tissue of the ovary and the seminiferous tubules of the testis concerned with hormonal secretion **islet c** a cell of the islets of Langerhans of the pancreas **juvenile c** the early developmental cell of a white blood cell **juxtaglomerular c** a modified smooth muscle cell found in the wall of the afferent arteriole leading to a glomerulus of the kidney. It secretes renin when there is a fall in blood pressure and activates the renin-angiotensin mechanism **killer T c** a type of T lymphocytes that directly kills organisms **Kupffer c** *see* Kupffer cell **L E** see LE cell **labile c** a cell which is continuously replicating, found in tissues which undergo high turnover such as gastrointestinal tract **Leydig c** see Leydig cell **littoral c** a macrophage found in the sinuses of lymphatic tissue **lutein c** a cell of the corpus luteum of the ovary, containing fatty yellowish granules **Lymph c** lymphocyte **mast c** see mast cell **mastoid c** one of the air spaces in the mastoid process of temporal bone **memory c** a cell derived from B or T lymphocytes that has the ability to recognise a foreign antigen to which the body has been previously sensitised. They stimulate plasma cells to produce antibodies **microglia c** a neuroglial cell found in the brain and spinal cord capable of phagocytosis **mother c** a cell that gives rise to similar cell through fission or budding **mucous c** a cell that secretes mucus, found in mucus secreting glands **myeloma c** a cell found in the bone marrow of patients with multiple myeloma **myoepithelial c** a spindle-shaped contractile epithelial cell found in the salivary, sweat and mammary glands **natural killer c** see NK cell **nerve c** see neuron **neuroglial c** cell of the supporting tissue of CNS and retina of the eye **null c** a lymphocyte exhibiting the features of neither a T cell nor a B cell **odontoblast c** a cell producing dentine **olfactory c** a special cell of the olfactory mucosa **osteoblast c** a mesodermal cell concerned with the production of bone matrix **osteocyte c** a cell found in bone matrix, concerned in its metabolic activity **oxyntic c** a parietal cell found in mucosa of the stomach concerned with secretion of hydrochloric acid **parent c** mother cell **pigment c** any cell containing pigment granules **plasma c** a cell derived from B lymphocytes concerned with the production of antibodies **prickle c** a cell having spine-like protoplasmic processes found in the stratum spinosum of the epidermis **primordial c** one of the original germ cells that is found in gonadal ridge in the embryo **Purkinje c** see Purkinje cell **pus c** a degenerated leucocyte found in the pus **Pyramidal c** Betz cell **quiescent c** a cell which replicates slowly **red c** erythrocyte; red-blood cell concerned with the transportation of oxygen to the cells of the body **reticular c** a cell that can develop into one of the several types of connective tissue cells or into a macrophage, found in the spleen, bone marrow or lymphatic tissue **reticuloendothelial c** a macrophage or phagocytic cell **rod c** a long and narrow sensory retinal cell that are stimulated in dim light **segmented c** neutrophil whose nucleus has two or more lobes **sensory c** a cell that on stimulation gives rise to nerve impulses that are conveyed to CNS **Sertoli c** see Sertoli cell **sickle c** an abnormal erythrocyte having shape like a sickle **signet ring c** a vacuolated cell with the nucleus at a side, often found in mucin secreting adenocarcinoma **smudge c** cell with a large, ovoid nucleus filled with a granular amphophilic to deeply basophilic mass of an indistinct nuclear membrane, seen in adenovius-infected cells **somatic c** body cells of different shapes and functions that possess two sets of chromosomes (diploid) **squamous c** a flat scale-like epithelial cell **stellate c** a star-shaped cell with processes extending from it **stem c** a cell capable of differentiation and self-renewal **stipple c** an RBC containing small basophilic staining dots, found in lead poisoning, malaria, severe anaemia and leukaemia **suppressor T c** a type of T lymphocyte that inhibits CD 4 + and B cell activity **T c** a lymphoid cell from the bone marrow that migrates to the thymus gland where it matures as a differentiated lymphocyte. These cells are antigen-specific responding to an antigen processed by a macrophage and are identified by surface protein markers called cluster of differentiation (CD) **target** c an erythrocyte with a rounded central area surrounded by lightly stained clear ring which in turn is encircled by a dense ring of peripheral protoplasm **tart** c a phagocytic cell that has ingested unaltered nuclear material of cells **taste** c a cell of a taste bud **totipotent** c an undifferentiated embryonic cell **undifferentiated** c a cell without any change into a mature cell of any type **wandering** c a macrophage capable of amoeboid movement **white** c white blood cell **zymogenic** c enzyme producing chief cell of the gastric glands

cell bank preservation of cells frozen at extremely low temperatures

cell block a paraffin-embedded specimen derived from mucus, sputum or debris found in fluids of pleural, pericardial and endobronchial sites.

cell counter an electronic instrument used to count cells

cell culture growth of cells *in vitro*

cell cycle cell sequence consisting of growth, reproduction and death

cell differentiation specialising of a cell into its mature form for a particular organ or function

cell-free pertaining to fluids and tissues that do not contain any cells

cell junction an intercellular region of adherence between, and contributed by, two cells

cell kinetics the study of cells and their growth and division

cell mass a collection of cells that develops into an organ or structure

cell-mediated immunity CMI immune mechanism that acts through the 'direct' cell action; T cell immunity

cellophane (sel'o-fan) a thin, transparent water proof membrane of cellulose acetate. It is used as a dialysis membrane

cellular (sel'u-lar) pertaining to, composed of or derived from cells c **immunity** *see*

immunity c **membrane** the envelope surrounding each cell that controls the passage of substances into and out of the cell

cellulitis (sel-u-li'tis) inflammation of the skin and the tissues beneath it from a bacterial infection. It may be localised or spreading through the tissues

cellulose (sel'u-los) a polysaccharide that forms plant fibre though it does not give any nutrients, it stimulates peristalsis of intestines

Celsius (sel'se-us) **scale** a temperature scale on which the boiling point of water is 100° and the freezing point is 0°. This centigrade scale is named after Anders Celsius, Swedish astronomer

cement (se'ment) a substance that hardens into a firm mass when prepared appropriately

cementitis (se'men-ti-tis) inflammation of the dental cementum

cementoblast (se'men-to-blast) a cell of the inner layer of dental sac of a developing tooth

cementoclasia (se-men'to-kla'se-a) decay of the cementum of a tooth root

cementogenesis (se-men'to-jen'e-sis) the development of cementum on the root of dentin of a tooth

cementum (se-men'tum) a thin layer of calcified tissue formed by cementoblasts which covers the tooth root

census the number of patients present in the hospital

center centre

centesis (sen-te'sis) puncture of a cavity

centigrade (sen'ti-grad) 1. having 100 degrees 2. pertaining to a thermometer divided into 100°.

centigram (sen'ti-gram) one hundredth of a gram

centilitre (sen'ti-le-tre) one hundredth of a litre

centimetre (sen'ti-me-tre) one hundredth of a metre. Inches are converted into centimetres by multiplying by 2.54.

centimorgan (sen'ti-mor-gan) a measure

of genetic distance that tells how far apart two genes are. 1 centimorgan is equal to a million base pairs; cM

centiped (sen'ti-ped) an arthropod having an elongated flat body of many segments

centrad (sen'trad) towards the centre

central (sen'tral) 1. situated at the centre 2. controlling site

central core myopathy an autosomal dominant myopathy causing hypotonia in infancy and non-progressive proximal muscle weakness

centre (sen'ter) 1. the mid-point of a body 2. a group of nerve cells within CNS that controls specific activity or function 3. a service facility in a particular field

central line a venous access devise inserted into and kept in the vein. It provides a route for administration of fluid and medicines and an access to the heart to obtain information about pressures in venous circulation

central nervous system CNS, the brain and the spinal cord

central venous pressure CVP, the pressure within the superior vena cava which reflects the pressure under which blood is returned to the right atrium. Normally it ranges from 5 to 40 cm H_2O. It is increased in circulatory overload and decreased in reduced blood volume

centre center

centrifugal (sen-trif-u-gal) away from the centre

centrifuge (sen-tri-fuj) a device that spins test tubes at high speeds, allowing heavy particles in the liquid to settle at the bottom and lighter liquid to go to the top

centrilobular (sen'tri-lob'u-lar) pertaining to the centre of a lobule

centring (sent'ring) any method of calming oneself physically, mentally and emotionally

centriole (sen'tre-ol) a minute organelle consisting of a hollow cylinder, closed

at one end and open at the other. It is found in the centre of a cell. It divides into two daughter centrioles before mitosis and migrate to opposite poles of the cell during mitosis

centripetal (sen-trip'e-tal) towards the centre

centromere (sen'tro-mer) a constricted region of a chromosome, joining point of two chromatids of a chromosome

centrosome (sen'tro-som) a region of the cytoplasm of a cell lying near the nucleus containing centrioles

centrosphere (sen'tro-sfer) the cytoplasm of the centrosome

centrum (sen'trum) 1. any centre 2. the body of a vertebra

cephalad (sef'a-lad) toward the head

cephalalgia (sef-a-lal'je-a) headache

cephalexin (sef'a-lek-sin) a cephalosporin antibiotic active against gram-positive and gram-negative organisms

cephalhaematoma (sef'al-he'ma-to'ma) a mass of clotted blood located between the periosteum and the skull of a new born. Characteristically limited to one skull bone

cephalic (se-fal'ik) 1. cranial 2. superior in position c index cranial capacity obtained by dividing the maximal length of the head into the maximum breadth of the head by 100

cephalocaudal related to central axis of the body

cephalodynia (sef'a-lo-din'e-a) headache

caphalogyric (sef'a-lo-ji-rik) pertaining to the rotation of the head

cephalomeningitis (sef'a-lo-men'in-ji-tis) inflammation of the cerebral meninges

cephalometry (sef'a-lom'e-tri) measurement of the head

cephalopathy (sef 'a-lop'a-the) any disease affecting the head or brain

cephalopelvic (sef'a-lo-pel' vik) pertaining to the relationship between the measurements of the foetal head and the diameter of the maternal pelvis

cephaloridin (sef'e-'or'i-den) a cephalosporin antibiotic

cephalosporin a group of antibiotics derived from a fungus that have a wide range of activity against many important gram-positive and gram-negative bacteria and are of value for treatment of serious infections. The historical classification is by generations (first to fourth)

Cephalosporium a genus of important fungi found in soil and cephalosporins are derived from them

cephalothin (sef'o-lo-thin) a semisynthetic analogue of the antibiotic cephalosporin

cephalothoracopagus (sef'a-lo-tho'ra-kop'a-gus) a conjoined foetus at the level of the head and thorax

cephalotome (sef'a-lo-tom) an instrument for cutting the head of the foetus to facilitate delivery

cephalotomy (sef'a-lo-to-me) cutting the foetal head to facilitate delivery.

cephapirin (sef'-a-pi'rin) a cephalosporin antibiotic

ceptor (sep'tor) receptor

cera (se'ra) wax

ceramics porcelain or porcelain-type materials

ceramide (ser'a-mid) a class of lipids devoid of glycerol

ceramodontia (se-ram'o-don'shee-a) porcelain-type material used in dentistry.

ceratotome (se-rat'o-tom) a knife for division of cornea.

cercaria (ser-ka're-a) pl cercariae a free swimming state in the development of a fluke.

cercaricide (ser-ka'-re-sid) an agent that is lethal to cercaria

cerclage (ser-klazh) encircling tissues with a ligature.

cercus (ser'kus) a hair-like structure

cerea flexibilitas waxy flexibility. The person can be moulded into a position which is then maintained

cereal an edible grain containing carbohydrates (70%-80%), protein (8%-15%) and fibre

cerebellitis (ser'e-bel-i-tis) inflammation of the cerebellum

cerebellospinal (ser'e-bel-o-spi'nal) pertaining to the cerebellum and spinal cord

cerebellum (ser-e-bel'um) little brain. The region of the back of the brain concerned with the maintenance of posture and balance and the coordination of movement. It consists of two lateral hemispheres united by a narrow middle portion, the vermis

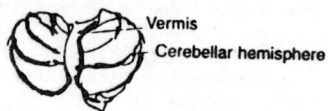

Vermis
Cerebellar hemisphere

Cerebellum

cerebral (ser-e-br'al) pertaining to the cerebral hemisphere c angiography radiologic examination of the blood vessels of the brain after injection of a contrast medium c cortex the outer surface of the brain concerned with mental functions, voluntary movement and sensation c dominance left cerebral hemisphere is dominant in 90 to 95% of individuals and are right handed c embolism blockage of one of the arteries to the brain by an embolus c gigantism an autosomal dominant disease with rapid early growth without endocrinopathy, accelerated bone maturation or precocious puberty c haemorrhage rupture of a sclerosed or diseased blood vessel in the brain c hemisphere one of the halves of the cerebrum c palsy disorders of movement and posture caused by brain damage that occurs before birth, during birth or in early life c thrombosis blockage of one of the arteries in the brain by a blood clot

cerebration (ser'e-bra'shun) thinking

cerebroside (ser'o-bro-sid) a lipid present in nerve and other tissues.

cerebrosidosis (ser'e-bro'si-do'sis) a form of lipoidosis with keratin in the fatty cells

cerebrospinal (ser'e-bro-spi'nal) pertaining to the brain and spinal cord **c axis** the central nervous system **c fever** meningococcal meningitis with acute onset of fever, head ache, neck rigidity, vomiting and photophobia **c fluid** the fluid flowing inside and around the brain and spinal cord that provides support and nutrition. It is formed in the cerebral ventricles by an active secretion from choroid plexus and it passes through the interventricular foramen to the third ventricle and then through a median and two lateral foramina to subarachnoid space. It is absorbed into intracranial venous sinuses over the convexity of the cerebral hemisphere through the arachnoid villi **c nerves** cranial nerves and spinal nerves **c puncture** a puncture for collection of cerebrospinal fluid or injection of contrast material or medication. The sites are lumbar, cisternal and open fontanelles

cerebrotomy (ser'e-brot'o-me) incision of the brain to evacuate an abscess

cerebrovascular (ser'e-bro-vas'ku-lar) pertaining to the blood vessels of the brain **c accident** any disease affecting suddenly an artery that supplies blood to the brain

cerebrum (ser'e-brum) the largest and most developed part of the brain . It performs the sensory and motor functions and various mental activities. It is derived from telencephalon and includes mainly cerebral hemispheres (cerebral cortex and basal ganglia)

ceroid (se'royd) a fatty pigment

ceroplasty (se'ro-plas'te) manufacture of anatomical models and pathological specimens in wax

certifiable (ser'ti-fi'a-bl) 1. pertaining to the infectious disease to be reported to the health authorities 2. a mentally incompetent person requiring the care by a guardian or institution

certification (ser'ti-fi-ka'shun) board certification in a speciality

ceruloplasmin (se'roo'lo-plaz'min) a glycoprotein carrying copper in the blood

cerumen (se-roo'men) ear wax. A substance secreted by the glands at the outer third of the ear canal

ceruminolysis (se-roo'min-nol'i-sis) a dissolution of the ear wax

ceruminous gland a modified sweat gland found in the skin lining the external auditory canal

cervical (ser'vi-kal) 1. pertaining to or in the region of the neck 2. pertaining to the cervix of an organ such as the cervix uteri **c cap** a flexible thimble-shaped device providing a covering to uterine cervix as a contraceptive **c dysplasia** changes in the cells on the surface of the cervix, that is considered precancerous **c factor** any quality in the mucus produced by the cervix that is hostile to the sperm, and cause inhibition of fertility **c incompetence** abnormal weakness of the cervix that can cause recurrent haemorrhage **c mucus method** a method of family planning that is based on observing changes in the mucus secreted by the cervix to determine the time of ovulation **c nerve** a nerve in the first eight pairs of spinal nerves **c osteoarthritis** a degenerative condition of the joints between the bones in the neck causing neck pain and stiffness **c plexus** a network of first four cervical nerves that supplies parts of the face, neck, shoulder and chest, and diaphragm **c rib** accessory cervical rib **c rib syndrome** compression of the brachial plexus by a cervical rib causing pain, and parasthesias of the hand, neck, shoulder or arms **c ripening** softening and dilatation of the uterine cervix in preparation for childbirth **c smear** a specimen of tissue removed from the cervix for examination under a microscope to detect cell abnormalities; pap smear **c spine** the uppermost part of the vertebral column consisting of seven vertebrae **c**

spondylosis disc degeneration with associated osteophyte formation and osteoarthritis of cervical vertebral joints **c stitch** a surgical stitch that is tied like a downstring around a weakened cervix to prevent recurrent miscarriage **c vertebra** one of the first seven bones of the vertebral column

cervicectomy (ser'vi-sek'to-me) operative removal of the cervix uteri

cervicitis (ser-vi-si'tis) inflammation of the cervix uteri

cervicobrachial (ser'vi-ko-bra'ke-al) pertaining to the neck and arm

cervicocolpitis (ser'vi-ko-kol-pi'tis) inflammation of the cervix uteri and vagina

cervicofacial (ser'vi-ko-fa'she-al) pertaining to neck and face

cervicovaginitis (ser'vi-ko-vaj'i-ni'tis) pertaining to cervix uteri and the vagina

cervicovesical (ser'vi-ko-ves'i-kal) pertaining to cervix uteri and the vagina

cervix (ser'viks) the neck or a part of an organ resembling a neck **cancer c** a malignant neoplasm of the cervix uteri **c uteri** the neck of the uterus. It is the small cylindrical lowest part of the uterus extending from the internal os to the external os, and protruding into the vagina. It separates the body of the uterus from the vagina. The menstrual flow and foetus escape through this canal **c vesicae** neck of the urinary bladder

cesium (se'ze-um) a metallic element with atomic number 55, whose isotopes are used for irradiation of cancerous tissue

cesspool septic tank

cestoda (ses-tod'a) a subclass of phylum platyhelminthes which includes tapeworms (taenia). They possess a scolex and a chain of segments (proglattids).

cestode (ses'tod) a tapeworm belonging to cestoda family

cestodiasis (ses'to-di'a-sis) infestation with tapeworms

cestoidea (ses-toy'de-a) a class of flat worms of the phylum platyhelminthes, that includes tapeworms

CFCs chlorofluorocarbons a family of stable, non-toxic non-flammable, non-corrosive chemicals used as coolants, foaming and cleansing agents and aerosol propellants

CFT abbreviation for complement fixation test

cGMP abbreviation for cyclic guanosine monophosphate

Chaddock's (chad'oks) **reflex** 1. extension of big toe on stroking the outer edge of the dorsum of the foot and is present in pyramidal tract lesions 2. flexion of the wrist and fanning of the fingers on pressing the tendon of palmaris longus muscle, named after Charles Chaddock, US neurologist

Chadwick's sign a deep blue-violet colouration of cervix uteri and vagina from increased vascularity seen by fourth week of gestation, named after James Chadwick, US gynaecologist

chafe (chaf) injury caused by rubbing or friction

chafing (chaf'ing) superficial erythema and masceration of skin when subjected to friction from clothing or adjacent skin

Chagas' (chag'as) **disease** American trypanosomiasis named after Carles Chagas, Brazilian physician

chain (chan) related series of events or things. **food c** the sequential transfer of the food energy from green plants to animals that eat plants, then to animals that eat the plant-eating animals **heavy c's** the large polypeptide chains of antibodies **kinematic c** a series of bones connected by joints **light c's** the small polypeptide chains of antibodies

chain termination method use of dideoxy bases to sequence DNA

Chakras(s) wheal,centers, focal points for receiving and distributing the life-force around the body and filtering incoming energies from the environment

Chakshu (s) eyes

chalasia (ka-la'ze-a) relaxation of sphincters

chalazion (ka-la'ze-on) a small hard cyst developing on the eyelids. It is due to distension of a meibomian gland with secretions

challenge (chal'enj) administration of a specific antigen to an individual known to be sensitive to that antigen to produce an immune response

chalone (kal'on) a protein that inhibits mitosis in the tissue in which it is produced.

chamber (cham'ber) a compartment or closed space **anterior** c the space between the cornea and iris of the eye. **aqueous** c the anterior and posterior chambers of the eye, containing the aqueous humour **hyperbaric** c an air tight enclosure with high internal pressure **posterior** c the space behind the iris and in front of the vitreous body. It contains the lens, the zonules and the aqueous humour **pulp** c the part of the pulp cavity within the crown of the tooth **vitreous** c the cavity behind the lens in the eyes containing vitreous humour

champ to chew noisily, to crunch, to bite upon repeatedly

champagne bottle legs marked distal peroneal muscle atrophy with tapering of the distal extremities and hypertrophy of the proximal muscles, seen in advanced peroneal muscular atrophy

chancre (shang'ker) a painless sore usually on the genitals, that develops during the primary syphilis **Huntarian** c primary syphilitic ulcer, a true ulcer which is hard ovoid with sloping edges, a blood-stained discharge, named after John Hunter, London surgeon

chancroid (shang'kroyd) a sexually transmitted disease caused by *Haemophilus ducreyi* that produces multiple, irregular tender ulcers on the genitals with tender unilateral, matted suppurative regional lymph nodes; erythromycin or co-trimoxazole are useful in the treatment

channel a conduit, groove or passage way enabling flow of different materials

character (kar'ak-ter) a person's pattern of thought and action

characteristic (kar'ak-ter-is'trik) a trait or character that is typical of an individual

characterise to describe the attributes of something

charcoal (char'kol) very fine powder prepared from soft charred wood. Activated charcoal is administered while treating persons who have ingested poisons except in those who have taken corrosive chemicals

Charcot's (shar-koz) **joints** a painless disorganisation of joints marked by hypermobility, encountered in tabes dorsalis, syringomyelia, or injury, named after Jean Charcot, French neurologist

Charcot-Bouchard anuerysm a microaneurysm in a small artery of the brain caused by hypertension, named after Jean Charcot and Charles Bouchard, French physicians

Charcot-Leyden (shar-ko'li-den) **crystal** a colourless, hexagonal, needle-like crystals found in sputum in asthma or in faeces in amoebiasis, named after Jean Charcot and Ernest Leyden, German physician.

Charcot-Marie-Tooth disease peroneal muscular atrophy named after Jean Charcot, Pierre Marie, French neurologists and Howard Tooth, British physician

Charcot's triad 1. a combination of nystagmus, intention tremor and scanning speech; seen in multiple sclerosis 2. a combination of intermittent fever, intermittent pain and intermittent jaundice seen in chronic cholecystitis

charlatan (shar'la-tan) quack

Charles' (sharl) **law** a given amount of gas expands its volume at constant pressure, in direct proportion to the absolute temperature described by Jacques Charles, French physicist

chart 144

chart 1. a paper documenting the course of a patient's illness. It includes the records of temperature, pulse, respiratory rate, blood pressure, weight and fluid intake and output. 2. to record on a graph the vital signs **dental c** a diagram of the teeth on which clinical and radiographic findings can be recorded

charting the process of making a tabulated record of a patient's progress during an illness

chartula (kar'tu-la) a paper folded to form a packet containing a dose of medicine

chasma (kaz'ma) an opening or gap

chaude-pisse (shod-pes) a burning sensation during micturition

chaulmoogra (caul'mugra) **oil** a vegetable oil used to treat leprosy, a Bengali name

Ch abbreviation for Chirurgeri (surgery)

CHD abbreviation for 1. coronary heart disease 2. congenital heart disease.

check 1. to verify 2. to arrest **c bite** hard wax used to make an impression of teeth

checkup clinical examination by a physician about status of health

Chediak-Higashi (she'de-ak-he-ga-she) **syndrome** a metabolic disorder inherited as an autosomal recessive trait wherein the neutrophils contain peroxidase-positive inclusion bodies. It is characterised by partial albinism, photophobia and pale optic fundi named after M. Chediak, French physician, and O. Higashi, Japanese physician

Chedini(s) expectorant

cheek 1. the side of the face forming the lateral wall of the mouth below the eye 2. the buttock

cheekbone malar bone; zygomatic bone

cheilitis (ke-li'tis) inflammation, cracking and dryness of the lips

cheilosis (ki-lo'sis) reddening and fissuring of the lips at the angles, often as a feature of riboflavin deficiency

cheiropompholyx (ki'ro-pom'fo-liks) blistering condition of hands and feet, related to excessive sweating

chelate (ke'lat) a compound inactivating a toxic substance

chelating agent a chemical used in the treatment of poisoning by metals such as lead, arsenic and mercury

chelation (ke-la'shun) combination of a metal with some heterocyclic structures

chemabrasion (kem-a-bra'shun) use of a chemical substance to destroy superficial layers of the skin

chemical (kem'i-k'l) 1. a substance containing chemical elements 2. pertaining to chemisty **c change** a process in which a substance breaks up or combines with other substances to produce a new substance **c colitis** an acute inflammatory colitis that develops following self-administration of a cleansing enema **c compound** a substance containing two or more chemical elements in a specific proportion **c diabetes mellitus** a preclinical or clinical form of diabetes mellitus characterised by diabetes mellitus-like response curves to glucose tolerance tests **c disaster** accidental liberation of large amounts of chemicals **c element** a chemical substance that can be further separated **c mumps** iodide mumps **c name** name used to describe the molecular structure of a drug **c pollutant** a chemical substance that enters environment through industrial or agricultural activities which poses a health hazard **c perit nitis** an early stage of perforated ulcer where acid is the main cause before infection takes over **c rhizotomy** relief of pain by partial damage to posterior nerve roots by injection of phenol **c warfare** the use of chemicals (in the form of gases) as weapons of war

chemistry (kem'is-tre) the science dealing with the various compounds of elements and the study of their structure

chemoattractant (ke'mo-atrak'tant) an agent that causes an organism or a cell to migrate towards it

chemocautery (kem'o-kaw'ter-e) cauterisation by application of a caustic substance

chemocoagulation (ke'mo-ko-ag'u-la'shun) coagulation by chemical substances

chemodectoma (ke'mo-dek-to'ma) a benign tumour of chemoreceptor system such as carotid body tumour or glomus jugulare tumour

chemokine any cytokine that induces chemotaxis

chemokinesis (ke'mo-ki-ne'sis) an increased activity of an organism in response to chemical stimuli

chemolysis (ke-mol'i-sis) destruction by chemical action

chemonucleolysis injection of chymopapain in certain cases of intervertebral disc rupture

chemopallidectomy (ke-mo-pal'i-dek'ta-me) chemical destruction of a part of globus pallidus of the brain

chemoprevention the use of diet or drugs to reduce the incidence of cancer

chemoprophylaxis (ke-mo-pro'fi-lak'sis) prevention of a disease by the use of a drug or chemical substance

chemopsychiatry (ke'mo-si-ki'a-tre) the use of drugs to treat psychiatric conditions

chemoradiotherapy (ke-mo'ra'de-o-ther'a-pe) the use of chemotherapy and radiotherapy in the treatment

chemoreceptor (ke'mo-re-sep'ter) a sense organ or sensory nerve ending sensitive to stimulation by chemical substances, such as oxygen receptors in carotid body

chemoreflex (ke'mo-re'fleks) any involuntary response to a chemical stimulus

chemoresistance (ke'mo-re-zis'tans) resistance of the cells or microorganisms to the effect of a drug

chemosensitive (ke'mo-sen'si-tiv) reactive to the changes in chemical composition

chemosensory (ke-mo-sen'sa-re) relates to the sensory perception of a chemical as in detection of odour

chemosis (ke-mo-sis) oedema of the conjunctiva producing a pronounced ring around the cornea

chemosterilant (ke-mo'ster'i-lant) a chemical compound causing destruction of microorganisms

chemosurgery (ke'mo-ser'je-re) destruction of tissue by chemical compounds; a technique used for excising locally invasive primary skin cancers

chemosynthesis (ke-mo-sin'the-sis) the production of new chemical compound from other chemical agents

chemotaxin (ke'mo-tak'sin) a substance attracting white blood cells to the site

chemotaxis (ke'mo-tak'sis) the movement of additional white blood cells to the site of inflammation in response to the chemical mediators released by neutrophils, monocytes and injured tissue

chemothalamectomy (kemo-thal-a-mek'to-me) destruction of a part of thalamus by chemical means

chemotherapy (ke'mo-ther'a-pe) treatment of disease by chemical agents most of which are toxic to cells undergoing division and to induce tumour cell lysis **combination c** use of two or more drugs simultaneously in order to enhance their effectiveness or to prevent development of drug resistance

chemzymes a group of small, soluble organic molecuies that catalyse chemical reactions in a fashion similar to that of natural enzymes catalysing biochemical reactions

chenodeoxycholic (ke-no-de-ok'se kol'ik) **acid** conjugated bile acid that facilitates fat absorption or cholesterol excretion

Chernobyl (cher'no-bil) **disaster** explosion of a nuclear reactor in the Ukranian city of Chernobyl in 1986 resulting in an increased incidence of thyroid cancer

cherry angioma senile angioma, a ruby

red papule surrounded by a pale halo, consisting of dilated thin capillaries on the trunk and extremities of elderly adults; de Morgan Spot

cherry red colour mucocutaneous discolouration seen in carbon monoxide poisoning

cherry red spots bright red macules in the optic fundus of patients with Tay-Sachs syndrome, and Niemann-Pick disease

cherubism (cher'u-bizm) facial deformity produced by cystic disease of jaw bones

chest thorax. The part of the body between the neck and diaphragm encased by ribs. It is divided into various regions as supraclavicular, suprasternal, clavicular, infraclavicular, mammary between the 3rd and 6th costal cartilages, inframammary between the 6th rib and the costal arch, sternal, axillary, infra-axillary, suprascapular, scapular, interscapular and infrascapular regions. alar c a long flat chest with scapulae standing prominently like wings on either side barrel-shaped c increase in anteroposterior diameter of the chest. The ribs are horizontal. The spine is unduly concave forwards and sternum is prominently arched, the chest appears circular and the subcostal angle is greater than 90° encountered in chronic airflow obstruction elliptical c bilaterally symmetrical chest with its transverse diameter being greater than the posteroanterior diameter in the ratio of 7:5. The subcostal angle is less than 90° flail c an unstable chest moving paradoxically following multiple fractures flat c shield-like chest with posteroanterior diameter being markedly decreased resulting in an increase in the transverse diameter funnel c pectus excavatum, a funnel-like depression of the lower two-thirds of the sternum with prominent costochondral junctions pigeon c pectus carinatum. The sternum is bulged forwards especially in its upper part. The ribs slope in to meet the sternum on either side, losing their curvature. Chest appears triangular rachitic c abnormalities of chest such as pigeon chest, funnel chest, Harrison's groove and rickety rosary, noted in those suffered from rickets and respiratory diseases in childhood c physiotherapy a rehabilitation programme consisting of postural drainage, cough facilitation, breathing exercises, clapping and vibration over the affected areas of the lungs

chest leads ECG V_1 to V_6 leads where V_1 is placed just to the right of sternum and V_6 in the mid-axillary line on left side and rest in between

chetana (s) consciousness

chewing gum diarrhoea an osmotic diarrhoea caused by excessive sorbitol in sugarless chewing gum

Cheyne-Stoke's respiration see respiration

CHF abbreviation for congestive heart failure

Chiari-Frommel (ke-ar'e-from-mel) syndrome continued lactation and amenorrhoea following child birth due to persistent prolactin secretion and decreased gonadotrophic hormone production, named after Hans Chiari, Austrian pathologist and Richard Frommel, German gynaecologist

chiasma (ki-az'ma) a decussation or crossing optic c an X-shaped crossing of the optic nerve fibres originating from the nasal half of the retina. Beyond this point in the brain the fibres travel in optic tracts

Chiba needle a flexible long needle used for percutaneous cholecystography, named after a Japanese University

chickenpox (chik'en-poks) varicella; a highly contagious disease caused by varicella zoster virus. It affects children. Rash appears on the second day of illness on the trunk, then spreads to the face and limbs. Macules are noted first which within a few hours become papular, then vesicular and within 24 hours pustular. They dry up in a few days to form scabs. As the spots appear in crops, the lesions of all stages of development can be seen in any area at the same time.

hief cells principal cell type of parathyroid gland and peptic cells of the stomach c hyperplasia a pathologic condition of primary or secondary increase in the production of parathyroid hormone

higgers (chig'ers) the six legged red larva of mites of the family Trombiculidae. Some species spread scrub typhus

hilblain (chil'blan) a cutaneous injury from exposure to cold or damp climate producing localised itching, swelling and painful erythema. The common sites are fingers, toes and ears

child human being between infancy and puberty c abuse physical, emotional and sexual injury to a child c bearing pregnant c birth the process of giving birth to a child.

chikitsa (s) treatment c tattva (s) therapeutic principles

chikungunya (chik'un-gun'ya) an acute alpha-virus infection transmitted by Aedes mosquitoes producing a dengue-like fever

chill (chil) a sensation of cold with shivering

chilomastix (ki'lo-mas'tiks) a parasite protozoa found as a commensal in the caecum and colon

chimera (ki'mera) mythical fire breathing monster with a mixture of animal and human

chimerical (ki-mer'I-kal) imaginary, unreal

chimerism (ki-mer'ism) the presence in a person of cells that are genetically different as they are derived from two different fertilised ova. It does not cause any ill health human c migration of foetal cells into the blood of the mother during pregnancy; the two-way migration of cells between transplanted organs and their recipients

chin the anterior prominence of the lower jaw below the lower lip

China clay kaolin

chinta (s) worry

chip a device that processes information at the most basic level within a computer

Chinese lantern site transillumination of infant skull with hydraencephaly and porencephaly demonstrating a lack of opacifiction as there are no cerebral hemispheres

Chinese restaurant syndrome an abrupt allergic reaction caused by sensitivity to monosodium glutamate, a seasoning used in Chinese restaurants. It is characterised by severe headaches, numbness, palpitations, thirst, abdominal and chest pains, sweating and flushing

chiragra (ki-rag'ra) pain in the hand

chiral (ki'ral) denoting an object, such as a molecule in a given configuration that possesses chirality

chiralgia (ki-ral'je-a) pain in the hand

chirality handedness; the three-dimensional conformation of a molecule. It may be a left handed, levo or L-orientation (a feature of most molecules in functioning biological systems) or right-handed, dextro or D-orientation

chiromegaly (ki-ro-meg'a-le) enlargement of the hands

chiropody (ki-rop'o-de) treatment of foot disorders

chiropractice a system of health care based on the concept that the nervous system is the single most important determinant of a person's state of health

chirospasm (ki'-ro-spazm) writers' cramps; a spasm of hand muscles

chistel (chis'l) a beveled-edge steel cutting instrument c fracture an incomplete fracture of the head of the radius where the fracture line extends distally from the centre of the articular surface

Chi-square (ki-skwar) x_2 a set of statistical procedures used to evaluate the relative frequency or proportion of events in a population that fall into well-defined categories

chitin (ki'tin) a horny covering of the body of certain invertebrates such as crabs

Chitta (s) mind

Chlamydiae (kla-mid'e-ae) small gram-negative organisms that only grow inside the cells. Unlike viruses they possess both DNA and RNA in their structure. They have a cell wall and divide by binary fission. There are three species such as *Chlamydia ˙pneumoniae, C. psittaci* and *C. trachomatis* **C pneumoniae** a human pathogen that makes a person to person spread. It presents with sinusitis, pharyngitis, laryngitis and pneumonia. It is sensitive to tetracyclines and macrolides **C psittaci** human infection is related to exposure to birds. It pursues a low grade course with malaise, high fever, cough and muscular pains **C trachomatis** causative agent of trachoma *see* trachoma

Chlamydiaceae (kla-mid'e-a'se) obligate intracellular bacteria belonging to the Chlamydiaceae family

chlamydiosis (kla-mid'e-o'sis) any infection or disease caused by Chlamydia

chloasma (klo-az'ma) melasma; presence of brown macules often seen symmetrically over the cheeks and forehead, mostly in women. May occur spontaneously or in association with pregnancy and oral contraceptive pill **c gravidarum** pigmentation over cheeks, forehead and around the eyes during pregnancy

chloral (klo'ral) an oily liquid with a pungent odour **c hydrate** a colourless crystalline substance used as a sedative and hypnotic

chlorambucil (klo-ram'bu-sil) an alkylating cytotoxic agent used in chronic lymphatic leukaemia and lymphomas

chloramine T an antiseptic used to irrigate wounds

chloramphenicol (klo'ram-fen'i-kol) the only naturally occurring broad spectrum antibiotic containing nitrobenzene

indicated in infections due to *Salmonella typhi, S. paratyphi, H. influenzae* infections

chlorcyclizine (klor-si'kli-zen) H_1 histamine receptor antagonist

chlordiazepoxide (klor'di-az'e-pok'sid) a benzodiazepine derivative used in the treatment of anxiety disorders and alcohol withdrawal syndrome

chloraemia (klo-re'me-a) increased level of chloride in the blood

chloretic (klo-ret'ik) an agent increasing the bile flow

chlorhydria (klor-hi'dre-a) an excess of hydrochloric acid in the stomach

chloride (klo'rid) a salt of hydrochloric acid. Serum level is 100 to 110 mEq/L. It is a major extracellular anion contributing to osmotic pressure and movement of water between fluid compartments **c channel** an ion channel in the plasma membrane of most cells. They participate in the regulations of cell volume, transepithelial transport and stabilisation of membrane potential in muscle **c shift** exchange of plasma chlorides with red cell bicarbonate in tissues producing CO_2 **ferric c** used as a reagent and topically as a styptic and astringent

chlorinated (klo'ri-nat'id) charged with chlorine **c lime** calcium hypochlorite and calcium chloride used as a bleaching agent and as an antiseptic

chlorination (klo'ri-na'shun) addition of chlorine and its compounds in a concentration of 1 part per million to the water to kill the bacteria

chlorine (klo'ren) a highly irritating gas, atomic number 17

chlorite (klo'rit) a salt of chlorous acid used as disinfectant and bleaching agent

chlorofluorocarbon CFC gaseous compound that contains chlorine and fluorine

chloroform (klo'ro-form) $CHCl_3$ a colourcess liquid with ethereal odour, used as solvent. Earlier it was used as an inhalation anaesthetic

chloroma (klor-o'ma) a malignant green coloured tumour arising from myeloid tissue; green cancer

chlorophyll (klor'o-fil) any of green magnesium complex of the phorbin derivative found in photosynthetic plants

chloroprivic (klor'o-pri'vik) deprived of chlorides from loss of chlorides

chloropsia (klor-op'se-a) a defect of vision in which objects appear green

chloroquin (klor'o-kwin) a 4-aminoquinoline antimalarial, schizonticidal agent used in treatment of malaria, also used in hepatic amoebiasis, and rheumatoid arthritis c resistant malaria Falciparum malaria increasingly resistant to the previously effective chloroquine

chlorosis (klo-ro'sis) green sickness, Virgin's disease; iron deficiency anaemia named for the yellow-green skin pallor in young females, associated with koilonychia

chlorthiazide (klor'o-thi'a-zid) first thiazid diuretic inhibiting renal tubular reabsorption

chlorphenesin (klor-fen'e-sin) a topical antifungal agent

chlorpheniramine (klor'fen-ir'a-men) a pyridine derived antihistaminic preparation

chlorpromazine (klor'pro'ma-zen) a phenothiazine derivative used as a tranquilliser and as an antiemetic

chlorpropamide (klor'pro'pa-mid) an oral sulphonyl-urea, long acting hypoglycaemic agent used in the treatment of non-insulin dependent diabetes mellitus

chlortetracycline (klor'te-tra-si'klen) original tetracycline, relatively unstable antibiotic active against a wide range of microorganisms

chlorthalidone (klor-thal'i-don) an orally effective diuretic

chloruresis (klor'ur-e'sis) excretion of chlorides in the urine

chloruria (klo-rur'ea) excretion of excess chlorides in the urine

choana (ko-a'na) funnel-shaped cavity or infundibulum

chocolate a preparation from ground and roasted beans of the cacao plant, Theobroma cacao c agar blood agar, a growth medium for bacteria such as H. influenzae Neisseria species and fastidious anaerobes c cyst endometrioma, an ovarian cyst filled with thick inspissated blood, grossly is likened to chocolate

choke (chok) to interrupt respiration by obstruction c urethrogram micturition against external pressure with contrast in the bladder to improve urethrogram picture

chokes sudden onset of respiratory distress in Caisson's disease. There is an increase in platelet adhesion to gas bubbles that release vasoconstrictors and platelet factor causing coagulopathy

choked disc papilloedema with swelling of nerve head. It is caused by raised intracranial tension. There is blurring of disc margins and obliteration of optic cup

cholagogue (ko'la-gag) a substance that stimulates contraction of gall bladder to promote bile flow

cholangiectasis (ko'lan'je-ek'ta-sis) dilatation of a bile duct

cholangiocarcinoma (ko-lan'je-o-kar'si-no-ma) an adenocarcinoma arising from the epithelium of the intrahepatic bile ducts

cholangioenterostomy (ko-lan'je-o-en'teros-ta-me) surgical anastomosis of a bile duct to the stomach.

cholangiography (kol-an'je-og'ra-fe) radiography of the bile ducts after they have been filled with a contrast medium

cholangiole (kol-an'je-ol) one of the terminal branches of the bile duct system

cholangiolitis (kol-aan'je-o-lit'is) inflammation of the cholangioles

cholangiotomy (kol-an'je-ot'a-me) incision into a bile duct

cholangitis (kol-an'ji-tis) inflammation of common bile duct cholate (ko'lat) cholic acid salt

chole-combining form, meaning bile

cholecalciferol (kol'e-kal-sef'er-ol) vitamin D2 and substance obtained from the diet or synthesised in the skin on irradiation of 7-dehydrocholesterol

cholecyst (ko'le-sist) the gall bladder

cholecystagogue (kol'e-sis'ta-gog) an agent promoting evacuation of the gall bladder

cholecystalgia (ko'le-sis'tel'je-a) distension of the gall bladder

cholecystectomy (ko'le-sis-tek'ta-me) surgical removal of the gall bladder

cholecystenterostomy (ko'le-sis'ten-ter-os'ta-me) surgical creation of a new communication between the gall bladder and intestine

cholecystitis (ko'le-sis'ti-tis) inflammation of the gall bladder **acute c** inflammation with variable infection, ulceration and neutrophilic infiltration of gall bladder wall, usually due to impaction of a stone in the cystic duct **chronic c** chronic inflammation of gall bladder, usually secondary to lithiasis and there is marked thickening of the wall **emphysematous c** infection with gas-producing organisms giving rise to gas in the gall bladder

cholecystoduodenostomy (ko'le-sis-to-doo'o-da-nos'ta-me) surgical anastomosis of the gall bladder and duodenum

cholecystogastrostomy (ko'le-sis-to-gas-tros'ta-me) surgical anastomosis between the gall bladder and stomach

cholecystogram (ko'le-sis'to-gram) a radiograph of the gall bladder obtained by cholecystography

cholecystography (ko'ale-sis'tog-ra-fe) radiographic study of the gall bladder after oral administration of a cholecysto-paque

cholecystojejunostomy (ko'le-sis'to-je-joo-nos'ta-me) an anastomosis between the gall bladder and jejunum

cholecystokinin (ko'le-sis'to-ki-nin) a polypeptide substance secreted in the small intestine that stimulates gall bladder contraction and secretion of pancreatic enzymes

choledochal (ko'le-do'kal) pertaining to the common bile duct

choledochitis (ko'le-do-ki'tis) inflammation of the common bile duct

choledochoduodenostomy (ko-led'o-ko-du'o-de-nos'to-me) surgical anastomosis of the common bile duct to the duodenum

choledochoenterostomy (-en'te-os'ta-me) surgical anastomosis of the bile duct to the stomach

choledochojejunostomy (-je-joo-nos'ta-me) surgical anastomosis of the bile duct to the jejunum

choledocholithiasis (-li-thia-sis) stone in the common bile duct

choledocholithotomy (-li-thot'o-me) surgical incision into common bile duct for removal of the stone

choledochorrhaphy (ko'le-do-ko-ra'fe) suture or repair of the common bile duct

choledochotomy (ko'le-do-kota-me) incision into the common bile duct

choledochus (ko'le-do-kus) the common bile duct

choleic (ko-la'ik) pertaining to the bile

cholelith (ko'le-lith) gall stone

cholelithiasis (ko'le-li-thi'a-sis) the presence or formation of gall stones

cholelithotomy (ko'le-li-thot'o-me) surgical incision of the biliary tract for removal of gall stone(s).

cholelithotripsy (ko'le-li'th'o-trip'se) crushing of a gall stone

cholaemia (ko-lo'me-a) presence of bile or bile pigment in blood

choleperitoneum (ko-le-per'i-ta-ne-um) the presence of bile in the peritoneum

cholepoisis (ko'le-poi-e'sis) the formation of bile in the liver **cholepoietic** adj

cholera (kol'er-a) a severe acute gastrointestinal infection caused by *Vibrio cholera.* It is transmitted through infected drinking water contaminated by stool or vomit of patients with cholera. Cholera vibrios multiply in the lumen of small intestine and are not invasive. They adhere to the intestinal mucosa and secrete a powerful exotoxin which by stimulation cAMP results in outpouring of fluid. It presents with severe diarrhoea without pain followed by vomiting of sudden onset. Later there is passage of rice water material consisting of clear fluid with flecks of mucus. There is severe dehydration with muscular cramps. The skin becomes cold and clammy and wrinkled. The eyes are sunken. There is fall in blood pressure and pulse becomes imperceptible and urine output diminishes. There is rapid improvement by replacement of water and electrolytes

choleragen (kol'er-a-jen) an exotoxin produced by cholera vibrio

choleraic (kol'a-ra'ik) of or pertaining to cholera

choleresis (kol'ler'e-sis) the secretion of bile by the liver

choleretic (ko'ler-et'ik) 1. stimulating the bile production by the liver 2. an agent stimulating production of bile

choleria (ko-ler'e-a) a hostile temperament

choleroid (kol'er-o-id) resembling cholera

cholestasis (ko'la-sta'sis) obstruction to the flow of bile inside the liver. **cholestatic** adj

cholesteatoma (ko'le-ste'a-to-ma) 1. a mass of keratinised squamous epithelium and cholesterol in the middle ear from chronic otitis media 2. an epidermoid cyst arising in CNS

cholesteatosis (ko'le-ste'a-to'sis) fatty degeneration due to cholesterol esters

cholesterol (ko-les'ter-ol) the most abundant steroid in animal tissues that is precursor of bile acids and steroid hormones and a key constituent of cell membranes. Most is synthesised in the liver, but some is absorbed from dietary sources, found in food rich in animal fat. It circulates in the plasma complexed to proteins of various

sities. It can accumulate or deposit abnormally and plays an important role in the pathogenesis of atheroma in the arteries

cholesterolesterase (ko-les'ter-ol-es'ter-as) an enzyme that catalyses the breakdown of cholesterol and other sterol esters and triglycerides

cholesterolosis (ko-les'ter-ol-o'sis) abnormal deposition of cholesterol in tissues

cholesteroluria (ko-les'ter-al-ur'e-a) the presence of cholesterol in the urine

cholesteryl (ko-les'te-ril) cholesterol radical formed by removal of the hydroxyl group

choletherapy (ko'le-ther'a-pe) treatment by administration of bile salts

cholic (kol'ik) one of the primary bile acids, usually exist conjugated with glycine or taurine. It helps in fat absorption and cholesterol excretion

choline (ko'len) 1. a quaternary amine 2. a member of B vitamin complex

choline acetyltransferase (ko'len-as'e-tel-trans'fer-as) an enzyme catalysing the synthesis of acetyl choline

cholinergic (ko'lin-er'jik) relating to nerve fibres that employ acetyl choline as their neurotransmitter

cholinesterase (ko'lin-es'ter-as) an enzyme that catalyses the hydrolysis of the acyl group from different esters of choline

cholinoceptor (ko'lin-o-sep'ter) cholinergic receptor

cholinolytic (-lit'ik) 1. blocking the action of acetyl choline or of cholinergic agents 2. an agent that blocks the action of acetyl choline in organs supplied by parasympathetic nerves and in voluntary muscles

cholinomimetic (-mi-met'ik) having an action similar to acetylcholine; parasympathomimetic

chol (o) combining word for bile

choluria (kol'u're-a) 1. presence of bile in the urine 2. discolouration of the urine with bile pigments. **choluric** adj

chondral (kon'dril) pertaining to the cartilage.

chondrectomy (kon-drek'ta-me) surgical removal of a cartilage

chondritis (kon-dri'tis) inflammation of a cartilage usually caused by mechanical pressure, stress or injury

chondroblast (kon'dro-blast) an immature cartilage producing cell

chondroblastoma (kon'dro-blas-to-ma) a benign tumour arising in the epiphyses of long bones of adolescents, consisting of highly cellular tissue resembling foetal cartilage

chondrocalcinosis (kon'dro-kal'si-no'sis) calcification of cartilage

chondrocostal (kon'dro-kos'tal) pertaining to the ribs and costal cartilages

chondrocranium (kon'dro-kra'ne-um) the cartilaginous cranial structures of the foetus

chondrocyte (kon'dro-sit) a mature cartilage cell

chondrodermatitis (kon'dro-der'ma-tit'is) an inflammation affecting the cartilage and skin as in the helix of the ear

chondrodynia (-din'e-a) pain in a cartilage

chondrodysplasia (-dis-pla'zah) a disturbance in the development of epiphyseal cartilage of the long bones resulting in arrested growth of the long bones and dwarfism

chondrodystrophy (-dis'tra-fe) a disorder of cartilage formation

chondoepiphysitis (-ep'i-fi-zit'is) inflammation affecting the epiphyseal cartilages

chondrofibroma (-fi-bro'ma) a fibroma with cartilaginous elements

chondrogenesis (-jen'i-sis) formation of cartilage

chondroid (kon'droid) 1. resembling cartilage 2. hyaline cartilage

chondroitin (kon-dro'i-tin) sulphate a glycosaminoglycan found in the ground substance of the connective tissue particularly cartilage, bone, blood vessels and cornea

chondroma (kon-dro'ma) a non-malignant tumour of cartilage cells on the surface of or inside the bones

chondromalacia (kon'dro-ma-la'sha) softening of the cartilage

chondromatosis (-ma-to'sis) presence of multiple tumour-like foci of cartilage

chondromyoma (-mi-o'ma) benign tumour of muscle and cartilage

chondromyxoma (-mik'so-ma) chondromyxoid fibroma

chondrosseous (-os'e-us) composed of cartilage and bone

chondropathy (-kon'drop'a-the) disease of cartilage

chondrophyte (kon'dro-fit) an abnormal cartilaginous mass developing at the articular surface of a bone

chondroplasia (kon'dro-pla'zha) formation of cartilage by chondrocytes

chondroplast (kon'dro-plast) chondroblast

chondroplasty (kon'dro-plas'ti) a debridement procedure to repair joint cartilage; abrasion arthroplasty

chondrosarcoma (kon'dro-sarcoma) a malignant growth of cartilage that usually affects the long bones, the pelvis and the clavicle

chondrosis (kon-dro'sis) cartilage formation

chondrotomy (kon-drot'a-me) surgical division of cartilage

CHOP a chemotherapeutic regimen used for treatment of lymphoma consisting of cyclophosphamide, adreomycin, oncovin and prednisone

chord (kord) cord pl chordae c dorsalis notochord c gubernaculum a portion of the gubernaculum testis or of round ligament of the uterus c magna tendo calcaneus c spermatica spermatic cord c spinalis spinal cord c tendina corditis tendinous strands running from the papillary muscles to the atrioventricular valves c tympani a nerve given off from the facial nerve in the facial canal and conveys taste sensation from anterior two thirds of the tongue and innervates submandibular, sublingual and lingual glands c umbilicalis umbilical cord c vocalis vocal cords

chorda (kor'da) pl. **chordae** a tendinous or cord-like structure

chordata (kor-dat-a) animals having a notochord during their developmental stage

chorde (kor'de) downward deflection of penis

chorditis (kor-dit'is) inflammation of the vocal or the spermatic cords

chordoma (kor-do'ma) a malignant tumour arising from the embryonic remains of the notochord, appears most commonly in fifth and sixth decade in sacrococcygeal region

chordotomy (kor-dot'a-me) cordotomy

chorea (kor-e'ah) irregular, purposeless, arrhythmic and asymmetric movements variable in type and location that constantly change in form and affecting different parts of the body at irregular intervals **c gravidarum** choreiform movements appearing in first trimester of pregnancy **Huntington's c** a progressive disorder noted in middle age with an autosomal dominant inheritance, choreoathetosis and dementia **senile c** chorea occuring in elderly age group **Sydenham's c** chorea occurring as a manifestation of rheumatic fever

choreiform (ko-re'i-form) resembling chorea

choreoathetosis (kor'e-o-ath'e-to'sis) a disorder exhibiting the features of choreic and athetoid movements

chorioadenoma (kor'e-o-ad'e-noma) adenoma of the chorion

chorioallantosis (kor'e-al-lan'to-is) extraembryonic membrane formed by union of the chorion and allantois, which forms the foetal portion of placenta in mammals

choriocarcinoma (kor'e-arkar'si-no-ma) a rare malignant tumour that develops inside the uterus from the placenta

choriogenesis (kor'e-o-jen'i-sis) the development of chorion

choriomeningitis (kor'e-o-men'in-jit'is) cerebral meningitis with lymphocytic infiltration of the choroid plexus

chorion (ka're-on) the outermost of the two membrane layers containing the aminotic fluid and the foetus. It gets attached to the placenta

chorionic gonadotropin human chorionic gonadotropin

chorionic villus sampling a prenatal diagnostic procedure in the ninth to 11th week of pregnancy under guidance of ultrasound scanning in which foetal cells are obtained from the placenta and studied for genetic abnormalities

chorioretinal (kor'e-o-ret'in-il) pertaining to the choroid and retina

chorioretinitis inflammation of the choroid and retina

chorioretinopathy (-ret'in-op'a-the) a disorder affecting both the choroid and retina

Christmas disease a rare inherited coagulation abnormality; it is also called haemophilia B disease, bears the surname of child in whom the disorder was recognised first

Christian's triad triad of symptoms in histiocytosis, consisting of lytic bony lesion, diabetes insipidus and exophthalmos, named after Henry Christian, US physician.

Christian syndrome an autosomal dominant digital dysmorphia characterised by shortened thumbs and distal phalanges

Christian-Weber disease relapsing nonsuppurative panniculitis. There is focal painful aggregates of subcutaneous fat necrosis with erythematous, ulcerating and eventually atrophic skin

choristoma (ko'ris-to'ma) a mass of histologically normal tissue located in an abnormal site

choroid (ko'roid) the middle vascular structure of the eye situated between the sclera and the retina. **choroidal** adj

choroiditis (ko'roi-dit'is) an inflammation of the choroid

choroidocyclitis (ko-roi'do-sik-lit'is) an inflammation of the choroid and ciliary body

chrom (o) combining word for colour

chromaffin (kro-maf'in) staining strongly with chromium salts, as some cells of the adrenal glands

chromaffinoma (kro-maf'i-no-ma) tumour containing chromaffin cells, such as pheochromocytoma

chromate (kro'mat) any salt of chromic acid

chromatic (kro-mat'ik) 1. pertaining to colour 2. pertaining to chromatin

chromatid (kro'ma-tid) **bodies** darkly staining, elongated relatively well circumscribed masses, 1-4 in number, found in amoebic cysts.

chromatin (kro'ma-tin) the material inside cells consisting of DNA and protein from which chromosomes are formed

chromatism (kro'ma-tizm) abnormal pigment deposits

chromatogenous (kro'ma-toj'e-nus) producing colour

chromatography (kro'ma-tog'ra-fe) a laboratory technique in which mixtures of complex molecules are separated along a gradient of pressure or solubility between a liquid or gas and solid or liquid phase. The molecules are separated by absorption, gel filtration, ion exchange or partitioning

chromatolysis (kro-ma-tol'i-sis) disintegration of the granules of chromophil substance, as in Nissl bodies of a neuron, which may occur after exhaustion of the cell or damage to its peripheral process.

chromatophil (kro-mat'o-fil) a cell staining easily **chromatophilic** adj

chromatophore (-for) 1. any pigmentary cell 2. colour producing plastid

chromatopsia (kro'ma-top'se-a) a visual defect in which colourless objects appear to be tinged with colour

chromatoptometry (kro'ma-top-tom'e-tre) measurement of colour perception

chromaturia (kro'ma-tur'e-a) abnormal colouration of the urine

chromhidrosis (kro'mi-dro'sis) secretion of coloured sweat

chromium (kro'me-um) chemical element with atomic number 24. An essential dietary trace element

chromoblast (kro'mo-blast) an embryonic cell which develops into a pigment cell

chromblastomycosis (kro'mo-blas'to-mi-ko'sis) a localised chronic mycosis of the skin and subcutaneous tissue, producing rough and irregular lesions as to present a cauliflower-like appearance.

chromoclastogenic (-klas'ta-jen'ik) causing chromosomal damage

chromocyte (kro'mo-sit) any pigmented cell

chromocystoscopy (kro'mo-sis-tos'ka-pe) cystoscopy of the ureteral orifices following oral administration of a dye

chromogen (kro'mo-jen) any agent producing colouring matter

chromogenesis (kro'mo-jen'e-sis) the production of colour or pigment

chromomere (kro'mo-mer) bead-like granular structures along a chromonema

chromonema (kro'mo-ne'ma) the central thread of a chromatid along which lie the chromomeres

chromophil (kro'mo-fil) any easily stainable cell or tissue. **chromophilic** adj

chromophobe (-fob) any cell or tissue that is not readily stainable

chromophobia (kro-mo-fo'be-a) the quality of staining poorly with dyes **chromophobic** adj

chromophore (kro'mo-for) 1. a coloured plastid in plants and in certain forms of protozoa 2. a pigment bearing phago-cyte

chromoscopy (kro-mos'ka-pe) diagnosis of renal functions by colour of urine following administration of dyes

chromosomal RNA oligonucleotide segments of RNA that serve to 'prime' the growth fork of DNA in the lagging strand after duplication of DNA

chromosome thread-like structures inside the nuclei of cells that consist of one or more (23 in humans) usually paired, very long DNA molecules that are associated with RNA and histones, and the complete complement of chromosomes contain the complete genetic information present in a living organism **c abnormality** an abnormality in the number or structure of chromosomes inside a person's cells, that can cause series of birth defects **c analysis** a laboratory procedure in which cells of foetal origin are obtained either in the first trimester by chorionic villus biopsy or later in pregnancy by amniocentesis and grown in a tissue culture medium to detect major chromosomal defects **c banding** a technique for identifying chromosome pairs and analyzing regions within chromosomes **c breakage syndromes** a group of inherited disorders in which the chromosomes have an increased fragility as in ataxia — telangiectasis, Fanconi syndrome. They exhibit an increased susceptibility to certain malignancies **human artificial c** HAC, a vector used to transfer or express large fragments of human DNA.

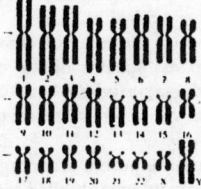

Chromosomes

chromotherapy (kro'mo-thera-pi) colour therapy

chronic (kron'ik) a disorder that is persisting for a long time **c active hepatitis** a type of hepatitis characterised by progressive inflammation and destruction of liver cells; it leads to cir-

rhosis of the liver **c fatigue syndrome** CFS a severe disabling illness characterised by a self-reported persistent or relapsing fatigue of ≥ 6 consecutive months duration accompanied by infections, rheumatologic and neuropsychiatric symptoms, which are not attributable to other known conditions and a symptom complex **c granulomatous diseases** (CGD) a heterogeneous group of immune system defects characterised by recurrent and potentially fatal pyogenic infections of early onset. The neutrophils though ingest pathogens fail to produce superoxide and related microbial oxygen intermediates **c obstructive pulmonary disease** COPD diffuse obstruction involving structural and functional changes in the parenchyma and also in the large and small airways. The airway obstruction is constant or makes slow progress and exists without a specific cause such as bronchiectasis, cystic fibrosis or obliterative bronchiolitis or localised disease in upper airways

chronobiology (kron'o-bi-ol-a-je) the scientific study concerned with the timing of biologic events, especially repetitive or cyclic phenomenon

chronograph (kron'a-graf) an instrument for recording small intervals of time

chronotropism (kro-not'ro-pizm) modification of the rate of a periodic movement such as a heartbeat.

chrys (o) combining form word for gold

chrysoderma (kris'o-der-ma) a slaty-gray discolouration of skin and sclera due to deposition of gold salts in the connective tissue of the skin and eye

chrysotile (kris'o-til) white asbestos as serpentine form with curly long fibres

chubby puffer syndrome a central sleep apnoea affecting obese, prepubescent males caused by primary hypoventilation

churna (s) powder

chylaemia (kile'me-a) presence of chyle in the blood

chyle (kil) a milky fluid taken up by the lacteals from intestine during digestion. It consists of lymph and chylomicrons in a stable emulsion, carried by the lymphatic system via the thoracic duct into the circulation

chylectasia (ki-lek-ta'ze-a) dilatation of a chylous vessel such as lacteal

chyliferous (ki-lif'er-us) 1. forming chyle 2. transporting chyle

chylocoele (kil'o-cel) scrotal elephantiasis

chylocyst (-sist) cisterna chyli

chyloderma (-der'ma) elephantiasis

chylomicron (-mi'kron) a class of lipoproteins that transport exogenous cholesterol, triglycerides and several apolipoproteins to tissues after meals

chylomicronaemia (ki'lo-mi-kron-e'me-a) an excess of chylomicrons in the blood. There is also an increase in the triglyceride level (> 2.25 mmol/L)

chylopericardium (-per'i-kar'de-um) presence of chyle in the pericardial cavity

chylothorax (-thor'aks) presence of chyle in the pleural cavity

chylous (ki'lus) pertaining to or of the nature of chyle

chyluria (kil-ur'e-a) the passage of chyle in the urine, giving a milky appearance

chyme (kim) the semi-digested food passed from the stomach into the duodenum

chymification (ki-mi-fi-ka'shun) conversion of food into chyme

chymotrypsin (-trip'sin) a serine proteinase produced in intestine by activation of chymotrypsinogen by trypsin

chymotrypsinogen (-trip'sin'o-jen) the precursor of chymotrypsin and converted to chymotrypsin by the action of trypsin

CI abbreviation for cardiac index; colour index

Ci abbreviation for curie

cib food

cicatrectomy (sik'a-trek'ta-me) surgical removal of a cicatrix

cicatrix (sik'a-triks) pl. cicatrices a scar

cicatrization (sik'a-tri-za'shun) the formation of a scar

cigarette paper skin markedly attenuated skin with a shiny velvety surface due to defective synthesis, processing of stability to type I and III collagen, seen Ehlers- Danlos syndrome type I

cilia (sil'e-a) tiny, hair-like projections from the surface of some cells of choroid plexus, trachea, bronchial passages, fallopian tubes and spermatozoa. They produce wave-like motion. They consist of a 9+2 pattern of nine peripherally placed doublets and a centrally placed doublet of microtubular filaments

ciliary (sil'e-e're) pertaining to any cilia or hair-like processes 2. relating to eye structures such as the ciliary body or muscle

ciliata (sil'e-a'ta) phylum ciliophora where members possess cilia throughout the life cycle, the examples are *Paramecium* or *Balantidium coli*

ciliate (sil'e-at) having cilia

ciliectomy (sil'e-ek'ta-me) 1. excision of portion of ciliary body. 2. surgical removal of a portion of the eyelid containing the eyelashes

cilium (sil'e-um) singular of cilia

ciliosis (sil-o'sis) spasms of the eyelid

cimbia (sim'be-a) a white band running across the ventral surface of the crus cerebri

cimetidine (si-met'i-den) an antagonist to H2 receptors which inhibits gastric acid secretion and used to treat peptic ulcer

cinchona (sin-ko'na) the dried bark of the root and stem of various species of cinchona; it is the source of quinine and quinidine and cinchonine and cinchonidine

cinchonism (sin'ko-nizm) toxic manifestation of cinchona characterised by flushed skin, tinnitus, blurred vision, dizziness, nausea, vomiting and diarrhoea. Very high levels of cinchona exhibit skin rashes, somnolence, blindness and marked hypotension

cine combining word for movement

cineangiocardiography (sin'e-an'je-o-karde-og'ra-fe) motion pictures of the passage of a contrast medium through chambers of the heart and blood vessels

cineangiography (- an'je-og'ra-fe) the photographic recording of the images of the heart and blood vessels by motion picture technique

cinerea (si-ne're-a) the gray matter of the nervous system **cinereal** adj

cingulectomy (sin'gu-lek'ta-me) electrolytic destruction of the anterior cingulate gyrus and corpus collosum

cingulum (sing'gu-lum) pl. **cingula** 1. a girdle or an encircling structure 2. a fibre bundle passing longitudinally in the cingulate gyrus

ciprofloxacin (sip'ro-flock'sa-sin) a synthetic fluoroquinolone antibiotic effective against many gram-positive and gram-negative organisms

circadian (ser'ka-de'an) denoting a 24-hour period **c rhythm** any biological pattern with a cycle of about 24 hours

circinate (ser-si-nat) resembling a ring or circle

circle (ser'kl) a round part. **c of Willis** a ring of blood vessels at the base of the brain

circling (ser'kling) movement in a circle

circuit (ser'kit) a course traversed by an electric current

circulation (ser'ku-la'shun) movement in a circle, usually referring to the movement of blood through the heart and blood vessels **allontoic c** foetal circulation through the arteries **blood c** the course of the blood through the capillaries and veins back again to the heart **capillary c** the course of the blood through the capillaries **collateral c** maintenance of blood flow in small anastomosing channels when main vessel is obstructed. **enterohepatic c** the cycle in which bile salts are absorbed from the intestine and returned to the liver, via the portal circulation and secreted into the bile and again enter the intestine **extracorporeal c** circulation of blood outside the body through a heart-lung machine or artificial kidney **foetal c** circulation propelled by foetal heart **hypophysioportal c** capillary network from the median eminence of the hypothalamus into the portal vessels to the sinusoids of anterior hypophysis **lesser c** the pulmonary circulation **lymph c** passage of lymph through the lymphatic vessels and lymph glands **placental c** circulation of blood through the placenta during intrauterine life **portal c** 1. any part of systemic circulation in which blood draining from one structure flows to supply capillary bed of another structure before reaching the heart 2. passage of blood from the small intestine, the right half of the colon and the spleen through the portal vein to the liver **pulmonary c** the flow of blood from the right ventricle through the pulmonary artery to the lungs and back through the pulmonary veins to the left atrium **systemic c** circulation of blood through the arteries, and returning venous blood to the right atrium. **thebesian c** system of smaller veins in the myocardium **vitelline c** the circulation through blood vessels of the yolk sac

circumcision (serk'um-siz'in) surgical removal of the foreskin of the penis

circumduction (-duk'shun) circular movement of the limb or of the eye

circumflex (serk'um-fleks) curved like a bow

circumference the outer boundary, especially of a circular area **chest c** measured at the level of nipples at mid-inspiration **c of arm** measured with a tape held firmly at the mid-point between the acromion and tip of the olecranon. It is a useful measure of nutritional status between age of 1 and 5 years as it is constant during those years. Normal is 16-17 cm **head c** circumference of the head at the level of supraorbital ridges in front and occiput behind, a useful parameter to assess the growth of the brain

circumscribed (serk'um-skribd) bounded, limited, confined to a limiting area.

circumstantiality (serk'um-stan'she-al'it-e) a disturbance in the thought process in which one makes an unnecessary elaboration of many trivial details

circumvallate (-val'at) referring to a structure surrounded by a wall as the papillae of the tongue

cirrhosis (si-rosis) progressive and widespread necrosis of liver cells associated with inflammation and fibrosis leading to loss of normal liver architecture. There is distortion and loss of normal hepatic vasculature with the development of portal systemic shunts and formation of nodules due to proliferation of surviving hepatocytes The condition makes a gradual onset with anorexia, dyspepsia, reduction in liver size, mild jaundice, ascites and signs of liver cell failure and portal hypertension **alcoholic c** cirrhosis developing in chronic alcoholism, which intially is associated with hepatomegaly due to fatty change and later by contraction of the liver **biliary c** cirrhosis due to biliary obstruction which may be primary resulting from destruction of intrahepatic bile ducts or secondary to large duct biliary obstruction **cardiac c** an extensive fibrotic reaction within the liver due to prolonged congestive heart failure; pseudocirrhosis **Laennec's c** portal cirrhosis, named after Rene Laennec, French physician and inventor of the stethoscope **micronodular c** presence of regenerating nodules of 1mm in diameter involving every lobule, surrounded by thick fibrous septa tends to evolve into macronodular cirrhosis **macronodular**

c nodules of variable size with many more than 3 mm in diameter and connective tissue septa varies in thickness **portal c** a chronic disease of liver where the normal liver lobules are replaced by small regenerating nodules separated by fibrous tissue strands **postnecrotic c** necrosis of whole lobules with collapse of reticular framework resulting in large scars, that may follow viral or toxic necrosis **cirrhotic** ad

cirsectomy (ser-sek'ta-me) excision of a portion of a varicose vein

cirsoid (ser'soid) resembling a varix.

cisplatin (sis'plat-in) a platinum chemotherapeutic agent with antitumour activity. It binds DNA and interferes with DNA synthesis

cistern (sis'tern) 1. any cavity or enclosed space serving as a reservoir for fluids such as chyle, lymph or cerebrospinal fluid 2. an ultramicroscopic space between the membranes of the flattened sacs of endoplasmic reticulum or the two membranes of nuclear envelope

cisterna (sis-ter'na) cistern **c basalis** interpeduncular cistern, dilatation of the subarachnoid space in front of the pons, where arachnoid membrane stretches across the two temporal lobes **c chyli** a dilated part of the thoracic duct at its origin in lumbar region into which the intestinal trunk and two lumbar lymphatic trunks open **c magna** cerebellomedullary cistern, the largest of the subarachnoid cisterns between the cerebellum and medulla oblongata **terminal c's** pairs of transversely oriented tubules of the sarcoplasmic reticulum occurring at regular intervals in skeletal muscle fibres

cisternography (sis'ter-nog'ra-fe) radiographic study of basal cistern of brain after subarachnoid injection of radioopaque contrast medium

cistron (sis'tron) the smallest unit of genetic material, considered synonymous with gene

citric (sit'rik) **acid** a tricarboxylic acid obtained from citrus fruits and functions as a key intermediate in intermediate metabolism

citrullinaemia (sit-rul'in-e'me-a) excess of citrulline in the blood

citrulline (sit'rul-en) an amino acid formed from ornithine in the course of urea cycle, which gets converted into arginine. It is also a product in nitric oxide biosynthesis

citrullinuria (-ur'e-a) presence of a large amount of citrulline in the urine

cittosis (si-to'sis) pica

civitte (si'vet) body necrotic keratinocyte, colloid body and hyaline body

CK abbreviation for creatine kinase

Cl chemical symbol for chlorine

clades (klay-dz) different subtypes of HIV

clamp (klamp) a surgical device for compressing a part or structure

clapotement (kla-pot'mawn) a splashing sound as in succussion splash

Clara cell a rounded, non-cilated cell protruding between ciliated epithelial cells in the bronchoiolar epithelium named after Max Clara, Austrian anatomist

clarificant (kar-if'i-kant) a substance which clears the turbidity of a liquid

clarithromycin (kal-rith'tro-mi'sen) a macrolide antibiotic effective against a wide range of gram-positive and gram-negative organisms

clasp (klasp) a device to hold something **c knife spasticity** in pyramidal lesions there is hypertonia offering increased resistance to passive movement. The resistance is greatest at the initial phase of movement and then suddenly it gives way during the latter phase. It is best appreciated in the flexor muscles of the upper limb and the extensor muscles of the lower limb

class (klas) a taxonomic category, the next division below the phylum and above the order

classification (klas'si-fi-ka'shun) a systematic arrangement into classes or groups based on certain common characteristics

clastic (klas'tik) undergoing division

clastogenic (klas'ta-jen'ik) causing breakage as of chromosomes

claudication (klaw'di-ka'shun) limping **intermittent c** attacks of pain and lameness brought on by walking chiefly in the calf muscle and the condition is seen in occlusive arterial disease

claustrophilia (klaws'tra-fil'e-a) an abnormal desire to be present in a closed room or place

claustrophobia (-fo'be-a) intense fear of closed places or crowded areas

clastrum (klaws'trum) an anatomical structure having a resemblance to a barrier, such as a thin layer of gray matter lying lateral to the external capsule, separating it from the white matter of insula

clavicle (klav'i-kl) the collar bone *see* table of bones **clavicular** adj

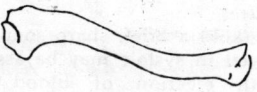

Clavicle

clavulanate (klav'u-la-nat) a beta lactamase antibiotic structurally related to the penicillins that inactivate B-lactamase in penicillin-resistant organisms

clavus (kla'vús) a corn caused by pressure over a bony prominence

claw foot (klaw'foot) a high arched foot with the toes hyperextended at the metacarpophalangeal joints and flexed at the distal interphalangeal joints

claw hand atrophy of the interosseous muscles of hand with hyperextension at the metacarpophalangeal joints and flexion at the interphalangeal joints.

clearance (kler'ans) 1. the act of removal of something from some place 2. removal of a substance from blood

creatinine c measurement of the clearance of endogenous creatinine, used to measure glomerular filtration rate **inulin c** determination of rate of filtration through the glomeruli by use of inulin that filters freely with water and it is neither excreted nor reabsorbed through tubules **mucociliary c** the clearance of mucus and foreign bodies from the airways by ciliary beating

cleavage (klev'aj) division into distinct parts

cleft (kleft) a fissure, especially noted during embryonic development **c lip** a birth defect characterised by a vertical, usually off-centre split in the upper lip **c palate** a birth defect characterised by a gap in the roof of the mouth, often associated with cleft lip

cleid (o) combining word for 'clavicle'.

cleidotomy (kli-dot'a-me) surgical division of the clavicle of the foetus to facilitate delivery during difficult labour

click (klik) a brief, sharp sounds produced in systole may be associated with ejection of blood across diseased semilunar valves into the great vessels as in aortic or pulmonary stenosis. They may occur due to sudden stretch of the arterial walls as in pulmonary hypertension or may be due to billowing action of the mitral valve in systole (mitral valve prolapse)

climacteric (kli-mak'ter-ik) the time span during which a woman moves from her reproductive to non-reproductive years

climatotherapy (kli-ma-to-ther'a-pe) treatment of disease by removing the patient to a region whose climate is conducive for recovery

climax (kli'maks) 1. the height of a disease exhibiting greatest severity 2. orgasm

clindamycin (kl'in-da-mi-sin) a semi-synthetic derivative of lincomycin active against gram positive organisms

clinic (klin'ik) 1. an institution where medical instruction is given to the medical students by means of demonstration of physical signs in a patient 2. an institution where ambulatory patients are taken care of

clinical (kl'in'i-kl) 1. pertaining to the bedside of a patient in a clinic where the patient is observed and treated 2. referring to the symptoms and course of a disease 3. pertaining to subjects like medicine, surgery etc that are concerned with patient care **c trial** a carefully monitored study on groups of people to evaluate the effectiveness and safety of treatment **controlled c trial** comparison of a new drug with the previously established therapy or placebo therapy under standard conditions **double-blind c trial** in clinical trials one group of patient receives treatment with the drug being tested whilst another receives a neutral substance. The patients do not know to which group they have been assigned, hence blind. Administrators of the treatment are also ignorant whether they are dispensing real substance or not **phase I c trial** the earliest stage of a clinical trial in human beings, designed to determine the safety of the drug or vaccine, and its maximum safe dose **phase I/II c trial** a stage in the clinical trial to determine the most effective dose of a drug **phase II c trial** a stage in the clinical trial to determine the effectiveness of the drug in short term **phase III c trial** a stage in the clinical trial when the experimental drug is given to a large number of people, at the dose determined in phase I or phase II clinical trial, often the trial drug is compared with a treatment already in vogue or with a placebo **single blind c trail** a type of clinical trial in which the participants do not know that treatment they are receiving but their doctors do **triple-blind c trial** in clinical trials, the evaluators of the treatment are unaware of the distribution of patients in two groups assigned in a double-blind trial

Clinical research method providing the essential understanding of why and how people become ill, characterising human diseases in detail and testing the response of patients to new therapies or methodologies

clinician (klin-nish'in) a health professional engaged in the care of the patients

clinicopathologic (klin'i-ko-path-loj'ik) pertaining to the clinical features manifested by a patient and the laboratory abnormalities, as they relate to the findings of gross and histologic abnormalities as revealed by biopsy or autopsy or both

clinistix (kl'in'i-stiks) glucose oxidase reagent strips used to test glucose in urine

clinitest (-test) copper sulphate reagent tablets used to test for reducing substances such as sugar in the urine

clinocephaly (klin'no-sefa-le) a developmental anomaly with a concave upper surface of the skull giving a saddle-shaped appearance

clinodactyly (-dak'til-e) permanent deflection or deviation of one or more fingers

clinoid (kli'noid) bed-shaped

clip (klip) a metallic device to hold the edges of a wound of skin incisions together with another

cliseometer (klis'e-omit-er) an instrument to measure the angles between the axis of the body and that of the pelvis

clitoridectomy (klit'a-ri-dek'ta-me) excision of the clitoris

clitorimegaly (-meg'a-le) enlargement of the clitoris; seen in excessive levels of androgenic hormones

clitoris (klit'o-ris) small sensitive female genital organ, partly enclosed in the labia, that swells in response to sexual stimulation

clitorism (klit'a-rizm) 1. hypertrophy of the clitoris 2. persistent erection of the clitoris

clitoritis (klit'a-rit'is) inflammation of clitoris

clivography (kli-vog'raa-fe) radiographic visualisation of posterior cranial fossa

clivus (kli'vus) 1. a downward sloping surface 2. the sloping surface in the posterior cranial fossa from the dorsum sellae to the foramen magnum

CLL abbreviation for chronic lymphocytic leukaemia

cloaca (klo-a'ka) an endodermal chamber in early embryos, into which the hindgut and allontois empty

cloacogenic (klo'a-ko-jen-ik) originating from the cloaca

clock (klok) a device to measure time **biological c** the physiologic mechanism governing the physiologic, biochemical and behavioural phenomenon in living organisms

clofibrate (klo-fi'brat) an antihyperlipidaemic agent to reduce serum lipids

clomiphene (klo'mi-fen) a non-steroidal oestrogen analogue used to stimulate ovulation. It is also used to study the relationship between the pituitary and gonads

clonality (klo-nal'I-te) the ability to form clones

clone (klon) an exact copy; often applied to a group of identical genes or a group of genetically identical cells or organisms

clonidine (klo'no-den) an antihypertensive agent that stimulates adrenergic receptors in the brain leading to a decrease in sympathetic outflow

clonism (klon'izm) a state of succession of clonic spasms

clonogenic (kllo'no-jen'ik) arising from or consisting of a clone

chlonorchiasis (klo'nor-ki-a-sis) a disease caused by the liver fluke *Clonorchis sinensis* affecting the biliary passages, acquired by eating raw or undercooked fish. There is inflammation of bile ducts and chronic infection, portal fibrosis and cirrhosis of the liver

clonospasm (klon'o-spasm) clonic spasm

clonus (klo'nus) rhythmic contraction and relaxation of the muscles from a sustained stretch of the tendon in a pyramidal lesion **ankle c** while a patient is lying supine, the hip and knee are semiflexed. The leg is held parallel to the bed giving support to the hip. The forepart of the foot is grasped and pushed suddenly backwards and the pressure is maintained. Clonus is exhibited by sustained repetitive flexion and extension of foot due to the contraction of the calf muscles, in presence of a pyramidal lesion **false c** an unsustained clonus noted in individuals who are tense or anxious. Clonus tends to diminish and becomes irregular **patellar c** while the knee is kept in extension, the patella held at its lateral borders is pushed downwards suddenly and the pressure is maintained. Clonus is revealed by repetitive jerky contractions and relaxation of quadriceps which pulls the patella upwards **true c** a sustained clonus that increases by dorsiflexion of foot **wrist c** elicited by suddenly hyperextending the wrist and maintaining the stretch on long flexors and the hand

closed fracture *see* fracture

Clostridium (klos-trid'e-um) pl **clostridia** a genus of anaerobic spore-forming, motile bacteria belonging to bacillaceae. They are found in soil and intestinal tract

clot (klot) 1. to coagulate, as of blood 2. a soft mass of coagulum as of blood or lymph

clotting factor one of several substances in the blood that are needed for blood to clot

clotrimazole (klo-trim'a-zol) an imidazole derivative used as an antifungal agent

clouding (klowd'ing) loss of clarity

cloxacillin (klok'sa-sillin) a semisynthetic penicillin useful in the treatment of staphylococcal infections due to penicillinase-positive organisms

clubbing (klub'ing) proliferation of soft tissues, especially nail beds affecting the fingers and toes. There is thickening of the terminal part of the digits and the nails are abnormally curved

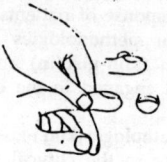

Clubbing

club foot *see* talipes

clumping (klump'ing) the aggregation of particles

clunis (kloo'nis) buttock

cluster headache a sudden severe pain on one side of the head involving the face and neck

Clutton's joint symmetrical arthrosis of knee joints, in congenital syphilis, named after Henry Clutton, British surgeon

clyster (klis'ter) an enema

Cm abbreviation for centimetre

Cm³ abbreviation for cubic centimetre

CMI abbreviation for cell mediated immunity

CMV abbreviation for cytomegalovirus

cnemial (ne-me-il) pertaining to the shin

CNS abbreviation for central nervous system

CoA abbreviation for coenzyme A

coaggulutination (ko'a-gloot-in-a'shun) the aggregation of antigens combined with agglutinins of more than one specificity

coagulability (ko-ag'u-la-bil'it-e) capability of forming c'ot

coagulant (ko-ag'u-lant) an agent that causes or stimulates coagulation, especially of blood

coagulase (-las) an antigenic substance especially that produced by staphylococci, may be related to the formation of thrombus

coagulate (-lat) 1. to cause to clot. 2. to become clotted

coagulation (ko-ag'u-la'shun) 1. the conversion of blood into a jelly-like clot 2. transformation of a sol into a semi-solid mass **blood c** the sequential process by which different coagulation factors or blood interact to result in the formation of clot **disseminated intravascular c** DIC a haemorrhagic condition which occurs following an uncontrolled activitation of clotting factors and fibrinolytic enzymes throughout small blood vessels **electric c** destruction of tissues by application of electric current

coagulopathy (ko-ag'u-lop'a-the) any disorder affecting blood coagulation **consumption c** disseminated intravascular coagulation

coagulum (ko-ag'u-lum) a clot or a curd; a soft insoluble mass formed when a sol undergoes coagulation

coalescence (ko'a-les'ens) the fusion of parts

coalition (ko-a-li'shun) fusion of parts that are originally separate

coapt (ko-apt) to approximate, as the edges of the wound

coarctate (ko-ark'tat) 1. to press together 2. to restrict

coarctation (ko-ark-ta'shun) a constriction, narrowing or stricture **c aorta** obstruction of the aorta in the region of the ductus arteriosus or ligamentum arteriosum just distal to the left subclavian artery. It is characterised by absence or delay of the femoral pulses, presence of high blood pressure in upper limbs, low blood pressure in the lower limbs and cardiac abnormalities **reversed c** aortoaortitis with absence of pulse in upper limbs and hypertension in lower limbs; Takayashu's disease.

coat (kot) tunic; 1. the outer covering of an organ or part 2. the protective layer of protein surrounding the nucleic acid in a virus 3. one of the layers of membrane or their tissue forming the wall of a canal or hollow organ **buffy c** the upper thin yellowish layer of leucocytes and platelets in a centrifuged, anticoagulated blood **muscular c** the muscular, middle layer of a tubular structure

Coats' (ko'tz) **disease** a variant of fascioscapulohumeral dystrophy associated with deafness, retinal telangiectasis and painless blindness

cobalamin (ko-bal'a-min) a compound containing the substituted ring and nucleotide structure characteristic of vitamin B_{12}

cobalt (co'ba-lt) a metallic element and a constituent of vitamin B_{12}

cobra (ko'bra) any of several highly venomous elapidae snakes. They have a spreading neck (hood) two short, erect, deep grooved fangs, and inject venom by biting or some spitting of spray of venom, which is primarily neurotoxic

cocaine (ko-kan) an alkaloid obtained from the leaves of *Erythroxylon coca* or by synthesis from ecgonine. It has topical anaesthetic activity and pronounced psychotropic effects. Its abuse leads to addiction

cocarcinogen (ko-kar-sin'o-jen) a substance that by itself cannot cause cancer, but increases the activity of a cancer causing substance

coccal (kok'al) pleural of coccus

coccidia (kok-sid'e-a) a subclass of protozoa in which mature trophozoites are intracellular; schizogony and sporogony occur in the same host

Coccidioides (kok-sid'e-oi'dez) a genus of fungi found in the soil of semi-arid areas, which includes pathogenic species *C. immitis*

coccidioidin (-din) a sterile solution containing the by-products of growth of *Coccidioides immitis*, used as an intracutaneous test for diagnosis

coccidioidoma (-do'ma) a residual granulomatous nodule in the lung seen radiologically following primary coccidioidomycosis

coccidioidomycosis (-oi'do-mi-ko'sis) a disease caused by *Coccidioides immitis* with lesions evolving like pulmonary tuberculosis, restricted to semi-desert areas of south-western US

coccidiosis (kok-sid'e-o'sis) an infection due to any species of coccidia *Isospora hominis* or *I. belli* may infect humans, which often remain asymptomatic and rarely cause watery mucus diarrhoea

coccidium (kok'sid'e-um) pl **coccidia** a protozoan parasite in which schizogony occurs within the epithelial cells

coccobacillus (kok'o-ba-sil'us) pl **coccobacilli** a short, thick bacterial rod having a shape of an oval or slightly elongated coccus

coccus (kok'us) pl **cocci** a round, spheroid or oval bacterium; **coccal** adj

coccygeal (kok-sij'e-il) pertaining to or located in the region of the coccyx

coccygodynia (-go-din'e-a) pain in the coccyx and neighbouring region

coccyx (kok'siks) *see* table of bones

cochlea (kok'le-a) a coiled structure in the inner ear; the organ responsible for hearing. It translates the sound vibrations into the electrical nerve impulses and transmits them to the brain via the auditory nerve

cochlear implant a device to treat deafness, consisting of electrodes implanted inside the cochlea to transmit sound generated nerve impulses to the brain

cochleariform (kok'le-ar'i-form) spoonshaped

cochleosacculotomy (kok'le-o-sak'u-lot'a-me) operative creation of a shunt between the cochlear duct and saccule, performed through the round window to relieve endolymphatic hydrops

cochleotopic (kok'le-o-top'ik) relating to the auditory pathways and auditory area of the brain.

Cockayne (ko-ken) **syndrome** a rare hereditary condition characterised by retinitis pigmentosa, hearing loss, dwarfism, mental retardation, premature senility, and photosensitive dermatitis

cocktail (kok'tal) a mixture that includes several ingredients or drugs

coctolabile (kok'ta-la'bil) capable of being changed or destroyed by heat

coctostabile (kok'ta-sta'bil) not changed by heating to the boiling point of water

code (kod) 1. a set of rules, or principles for regulating conduct 2. a system by which information can be communicated **genetic c** the genetic information carried by specific DNA molecules of the chromosomes

codeine (ko'den) a narcotic alkaloid obtained from opium or prepared from morphine; acts as an analgesic and antitussive

cod fish vertebra progressive decrease in vertebral mineral density causing the vertebral bodies biconcave with expansion of the intervertebral disc

codependency the stress of living in close association with a dependent person

coding system a system of classification of diseases, which are grouped according to certain common characteristics thus facilitating the statistical study of disease phenomenon, as International Classification of Diseases (ICD) produced by WHO and accepted for national and international use

cod liver oil oil from fresh cod fish livers, a rich source of vitamins A and D

codocyte (ko'do-site) red cell having a target-like appearance

codominance (ko-dom'i-nins) a clinical state in which each allele of a gene expresses an effect in a heterozygous individual

codon (ko-don) three adjacent nucleotide bases in DNA/RNA that encode for an amino acid

coefficient (ko'e-fish'ent) 1. an expression of the amount or degree of any quality possessed by a substance 2. an expression of a ratio between two different quantities or the effect produced by altering certain factors

coelenterata (se-len'ter-a'-ta) a phylum of Cnidaria to which hydras, jelly fish and sea anemones belong

coeliac disease a gluten sensitive enteropathy characterised by chronic diarrhoea, growth failure, anaemia and other nutritional deficiencies, seen in infants, and children following introduction of wheat or other gluten containing cereals, also seen in adults

coelom (se'lom) the cavity between the splanchnic and somatic mesoderm in the embryo. It develops into the pleural, peritoneal and pericardial cavities

coelosomy (sel'a-so'me) a developmental abnormality with protrusion of the viscera outside the body cavity

coenocyte (se'no-sit) a multinucleated mass of protoplasm

coenzyme (ko-en'zim) dialysable and relatively heat stable organic substance of low molecular weight that enhances or necessary for the action of enzymes **cA** a coenzyme containing pantothenic acid, involved in transfer of acyl groups, especially in transacetylations

coeur en sabot (ker-en-sa-bo) radiologic appearance of heart in tetrology of Fallot, in which elevated apex is associated with a transverse rectangular enlargement

coexcitation (ko-ek'si-ta'shun) simultaneous excitation of two parts

cofactor (ko'fak-tor) an element essential for enzyme action, such as haeme, coenzymes and magnesium ions

coffee the beverage made from dried, roasted beans of coffee tree, *Coffea arabica* It contains many volatile and non-volatile compounds and is a moderate stimulant **c bean sign** abdominal radiograph exhibiting a greatly distended, air-filled, oval loop of sigmoid colon, where the apposed medial wall's of the dilated bowel form a distinct oblique line that resembles the cleft of a coffee bean **c ground appearance** colour and consistency of gastric haemorrhage

Cogan's (ko'gans) **syndrome** interstitial keratitis, with tinnitus, vertigo and deafness, named after David Cogan, US ophthalmologist

cognisant aware, conscious, taking notice

cognition (kog-nish'un) a mental process of knowing which includes perceiving, recognising, conceiving, judging, sensing, reasoning and imagining

cogwheel rigidity circular jerking rigidity in flexion and extension in a background of a tremor that continues throughout the entire range of movement, as in Parkinsonism

coherent (ko-her'ent) 1. sticking together 2. consistent

cohesion (ko-he'zhun) adhering together

cohesive (ko-he'sis) adhesive, sticky

cohort a population group who share a common characteristic or experience within a defined period of time **birth c** a group of people born on the same day or in the same period of time **c study** an observational study undertaken to obtain additional evidence to support or refute the existence of an association between suspected cause and disease, which can be done prospectively or retrospectively

coil (koyl) a winding structure such as spiral or loop

coilonychia (koy'lo-nik'e-a) *see* koilonychia

coin counting a sliding movement of the tips of the thumb and index finger over each other, may be seen in paralysis agitans

coin lesion presence of a single, small round or oval shadow in the lung parenchyma noticed while performing chest roentgenographic examination of asymptomatic individuals

coin test a special auscultatory sign where the chest is percussed at the back or front using two coins and examiner auscultates from the opposite side.

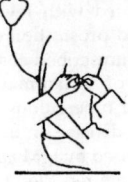

Coin test

When there is air between the areas as in pneumothorax, large pulmonary cyst or bullous emphysema, the sounds are heard with a ringing metallic quality

coinfection a simultaneous infection by two different microorganisms

coitorche age at first sexual intercourse

coition (ko-ish'un) coitus

coitophobia (ko'i-to-fo'be-a) unusual fear of sexual intercourse

coitus (ko'i-tus) sexual union between male and female by insertion of the penis into the vagina **c interruptus** a method of voluntary fertility control where male withdraws before ejaculation thereby prevents deposition of semen into the vagina. **c reservatus** coitus in which ejaculation is delayed or suppressed

col (kol) gingival tissue found between adjacent teeth

colation (ko-la'shun) straining; filtering.

colchicine (kol'chi-sin) an alkaloid from *Cochicum autumnale*, used in the treatment of gout

COLD abbreviation for chronic obstructive lung disease.

cold 1. catarrhal disorder of the upper respiratory tract 2. low temperature; the opposite of hot 3. spiritless; indifferent **common c** acute illness of short duration presenting as an acute inflammation of the upper respiratory passages and it is frequently due to rhinoviruses. It is characterised by nasal irritation, nasal stuffiness, sneezing, sore throat conjunctival irritation and watery nasal discharge, usually afebrile **feverish c** infection from rhinovirus, adenovirus and influenza virus associated with fever, weakness and profound prostration **c abscess** focal, well-circumscribed abscess without usual signs of inflammation, seen in paravertebral tuberculous cold abscess **c agglutinin disease** an immune disorder characterised by IgM autoantibodies that agglutinate red blood cells at very low temperatures **c chain** a system of

storage and transport of vaccines at low temperature from the manufacturer to the actual vaccination site **c sore** infection by herpes simplex virus on the lips and adjoining skin; herpes labialis **c cream** a water-in-oil emulsion ointment base applied to the skin **c hypersensitivity** exaggerated response of autonomic nervous system to low environmental temperature characterised by bradycardia and a local wheal-and-flare reaction **c nodule** a focus of reduced radio-isotope uptake on a ^{131}I or 99m Tc scintillation scan of thyroid, seen in cystic or solid non-functional thyroid swellings **c pack** covering a patient or an area in towel dipped in cold water and used to reduce fever, pain or swelling **c pressor test** a test to measure blood pressure response to the immersion of one hand in ice cold water **c stress** hypothermia

colectomy (ko-lek'to-me) surgical removal of part or whole of the colon

coleoptosis (ko'le-op-to'sis) prolapse of the wall of the vagina

coleotomy (ko-le-ot'o-me) colpotomy

colibacillosis (ko'li-bas-i-lo'sis) infection with *Escherichia coli*

colibacilluria (ko'li-bas-il-u're-a) presence of *E. coli* in the urine

colibacillus (ko'li-ba-sil'us) the colon bacillus, *Escherichia coli*

colic (kol'ik) 1. painful spasm in any hollow organ or tubular structure 2. pertaining to the colon **biliary c** colic due to passage of gall stones along the bile duct **infantile c** paroxysms of pain with crying and irritability occurring in infants **intestinal colic** severe abdominal pain **lead c** severe abdominal pain due to lead poisoning **menstrual c** dysmenorrhoea **renal c** pain in the lumbar region radiating over to the abdomen into the groin associated with the passage of renal calculi **uterine c** severe colic arising in the uterus during menstrual period

colicky (kol'ik-e) pertaining to colic or affected by it

colicolitis (ko'li-ko-li'tis) inflammation of colon due to infection from *E. coli*.

coliform (ko'li-form) 1. cribriform; sieve-like 2. some species of the family enterobacteriaceae including *Escherichia coli*, *Enterobacter* and *Klebsiella* species. Presence of *E. coli* in water implies faecal contamination

colipase a trypsin-activated proenzyme secreted by the exocrine pancreas that acts on fat droplets

coliplication (ko'li-pli-ka'shun) operation to correct a dilated colon

colistin (ko-lis'tin) an antibiotic effective against some gram-negative microorganisms, especially pseudomonas, that are resistant to other antibiotics

colitis (ko-li'tis) inflammation of the colon **amoebic c** colitis due to *Entamoeba histolytica* **antibiotic associated c** antibiotic induced diarrhoea **granulomatous c** granulomas involving the colon giving rise to colitis **ischaemic c** acute vascular insufficiency of the colon in the territory of inferior mesenteric artery giving rise to pain in left iliac fossa, bloody diarrhoea and abdominal distension **mucous c** irritable bowel syndrome **pseudomembranous c** colitis associated with antibiotic therapy, usually due to a toxin produced by *Clostridium difficile*. Characterised by formation of pseudomembrane on the mucosa of the colon with diarrhoea, passage of blood and mucus, abdominal pain and fever **radiation c** colitis developing from radiation therapy **ulcerative c** *see* ulcerative colitis

collagen (kol'a-jen) the protein substance of white fibres of connective tissue, cartilage and bone. It contains glycine, alanine, proline and hydroxyproline **collagenous** adj. **c vascular diseases** a group of disorders characterised by arthropathies, immune complex deposition, renal involvement and partial or temporary response to corticosteroids

collagenase (kol-laj'e-nas) an enzyme that acts on collagen to bring about its degradation

collagenic (kol'a-jen'ik) producing or containing collagen

collagenoblast (kol-laj'e-no-blast) a cell developing from a fibroblast which on maturation is concerned with the production of collagen

collagenolysis (kol'a-jen-ol'i-sis) degradation of collagen

collagenosis (kol-laj''e-no'sis) a connective tissue disorder

collapse (ko-laps) 1. a condition of extreme prostration 2. a falling together of the walls of a structure or the failure of a system **circulatory c** shock due to circulatory insufficiency **c of lung** loss of volume of a lobe, segment or whole lung and it may result from bronchial obstruction (resorption), fibrosis (cicatrization), extrinsic pressure such as pleural effusion or pneumothorax (relaxation) or abnormality of surfactant (adhesive)

collapsing pulse pulse with a rapid upstroke due to a markedly increased stroke volume and a fall due to regurgitation of blood back into the left ventricle during diastole and to decreased systemic vascular resistance. Seen in aortic incompetence and other hyperdynamic circulatory states

collapsotherapy (ko-lap'so-ther'a-pe) artificial pneumothorax and thoracoplasty to give rest to diseased lung with tuberculosis, practised before introduction of antituberculosis drugs

collar (kol'ar) an encircling band generally around the neck **cervical c** a rigid or soft collar around the neck to restrict the movements of the neck in cervical spondylosis or cervical injuries **c bone** clavicle

collateral (ko-lat'er-al) 1. accessory or subsidiary to main thing 2. a side branch of a vessel or nerve accompanying side by side **c damage** the undesired, but unavoidable collateral damage associated with a treatment modality

collecting tubule one of the many relatively, large straight tubules of the kidney that drain urine from distal convoluted tubules into the renal pelvis. Antidiuretic hormone makes the collecting tubules of the kidney permeable to water and thus they help in maintenance of fluid balance

Colles' fracture a transverse fracture of the distal end of the radius with displacement of the hand backward and outward named after Abraham Colles, Irish surgeon

colliculitis (kol-lik'u-li'tis) inflammation of seminal colliculus

colliculectomy (kol-lik'u-lek'to-me) surgical removal of seminal colliculus

colliculus (kol-lik'u-lus) pl. **colliculi** a small eminence above the surrounding parts **seminal c** an elevated portion of male urethral crest upon which open the prostatic utricle and two ejaculatory ducts

collimation (kol'i-ma-shun) 1. the process of making light rays parallel 2. restricting and containing the x-ray beam to a given area

collimator (kol'i-ma'tur) a radiographic device that restricts the scatter and extent of the x-ray beam

colliquation (kol'i-kwa'shun) 1. excessive discharge of a body fluid 2. softening of tissues 3. degeneration of tissue

colliquative (ko-lik'wa-tiv) denoting an excessive discharge of liquid or liquefaction of tissues

collision tumour extremely rare merging of two originally seperate tumours from two organs, seen at gastrooesophageal junction

collodion (ko-lo'de-on) a liquid prepared by dissolving pyroxylin in ether and alcohol, which on evaporation gives a glossy, contractile film. It is used topically to the skin on wounds, cuts and abrasions, and to hold surgical dressings in place and to keep medications in contact with the skin

colloid (kol'oyd) 1. a glue-like substance 2. aggregates of atoms or molecules in finely divided state dispersed uniformly in a solvent 3. a homogeneous gelatinous substance containing thyroid hormones found in the follicles of thyroid gland

colloidin (kol-loy'din) a jelly-like substance in colloid degeneration

colloidoclasia (kol-oyd'o-kle'se-a) entry of colloids into the blood stream producing an anaphylactic shock

colloma (ko-lo'ma) a colloid degeneration of a malignancy

collopexia (kol'opek'se-a) fixation of cervix uteri

collum (kol'lum) 1. the neck 2. neck-like structure of an organ

collyrium (ko-lir'e-um) a lotion for the eye

coloboma (kol'o-bo'ma) any defect of the eye. It may affect the choroid, ciliary body, eyelid, iris, lens, optic nerve or retina. It may be congenital, pathological or surgical

colocecostomy (ko'lo-se-kos'to-me) surgical anastomosis of the colon and caecum

colocentesis (ko'lo-sen-te'sis) surgical puncture of the colon to relieve distension

colocolostomy (ko'lo-ko-los'to-me) surgical creation of a passage between two portions of the colon

colon (ko'lon) the division of large intestine extending from caecum to the rectum. It is 1.5 m long and it mixes the intestinal contents. No digestive enzymes are secreted by colon. As more water is absorbed in the colon, the contents get dehydrated **colonic** adj **ascending c** the portion of the colon between caecum and the right colic flexure **descending c** the part of the colon extending from left colic flexure to the sigmoid colon **iliac c** the part of the descending colon lying between the crest of left ilium and the pelvic brim **irritable c** a functional disorder characterised by abdominal pain associated with defecation and it develops in response to psychological factors, altered gastrointestinal motility and increased sensitivity to intestinal distension **sigmoid c** colon having an S-shaped curve found in the pelvis and it extends from descending colon to the rectum **spastic c** irritable bowel syndrome **transverse c** the part of large intestine extending transversely across the abdomen between the right and left colic flexures

colonic (ko'lon-ic) pertaining to the colon **c irrigation** colonic wash by injection of a large amount of fluid into the colon through a tube

colonitis (ko-lon-i'tis) inflammation of the colon

colonization (kol'o-ni-za'shun) 1. a group of organisms living together 2. a group of cells growing together

colonopathy (ko'lo-nop'a-the) any disorder of the colon

colonopexy (ko'lon'o-pek'se) attachment of a part of the colon to the abdominal wall by suture

colonorrhagia (ko'lon-o-ra'je-a) bleeding from the colon

colonorrhoea (ko'lon-o-re-a) discharge of watery fluid from the colon

colonoscope (ko'lon'o-skop) a lighted instrument for examining the colon

colonoscopy (ko'lon-us'ko-pe) visualisation of the large intestine using a colonoscope

colony (kol'o-ne) a growth of microorganisms in a culture media; a group of cells **c stimulating factor-1**, CSF-1, a serum protein that promotes the differentiation of monocytes

colopexostomy (ko'lo-peks-os'to-me) resection of the colon and establishment of an artificial anus by opening into the colon after its fixation to the abdominal wall.

colopexy (ko'lo-pek'se) surgical attachment of a part of the colon to the abdominal wall

coloplication (ko'lo-pli-ka'shun) surgical creation of a fold in the colon so as to reduce its lumen

coloproctectomy (ko'lo-prok-tek'to-me) surgical removal of the colon and rectum

coloproctitis (ko'lo-prok-ti'tis) inflammation of colon and rectum

coloptosis (ko-lop-to'sis) a downward displacement of the colon

colorectal carcinoma tumours of the large intestine developing from malignant transformation of a benign adenomatous polyp. Rectosigmoid colon is a common site. The tumour may be polypoid and fungating or annular and constricting. Lymphatic spread is common. It is characterised by fresh rectal bleeding and obstruction (left colon) and anaemia or altered bowel habit (right colon); early bleeding, mucus discharge or a feeling of incomplete emptying (rectum). Tumour has to be removed with adequate resection margins and pericolic lymph nodes

colorectostomy (ko'lo-rek-tos'to-me) surgical creation of a passage between the colon and rectum

colorimeter (ka'lor-im'e-ter) an instrument for measurement of the intensity of colour in a fluid such as amount of haemoglobin in the blood

colorimetry a photometric procedure that compares the absorption of light by the colour developed in a test solution with that of a standard solution

colorrhaphy (ko-lor'a-fe) suture of the colon

coloscopy (ko-los'ko-pe) inspection of the colon through a sigmoidoscope

colosigmoidostomy (ko'lo-sig'moy-dos'to-me) surgical anastomosis between the descending colon and sigmoid colon

colostomy (ko-los'to-me) the surgical creation of an opening of a portion of the colon through the abdominal wall to its outside surface

colostrum breast fluid secreted in the first 2 to 3 days after birth. It is a thin yellowish fluid rich in protein and other nutrients for the needs of the body and it contains anti-infective factors which protect the baby against infections

colotomy (ko-lot'o-me) incision of the colon

colour (kul'ur) a sensation of light induced in the eye by waves of certain frequency of colour to a particular colour being determined by the frequency **c additive** any dye or pigment that impart colour on addition or application of colour to food, drug or cosmetic **c blindness** inability to distinguish certain colours, and occurs as a genetically determined condition **c index** amount of haemoglobin present in each red cell **primary c** any of the three (red, green or violet) colours of light

colovaginal (ko'lo-vaj'i-nal) pertaining to the colon and vagina or a communication between the two

colovesical (ko'lo-ves'i-kal) pertaining to the colon and the urinary bladder or a communication between the two

colpalgia (kol-pal'je-a) pain in the vagina

colpectomy (kol-pek'to-me) surgical removal of the vagina

colpeurysis (kol-pu'ris-is) surgical dilatation of the vagina

colpitis vaginitis

colpoceliotomy (kol'po-se'le-ot'o-me) an incision into the abdomen through the vagina.

colpocleisis (kol'po-kli-sis) surgical closure of the lumen of the vagina.

colpocoele (kol'po-sel) herniation into the vagina

colpocystitis (kol'po'sis-ti'tis) inflammation of the vagina and bladder

colpocystocoele (kol'po-sis'to-sel) prolapse of the bladder into the vagina

colpocystoplasty (kol'po-sis'to-plas'te) surgical repair of a vesicovaginal fistula

colpocystotomy (kol'po-sis-tot'o-me) an incision into the bladder through the vagina

colpohyperplasia (kol'po-hi-per-pla'ze-a) vaginal mucosal overgrowth

colpomicroscope (kol'po-mi'kro-skop) a special optical device to observe and study the cells in vagina and cervix magnified.

colpomyomectomy (kol'po-mi'o-mek'to-me) surgical removal of an uterine fibroid through the vagina

colpomyomotomy (kol'pomi'o-mot'o-me) incision of the uterus through the vagina for removal of a fibroid

colpoperineoplasty (ko'po-per'in-e-o-plas'te) plastic repair of the vagina and perineum

colpoperineorrhaphy (kol'po-per'in-e-or-ra-fe) surgical repair of the perineal tears in the vagina

colpopexy (kol'po-pek'se) suture of a prolapsed vagina to the abdominal wall

colpoplasty (kol'po-plas'te) plastic repair of the vagina.

colpoptosis (kol'pop-to'sis) proplapse of the vagina

colporrhexis (kol'po-rek'sis) laceration of the vagina.

colposcope (kol'po-scop) an endoscope for visualisation of tissues of the vagina and cervix through a magnifying lens

colposcopy (kol-pos'ko-pe) examination of the vagina and cervix by an endoscope

colpostenosis (kol'po-sten-o'sis) narrowing of the vagina

colpotomy (kol-pot'o-me) an incision into the wall of the vagina.

columella (kol'u-mel'la) 1. a small column 2. a portion of the sporangiophore on which the spores develop

column (kol'um) a pillar or cylindrical supporting structure **anal c** vertical folds of the mucous membrane in the upper half of the anal canal **anterior c** the anterior or ventral portion of the gray matter on either side of the spinal cord that appears like a horn in transverse section **c of Bertin** renal column **c of Burdach** fasciculus cuneatus of the spinal cord **Clarke's c** collection of large cells in the posterior gray column of the spinal cord extending from the eighth cervical segment to the third or fourth lumbar segment **c of Gall** gray columns of the anterior, posterior and lateral masses of gray matter extending longitudinally through the lateral half of the spinal cord. In transverse sections the columns appear as gray horns; fasciculus gracilis **gray c** the longitudinally oriented anterior and posterior horns of gray matter of spinal cord **lateral c** lateral portion of the gray matter of spinal cord projecting into the lateral funiculus or white matter between the roots of the spinal nerves on either side especially marked in the thoracic region. It contains the cell bodies of preganglionic neurons of the sympathetic nervous system **c of Gowers** the tract of ascending fibres anterior to direct cerebellar column and on the lateral surface of the spinal cord **c of Morgagni** anal column **posterior c** 1. posterior or dorsal portion of gray matter of the spinal cord 2. palato-pharyngeal arch **rectal c's** anal columns **renal c** the inward extension of the cortical material of kidney separating the pyramids of the kidney **spinal c** vertebral column **vertebral c** 1. spinal column; spine 2. backbone, the axial skeleton consisting of vertebrae from cranium to the coccyx giving the support to the axis of the body and offering protection for the spinal cord

columna (ko-lum'na) pl **columnae** a column or pillar

columnar layer tall narrow epithelial cell layer

coma (ko'ma) profound degree of unconsciousness with an unarousable psychological unresponsiveness in which the subjects lie with eyes closed **comatose** adj **diabetic c** coma due to severe diabetic ketoacidosis **hepatic c** coma accompanying hepatic encephalopathy noted in advanced cirrhosis, fulminant hepatitis or poisoning **irreversible c** brain death **metabolic c** coma resulting from metabolic abnormalities **uraemic c** coma due to disturbances in

kidney function with retention of metabolic end products **c vigil** coma in which the patient appears to be in sleep but ready to be aroused

comatose (ko'ma-tos) in a state of coma

combustion (kom-bust'yun) 1. burning 2. oxidation of food with production of heat

comedo (kon-e-do) pl **comedos, comedones** a plug of sebaceous material and epithelial debris in the pilosebaceous orifice **closed c** white head; comedo appearing as a papule from which the contents are not easily expressed as the orifice is narrow **open c** blackhead; a comedo with a dilated orifice from which the debris can be easily expressed.

comes (ko'mez) a blood vessel accompanying a nerve or another blood vessel

command automatism automatic following of suggestions

commensal (ko-men'sal) an organism living on or within another organism and deriving benefit and host is not harmed

commensalism (ko-men'sal-izm) a symbiotic relationship in which one organism gets benefit and other is unharmed

commentary critical or explanatory remarks

comminute (kom'i-nut) to break into pieces

comminution (kom'i-nu-shun) the reduction of a solid to varying sizes

commissura (kom'mi-su'ra) pl **commissurae** a commissure

commissure (kom'i-shur) 1. a bundle of nerve fibres passing from one side to another in the brain or spinal cord 2. a site of union of corresponding parts such as the sites of junction between adjacent cusps of heart valves 3. angle or corner of the eye, lips or labia **anterior cerebral c** a band of fibres that pass through lamina terminalis connecting the two cerebral hemispheres **anterior gray c** the commissure lying in front of the central canal of the spinal cord **anterior white c** the band of fibres lying in front of the central canal and the anterior gray commissure of the spinal cord **c of cerebral hemispheres** corpus callosum **hippocampal c** a thin sheet of fibres connecting the medial margins of the crura of the fornix **posterior cerebral c** a thin band of white matter just above the mid-brain connecting superior colliculi **posterior gray c** the 'gray commissure lying behind the central canal of the spinal cord and connecting both halves of the spinal cord **supra optic c's** commissure crossing the midline of the brain dorsal to the caudal border of optic chiasma

commissurorraphy (kom'i-shur-or'a-fe) suture of the parts of a commissure to decrease the size of the orifice ·

commissurotomy (kom'i-shur-ot'o-me) surgical division of any commissure to increase the size of the orifice

commode a toilet that enables a person to sit comfortably while using it

communicable 1. to send across to another person 2. capable of being transmitted **c disease** an illness due to a specific infectious agent or its toxic products capable of being directly or indirectly transmitted from man to man or from the environment to man **c period** the time during which an infectious agent may be transmitted directly or indirectly from an infected individual to another individual, from an infected animal to man or from an infected individual to an animal, including arthropods

communicans (ko-mu'ne-kanz) one of the several communicating nerves or arteries

communication a joining structure in anatomy such as tendons and nerves

community a contiguous geographic area composed of people living together, and co-operate to satisfy their basic needs. It is a network of human relationships and a functioning unit of society **c health** personal health and environmental services in any community **c medicine** the practice of medicine concerned with groups or populations rather than with individual patients

comorbid disease a disease coexisting with the primary disease

compact tightly packed together

compaction (kam-pak'shun) 1. simultaneous engagement of the presenting parts of twins in the pelvis preventing their descent during labour 2. filling the dental cavity with gold

compatibility 1. suitability of mixing or taking without any adverse effects, as drugs 2. ability of two persons or groups living in harmony

compatible ability to combine two medicines without interfering with their action

compensating making up for a deficiency

compensation 1. making up for any defect as in valvular defect 2. a mechanism by which a person tries to make up for real or imagined physical and psychologic deficiencies

competence (kom'pe-tens) the ability of the immune system to mount a response to an antigen 2. a set of abilities needed for adequate decision making 3. ability of a physician to perform procedures and practice his specialty in a skilled manner

competition (kom'pe-tish'un) an attempt made by similar substances simultaneously to get attached to the receptor site of a cell membrane

compilation collection of material from various sources or documents

complaint (kom-plant) reason to seek medical assistance **chief c** the symptoms representing the primary reason to seek medical assistance by a patient

complement (kom'ple-ment) 1. globulins found in varying proportion in the serum. They have been named as Clq, Clr, Cls and C_2 to C_9. The complement

173   **compulsory**

system is activated sequentially when antibody attaches to antigen components on the cell surface. Some microbial polysaccharides activate an alternate pathway bypassing the initial complement components, and it does not require specific antibodies

complemental supplying a material that is not present in another system

complement fixation a test to determine occurrence of antigen-antibody disorder by using complement

complex (kom'pleks) 1. a combination of ideas, feelings, thoughts and perceptions 2. a composite of chemical or immunological structure 3. an entity consisting of three or more interrelated components 4. an electrocardiogram showing atrial or ventricular systole 5. a group of related structures. **AIDS dementia c** affective disorders with depression in HIV infection **AIDS related c** ARC patients exhibiting symptoms but do not have AIDS-defining condition. These patients are relatively immunosuppressed **atrial c** P wave in ECG representing atrial electrical activity **antigen-antibody c** a complex formed by binding of antigen to antibody **Eisemenger's c** increased pulmonary flow due to an initial left-to-right shunt causes severe pulmonary hypertension and reversal of the shunt with central cyanosis and digital clubbing. **Ghon's c** primary complex **Golgi c** a complex cellular organelle consisting of flattened saccules, vesicles and vacuoles lying adjacent to the nucleus and are concerned with formation of secretory products **immune c** antigen combined with a specific antibody to which complement may also be fixed **inferiority c** a feeling of inferiority causing shyness or timidity or as a compensatory reaction in aggressiveness or exhibitionism **primary c** lesions of primary tuberculosis consisting of a subpleural focus of infection with hilar lymph node involement.

QRS c the main deflection in ECG representing ventricular depolarisation **superiority c** an increased conviction of one's own superiority **symptom c** clinical manifestations **ventricular c** the QRST complex in ECG.

complex disorder a disorder resulting from the inheritance of more than one genetic locus, environmental factors and/or genotype interactions

complexion (kom-plek'shun) the colour, texture and appearance of the skin of the face

compliance (kom-pli'ans) 1. the quality of alteration in size and shape without disruption 2. the degree of adherence by a patient to a prescribed regimen or advice

complication the development of a fresh symptom in a proportion of those suffering from a particular disease and which deteriorates the clinical condition of the patient further

component constituent part **c blood therapy** blood component therapy

compos mentis (kom'pus-men'tis) sound mind

Composure calmness, tranquility, serenity

compound (kom'pownd) 1. a preparation containing several ingredients 2. a substance made up of two or more elements.

comprehend to understand something

compress (kom'pres) a pad of gauze or other material applied with pressure. It may be hot or cold; wet or dry

compression (kom-presh'un) exertion of pressure on a body so as to press together

compressor contraction of a muscle causing compression of any structure

compromised host a person who lacks resistance to infection due to a deficiency in any of the host defences

compulsion (kom-pul'shun) uncontrollable impulse to perform an act repetitively

compulsory (kom-pul'sor-e) compelling action against one's will.

conarium (ko-na're-um) the pineal body

conation (ko-na'shun) an initiative, drive and an impulse to act

concave (kon'kav) having a depressed surface

concavity (kon-kav'i-te) a depression with evenly curved edges on any surface

concavoconcave (kon-ka'vo-kon'kav) concave on opposing sides

concavoconvex (kon-ka'vo-kon'vexs) concave on one side and convex on the opposite side

conceive (kon-sev) 1. to become pregnant 2. to form a mental image 3. to form an idea

concentration (kon-sen-tra'shun) 1. increase in strength of a fluid by evaporation 2. preparation obtained by extracting a crude drug 3. quality of substance per unit volume or weight **hydrogen ion c** the degree of concentration of hydrogen ions in a solution **mean corpuscular haemoglobin c** MCHC concentration of haemoglobin in individual red blood cells as Hb in grams per 100 ml blood/packed cell volume in ml of blood $\times$ 100 **minimum inhibiting c** MIC, minimum concentration of antibiotic required to cause 99% reduction in colony-forming units on a culture medium

concentric (kon-sen'trik) having a common centre

concept (kon'sept) an idea

conception (kon-sep'shun) 1. a mental process of forming an idea 2. the union of sperm and ovum; fertilisation

conceptus (kon-sep'tus) the products of conception

concha (kong'ka) pl conchae 1. the outer ear; pinna 2. one of the three nasal conchae **c auriculae** the hollow of the auricle of the external ear between the anterior portion of the helix and antihelix **nasal c** a thin bony plate with curved margins projecting from the lateral wall of nasal cavity, and separating the middle from inferior meatus (inferior), the superior from middle meatus (middle) and superior

meatus from the sphenoethmoidal recess (superior) **sphenoidal c** one of the two curved plates forming the roof of the nasal cavity

conchoidal (kong-koy'dal) shell-shaped

conchoscope (kong'ko-skop) an instrument for examining nasal cavity

conchotome (kong'kom-tom) a device for excising the middle turbinate bone

concoction (kon-kok'shun) a mixture of two medicinal substances prepared by heating

concomitant (kon-kom'i-tant) occurring at the same time

concordance (kon-kor'dans) 1. occurrence of a given trait in both members of a twin pair 2. agreement ; harmony

concrement (kon'kre-ment) a concretion made of protein and other substances It turns to be a calculus on calcium deposition

concrescence (kon-kres'ens) coalescence; the union of two separate parts

concrete (kon'kret) solidified or hardened **c thinking** literal thinking; one-dimensional thought

concretio cordis (kon-kre'she-o-kor'dis) extensive adhesion between parietal and visceral pericardium with obliteration of pericardial cavity

concretion (kon-kre'shun) formation of solid material; a calculus

concussion (kon-kush'un) transitory loss of consciousness, accompanied by a variable period of amnesia for events before and after the injury as a result of head trauma

condensation (kon'den-sa'shun) 1. fusion of various concepts into one 2. compression making it dense 3. change of a gas to a liquid or of a liquid to a solid 4. the process of packing a filling material into a cavity in a tooth

condenser (kon-den'ser) 1. an apparatus used to cool a gas to a liquid or a liquid to a solid 2. an instrument to pack material into a cavity of a tooth 3. a lens on a microscope used to supply the illumination required for visibility of the specimen under observation

condiment (kon'di-ment) a seasoning used to give a flavour to the food

condition (kon-dish'un) 1. a state in which things exist 2. to train a person to respond in a predictable way 3. a state of health

conditioning (kon'dish'un-ing) 1. improvement of the physical capability of a person 2. a change in the behaviour due to an influence of the environment

condom (kon'dom) a sheath or covering made to fit over a man's erect penis. It is also called rubbers, sheaths, skin, made of thin latex rubber, some condoms are coated with a dry lubricant or with spermicide. It helps in protecting both pregnancy and sexually transmitted diseases **female c** a thin, transparent, soft plastic sheath inserted into a woman's vagina

conductance (kon-duk-tans) the capacity for conducting a gas or fluid

conduction (kon-duk'shun) transmission of energy as of heat sound or electricity through air, bone or nerve

conductivity (kon'dak-tiv'i-te) capacity for conduction.

conductor (kon-duk'tor) 1. a probe or sound with a groove along which a knife is passed to slit open a sinus or fistula 2. that which is having conductivity

conduit (kon'doo-it) a channel for passage of fluids

condylar (kon'di-lar) pertaining to a condyle

condylarthrosis (kon'dil-ar-thro'sis) a joint formed by condylar surfaces

condyle (kon'dil) pl **condyles** the rounded articular surface at the end of a bone

condylectomy (kon'di-lek'to-me) surgical removal of a condyle

condyloid (kon'di-loyd) pertaining to or resembling a condyle

condyloma (kon'di-lo'ma) a wart-like growth on the skin **c accuminatum** an epithelial proliferation like a 'cauliflower' induced by human papilloma viruses of low malignant potential

condylomatous (kon'di-lo'ma-tus) pertaining to a condyloma

condylotomy (kon'di-lot'o-me) division of a condyle

condylus (kon'di-lus) pl **condyli** condyle

cone (kon) 1. a figure or body having a circular base and tapering to a point 2. one of the photoreceptors of the retina 3. a conical open ended cylindrical structure used as an aid in centering the radiation beam **c cutting** failure to expose whole area of a radiograph

connexus (ko-nek'sus) a connecting structure

confabulation (km-fab'u-la'shun) unconscious filling of gaps in memory by imaginary experiences that patient believes but that have no basis at all

confection (kon-fex'shun) a pharmaceutical preparation consisting of a drug mixed with a sweetener

confidentiality the right a person has not to have information about his circumstance revealed publicly by professionals whose advice and aid he has sought in confidence

configuration (kon-fig'u-ra'shun) 1. the general form of the body and its parts 2. the spatial arrangement of atoms in a molecule

confinement (kon-fin'ment) giving birth to a child; lying in

conflict (kon'fli-kt) a clash between two or more courses of action or between opposing ideas, which often generates painful emotions **extrapsychic c** that between the person and the external environment **intrapsychic c** that between forces within the personality

confluence a flowing or running together; a joining

confluent (kon'floo-ent) relating to or characterised by confluence.

conformation (kon'for-ma'shun) 1. the form or shape of a part, body or material 2. the three-dimensional configuration of a molecule in space confrontation (kon'frun-ta'shun) 1. to bring face to face 2. method to determine visual fields 3. a feedback procedure c method a bedside method in which the examinar compares the field of vision of the patient with his own

confusion (km-fu'shun) a state in which a person lacks clarity in mental processes

congener (kon'jen-er) any member of a family of related molecules

congenital (kon-jen'i-tal) present at birth c anomaly biochemical, structural and functional disorders present at birth c disorders those diseases that are substantially determined before or during birth and generally are recognisable in early life c malformations anatomical defects

congested (kon-jes'ted) denoting congestion

congestion (kon-jee'chun) an abnormal amount of fluid in a part active c congestion due to an increased blood flow to a part hypostatic c congestion due to pooling of venous blood in a dependent part passive c congestion due to stagnation of blood pulmonary c engorgement of the pulmonary vessels with transudation of fluid into alveolar and interalveolar spaces

conglobate (kon'glo-bat) formed into a single, round mass

conglobation (kon'glo-ba'shun) an act of formation into a round mass

conglomerate (kon-glom'er-at) composed of several parts aggregated into a single mass

conglutinant (kon'gloo'ti-nant) adhesive, promoting the union of a wound

conicotine a metabolite of nicotin that may remain at detectable levels in the circulation for upto a week after a last cigarette

conidia (ko-nid'e-a) spores of fungi

conidiophore (kon-id'e-op-for) the stalk supporting conidia

coniology (ko-ne-ol'o-je) the study of dust and its effects

coniosis (ko'ne-o'sis) any disease caused by dust

coning displacement of parts of the brain between its various compartments due to rise in intracranial pressure from a mass lesion temporal c downward displacement of the temporal lobes through the tentorium tonsillar c downward movement of the cerebellar tonsils through the foramen magnum

coniofibrosis (ko'ne-o-fi-bro'sis) pneumoconiosis produced by dust and there is development of pulmonary fibrosis

conization (kon'i-za'shun) removal of a cone of tissue

conjugata (ko'ju-ga'ta) conjugate

conjugate (kon'ju-gat) 1. paired or joined 2. a product of chemical conjugation 3. a conjugate diameter of the pelvic inlet, the distance from the premontory of the sacrum to the upper edge of the pubic symphysis

conjugation (kon'ju-ga'shun) 1. the union of two unicellular organisms or of the male and female gametes 2. the combination by which the biologic effects of some chemical substances are terminated 3. transfer of genetic material from a donor bacterial strain to a receptor strain

conjunctiva (kon'junk-ti'va) the delicate mucous membrane covering the anterior surface of the eyeball and lining the eyelids bulbar c covering of the anterior eyeball palpebral c cover of the undersurface of the eyelids conjunctival adj c reflex closure of the eyelids on touching the conjunctiva with a wisp of cotton and it gives information on integrity of the upper cervical sensory neurones.

conjunctivitis (kon-junk'ti-vi'tis) inflammation of the conjunctiva acute contagious c acute epidemic conjunctivitis. Pink eye. highly contagious condition with intense hyperaemia and profuse mucopurulent discharge, caused by *Haemophilus aegypticus* acute

haemorrhagic c a contagious viral infection characterised by pain, swollen eyelids, hyperaemia and subconjunctival haemorrhage **allergic c** a conjunctival reaction to a substance causing an allergic reaction **catarrhal c** conjunctivitis due to bacteria, foreign bodies or *Chlamydia trachomatis*. **gonococcal c** intensely swollen, congested conjunctiva, profuse purulent discharge and swollen eyelids caused by *Neisseria gonorrhoeae* **granular c** trachoma **phlyctenular c** marked nodules that may ulcerate **vernal c** conjunctivitis occurring in spring

conjunctivoplasty (kon'junk-ti'vo-plas'te) plastic repair of conjunctiva

Conn's syndrome primary hyperaldosteronism due to adrenocortical adenoma. There is hypersecretion of aldosterone leading to sodium retention and loss of potassium and hydrogen. There is muscle weakness, hypertension, polyuria and hypokalaemia, named after J. Conn, US physician

conoid (ko'noyd) resembling a cone; conical

consanguinity (kon'san-gwin'i-te) a state of close genetic relationship and marriage between close blood relatives, associated with an increased risk in the offspring of traits controlled by recessive genes and those determined by polygenes

conscience (kon'shunz) the knowledge of our own acts and feelings, as right or wrong

conscious (kon'shus) having the feeling; being aware

consciousness (-ness) the working state of the mind; state of being conscious **clouding of c** incomplete clear-mindedness with disturbance in perception and attitude.

consensual (kon-sen'shu-al) refers to the thing done in response to a stimulus without the participation of the will **c light reflex** indirect light reflex. When bright light is shone in one eye, opposite pupil not exposed to light contracts as quickly as the pupil on which the light is shone

consent a document or verbal agreement by the patient that gives permission to undertake a therapeutic or diagnostic procedure

conservative (kon-ser'va-tiv) pertaining to treatment by simple, well-established procedures as opposed to the radical **c therapy** the management of a clinical condition with the least aggressive therapeutic options.

conservation 1. the act of keeping, 2. keeping the entire **c chemotherapy** a phase of chemotherapy for leukaemia that follows the initial intensive phase of chemotherapy

consolidation (kon-sol-i-da'shun) the process of becoming solid, especially in pneumonia from an acute inflammatory exudate into the alveolar spaces. It is characterised by dull percussion note and tubular breathing.

constant (kon'stant) unchangeable; fixed. **c region** a highly conserved part of an immunoglobulin molecule that can be separated from the whole molecule by partial digestion

constellation (kon'ste-la'shun) a cluster, a group or configuration of objects, individuals or conditions

constipation (kon'sti-pa'shun) infrequent passage of hard stools, often associated with straining, a sensation of incomplete evacuation

constitution (kon-sti-tu'shun) 1. the natural condition of the body and mind; disposition 2. the arrangement of atoms in a molecule

constriction (kon-strik'shun) 1. a pressing together; contraction 2. a narrowing of a part

constrictor (kon-strik'tor) 1. that which constricts or draws together 2. a muscle action to narrow a canal as a sphincter

consultant a physician or a surgeon acting in an advisory capacity

consultation meeting of two or more health professionals to evaluate the disease in a particular patient and to establish the diagnosis and management

consumer protection act, CPA, provision of a forum to the consumer for speedy redressal of their grievances against medical services

consummation to make marriage legally complete by sexual intercourse

consumption (kon-sump'shun) 1. using of something 2. wasting of the tissues of body, usually tuberculosis **c coagulopathy** disseminated intravascular coagulation

consumptive pertaining to or related to tuberculosis

contact (kon'takt) 1. touching of two bodies 2. an individual who has been exposed to a contagion **c dermatitis** a disorder of skin as a result of the skin coming in contact with irritants which cause an altered state of sensation and morphologic changes **c inhibition** ability of a tissue, on reaching its mature size, to suppress additional growth **c lens** a transparent devise that fits over the cornea or part of the cornea to bring changes in refractive ability of the cornea or lens of the eye **c range** a funnel-shaped depression of the skin with marginal abrasion and bruising of epidermis caused by a zero range gun shot wound **c surface** a proximal tooth surface

contactant (kon-tak'tant) an allergen capable of eliciting hypersensitivity by direct contact with skin or mucosa

contagion (kon-ta'jun) 1. the spread of disease by contact with the sick 2. a contagious disease

contagious (kon-ta'jus) a disease that is transmitted through contact such as scabies and sexually transmitted disease

contagium (kon-ta'je-um) the agent causing an infection

container (kon-ta'ner) a receptacle to store a medical specimen or supply material

contaminant (kon-tam'i-nant) something that causes contamination

contamination the presence of an infectious agent on a body surface, and also on clothes, bedding, instrument or dressings or other articles, or substances including water, milk and food.

contig (kon'tig) a chromosome map depicting the location of those regions of a chromosome where contiguous DNA segments overlap.

contiguity (kon'ti-gu'i-te) contact without actual continuity

continence (kon-ti'nens) 1. ability to control natural impulses 2. self-restraint

continent (kon'ti-nent) 1. able to control, such as urination and defecation 2. restraining the indulgence of pleasure, especially sexual

continuing extending **c medical education** (CME) **programme** formal, organised, educational programmes designed to promote the knowledge, skills and professional attitude

continuity (kon'ti-no'i-te) state of being continuous; uninterrupted connection

continuous joined together; without interruption **c ambulatory peritoneal dialysis** CAPD, a maintenance system of peritoneal dialysis wherein an indwelling catheter allows fluid to drain into and out of peritoneal cavity **c anaesthesia** maintenance of regional nerve block by allowing anaesthetic agent to drip at intervals or at a low rate of flow **c cycling peritoneal dialysis** CCPD, a dialysis method in which the patient is attached to an automatic cycler for short exchanges while sleeping **c fever** raised temperature persisting for many days without marked fluctuation **c murmur** murmur due to the continuous flow of blood through an abnormal communication from a high pressure to a region of low pressure with a large pressure gradient between the two regions **c positive airway pressure** CPAP ventilation assisted by a flow of air delivered at a constant pressure throughout the respiratory cycle

contour (kon'toor) the outline

contra- prefix indicating opposite or against

contra-aperture counter-opening to facilitate discharge

contraception (kon'tra-sep'shun) prevention of conception or impregnation

contraceptive (kon'tra-sep'tive) relating to measure or agent used to prevent conception **c methods** preventive methods to help woman to avoid unwanted pregnancies resulting from coitus

contract (kon-trakt) to shorten; to become reduced in size

contractile (kon-trak'til) having the property of contracting

contractility (kon-trak-til'i-te) the ability of shortening or becoming reduced in size

contraction (kon-trak'shun) 1. a shortage or shrinkage 2. increase in tension

contracture (kon-trak'chur) fibrosis of connective tissue in skin, fascia, muscle or a joint capsule that hinders normal mobility of the related tissue or structure

contrafissura (kon'tra-fi'shu'ra) fracture of a bone, as in the skull, at a point opposite the site of blow

contraindication (kon'tra-in-di-ka'shun) any condition or circumstance that renders a particular mode of treatment improper or inadvisable

contralateral (kon'tra-lat'er-al) occurring on the opposite side

contrast (kon'trast) opposition or unlikeness in things compared **c agents** substances used in radiology to provide a difference in density or organs. The substances can be radioopaque and positive such as barium sulphate, and iodinated compounds or radiolucent and negative such as air

contravolitional (kon'tra-vo-li'shun-al) without will; involuntary

contrecoup (kon-tr-koo) an injury as in the skull or brain occurring at a site opposite to the point of impact

control (kon-trol) 1. to regulate or main-

tain certain objects or events 2. a standard against which experimental observations are evaluated **aversive c** use of unpleasant stimuli to change the undesirable behaviour **birth c** deliberate limitation of child bearing by use of contraceptive methods **disease c** operations aimed to reduce the incidence and duration of disease

contrude (kon-trood) to crowd together, as in teeth

contrusion (kon-troo'shun) 1. abnormal line of dental arch 2. having the teeth crowded together

contuse (kon-tooz) to bruise

contusion (kon-too'zhun) a bruise; an injury without a break in the skin

conus (ko'nus) 1. a cone or cone-shaped structure 2. posterior staphyloma of a myopic eye **c arteriosus** the anterior part of the right ventricle which terminates in the pulmonary artery **c medullaris** the cone-shaped lower end of the spinal cord

convalescence (kon'val-es-ens) the period that elapses between the end of an illness, operation or injury and the recovery of the patient

convalescent 1. pertaining to convalescence 2. a patient recovering from a disease or operation

convection (kon-vek'shun) transference of heat in liquids or gases by movement of the heated particles

converge to move towards one point, to come together gradually

convergence (kon-ver'jens) movement of two objects towards a common point as in turning the eyes medialward

convergent (kon-ver'jent) tending towards a common point **c squint** a visual defect in which a deviating eye looks inward towards the nose.

conversion (kon-ver'zhun) 1. changing from one form to another 2. correction of foetal position during labour 3. *psy* transformation of emotional conflicts into physical symptoms without any organic basis **c disorder** a syndrome characterised by a loss or distortion of neurologic function not fully explained by organic disease and it presents with gait disturbance; dissociative disorder **c symptom** common presentation of conversion disorder are gait disturbances, loss of function in the limbs, aphonia, pseudoseizures, sensory loss and blindness

convex (kon'veks) a surface that is evenly curved; bulging outwards

convexoconcave (kon-vek'so-kon'kav) having one convex and one concave surface

convexoconvex (kon-vek'so-kon-veks) convex on two opposite surfaces

convoluted (kon-vo'loot'ed) rolled

convolution (kon'vo-loo'shun) 1. a rolling of an organ by infolding upon itself 2. a gyrus, one of the many folds on the surface of cerebral hemisphere

convulsant (kon-vul'sant) an agent producing convulsion

convulsion (kon-vul'shun) an involuntary muscular spasms of voluntary muscles occurring in paroxysms; seizure **clonic c** a convulsion in which muscles contract and relax alternately **febrile c** convulsions associated with high fever especially in infancy and early childhood **hysterical c** convulsions noted in hysteria **mimic c** facial muscle spasm **puerperal c** an eclamptic convulsion in pregnancy or puerperium **salaam c** a nodding spasm **tonic c** sustained muscle contraction

convulsive (kon-vul'siv) relating to convulsions

Cooley's anaemia thalassemia major, named after Thomas Cooley, US paediatrician

cooling reducing the temperature, such as body temperature by ice packs or cold moist dressing

Coomb's test in acquired haemolytic anaemia antibodies are formed against red cell antigens and cause inappropriate destruction of red blood cells. The presence of antibody on red cells is estab-

lished by direct antiglobulin test using an antihuman globulin antiserum which causes agglutination of erythrocytes (direct test) and when antibodies are present in the serum they have to get attached to red cells with appropriate antigen before they can be detected (indirect test) named after R. Coomb, British immunologist

Cooper's ligament the supporting fibrous structures found in the breast named after Sir Astley Cooper, British surgeon

coordination (ko-or'din-a'shun) the harmonious functioning of interrelated organs, applied to muscular movements

COPD abbreviation for chronic obstructive pulmonary disease

cope (kop) 1. *psy* to deal effectively with the challenge or conflict 2. the cavity side of a denture flask

coping (kop'ing) 1. a process by which an individual deals with the stress, finds a solution to the problem and takes a decision 2. a thin metal covering applied over a crown or root of a tooth

copodyskinesia (ko'po-dis'kin-e-se-a) fatigue of the muscles used in working

copper a metal, Cu (cuprium) atomic no. 29 necessary in small amounts to utilise iron

copper sulphate $CuSO_4$ deep blue crystals used as astingent

copremesis (kop'rem'e-sis) vomiting of faecal material

coproantibody (kop'ro-an'ti-bod'e) IgA antibody occurring in the intestinal contents and are formed by the plasma cells in the intestinal mucosa

coprolagnia (kop'ro-lag'ne-a) a sexual perversion in which thought or sight of a excreta causes pleasurable sensation

coprolalia (kop'ro-la'le-a) use of obscene language

coprolith (kop'ro-lith) a hard mass of inspissated faecal material

coprology (kop-rol'o-je) study of faeces

coprophagy (kop-rof'aje) eating of faecal material

coprophilia (kop'ro-fil'e-a) 1. *psy* an abnormal attraction to faecal material 2. attraction of microorganisms for faecal material

coprophobia (kop'ro-fo'be-a) abnormal fear of defecation of faeces

coproporphyria (kop'ro-por'fir'e-a) an inherited disorder of porphyria associated with excretion of an increased amount of coproporphyrin in the faeces

coproporphyrin (kop'ro-por'fir-in) one of two porphyrin compounds found normally in the urine and faeces as a decomposition product of bilirubin

coproporphyrinuria (kop'ro-por'fir-in-u-re-a) excess amount of coproporphyrin in the urine

copula (kop'u-la) 1. a narrow part connecting two structures 2. a median elevation on the floor of embryonic pharynx forming the roof of the tongue

copulation (kop'u-la'shun) sexual intercourse

cor 1. the heart 2. relating to the heart **c bovinum** markedly enlarged heart due to hypertrophied or dilated left ventricle **c pulmonale** pulmonary heart disease **c triatrium** heart with three atrial chambers with pulmonary veins emptying into an accessory chamber above the true left atrium

coracoacromial (kor'a-ko-a-kro'me-al) relating to coracoid and acromial processes

coracoid (kor'a-koyd) scapular process shaped like a crow's beak

cord (kord) any long, cylindrical, firm structure **nuchal c** the umbilical cord wrapped around the neck of foetus **spermatic c** the cord consisting of pampiniform plexus, nerves, vas deferens, testicular artery, extending from the abdominal inguinal ring to the testis **spinal c** the portion of CNS contained in vertebral canal **umbilical c** the structure connecting the circulatory system of the foetus to the placenta **vocal c** folds of mucous membrane in the larynx; superior pair is false and inferior pair is true vocal cord

cordal (kor'dal) pertaining to a cord

cordate (kor'dat) heart-shaped

cordectomy (kor-dek'to-me) surgical removal of a cord as of a vocal cord

corditis (kor-di'tis) inflammation of the spermatic cord

cordocentesis percutaneous umbilical venepuncture under ultrasonographic guidance to obtain a foetal blood sample

cordotomy (kor-dot'o-me) division of lateral spinothalamic tracts of the spinal cord

core (kor) 1. the centre of a structure 2. a plaster mold in dentistry, made over assembled parts of a dental restoration **c temperature** the temperature of deep structures of the body

coreclisis (kor'e-kli'sis) occlusion of the pupil

corectasia (kor'ek-ta'ze-a) dilatation of the pupil due to disease

corectomy (ko-rek'to-me) iridectomy

corectopia (kor-ek-to'pe-a) eccentric location of the pupil instead of being in the centre of the iris

core dialysis (ko're-di-al'i-sis) surgical separation of the outer margin of the iris from the ciliary body

corelysis (kor-el'i-sis) separation of adhesions between the capsule of the lens and the iris

coremorphosis (kor'r-mor-fo'sis) surgical formation of an artificial pupil

coreometer (ko're-om'e-ter) an instrument for measuring the pupil

coreometry (ko're-om'e-tre) measurement of the pupil

coreoplasty (ko-re-o-plas'te) operative correction of a deformed or occluded pupil

corestenoma (kor'e-sten-o'ma) narrowing of the pupil

Cori cycle the cycle in the carbohydrate metabolism in which muscle glycogen gets converted into lactic acid, and reaches the liver to get converted into liver glycogen. It is then broken down into glucose and carried to the muscle for reconversion into muscle glycogen, described by Carl Cori and Gerty Cori, Czech born US biochemists

corium (ko're-um) pl **coria** the dermis, layer of skin deep to the epidermis, the superficial thin layer interdigitates with the epidermis and the deeper thick layer of dense irregular connective tissue, contains blood vessels, nerves, nerve endings and glands

corn (korn) a horny induration and thickening of the skin caused by friction and pressure **hard c** located on the outside of little toe or the anterior surface of other toes **soft c** located between the toes, kept soft by moisture

cornea (kor-ne'a) the transparent circular anterior part of the eye, whose curvature is greater than that of other parts of the eye, hence functions as a refractive medium. It continues at its periphery with the sclera **corneal** adj **conical c** keratoconus **c reflex** reflex dependent on integrity of the ophthalmic branch of trigeminal nerve and the facial nerve with centre at pons. It is tested by an elongated wisp of cotton brought from the side, touching the lateral edge of the cornea. It causes blinking of both eyes **c transplant** implantation of a cornea from a healthy donor eye

corneitis (kor'ne-i-tis) keratitis

corneoblepharon (kor'ne-o-blef'a ron) adhesion of the eyelid to cornea

corneosclera (kor'ne-o-skle' ra) cornea and sclera forming the external coat of the eye ball

corneous (kor'ne-us) horny

corneum (kor'ne-um) stratum corneum

corniculum (kor-nik'u-lum) a small hornlike process

cornification (kor'ni-fin-ka'shun) keratinisation

cornified (kor'ni-fid) altered into horny tissue

cornu (kor'nu) pl **cornua** any structure resembling a horn **c ammonis** the hippocampus major of the brain **c anterius** 1. the anterior horn of the lateral ventricle of the brain 2. anterior gray column of the spinal cord in cross section **c cutaneum** a horn-like excrescence in the lateral ventricle of the brain **c inferius** the inferior horn of the lateral ventricle of the brain **c posterius** 1. the posterior horn of the lateral ventricle of the brain 2. the posterior gray column of the spinal cord in cross section

corona (ko-ro'na) a structure resembling a crown **c capitis** the crown of the head **c dentis** the crown of a tooth **c glandis** the prominent posterior border of the glans penis **c radiata** the radiating fibres from internal capsule to every part of the cerebral cortex

coronary (kor'o-na-re) 1. resembling or relating to a crown 2. encircling, referring to the arteries of the heart **c angiography** procedure useful to detect stenosis and guide revascularisation procedures in patients with coronary artery disease, and the procedure is accomplished by cannulating the right femoral or brachial artery **c angioplasty** undertaken by passing a fine guidewire across a coronary stenosis under radiographic control and using it to position a balloon which is then inflated to dilate the stenosis **c artery bypass surgery** CABG surgical establishment of a shunt that enables blood to travel from the aorta to a branch of coronary artery at a point past obstruction. The reversed segments of saphenous vein or internal mammary arteries are used to bypass the obstruction **c artery disease** most common form of heart disease. There is narrowing of the coronary arteries due to atheroma and its complications, particularly thrombosis to prevent adequate blood supply to the myocardium. The condition can manifest with stable angina, unstable angina, myocardial infarction, heart failure, arrhythmia or sudden death c **care unit** a specially equipped ward of a hospital giving intensive nursing and medical care for patients of coronary heart disease c **circulation** the left main and right coronary arteries arise from left and right coronary sinuses respectively just distal to the aortic valve. The left main coronary artery within 2.5cm of its origin divides into left anterior descending (LAD) artery and circumflex artery. LAD supplies the front wall and apex of the heart and circumflex artery, the posterior wall of the heart and a part of the inferior wall. The right coronary branches supply the right atrium, right ventricle and inferoposterior aspects c **stent** a piece of coated metallic 'scaffolding' that can be sent on a balloon and used to dilate a stenosed vessel after coronary angioplasty c **thrombosis** occlusion of one or more of the coronary arteries by a thrombus

coronavirus (kor'o-na-vi'rus) a single stranded RNA virus belonging to the family of coronaviridae, that causes upper respiratory tract infections

coroner (kor'o-ner) a person to investigate and provide official interpretation regarding the manner and possible cause(s) of deaths occurring suddenly, violently, without natural cause, with conflicting findings between stated cause and postmortem findings and foul play

coronoid (kor'o-noyd) shaped like a crown

coronoidectomy (kor'o-noy-dek'to-me) surgical removal of the coronoid process of the mandible

corpora (kor'po-ra) pleural of corpus, body c **arantil** small fibrous nodules at the centers of the semilunar valve cusps along the lines of closure

corporeal (kor-po're-al) pertaining to the body or to a corpus

corpse (korps) the dead human body; cadaver

corpulence (kor'pu-lens) obesity **corpulant** adj

cor pulmonale a heart affected secondarily to pulmonary disease resulting in right ventricular hypertrophy **acute** c develops when pulmonary embolus is sufficiently massive to obstruct more than two-thirds of pulmonary circulation. There is obstruction to the right ventricular outflow. **chronic** c hypertrophy of the right ventricle resulting from diseases affecting the function and/or the structure of the lung except when these pulmonary manifestations are the result of diseases that primarily affect the left side of the heart, or of congenital heart disease

corpus (kor'pus) pl **corpora** 1. a human body consisting of head, neck, trunk and limbs 2. any body or mass 3. the principal part of any organ or body c **albicans** a white fibrous tissue replacing the regressing corpus luteum in the ovary c **amygdaloideum** a rounded mass of gray matter in the anterior portion of temporal lobe of the cerebrum c **amylacea** one of a number of small ovoid bodies resembling a grain of starch found in nervous tissue, prostate and lungs c **calloşum** an arched mass of white matter in the longitudinal fissure composed of nerve fibres interconnecting the cortical hemispheres c **cavernosum clitoridis** one of the two columns of erectile tissue in the body of clitoris c **cavernosum penis** one of the two parallel columns of erectile tissue forming the dorsal part of the penis c **ciliaris** ciliary body c **coccygeum** coccygeal body c **geniculatum** the medial and lateral geniculate body lying in the thalamus c **haemorrhagicum** corpus luteum containing a blood clot c **luteum** small yellow endocrine body formed in the ovary at the site of ruptured ovarian follicle following ovulation c **mamillare** mamillary body protruding into the interpeduncular fosssa from hypothalamus c **quadrigemina**

quadrigeminal bodies **c spongiosum penis** the medial column of erectile tissue located between and the ventral to the two corpora cavernosa of the penis **c striatum** a striate body consisting of caudate and lentiform nuclei in the cerebral hemisphere **c ventriculi** body of the stomach **c vitreum** vitreous

corpuscle (kor′pus-el) 1. any small mass 2. a blood cell 3. an encapsulated nerve ending **corpuscular** adj **blood c** a red or white blood cell **corneal c** star-shaped connective tissue cell found between the laminae of fibrous tissue in the cornea **genital c** an encapsulated sensory nerve ending found in the skin of external genitalia and nipple **ghost c** achromocyte **Golgi-Mazzoni c** an encapsulated sensory nerve ending in the skin of the finger tips **Hassall′s c** flat epithelial cells arranged around a granular nucleated cell found in the medulla of thymus **lamellated c** large encapsulated nerve ending found throughout the body **lymph c** a lymphocyte **Malpighian c** renal corpuscle **Meissner′s c** tactile corpuscle **red c** erythrocyte **Ruffinis c′s** ovoid capsule with sensory nerve endings in subcutaenous tissues of the fingers **white c** any type of leucocyte

corpuscular (kor-pus′ku-lar) pertaining to corpuscles

correction altering of a condition that is abnormal

corrective (ko-reck′tiv) a drug that brings about a change in action of other

correlation (kor′e-la′shun) a statistical index of the relationship between variables

correspondence 1. act of corresponding 2. the condition of being in agreement 3. the point on each retina that has the same visual direction; when stimulated produces a single image.

Corrigan′s pulse water hammer pulse, named after Sir Dominic Corrigan, Irish physician

corroborating (kor-ob′o-ra-ting) confirming or supporting with evidence

corrosion (ko-ro′zhun) gradual disintegration of something by a destructive agent

corrosive (ko-ro-siv) producing corrosion

corrugator (kor′u-ga′tor) a muscle that draws together the skin causing it to wrinkle

cortex (kor′teks) pl **cortices** the outer part of an organ as distinguished by inner medulla **adrenal c** the outer larger part of the adrenal gland consisting of three zones: zona glomerulosa, zona fasciculata and zona reticularis, secreting corticosteroids and androgens. **auditory c** auditory area in cerebral cortex **cerebellar c** the thin layer of gray matter in the surface of cerebellum that contains Purkinje′s cells **cerebral c** the layer of gray matter covering the entire surface of cerebral hemisphere. There is a laminar organisation of its cellular and fibrous components **motor c** the region of cerebral cortex influencing the movements of the body **renal c** the part of the kidney containing the glomeruli and the proximal and distal convoluted tubules **sensory c** cerebral cortex refelecting to somatic, sensory, auditory, visual and olfactory regions

cortical (kor′ti-kal) pertaining to a cortex **c bone** the hard dense part of the bone that surrounds inner, soft bony tissue

corticectomy (kor′ti-sek′to-me) surgical removal of a part of cerebral cortex

cortices (kor′ti-sez) plural of **cortex**

corticifugal (kor′ti-sif′u-gal) conducting impulses away from the cortex

corticipetal (kor′ti-sip′e-tal) conducting impulses towards the cortex

corticobulbar (kor′ti-ko-bul′bar) pertaining to the cerebral cortex and upper part of the brain stem

corticoid (kor′ti-koyd) corticosteroid, a steroid hormone of the adrenal cortex

corticopontine (kor′ti-ko-pon′tin) pertaining to the cerebral cortex and pons

corticospinal (kor'ti-ko-spi'nal) **tract** one of the descending tracts of the spinal cord, which consists of fibres arising from pyramidal cells of Betz present in the motor cortex

corticosteroid (kor'ti-ko-ster'oyd) any of the steroids produced by the adrenal cortex or any synthetic equivalents. They are classified into two major groups based on their biologic activity: glucocorticoids involved in carbohydrate metabolism, increased gluconeogenesis and increased protein catabolism. It is also involved in immunomodulation and regulation of blood pressure; and mineralocorticoids concerned with the regulation of electrolyte and water balance used in hormone replacement therapy, as anti-inflammatory agents to suppress immune response and for suppression of ACTH secretion

corticosterone (kor'ti-kos'te-ron) a natural corticoid from the adrenal cortex that induces glycogen deposition in the liver, retention of sodium and excretion of potassium

corticothalamic (kor'ti-ko-tha-lam-ik) pertaining to the cerebral cortex and thalamus

corticotrophic (kor'ti-ka-trop'ik) pertaining to corticotropin

corticotropin (kor'ti-ko-tro'pin) **corticotrophin** (-tro'fin) adrenocorticotropic hormone secreted by the anterior pituitary gland having a stimulatory effect on adrenal cortex

cortisol (kor'ti-sol) major glucocorticoid in humans and its levels are highest in the morning on waking and lowest in the middle of the night. The level increases during stress and illness. 95% is bound to protein (cortisol-binding globulin) and free fraction is biologically active and it acts through glucocorticoid receptors.

cortisone (kor'ti-son) a natural glucocorticoid secreted by the adrenal cortex and also prepared synthetically.

It becomes active on conversion to cortisol. It is used as an anti-inflammatory, and immunosuppressive agent and for adrenal replacement therapy

coruscation (ko-rus-ka'shun) a sensation of flashes of light before the eyes

Corynebacterium (ko-ri'ne-bak-te're-um) a genus of non-motile rod-shaped gram-positive bacteria belonging to the family of Corynebacteriaceae. The important species is *C. diphtheriae* and it causes diphtheria

coryza (ko-ri'za) an acute catarrhal inflammation of nasal mucous membrane with profuse nasal discharge; acute rhinits

cosensitize (ko-sen'si-tiz) to sensitise to more than one infection

cosmesis (koz-me'sis) concern in surgical procedures about the appearance of the patient

cosmetic (koz-mat'ik) 1. relating to preservation and restoration of bodily beauty 2. a beautifying preparation **c surgery** an operation to improve appearance

costa (kos'ta) pl **costae** 1. one of the 24 elongated curved bones forming the bony thoracic cage 2. a rod-like supporting structure along the base of undulating membrane of certain flagellates

costal (kos'tal) pertaining to a rib **c cartilage** flexible cartilage that connects ribs to the sternum

costalgia (kos-tal'je-a) pleurodynia

cost benefit comparison of the costs of treatment and cost savings resulting from benefits of the treatment in rupees

cost effectiveness management technique where the economic benefits of any programme are compared with the cost of the programme. The benefits are expressed in terms of results achieved, as number of lives saved or the number of days free from disease

costectomy (kos-tek'to-me) excision of a rib

cost-identification cost of applying a treatment to a specified population under a particular set of conditions

costochondritis inflammation of costochondral junctions presenting with dull localised pain and tenderness over the costochondral junctions

costocervical (kos'to-ser'vi-kal) relating to the ribs and neck

costosternal (kos'to-ster'nal) relating to the ribs and sternum

costotome (kos'to-tom) knife to cut through a rib or cartilage

costotomy (kos'tot'o-me) division of a rib

costotransverse (kos'to-trans-vers) pertaining to the ribs and transverse processes of the vertebrae articulating with them

costovertebral (kos'to-ver'te'bral) pertaining to the ribs and the bodies of the thoracic vertebrae with which they articulate

costoxiphoid (kos'to-zi'foyd) pertaining to the ribs and the xiphoid cartilage of the sternum

cost-utility comparison of the cost and benefits of a treatment

cottage loaf sign MR image or US images giving an appearance of a cottage loaf of bread prepared with wheat flour and yeast, seen in partial herniation of liver through the diaphragmatic defect due to trauma to the right hemidiaphragm

cotton a soft, white fibrous material from the seeds of *Gossypium* **c wool appearance** multiple rounded fluffy nodular shadows on a plain chest film in patients with pulmonary tuberculosis **c wool exudates** fluffy exudates in the retina that accumulate after microinfarcts in retinal nerve fibre layer, seen in grade III hypertensive retinopathy, and diabetes mellitus

cotyledon (kot'i-le'don) a subdivision of the uterine surface of the placenta.

cotyloid (kot'i-loyd) cup-shaped, relating to acetabulum

cough (kawf) a protective reflex mechanism induced reflexly or consciously to get rid of foreign material or accumulated secretions in the airways **bovine c** cough that has lost its explosive nature as in vocal cord paralysis **brassy c** cough of metallic and hard quality as in tracheal obstruction especially caused by intrathoracic tumours **dry c** without expectoration, as in initial stages of acute bronchitis **hacking c** a short, frequent, shallow cough **laryngeal c** harsh, irritative and repetitive cough that may be accompanied by stridor **pharyngeal c** short and dry irritative cough accompanied by pain behind jaw or in the neck **postural c** cough brought on by adopting particular attitudes or changing posture as in bronchiectasis or lung abscess **productive c** accompanied by expectoration of sputum **reflex c** cough due to irritation of some remote organ **tracheal c** dry cough accompanied by retrosternal discomfort **wet c** productive cough **whooping c** *see* whooping cough **winter c** attacks of cough during cold seasons as in initial phases of COPD

Coulomb (koo'lom) the amount of electricity delivered by a current of 1 ampere in 1 second, named after C. Coulomb, French physicist

coumarin (koo'ma-rin) one of the natural or synthetic compounds containing dicumarol that inhibits hepatic synthesis of vitamin K-dependent coagulation factors.

Councilman's (kown'sil-man) **body** deeply stained acidophilic bodies due to dead shrunken liver cells in acute hepatitis and yellow fever named after William Councilman, US pathologist

counselling providing advice and guidance to a patient

count (kownt) an enumeration. The numerical computation of units of object per unit of volume, such as bacterial count, blood cell count, platelet count, reticulocyte count, absolute cell count, and differential white blood cell count. The emission of radiation is counted per unit of time

counter (kown'ter) a device that counts **coulter c** an electronic device that can rapidly identify and count the red and white blood cells in a sample of blood **Geiger-Muller c** an instrument for measuring radioactivity by counting the emission of radioactive particles **scintillation c** a device for detecting and counting radiation **whole body c** detectors designed to evaluate the total-body burden of different gamma-emitting nucleids

counteract (kown'ter-akt) to act against

counteraction (kown'ter-ak'shun) the action of a drug having an action opposing that of another agent

counterextension (kown'ter-eks-ten'shun) traction in a proximal direction offering resistance to extension

counter immunoelectrophoresis (kown'-ter-im'u-no-e-lek'tro-fo-re'sis) an immunoassay capable of detecting minute quantities of an antigen by the formation of a precipitin line in a gel between an antibody and antigen of different electrophoretic mobilities

counterincision (kown'ter-in-sizh'un) a second incision made to promote drainage and sometimes to relieve tension on the edges of a clean wound during closure

counterirritant (kown'ter-ir'i-tant) 1. producing a counterirritant 2. any agent causing counterirritation

counterirritation (kown'ter-ir'i-ta'shun) an irritation that is intended to relieve some other irritation

counteropening (kown'ter-o'pen-ing) a second incision made across an earlier one to facilitate drainage

countershock delivery of a high intensity direct current shock to the heart to interrupt ventricular fibrillation and to restore regular electrical activity

counterstain (kown'ter-stan) a stain applied to render the effects of the earlier stain more prominent

countertraction (kown'ter-trak'shun) traction opposed to another traction used in the reduction of fracture

couplet a pair of successive premature ventricular contractions

couple 1. to join together 2. to copulate **c protection rate** the percent of eligible couples effectively protected against childbirth by one or other approved methods of fertility regulating methods

coupling (kup'ling) 1. pairing or joining 2. bigeminal rhythm from repeated pairing of a normal sinus beat with a ventricular extrasystole

Courvoisier's (koor-vwa'ze-az) **law** if in a jaundiced patient, gall bladder is enlarged, it is not a case of stone impacted in the common bile duct, for previous cholecystitis, which existed when the stone was in the gall bladder must have rendered the gall bladder fibrotic and incapable for dilatation, described by Ludwig Curvoisier, Swiss surgeon. The law has lost its significance

Couvelaire (koo'vel-or) **uterus** extravasation of blood into the uterine musculature in *abruptio placentae*, named after Alexandre Couvelaire, French obstetrician

covalence (ko-val'ens) the sharing of electrons between two atoms

cover prophylactic treatment of a patient with antibiotics who is at risk for a bacterial infection following trauma or surgery.

Cowper's glands bulbourethral glands situated on either side of the membranous urethra, that secrete fluid into the urethra during sexual stimulus, named after William Cowper, English surgeon

cowperitis (kow'per-i'tis) inflammation of Cowper's gland. They are felt on passing the forefinger into the rectum and placing the thumb first on one side and then on the other of the median-raphe of the perineum

cowpox (kow'poks) a mild eruptive skin

disease caused by vaccinia virus, affects the udder and teats of cows and may be transmitted to man by inoculation and contact

coxa (kok'sa) the part of the body lateral to and including the hip joint

coxalgia (kok-sal'je-a) 1. hip joint disease 2. pain in the hip

coxarthrosis (koks'arth-ro'sis) osteoarthiritis of hip joint

Coxiella (kok'se-el'la) a genus of bacteria of the order Rickettsiales, named after Herald Cox, US bacteriologist; *C. burnetii* is responsible for Q fever.

coxitis (kok-si'tis) inflammation of the hip joint

coxodynia (kok'so-din'e-a) coxalgia

coxofemoral (kok'so-fem'or-ral) pertaining to the hip and thigh

Coxsackievirus (kok-sak'e-vi'rus) a family of picornaviruses named after a city in New York State, which may produce herpangina, aseptic meningitis, epidemic pleurodynia, acute nonspecific pericarditis and myocarditis

cozymase (ko-zi-mas) nicotinamide- adenine-dinucleotide (NAD)

C- peptide a biologically inactive proinsulin stored within secretory granules

CPAP abbreviation for continuous positive airway pressure

CPC abbreviation for clinicopathological conference

CPK abbreviation for creatine phosphokinase

CPPV abbreviation for continuous positive pressure ventilation

CPR abbreviation for cardiopulmonary resuscitation

CPU Central Processing Unit. It forms the brain of PC, carrying out millions of arithmetic and control functions every second. Its power is defined by its speed in MegaHertz, which is the number of times it 'thinks'a second

Cr symbol for element chromium

crab louse pubic louse

crack a crystalline form of cocaine that is smoked

craked pot sign increased intracranial pressure leads to separation of the cranial sutures and percussion of the skull gives a sound likened to a 'cracked vessel'

cracker sign marked difficulty in eating dry foods as in xerostomia

crackle (krak'l) discontinuous explosive crackling sounds produced in the alveoli, proximal and distal airways and sometimes in the cavities **early inspiratory** c heard in widespread airflow obstruction attributed to early opening of proximal and larger airways prematurely closed during previous expiration **late inspiratory** c originate in the peripheral airways begin in mid inspiration and continues to the end of inspiration, profuse in number, heard in restrictive lung diseases

cradle (kra'dl) a light weight frame placed over part of bed for protection of injured parts, or for application of heat or cold **c cap** thick yellow scales occurring in patches over the scalp in infants

cramp (kramp) a painful spasmodic muscular contraction, often noted during or after exercise

cranial vault the frontal, parietal and occipital bones form the movable part of the foetal skull and they get moulded to female birth canal facilitating passage of the caphalic-presenting infant

crani (o) combining word for skull

craniad (kra'ne-ad) in a cranial direction; superior end of the body

cranial (kra'ne-al) pertaining to the cranium

cranialis (kra'ne-a-lis) pertaining to the cranium or the superior end of the body

craniofenestra (kra'ne-o-fen-es'tre-a) a defective development of foetal skull with areas in which no bone is formed

craniolacunia (-la-ku'ne-a) a defective development of foetal skull with depressed areas on the inner surface

craniomalacia (-ma-la'she-a) markedly soft bones of the skull

craniopharyngeoma (kra'ne-o-fa-rin'je-o'ma) a tumour arising from cell rests derived from the hypophyseal stalk or Rathke's pouch. There is raised intracranial tension and calcium deposits

cranioplasty (kra'ne-o-plas'te) any plastic surgery on the skull

craniorhachischisis (kra'ne-o-ra-kis'ki-sis) congenital fissure of the skull and vertebral column

cranioschisis (kra'ne-os'ki-sis) congenital fissure of the skull

craniosclerosis (kra'ne-o-skle-ro'sis) thickening of the bones of the skull

craniostenosis (-ste-no'sis) deformity of the skull caused by premature closure of the cranial sutures

craniosynostosis (-sin'os-to'sis) premature closure of the sutures of the skull

craniotabes (-ta'bez) softening of the cranial bones noted in premature infants and in those exposed to abnormal intrauterine pressures

craniotomy (kra'ne-ot'a-me) 1. any operation on the cranium 2. an operative procedure to decrease the size of the head of a dead foetus to facilitate delivery

cranium (kra'ne-um) the skeleton of head that includes all the bones of the head except mandible, and it acts as a vault to contain brain

crater (krat'er) a circular area of depression surrounded by an elevated margin

cravat (kra-vat) a triangular bandage

crazy pavement appearance mottled zones of pigmented and depigmented skin in infants with protein calorie malnutrition

cream (krem) 1. the upper fatty layer which forms in milk 2. a-semi solid emulsion of oil and water, for topical use

crease (kres) a line with slight depression

creatine (kre'a-tin) an amino acid occurring in vertebrate tissues **c kinase** (ck) an **enzyme** that catalyses the phosphorylation of creatine by ATP to form phosphocreatine. It occurs in three isozymes specific to brain (CK-BB), cardiac muscle (CK-MB) and skeletal muscle (CK-MM)

creatinine (kre-at'i-nin) the final product of creatine catabolism

creatinuria (kre-a-tin-nu'ar-a) excretion of increased amount of creatine in urine

creatorrhoea (kre-a-to-re'a) presence of muscle fibres in the stools in chronic pancreatitis, demonstrable by microscopy

Crede's (kra-daz) **method** a technique to expel placenta wherein downward pressure is applied on the uterus through the abdominal wall. Such a technique is also adapted to empty a flaccid bladder, named after Karl Crede, German gynaecologist

cremasteric (krem'as-ter'ik) relating to the cremaster muscle

crena (kre'na) a notch or cleft

crenate, crenated (kre'nat; kre'nat-ed) notched; scalloped

crenation (kren-a'shun) abnormal notching in the edge of an erythrocyte

crenocyte (kre'na-sit) a red blood cell with serrated edges

crepitation (krep'i-ta'shun) 1. crackles; the discontinuous explosive sounds heard in either phases of respiratory cycle, may be fine or coarse **coarse c** low pitched, loud adventitious sounds appear bubbling in bronchiectasis **fine c** crackles, sounds simulated by rubbing of a lock of hair between the thumb and finger near ear. They may be heard either in early (widespread airflow obstruction) or late (restrictive lung diseases) inspiration and also during expiration **post tussive c** a deep inspiration after coughing, often heard over minimal lesions of tuberculosis or cavities

crepitus (krep'i-tus) 1. a grating sensation felt by hand kept on knee joint when it is moved passively as in osteoarthropathy 2. a crackling sensation felt on palpation of the skin in subcutaneous emphysema or in gas gangrene

crescent (kres'int) shaped like a sickle or new moon **articular c** a crescent-shaped cartilage as the menisci in knee joint. **epithelial c** presence of macrophages, epithelial cells and fibroblasts in the Bowman's space in acute glomerulonephritis **malarial c** male and female gametocytes of *Plasmodium falciparum* in the red blood cells **myopic c** a greyish white crescentic area in the fundus of eye due to atrophy of choroid allowing the sclera to become visible

cresol (kre'sol) yellow-brown liquid from coal tar, used as a disinfectant

crest (krest) a ridge, or an elongated prominence especially on a bone

cretin an individual exhibiting cretinism

cretinism (kret'n-izm) a congenital condition due to lack of thyroid hormone causing arrest of physical and mental development **endemic c** nervous cretinism noted in Himalayas. Intellectual functions are impaired and there is hearing defect **myxoedematous c** a sporadic type of cretinism **sporadic c** occurs from dysgenesis of thyroid gland, inadequate hormone synthesis due to enzyme defect and damaged gland

CREST complex the pentad of clinical signs with mixed connective tissue disease, calcinosis, Raynaud's phenomenon, oesophageal dysmotility, sclerodactyly and telangiectasia

crevice (kervis) a small fissure in a solid structure **gingival c** the space between the surface of a tooth and the free gingiva

crevicular (kre-vik'u-ler) relating to a crevice, especially the gingival crevice

Creutzfeldt-Jakob (kroits'felt yak'ob) **disease** (CJD) a prion disease characterised by rapidly progressive dementia with myoclonus. It is transmissible experimentaily to chimpanzees, named after Gerhard Creutzfeldt and Alfons Jakob, German psychiatrists

CRF chronic renal failure

CRH corticotropin releasing hormone

crib death sudden infant death syndrome

cribration (kri-bra'shun) a pitted or perforated condition

cribriform (krib'ri-form) containing multiple perforations; sieve-like histological pattern, in which sheets of epithelial cells are punctuated by gland-like space **c plate of ethmoid** forms the roof of the nose that is pierced by the branches of olfactory nerve

cribrum (krib'rum)cribriform plate of ethmoid bone.

cricoid (kri-koid) 1. ring-shaped 2. the cricoid cartilage

cricopharyngeal (kri'ko-fa-rin'ge-al) relating to the cricoid cartilage and pharynx

cricothyroid (kri-ko-thi'royd) relating to the cricoid and thyroid cartilage.

cricothyreotomy (kri'ko-thi're-ot-a-me) incision through the cricoid and thyroid cartilages

cricothyreotomy (-thi-rot'a-me) incision through the skin and cricothyroid membrane, undertaken to relieve respiratory obstruction

cricotracheotomy (-tra'ke-ot'o-me) incision of trachea through the cricoid cartilage

cri du chat (kre-doo-shah') a condition with loss of short arm of chromosome 5 with mental retardation and cat-like cry

Criggler-Najjar jaundice a recessive defect of bilirubin conjugating enzyme in the liver leading to unconjugated hyperbilirubinaemia

crinophagy (krin-of'a-je) elimination of excess granules by lysosomes

crisis (kris'sis) 1. any acute exacerbation of a clinical condition **Addisonian c** acute adrenocortical insufficiency **Dietl's c** paroxymal attacks of lumbar and abdominal pain due to kinking of ureter in persons with wandering kidney **identity c** a disorientation concerning one's sense of self and role in society, occurring acutely **sickle cell c** recurrent acute symptoms in patients with sickle cell anaemia due to vascular occlusion or haemolysis. **thyrotoxic c** thyroid storm, aggravation of symptoms of thyrotoxicosis following surgery, shock or thyroidectomy

crista (kris'ta) crest, a projection or projecting structure

criterion standard used in formulating a conclusion

cRNA complementary RNA

crocodile tears lacrimation while eating especially after recovery from facial palsy, due to faulty regeneration of the nerve

crocidolite (kro'sid'o-lit) blue asbestos

Crohn's disease regional ileitis; common sites of involvement are terminal ileum, right side of colon; entire wall of bowel is oedematous and thickened; deep ulcers occur like linear fissures and are patchy. Presents with bloody diarrhoea, passage of mucus and constitutional symptoms, named after B. Crohn, US physician

cromolyn (kro'mol-in) a kellin compound, that acts on tissue mast cell and stabilises its cell membrane and prevents its degranulation, thus of release of histamine and other tissue mediators involved in asthmatic attack. It is used as a prophylactic

cross (kross) any figure or structure in the shape of a cross

cross bite (kros'bit) an abnormal relation of one or more teeth of upper and lower jaw due to deviation of teeth or to abnormal position of jaw

cross breeding (-bred-ing) the mating of animals or plants of different strains and species

cross eye (-i) strabismus in which there is deviation of a visual axis of one eye toward that of the other eye to result in diplopia

cross matching (kros-mach'ing) 1. test to determine the compatibility between donor and recipient blood undertaken prior to transfusion 2. to determine the presence of antibody in an allograft

recipient against lymphocytes of the allograft donor and their presence contraindicates transplantation

cross leg flap use of flap from other leg while doing plastic repair

cross reactivity reaction of antibody with several antigens or *vice versa*, indicative of similarity of antigen determinants

cross resistance organisms developing resistance to one drug, become automatically resistant to other similar drugs

cross section studies examination of a large number of persons at one time

crossing over (kros'ing o'ver) exchange of lengths of DNA between members of each chromosome pair during prophase of first meiotic division

crotalid (krot'a-lid) any snake of the family Crotalidae, a pit viper

Crotalidae (kro-tal'i-de) a family of venomous snakes; pit vipers have front, movable hollow fangs and a pit between the nostril and eye

crotalus (krot'a-lus) rattle snake of the family Crotalidae

crotamiton (krot'a-mi'ton) a light yellow oily liquid useful in scabies

crotonic acid butyric acid with a double bond

croton oil an extract from seeds of *Croton tiglium*, a violent purgative and vesicant

croup (kroop) 1. laryngotracheobronchitis in infants and young children by parainfluenza virus

Crouzon's (kroo-zonz) **disease** a congenital condition characterised by hyperteleorism, craniofacial dysostosis, exophthalmos, and optic atrophy, named after Octave Crouzon, French neurologist

crowding 1. altered position of teeth making them crowded 2. crowding of ribs in collapse or fibrosis of the lung

crown (krown) 1. corona 2. the part of teeth covered with enamel

crowning (krown'ing) first sight of vertex at vulva during labour

CRP C-reactive protein

CRST syndrome calcinosis, Raynaud's syndrome, sclerodactyly and telangiectasis exhibiting a slower progress than scleroderma

cruciate (kroo'she-at) shaped like a cross c ligaments 1. anterior and posterior ligaments forming central link in knee joint 2. ligament separating dens of axis from vertebral canal in atlantoaxial joint

cruciform (kroo'si-form) cross-shaped

crude rate simple enumeration of cases, death etc. in a population without making any adjustment for nature of population

crunch a crunching sound audible in pneumomediastinum

crura (kroo'ra) pleural of crux

crus (krus) 1. the leg, the part between the knees and the ankle 2. any structure resembling a leg, as elongated masses or a pair of diverging bands

crust (krust) 1. a scab 2. an outer layer or covering

crustacea (krus-ta'she-a) a class of arthropods, such as crabs and shrimps

crutch (kruch) a device used singly or in pairs to assist walking c palsy pressure in axilla causing ischaemic radial palsy

Creveilhier-Baumgarten (kroo-val-ya'bom-gar'ten) syndrome portal hypertension with a large umbilical collateral vessel with a marked blood flow giving rise to a venous hum on auscultation, named after Jean Cruveilhier, French pathologist and Paul Baumgarten, German pathologist

crux (kruks) cross

cry (o) combining word for cold

cryoablation (kri'o-ab-la'shun) removal of the tissue by destroying it with extreme cold

cryalgesia (kri'al-je'ze-a) pain on application of cold

cryesthesia (-es-the'zhah) 1. subjective sensation of cold 2. sensitivity to cold

crymodynia (kri'mo-din'e-a) pain caused by cold

cryoanalgesia (kri'o-an'al-je'ze-a) the relief of pain by application of cold

cryobank (kri'o-bank) a place for storage of biological tissues at very low temperatures

cryobiology (kri'o-bio-logi) the science of freezing tissue

cryoextraction (-eks-trak'shun) removal of cataract by freezing contact

cryofibrinogen (-fi-bin'o-jen) an abnormal type of fibrinogen precipitated upon cooling, but redissolves when warmed to room temperature

cryofibrinogenaemia (-fi-brin'-a-jen-e'me-a) presence of cryofibrinogen

cryogenic (-jen'ik) concerned with or producing low temperature

cryoglobulin (-glob'u-lin) precipitation of plasma protein especially IgM-IgG complex when cold

cryoglobulinaemia (-glob'u-lin-e'me-a) presence of abnormal amount of cryoglobulin within the blood

cryohypophysectomy (-hi'po-fiz-ek'ta-me) destruction of hypothalamus by cold

cryopathy (kri-op'a-the) disorder caused by cold

cryoprecipitate (-pre-sip'i-tat) a soluble material from plasma getting precipitated on cooling, and the material is rich in factor VIII

cryopreservation (-pre'zer-va'shun) preservation of cells at very low temperatures, often in liquid nitrogen

cryoprobe (kri-o-prob) an extremely cold instrument used in cryosurgery

cryoprotein (-pro'ten) a protein that precipitates from solution when cooled, and redissolves upon warming

cryostat (kri'o-stat) refrigerator working at temperatures below freezing

cryosurgery (kri'o-ser'jer-e) treatment by local freezing

cryothalamectomy (-thal'a-mek'ta-me) destruction of a portion of thalamus by application of extreme cold

cryotherapy (-ther'a-pe) use of cold in the treatment

crypt (kript) 1. a pit-like depression 2. a recess in tubule **c of Lieberkuhn** a tubular gland of intestine concerned with secretion of intestinal juice **tonsillar c** a deep invagination of the stratified epithelium and substances of tonsils

crypt (o) combining word for concealed; crypt

crypta (krip'ta) pl **cryptae** crypt

cryptitis (krip-tit'is) inflammation of a follicle or glandular tubule

crytococcosis (krip'to-kok-o'sis) caused by *Cryptococcus neoformans;* it is characterised by granulomatous lesion of the lung, bones, brain and meninges. Immunocompromised persons are at special risk. Amphotericin B and flucytosine are useful in the management

Cryptococcus (-kok'us) a genus of yeast-like fungi that reproduces by budding. *C. neoformans* is a ovoid and thick- walled. It contains a mucinous capsule with large amounts of polysaccharide demonstrable by India ink

cryptogenic (krip'to-jen'ik) of undetermined aetiology; obscure

cryptolith (krip'to-lith) a concretion in a gland follicle

cryptomenorrhoea (krip'to-men'ore-a) absence of menstrual flow

cryptophthalmos (krip'tof-thal'mos) congenital absence of eyelids

cryptopyic (krip'to-pi'ik) hidden suppuration

cryptorchid (krip-tor'kid) a person with undescended testes

cryptorchidectomy (krip'tor-kid-ek'ta-me) surgical removal of an undescended testis

cryptorchidopexy (krip'tor-kid-a-pek'se) orchipexy

cryptorchism (krip-tor'kim) failure of descent of a testis

cryptosporidiosis (krip'to-spo-rid'e-o'sis) infection with Cryptosporidium presenting with chronic watery diarrhoea and abdominal cramps. The disease is se-

vere in immunocompromised patients

Cryptosporidium (krip-to-spo-rid'e-um) a coccidian protozoa of humans and domestic animals found in intestinal tract. *C. parvum* is an example

crystal (kris'tl) an angular solid of definite form **Charcot-Leyden c** protein crystals in situations of fragmentation of eosinophils, in bronchial secretion of asthmatics and in stools in certain intestinal parasitic infestation

crystalline (kris'til-in) 1. clear or transparent 2. relating to a crystal or crystals

crystallise to firm up, give a definite form to something vague

crystalluria (kris'til-ur'e-a) excretion of crystalline substances

CSF 1. cerebrospinal fluid 2. colony stimulating factor **CSF rhinorrhoea** escape of CSF in skull fracture through nose

CSOM chronic suppurative otitis media

CT computed tomography

Cu chemical symbol, copper

cubital (ku'bi-tal) relating to the elbow or to the ulna

cubital tunnel syndrome compression of ulnar nerve at elbow with pain and numbness, and later muscle weakness

cubitus (ku'bi-tus) 1. elbow 2. ulna **c valgus** deviation of the extended forearm outside of the axis of the limb **c varus** deviation of the extended forearm inside of the axis of the limb

cubulin (ku'bu-lin) gene on chromosome 10 responsible for the uptake of vitamin B12 and related molecules in the intestine

cuff (kuf) a band-like structure **rotator c** a musculotendinous structure surrounding the shoulder joint **sphygmomanometer c** a bladder containing cuff that encompasses at least two-thirds of the circumference of the arm

cul-de-sac (kul-de-sak) 1. a blind pouch 2. a tubular cavity closed at one end

culdocentesis (kul'do-sen-te'sis) aspiration of fluid from rectouterine pouch

culdoscopy (kul-dos'ka-pe) visualisation of the rectovaginal pouch and pelvic viscera by an endoscope introduced through the posterior vaginal wall

Culex (ku'leks) a genus of mosquitoes belonging to the family of culicidae which transmit diseases to man

culicide (ku'li-sid) an agent that destroys mosquitoes

culicifuge (ku-lis'i-fuj) mosquito repellant

Cullen's (kul'enz) sign bluish discolouration of the periumbilical region in intraperitoneal haemorrhage, named after Thomas Cullen, US gynaecologist

culmen (kul'men) the summit

cultivation (kul'tiva'shun) culture, propagation of organisms in an artificial medium

culture (kul'cher) 1. growth of microorganisms on or in a media 2. a mass of microorganisms on or in a medium

culture medium (kul'cher med'e-um) propagation of microorganisms in a media such as bile broth, glucose, serum broth or cooked media

cumulative steadily increasing in volume, value or strength by addition or repetition

cumulus (ku'mu-lus) a small elevation

cuneate (ku'ne-at) cuneiform

cuneiform (ku-ne'form) wedge-shaped

cuneus (ku'ne-us) pl. cunei region of the medial aspect of the occipital lobe on either side of cerebral hemisphere bounded by parietooccipital and calcarine fissures

cuniculus (ku-nik'u-lus) a burrow of itch mite in the epidermis

cunnilingus (kun'i-ling'gus) an oro-genital sexual act of licking the vulva or clitoris

cunnus (kun'us) the vulva

cup (kup) a cup-shaped or an excavated structure optic c slight depression observed in optic disc

cupola (ku'pa-la) cupula

cupping (kup'ing) 1. occurrence of a cup-shaped excavation 2. application of cupping glass

cuprophane (koo'pro-fan) a cellulose membrane used in haemodialysis

cupruresis (ku'proo-re'sis) excretion of copper in urine

cupruretic (ko'proo-ret'ik) pertaining to or promotion of urinary excretion of copper

cupula (koo'pu-la) a dome-like structure closing ampulla of semi-circular canals

cupulometry (ku'pu-lom'i-tre) a method of testing vestibular function. The patient is accelerated in a rotational chair. The post-rotational vertigo and nystagmus are graphically represented against the speed of angular movement

curare (koo-ra're) an extract of Strychnos toxifera that produces paralysis of skeletal muscles by blocking transmission at the myoneural junctions

curarisation (ku'rar-i-za'shun) administration of curare to induce muscle relaxation

curarimimetic (koo-ra're-mi-met-ik) producing effects similar to those of curare

cure (kur) 1. to make well; to heal 2. a restoration to health 3. a medicine effective in treating a disease

curettage (ku're-tazh) scraping, usually of the interior of a cavity or tract to obtain material for tissue diagnosis and to remove abnormally looking tissues

curie (ku're) radioactivity unit, named after Pierre and Marie Curie, French scientists

Curling's (kur'lingz) ulcer acute peptic ulcer with bleeding noted in patients with severe burns, named after Thomas Curling, British physician

current (kur'ent) a stream or flow of fluid, air or electricity

Curschmann's (koorsh'manz) spirals twisted strips of cell debris in the sputum of asthmatic patients, named after G. Curschmann, German physician

curvatura (ker'va-tu'ra) curvature

curvature (ker'va-chur) a blending or flexure angular c a sharp angulation of the spine greater c of stomach the border of stomach to which the greater omentum is attached **lesser c of stom-ach** the border of the stomach to which lesser omentum is attached

curve (kerv) 1. a curvature 2. a graphic representation by lines

curvularia (kur-vu-lar'e-a) a genus of fungi of the class Hyphomycetes

Cushing's disease Cushing's syndrome produced by ACTH secreting basophil adenoma of pituitary, named after Harvey Cushing, US surgeon

Cushing's syndrome a syndrome caused by pituitary dependent bilateral adrenal hyperplasia, ectopic ACTH production, iatrogenic (ACTH and glucocorticoid therapy), adrenal adenoma, and adrenal carcinoma characterised by moon face, psychosis, acne, plethora, centripetal obesity, hypertension, striae, osteoporosis, bruising, hyperglycaemia, peptic ulcer, menstrual disturbances, tendency to infection and poor wound healing

cushion (koosh'in) a pad-like structure.

cusp (kusp) 1. a leaflet of one of the heart's valves 2. a conical elevation arising on the surface of a tooth

cuspid (kus'pid) 1. having one cusp or point 2. a canine tooth

cuspis (kus'pis) a cusp

cutaneous (ku-ta'ne-us) pertaining to the skin

cutdown (kut'down) dissection of a vein for insertion of a cannula or needle to administer intravenous fluids or medication

cuticle (ko'ti-k'l) 1. epidermis 2. an outer thin layer

cuticula (ku-tik'u-la) cuticle

cutireaction (kut'i-re-ak'shun) an inflammatory or irritative reaction on the skin

cutis (ku'tis) skin; protective covering of the body consisting of epidermis and dermis

cuvette (ku-vet) a transparent glass container to examine solutions photometrically

CVA cerebrovascular accident

CVC chronic venous congestion

CVP central venous pressure

CVS cardiovascular system

CWP coal workers' pneumoconiosis

CXR Chest X-ray

cyan (o) combining word for blue

cyanhaemoglobin (si'an-he'mo-glo'bin) a compound of cyanide and methaemoglobin formed after administration of methylene blue in cyanide poisoning.

cyanobacteria (si'a-no-bak-ter'e-a) chlorophyll-containing bacteria

cyanocobalamin (-ko-bal'a-min) vitamin B_{12}, a complex of cyanide and cobalamin, used in the treatment of pernicious anaemia

cyanophil (si-an'a-fil) a cell taking blue colour after staining

cyanophyceae (si'a-no-fi'se-e) cyanobacteria

cyanopsia (si'a-nop'se-a) a condition where all objects appear blue; it may be temporarily seen following cataract extraction

cyanosed (si'a-nosed) cyanotic

cyanosis (si'a-no'sis) bluish discolouration of the skin and mucous membranes due to presence of excess amounts of reduced haemoglobin in the arterial blood. Cyanosis becomes visible when the amount of reduced haemoglobin exceeds 5 G/dl. **central c** occurs due to mixing of arterial and venous blood at the level of heart or great vessels and to defective oxygenation in the lungs. The central parts such as tongue and peripheral parts such as nail beds, tip of the nose, finger and toes are cyanosed. The extremities are warm **differential c** occurrence of Eisenmenger's reaction in a patent ductus arteriosus, causes cyanosis in the lower limbs with sparing of upper limbs **peripheral c** extremities such as tips of the fingers and toes, nail bed and tip of the nose are cyanosed. It is caused by excess extraction of oxygen by the tissues from capillaries, which is secondary to impaired circulatory state either due to reduction in cardiac output or vasospasm. The extremities are cold to feel **regional c** noted in Raynaud's disease, arterial occlusion and thrombophlebitis

cybernetics (si'ber-net'iks) 1. a comparative study of computers and nervous system 2. the science of control and communication

cybrid (sa'i-brid) cytoplasmic hybrid

cycl(o) combining word for round, recurring; ciliary body of the eye

cyclamate (si'kla-mat) a salt of cyclamic acid, a sweetening agent

cyclarthrosis (si'klar-thro'sis) a rotary joint

cyclase (si'klas) an enzyme that forms a cyclic compound

cycle (si'k'l) 1. recurrent series of events 2. a recurring period of time. **cardiac c** the period from the commencement of one heart beat to the beginning of next beat includes systole, the contraction of atria and ventricles to move blood forwards and diastole, the period during which the cavities are refilled with blood **cori c** the phases in the metabolism of carbohydrate **krebs c** tricarboxylic acid cycle, the final common pathway for oxidation to CO_2 of carbohydrate, fat and protein **menstrual c** a series of periodically recurring changes in the hormonal status and in the endometrium of uterus, which in the absence of fertilisation leads to menstruation **nitrogen c** the series of events in which nitrogen of atmosphere is taken by plants and animals and then returned to atmosphere

cyclectomy (si'klek'ta-me) cutting of the ciliary muscle

cyclic (sik'lik) 1. occurring periodically 2. continuous

cyclitis (si-klit'is) inflammation of ciliary body

cyclazine (si'kli-zen) antihistamine with sedative effect chiefly used in motion sickness

cyclochoroiditis (si'klo-ko'roid-i'tis) inflammation of the ciliary body and the choroid of the eye

cyclocryotherapy (-kri'o-the'ra-pe) application of a freezing probe to the sclera near the region of ciliary body in glaucoma

cyclodialysis (-di-al'i-sis) creation of a communication between the anterior chamber and suprachoroidal space to decrease intraocular tension in glaucoma

cyclodiathermy (-di'a-ther'me) application of diathermy to the ciliary body in the treatment of glaucoma

cycloid (si'kloid) 1. resembling a circle 2. a ring of atoms 3. marked variation in mood

cyclokeratitis (si'klo-ke'ra-tit'is) inflammation of cornea and ciliary body

cyclophoria (-for'e-a) tendency of the eyes to rotate around their anteroposterior axis due to weakness of oblique muscles

cyclophosphamide (-fos'fa-mi-de) alkylating cytotoxic agent

cyclopia (si-klo'pe-a) a developmental defect in which both orbits merge to form a single cavity and contain one eye

cycloplegia (si'klo-ple'je-a) paralysis of ciliary muscle and accommodation

cyclops (si'klops) 1. a genus of minute crustaceans that act as host to Dracunculus 2. a foetal abnormality with one eye

cyclorotation (si'klo-ro-ta'shun) torsion

cycloserine (-se'ren) a weak bacteriostatic antituberculosis agent that acts by inhibiting the D-alanine enzymes leading to defective cell wall synthesis

cyclosis (si-klo'sis) movement of protoplasm within the cell

cyclosporin A (si'klo-spor'in) cyclosporine

cyclosporine (-spor'en) an agent obtained from a soil fungus used to suppress the rejection of allografts

cyclothiazide (si'klo-thi'a-zid) a thiazide diuretic

cyclothymia (-thi'me-a) alternating between maniac and depressive phases.

cyclotomy (si-klot'a-me) incision of the ciliary muscle

cyclotron (si'kla-tron) an apparatus for accelerating protons or deutrons to high energies. It is done by rotation between magnets

cyclotropia (si'klo-trop'e-a) permanent deviation of an eye around its anteroposterior axis, resulting in diplopia

cyesis (si-e'sis) pregnancy

cylinder (sil'in-der) 1. a hollow tubular structure 2. a cylindrical lens.

cylindroid (sil'in-droid) 1. cylinder-shaped 2. a urinary cast

cylindroma (sil'in-dro-ma) glandular tumours with darkly staining small cells and hyaline stroma

cylindruria (sil-in-dru'ri-a) presence of renal casts in the urine

cynanche (si-nan'ke) sore throat

cyanophobia (sin'o-fe'be-a) morbid fear of dogs

cyproheptadine powerful antagonist of histamine and 5 hydroxytryptamine

cyrtometer (sir-tom'e-ter) an instrument to measure curved surfaces of the body

cyrtosis (sir-to'sis) kyphosis

cyst (sist) 1. a swelling containing fluid or semisolid material, which is lined by epithelium, endothelium or granulation tissue. It may be true or false 2. a stage in the life cycle of some parasites during which they are enveloped in a protective wall **congenital c** may arise from the foetal remnants of buried epithelium along the lines of fusion (sequestration dermoid) or from collection of fluid in an ectodermal tube (tubuloembryonic or tubulodermoid) or from remnants of embryonic tubúles and ducts **degenerative c** a false cyst occurring due to collection of fluid in the centre of a degenerating tumour from haemorrhage or necrosis **distension c** cyst occurring from dilatation of acini as in thyroid gland or from distension of the follicles as in ovary **dental**

c occurs in connection with a carious tooth, epithelial in origin and produces an elevation of the alveolus especially in the upper jaw and contains sterile, clear fluid with cholesterol crystals **dentigerous c** arises at the site of an unerupted permanent tooth in young adult (especially the third molar) and may cause expansion of bone. Cyst contains viscid fluid and maldeveloped unerupted tooth **exudation c** cyst occurring due to exudation of fluid in a normal anatomical space which is lined by endothelium as in hydrocoele of tunica vaginalis, or a false cyst due to encysted collection of exudate **false c** pseudocyst devoid of an epithelial lining which usually contains exudative or degenerative fluid as in pseudocyst of pancreas, or cystic degeneration of the tumour **ganglionic c** a localised round cystic swelling occurring in relation to a tendon sheath or a joint capsule, contains gelatinous fluid under tension **haemorrhagic c** a cyst resulting from a resolving haematoma of muscle and is lined by endothelium, contains straw- coloured fluid **infestation c** cyst occurring in any organ of the body but commonly in liver as hydatid cyst **c lens** a transparent device that fits over the cornea or part of the cornea to bring change in refractive ability of the cornea or lens of the eye **mesenteric c** a spherical smooth, soft or firm swelling along the course of the mesentery **neoplastic c** benign or malignant cystadenoma of ovary or cystic teratoma of ovary and testis **parasite c** infestation cyst **retention c** cyst occurring due to accumulation of secretion common in the scalp, face and scrotum **sebaceous c** an epidermal cyst containing desquamated cells due to obstruction of duct of the sebaceous gland. The obstructed opening is seen as a blue spot (punctum) which is fixed to the skin **true c** a cyst usually lined by epithelium, endothelium or granulation tissues, containing fluid that may be watery, serous, mucous, blood stained or seropurulent **thyroglossal c** an elongated swelling along the course of the thyroglossal tract in the upper neck that moves up on protrusion of the tongue **urachal c** an immobile swelling of variable size in the hypogastrium deep to the abdominal muscles developing from the persistence of middle segment of urachus (remnant of allontois extending from the urinary bladder to the umbilicus)

cystadeno carcinoma (sis-tad'e-no-kar'si-no'ma) a malignant tumour from glandular epithelium in which there are cystic accumulations of retained secretions, seen in ovary

cystadenoma (sis-tad'e-no-ma) a benign tumour derived from glandular epithelium, containing cystic accumulations of retained secretions

cystalgia (sis-tal-ja) pain in the bladder

cystathionine (sis'ta-thi'o-nen) an intermediate in the conversion of methionine to cysteine

cystathioninuria (sis'ta-thi'o-ne-nu're-a) a heritable disorder exhibiting an inability to metabolise cystathionine leading to its increased levels in the blood, tissue and urine. It is associated with mental retardation

cystectasia (sis'tek-ta'zhah) dilatation of the bladder

cystectomy (sis-tek'ta-me) removal of cyst or bladder

cysteic (sis-te'ik) **acid** an oxidation product of cysteine.

cysteine (sis'te-en) sulphur-containing amino acid derived from methionine in the body

cystic (sis'tik) 1. relating to a cyst 2. containing cysts 3. relating to bladder **c fibrosis**, CF, an autosomal recessive genetic disease characterised by a defect in electrolyte transport in the airway lumen and an increase in reabsorption of sodium from the airway lumen leading to a decrease in water content and an increase in viscosity of airway secretions. It is responsible for thick and poorly cleared inspissated airway secretion, impaired mucociliary clearance, chronic bacterial infections, bronchiectasis, and progressive respiratory failure. Lung is predominantly involved and there is also involvement of epithelial tissues of pancreas, sweat duct and gastrointestinal tract **c hygroma** the only brilliantly translucent swelling of the neck, a lymph cyst occurring in early childhood, that can be reduced in size by steady pressure

cystic fibrosis transport regulator CFTR gene on chromosome 7 regulating sodium and chloride transporter found on surface of cells lining lungs and other organs. It mutation causes cystic fibrosis

cysticercosis (sis'ti-ser-ko'sis) disease caused by encystment of cysticercus larvae of *Taenia solium* in the subcutaneous tissue, skeletal muscles and brain. They present with pea-like ovoid bodies under the skin or epileptic fits. Praziquantel and albendazole are used in the treatment

cysticercus (-ser'kus) larval form of *Taenia solium*

cystigerous (sis-tij'er-us) containing cysts

cystine (sis'ten) an oxidation product of cysteine

cystinosis (sis'ti-no'sis) a hereditary disorder of early childhood characterised by deposits of cystine crystals throughout the body due to abnormality in the metabolism of cysteine. It is accompanied by aminoaciduria, glycosuria, polyuria and vitamin D resistant rickets

cystinuria (sis'ti-nu're-a) a defect in renal tubular function associated with excess excretion of cystine in the urine

cystitis (sis-tit'is) inflammation of the bladder

cystitomy (sis-tit'o-me) 1. surgical incision of a cavity 2. incision into the lens capsule cyst (o) combining word for cyst, sac, bladder

cystocoele (sis'to-sel) herniation of urinary bladder into the vagina

cystoelytroplasty (-el'i-tro-plas'ta) surgical repair of a vesicovaginal fistula

cystogenetics study of chromosomes

cystography (sis-tog'ra-fe) radiography of the bladder after injection of a radioopaque substance.

cystoid (sis'toid) resembling a cyst

cystojejunostomy (sis'to-je'joo-nos'ta-me) surgical anastomosis of a cyst to the jejunum

cystolithectomy (sis'to-li-thek-ta-me) removal of a stone from the bladder through an incision in its wall

cystolithiasis (-li-thi'a-sis) presence of a vesical calculus

cystometer (sis-tom'it-er) a device useful in the study of bladder function such as its capacity, intravesical pressure and residual urine

cystometrography (sis'to-me-trog'ra-fe) measurement of bladder function by a cystometer

cystomorphous (-mor'fis) cyst-like

cystopexy (sis'to-pek'se) surgical attachment of gall bladder or of urinary bladder to the abdominal wall or other supporting structures

cystoplasty (sis'to-plas'te) surgical repair of a defect in the urinary bladder

cystoplegia (sis'to-ple'jah) paralysis of the bladder

cystoproctostomy (sis'to-prok-tos'to-mi) creation of a connection between the urinary bladder and the rectum

cystopyelitis (sis'to-pi'il-it'is) inflammation of the urinary bladder and renal pelvis.

cystorrhaphy (sis'tor'e-fe) suture of the bladder

cystorrhoea (sis'tor-e-a) mucous discharge from the bladder

cystosarcoma (sis-to-sar-ko'ma) a s+1 sarcoma containing cysts or cyst-like foci

cystostomy (sis-tos'ta-me) suprapubic drainage of bladder

cystoureteritis (sis'to-ur-et'er-it'is) inflammatioon of the urinary bladder and ureter

cystourethrography (-u're-throg'ra-fe) radiography of the bladder and urethra by means of radioopaque substance

cystourethroscope (-ur-eth'rah-skop) an instrument for examining the posterior urethra and bladder

cyt (o) combining word for a cell

cytarabine (si-tar'ah-ben) an antimetabolite inhibiting DNA synthesis

-cyte a combining word for a cell

cytidine (si'ti-den) a purine nucleoside consisting of cytosine and ribose, a constituent of RNA

cytoarchitectonic (si'to-ar'ki-tek-ton'ik) pertaining to cellular structure or arrangement of cells in a tissue

cytochemistry (si'to-kem'is-tre) study of intracellular distribution of chemical compounds and their activities.

cytochrome (si'to-krom) a class of haemoprotein found in the mitochondria that transport electron and/or hydrogen.c oxidase an enzyme complex containing cytochrome and copper found in the mitochondria

cytocide (-sid) an agent destructive to the cells

cytoclasis (si-tok'la-sis) fragmentation of the cells

cytodiagnosis (si'to-di'ag-no'sis) diagnosis of pathologic conditions by studying cells in the fluids or exudates

cytodifferentiation (si'to-dif'er-en'she-a'shun) development of specialised structures in the embryonic cells

cytodistal (-dis't'l) 1. denoting to the part of an axon remote from cell 2. pertaining to a neoplasm away from the cell of origin

cytogenetic map the visual appearance of a chromosome when stained and examined under a microscope. It exhibits visually distinct regions called light and dark bands . which give each of the chromosomes a unique appearance.

cytogenetics (-je-net'iks) the branch of genetics concerned with the structure and function of the cells, with special reference to the chromosomes

cytogenous (si-toj'in-is) producing cells

cytoglycopaenia (sis'o-gli'ko-pe'ne-a) deficient amount of glucose in the body or blood cells

cytohistogenesis (-his'to-jen'is-is) the development of the structure of the cell

cytoid (si'toid) resembling a cell

cytokines a range of secreted proteins (monokines and cytokines) from macrophages, lymphocytes (T and B) monocytes and stromal cells that regulate the host defence systems to inflammation. They are chemoattractants for neutrophils, monocytes and T cells. They act by binding to more than one receptors

cytokinesis (si'to-ki-ne'sis) changes that occur in the the protoplasm of a cell during cell division

cytology (si-tol'a-je) the study of a cell **exfoliative c** examination for diagnosis, of the cells denuded from a lesion and recovered from the sediment of exudate, secretions or washings from the tissue

cytolysin (si-tol'i-sin) an antibody causing destruction of a cell in association with a complement

cytolysis (-sis) dissolution of a cell

cytolysosome (sit'o-li'so-som) a lysosome that contains mitochondria, ribosomes or other organelles

cytomatics (si'to-mat'riks) study of the effects of sound waves on physical matter

cytomegalic (-me'gal'ik) referring to the markedly enlarged cells with nuclear inclusions seen in cytomegalovirus infections.

cytomegalovirus (sit'o-meg'a-lo-vi'rus) (CMV) a herpes virus that inhibits salivary glands, causes characteristic giant cells with large intranuclear inclusions. It is transmitted from mother with a latent infection to her foetus either transplacentally or at the time of birth, or by blood transfusion. **CMV infection** CMV infection may be congenital (hepatosplenomegaly, encephalitis, mental retardation) or acquired in immunocompetent (asymptomatic, mononucleosis-like illness) in immunosuppressed (retinitis, pneumonia, enteritis) individuals

cytometaplasia (-met'a-pla'zhah) alteration in the form and function of the cell

cytometer (si-tom'e-ter) an instrument for counting and measuring cells

cytometry (-tre) the measurement of cells and their constituents

cytomorphology (sit'o-mor-fol'a-je) the study of the structure of the cells

cytopathic (-path'ik) pertaining to pathologic changes in the cells

cytopathogenesis (-path'o-jen'is-is) production of pathologic changes in the cells

cytopathogenic (-jen'ik) capable of bringing about pathologic changes in the cells

cytopathologist (-pa-tho'lo-jist) a medical specialist specialised in the study of cells in disease

cytopathology (-pa-thol'o-ji) a medical speciality concerned with the study of disease states by microscopic examination of cellular specimens

cytopaenia (-pe'ne-a) decrease in the number of cellular elements in the blood

cytophagocytosis (-fag'o-si-to'sis) ingestion of cells by phagocytes.

cytophagy (si-tof'a-je) ingestion and destruction of other cells by phagocytes

cytophilic (sit'a-fil'ik) an affinity for cells

cytophylaxis (-fi-lak'sis) protection of cells against lysis

cytoplasm (sit'o-plazm) the protoplasm of a cell

cytoproximal (sit'o-prok'si-mal) denoting to the portion of axon nearer to the cell body

cytoreductive (-re-duk'tiv) decreasing the number of cells.

cytosine (si'to-sen) a pyrimidine base condensed with ribose or deoxyribose to form the nucleosides, cystidine and doxycystidine in the nucleic acids

cytoskeleton (-skel'it-on) internal structural framework of a cell to maintain the shape of the cells and consists of 3 types of filaments: microfilaments, microtubules and intermediate filaments

cytosol (sit'o-sol) the cytoplasm without mitochondria and endoplasmic reticulum

cytosome (-som) the cell body exclusive of its nucleus

cytostasis (si-tos'ta-sis) accumulation of white blood cells at the site of inflammation

cytostatic (sit'o-stat'ik) preventing the growth and multiplication of cells

cytotaxis (sit'o-tak'sis) attraction or repulsion of cells

cytothesis (si-toth'is-is) restoration of cells

cytotoxin (si'to-tok'sin) an antibody or a toxin inhibiting the functions of cells or cause destruction of cells or both

cytotrophoblast (-trof'o-blast) the inner layer of the trophoblast

cytotropism (si-to'tra-pism) 1. movement of cells towards or away from a stimulus 2. tendency of viruses, bacteria or drugs exerting their effect upon certain cells of the body

cytozoic (sit'o-zo'ik) living within or attached to the cells, denoting certain parasites

cyturia (si-tu're a) presence of any kind of cells in the urine

D

d symbol for dalton, deciduous, diopter, distal, dorsal vertebrae, dose, duration

δ delta, fourth letter of Greek alphabet, day, density, diameter, dextrorotary

daboya (da-boy'a) Russel's viper, a large poisonous snake

Dacosta's syndrome neurocirculatory asthenia, named after J. DaCosta, US physician

dacrocyte (da'cr-o-site) a distended red blood cell which looks like a tear drop, seen in myelofibrosis

dacryadenalgia (dak're-ad-en-al'je-a) pain in a lacrimal gland

dacryadenectomy (dak're-o-ad'e-nek'to-me) surgical removal of a lacrimal gland

dacryagogue (dak're-a-gog) an agent that stimulates the secretion of tears

dacryoadenitis (dak-re-ad-e-ni-tis) inflammation of the lacrimal gland

dacryoblennorrhea (dak're-o-blen'o-re'a) discharge of mucus from a lacrimal sac

dacryocoele (dak're-o-sel) protrusion of a lacrimal sac

dacryocyst (dak're-o-sist) the cystic swelling of the lacrimal sac at the medial end of the eye

dacryocystalgia (dak're-o-sis-tal'je-a) pain in lacrimal sac

dacryocystectomy (dak're-o'sis-tek'to-me) surgical removal of the lacrimal sac

dacryocystitis (dak're-o-sis'ti'tis) inflammation of the lacrimal sac caused by obstruction of the nasolacrimal duct. It is associated with excessive tears, redness and swelling in the area of lacrimal sac. It requires hot compresses, antibiotic therapy and incision and drainage of the sac

dacryocystocoele (dak'ri-o-sis'to-sel) protrusion of the lacrimal sac

dacryocystorhinostomy (dak're-o-sis'to-ri-nos'to-me) creation of a fistula between lacrimal sac and nasal cavity for lacrimal duct obstruction

dacryocystotomy (dak'ri-o-sis-tot'o-mi) incision of the lacrimal sac

dacryo-relating to tears or to the lacrimal sac or duct

dacryolith (dak'ri-o-lith) lacrimal calculus; a concretion in the lacrimal apparatus

dacryoma (dak're-o'ma) a lacrimal tumour

dacryops (dak-re-ops) a watery state of the eye

dacryorrhoea (dak're-o-re'a) excessive flow of tears

dacryostenosis (dak're-o-ste-no'sis) stricture of any lacrimal passage

dactyl (dak'til) a digit, a finger or toe

dactylalgia (dak'til-al-gea) pain in the fingers or toes

dactylitis (dak'til-itis) inflammation of a digit **tuberculous d** commonly involves metacarpals or phalanges and bone is enlarged as a fusiform swelling due to thickened and raised periosteum and there is destruction of original bone **syphilitic d** there is infiltration of the bones of hands or foot with syphilitic granulation tissue which may undergo central necrosis

dactylography (dak'ti-log'ra-fe) the study of fingerprints

dactylogryposis (dak'ti-lo-gri-po'sis) permanent contraction of the fingers or toes

dactylology (dak'ti-lol'a-je) hand and finger movements for communication

dactylolysis (dak'ti-lol-i'sis) surgical correction of syndactyly; amputation of a digit

dactylus (dak'ti-lus) a digit

dagger sign ossification of the posterior longitudinal ligament with spinal cord compression due to a dense vertical ossified plaque at the posterior margin of the vertebral body and intervertebral discs, noted in cervical spine or upper thoracic spines

is traditional birth attendant

aisy form a rosette-like intraerythrocytic pattern of mature schizonts of *Plasmodium malariae*

ale's reaction an *in vitro* test for anaphylactic sensitisation in a guinea pig named after Sir Henry Dale, British physiologist

alkon shield an intrauterine contraceptive device

allas criteria standards for the diagnosis of myocarditis from endomyocardial biopsy. Subdivided as no myocarditis, border line myocarditis or lymphocytic myocarditis established by a group of cardiac pathologists in Dallas

alrymple's sign abnormal widening of the palpebral tissues noted in exophthalmic goitre named after J. Dalrymple, UK ophthalmologist

alton a unit of a molecular weight equivalent to the weight of a hydrogen atom named after John Dalton, UK chemist

alton's law the partial pressure of gas in mixture equals that which it would exert if alone in same total volume

am a thin sheet of rubber used in dentistry and surgery to isolate a part from surrounding tissues and fluids

amocles' syndrome long term uncertainty experienced by the patients and families of those successfully treated for childhood leukaemia due to chance of future malignancy and is likened to the situation where Damocles was seated beneath a naked sword suspended by a horsehair

amp moist or humid

anazol (dah'nah'zol) a non-virilising androgen useful in treatment of endometriosis

nce signe de a feeling of emptiness in the right iliac fossa in intussusception

ncing eyes prominent nystagmus with rapid changes in all directions

D and C dilatation and curettage, dilatation of the uterine cervix and scrapping of the endometrium of uterus with a curette

dander (dan'der) a mixutre of desquamated epithelium and hairs shred by domestic animals such as dogs and cats that evokes an allergic response in atopic persons

dandruff (dan'druf) an excess amount of scaly material composed of dead keratinised epithelium shed from scalp

Dandy-Walker (dan'de-wawk'er) **syndrome** congenital hydrocephalus in infants characterised by cerebellar hypoplasia and obstruction to the outflow of cerebrospinal fluid through the foramina of the fourth ventricle named after Walter Dandy, US neurosurgeon and Arthus Walker, US surgeon

Dane particle a particle seen by electron microscopy in acute stage of hepatitis B composed of DNA polymerase named after David Dane, British virologist

danger space a region posterior to retropharyngeal space descending in the posterior mediastinum directly to the diaphragm which can become seat of potentially life-threatening infection. **d infection** a potentially life threatening infection of the danger space by extension from the nasopharynx

danta(s) tooth *d. sanku* tooth scaler

dapsone (dap'son) **4, 4**-diaminodiphenyl sulphone (DDS) compound used in treatment of leprosy and dermatitis herpetiformis

darshana (s) observation

dark adaptation the time required for the retina to get adapted to low illumination after exposure to bright light

dark field microscopy a method to identify spirochaetes where they are illuminated at an oblique angle. The organisms appear bright against a dark background

dark reactivation the enzymatic repair of DNA damaged by ultraviolet light

Darling's disease histoplasmosis named

after Samuel Darling, Panama physician

darting motility 'falling leaf' pattern of movement of flagellate parasites such as *Trichomonas vaginalis*

dartos (dart'-os) the contractile tissue under the scrotum, which helps in the regulation of temperature of testes

Darier's (dar-e-az') **disease** a rare hereditary disorder characterised by verrucous papular growths that coalesce into plaques and are found on the scalp, face, neck, trunk and axillae, named after J Darier, French dermatologist

Darwinian tubercle a blunt point projecting from the upper part of the helix of the ear, named after Charles Darwin, British naturalist

Darwinism (dar'win-izm) the theory of evolution propounded by Charles Darwin; it states that evolution of species, results from mutation and selection of organisms that are best adapted to survive in their environment

dash board fracture a shear fracture with hip dislocation occurring in a person seated in front seat thrown forward

data 1. factual information in the form of measurements or statistics 2. any information processed by, or stored on, a computer

database a programme used for storing, organising and sorting information

Dathu samya (s) homeostasis

datura (da-tu'ra) extract from plant *Datura stramonium* containing hyoscyamine and scopalamine which possess anticholinergic properties

daunorubicin a cytotoxic antibiotic used for leukaemia

daughter (dawt'er) **cell** cell arising from cell division; a nuclide formed from the radioactive decay of parent molecule

Davis gag clamp to hold mouth wide open xpecially for tonsillectomy

Dawakhana dispensary

dawn phenomenon occurrence of ear morning hyperglycaemia that is re lated to increased insulin requiremen in insulin dependent diabetics poss bly due to nocturnal pulses of grow hormone

day blindness hemaralopia, inability see clearly in a bright light

day care a facility in which infants an pre-school children are supervised an their needs attended to while the pa ents work

day frame device to maintain traction c fractured bone by pins

dB decibel

dBA decibels as read by noise meter s to A scale

D-Dimer a marker of fibrin turnove and is produced when plasmin lys cross-linked fibrin

DDS syndrome a hypersensitivity rea tion encountered in leprosy patien treated with dapsone (diaminodiphen sulphone) and it requires discontinu tion of dapsone

ddvap 1-deamino, 8d-arginin vasopressin; a long acting antidiuret analogue of vasopressin administere as a nasal spray in treating diabet insipidus

DDT dichloro-diphenyl-trichloroethane, highly hepatotoxic and potentiall neurotoxic insecticide. It is effectiv against a wide variety of insects suc as flea, fly, louse, mosquito, bedbu and cockroach

dead birth birth of a viable foetus i which respiration does not occur an there is no other sign of life; still bir

dead foetus syndrome a clinical comple due to intrauterine death with rete tion of the foetus for more than 4 hours

deadly night shade *Atropa balladonna*

dead space non air exchanging spac that portion of a syringe's tip an needle that contains medication tha cannot be administered **alveolar**

noted in ventilation and perfusion imbalance wherein there is ventilation of alveoli which are not perfused or inadequately perfused with blood or hyperventilation of alveoli with normal perfusion resulting in diminished volume of air available for gas exchange **anatomical d** the air in the conducting system from nose to the bronchioles that does not participate in the gas exchange and considered wasted ventilation **physiologic d** the tidal volume which does not participate in gas exchange. It includes anatomical and alveolar dead spaces

deaf (def) 1. inability to hear 2. unwilling to hear

deaf mute (def'mut) a person who can neither hear nor talk

deaf mutism the state of being both deaf and unable to speak

deafness (def'nes) loss of sense of hearing either completely or partially **conduction d** impaired hearing due to middle ear disease **nerve d** impaired hearing due to the diseases of the auditory nerve **perception d** nerve deafness

deaminase (de-m'i-nas) an enzyme that promotes the removal of the amino group from amino compounds

deamination (de-am'i-na'shun) removal of the amino group

dearticulation (de'ar-tik'u-la'shun) dislocation of a joint

death (deth) the cessation of life A person is dead if there is irreversible cessation of circulatory and respiratory functions or irreversible cessation of all functions of brain, including the brain stem **black d** bubonic plague **brain d** irreversible brain damage with unresponsiveness to all stimuli, absence of all spontaneous muscle activity **cot d, crib d** sudden infant death syndrome **d certificate** certificate giving the immediate cause of death and the underlying cause of death which initiated the train of morbid events

leading directly to death. It also contains record of any significant associated diseases **d rate** the number of deaths per 1000 population per year in a given community, indicative of the rate at which people are dying **d rattle** a sound characteristic of end-stage lung disease, wherein the clearance of large airway secretions becomes impossible **d star** rounded aggregation of malignant cells obtained from fine needle aspiration biopsies from breast cancer and it implies poor prognosis

debilitate (de-bil'i-tate) produce weakness or debility

debility (de-bil'i-te) loss of strength

debranching normal mode of breakdown of glycogen

debridement (da-bred-mon) surgical removal of foreign material and/or devitalised, infected tissue and all foreign materials from a wound surface or burn. It facilitates exposure of healthy tissue and promotes healing process

debris (de-bre') fragments of devitalised tissue or foreign material

debrisoquine (deb-ris'o-kwin) adrenergic blocking antihypertensive agent

debt (det) deficit **oxygen d** oxygen requirement following a strenuous exercise to oxidise the excess lactic acid and to replenish depleted stores of ATP

debulking operation excisional reduction of large malignant tumour masses

DEC diethyl carbamazine

decalcification (de'kal-si-fi-ka'shun) loss of calcium salts from bones or teeth

decannulation (c 2-kan'nu-la'shun) the removal of a cannula

decant (de-kant) to pour off the liquid allowing the sediment to remain in the bottom

decapitate (de-kap'i-ta-te) to remove the head

decapitation (de-kap'i-ta'shun) the separation of the head from the body; beheading; separation of the head from the shaft of the bone

decarboxylase (de′kar-bok′si-las) an enzyme that catalyses the release of carbon dioxide from compounds such as amino acids

decarboxylation (de′kar-boks-i-la′shun) a chemical reaction where a carboxyl (-COOH) is removed from in organic compound

decay (de-ka′) decomposition of organic matter; radioactive disintegration of an atom

deceleration (de-sel′e-ra′shun) decrease in speed or velocity of an object or reaction; the periodic and transient slowing of the foetal heart rate in response to uterine contraction **d injury** a motor vehicle accident-related injury when the heart in the pericardial cavity is thrown forwards causing either tears in the *ligamentum arteriosum* or rupture of the aorta

decerebrate position position of a patient who is comatose due to compression of brain stem at its lower level, in whom arms are extended and internally rotated and hips are extended with feet plantar flexed

decerebration (de-sēr-e-bra′shun) removal a portion of the brain

decibel (des′i-bel) a unit to measure the ratio of two powers such as electric or acoustic powers equal to one-tenth of a bel, db, dB.

decidua (de-sid′u-a) the endometrium of the uterus which undergoes modification preparing for and during pregnancy and it gets cast off at the time of parturition or during menstruation **d basalis** the layer immediately external to the embryo constituting the maternal vascular socket **d capsularis** the layer that covers the endometrium around the remainder of non basalis portion of embryonic sac **d parietalis** that portion of the decidua seen at the fallopian tube junction with the endometrium

decidual space uterine cavity remaining during early pregnancy

deciduoma (de-sid′u-o′ma) a uterine tumour containing decidual tissue

deciduous (de-sid′u-us) temporary **d teeth** primary dentition which is replaced by permanent teeth

decilitre (des′i-let′er) one-tenth of a litre one hundred millilitres

decinormal (des′i-nor′mal) having one tenth the strength of a normal solution

decision making arrival of decision regarding the treatment plan by using all available information

declinator (dek′lin-a′tor) an instrument used to hold apart the dura mater during trephining

declive (de-kliv′) a slanting surface

decoction (de-kok′shun) a liquid medicinal preparation made by boiling vegetable substances with water

decolouration (de-kul′er-a-shun) removal or loss of colour or pigment, bleaching

decomposition (de-kom-po-zish′un) 1. decay, putrefactive process 2. reducing a compound to its simpler constituents

decompression technique to readjust an individual to normal atmospheric pressure after exposure to high pressures **d sickness** a painful, sometimes fatal disorder that results from formation of gas bubbles in body tissues; this is especially noticed when a diver ascends too rapidly to the surface **d laminectomy** removal of spine and laminae on either side so as to allow the spinal cord to move backwards **d sickness** condition produced by rapid ascent to high altitude. It is due to supersaturation of tissues with nitrogen and present with limb pains (the bends), respiratory disturbances (the chokes), skin irritation (the creepers), CNS disturbances (the staggers) and cardiovascular collapse (syncope) and it has to be treated by descent to the ground level as rapidly as possible

deconditioning a loss of physical fitness due to failure to maintain an optimal level of physical training

decongestant (de-kon-jes′tant) an agent

that relieves congestion or swelling.

decontamination (de-kon-tam-i-na'shun) removal of harmful agents

decortication (de-kor'tika'shun) removal of the cortical substance **pulmonary d** removal of the thickened pleura **renal d** removal of renal capsule

decrement (dek're-ment) 1. a decrease in the quantity or force of an entity 2. a reduction in response of the nervous system to repeated stimulation 3. fall in the temperature in the course of a febrile illness

decubitus (de-ku'bi-tus) lying down, recumbent or horizontal position **d ulcer** *see* pressure sore

decussate (de-kus'at) to cross in the form of X

decussation a crossing of structures in the form of an X

dedifferentiation (de-dif'er-en'she-a'shun) the reversal of specialised to a more primitive forms

deep below the surface **d reflex** muscle or monosynaptic stretch reflex. A single sharp tap on the tendon of a slightly stretched muscle results in a brief contraction of the muscle **d vein thrombosis** (DVT) clotting of blood inside deep-lying veins, usually in the legs or pelvis

defecation (def-e-ka'shun) the elimination of faeces through the anus **d syncope** syncope occurring during or immediately after defecation

defect (de'fekt) malformation or imperfection

defense 1. resistance to disease 2. protective action against injury

deferens (def'er-enz) deferent

deferent (def'er-ent) conveying something away from or downward

deferiprone DFP, an oral iron chelator

deferoxamine (de-fer-oks'a-men) **mesylate** a drug having a marked affinity for iron and is used parenterally to reduce the iron store in the body

defervescence (def'er-ves'ins) bodily defenses begin to take an upper hand

over the infecting agent and the patient begins to feel better. It marks the subsidence of fever

defibrillation (de-fib'ril-a'shun) giving a brief electric shock to the heart to reverse some types of irregularities in the rhythm

defibrillator (de-fib'ri-la'tor) a machine utilised to restore normal cardiac rhythm by delivery of an electric shock at a preset voltage to the myocardium through chest wall by means of two metal plates applied to the chest

defibrination (de-fi'bri-na'shun) the removal of fibrin from the blood **d syndrome** persistent bleeding as the blood fails to clot. It may be associated with circulatory collapse and it requires restoration of fibrinogen level to a safe level

deficiency (de-fish'en-se) a shortage; lack **d disease** any clinical condition that results from the inadequate availability of an essential nutrient such as proteins, vitamins or minerals

deficit (def'i-sit) a deficiency

definition 1. the precise determination of limits especially of a disease process 2. recording of images on radiographic film

definitive clear, conclusive, sharply defined, final, complete

deflection (de-flek'shun) the act of turning aside

defloration (def'lo-ra'shun) rupture of the hymen

deflorescence disappearance of an eruption of the skin

deformity (de-for'mi-te) disfigurement; alteration in the normal form of a part or organ

deflurium hair loss

defurfuration (de-'fer-fu-ra'shun) shedding of epidermis in scales as in dandruff, psoriasis or ichthyosis

degeneration (de-jen'er-a'shun) deterioration or an impairment of an organ or part of the body

degenerative arthritis *see* osteoarthritis

degloving traumatic separation of skin from underlying tissue

deglutition (de'gloo-tish'un) the act of swallowing

degradation (deg're-da'shun) physical, metabolic, or chemical change to a less complex form

degranulation (de'gran-u-la'shun) the loss of granules

degree 1. a unit of measurement on a scale 2. a unit of angular measure 3. a stage of severity of a disease 4. academic recognition by an University

degustation (de'gus-ta'shun) the taste sensation

deha (s) human body *dehabhanda* binding the body *dehasvabhava* human nature *deha tatva* body constitution

dehiscence (-le-his'ens) rapture of a wound closure, separation of a surgical incision

dehumidifier (de'hu-mod'i-fi'er) a device for removing moisture from air

dehydration (de'hi-dra'shun) a dangerous fall in water content of body or tissues **d fever** raised temperature in a neonate due to inadequate fluid intake especially in high ambient temperatures

dehydrocholesterol (de-hi'droko-les'ter-ol) a sterol found in the skin that forms vitamin D after activation by irradiation

dehydrocholic acid a bile salt that stimulates production of bile from the liver

dehydrocorticosterone (de-hi'dro-kor-ti-kos'ter-on) a physiologically active steroid isolated from the adrenal cortex

dehydrogenase (de-hi-droj'e-nas) an enzyme that catalyses the oxidation of a specific substance

deionisation (de-i'on-i-za'shun) removal of ions from a substance

Deiters (di'terz) **cells** supporting cells in organ of Corti, named after Otto Deiters, German anatomist

de'ja (f) a group of paramnesias in which there is a perception of being familiar or having had previous experience which have not occurred **de'ja entendu** illusion of auditory recognition **de'ja eprouve** intense feeling of having previously experienced something **de'ja pense** illusion that a new thought is recognised as a thought previously felt or expressed **de'javu** illusion of visual recognition in which a new situation is incorrectly considered as a repetition of a previous event

Dejans' syndrome pain and anaesthesia in cheek, exophthalmos and diplopia indicating a lesion of the floor of orbit, named after M.C. Dejans, French ophthalmologist

dejecta (de-jek'ta) faeces

dejection (de'jek'shun) a state of mental depression

Dejerine's (de'zher-en) **sign** nerve root pain that increases on coughing named after Joseph Dejerine, French neurologist

Dejerine-Klumpke (-klump'ke) **paralysis** paralysis of the muscles of the arm and hand from lesion of the eighth cervical and first dorsal nerves. It often occurs in infants delivered by breech extraction, named after Joseph Dejerine and Madam Augusta Klumpke, wife of Dejerine

Dejerine-Roussy (-roo'se) **syndrome** thalamic syndrome characterised by ipsilateral hemianaesthesia and contralateral pain named after Joseph Dejerine and Gustav Roussy, French pathologist

Dejerine-Sottas (-sot'tahz) **syndrome** progressive hypertrophic interstitial neuropathy with gross thickening of nerves and muscle weakness, named after Joseph Dejerine and Jules Sottas, French neurologists

del Castillo syndrome germ cell aplasia in which the seminiferous tubules are devoid of spermatogonia and contain only Sertoli cells. It results in infertility

delayed flap pedicled skin flap dissected out and then resutured in place, to give time for blood supply to readjust before use

delead (de-led) to remove lead from the body or tissues

deleterious (del'e-te're-us) harmful

deletion (de-le'shun) loss of genetic material from a single base for RNA or base pair for DNA to a large piece of chromosome **d syndromes** hereditary disease complexes due to the loss of major chromosome segments

Delhi boil oriental sore infestation by *Leishmania tropica* results in an indurated papule on face or hand which breaks down to form an indolent ulcer and on healing an ugly pigmented scar

Delilah syndrome *psy* a clinical complex seen in the daughters of dominating aggressive fathers, characterised by marked sexual promiscuity, who seduce and overcome men as the biblical Delilah seducing the powerful Samson

delirious a state of mental confusion, restlessness, and disoriented reaction

delirium (de-lir'e-um) a delirious state due to physical illness **d tremens** a state of confusion accompanied by trembling and hallucinations noted in chronic alcoholics when they abstain drinking **puerperal d** the mental manifestations of a severe toxic infection such as puerperal sepsis. It is characterised by confusion, drowsiness alternating with excitement and visual illusions and hallucinations

deliver to aid in childbirth; to remove or extract

delivery 1. child birth 2. making available of health services to those who need it **abdominal d** delivery of an infant through an incision made into intact uterus through abdominal wall **breech d** delivery of an infant in breech presentation **forceps d** extraction of child from maternal passages by application of forceps to the child's head **postmature d** delivery of a postmature

infant **postmortem d** birth of a child after death of the mother **premature d** birth of a premature infant **spontaneous d** birth of an infant without any aid **vaginal d** delivery of an infant through the normal opening of the uterus and vagina

dell the central clear area of an erythrocyte

dellen (del'en) pits in corneal surface

Delphi method a multi-stage survey technique intended to produce a consensus from a target group of experts regarding therapy

Delta agent, hepatitis D virus (HDV) a circular single-stranded non-enveloped incomplete RNA virus, that depends on hepatitis B virus (HBV) for packaging its genome into viral particles. It requires that the patient be previously infected by HBV

delta cell tumour *see* somatostatinoma

delta hepatitis infection with hepatitis D virus

delta osmolality difference between the calculated and the measured osmolality.

delta sign a filling defect in cerebral venous sinus thrombosis seen by CT

delta wave 1. the slowest of the four brain waves 2. *ECG* a slow upstroke of the QRS wave in a background of short PR interval in ECG of WPW syndrome

deltoid (del'toid) a triangular shaped **d ligament** internal ligament of ankle joint **d muscle** a large triangular muscle covering the shoulder prominence **d ridge** ridge on humerus where deltoid muscle is attached

delusion (de-loo'zhun) false belief based on incorrect inference about external reality. It is not consistent with patient's intelligence and cultural background. Reasoning fails to correct it **bizarre d** an absurd, very strange false belief **d of accusation** false feeling of remorse and guilt **d of control** false feeling that one's will, thoughts or feelings are being controlled by external forces **d of infidelity** false belief got from pathologic jealousy that one's lover is unfaithful **d of grandeur** exaggerated conception of one's importance, power or identity **d of persecution** false belief that one is being harassed, cheated or persecuted **d of poverty** false belief that one is bereft or will be, of all material possessions **d of reference** false belief that the behaviour of others refers to oneself **d of self accusition** false feeling of remorse and guilt **mood-congruent d** delusion whose content is mood-appropriate **mood-incongruent d** delusion whose content has no association to mood or is mood-inappropriate **nihilistic d** false feeling that self, others or the world is non-existent or ending **paranoid d** delusions of persecution and delusions of references, control and grandeur **somatic d** false belief involving functioning of one's body **systematised d** false belief or beliefs united by a single event or theme

demand something that is needed

demarcate (de'mar-ka't) to set, mark off or limit the boundaries of

demarcation (de'mar-ka'shun) a limit or boundary

demeanour behaviour bearing

dementia (de-men'she-a) organic and global deterioration of the intellectual functioning without clouding of consciousness

demethyl chlortetracycline broad-spectrum antibiotic with antidiuretic activity

demineralisation (de-min'er-il-iz-a'shun) a reduction in the mineral content of the tissues

demise (de'miz) death

demographic process the size, composition and distribution of population is determined by fertility, mortality, marriage, migration and social mobility

demography (de-mog'ra-fe) the scientific study of human population especially the changes in population size, the

composition of the population and distribution of population in space

de Morgan's (de-mor'ganz) **spots** small angiectasis of skin noted in elderly especially on the face named after camp bell de Morgan, English physician

demorphobia morbid fear of crowds

demulcent soothing agent.

de Musset's (de-mu-saz') **sign** head nodding with each heart beat noted in aortic incompetence named after Alfred de Musset, French poet

demyelination (de-mi'e-li-na'shun) destruction of myelin from the sheath of the nerve fibres

denaturation (de-na'chur-a'shun) alteration of proteins by moderate heat that leads to loss of function

dendrite (den'drit) a short thread-like extension of a neuron which conducts impulses received from the terminal of other neurones **d ulcer** a corneal ulcer exhibiting thread-like extension

dendritic tree-like in form **d keratitis** linear, arborescent lesions on the cornea caused by *Herpes simplex* **d reticular cells** cells of mononuclear phagocytic system located in the skin, lymph nodes, and spleen. **d ulcer** herpetiform corneal ulcers seen in the autosomal recessive tyrosinaemia

denervation excision or blocking of a nerve supply

dengue (deng'ge) breakbone fever derived from Spanish language a flavi viral infection (group B virus) carried by aedes mosquito. It is characterised by abrupt onset of fever, malaise, headache, severe backache, conjunctival suffusion and a morbilliform of rash. The fever is biphasic. Convalescence is protracted. Treatment is symptomatic **d haemorrhagic fever** a severe form of dengue fever associated with spontaneous haemorrhage into the skin, epistaxis, haematemesis and malaena and hypotension **d shock syndrome** more severe form of dengue with vascular leakage. There is rapid onset of circulatory failure

denial (de-ni'al) *psy* unaware of something that a person might reasonably be expected to know; an ego of defense mechanism in which a person consciously or unconsciously negates the existence of a disease or other stress producing factor in his environment

denitrogenation removal of nitrogen from the body of a person preparing to fly by breathing 100% oxygen for variable period of time

Denny-Brown neuropathy neuropathies and myopathies related to malignancy without direct involvement of nervous system, named after N. Denny-Brown, British neurologist

dens (denz) 1. a tooth 2. the odontoid process of the axis

dense deposit disease type II membranoproliferative glomerulonephritis. There is deposition of electron dense material such as complement C_3, in the glomerular capillary basement membrane and patchy mesangial proliferation in Bowman's capsule

dense granule a round storage site in platelets that contains ADP, ATP, calcium, pyrophosphate and serotonin

dens in dente a malformed tooth with invaginated outer enamel epithelium of the odontogenic germ layer; *dens invaginus*

densitometer (den'si-tom'e-tre) 1. an instrument that measures bacterial growth 2. an instrument that measures the optical density of a radiograph

densitometry (den'si-tom'e-tre) 1. the measurement of the density of a substance 2. determination of the amount of ionising radiation to which a person has been exposed

density the relative weight of a substance compared with a reference standard

dental relating to teeth **d arch** arch formed by the cutting and chewing surfaces of the teeth **d assistant** person assisting in the care and treatment of dental patients. **d caries** a pathologic process of localised destruction of the teeth **d chart** a diagrammatic representation of the mouth on which the clinical and radiographic findings can be recorded **d consonant** a consonant pronounced with the tongue at or near the front of upper teeth **d curve** curve of the line of teeth in the jaw **d disk** a thin circular piece of paper cloth charged with abrasive powder for cutting or polishing teeth and fillings **d dysfunction** malfunctioning of the parts of the dental structures **d fossa** thread or tape used for cleaning and removing plaques between teeth and testing for defects in the teeth **d formula** expression of dentition **d hygienist** a professionally trained person who cleans teeth **d material** any of several types of colloids, plastics, resins and metal alloys used in dentistry. They are useful to take impressions, restore teeth or duplicate dentition **d plaque** dense aggregate of debris and bacteria on tooth surface **d prosthesis** an artificial part used in mouth to replace missing teeth **d pulp** narrow core of tooth, of vascular connective tissue with nerve fibres and odontoblasts

dentalgia (den-tal'je-a) tooth ache

dentate (den'tat) notched **d nucleus** largest cerebellar nucleus

denticulate finely toothed or serrated

dentiform shaped like a tooth

dentifrice (den'ti-fris) a paste, liquid, gel or powder for cleaning teeth

dentigerous (den-tij'er-us) containing teeth **d cyst** cyst surrounding an unerupted normal tooth

dentilabial (den-ti-la'be-al) pertaining to teeth and lips

dentine (den'tin) the hard tissue forming the main substance of teeth. It surrounds the pulp chamber, covered by enamel in the crown and cementum in the root area

dentist (den'tist) a person practising dentistry

dentistry (den'tis-tre) the science concerned with the prevention, diagnosis and treatment of diseases of teeth and gums

dentition the type, number and arrangement of teeth in the dental arch

dentoid tooth-shaped

denture (den'chur) a partial or complete set of artificial teeth set **d mouth** chronic atrophic candidiasis

denudation removal of a protective layer or covering through surgery or pathological condition

Denver developmental sereening test a psychological test for assessment of child's neuro-developmental maturation

Denver shunt a peritoneovenous shunt that relieves ascites and improves renal function

deodourant (de-o'dor-ant) a substance which suppresses or neutralises bad odour such as lime, bleaching powder

deontology (de'on-tol'o'je) medical ethics

deorsum (de-or'sum) downward

deossification (de-os'i-fi-ka'shun) loss or removal of mineral matter from bone

deoxygenation (de-ok'si-jen-a'shun) removal of oxygen from a chemical substance or tissue

deoxyhaemoglobin reduced haemoglobin

deoxyribonuclease (de-ok'se-ri'bo-nu'kleas) (DNase) an enzyme that depolymerises DNA

deoxyribonucleic (de-ok'se-ri'bo-nu-kle'ik) **acid** (DNA) a complex nucleic acid consisting of deoxyribose, phosphoric acid and four bases (two purines - adenine and guanine and two pyrimidines - thymine and cytosine) which are arranged as two long chains that twist around each other to form a double helix. It forms the chemical basis of heredity and carries genetic information for all organisms except RNA virusus

deoxyribose (de-ok'se-ri'bos) a pentose sugar that is part of DNA

dependence (de-pen'dens) substance abuse. A psychological compulsion for a person to use a substance such as

narcotic on a chronic and repeated basis

dependent the lower most aspect of a body part or cavity, such as feet, sacrum

dependents individuals who rely on someone else for financial support

depersonalisation *psy* a subjective sense of being unreal, strange or unfamiliar to one-self

dephosphorylation (de-fos'for-i-la'shun) removal of a phosphate group from a compound

depigmentation (de'pig-menta'shun) loss of normal pigment as in vitiligo or removal of pigment

depilation (dep'il'a-shun) the process of removal of hair

deplete (de-plat) to empty, to exhaust, to reduce or lessen

depletion (de-ple'shun) removal of substances, such as blood, fluids, iron, fat or protein from the body

depolarisation (de-po'lar-i-za'shun) reversal of normal potential across cell membrane, leading to inflow of sodium

deposit (de-poz'it) 1. a sediment or precipitate 2. matter collected in any part of the body

depot preparation a drug designed for slow release from site of injection such as methyl prednisolone, or medroxyprogesterone

depressant an agent that decreases the level of a body function or nerve activity

depression 1. psychopathologic feeling of sadness 2. a hollow region 3. a decrease in vital functions

depressor an instrument for drawing down a part of the body **tongue d** a device used to bring down the tongue to facilitate visual examination of the throat

deprivation (dep'ri-va'shun) loss or absence of a necessary part or function

depth intensity; the quality of being deep

de Quervain's tenovaginitis pain over

the styloid process of the radius and a palpable nodule in the course of the abductor pollicis longus and extensor pollicis brevis tendons named after Fritz Quervain, Swiss surgeon

derailment gradual or sudden deviation in train of thought without blocking; there is losening of associations

Dercum's disease multiple painful subcutaneous lipomata, named after Francis Dercum, US neurologist

derealidation (d'real'i-shun) an alteration in the perception or experience of the external world that it seems strange or unreal

dereism (de're-izm) *psy* mental activity not concordant with logic or experience

derivation (der'i-va'shun) the source or origin of a substance

derivative (de-riv'a-tiv) 1. something that is not original 2. something derived from another body 3. anything that develops from a preceding structure

dermabrasion (derm'bra'zhun) a surgical procedure for removal of scars, naevi, tattoo on the skin by sandpaper or mechanical methods

dermatatrophia (derm'at-a-tro'fe-a) atrophy of the skin

dermatitis (der'ma-ti'tis) pl **dermatitides**. inflammation of the skin characterised by itching, redness and various skin lesions **actinic d** reaction of skin to sunlight or x-rays **d artifacta** factitial dermatitis **atopic d** an allergic disorder of the skin where the patient inherits an increased tendency of getting sensitised to various antigens in his environment **contact d** allergic reaction of the skin mediated by delayed hypersensitivity to a substance which comes in contact with the surface of the skin **diaper d** irritation of the skin in contact with a diaper such as soap, powder, urine and faeces **exfoliative d** an erythematous condition characterised by erythema and scaling **factitial d** a skin injury that is self-inflicted **d**

herpetiformis a chronic inflammatory condition characterised by erythema, papules, vesicles, and pustules. These lesions may coalesce and produce itching and burning sensation **d mediacamentosa** a skin eruption due to medicinal preparation ingested or applied **photo contact d** application of a photosensitiser substance to the skin and subsequent exposure to sunlight resulting in skin lesions **seborrhoeic d** an inflammation of the sebaceous glands manifesting in the form of diffuse scaling and erythema **stasis d** impaired circulation resulting in eczema of the legs **d verrucosa** a chronic fungal infection of the skin manifesting with wartlike nodules

dermatocellulitis (der'ma-to-sel'u-li'tis) inflammation of subcutaneous connective tissue

dermatocoele (der'ma-to-sel) a tendency of hypertrophied skin and subcutaneous tissue to hang loosely in folds

dermatologist (der'ma-tol'o-jist) a specialist in the diseases of the skin

dermatology (der'ma-tol'o-je) the medical speciality of the skin and its diseases

dermatoma (der'ma-to'ma) the circumscribed thickening of skin

dermatomycosis (der'ma-to-mi-ko'sis) pl **dermatomycoses** a skin infection caused by fungi belonging to the genera *Trichophyton, Epidermophyton* and *Microsporan*

dermatomyositis (der'ma-to-mi'o-si'tis) an auto-immune disease in which skeletal muscle is damaged by a non-suppurative inflammatory process dominated by lymphocytic infiltration. There is heliotrope (lilac) discolouration of the eyelids, erythematous rash over the face, neck and upper part of the body. The condition may coexist with other connective tissue disorders

dermatopathy (der'ma-top'a-the) any skin disease

dermatophagoides (der'ma-tof'a-goi'des) mites found in house dust live on human skin scales and are concentrated on a bedding and mattresses especially in damp places. *D pteronyssimus* and *D culinae* are important examples which can provoke asthma

dermatophytes (der'ma-to-fit's) fungi that live on keratinous structures and can infect the epidermis, the hair and nails. Those responsible for human infections belong to three genera - *Microsporan, Trichophyton* and *Epidermophyton* **anthropophilic d** dermatophytes living only on the humans **geophilic d** dermatophytes thriving in the soil **zoophilic d** dermatophytes infecting animals

dermatoplasty (der'ma-to-plas'te) transplantation of living skin to cover cutaneous abnormality caused by injury, operation or disease

dermatoscopy (der'mat'o-sko-pi) a noninvasive technique that allows *in vivo* microscopic examination of skin lesions at 10x magnification

dermatosis (der'ma-to-'sis) pl **dermatoses** any disease of the skin in which inflammation may not be a feature

dermatotherapy treatment of skin diseases

dermatotome (der-ma-to-tom) 1. a knife for incising the skin or small lesions 2. area of skin corresponding to one posterior nerve root

dermatotropic (der'ma-to-trop'ik) acting preferentially on the skin

dermatozoon (-zo'on) an animal parasite of the skin

dermatozoonosis (der'ma-to'zoo-no'sis) any skin disease caused by an animal parasite

dermis (der'mis) the layer of the skin lying below the epidermis; true skin. It is composed of fibrous connective tissue composed of collagen and elastin. It consists of numerous capillaries, lymphatics and nerve endings. The hair follicles, sebaceous glands and sweat glands and their ducts are hidden in dermis

dermoglyphics the study of the combined patterns of skin ridges on the fingers and toes, palms and soles

dermographia a form of urticaria due to allergy

dermoid a cyst lined by an epidermis containing various epidermal appendages. Such lesions are found along embryonal fusion planes such as lateral third of eyebrows, nose and scalp. They can be inflamed and infected necessitating excision

dermomycosis (der'mo-mi-ko'sis) a skin disease caused by a fungus; dermatomycosis

desaturation a process by which a saturated organic compound is converted into an unsaturated one

descematocoele herniation of a minute portion of corneal endothelial layer forward into cornea

Descemet's membrane basement membrane of endothelium lining posterior surface of cornea named after Jean Descemet, French anatomist

descendens (de-sen'dens) descending

descriptive statistics methods used to summarise, organise and describe observations

desensitisation a therapeutic modality that attempts to reduce IgE-mediated hypersensitivity to various substances by administering ever increasing amounts of an antigen to form blocking antibodies

desert fever coccidioidomycosis

desferrioxamine chelating agent used to remove excess iron

desi native

desicant (des'i-kant) causing dryness

designer antibody an immunoglobulin that has been genetically engineered for a specific purpose

designer drug an abuse substance

Desjardin's (da'zhar-danz) **forceps** forceps for removing the stones from bile ducts, named after Abel Desjardin, French surgeon

desktop hypoglycaemia erroneous diagnosis of hypoglycaemia due to errors in collection or handling of a blood specimen

desktop workspace on the computer screen. It presents a set of icons on screen

desmitis (des-mi'tis) inflammation of a ligament

desmocyte (des'mo-sit) a supporting tissue cell

desmoid (des'moid) 1. fibromatosis of striated muscle especially rectus abdominis 2. fibroma or fibroid

desmolase (des'mo-las) an enzyme that catalyses the addition or removal of some chemical groups to or form a substrate **d enzyme** an enzyme converting cholesterol to pregnenolone, necessary step in steroid synthesis

desmoplasia a dense stromal reaction in which malignant epithelial cells are compressed into single layer of cells, a feature noted in infiltrating ductal carcinoma of the breast

desmopressin vasopressin

desmosis (des'mo'sis) any disease of connective tissue

desmosome an area of close contact and attachment between epithelial cells

desmotomy (des-mot'o-me) dissection of a ligament

desoxycorticosterone (des-ok'se-kerti'kos'ter-on) an active steroid hormone produced by the adrenal cortex

d'Espine's (des-penz) **sign** normally whispering pectoriloquy is heard on the back up to T4 spine due to trachea. It may be heard lower down due to enlarged lymph nodes named after Jean d'Espine, French physician

desquamation abnormal shedding or an accumulation of stratum corneum in perceptible flakes

desquamative interstitial pneumonia (DIP). An interstitial pneumonia characterised by filling of alveoli with large mononuclear cells, minimal interstitial changes and no necrosis. Radiologically it gives a ground glass appearance and treated with corticosteroids

destructive causing destruction

desynchronosis (de-sin'kro-no'sis) derangement of internal biological clock caused by the difference between the time at a person's present location and the time to which the person is accustomed, noted in long distance travellers who pass through several time zones in a short period; jet lag

detector a device for determining the presence of something

detergent a cleansing agent which acts by lowering surface tension such as soap; *mol* a surface active emulsifying agent used to lyse cells and solubilise membranes

deterioration impairment of physical or mental functions

determinant (de-ter'mi-nant) that which determines the character of something

determination establishing the nature of substance

detortion correction of any deformity

detoxification removal of a toxic excess of any agent, including overdosage of a therapeutic agent, drug of abuse or toxic agent (pesticides) and heavy metals from the body by inducing vomiting, administrating activated charcoal, dialysis or metabolic interference

detrusor thruster down or out

detumescence (de'tu-mes'ens) 1. subsidence of a swelling 2. subsidence of swelling of erectile tissue of genitalia (penis or clitoris) following erection

deturgescence removal of turgidity

deutoscolex (du'to-sko'leks) a secondary daughter cyst that develops on the inner wall of a hydatid cyst

deuteranopsia (du'ter-an-o'pse-a) colour blindness in which there is defect in perception of green colour

devascularisation (de-vas'kular-iza'shun) a decrease in blood supply to a part of the body or tissue

developer the solution used to make latent image visible on radiographic or photographic film

development growth to full size or attain maturity

developmental milestone any of a series of activities such as raising the head, rolling over, walking or other important points in a child's physical and/or maturation and to detect developmental delay

deviance a variation in the accepted norm

deviation 1. *stat* distance of value from mean 2. to move steadily away from an accepted norm

device (di-vis) an apparatus or instrument constructed to perform a special function

Devic's disease neuromyelitis optica, named after M.E. Devic, French neurologist

devil's grip epidemic pleurodynia *see* Bornholm's disease

devitalisation (de-vi'tal-iza'shun) the deprivation of vitality of life

dewdrop appearance minute round nodules of amyloid seen on the heart

deworming (de-werm'ing) the destruction and removal of worms from an infected individual

dew point humidity (moisture) is always present in air. The amount of moisture which air can hold depends on its temperature. If air is cooled, excess moisture precipitates for a particular temperature

dexamethasone synthetic glucocorticoid with minimal mineral activity **d suppression test** dexamethasone suppresses production of cortisone in low doses in normals, and in moderate doses in Cushing's disease. But it fails to suppress cortisone secretion in adrenal tumours or ectopic ACTH

dexter (dek'ster) right hand side

dextral (dek'stral) pertaining to the right side

dextran (dek'stran) a high molecular weight, branched-chain polysaccharide polymer of glucose

dextrase (deks'tras) an enzyme that splits dextrose and converts it into lactic acid

dextrin (dek'strin) partially hydrolysed starch or glycogen

dextrocardia (dek'stro-kohr-de-ah) abnormal location of the heart on the right side of the chest **mirror–image d** dextrocardia with concomitant situs inversus of the abdominal organs

dextroposition (dek'stro-po-zish'un) abnormal right sided location of an organ normally located in the left side

dextrorotatory (deks'tro-ro'ta-tor'e) causing a rightward turn

dextrose (dek'stros) glucose, a simple sugar of the monosaccharide group

DF-2 dysgonic fermenter. A fastidious gram-negative bacillus found in canine oral flora that causes infections of dog-bite wounds now classifed as Capnocytophaga species

DGHS Director General of Health Services

dhairya (s) courage

dhamani (s) artery

dhanurvata (s) tetanus

Dhanvantari the God of healing

dhat (s) passage of semen in the urine d *syndrome* undue concern about the debilitating effects of loss of semen

dhatu (s) body constituents that support the body; metal *dvaishamya* imbalance of bodily constituents resulting in disease *d samya* state of equilibrium of dhatus *d vaisamya* increase or decrease of dhatus upsetting the equilibrium

dhobie itch contact dermatitis associated with the use of laundry marking fluids

dhumapana (s) inhalation of smoke

diabesity a common clinical association of adult-onset diabetes mellitus and obesity

diabetes (di'a-be'tes) a term applied to diseases marked by an increased amount of urination, usually refers to diabetes mellitus **brittle d** a condition exhibiting frequent episodes of hypoglycaemia followed by hyperglycaemia necessitating constant adjustment of dietary intake and insulin dosage **bronzed d** damage to several organs from excess iron deposition with features of diabetes mellitus associated with leaden-grey skin pigmentation; haemochromatosis **chemical d** altered glucose metabolism without obvious features of diabetes mellitus **endocrine d** diabetes mellitus associated with diseases affecting pituitary, thyroid or adrenal cortex **gestational d** onset or first recognition of diabetes mellitus during pregnancy, most commonly during the third trimester. They exhibit insulin resistance and impaired insulin secretion **d insipidus** a condition characterised by persistent excretion of excessive quantities of dilute urine, and thirst. There are two types as Cranial (deficient production of ADH due to a genetic defect or lesions of hypothalamus on high stalk or idiopathic) and Nephrogenic (renal tubules are unresponsive to ADH, as in genetic defect, hypokalaemia, hypercalaemia, lithium or heavy metals poisoning) diabetes insipidus. Cranial type is treated with des-amino-des-aspartate–arginine vasopressin and peripheral type with thiazide diuretics **fibrocalculous pancreatic d** (FCPD) diabetes mellitus associated with presence of stones in the pancreatic duct and its main branches. Consumption of tapioca (cassava) rich in cyanoglucosides leads in diabetes mellitus especially in Kerala, India. **insulin dependent d** (IDDM) diabetes mellitus usually having its onset before the age of 30 years in which the essential abnormality is related to absolute insulin deficiency whose pathogenesis is due to genetic, environmental or immunological factors **juvenile onset d** type 1 diabetes **latent d** diabetes mellitus manifesting during times of stress such as pregnancy, obesity, infections or trauma **d mellitus** a metabolic disorder characterised by disturbances in carbohydrate, lipid and protein metabolism. These metabolic derangements result from a combination of insulin deficiency and/or insulin resistance and lead to a variety of acute and chronic complications. **malnutrition related d** (MRDM) young persons with age of onset of diabetes mellitus below 30 years and evidence of past or present malnutrition. It includes protein deficient diabetes mellitus and fibrocalculous pancreatic diabetes **maturity-onset d of the young** (MODY) NIDDM with age of onset less than 25 years. It has an autosomal mode of inheritance **non-insulin dependent d** (NIDDM). diabetes with resistance to ketoacidosis in the absence of hepatic production of glucose and resistance to the action of insulin in muscle **type I d** all causes of diabetes that result from destruction of the pancreatic beta cells. This may be immune mediated or idiopathic. Immune mediated type I diabetes mellitus (IDDM or juvenile onset diabetes) is caused by an autoimmune cell-mediated destruction of pancreatic beta cells. Idiopathic type is characterised by insulinopaenia without any evidence of autoimmune beta-cell destruction. **type II d** all forms of diabetes that are characterised by the combination of insulin resistance and deficient secretion of insulin. This condition previously known as NIDDM, has a strong genetic disposition, typically has its onset later in life and is associated with insulin resistance syndrome (dyslipidaemia, hypertension, atherosclerotic cardiovascular disease)

diabetic (di-abet'ik) 1. pertaining to diabetes 2. a person suffering from diabetes mellitus **d coma** loss of consciousness due to severe diabetes mellitus **d foot** ulceration due to neuropathy and peripheral vascular insufficiency in diabetics. Superimposed infections and trauma often contribute to the development of foot ulcers **d ketoacidosis** occurrence of ketoacidosis, usually accompanied by hyperglycaemia, as a result of diabetes mellitus. It represents as a state of absolute or relative insulin deficiency and occurs in association with counter-regulatory or stress hormone excess, such as glucagon, catecholamines, cortisol and growth hormones **d nephropathy** renal insufficiency with evidence of poor glycaemic control in diabetics. The condition makes its onset with microalbuminuria. There is clinically detectable albuminuria at the time of diagnosis. Nephropathy is an important cause of end-stage renal failure **d neuropathy** a group of clinical and subclinical syndromes each of which is characterised by diffuse and focal damage to peripheral somatic or autonomic fibres resulting from diabetes mellitus such as mononeuropathy with isolated cranial or peripheral nerve involvement, radiculopathy, polyneuropathy and autonomic neuropathy. Distal, symmetric, primarily sensory polyneuropathy is the common presentation **d retinopathy** a leading cause of blindness and the condition has been categorised into nonproliferative retinopathy, proliferative retinopathy, advanced diabetic eye disease and maculopathy. Microaneurysms representing haemorrhages and exudates, appearance of new vessels (neovascularisation) on the retina or optic disc, and macular oedema (collection of intraretinal fluid in the macular area) are the features of diabetic retinopathy

diabetogenic (di'a-bet'o-jen'ik) causing diabetes

diabetogenous (di'a-be-toj'en-us) caused by diabetes

diabetologist (di'a-be'to-lo-gist) a specialist in the study and treatment of diabetes

diadochokinesia (di-ad'ah-ko-ki-ne'zha) normal ability of alternating opposite muscular action such as pronation and supination in quick succession

diethylstilboestrol a synthetic oestrogen that is more potent than natural oestrogens

diagnose (di'ag-nos) to identify the name of a disease

diagnosis (di'ag-no'sis) the determination of nature of a disease based on signs and symptoms **antenatal d** determination of health status of a foetus **clinical d** identification of disease by history and physical signs, and laboratory studies **community d** the pattern of disease in a community described in terms of the important factors which influence this pattern **cytologic d** identification of a disease based on cells present in body tissues or exudates **differential d** identification of a disease by comparing the symptomatology of two or more similar diseases **pathologic d** identification of an illness based on structural lesions **physical d** recognition of disease by physical examination **preimplantation genetic d** a technque for evaluating the genes of an embryo that has undergone in vitro fertilization before it is implanted in the uterus **radiologic d** recognition of a disease by interpretation of radiographic findings **serologic d** identification of a disease through serologic test

Diagnostic and statistical manual of mental disorders, DSM a manual to diagnose mental disorders published by the American Psychiatric Association since 1952

diagnostician (di'ag-nos-tish'un) person skilled in making diagnosis

diakinesis (di'a-ki-ne'sis) the homologous chromosomes becoming thick and short in the final stages of cell division

dial-up connection the process of accessing another computer via a telephone line

dialysate (di-al'l-is-at) fluid used in dialysis

dialysis (di-al'l-sis) the separation of crystalloids from colloids in a solution by selective diffusion through a semipermeable membrane **continuous ambulatory peritoneal d** (CAPD). drainage of fluid into and peritoneal cavity through an implanted catheter by gravity **continuous cyclical peritoneal d** (CCPD) dialysis every night wherein the fluid remains in the peritoneal cavity until next night **intermittent peritoneal d** (IPD) dialysis performed overnight where the fluid is drained from peritoneal cavity at the end of treatment **d ascites** exudative peritonitis related to chronic dialysis **d dementia** dialysis encephalopathy due to aluminium present in dialysate solutions and is noted in those with terminal renal failure **d equilibrium** a disturbance with features of nausea, vomiting, drowsiness, headache and seizures developing shortly after beginning haemodialysis or peritoneal dialysis. It is due to rapid changes in pH in the blood, and fall in the osmolarity of the extracellular fluid **d osteodystrophy** bone changes in long term dialysis patients **peritoneal d** dialysis wherein the lining of the peritoneal cavity is used as the dialysing membrane. The dialysing fluid introduced into the peritoneal cavity is left there for 1 to 2 hours and is then removed. This procedure is used to remove toxic substances from the body by perfusing warm sterile fluid through the peritoneal cavity

diameter (di-am'e-ter) the distance from any point in periphery of a surface or body to the opposite point

Diana complex masculine tendencies in female named after Roman mythologic goddess of moon, hunting and chastity

dianetics (di'a-net'ikz) Science that considers the mind to be real, although separate from the body and superior to the brain

diapedesis (di'a-pe-de'sis) the passage of blood or any of its cells through the pores of blood vessels

diaphoretic (di'a-for-et'ik) an agent that causes sweating

diaphragm (di'af-fram) 1. the muscular membranous structure separating thorax and abdominal cavity 2. any dividing membrane 3. a soft rubber cap that covers the uterine cervix and used for contraceptive purpose 4. an apparatus located beneath the opening in the stage of microscope and permitting the amount of light passing through the object **slit-pore d** the gap between adjacent foot processes in the glomerulus

diaphragmatic pertaining to the diaphragm **d fatigue** occurs when energy expenditure of the diaphragm exceeds the capacity of the blood supply **d flutter** rapid, rhythmic diaphragmatic contractions lasting for a period of seconds to weeks **d hernia** herniation of abdominal contents through the congenital defect or weakness in diaphragm **d paralysis** paralysis of diaphragm from interruption or dysfunction of the phrenic nerve

diaphysis (di'ah-f'i-sis) the shaft of a long bone

diapophysis (di'ah-pof'i-sis) the upper anterior surface of a transverse vertebral process

diarrhoea (di'ah-re'ah) abnormal frequent passage of loose stools **chewing gum d** an osmotic diarrhoea caused by excessive intraluminal sorbitol in chewing gum **dysenteric d** diarrhoea due to dysentery characterised by passage of blood and mucus **fatty d** diarrhoea with stools containing undigested fat **infantile d** diarrhoea in infants with increased frequency and amount of stools with change of colour and consistency and signs of dehydration **mucous d** diarrhoea with mucus **osmotic d** diarrhoea caused by retention of osmotically active solutes in the small intestine which facilitates the fluid to be drawn into the intestinal lumen **secretory d** a large volume of faecal output from abnormalities of the movement of fluid and electrolytes into the intestinal lumen **summer d** diarrhoea occurring in children during summer **traveller's d** diarrhoea experienced by travellers who move from an area in which organisms that commonly cause diarrhoea are endemic

diarthrosis joint with synovial cavity

diascopy examination of skin lesions by pressure with glass slide causing blanching

diastalsis (di-as'tal-sis) peristalsis of the small intestine in which wave of inhibition precedes the wave of contraction

diastate starch-splitting enzyme

diastasis separation especially of sutures of the skull by raised intracranial pressure in children

diastole (di-as'tah-le) rhythmic relaxation of the heart chambers during which time they fill with blood

diastolic gallop the triple rhythm produced by the development of the third heart sound **d shock** palpable pulmonary component of second sound in presence of pulmonary hypertension

diathermy (di'ah-therm'e) local generation of heat in the body tissues by a high frequency electric current

diathesis (di'ath'i-sis) an inherited or congenital bodily predisposition to a disease

diatrozoic acid water-soluble contrast medium, as sodium and meglumine salts for urograms and myelograms

diazepam benzodiazepine anxiolytic agent used as hypnotic, preoperative sedative and intravenously in status epilepticus

diazoxide direct acting vasodilator

antihypertensive used intravenously in hypertensive crisis

DIC disseminated intravascular coagulation

dichotomy (di-kot'o-me) division into two parts

dichromatism (di-kro'ma-tizm) the ability to distinguish only two primary colours

Dick test a test to determine the susceptibility or immunity to scarlet fever following injection of the erythrogenic toxin from streptococcus, named after George Dick and Glady Dick, US bacteriologists

dicloxacillin (di-kloks-sil'in) a semisynthetic penicillinase-resistant penicillin

dicoumarol (di-koo'ma-rol) an anticoagulant that acts in the liver to impair synthesis of vitamin K dependent coagulation factors including prothrombin. It is used in the prophylaxis and treatment of intravascular thrombosis and in postoperative thrombophlebitis, pulmonary embolism, and acute coronary thrombosis

dicrotic (di'krot'ic) having double beat **d notch** slight hesitation on downward stroke of normal pulse tracing due to AV closure **d pulse** pulse with two separate peaks and the term applies to subsidiary peak on down-stroke. It is encountered in low peripheral resistance

dictum authoritative or dogmatic statement

Dictyostelium discoideum (dik'teo-stel'ium-dys-koid'um) a soil dwelling organism that exists as a free-living amoeba feeding on bacteria. It can aggregate into multicellular organism just about visible to naked eye. It is a useful model to investigate cell differentiation and development

didactic (di-dak'tik) instructions by lectures

didactylism (di-dak'ti-lizm) a congenital condition with two digits in a hand or foot

DIDMOAD syndrome disease complex characterised by diabetes insipidus, diabetes mellitus (insulin-dependent), optic atrophy and deafness

didymitis (did-i-mi'tis) inflammation of a testicle

didymus (did-i-mus) 1. a twin 2. a testicle

die 1. death 2. a positive duplicate made from an impression of a tooth

diencephalon (di-en-sef'a-lon) midline structure from which cerebral hemispheres arise

dienoestrol (di'en-es'trol) synthetic oestrogen

dientamoeba (di'en-ta-me'ba) protozoa possessing two similar nuclei

diet (di'it) bodily nourishment

dietary fibre skeletal remains of plant cells including cellulose and cell wall polymers that are resistant to digestion by enzymes in man

dietetics (di'atet'iks) the study of diet in relation to health and disease

diethyl carbamazine a piperazine derived anthelmintic drug used in the control and treatment of lymphatic filariasis and treatment of tropical eosinophilia, effective in onchocerciasis and loiasis

Dietl's (de'tiz) crisis relief of pain and disappearance of swelling on drinking large quantity of water in intermittent hydronephrosis due to reflex polyuria named after Jozef Dietl, Polish physician.

differential (dif'er-en'shal) pertaining to a difference or differences **d count** tabulation of frequencies of different kinds of cells especially WBC in a blood film **d diagnosis** list of conditions which could explain the signs and symptoms known at the time **d ophthalmodynamometry** comparison of pressure in retinal arteries on two sides as an evidence of carotid block

diffusion (di-fu'zhun) process of uniformly spreading out **d capacity** transfer factor of gas. It measures the amount of oxygen or other gas in ml. transferred per minute for each mm. pressure difference for oxygen or other gas across the pulmonary membrane. It is expressed as ml. of volume of gas uptake per minute per alveolar to mean pulmonary capillary pressure difference (ml/min/mmHg)

digastric (di-gas'trik) having two bellies. **d triangle** submaxillary triangle

DiGeorge syndrome congenital absence of thymus leading to T-lymphocyte deficiency and parathyroids, named after G. DiGeorge, US paediatrician

digestion (di-jes'chun) to break up food into simpler, assimilable compounds

digestive (di-jes'tiv) pertaining to digestion **d juice** one of the several secretions that aid in the digestive process **d system** all structures associated with ingestion and digestion of food

digit (dij'it) a finger or toe **sausage d** a clinical and radiologic appearance of diffuse fusiform swelling of a digit due to soft-tissue inflammation from underlying arthritis or dactylitis

digital (dij'i-tal)1.data that exists in binary number form 2. relating to or resembling a digit or digits or an impression made by them **d image** an image stored in number format, that can be transferred to hard disks or removable storage disks, displayed on screen or printed

digital index the perimeter of each finger at the nail bed (NB) and the distal interphalangeal joint (DIP) is measured by a non-elastic string. If the sum of the 10 NB/DIP ratio becomes >10 it indicates probably clubbing is present

digitalis (dij'i-tal'is) a preparation from dried leaves of *Digitalis purpura*. It has a positive inotropic and negative chronotropic effect on heart. It reduces the heart rate which is useful in atrial fibrillation and atrial flutter. It increases cardiac output with secondary increase of renal flow and glomerular filtration rate

digitalisation (diji'i-tal-i-za'shun) administration of sufficient amount of digoxin to have its effect, can be achieved by intravenous route

digital radiography radiography using computerized imaging

digital subtraction angiography study of arterial blood circulation using computer. Computer subtracts the image produced by surrounding tissues

digitate having finger-like process or impression

digitation (dij-i-ta'shun) a finger-like process

digitoxin (dij-i-tok'sin) a cardiac glycoside used as a heart stimulant

digitus a finger or toe pl. **digiti**

digoxin (di-gok'sin) commonly used cardiac glycoside, used in cardiac failure, atrial fibrillation and flutter

dihydrocodeine (di-hi'dro-ko'de-in) an opioid analgesic

dihydroergotamine (di-hi'dro-er-got'a-min) a vasoconstrictor useful in migraine

dihydrotachysterol (di-hi'dro-tak-is'ter-ol) a steroid obtained by irradiation of ergosterol

dihydroemetine emetine preparation with less cardiotoxicity used in the treatment of amoebiasis

dilatation (dil'a-ta'shun) the condition of being enlarged; act of stretching

dilatation and curettage *see* D and C

dilatation and evacuation D and E removal of production of conception during second trimester by suction curettage and by use of forceps

dilation expansion of organ, orifice or vessel

dilator an instrument for dilating muscles or for stretching cavities or openings

dildo dildoe, an object having shape and size of an erect penis

diluent (dil'u-ent) an agent that dilutes the substance

dilution (di-loo'shun) process of weakening a substance

dimer (di'mer) a capsomer containing two subunits

dimercaprol (di-mer-kap'rol) an antidote in poisoning from heavy metals such as arsenic, gold and mercury

dimethicone (di-methi'i-kon) a silicone oil used as a protective of skin against water soluble irritants

dimethyl phthalate (di-meth'il-thal'at) an insect repellant

dimetria (di-me'tre-a) a double uterus

dimorphic anaemia presence of both microcytic hypochromic and normocytic macrocytic red cells in the peripheral blood smear due to iron deficiency and B_{12}/folic acid deficiency

dimorphous (di-mor'fus) a property of fungi that may produce two different forms such as yeasts or mycelia depending on whether the organism is cultuted at 25°C or is at body temperature (37°C)

dimple a small depression in the skin

dinacharya (s) daily routine

dinner fork deformity deformity of the hand in Colles' fracture

dionosil a contrast medium used in taking bronchogram or to determine the lower limit of empyema cavity

diopter (di-op'ter) the unit (d) used to designate the refractive power of a lens

dioptometer (di-op-tom'i-tre) an instrument for measuring refraction and accommodation of the eye

diovulator (di-ov'u-la-to're) producing two ova in the same ovarian cycle

dioxide (di-ok'sid) a compound having two oxygen atoms per molecule

dipalmitoylphosphatidylcholine (DPPC) principal phospholipid component of surfactant. It provides both the stability and the very low surface tension of the monomolecular film

Dipani (s) gastric stimulant

dipeptide (di-pep'tid) a protein obtained by hydrolysis of the proteins

dipeptidase (di-pep'ti-das) an enzyme that catalyses the hydrolysis of dipeptides to aminoacids

diphasic (di-fa'sik) having two phases

diphenhydramine H_1-receptor blocking antihistamine

diphenoxylate (di'fen-ok-si-lat) a smooth muscle relaxant used with atropine to treat diarrhoea

diphenylhydantoin (di-fen'il-hi-dan'to-in) an anticonvulsant used in generalised tonic-clonic seizures, partial and secondary epilepsy

diphonia (di-fo'ne-a) simultaneous production of two diffent voice tones

diphtheria (dif-ther'e-a) an acute contagious disease caused by *Corynebacterium diphtheriae*. It spreads by droplet infection. The organisms remain localised at the site of infection-upper respiratory tract. The serious consequences are from the absorption of a soluble exotoxin. The disease begins insidiously and presents with membranous tonsillitis, nasal or laryngeal infection. It may lead to complications due to damage to the heart muscle or nervous system with features of laryngeal obstruction or paralysis, myocarditis and peripheral neuropathy. The condition is treated by administration of antitoxin and penicillin. Prevented by active immunisation

diphtheroid (dif'ther-oid) 1. resembling diphtheria 2. a false membrane not due to the diphtheria bacillus

diphylline a theophylline preparation that is stable in acidic medium and less irritant to gastric mucosa

diphyllobothriasis (di-fil'o-both-ri'a-sis) infestation with *Diphyllobothrium latum* (fish tapeworm), presents with megaloblastic anaemia, treated with niclosamide or praziquantel

Diphyllobothrium latum the broad or fish tape worm, of 15 to 18 metres, acquired from eating uncooked fish

diplegia (di-ple-je-a) paralysis of corresponding parts of both sides of the body.

diplococcus (dip'lo-kok'us) spherical gram- positive bacteria joined together in pairs *D(Streptococcus) pneumoniae* is an example pl **diplococci**

diploe (dip'lo-e) spongy bone with a limited marrow cavity between the two tables of the cranial bones

diploid (dip'loid) having two sets of chromosomes in the somatic cells

diplopia (di-plo'pe-a) double vision

dipping 1. a special technique to palpate organs and tumours in case of ascites. The pads of the fingers are placed on the abdomen, then by a quick push the abdominal wall is depressed 2. immersion of an object in a solution

dipsomania an insatiable uncontrollable desire for alcoholic drinks

dipsosis (dip-so'sis) abnormal thirst

dipstic reagent strip a blotting paper impregnated with enzymes or chemicals sensitive to various substances, undergoes a change in colour enabling measurement of the substance semiquantitatively

diptera (dip'ter-a) insects characterised by sucking or piercing mouth parts and a pair of wings, flies and mosquitoes are examples

dipyridamole an antiplatelet agent, which in combination with aspirin reduces thrombosis in patients with thrombotic diseases. It inhibits embolisation from prosthetic valves

direct contact transmission of a disease agent directly from the infected person to a susceptible host during physical contact such as infections, STD, or neonatal infections

directly observed therapy (DOT) oral administration of a drug(s) to a patient and making him swallowed in presence. It is of importance in treating tuberculosis in which development of drug resistant organisms is more likely to occur, if the drug is not taken properly

Dirofilaria (di'ro-fi-la're-a) a genus of filaria known to infect mammals, rarely found *D immitis* a filarial nematode causing pulmonary dirofilariasis, and tropical pulmonary eosinophilia

dirofilariasis a zoonotic disease due to *D. immitis*. The infective larvae inoculated into dermis and subcutaneous tissue die before attaining sexual maturity and causes granulomatous reaction in the lungs

disability (dis'a-bil'i-te) any restriction or lack of ability to perform an activity in the manner or within the range considered normal for a person **d limitation** preventing or halting the transition of the disease process from impairment to handicap when a patient reports late in the pathogenesis phase **d prevention** reduction of the occurrence impairment by immunisation (primary), by treatment (secondary) and by preventing the transition of disability into handicap (tertiary)

disaccharidase (di-sak'a-ri-das) enzyme that splits disaccharides into monosaccharides

disaccharide (di-sak'i-rid) a carbohydrate containing two monosaccharides

disarticulation (dis'ar-ti-ku-la-shun) separation of the bones at the joint

disaster any unusually unanticipated event requiring urgent response, such as earthquakes, floods, fires, explosions, bomb attack, poison gas, toxic spill etc. **d planning** a comprehensive plan of action to cope with a sudden, unexpected event

disc (disk) a platelike structure **d diffusion test** measure of susceptibility of organism by width of clear zone of inhibition of agar culture round disc impregnated with antibiotic **d lesion** herniation of intervertebral disc

discern to see clearly with the mind or eye

discharge (dis'charj) 1. release of material 2. to release from care 3. flowing away of secretions, or excretion of faeces, urine or pus 4. escape of pentup energy **d summary** a summary of hospi-

tal record of a patient, and it is prepared at the time of discharge

discharging the flowing out of material as of pus from a lesion

discission (dis-sizh'un) rupture of the capsule of lens in cataract surgery.

discography x-rays (AP and lateral) taken after injecting water soluble dye into lower lumbar discs using a very fine injection needle and it is undertaken in prolapsed intervertebral disc with normal myelogram

discitis (disk-itis) infection affecting the disc

discoid (disk'oi-d) having shape like a disc

discordance (dis-kor-dans) expression of a trait in only one of a twin

discrete (dis-kret) separate

discriminant analysis a multivariate method to find the relationship between a single discrete outcome and a linear combination of two or more predictions

discrimination the process of differentiating or distinguishing

didiadochokinesia (di-di'a-do-ko-ki-neze-a) the inability to make finely coordinated antagonist movements.

disease (di-zez) without ease, a physiological/psychological dysfunction resulting from a complex interaction between man, agent and the environment **acute d** a disease with a rapid onset and relatively of short duration **autoimmune d** a disease produced when the body's normal tolerance of antigens on its own cells disappears **chronic d** a disease with a slow onset and lasting for a long duration **chronic obstructive pulmonary d** (COPD) a disease state characterised by the presence of air-flow obstruction due to chronic bronchitis or emphysema; the air-flow obstruction is generally progressive may be accompanied by air-flow hyperreactivity which may be viewed as partially reversible **communicable d** a disease in which the causative organism is transmissible from one person to another either directly or indirectly through a carrier or vector **congenital d** a disease that is present at birth **connective tissue d** a group of diseases that affect connective tissue. It includes muscle, cartilage, tendons, vessels, skin and ligaments **contagious d** an infectious disease readily transmitted from one person to another **deficiency d** a disease resulting from inadequate intake or absorption of essential dietary factors **degenerative d** a disease resulting from deterioration of tissues and organs **degenerative joint d** osteoarthritis **demyelinating d** a disorder of nerve fibres due to destruction of their myelin sheath **endemic d** a disease present continuously in a community and it may recur frequently **epidemic d** a disease affecting a large number of persons in a community at the same time **epizootic d** an epidemic affecting animals of a particular region, usually in a short period of time **extrapyramidal d** degenerative disease of nervous system involving the extrapyramidal system and basal ganglion of the brain. Parkinsonism is a classic example **familial d** a disease occurring in several members of the same family **focal d** a disease confined to a specific area such as tonsils, adenoids or a boil **foot and mouth d** a viral disease noted in cattle and horses, that is rarely transmitted to humans **functional d** a disease in which no anatomic changes can be seen to account for the symptomatology **heavy chain d** a group of diseases involving serum immunoglobulins **hereditary d** a disease due to genetic factors transmitted from parent to offspring **hookworm d** ankylostomiasis **hydatid d** the disease produced by larval stage of *Echinococcus granulosus* **iatrogenic d** a disease produced by medical or surgical intervention **idiopathic d** a disease for which no causative agent can be recognised **infectious d** any disease caused by growth of pathogenic organisms in the body **intercurrent d** a disease developing during the course of another, unrelated disease **iron storage d** haemochromatosis **lysosomal storage d** a disease caused by deficiency of specific lysosomal enzymes that normally degrade glycoproteins, glyocolipids or mucopolysaccharides, and such substances accumulate in lysosomes **malignant d** 1. cancer 2. a disease not necessarily cancer making rapid progress and is life threatening **metabolic d** a disease occurring from under-production or overproduction of substances needed by the body in the metabolic process **mixed connective tissue d** a connective tissue disorder exhibiting features of SLE, progressive systemic sclerosis and polymyositis **motor neuron d** neurologic disease characterised by degeneration of anterior horn cells of the spinal cord, the motor cranial nerve nuclei and corticospinal tracts **natural history of d** the way in which a disease evolves over time from earliest stage of its prepathogenesis phase to termination as recovery, disability or death in the absence of treatment or prevention **occupational d** a disease resulting from factors associated with occupation **organic d** a disease resulting from anatomical alteration in an organ or tissue of the body **pandemic d** a widespread epidemic affecting the population of several countries as in influenza **parasitic d** a disease resulting from the growth and development of parasites in or on the body **psychosomatic d** an organic disease caused or exacerbated by psychological factors **reactive airway d** persistence of airway reactivity after acute exposure to respiratory irritants **restrictive lung d** any chest disease that results in a reduced lung volume **secondary d** a disease caused by another condition such as obesity **self limited d** a disease that recedes of its own **storage d** a disorder involving abnormal deposition of a substance in body tissues **subacute d** an intermediate between acute and chronic disease **systemic d** a generalised disease **venereal d** a disease acquired through sexual contact

disengagement 1. emergence of foetal head from within the maternal pelvis 2. *Psy* autonomous functioning without any emotional attachment

disentaglement a rescue technique adapted to free a trapped victim from the wreckage

disequilibrium (dis-e'kwi-lib're-um) an unequal and unstable equilibrium **d syndrome** a complication of renal dialysis characterised by irritability, muscle cramps, headache, nausea, drowsiness, convulsions and raised intracranial tension, due to rapid lowering of levels of urea in the blood

disinfectant a substance which destroys harmful microbes with the object of preventing transmission of diseases

disinfection (dis-in-fek'shun) the destruction of infectious agents by direct exposure to chemical or physical agents **concurrent d** application of disinfection measures as soon as possible after the discharge of infectious material from the body of an infected person or after soiling of articles with such infectious discharges **prophylactic d** disinfection to prevent acquiring infectious agents like chlorination of water, pasteurisation of milk and hand washing **terminal d** application of disinfectious measures after the death of the patient or after moving the patient to the hospital

disinfestation (dis'in-fes-ta'shun) killing of infested insects and parasites

disinhibition (dis'in-hi-bish-un) 1. abolistion of inhibition 2. *Psy* freedom to act without any social or cultural inhibitions

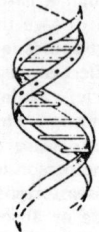

DNA

disintegration (dis-in'ti-gra-shun) breakdown

disjunction (dis-junk'shun) separation of homologous pairs of chromosomes during anaphase of the first meiotic division

disk a device for storing digital data **hard d** a stack of high-speed rigid disks. It contains the operating system, the programmes and all created files. **floppy d** a portable, flexible plastic disk. Each 3.5 inch disk can hold up to 1.44 Mb of information **jaz d** a portable storage device that is capable of storing up to 2 Gb of data **super d** a portable storage device similar to that of a floppy disk, wherein each disk can store up to 200 Mb of data **zip d** a portable storage device that stores up to 100 Mb of information

dislocation (dis'lo-ka'shun) displacement of a limb or organ from the normal position **joint d** total displacement of articular surfaces causing a loss of apposition between them. The dislocation may occur spontaneously at any joint in consequence of a structural defect or of destructive disease, or trauma

dismutase (dis-mu'tas) an enzyme that acts on two molecules of the same substance, where one is oxidised and other reduced **superoxide d** an enzyme found in aerobic bacteria that destroys highly reactive free radicals form of oxygen superoxide

disocclusion loss of contact between opposing teeth .

disodium cromoglycate (DSC) a khellin compound acting on tissue mast cell and stabilises its cell membrane. It prevents the degranulation and prevents release of histamine and other tissue mediators involved in the pathogenesis of asthmatic attacks. It is effective in preventing asthmatic attack noted on exercise or hyperventilation

disomy the inheritance of both haploid chromosomes from one parent

disorder (dis-or'der) a disturbance of a function of the body or mind

disorganisation alteration in an organ causing loss of its distinct features

disorientation (dis-or're-enta'shun) loss of sense of direction or location; a state of mental confusion as to time, place or person.

dispensary (dis-pen'ser-e) any place where drugs and medicines are dispensed

dispensatory (dis-pen'sa-tor'e) a book describing medical preparations and uses

dispense (dis'pens) to prepare medicines and distribute

disperse (dis-pers) 1. to scatter 2. cause to disappear

dispersonalisation (dis-per'son-al-i-za'shun) *Psy* a mental state in which the individual denies the existence of his or her personality or parts of the body

displacement activity a set of behaviour patterns occurring alongside an unrelated set of behaviour patterns

Disposition a person's built-in tendency to react to a given situation in a characteristic way

disproportion a state of wrong proportion **cephalopelvic d** a disproportion due to the pelvis being too small for the head, or head too large for the pelvis

dissect (di-sekt) to cut apart and expose the structures of a cadaver

dissection (di-sek'shun) the act of dissecting

disseminated intravascular coagulation (DIC) a consumptive coagulopathy, noted in critically ill patients and often heralds the onset of multi-organ failure. It is characterised by an increase in prothrombin time, partial thromboplastin time and fibrin degradation products and a fall in platelets and fibrinogen. There is either widespread bleeding from vascular access points or widespread microvascular and even macrovascular thrombosis. It is treated with fresh frozen plasma, platelets and low dose heparin

dissipation (dis-i-pa'shun) dispersion of matter

dissociation (dis-so'se-a'shun) 1. separation 2. ability to move one body segment independently of another 3. not going together 4. *Psy* the breaking off of normal thought processes from consciousness

dissolution 1. death 2. resolution 3. breaking up of the integrity of anatomical structure

dissolve (di-zolv) to cause absorption of a solid by a liquid

distal (dis'-t'l) farthest from a point of reference

distance the space between two objects

distension the state of being stretched or distended

distillation condensation of a vapour that has been obtained from a liquid heated to a volatilisation point

distortion 1. a twisting or bending out of a regular shape. 2. a twisting movement 3. a deformity in which the part or structure is altered in shape

distractibility inability to concentrate attention; attention drawn to unimportant or irrelevant external stimuli

distraction (dis-trak'shun) 1. a state of mental confusion 2. separation of joint surfaces by extension

distraught (dis-trawt) deeply troubled with conflicting thought

distress (dis-tres) physical or mental suffering

distribution 1. dividing and spreading of anything 2. presence of entities at different locations 3. the location pattern of particular persons who are ill or of events

disturbance 1. interruption of the normal sequence 2. departure from the norm

disulphate (di-sul'fat) a compound containing two sulphate radicals

disulphiram (di-sul'fi-ram) a drug used in the treatment of alcoholism. It prevents degradation of toxic substance acetaldehyde, a product of metabolism of alcohol

disuse musculoskeletal inactivity **d atrophy** wasting from disuse especially after paralysis or joint disease

Dittrich's (dit'riks) **plugs** small particles of foetid sputum named after Franz Dittrich, German pathologist

diuresis (di'u-re'sis) discharge of increased amounts of urine

diuretic (di'u-ret'ik) agent that increases amount of urine

diurnal 1. daily 2. happening in daytime

divarication wide separation.

diverge (di-verj) to spread apart, to lead away from each other

divergence (di-verj'ens) moving apart or moving away from a common point

diverticulitis (di'ver-tik'ul'it-is) inflammation of a diverticulum

diverticulosis (di'ver-tiku-lo'sis) diverticula in the colon develop in individuals who are on a life long refined diet with relative deficiency of fibre and symptoms are result of associated constipation or spasm, generally asymptomatic

diverticulum (di'ver-tik'u-lum) a sac-like protrusion of mucosa covered by peritoneum from a tubular organ, most common in the sigmoid and descending colon and is acquired pl. **diverticula**

dizziness (diz'e-nes) unsteadiness characterised by a feeling of movement within the head with actual motion

DNA deoxyribonucleic acid **DNA fingerprint** a distinctive pattern of bands formed by repeating sequences of base pairs of satellite DNA which are different in every individual **DNA ligase** the enzyme that joins two DNA ends together **DNA polymerase** the enzyme that replicates DNA **DNA probe** labelled segment of single-strand DNA of known type used to identify similar sequences on DNA chain **DNA sequencing** the process of determining the exact order of the bases-A,T,C and G- in a piece of DNA **mitochondrial DNA** DNA founding mitochondria; mDNA

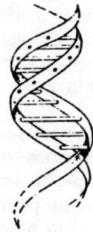

DNA

DNase deoxyribonuclease

dobutamine a synthetic beta agonist increasing cardiac contractility with little effect on systemic vascular resistance. Useful in cardiogenic shock as a vasoactive agent

dolichocephalic (dol'i-ko-se-fal'ik) long headed

dolichocephaly (do'i-ko-se-fal-e) long head

doll's eye sign movement of the eyes in a direction opposite to a sudden movement of the head caused by a lesion in the central mechanism for voluntary eye movement

dolor (do'lor) pain, one of the cardinal signs of inflammation

domiciliary (dom'i-sil'e-are) pertaining to or carried in a house

dominant a trait expressed in individuals who are heterozygous for a particular gene

donee (do'ne) a person who receives something from a donor

donor one who donates tissue, an organ, blood or blood products

do not resuscitate (DNR) an order stating that a patient should not be revived

Donovan body causative agent of granuloma inguinale, named after Charles Donovan, Irish physician who worked in India

donut sign resemblance to a donut, an imaging finding on ultrasonography or axial abdominal magnetic resonance. It is due to a circumferential bowel wall thickening seen in colon carcinoma, inflammatory bowel disease and intussusception

DOPA 3, 4 dihydroxy phenylalanine produced by exudation of tyrosine. It is a precursor of catecholamines and melanin

dopamine a sympathomimetic agent which is the immediate metabolic precursor of norepinephrine and epinephrine. Useful in treatment of shock with oliguria and low or normal peripheral vascular resistance, also useful in the treatment of cardiogenic and septic shock

dopaminergic (do'pa-men-er'jik) 1. tissues influenced by dopamine 2. caused by dopamine

dope narcotic drug

doping use of a drug or blood product by an athlete to improve performance

Doppler echocardiography see echocardiography

dopper effect variation of the apparent frequency of waves; wavelength of signal appears longer if source or reflector is moving away from observer and shorter if approaching, named after Johann Doppler, Austrian physicist. Doppler flowmeter measures rate of flow in vessels from reflection of ultrasound by moving blood cells

dormancy 1. condition of markedly reduced metabolic activity 2. a state in which the disease process is not active. adj **dormant**

dorsal (dor'sal) relating to the back

dorsalgia (dor-sal'je-a) pain in the back.

dorsalis (dor-sa'lis) pertaining to the back

dorsiflexion movement of a part at a joint to bend the part toward the dorsum

dorsum the posterior surface or back of a part

dosage the determination of the amount, frequency and number of medication for a patient

dose (dos) the amount of medicine or radiation to be administered at one time **bolus d** an amount of medicine given intravenously rapidly at the beginning of treatment **booster d** an additional dose of an immunising agent to increase the protection afforded by original series of injections **cumulative d** 1. amount of drug present in the body after repeated exposure 2. total dose resulting from repeated exposure to radiation **divided d** fractional portions of drug administered at short intervals **fatal d** a dose resulting in death **infective d** the amount of microorganisms that will cause disease **loading d** initial administration of a drug in doses that exceed the elimination rate of the drug from the body **maintenance d** the dose required to maintain the desired effect **maximum d** the largest dose that is safe to administer **minimum d** the smallest effective dose **therapeutic d** the dose required to produce desired effect **toxic d** a dose that causes signs and symptoms of drug toxicity

dosha - vaishmya (s) pathologic features

dosimetry (do'sim'e-tre) measurement of doses

DOT directly observed therapy

DOTs directly observed therapy, short course with reference to the treatment of tuberculosis

double (dub'l) twofold **d-blind technique** a method of scientific investigation in which neither the subject nor the investigator knows what treatment the subject is receiving. On completion of the investigation the 'code' is broken and data is analysed. It eliminates the bias **d vision** two images of an object seen at the same time **d helix** shape of a DNA molecule, like a spiral staircase

doublet a condition of two similar structures

doubling time a period required for the diameter of the lesion to increase. 1. 25 times, eg. from a 2 cm to lesion to become 2.5 cm in diameter, an important way of evaluating nodules for potential malignancy

douche (doosh) a stream of liquid directed into a cavity of body

Douglas bag a portable large bag to collect expired air for measuring oxygen use and CO_2 output, named after Claude Douglas, British physiologist

Douglas pouch rectovesical pouch named after James Douglas, Scottish physician

down lanugo; fine hairs of the skin of newborn

down growth (down groth) a growth downwards

download to copy a file or programme from one computer to another computer by using a modem or a network connection

down regulate to suppress the normal response of an organ or system

Down's (downz) **syndrome** a chromosomal abnormality having 3 chromosomes instead of normal two in the pair no. 21 (47XY) resulting in many congenital defects described by an English physician John Down; mongolism. It is characterised by dwarfed physique, low set ears, a flat nose, short broad hands with a single palmar crease, a sloping forehead and small ear canals

doxapram (dok's'a-pram) analeptic used as a respiratory stimulant

doxorubicin an anthracyclic antibiotic, is effective in acute leukaemias and malignant lymphomas and is administered intravenously. Myelosuppression is a major complication

doxycycline an antimicrobial agent belonging to tetracycline group has antimicrobial activity against aerobic and anaerobic, gram-positive and gram-negative bacteria especially useful in diseases caused by rickettsiae, mycoplasma and chlamydiae

DPT vaccine diphtheria, pertusis and tetanus vaccine used to immunise infants against three infectious diseases such as diphtheria, pertusis and tetanus

drab dull, colourless

dracantiasis (drak'on-ti'a-sis) infection with *Dracunculus medinensis*

dracunculosis (dra-kung'ku-lo'sis) dracantiasis, dracunculiasis infection acquired by ingesting a small crustacean, cyclolps which inhabits step wells and ponds and which contain infective larval stages of *D. medinensis*. They penetrate intestinal wall and migrate through connective tissue. The fully mature female surfaces under skin to discharge its larvae externally. There is painful vesicle, ulcer, cellulitis usually on leg and secondary infection. The disease has been eradicated

Dracunculus (drah-kung'ku-lus) *medinensis* a thread-like long nematode worm, guinea worm; serpent worm

drain (dran) provision of exit for the fluid

drainage (dran'ij) the free flow or withdrawal of fluids from a wound or cavity **d tube** a device for allowing escape of fluid, pus, serum from a wound

draught (draft) liquid medicament prescribed as a single dose

drava(s) fluid

dravya (s) drug, substance employed in medicine *dravyaguna* pharmacology dealing with identification, classification and description of drugs *dravykalpa* medicinal properties

Drawer's sign useful in the diagnosis of tear of cruciate ligaments when the patient lying on the back with the knee to be tested flexed the upper end of tibia is grasped and pushed backwards and pulled forwards and a free movement of tibia over the lower end of the femur. There is abnormal mobility of tibia on femur in tear of cruciate ligaments which can even be demonstrated on the extended knee

draw sheet a rubber or plastic sheet to protect the mattress and bed sheet from drainage and soilage

dream occurrence of ideas and sensations during sleep. Dream activity is seen during rapid eye movement sleep

dressing (dres'ing) bandage applied to a wound or lesion to prevent external infection

Dressler's syndrome post-myocardial infarction syndrome characterised by persistent fever, pericarditis and pleurisy and is probably due to auto-immunity named after William Dressler, US physician

dribble to flow in drops

drift movement due to external force

drip to fall in drops **intravenous d** slow injection of a solution into a vein a drop at a time **postnasal d** flow of discharge from the postnasal region into the pharynx by aerosol route

drive the force or impulse to act

drop 1. a minute spherical mass of liquid 2. failure of a part to maintain its normal position **d attack** sudden fall without warning, with loss of consciousness or dizziness **d-out** cases lost the followup **foot d** paralysis of anterior tibial muscles making the foot to hang **hanging d** application of a drop on coverslip, which is inverted over a glass slide with a central depression. The suspended solution is examined under a microscope **nose d** medication instilled in or sprayed into nose **wrist d** paralysis of extensor muscles causing wrist to hang

droplet a very small drop **d infection** invasion of a micro-organism, conveyed by particles

dropper a tube with a narrowed end on one side for dispensing drops of liquid

dropsy (drop'se) hydrops; generalised accumulation of fluid in the body

drowning asphyxiation due to immersion in liquid

drowse partially asleep

drowsiness the state of almost falling asleep

drug substance used as medicine, narcotic or hallucinogen **d abuse** self-administration of a drug for non-medical reasons in quantities and frequencies which may impair an individual's ability to function effectively and which result in social, physical or emotional harm **d addict** a person exhibiting psychological dependence with an overpowering desire to take the drug and obtain it by any means, physical dependence when the drug is withdrawn exhibiting withdrawal symptoms and a tendency to increase the dose due to development of tolerance **d addiction** a state of periodic or chronic intoxication detrimental to the individual and society produced by the repeated intake of habit forming drugs **d dependence** a state of psychic and sometimes also physical resulting from the interaction between an individual and a drug, characterised by behavioural and other responses that always include a compulsion to take the drug on a continuous or periodic basis in order to experience its psychic effects and sometimes to avoid the discomfort of its absence **d resistance** situation where patient fails to show response to chemotherapy. It may be primary when the patient has been infected with organisms that are resistant to one or more drugs or secondary wherein the infection is acquired either from a patient who has received inadequate chemotherapy or from a naturally resistant organism (wild strain) **d synergism** enhancement of a drug's effect as a result of the presence of additional drugs within the system **d tolerance** progressively decreased sensitivity to a drug that a person has taken repeatedly requiring high doses to produce the desired effect **d withdrawal** unpleasant symptoms experienced by a person stopping the drug on which he or she had become physically dependent

DSM diagnostic and statistical manual of mental disorders, produced by the American Psychiatric Association that standardise the criteria required to establish the diagnosis of psychiatric conditions

DUB dysfunctional uterine bleeding

Dubin-Johnson syndrome familial conjugated bilirubin excess in blood due to transport defect in liver cells. Patient remains asymptomatic, named after Isadore Dubin and Frank Johnson, US pathologists

dubious doubtful, uncertain

Duchenne's muscular dystrophy a sex-linked recessive disease and most common of the mascular dystrophies. It occurs after age of 2 years and affects proximal limb muscles causing pseudohypertrophy and cardiac involvement is common, named after Guillaume Duchenne, French neurologist

duct (dukt) a tube to convey the products of a gland to another part of the body **alveolar d** a branch of respiratory bronchiole that leads to the alveolar sacs. The duct contains alveoli in their walls **Bartholin's d** *see* sublingual duct **biliary d** a canal that carries bile **common bile d** the duct that carries bile and pancreatic juice to the duodenum. It is formed by the union of the cystic duct of the gall bladder and the hepatic duct of the liver and is joined by the pancreatic duct **cystic d** the secretory duct of gall bladder **efferent d** one of a group of small tubes from the testis, and lie within the epididymis **ejaculatory d** the duct conveying semen from the vas deferens and semi-

nal vesicle to the urethra **hepatic d** a duct receiving bile from liver and carrying it to the common bile duct **interlobular d** a duct passing between lobules within a gland **lacrimal d** one of two short ducts (inferior and superior) that convey tears from the lacrimal lake to the lacrimal sac. They open on the margin of upper and lower eyelids **lactiferous d** one of several ducts draining the lobes of the mammary gland. They open in a slight depression in the tip of the nipple **lymphatic d** one of two main ducts conveying lymph to the blood stream. The right lymphatic duct drains lymph from the region above the diaphragm and discharges into the right subclavian vein **mesonephric d** an embryonic duct connecting the mesonephros with the cloaca **Mullerian d** one of the bilateral ducts in the embryo that forms the uterus, vagina and fallopian tubes named after Johannes Muller, German physiologist **nasolacrimal d** a duct that conveys tears from the lacrimal sac to the nasal cavity. It opens beneath the inferior nasal cavity **pancreatic d** a duct that conveys pancreatic juice to the duodenum called Wirsung's duct, named after Johann Wirsung, German physician **parotid d** a duct carrying secretions from the parotid gland to the oral cavity. It opens opposite the second upper molar tooth also called Stensen's duct, named after Niels Stensen, Danish physician **prostate d** one of about 20 ducts that discharge prostatic secretions into the urethra **semicircular d** one of three (anterior, posterior and lateral) membranous tubes forming a part of the membranous labyrinth of the inner ear. They are present within the semicircular canals **Skene's d** one of two slender ducts of Skene's gland that open on either side of the urethral orifice in women, named after Alexander Skene, American gynaecologist **Stensen's d** *see* parotid duct **sublingual d** any of the secretory ducts of sublingual gland, also called Bartholin duct, named after Casper Bartholin Jr., Danish anatomist **submandibular d** a duct of the submandibular gland that opens on a papilla at the side of frenum of the tongue, also called Wharton's duct, named after Thomas Wharton, British anatomist **thoracic d** lymphatic duct draining the left side of the body above the diaphragm and all of the body below the diaphragm and it opens into the left subclavian vein **utriculosaccular d** a narrow tube arising from the utricle connecting it into the saccule and open into the endolymphatic duct of the inner ear **vitelline d** a narrow duct, in the embryo connecting yolk sac with the intestine **Whorton's d** see submandibular duct **Wirsung's d** see pancreatic duct **Wolffian d** see mesonephric duct

duct ectasia an inflammatory condition of lactiferous ducts of breast

duction rotation of an eye about an axis

ductless having no duct **d gland** gland lacking in an external duct; endocrine gland

ductule (duk'tul) a very small duct

ductus arteriosus a vessel leading from the bifurcation of the pulmonary artery to the aorta just distal to the left subclavian artery. Normally the vascular channel closes immediately after birth

Duffy (duf'e) **system** a blood group consisting of two antigens determined by allelic genes

Dugas test normally with the elbow by the side of the trunk it is possible to touch the opposite shoulder with the hand. A patient with dislocation of the shoulder is unable to touch the opposite shoulder, named after Louis Dugas, US physician

dukha (s) unplesant, misery, sorrow

dullness percussion note when there is consolidation, tumour, pleural effusion, pleural thickening or empyema **stony d** absolute dullness as in pleural effusion **woody d** note over a consolidated lobe where chest offers greater resistance

dumb lacking the power to speak

dumbness muteness

dumbbell a tubular structure with terminal bulbous enlargement and central constriction **d bones** shortened and terminally enlarged long bones **d gall bladder** a transverse septation between the body and fundus of gall bladder **d tumours** benign tumours with central constriction such as neurofibroma located on either side of intervertebral foramina impinging on the spinal cord

dumping syndrome post-gastrectomy syndrome **early d s** in patients with gastrectomy, rapid gastric emptying leads to distension of the proximal small intestine. There is abdominal discomfort and diarrhoea after eating and vasomotor features such as flushing, palpitations, sweating, tachycardia and hypotension. The patients should avoid large meals with high carbohydrate **late d s** symptoms develop 90 to 180 minutes after eating. There is reactive hypoglycaemia from exaggerated release of insulin causing mental confusion

Duncan mechanism during separation of placenta, the detachment begins at the lower pole and whole organ is gradually forced into the cervix, the upper pole being the last to leave the uterine cavity, described by James Duncan British gynaecologist

duodenal (du-o-de'nal) pertaining to the duodenum **d bulb** the area of duodenum just beyond the pylorus **d ulcer** ulcer in the first part of the duodenum. The patients have a greater number of parietal cells and a tendency to higher gastric acid secretion, noted in age group 20-40 years. Presents with pain on an empty stomach with a clock-like regularity with relief on food intake

duodenectomy (du'o-den-ek'to-me) excision of part or all of duodenum

duodenitis (du'od-e-nitis) inflammation of the duodenum

duodenocholecystostomy(du'o-de'n'o-ko-li-sis-tos'to-mi) surgical formation of a passage between the duodenum and gall bladder

duodenoenterostomy (du'o-de-no-en'ter-os'to-me) surgical formation of a passage between the duodenum and intestine

duodenography (du'o-de-nog-ra-fe) radiographic examination of the duodenum

duodenoileostomy (du'o-de'no-il'e-os'to-me) surgical formation of a passage between the duodenum and the ileum

duodenojejunostomy (du'o-de'no-je-joo-nos'to-me) surgical formation of a passage between the duodenum and jejunum

duodenoscopy (du'o-de'-nos'ko-pe) inspection of the duodenum with an endoscope

duodenostomy (du'od-e-nos'to-me) surgical creation of a permanent opening into the duodenum through the wall of abdomen

duodenum (doo'o-de'num) the first part of the small intestine shaped like a horse shoe, between the stomach and jejunum. It is 20-28 cm long. It receives the hepatic and pancreatic secretions through a common bile duct at the ampulla of Vater, named after Abraham Vater, German anatomist

duplication doubling; folding of a part or an organ

dupp (dup) the second heart sound audible through stethoscope. It is shorter and of higher pitch than the first heart sound

Dupuytren's (du-pwe-tranz) **contracture** thickening and contracture of palmar fascia, typically affects the ring finger and may involve years later incompletely, little finger. The finger resists extension, described by Baron Dupuytren, French surgeon

Dupuytren's fracture a fracture dislocation of the ankle. The talus is displaced upwards

dura mater a tough fibrous white membrane forming the outermost of the three coverings of the brain and spinal cord

duration 1. the average length of time a disorder is present 2. the time interval between the beginning and the end of one uterine contraction

durgandha (s) nauseating

Duroziez (du-roz'e-az) **murmur** presence of systolic and diastolic murmur audible on the femoral artery in patients with aortic insufficiency. The murmur is audible when pressure is applied to the area just distal to the stethoscope, named after Paul Duroziez, French physician

dust minute, fine particles of earth, powder or extraneous particles **d cell** alveolar macrophage that engulfs the pathogens and particulate material **house d** particles found in the air in a house which includes mites, fibres, pollens and smoke

dusting powder any fine powder for dusting on skin

DVT deep vein thrombosis

dwarf (dworf) person with abnormally short stature **d tapeworm** *Hymenolepis nana* the only human tapeworm that has no intermediate host. Spreads by direct person to person, eggs hatch in stomach and intestine, penetrate the villi and metamorphose into cercocysts. Presents with irritability, anorexia, convulsions, weight loss and treated with praziquantel or niclosamide

dwarfism (dwarf'izm) failure to attain full growth potential

dyad a pair

dye any substance that is of itself coloured or that is used to impart colour to another material

dying the condition in which death is inevitable

dynamic (di-nam'ik) an inherent power

dynamometer (di′na-mom′e-ter) a device for measuring muscular strength or magnifying power of a lens

Dyne (din) the force needed for imparting an acceleration of 1 cm per second to a gram mass

dynein a 500 kd ATPase that forms the arms of the axoneme in cilia and flagella and is responsible for movement of cilia **d arms** short diverging arms of the outer doublet of the cilia, that act as temporary cross bridges for the sliding of the microtubules of the axoneme

dys- a prefix meaning difficult or painful

dysacusis (dis′a-koo′sis) 1. discomfort caused by loud noise 2. difficulty in hearing

dysarthria (dis-ar′thre-a) difficulty in articulation

dysarthrosis (dis-ar′thro′sis) malformation of a joint

dysautonomia (dis′au-to-no-me-a) dysfunction of the autonomic nervous system

dysbasia (dis-ba′ze-a) difficulty in walking due to diseases of CNS

dyschezia (dis-ke′ze-a) difficult or painful defecation

dyschondroplasia (dis′kon-dro′pla′ze-a) a congenital condition where masses of unossified cartilage persist within the metaphyses of certain long bones and the growth of the bone is retarded; multiple chondromatosis.

dyschromia (dis-kro′me-a) disorder of pigmentation of skin or hair

dyscoria (dis-ko′re-a) abnormality of the pupil

dyscrasia (dis′kra-zhah) a morbid condition

dysdiadochokinesia (dis′di-ad′o-ko-ki-ne-se-a) inability to make alternate movements in rapid succession

dysentery (dis′in-te′re) frequent watery stools with blood and mucus accompanied by abdominal pain **amoebic d** infection of intestine by *Entamoeba histolytica* presents with bloody motions, lower abdominal pain, the motions have more stool, less blood. Stools reveal presence of amoebic trophozoites **bacillary d** Shigellosis, named after Kiyoshi Shiga, Japanese physician, an infection of intestine by bacteria of shigella, such as *S. dysenteriae, S. boydii, S. flexneri* and *S. sonnei*, characterised by abrupt onset of fever, malaise, abdominal pain, bloody diarrhoea with mucus and faecal urgency **balantidial d** dysentery caused by ciliate protozoa, *Balantidium coli*

dysergia (dis-er′je-a) motor inco-ordination

dysethesia (dis′es-the′ze-a) abnormal sensations on the skin that may be in the form of tingling, numbness, burning, cutting or pricking

dysfunction (dis-funk′shun) impaired, inadequate or abnormal function of an organ or part

dysfunctional inability to function normally **d uterine bleeding** (DUB) excess menstrual haemorrhage of hormonal origin

dysgenesis (dis-jen′i-sis) defective embryonic development **gonadal d** a disorder due to failure of ovaries to respond to pituitary gonadotrophins resulting in amenorrhoea, short stature and failure of sexual maturation

dysgerminoma (dis-jerm′in-o-ma) a rare malignant ovarian tumour originating from primordial germ cells of the sexually undifferentiated embryonic gonad

dysgeusia (dis-gu′ze-a) distortion of normal taste perception

dysgnathia (dis-na′the-a) abnormality of the mandible and maxilla

dysgonesis (dis′go-ne′sis) 1. sparse growth of bacterial culture 2. a functional disorder of genital organs

dysgraphia (dis-graf′e-a) difficulty in writing

dyshidrosis (dis′hi-dro′sis) an abnormality of sweat production

dyskaryosis (dis-kar′e-o′sis) abnormality of the nucleus of a cell

dyskeratosis (dis′ker-a-to′sis) alteration in

the keratinisation of the epithelial cells of the epidermis

dyskinesia a movement disorder after chronic exposure to dopamine receptor antagonists characterised by stereotyped orolingual and masticatory movements such as lip smacking, lip pursing, tongue protrusion, licking and chewing

dyskinesis (dis'ki-ne'se-a) difficulty in performing voluntary movements

dyslalia (dis-la'le-a) impaired speech due to defective speech organs

dyslexia (dis-lek'se-a) a learning disability wherein the individual experiences difficulty with written symbols

dyslipidaemia abnormalities of plasma lipids and lipoprotein concentrations

dysmelia (dis-mel'e-a) congenital abnormality of a portion of one or more limbs

dysmnesia (dis-ne'ze-a) any impairment of memory

dysmenorrhoea (dis'men-or-e'a) pain or discomfort experienced just before or during menstrual periods

dysmetria (dis-me'tre-a) inability to stop a muscle movement at a desired point

dysmorphology the systemic study of structural defects of prenatal onset

dysostosis (dis'os-to-sis) defective bone formation

dysoxia (dis-ok'se-a) inability of tissues to make full use of available oxygen

dyspareunia (dis'pa-ru'ne-a) pain or discomfort in vaginal or pelvic area experienced by a woman during sexual intercourse

dyspepsia (dis-pep'se-a) indigestion. Often a symptom of other diseases and characterised by vague abdominal discomfort, a sense of fullness after eating, eructation, nausea, vomiting and loss of appetite

dysphagia (dis-fa'je-a) difficulty in swallowing **d lusoria** dysphagia from pressure exerted on oesophagus by an anomalous subclavian artery **d paralytica** dysphagia due to paralysis of pharyngeal or oesophageal muscles

dysphasia (dis-fa'zha) impairment of co-ordination in speech and inability to arrange words in their proper order.

dysphoric unpleasant **d mood** unpleasant mood

dysplasia (dis-pla'zha) a defective growth of tissues; a histologic lesion with premalignant potential **dysplasia associated lesion or mass** (DALM) presence of dysplasia histologically and a mass by endoscopy as in adenocarcinoma of colon with ulceratrive colitis

dysplastic naevus a skin lesion characterised by irregular macules with a central papule variegated dark colour and lenticular changes. It is generally regarded as premalignant

dyspnoea (disp-ne'a) difficulty or laboured breathing and is a subjective complaint. **acute d** sudden onset of shortness of breath from pulmonary oedema, asthma, spontaneous pneumothorax, pulmonary embolism, ARDS, pleural effusion, or injury to chest wall and intrathoracic structures **chronic d** progressive breathlessness is a feature of left ventricular failure, diffuse interstitial fibrosis, COPD, asthma, pleural effusion, and pulmonary thromboembolic disease

dysthymia a mood disorder with depressive neurosis

dyspraxia (dis-prak'se-a) impaired functioning of an organ or a part

dysprosody loss of normal speech melody

dysraphism (dis'rah-fizm) failure of normal fusion of the foetal neural tube

dysrhythmia (dis-rith-me-a) arrhythmia. Abnormal, disordered rhythm

dyssomnia sleep disorders characterised by a disturbance in the amount, quality and timing of sleep

dysstasia difficulty in standing

dysthymia (dis-thi'me-a) depressed mood

dystocia (disto-se-a) difficult childbirth

dystonia (dis-to'ne-a) rigidity of muscles causing painful spasms or abnormal movement patterns

dystrophia (dis-tro'fe-a) dystrophy

dystrophin (dis'tro-fin) a large 427-kD subsarcolemmal cytoskeletal protein, controlled by the largest gene in the genome. Its mutation causes Duchenne muscular dystrophy and Becker type muscular dystrophy

dystrophy (dis'trof-e) any disorder caused by faulty nutrition

dysuria (dis-u-re-a) difficulty or pain in urination

dyszoospermia (dis'zo-o-sperm'e-a) imperfect formation of spermatozoa

E

EAEC Enteroadherent *Escherichia coli*. A bacteria causing a rare chronic diarrhoea in infants and they fail to thrive

Eale's (elz) disease recurrent haemorrhages into the retina and vitreous noted in males in second and third decades of life, named after Henry Eales, British ophthalmologist

e-antigen hepatitis B virus e antigen.

ear the organ of hearing and balance. It consists of the external, middle and internal ear. The external ear has the skin covered cartilaginous auricle and the external auditory canal. They form a funnel directing sound waves towards the tympanic membrane or ear drum. On the other side of the ear drum is the air-filled middle ear. It contains three very small bones, the malleus, incus and stapes which transmit the vibrations caused by the sound waves reaching the tympanic membrane to the oval window of the inner ear. The inner ear consists of two separate organs. The vestibular apparatus providing the sense of balance and the organ of Corti which translates the vibrations received from the middle ear into nerve impulses which are interpreted by the brain cells as specific sounds **bladder e** *uro* transient bilateral extraperitoneal herniation of the bladder in infants **earache** (ir'ak) pain in the ear **e drops** a topical liquid medication for the local treatment of infection of the lining of external auditory canal or impacted cerumen **e drum** a thin oval membrane separating the middle ear from external ear that transmits sound waves **e oximeter** a device helping to measure the level of saturated haemoglobin in the blood **e speculum** a short funnel-shaped tube attached to an otoscope for examination of the ear canal **e wax** a waxy secretion produced by sweat glands in the external ear canal, cerumen

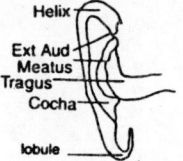

External ear

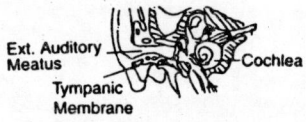

Middle ear

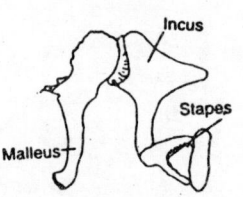

Ear osscicles

early gene *vir* a gene produced by a host cell shortly after integration of a virus into the host's genome. It encodes enzymes of interest to the virus

early intervention starting treatment relatively early in the course of the disease

Eaton-Lambert (e'ton-lam'bert) **syndrome** myasthenic myopathic syndrome, occurs in association with small cell carcinoma of the lung. There is weakness of the pelvic and shoulder gridle muscles, loss of tendon reflexes, and improvement of weakness after exercise named after Lealdes Eaton, American neurologist and Edward Lambert, American Physiologist.

Ebola disease a haemorrhagic fever caused by an RNA virus, first recognised in Zaire on the banks of Ebola river. It presents with gastrointestinal symptoms, arthralgias, and severe diarrhoea, infection spreads by direct contact

ebonation (e'bo-na'shun) removal of bony fragments after injury

ebriety drunkenness

Ebstein's (eb'stinz) **anomaly** tricuspid valve is dysplastic and displaced into right ventricle and right ventricle is atrialised. There is tricuspid regurgitation and there is right atrium to left atrium shunt, named after Wilhelm Ebstein, German physician

ebullism (eb'u-lizm) air embolism at high altitude where the ambient pressure is 47 mmHg or less. There is acute hypoxia and evaporation of body fluids causing widespread air bubble formation in the vessels and tissue

eburnation (eb'ur-na'shun) ivory-like appearance of weight bearing joints with erosion of cartilages, leaving polished, sclerotic bone as the new articular surface

EB virus *see* Epstein-Barr virus

eccentric (eksen'trik) 1. pertaining to an object or activity that departs from usual course or practice 2. pertaining to a behaviour that is odd

eccentricity (ek'sentris'ite) behaviour that is odd for a particular culture

ecchondroma (ek-on-dro'ma) overgrowth of cartilage on a normally situated cartilage

ecchymosis (ek-i-mo'sis) a purplish discolouration from extravasated blood into the skin or mucous membrane. It follows bleeding from a large vessel

ecchymotic (ek-i-mo'tik) pertaining to a discoloured area on the skin or mucous membrane caused by extravasation of blood into the tissue

eccrine (ek'rin) exocrine secretion by cells which remain intact **e gland** sweat glands found in the corium of the skin. They secrete outwardly through a duct to the surface of the skin. They promote cooling by evaporation of their secretions

eccyesis (ek'i-sis) ectopic pregnancy

ECF abbreviation for extracellular fluid

ECF-A abbreviation for eosinophilic chemotactic factor of anaphylaxis

ECG abbreviation for electrocardiogram or graph

echino pertaining to spiny or spines

echinococcosis (e-ki'no-kok-a'sis) echinococcal infestation, hydatid disease

Echinococcus (e-ki'no-kok'us) a small tapeworm whose larval infection forms hydatid cysts. *E. granulosus Taenia echinococcus.* By handling a dog or drinking contaminated water man may ingest eggs. The embryo liberated from the ovum in small intestine reaches the liver sometimes lung and the resultant cyst grows slowly. *E. multilocularis* tapeworm producing multilocular hydatid cysts

echinocyte spiny red cell

echo (ek'o) a repetition of sound produced by reflection of sound waves from an obstructing surface **echo virus** enteric cytopathogenic human orphan virus. An RNA virus belonging to picorna virus family which produces cytopathic effect in cell culture. It presents with upper respiratory tract infections, exanthema and diarrhoea

echocardiogram (ek'o-kor'do-o-gram) the ultrasonic record of the movement of the heart produced by echocardiography

echocardiography (ek'o-kar'de-og'ra-fe) a two-dimensional imaging technique using Doppler ultrasonography that provides information on pressure differences and blood flow in the heart and great vessels. The blood flowing through the heart produces sound, some of which is reflected back by each acoustic interface the blood encounters (Doppler effect) which is received by a transducer; the time elapsed between the sound transmission to the time that the echo is received is converted to a display and there is production of an imaging plane with construction of two-dimensional echocardiogram which is useful in evaluating cardiovascular disorders

echoencephalogram (ek'o-en-sef'a-logram) recording of the ultrasonic echoes of the brain, useful in determining the cause of shift in midline structures of the brain

echogenic (ek'o-gen'i-k) surface reflecting high frequency sound waves

echolalia (ek'o-la'le-a) the repetition by a person of words or phrases spoken by others. It may be spoken with a mocking or staccato intonation

echopraxia pathological imitation of movements of one person by another

eciectic selecting what seems best available treatment

Eck's (eks) **fistula** an artificial communication between the portal vein and the inferior vena cava, named after N. Eck, Russian physiologist

eclabium (ek-la'be-um) eversion of a lip or lips

eclampsia (e-klamp'se-a) toxaemia of pregnancy noted in late pregnancy, labour or the immediate puerperium, characterised by convulsions, hypertension albuminuria, hypoproteinaemia, raised blood urea nitrogen, haemoconcentration and sodium retention with oedema

eclipse the period between the time a cell is infected by a virus and the production of intracellular progeny

ecmnesia (ek-ne'ze-a) loss of memory for recent events

ECMO abbreviation for extracorporeal membrane oxygenation

eco- referring to environment

ecology (e-kol'o-je) biologic science concerned with the inter-relationship between organisms, and environment **e of health** health as a state of dynamic equilibrium between man and his environment

econozole an imidazole antifungal agent useful for the topical therapy of superficial fungal infections

ecosphere (ek'o-sfer') the portions of the universe habitable by living organism and plant life

ecstasy (ek'sta-se) a feeling of intense rapture.

ECT electroconvulsive therapy; electric shock treatment

-ectasia a suffix to refer dilatation of any tubular structure.

-ectasis a suffix to refer dilatation especially of tubular structures

ecthyma (ek-thi'ma) a pyogenic infection of the skin with ulcers covered by adherent crusts

ecto-combining word for outer; outside

ectocardia (ek'to-kar'de-a) congenital displacement of the heart

ectoderm (ek'to-derm) the outermost germ layer of cells in the embryo. It gives rise to epidermis, teeth, tongue, palate, salivary glands, anogenital region, hypophysis, nervous system and sensory organs such as eyes, ears and nose

ectodermal relating to or derived from the ectoderm **e dysplasia** a familial defect of multiple ectodermal tissues such as teeth, hair, sweat glands and skin associated with mental defect

ectomorph (ek'to-morf) a body constitution or build where the tissues that originated from the ectoderm are prominent such as limbs over the trunk and the individual is long, lean and lanky. Diseases such as peptic ulcer, mental disorders, ulcerative colitis, irritable colon and neurologic disorders are more common in such individuals

-ectomy a suffix to refer removal of any structure or excision

ectopagia (ek-op'-agea) conjoined twins which are united along the side of the body

ectoparasite (ek'to-par'a-sit) a parasite that lives on the surface of the host's body

ectopia (ek-to'pe-a) congenital displacement or of malposition of any organ or part of the body **e lentis** displacement of lens of the eye **e vesicae** extroversion of the bladder

ectopic (ek-top'ik) aberrant; located away from normal place **e beats** extrasystoles **e hormone** a hormone is considered ectopic if there is an abnormal endocrine function demonstrable by biochemical and clinical evidence and coexistence of a tumour. It is considered as a paraneoplastic syndrome **e pregnancy** the implantation of an embryo in sites anywhere outside the uterus not designed to accommodate the massive vascular supply needed by a growing foetus **e secretion** the secretion of a hormone by a tumour arising from tissues that do not normally secrete the hormone. **e testis** maldescended testis

ectopiotomy removal of ectopic pregnancy by laparotomy

ectostosis (ek-tos-to'sis) ossification of cartilage beneath the perichondrium

ectothrix (ek'to-thriks) a form of tinea capitis with presence of fungal spores as a sheath outside the hair and their growth within the hair

ectozoon (ek-to-zo'on) ectoparasite

ectrocheiry partial or total absence of a hand

ectrodactyly (ek'-ro-dak-til-e) congenital absence of one or more digits or of only part of a digit

ectrogeny (ek-troj'e-ne) congenital absence of any part

ectromelia (ek'tro-me'le-a) congenital absence of one or more limbs

ectropion (ek-tro'pe-on) the abnormal eversion of the margin of a part especially of an eyelid

ectropody (ek-tro'pode) partial or total absence of a foot

eczema (ek'ze-ma) a superficial inflammation affecting the epidermis which manifests in redness, itching, weeping, oozing and crusting **asteatotic e** 'crazy paving' pattern of fine fissuring on an erythematous background in the legs in elderly with dry skin **atopic e** a generalised and prolonged hypersensitivity to common environmental antigens. The individuals exhibit a genetic predisposition to form excessive IgE **discoid e** discrete coin-shaped lesions of eczema on the limbs of young one **dyshidrotic e** recurrent vesicles and bullae over palms, palmar surface of the fingers and soles, that is very itchy **gravitational e** eczema on the legs and is often associated with signs of venous insufficiency; stasis eczema **irritant e** detergents, alkalis, acid and solvents producing reaction at the site of contact **napkin e** eczema in babies due to irritant ammoniacal urine and faeces **seborrhoeic e** eczema unrelated to seborrhoea, affects the scalp, ears, central face and nasolabial folds

eczematoid (ek'ze-ma-toyd) resembling eczema

eczematous (ek-zem'a-tus) affected with eczema

edema oedema.

edentate (e-den't-ate) toothless

edentulous (e-dent'u-lus) without teeth

edge a border at which a surface ends

edible (ed'i-bl) fit to eat

Edinger-Westphal (ed'ing-ger-vest'fahl) **nucleus** nucleus of the oculomotor nerve in the midbrain from which parasympathetic supply to pupils and ciliary muscles arise, named after Edinger Carl Westphal, German neurologist

EDRF endothelium-dependent relaxing factor. It is the nitric oxide produced by endothelium

edrophonium bromide a short-acting anticholinesterase useful as a diagnostic aid in myasthenia gravis. There is improvement in muscular power following its intravenous administration

EDTA ethylene diaminetetraacetic acid. A chelating agent that binds substances like calcium, lead, magnesium and arsenic. It is used to treat lead and other heavy metal intoxication. It is added to specimen tubes in the laboratory to transport specimens

Edward's syndrome chromosomal disorder with trisomy 18(47 XY) with characteritic skull and facies, malformations of heart, kidney and other organs, named after J. Edward, UK genetist

EEC syndrome an autosomal dominant dysplastic syndrome characterised by ectodactyly, ectodermal dysplasia and cleft lip and/or palate

EEG abbreviation for electroencephalogram

EFA abbreviation for essential fatty acid

efface (e-fas') to wipe out; destroy

effacement a thinning and pulling back of cervical opening to facilitate movement of the foetus from the uterus

effect (e-fekt') the result produced by an action; result

effector a muscle or a gland which contracts or secretes respectively in response to a nerve impulse

effemination (e-fem'i-na'shun) feminisation

efferent conveying from a centre e nerve a nerve that conveys impulses away from the brain or spinal cord to muscles or glands

efflorescence (ef'flore-res'ens) a rash or eruption of the skin

efflorescent becoming powdery

effluvium (ef-loo've-um) disagreeable emanation

effuse (e-fus') spread out; to pour out

effusion (e-fu'zhun) the escape of a fluid into a cavity or space

egesta (e-jes'ta) undigested material thrown out from the body

egg female reproductive cell; ovum

egg-shaped heart globoid heart shadow on a chest radiograph of young children with transposition of great vessels. There is a large venticular shadow and a small 'waist' due to the abnormal location of the aorta directly in front of the pulmonary artery, with a ventricular septal defect

egg shell calcification a radiologic abnormality wherein mediastinal and hilar lymph nodes exhibit a thin wall of calcium, seen in silicosis and sarcoidosis

ego (e'go) the conscious sense of the self

egoism (e'go-izm) over-evaluation of the self

egomania (e'go-ma'ne-a) pathological-preoccupation

egress exit, going our

Ehrlichia an obligate intracellular coccobacillus that has a tropism for either macrophages or granulocytes where it grows within cytoplasmic membrane-bound vacuoles. The genus bears the name of German chemist Paul Ehrlich

ehrlichiosis a tick-borne zoonosis a mild to severe multisystem illness from *E. chaffensis* or granulocytic ehrlichiosis sp. Responds to tetracycline or doxycycline

Ehrlich's test test to demonstrate urobilinogen in the urine

EHEC Enterohaemorrhagic *Escherichia coli* producing toxin to cause bloody inflammatory diarrhoea and a haemolytic uraemic syndrome

Ehlers-Danlos (a'lerz-dan'los) **syndrome** an inherited autosomal dominant trait characterised by skin laxity, hypermobility of joints, scoliosis, skin bruising and visceral vascular catastrophies, named after Edvard Ehlers, Danish dermatologist and Henri Danlos, French dermatologist

EIA abbreviation for enzyme immunoassay.

eicosanoid A 20-carbon cyclic fatty acid derived from arachidonic acid synthesised from membrane phospholipids

eicosapentaenoic acid fatty acid of fish oil, prostaglandin precursor

eidatic images visual memories of almost hallucinatory vividness

EIEC Enteroinvasive *Escherichia coli* a serotype of *E. coli* producing inflammatory dysentery

eighth cranial nerve *see* vestibulocochlear nerve

eiknometry determination of the distance of an object by measuring the image produced by a lens of known focus

Einstein (in-stin) **sign** a ruptured aortic aneurysm mimicking biliary colic as in Albert Einstein's case

Eisenmenger's (i'sen-meng'erz) **syndrome** a condition that develops when increased pulmonary flow due to an initial left-to-right shunt produces severe pulmonary hypertension and reversal of the shunt. On establishment the raised pulmonary resistance is irreversible. There is development of central cyanosis and digital clubbing. ECG shows right ventricular hypertrophy, named after Victor Eisenmenger, German physician

eisodie (i-sod'e) afferent

ejaculation (e-jak'u-la'shun) 1. a sudden act of expulsion 2. an abrupt exclamatory utterance 3. the release of semen from penis at orgasm **electro-e** a technique for inducing ejaculation by direct electrical stimulation of the efferent nerves innervating the seminal vesicles and the terminal vas **premature e** persistent or recurrent ejaculation with minimal sexual stimulation that occurs before, during or shortly after penetration and before person wishes it **retrograde e** failure of reflex closure of the internal urethral sphincter enabling backward ejaculation

ejaculatory duct the terminal portion of seminal duct

ejection click a cardiac sound heard in early systole that may be so close to the first heart sound that simulates a splitting **aortic ec** best heard at left lower sternal border in aortic stenosis, Fallot's tetrology and truncus arteriosus **midsystolic ec** heard at the apex preceding a late systolic murmur in mitral valve prolapse **pulmonary ec** best heard at the left mid-sternum and disappears with inspiration, in pulmonary stenosis

ejection fraction the volume of the blood in the ventricles that is effectively ejected forward during systole

ejaculate to eject suddenly and swiftly

ELAM endothelial leucocyte adhesion molecule. An endothelial glycoprotein that mediates neutrophil adhesions

elapid any of the snakes of the family Elapidae which have erect fangs in front of the upper jaw

elastance elastic resistance of the lung, reciprocal expression of compliance expressed as cm of water pressure change per litre of volume change

elastase (e-las'tas) an enzyme catalysing the digestion of elastic tissue

elastic (e-las'tik) resilient, capable of returning to its original shape and length after being stretched **e bandage** a bandage that can be stretched on application to exert continuous pressure **e cartilage** yellow cartilage seen in external ears, epiglottis, and pharynx **e skin** unusually elastic skin **e stocking** a stocking worn to apply pressure to the extremity facilitating return of blood to the heart **e tissue** connective tissue with elastic fibres.

elasticity (e'las-tis'i-te) a quality of being elastic

elastin (e-las'tin) a fibrous protein similar to collagen, this rubbery substance is found in arterial walls, vocal cords, alveolar septa and ligaments

elastolysis digestion of elastic tissue

elastoma (e'las-to'ma) hypertrophy or tumour of elastic tissue

elastosis (e-los-to'sis) local overgrowth of elastic tissue

elation (e-la'shun) joyful emotion

elbow (el'bo) the bend of the arm; connection between the arm and forearm; cubitus **e joint** the joint between the arm and the forearm; it consists of humeroulnar, humeroradial and proximal radioulnar articulations

elective a procedure that is not an emergency **e surgery** any surgical procedure that can be undertaken with advanced planning

electra complex *Psy* the daughter perceives the mother as a rival, Electra of Greek mythology killed both her mother and her mother's lover as a retaliation for the murder of her father.

electrical alternans marked swings in the amplitude of the QRS complex in the electrocardiogram that occurs every second or third beat from a circus movement in the myocardium

electrical shock therapy *see* electroconvulsive therapy

electric shock injury from electricity

electroanatomic mapping a nonfluoroscopic mapping system using a special catheter to generate 3-D electroanatomic maps of the heart chamber

electrocardiogram (e-lek'tro-kar'de-o-gram) a graphic record of the electric current produced by the excitation of the cardiac muscle; ECG, EKG

ECG

electrocardiograph (e-lek'tro-kar'de-o-graf) an instrument to make electrocardiograms

electrocardiography producing graphic records of the electrical activity of the heart muscle **ambulatory e** recording of the electrical activity of the heart over extended period with the patient engaged in all his routine activity **dynamic e** ambulatory electrocardiography **exercise e** the recording of the electrical activity of the heart while the individual is subjected to the stress of graded exercises performed by bicycle ergometer or the treadmill

electrocautery (e-lek'tro-kaw'ter-e) a platinum wire which when heated by an electric current cauterises the tissues

electrocoagulation (e-lek'tro-ko-ag'u-la'shun) coagulation of a tissue by high frequency electric current. It seals blood vessels to prevent bleeding

electrocochleography (e-lek'tro-kok-le-og'ra-fi) recording of action potentials of cochlea using needle electrode on round window

electroconvulsive (e-lek'tro-kon-vul'siv) inducing convulsions by electric shock **e therapy** ECT *Psy* iatrogenic induction of generalised tonic-clonic seizures for treating depression

electrocution (e-lek'tro-ku'shun) to kill by passage of electric current through the body

electrode (e-lek'trod) a medium between an electric conductor and the part to which the current is to be applied

electroencephalogram (e-lek'tro-en-sef'a-lo-gram) EEG, a graphic record of the electrical activity of the brain

electroencephalograph (e-lek-tro-en-sef'a-lo-graf) an instrument to undertake electroencephalography

electroencephalography the recording and study of the electrical activity of the brain

electroimmunodiffusion an enzyme immune assay in which an antigen containing fluid is electrophoresced through agarose containing antiserum to the antigen of interest

electrolysis (e'lek-trol'i-sis) destruction by passage of an electric current, used in permanent removal of unwanted hair

electrolyte (e-lek'tro-lit) 1. a solution that conducts electricity 2. an ionised salt in the blood, tissue fluids and cells which include sodium, potassium and chlorine

electromyogram (e-lek'tro-mi'o-gram) (EMG) a graphic record of the electric currents associated with muscular action

electromyography (e-lek'tro-mi-og'ra-fe) recording and study of the electrical activity in muscle

electron an elementary particle with a negative electrical charge

electron-dense a density preventing penetration of electrons

electronic foetal monitoring use of electronic or pressure sensitive devices for the measurement of the foetal heart rate and woman's uterine contractions during labour

electro-oculogram (e-lek'tro-ok'u-lo-gram) a graphic recording of the movement of the eyes; EOG

electrophoresis (e-lek-tro-for-e'sis) the motion of the colloid particles suspended in a liquid under the influence of an applied electric field, useful in identification of proteins

electrophoretic relating to electrophoresis

electroporation the use of a pulsed electric field to introduce DNA into cells in culture

electroretinogram tracing of retinal potential response to light using one electrode on cornea or conjunctiva and another on forehead

electrotherapy (el'ek-tro'the-ra-pi) treatment procedures that use electromagnetic energy either by direct application to the body or by placing the relevant part of the body in an electromagnetic field

elemental diet a basic diet consisting of oligopeptides and aminoacids, disaccharides and minimum amount of fat, used in patients with severe burns

elementary body Chlamydia species on entry into the cell, the perinuclear elementary bodies attach to specific membrane receptors on the host cell

elephantiasis (el'e-fan-ti'a-sis) cutaneous induration due to lymphatic obstruction. It may occur in legs or scrotum due to filariasis, in the penis and scrotum due to lymphogranuloma venereum or in the arms following axillary lymph node dissection in radical mastectomy

elevator an instrument for elevating tis-

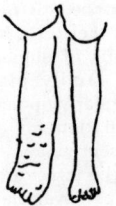

Elephantiasis

sues **e testicle** migrating testicle that is highly mobile in the inguinal canal and it may even migrate into the abdominal cavity **e neuromatosa** neurofibromatosis associated with deep, diffuse and massive lesions causing broad-based hanging of tissue filled with neurofibromas **e nostra** pseudoelephantiasis; an inflammation, oedema or obstruction of the scrotal lymphatics in temperate climate due to non-filarial infections such as granuloma inguinale, lymphogranuloma venereum, syphilis, tuberculosis or streptococcal infections

elevated mood air of confidence and enjoyment: a mood more cheerful than normal

eleventh cranial nerve *see* spinal accessory nerve

elfin face syndrome an idiopathic hypercalcaemic disorder with possibly hypovitaminosis D exhibiting a characteristic facies such as small mandible, prominent maxilla, an upturned nose, depressed nasal bridge, anteverted nares, medial eyebrow flare, a 'cupid's bow' upper lip, short palpebral fissures, carious peg teeth. It is associated with feeding difficulties, failure to thrive, supravalvular aortic stenosis and septal defect

elicit to draw forth, to evoke

elimination the act of expulsion

eligible couples a currently married couple wherein the wife is in the reproductive age (between ages of 15 to 45) who are in need of family planning services **e c register** a basic document giving details of eligible couples for organising family planning works which is regularly updated for the area

ELISA abbreviation for enzyme-linked immunosorbent assay

elixer (e-lik'ser) a sweet aromatic solution which acts as a vehicle for medicinal substances

ellipsoid (e-lip'soyd) a spindle shape

elliptocyte (e-lip-to-sit) a red blood cell with elliptical or ovoid shape

Embden-Meyerhof pathway major source of energy in the form of ATP in cells which involves conversion of glucose 6-phosphate via triose phosphates to pyruvate, named after Gustav Embden and Otto Meyerhof, German biochemists

embedding the process by which a piece of tissue is placed in paraffin, it is used to cut into thin section for microscopic examination

Ellis plate plate for internal fixation of fractures of long bone, named after J. Ellis, British orthopaedic surgeon

Ellis's (el'i-sez) **curve** the level of dullness in pleural effusion, is highest in the axillary region from which it slopes down in front and back assuming an S-shape, named after Calvin Ellis, US physician

Ellis-van Creveld (el'is-vahn-kre'veld) **syndrome** a rare autosomal disorder exhibiting dwarfism, extra fingers and malformations of the heart named after Richard Ellis, Scottish paediatrician and Simon van Creveld, Dutch paediatrician

elongation (e'long-ga'shun) the process of lengthening

El tor subtype of cholera vibrio first isolated in eltro quarantine station, Egypt.

elute (el'u-at) the substance separated out

emaciation a wasting of the body

e-mail electronic mail. Electronic messages sent from one computer to another through the Internet or a network.

emanation that which is given of

embalming (em'bam'ing) the treatment of the dead body with preservatives and antiseptics so as to preserve it

embole (em'bo-le) reduction of a dislocation

embolectomy (em'bo-lek'to-me) surgical removal of an embolus from a blood vessel

embolisation therapy use of emboli introduced by selective arteriography catheter to treat bleeding points, AV fistulas and vascular tumours

embolism (em'bo-lizm) the sudden obstruction of an artery by a clot or foreign material which has been brought by circulation from a different side **air e** presence of gas in the coronary or cerebral arteries and 100 ml of gas can kill a person. There is bubbling when the organ is opened under water during autopsy **amniotic fluid e** embolism of amniotic fluid through the communication in the maternal circulation **fat e** long bone fractures leads to the entry of fat into the lungs causes ARDS, and to the brain causes coma **nitrogen e** noted in divers who surface too rapidly where the nitrogen boils in the vessels causing joint and abdominal pain **paradoxical e** an embolus that migrates in the direction opposite to the blood flow, a complication of right-to-left shunt in congenital heart disease, especially through a patent foramen ovale **pulmonary e** condition associated with the obstruction of pulmonary artery by thrombus arising from an extrapulmonary source. It occurs as a potential lethal complication of deep vein thrombosis in the legs or pelvis

embolus (em'bo-lus) a clot or other material carried by the blood stream and impacted in some part of the vascular system

embolysis (em-bol'i-sis) the dissolution of an embolus, especially a blood clot

embryo (em'bre-o) the entity prior to the time at which all organs are developed, at about the eighth week after conception

embryogenesis (em'bre-oj'e-ne-sis) the process of embryo formation

embryoid body a germ cell tumour containing an embryonal disk, an amniotic sac and an amniotic cavity

embryology the science dealing with the study of development of the individual during the embryonic stage

embryoma (em-bre-o'ma) neoplasm derived from embryonic cells

embryonic (em'bre-on'ik) of or pertaining to the embryo

embryopathy (em'bre-op'a-the) developmental anamolies from interference with normal embryonic development

embryotome (em'bre-o-tom) a cutting instrument used in embryotomy

embryotomy (em'bre-ot'o-me) the dismemberment of the foetus in the uterus or vagina

emergency an accident; urgent; sudden unforeseen incident requiring immediate action **e oral contraception** combined oral contraceptives used soon after unprotected sexual intercourse to prevent pregnancy

Emery-Dreifuss (em'e-re-dri'fes) **dystrophy** an X-linked muscular dystrophy characterised by slowly progressive muscular weakness, contractures and cardiomyopathy named after Alan Emery, British geneticist and F.E. Dreifuss, British physician

emesis (em'e-sis) vomiting; act of vomiting

emetic (e-met'ik) an agent that induces vomiting

emetine (em'e-ten) alkaloid from ipecacuanha root, used as amoebicide and emetic

EMG abbreviation for electromyogram

eminence a prominence; projection

eminentia (em'in-en'she-a) an eminence

emissary (em'i-sa-re) an outlet **e vein** a small vein that pierces the skull. It carries blood from the sinuses within the skull to the veins outside it

emission (e-mish'un) a discharge

emit to utter, to voice, to give out

emmenia (e'me'ne-a) menstruation

emmeniopathy (e-me'ne-op'a-the) any disorder of menstruation

emmetropia (em'e-tro'pe-a) normal refraction of the eye

emollient (e-mol'yent) having softening or soothing effect

emotion (e-mo'shun) a mental state experiencing joy, sorrow, fear, hate, love or the like

emotional pertaining to the emotions

empathy (em'pa-the) ability to see the world from the client's perspective

emphysema (em'fi-se'ma) inflation, abnormal distension of an organ or part **centriacinar e** destruction of the wall of respiratory bronchioles of the first or second order and of peribronchiolar alveoli and the alveolar duct and they are converted into abnormal airspaces. Changes seen in men and associated with chronic bronchitis and cigarette smoking **distal acinar e** predominant involvement of distal part of the acinus, alveolar ducts and sacs in emphysematous changes **mediastinal e** air inside the mediastinal space following chest injury or secondary to rupture of an emphysematous bulla, usually associated with surgical emphysema. There is pain or feeling of tightness over the sternum **e lung** abnormal permanent enlargement of the airspaces distal to the terminal bronchioles accompanied by destructive changes of the alveolar walls and without fibrosis **panacinar e** destruction of the wall of alveolar ducts and alveoli and there is involvement of all components of the acinus in a uniform manner, commonly assoicated with alpha-1 antiprotease deficiency **senile e** with age there is thinning of the alveolar walls resulting in the enlargement of alveoli and bronchioles, not associated with airway obstruction **subcutaneous** (surgical) **e** a crackling sound and crepitus due to displacement of gas bubbles or air in the subcutaneous tissue or in the underlying muscles

emphysematous bullae small air-filled cysts often seen in the lungs of patients with emphysema

empiric (em-pir'ik) conclusions derived from or other's self-experience

empirical (em-pir'ik-al) acceptance of observed fact

empty calorie a unit of food-derived energy, usually in the form of carbohydrates, devoid of protein, vitamins, or dietary fibres. The junk foods are examples

empty sella syndrome a moderately enlarged sella turcica due to a partial or complete absence of the sellar diaphragm. Clinically it may present with headaches, systemic hypertension, pseudotumour cerebri or it may remain asymptomatic

empyema (em'pi-e'ma) a collection of pus in a body cavity **e thoracis** a collection of suppurative material in the pleural space characterised by opaque appearance, foul odour or demonstration of organisms in Gram stain **e necessitans** a swelling in the side of the chest in conditions of empyema which exhibits an impulse on coughing

empyesis (em'pi-e'sis) any skin eruption with accumulation of pus.

emulsification (e-mul'si-fi-ka'shun) 1. the process of making an emulsion 2. the breaking down of large fat globules in the intestine into smaller uniformly distributed particles

emulsifier an agent used to produce an emulsion

emulsion a preparation of one liquid distributed in small globules in another liquid

emulsive capable of emulsifying a substance

enalapril an angiotensin-converting enzyme inhibitor with a vasodilator activity useful in improving haemodynamic indices and the symptoms of congestive heart failure

enamel (en-am'el) white, hard calcareous substance that covers and protects the corner of a tooth

enanthema (en-an'thema) an eruption upon a mucous membrane

enantiodromia (en'anti'o-dro-mia) inherent tendency of all homoeostatic systems to transform into its opposite; spontaneous reversal

enarthrosis (en'ar-thro'sis) ball and socket joint.

en bloc (en block) as a whole; entirety **e resection** surgical removal of the entire primary lesion, the contiguous draining lymph nodes and other structures lying in between, in certain malignancies

encapsulated enclosed within a capsule

encelialgia (en-sel-i-al'jea) pain in the abdominal viscera

encephalalgia (en-sef'al-al'je-a) headache

encephalatrophy (en-sef'a-lat'ro-fe) atrophy of the brain

encephalaemia (en-sef'a-le-mia) congestion of the brain

encephalitis (en-sef'a-li'tis) inflammation of the substance of the brain **Japanese B e** caused by a specific arbovirus, transmitted to man by bite of infected culecine mosquitoes (*Culex tritaenorhynchus*) and the reservoir of infection is pigs. Children are more prone and may present with febrile headache type, meningitic type and encephalitic type with severe headache, fever, vomiting, twitchings, muscular rigidity, convulsions, carries high mortality and corticosteroids are useful

encephalocoele (en-sef'a-lo-sel) a gap in the skull leading to hernia of the brain

encephalogram (en-sef'a-lo-gram) a roentgenogram of the head

encephalomalacia (en-sef'a-lo-ma-la'se-a) softening of the brain

encephalomeningitis (en-sef'a-lo-men'in-ji'tis) inflammation of the brain and its membranes

encephalomeningocoele (en'sef'a-lo-mening'go-sel) protrusion of the meninges and brain.

encephalomyelitis (en'sef'a-lo-mi'el-i-tis) inflammation of the brain and spinal cord **acute demyelinating e** may develop in association with viral diseases (measles, chickenpox, mumps) or follow vaccination against rabies. There is massive and widespread demyelination of white matter and is probably caused by immunologic damage. It presents with headache, vomiting, fever, clouding of consciousness, meningeal irritation, convulsions and coma, flaccid paralysis of limbs and cranial nerve palsies. Treatment is supportive

encephalomyelocoele herniation of the meninges, brain and spinal cord

encephalomyelopathy (en-sef'a-lo-mi'el-op'a-the) any disease of the brain and spinal cord

encephalomyeloradiculitis (en-sef'a-lo-mi'e-lo-ra-dik'u-li'tis) inflammation of the brain, spinal cord and spinal nerve roots.

encephalomyeloradiculopathy (en-sef'a-lo-mi'e-lo-ra-dik'u-lop'a-the) any disease affecting the brain, spinal cord and spinal nerve roots

encephalon (en-sef'al-on) the brain

encephalopathy (en-sef'a-lop'a-the) any disorder of the brain that involves widespread destruction or degeneration of brain tissue

encephalorrhagia (en-sef'a-lo-ra'je-a) haemorrhage within the brain

encephalotomy (en-sef'a-lot'o-me) the destruction of the foetal head to facilitate delivery

enchondroma (en'kon-dro'ma) a benign hypertrophy of a cartilage arising in the metaphysis of a bone

enchondromatosis (en'kon-dro'ma-to'sis) proliferation of the cartilage within the metaphyses of several bones

encode *mol* the process of reading a message from a segment of DNA nucleotides, transcribing that message into code for a messenger RNA from a structural gene in the process to obtain a mature protein

encopresis (en'co-pres'is) repeated passage of faeces into inappropriate places

encysted (en-sist'ed) enclosed in a sac or cyst **e effusion** collection of fluid which is walled off in the pleural space

end point an event used by a clinical trial to evaluate whether a trial therapy is working

endarterectomy (end'ar-ter-ek'to-me) surgical removal of the thickened, atheromatous *tunica intima* of an artery to restore normal blood flow

endarteritis (end-ar-ter-i'tis) an inflammation of the innermost layer of an artery.

endarterium (end-ar-ter-i'um) the innermost layer (*tunica intima*) of an artery

end-artery the artery having no anastomosis

end-bulb the terminal portion of a sensory nerve

endemic constant existence of a disease or infectious agent in a locality at all times, without importation from outside **e goitre** thyroid swelling in areas of iodine deficiency

Enders's (en'derz) **nail** nail for internal fixation of intertrochanteric hip fractures, ,named after J. Enders', Austrian orthopaedic surgeon

ending a termination

endobronchitis (en'do-brong-ki'tis) inflammation of the epithelial lining of the bronchi

endocardial situated within the heart

endocarditis (en'do-kar-di'tis) infection of the endocardium and heart valves. **infective e** caused by bacteria **non-bacterial e** sterile platelet or fibrin thrombi on damaged cardiac valve. There is sterile emboli, negative blood culture and valvular vegetations in chronically ill-patient, requires anticoagulants

endocardium the serous membrane that lines the cavities of the heart

endocervical (en'do-ser'vi-kal) referring to the interior of the uterine cervix

endocervicitis (en'do-ser'vi-si'tis) inflammation of the uterine cervix

endocervix (en'do-ser'viks) the mucous membrane lining uterine cervical canal

endochondral (en'do-kon'dral) occurring within cartilage

endocommensal an organism living inside the body

endocranial (en'do-kra'ne-al) situated within the cranium

endocranium (en'do-kra'ne-um) duramater, the inner lining membrane of the skull.

endocrine (en'do-krin) secreting internally **e gland** a gland that secretes hormones directly into the blood stream **e system** a group of ductless glands and tissues that secrete hormones directly into the blood stream to regulate the function of specific tissues or organs or of the entire body

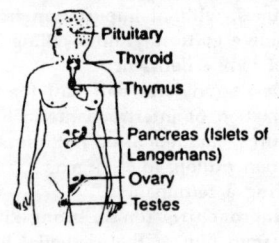

Pituitary
Thyroid
Thymus
Pancreas (Islets of Langerhans)
Ovary
Testes

Endocrine Glands

endocrinologist a specialist in endocrinology

endocrinology (en'do-krin-ol'o-je) branch of medical science dealing with the endocrine glands and their secretions

endocyst (en'do-sist) the inner germinative layer of the hydatid cyst

endocyte any cell inclusion

endoderm (en'do-derm) entoderm. The innermost of the embryo's primary germ layers. It develops into the lining of the mouth, pharynx, gastrointestinal and respiratory tracts, liver, gall bladder and pancreas

endodermal sinus tumour an ovarian tumour of female children and adoles-

cents characterised by a large tumour mass composed of a meshwork of cuboidal cells recapitulating the embryonic yolk sac and elevated levels of alpha-fetoprotein; yolk sac tumour

endodontics (en'do-don-tik's) the branch of dentistry concerned with disorders affecting the dental pulp, and root

endodontist a dentist specialised in endodontics

endodontitis (en'do-don-ti'tis) pulpitis

endogamy (en-dog'a-me) inbreeding

endogastric (en'do-gas'trik) pertaining to the interior of the stomach

endogenous (en-doj'e-nus) originating within; arising from inside the body

endolymph (en'do-limf) the fluid within the membranous labyrinth of the ear

endometrial polyp a growth arising from the lining of the uterus

endometriosis (en'do-me-tre-o'sis) a disorder in which fragments of uterine mucous membrane occurs in locations outside the uterus

endometritis (en'do-me-tri-tis) inflammation of the endometrium

endometrium (en-do-me'tre-um) the mucous membrane lining the inner surface of the uterus. It increases in thickness during each menstrual cycle and is shed during menstruation

endometroid tumour an adenocarcinoma that histologically mimics that of primary endometrial carcinoma. It develops in the ovary and prostate

endometry (en-dom'e-tre) the measurement of the capacity of a cavity

endomorph (en'do-morf) a body configuration with soft round contours and well-developed cutaneous tissue. The extreme variety is considered obese. Certain diseases like diabetes mellitus, hypertension, gall stones and osteoarthritis are more common in such individuals

endomyocardial biopsy a biopsy of the endocardium and subjacent myocardium

endomyocardial fibrosis EMF a distinct form of heart disease leading to restrictive filling of the ventricles and cardiac failure. There is marked thickening of the endocardium due to the deposition of dense fibrous tissue composed of waxy bundles of collagen causing tricuspid and mitral regurgitation

endonasal within the nose.

endoneural referring to or situated within a nerve

endonuclear within a cell nucleus

endonuclease (en'do-nu'kle-as) any of a group of hydrolytic enzymes that attack specific internal DNA and RNA oligo-nucleotide sequences

endoparasite a parasite living within the body of the host

endophthalmitis (en'dof-thal-mi'tis) inflammation of the inside of the eye and its adjacent structures

Endophytic (en'do-fy-tik) growing inward from the skin surface

endoplasm the central portion of the cytoplasm of a cell

Endoplasmic reticulum cytoplasm membrane that holds ribosomes

endoplast the nucleus of a cell

end-organ large encapsulated ending of the sensory nerves

endorphins (en-dor'fins) endogenous opioid peptides such as endorphin, leuencephalin, met-encephalin and dynorphin produced in the brain that help in controlling response to pain and stress and improve mood

endosalphinx (en'do-sal'pinks) the mucous membrane of the uterine tube

endoscope (en'do-skop) slender tubular lighted viewing instrument to examine the interior of a hollow viscus or a body cavity

endoscopic retrograde cholangio pancreatography (ERCP) a procedure in which flexible endoscope is inserted through the ampulla of Vater with the injection of radio contrast material to delineate the bile and pancreatic ducts

endoscopy (en-dos'ko-pe) visual inspection of any cavity of the body by an endoscope

endosteitis (en'dos-ti'tis) inflammation of the endosteum

endosteum (en-dos'te-um) the membranous lining of the medullary cavity of a bone

endosteoma (en-dos'te-o'ma) a tumour in the medullary cavity of the bone

endostosis (en'dos-to'sis) bone formation beginning in the cartilage

endothelial (en'do-the'le-al) pertaining to or consisting of endothelium **e leucocyte adhesion molecule** (ELAM) an endothelial glycoprotein that mediates neutrophil adhesion

endothelin one of several peptides obtained from the vascular endothelium, most powerful vasoconstrictor causing prolonged pressor response, stimulating aldosterone release and inhibition of renin release

endotheliosis (en'do-the'le-o'sis) increased growth of endothelium

endothelium (en'do-the'le-um) the single layer of flattened cells lining the cavities of the heart, and of the blood and lymphatic vessels and the serous cavities of the body

endothelioma (en'do-the-le-o'ma) a tumour originating from the endothelium

endothoracic within the thorax.

endothrix (en-do'-thriks) a dermatophyte whose growth and spore formation chiefly occurs within the shaft of the hair.

endotoxin toxin present within the bacterial cell of gram-negative bacteria which is liberated when the microorganism dies and disintegrates. It is a heat-stable lipopolysaccharide which induces release of pyrogens from neutrophils, potentially causing haemorrhagic shock and altering resistance to infection.

endotracheal within or through the trachea **e tube** a narrow plastic tube surrounded by an inflatable cuff that is introduced through the mouth or nose into the trachea to maintain breathing in an unconscious or anaesthetised person

end-plate a flattened discoid expansion at the neuromuscular junction where a myelinated motor nerve fibre joins a skeletal muscle fibre

end-stage renal disease (ESRD), the decompensated stage of chronic renal disease

endurance the ability to withstand extraordinary mental or physical stress for a prolonged period of time

enema (en'e-ma) the introduction of a liquid into the rectum, to stimulate bowel activity **air contrast e** an enema in which thick barium sulphate and air are introduced simultaneously to obtain multiple radiographs of the colon **barium e** introduction of barium sulphate to visualise colon **cleansing e** an enema containing soap water to empty the colon **nutrient e** an enema containing predigested food material **retention e** a small amount of solution (100-200 ml) administered to provide medication, which will not stimulate nerve endings

energy (en'er-je) capacity to work

enervation a section of a nerve

enflagellation (en'flaj-el-la'shun) the formation of flagella

enfleurage (en'flu-raj) a process of producing oils from flowers, used in aroma therapy

engagement entry of the foetal head or presenting part into the pelvis prior to delivery

Englishman's disease chronic bronchitis

engorged (en-gorjd) distended with fluid

engorgement congestion; illness due to accumulation of blood **breast e** condition resulting when more milk accumulates in the breasts than the infant consumes. It may cause the breasts to feel hard, painful and hot

Engram (en'gram) memory traces in the unborn foetus from impressions received from the outside world

engulf to swallow up

enhancement (en-hans'ment) to increase the level of response

enkephalins (en-kef'a-lin) a family of endogenous opioids that are produced in the central nervous system and gastrointestinal tract

enlargement (en-larj'ment) an increase in the size

en masse all together

enolase (e'no-las) a neuroendocrine enzyme that catalyses the formation of high energy phosphoenolpyruvic acid during glycolysis

enophthalmos (en'of-thal'mus) a backward displacement of the eyeball into the orbit

enostosis (en'os-tosis) a bony growth within the cavity of a bone

en plaque a flat, white, fibrous lesion located on the surface of an organ

enriched food fortification of food with vitamins and minerals to compensate for their loss during the refinement

enrichment the addition of nutrients

ensiform (en'si-form) sword-shaped; xiphoid

enstrophe (en'stro-fe) inversion

ENT abbreviation for ear, nose and throat, refers to otorhinolaryngology

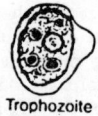
Trophozoite

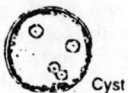
Cyst

Entamoeba histolytica

Entamoeba (en'ta-me'ba) a genus of amoebae. *E coli* common non-pathogen of gut *E. hartmonni* small amoeba related to E histolytica but non-pathogenic E histolytica passes its life cycle in one host-human being. Cysts reach intestine where its encystation occurs as the cyst wall is digested by trypsin. Some mature and burrow their way into submucosa of large and small intestine and cause amoebic ulcers. Some of them enter the portal radicals and reach liver and cause amoebic hepatitis with or without ulcer formation. It may rarely metastasise to lungs or brain. Amoebae are passed in the stools as cysts

enteral (en'ter-al) within, by way of or referring to the small intestine

enterectasis (en'ter-ek-ta-sis) distension of the intestines

enterectomy (en'ter-ok'to-me) resection of the intestine

enteric (en'ter'ik) relating to the small intestine. **e coated** a special coating applied to the tablets whose contents are released only in the intestine **e fever** typhoid and paratyphoid fever

enteritis (en'ter-i'tis) the inflammation of the intestines

enteroanastomosis (en'ter-o-an-as'to-mo'sis) formation of an anastomosis between two portions of the intestine

enterobacter an aerobic gram-negative organism that can produce pneumonia in debilitated persons

enterobacteriaceae (en'ter-o-bak-te're-a'se-e) a genus of gram-negative non-spore forming aerobes. It includes organisms such as shigella, salmonella, klebsiella, prcteus, enterobacter, escherichia and yersinia

enterobiasis (en'ter-o-bi'a-sis) infestation of the intestines by nematodes of the genus Enterobius

Enterobius (en'ter-o'be-us) a genus of intestinal nematodes E. *vermicularis* pinworm, threadworm, or seatworm common small nematode of caecum, gravid female migrates to anus to lay eggs, which after ingestion hatch in duodenum

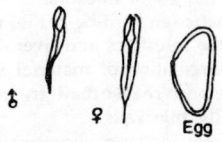

Enterobius vermicularis

enterocoele (en'ter-o-sel) hernia of the intestine through vagina

enterocholecystostomy (en'ter-o-kol'le-sis-tos'to-me) formation of an opening from the gall bladder into the small intestine

enterocinesia (em'ter-o-sin-e'se-a) peristalsis

enteroclysis (en'ter-ok'li-sis) a small bowel radiocontrast study following its administration as an enema

enterococcus (en'ter-o-kok'us) any streptococcus of human intestine

enterocoele (en'ter-o-sel) the body cavity formed by the outpouchings from the primitive gut

enterocolectomy (en'ter-o-ko-lek'to-me) resection of the terminal ileum, caecum and ascending colon

enterocolitis (en'ter-o-ko-li'tis) inflammation of the small intestine and colon

enterocolostomy (en'ter-o-ko-los'to-me) the surgical communication between the small intestine and the colon

enterocyst (en'ter-o-sist) a cyst arising from the peritoneum

enteroenterostomy (en'ter-o-en'ter-os'to-me) surgical anastomosis between two segments of the intestine

enterogastric of or pertaining to the intestine and stomach

enterogastritis (en'ter-o-gas-tri'tis) inflammation of the stomach and the intestines

enterogastrone (en'ter-o-gas'tron) a hormone secreted by the intestinal mucosa which controls the emptying of food from the stomach into the duodenum by depressing gastric motility and secretion

enterogenous (en'ter-oj'e-nus) originating within the small intestine

enterohepatic (en'ter-o-he-pat'ik) pertaining to the intestines and liver. **e circulation** circulation of material secreted in bile and reabsorbed in intestine especially bile salts

enterokinetic (en'ter-o-ki-ne-tik) pertaining to or stimulating peristalsis

enterolith (en'ter-o-lith) an intestinal calculus

enterolysis (en'ter-ol'i-sis) the operative division of adhesions between loops of intestine or between intestine and abdominal wall

enteromegaly (en'ter-o-meg'a-le) enlargement of the intestine

enteron (en'ter-on) alimentary canal or gut

enteropathogen (en'ter-o-path'o-jen) any microorganism which produces a disease of the intestines

enteropathogenic pertaining to production of the disease of the intestines

enteropathic arthritis seronegative polyarthritis associated with ulcerative colitis and Crohn's disease, involves weight bearing joints

enteropathy (en'ter-op'a-the) any disease of the intestine

enteroplegia (en'ter-o-ple'je-a) paralysis of the intestines

enteropexy (en'ter-o-peks'e) surgical fixation of the intestine to the abdominal wall

enteroproctia (en'ter-o-prok'she-a) an artificial anus

enteroptosis (en'ter-op-to'sis) downward displacement of the intestines in the abdominal cavity

enterrhagia haemorrhage from the intestine

enterorrhaphy (en'ter-or'a-fe) repair of the intestine

enterorrhexis (en'ter-o-reks'is) rupture of the intestine

enteroscope (en'ter-o-skop) an endoscope to visualise the lumen of the intestine.

enterostenosis (en'ter-o-ste-no'sis) stricture of the intestine

enterostomy (en'ter-os'to-me) the making of an artificial opening into the intestine which opens into the abdominal wall

enterotome (en-ter-o-tom) cutting forceps.

enterotoxin (en'ter-o-tok'sin) a toxin arising in the intestine; a toxin specific for the cells of intestinal mucosa

enterotropic having an affinity for intestine

enterovaginal communication between intestine and vagina

enterovesical communication between intestine and urinary bladder

enterovirus virus infecting the gastrointestinal tract, belonging to genus of picornoviruses which includes polio-, coxsakie- and echoviruses

enthesis (en'the-sis) utilisation of an artificial material in the repair of a defect; zone of a ligament insertion into the bone

enthesopathy inflammation at the zone of a ligament's insertion into the bone often encountered in HLA-B27-linked ankylosing spondylitis

entity (en'ti-te) an independently existing thing

entoderm (en'to-derm) the innermost primary germ layer of the embryo

entodermal pertaining to or derived from entoderm

entomology (en'to-mol'o-je) the branch of zoology concerned with the study of insects

entoptic (en-top'tik) pertaining to the interior of the eye

entotic (en'to'tik) pertaining to the interior of the ear

entozoon (en'to-zo'on) an animal parasite living within the body of the host

entrain to alter the biologic rhythm

entrapment syndromes a group of neuromuscular syndromes caused by anatomic restriction or compression of peripheral nerve(s). It produces pain, parasthesia, muscle weakness which may progress to muscle atrophy. The important examples are carpal tunnel and tarsal tunnel syndromes

entripsis rubbing

entropion (en-tro'pe-on) a turning inward of an edge or margin such as eyelid margins

enucleate (e-nu'kle-at) to remove in entirety from its enveloping cover; to remove the eyeball surgically

enucleation (e-nu'kle-a'shun) the removal *in toto* from its enveloping capsule, sac or covering.

enunciate to state formally and exactly

enuresis (en'u-re-sis) involuntary discharge of urine; bed-wetting

env a retroviral gene that encodes envelope glycoprotein

envelope (en've-lop) a membranous coat **e appearance** appearance of *Pneumocystis carinii* when stained with Gomori-methenamine silver. The flap of the envelope corresponds to the organism's folded membrane

envenomation (en-ven'o-ma'shun) the introduction of venomus poisons by bites or stings

environment the aggregate of surrounding things, conditions which have influence on existence or development

enzootic (en'zo-t'ik) an endemic occurring in animals

enzymatic relating to or of the nature of an enzyme

enzyme (en'-zim) a complex organic substance having capacity to accelerate or promote chemical changes in a substrate. The examples are oxidoreductases (catalyse oxidation/reduction), transferase (catalyse transfer of one molecular species to another), hydrolase (catalyse hydrolytic cleavage), lysase (catalyse removal or addition of a group to a double bond), isomerase (catalyse intramolecular rearrangement and ligase (catalyse a reaction that joins two molecules) **e blocker** a drug that inhibits the action of an enzyme **e induction** stimulation of increased production of an enzyme

e replacement therapy any of therapeutic modality in which a congenitally defective enzyme is administered, by coupling the enzyme to a carrier molecule or by introducing the gene into the recipient **restriction e** a chemical that snips a specific point on a DNA molecule **e the apy** supplementation of an enzyme such as streptokinase, tissue plasminogen activator or urokinase

enzyme-linked immunosorbent assay (ELISA), a heterogeneous immunoenzyme assay that can be used to measure any antigen and antibody. An antigen of interest is incubated in a medium containing an antibody usually monoclonal, raised against the antigen and bound to a solid phase. A second incubation is carried out with a detector antibody raised against the monoclonal antibody, often with an attached indicator enzyme such as peroxidase or alkaline phosphatase. On addition of a substrate, it is digested by the detector enzyme producing a colour measured by spectrophotometry

eosin (e'o-sin) a red coloured synthetic dye used to stain tissues for microscopic examination

eosinopaenia (e'o-sin-o-pe'ne-a) an abnormal decrease in the number of eosinophils in the blood

eosinophil (e'o-sin'o-fil) a granular leucocyte with a bilobed nucleus and cytoplasm containing coarse round granules. It forms less than 3 per cent of the circulating leucocytes. There is marked affinity for acidic dyes. The granules in mature eosinophils are heterogeneous in their densities. The core of the granules contain the highly toxic cationic proteins

eosinophilia (e'o-sin-o-fil'e-a) an abnormal increase in the number of eosinophils in the blood and it may develop in a variety of conditions (Table 3).

eosinophilic (e'o-sin-o-fil'ik) readily

stainable with eosin e **fasciitis** hardening of the skin and marked thickening of the deep fascia of the extremities, peripheral eosinophilia and hypergamma globulinaemia. The condition may follow strenuous physical exertion and trauma e **granuloma** an abnormal organ infiltration of Langerhans cells seen in young and middle aged adults affecting bones and lungs. There may be osteolytic skull lesions, recurrent pneumothorax and diabetes inspidus; histiocytosis X

eosinophil-myalgia syndrome A syndrome characterised by myalgia, myopathy, arthralgia, angioedema, rash, oral ulcers, dyspnoea, fever, restrictive lung disease, lymphadeno-

Table 3. Conditions associated with peripheral blood eosinophilia

1. Allergic diseases
   Bronchial asthma
   aspirin-sensitive asthma
   Bronchopulmonary aspergillosis
   allergic angiitis and granulomatosis
   atopic dermatitis
   allergic urticaria
   drug hypersensitivity
2. Parasitic infestation
   Tropical pulmonary eosinophilia
   Loffler's syndrome
   Helminthic infestations
   Visceral larva migrans
3. Respiratory disorders
   Chronic eosinophilic pneumonia
   Acute eosinophilic pneumonia
4. Lymphoreticular and neoplastic conditions
   Hodgkin's disease
   Chronic myeloid leukaemia
   Eosinophilic leukaemia
   Ovarian carcinoma
5. Miscellaneous conditions
   Hypereosinophil. syndrome
   Selective IgA deficiency
   Addison's disease
   Eosinophil-myalgia syndrome

pathy and eosinophilia due to an altered amino acid-di-tryptophan aminal acetaldehyde contaminating L-tryptophan

EPA eicosapentanoic acid, a polyunsaturated fatty acid predominantly omega-3 fatty acid

eparterial (ep'ar-te're-al) over an artery

EPEC Enteropathic *Escherichia coli* a serotype of *E. coli* causing epidemic diarrhoea

epencephalon (ep'en-sef-a-lon) the hind brain

ependyma (ep-en'di-ma) a membrane lining the ventricles of the brain and the central canal of the spinal cord

ependymal (ep-en'di-mal) pertaining to or composed of ependyma

ependymoblast (ep-en'di-mo-blast) an embryonic ependymal cell

ependymoblastoma (ep-en'di-mo-bast'oma) a malignant tumour composed of ependymoblasts

ependymoma (ep-en'di-mo'ma) a tumour arising from ependymal cells

ephedrine a sympathomimetic agent, used as a bronchodilator

ephelis (ef-e'lis) freckle, light brown macule that fades in winter and becomes accentuated in summer

ephemeral (e'fem'er-al) short-lived

epiblepharon (ep'i-blef'a-ron) a condition wherein a fold of skin extends along the border of the lower eyelid and presses the eyelashes against the eyeball

epicanthal overlying the canthus

epicanthic fold a fold of skin along the upper eyelid, noted in mongolism

epicanthus a vertical fold of skin on either side of the nose which sometimes covers inner canthus

epicardia (ep'i-kard'e-a) the abdominal portion of the oesophagus

epicardium the inner serous layer of the pericardium on the surface of the heart

epichorion (ep'i-ko're-on) the portion of the decidua of the placenta that covers the ovum

epicondyle (ep-i-kon′di′l) either of the bony eminences above its condyles at the distal end of the humerus

epicondylitis (ep′i-kon′di-li′tis) inflammation of the epicondyle

epicostal situated upon a rib

epicranium the soft tissue covering of the cranium

epicritic (ep-i-krit′ik) discriminative responsiveness to small variations of touch or temperature stimuli

epicystitis inflammation of the structures above the bladder

epicystostomy (ep′i-sis-tot′o-me) suprapubic cutting in the bladder

epidemic (ep′i-dem′ik) affecting a large number of persons in a community at the same time suddenly by disease, or specific health-related behaviour such as smoking or other health-related events such as traffic accidents **e dropsy** contamination of mustard oil with argemone oil. The toxic alkaloid, sanguinarine from argemone oil interferes with the oxidation of pyruvic acid which accumulates in the blood. The condition presents with sudden bilateral swelling of legs, diarrhoea, dyspnoea, glaucoma and cardiac failure. On addition of nitric acid to a sample of oil in the test tube and shaking, there is appearance of brown or orange-red colour in presence of argemone oil **e investigation** investigation to define the magnitude of the epidemic outbreak, to determine the factors responsible and to identify the cause, source of infection and modes of transmission, to determine measures to control the epidemic and to make recommendations to prevent recurrence

epidemiological concerned with epidemiology **e triad** a broader concept of disease causation based on agent, host and environment

epidemiology (ep′i-de-me-ol′o-je) the branch of medical science concerned with the study of the distribution and determinants of health-related states or events in specified populations and the application of this study to the control of health problem

epidermal pertaining to the epidermis

epidermis (ep′i-der′mis) the thin outermost non-sensitive nonvascular layer of the skin

epidermoid (ep′i-der′moyd) resembling epidermis **e cyst** cyst lined by squamous epithelium **e pearl** a compact round cluster of curved and flattened keratinocytes seen in well differentiated squamous cell carcinoma

epidermolysis (ep′i-der-mol′i-sis) a loosened state of the epidermis

epidermomycosis (ep′i-der′mo-mi-ko′sis) dermatophytosis

epidermopoiesis (epi′der-mo′poi-sis) the process of maturation whereby epidermal basal cells become transformed into cornified cells

epidermotropism (epi′der-mo-tro′pizm) the movement of cells toward and into the epidermis

epididymal pertaining to the epididymis

epididymis (ep′i-did′i-mis) the elongated coiled tube at the back of each testes in which sperms mature, and develop their swimming capabilities

epididymitis (ep′i-did′i-mi′tis) inflammation of the epididymis

epididymo-orchitis (ep′i-did′im-o-or-ki′tis) inflammation of the epididymis and testis

epidural situated upon or outside the dura **e anaesthesia** injection of anaesthetic into the epidural spaces to block the nerves for pain relief **e haemorrhage** bleeding between dura mater and the inner suface of the skull **e space** the space outside the dura mater of the brain and spinal cord

epigastric hernia a protrusion through a weakness in the muscles of the epigastrium

epigastrium (ep′i-gas′tre-um) the upper and middle portion of the abdomen lying over the stomach

epigastrocoele (ep′i-gas′tro-sel) hernia of the epigastric region

epigenetic changes which influence the phenotype but have not arisen from alterations in gene structure

epiglottiditis (ep'i-glot'tid-i'tis) inflammation of the epiglottis

epiglottis (ep'i-glot'is) the flap of cartilage structure behind the tongue that covers the entrance to the larynx and helps to prevent food or liquid from being inhaled

epiglottitis inflammation of the epigloitis.

epilate (ep'i-lat) to remove hairs by physical, chemical or radiologic agents

epilation (ep-i-la'shun) the removal of hair by the roots

epilepsy (ep'i-lep'se) a disorder of the brain caused by abnormal electrical activity, characterised by seizures and is a symptom rather than a disease itself **childhood absence e** frequent brief loss of consciousness in childhood **juvenile absence e** less frequent loss of consciousness than childhood absence **juvenile myoclonic e** generalised tonic clonic seizures with loss of consciousness and morning myoclonus in the age 15-20 years **partial e** partial seizures may arise from any disease of cerebral cortex and frequently generalise. The condition implies presence of focal cerebral pathology **primary generalised e** idiopathic epilepsy with onset in childhood or adolescence. There is no structural abnormality and exhibits greater genetic predisposition **secondary generalised e** generalised epilepsy may arise from spread of partial seizures. It is due to structural disease or secondary to drugs or metabolic disorders

epileptic (ep'i-lep'tik) pertaining to or symptomatic of epilepsy

epileptiform (ep'i-lep'ti-form) resembling epilepsy or its manifestations

epileptogenic (ep'i-lep-to-jen'ik) producing epileptic attacks

epiloia (ep'i-loy'a) tuberous sclerosis

epimandibular (ep'i-man-dib'u-lar) situated upon the lower jaw

epimenorrhagia too frequent and too excessive menstruation

epimenorrhoea abnormally frequent menstruation

epinephrine (ep'i-nef'rin) adrenaline. A hormone produced by the adrenal glands. It accelerates heart rate and blood flow, improves breathing and helps the body to cope with demands of exercise.

epineural (ep'i-nu'ral) situated upon a neural arch

epineurium (ep'i-nu're-um) the connective tissue covering of a peripheral nerve

epinychia purulent blister involving the epidermis at the groove of the nail

epinychium cuticle, the narrow band of epidermis that extends from the nail wall onto the nail surface

epiphenomenon (ep'i-fe-nom'e-non) an accidental occurrence during the course of any disease

epiphora (e-pif'o-ra) an abnormal overflow of tears down the cheeks due to stricture of the lacrimal duct

epiphyseal (ep'i-fiz'e-al) pertaining to or of the epiphysis **e cartilage** disc of cartilage at the end of the shaft of long bones during growth which helps in lengthening

epiphysis (e'pif'i-sis) either of the two growing wider ends of the long bones of the upper or lower extremities

epiphysitis (e-pif'i-si'tis) inflammation of an epiphysis

epiplocoele (e-pip'lo-sel) a hernia containing omentum

epiploectomy omentectomy

epiploenterocoele (e-pip'-lo-en'ter-o-sel) a hernia consisting of omentum and intestine

epiploic (ep'i-plo'ik) omental **e foramen** the opening between the greater and lesser omentum

epiploon (e-pip'lo-on) the omentum

episclera (ep'i-skle-ra) the loose connective tissue forming the outer surface of the sclera

episcleral (ep'i-skle'ral) overlying the sclera

episcleritis (ep'i-skle-ri'tis) inflammation of tissues overlying the sclera

episioperineoplasty (e-pis'e-o-per'a-ne'o-plas'te) surgical repair of the vulva and perineum

episioplasty (e-pis'e-o-plas'te) surgical repair of the vulva

episiorrhapy the suturing of the labia majora

episiotomy (e-pis'e-ot'o-me) surgical incision of the vulva to facilitate childbirth

episode a noteworthy incident

epispadias (ep'i-spa'de-as) a congenital defect wherein the urethra opens on the dorsum of the penis, rather than at its tip

episome (ep'i-som) plasmid or plasmid like extrachromosomal DNA which can integrate into the host's chromosome

episplenitis (ep'i-sple-ni'tis) inflammation of the capsule of the spleen

epistaxis (ep'i-stak'sis) haemorrhage from the nose; nose bleed

episternal (ep'i-ster-nal) situated on or over the sternum

epitarsus a fold of conjunctiva passing from the fornix to near the lid margin.

epitendineum (ep'i-ten-din'e-um) the fibrous sheath covering a tendon

epithalamus (ep'i-thal'a-mus) the region above and behind the thalamus

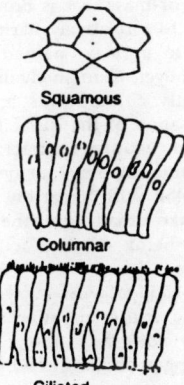

Squamous

Columnar

Ciliated

Epithelial cells

epithelial (ep'i-the'le-al) pertaining to or composed of epithelium

epithelialisation (ep'i-the-le-al-i-za'shun) healing by the growth of epithelium

epithelialise to cover with epithelium

epitheloid (ep'i-the'le-oyd) resembling epithelium **e cells** histiocytes whose morphology mimics large epithelial cells **e granuloma** a granuloma in which multiple histiocytes fuse into giant cells in the background of mononucleated histiocytes and chronic inflammatory cells **e haemangioendothelioma** a tumour of medium-to-large veins composed of endothelial cells that bulge into vascular spaces in a tombstone like fashion **e sarcoma** a low grade soft tissue sarcoma noted in the upper extremity

epithelioma (ep'i-the'le-oma) any tumour derived from epithelium

epithelium (ep'i-the'le-um) the covering of the internal and external surfaces of the body

epitope (ep'i –top) any site on an antigenic determinant that is capable of eliciting antibody formation

epitrochlea (ep'i-trok'le-a) the inner condyle of the humerus

epituberculosis collapse of middle lobe occurring from enlarged glands in tuberculosis. The lobe reexpands following subsidence in the size of the glands. It may lead to stricture of the bronchi

epiturbinate (ep'i-ter-bin-at) the soft tissue covering of a nasal concha

epitympanic situated upon or over the tympanum

epityphlitis (ep'i-tif-li-tis) appendicitis

epityphlon (ep'i-tif-lon) the vermiform appendix

epiozoon (ep'i-zo'on) an animal parasite living upon the surface of the body of the host

epizootic a disease affecting many animals in any region at the same time

epomithic an outbreak of disease in a bird population

eponym (ep'o-nim) any syndrome, lesion, clinical sign, diagnostic or treatment procedure that bears the name of the author who first described the entity or less commonly the name of the index patient in whom the lesion was first described or the place where the disease entity was recognised

epiphoron (ep'o-of'o-ron) a vestigeal structure consisting of mesonephric tubes associated with the ovary

Epstein-Barr virus (EBV) a DNA herpes virus associated with aplastic anaemia, infectious mononucleosis, Burkitt's lymphoma, hairy cell leukaemia histiocytic sarcoma in renal transplantation and immune compromise, named after M.A. Epstein, British physician and Y.M. Barr, Canadian physician

equilibrium constant a value that reflects the concentrations of the reactants and products of a chemical reaction when it has reached a steady state, expressed as 'K' value

epulis (ep-u'lis) a growth on the gingiva

Epworth sleepiness scale subjective measure of sleep propensity

equilibrium a state of balance

equine (e'kwin) pertaining to or derived from the horse

equinovarus (e'kwi'no-va'rus) a form of club foot, walking without touching the heel to the ground and with the sole turned inwards

equivalent (e'kwi'v-lent) equal in power, force or value

equivocal of uncertain significance

era a period in time

eradication termination of transmission of infection by extermination of the infectious agent through surveillance and containment

Erb's area the third left interspace lateral to the sternum, often referred as second aortic or the early neoaortic area, named after Wilhelm Erb, German physician. The early diastolic murmur of aortic incompetence is better heard in this location

Erb's paralysis paralysis of the group of shoulder and arm muscles involving the cervical roots of fifth and sixth spinal nerves. The arm hangs limp and the hand is rotated inwards with loss of normal movements, named after Wilhelm Erb, German neurologist

ERCP abbreviation for endoscopic retrograde cholangiopancreatography

erectile dysfunction inability to achieve erection

erectile tissue spongy tissue capable of erection. It becomes stiff and raised when filled with blood in response to stimulation

erection becoming rigid and distended

erepsin (e-rep'sin) a group of enzymes in the small intestine which catalyse hydrolysis of partially digested proteins

erg a human oncogene located in chromosome 21

ergot a fungus whose derivatives are used to make the uterus to contract after childbirth or in the treatment of migraine

ergotism (er'go-tizm) poisoning from excess of ergot. It presents with vomiting, abdominal cramps, excessive thirst, profound weakness, diarrhoea and dilated pupils

Erlenmeyer flask deformity a deformity, lesion or mass that is broadbased and tapers to a relatively narrow neck likened to a flask, named after Emil Erlenmeyer, German chemist. 1. radiologically corresponds to an under-tubulisation of the distal femur and a loss of usual constriction due to ischaemic necrosis 2. amoebic ulcers in the colon with a narrow neck and a flask-like broad base, the submucous lesion being covered with an intact mucosa

erode (e-rod) to wear away.

erogenous (er-oj'e-nus) arousing erotic feelings **e zone** any part of the body, touching or stroking of which can cause sexual excitement

ergograph (er-go-graf) an instrument that

records the amount of work done when muscle contracts

ergometrics measurement of work output

ergosterol precursor of Vitamin D_3

E rosette test a laboratory test performed to identify T lymphocytes

erosion (e-ro'shun) an eating away; ulcerate

erosive (e-ro'siv) an agent causing erosion **e gastritis** an inflammatory condition with multiple raw areas in the stomach which usually bleed

erotic (e-rot'ik) stimulating sexual desire

eroticism (er'o-tizm) a sexual desire or instinct

erotogenic (e-ro'to-jen'ik) producing erotic excitement

error a mistake, miscalculation, an erroneous result from a patient sample

eructation (e-ruk-ta'shun) belching

eruption (e-rup'shun) breaking out as in the emergence of a new tooth or the sudden appearance of a skin rash

Erysichthon syndrome a condition of overeating, insatiable hunger and indiscriminate dietary indulgence, named after a Greek mythology character who had an unsatiable hunger that led him to eat himself

erysipelas (er'i-sip'e-las) a contagious disease of skin and subcutaneous tissue with diffuse deepened inflammation due to infection with *Streptococcus pyogenes*. It has an acute onset of fever, malaise, skin lesions with cellulitis, brawny induration and a butterfly rash on the face

erysipeloid (er-i-spi'e-loyd) an infection by microaerophilic gram-positive *Erysipelothrix rhusiopathiae* noted in persons handling animal products. It is associated with sharply-demarcated red maculopapular lesions of the hands

erythema (er'i-the'ma) abnormal redness of the skin due to congestion of the capillaries **e gyratum** dusky red macular itchy rash over face, trunk and limbs noted in lung cancer **e multiforme** a macular eruption with

dark red papules, vesicles, on the extremities, which may appear as rings, patches, elevations or figures, occurs as immune reaction to antigens **e nodosum** red, painful nodules on the legs due to streptococcal infections and sarcoidosis

erythematous (er'i-the'ma-tus) characterised by erythema

erythraemia (er'i-thre'me-a) *see* polycythaemia vera

erythralgia (er'i-thral'je-a) a condition characterised by pain and redness of the skin

erythrityl (e-rith'ri-til) **tetranitrate** a coronary vasodilator

erythroblast (e-rith'ro-blast) immature red blood cell; nucleated red cell

erythroblastaemic (e-rith'ro-blas-te'mi-k) presence of a large number of nucleated red cells

erythroblastoma (e-rith'ro-blast-oma) a tumour like mass consisting of nucleated red blood cells

erythroblastosis (e-rith'ro-blas-to'sis) erythroblastaemia **e foetalis** a haemolytic disease of newborn characterised by anaemia, jaundice, hepatosplenomegaly and oedema

erythrocyte (e-rith'ro-sit) red blood cell or corpuscle

erythrocyte sedimentation rate *see* ESR.

erythrocytic (e-rith'ro-sit'ik) pertaining to erythrocytes

erythrocytometer (e-rith'ro-si-tom'e-ter) an apparatus useful for counting red blood cells

erythrocytosis (e-rith'ro-si-to'sis) increase in the total red cell mass

erythroderma (e-rith'ro-der'ma) abnormal redness of the skin over a wide area

erythrodontia (e-rith'ro-don'she'a) reddish brown pigmentation of the teeth

erythrogenesis (e-rith'ro-jen'e-sis) production of erythrocytes

erythroid (er'i-throyd) reddish; referring to the developmental series of cells which produce erythrocytes

erythromelalgia (e-rith'ro-mel'al-gia) red, painful extremities

erythromelia (e-rith'ro-ma'le-a) a condition noted in elderly women, with episodic vasodilation induced erythema of the acral parts accompanied by burning pain. Aspirin is used to get relief

erythromycin a macrolide antibiotic that binds to ribosomal subunits of bacteria and suppress protein synthesis, used in treatment of respiratory infections, and in infections where patient is sensitive to penicillin

erythroplasia (e-rith'ro-pla'ze-a) patches of red discolouration in the mucous membrane

erythropoiesis (e-rith'ro-poy-e'sis) the production of erythrocytes

erythropoietin (e-rith'ro-poy'e-tin) a hormone that stimulates red blood cell production in the bone marrow. It is a glycoprotein growth factor produced by cells adjacent to the proximal renal tubules in response to hypoxia

escape the act of becoming free **e beat** an automatic heart beat occurring after an interval longer than the dominant cycle length

eschar (es'kar) a slough produced by a thermal burn or by application of corrosive or by gangrene

Escherichia (esh-er-ik'e-a) gram-negative microorganisms of the family Enterobacteriaceae *E. coli* gram-negative non-spore forming motile bacilli found in the alimentary tract. They are normally non-pathogenic, may be responsible for urinary tract infection

escutcheon (es-kuch'an) the patch of pubic hair like a shield. In female it is a triangle pointing downward sharply cut off at the level of pubic symphysis, and in male it is diamond shaped with both downward and upward angles. A male pattern in the female indicates an excess of androgen

Esmarch's (es'markz) **bandage** a triangular bandage to control bleeding, named after Johannes Esmarch, German surgeon

ESR erythrocyte sedimentation rate. A test that measures the rate at which red cells in the venous blood mixed with sodium citrate settle to the bottom of a special tube. It is a non-specific indicator of inflammation. It is raised in collagen vascular diseases, neoplasia, anaemia, pregnancy and is decreased in polycythaemia, microcytosis and in sickle cell anaemia

ESRD *see* end stage renal disease

esotropia (es-o-tro'pe-a) a cross-eye wherein one of the eyes is directed inward

essential idiopathic; indispensable **e aminoacids** a group of eight amino acids – isoleucine, leucine, lysine, methionine, phenylalanine, threonine, tryptophan and valine – that are essential for normal growth and development. A negative nitrogen balance is produced in their absence. Premature infants need histidine, arginine and cystine **e dietary component** a requirement in the diet without which a deficiency state will develop. The components are carbohydrates, fat, protein, vitamins, minerals and water **e fatty acids** fatty acids that humans cannot synthesise. They include linoleic acid, and linolenic acid **e haematuria** episodic gross haematuria in male children **e hypernatraemia** a disorder associated with an increased secretion of anti-diuretic hormone in response to volume contraction **e hypertension** primary hypertension where an aetiology of hypertension is not established and it accounts for 95% of cases of hypertension **e thrombocythaemia** a primary myeloproliferative disorder with raised platelet count exhibiting features like polycythaemia vera and splenomegaly **e thrombocytopaenia** low platelet count with clinically significant bleeding

estropia a type of cross-eye in which only one of the eyes is directed inward

et al and others, et alit; and elsewhere, et alibi

ETEC enterotoxic *Escherichia coli* a serotype of *E. coli* causing secretory or traveller's diarrhoea

ethacrinic acid a diuretic

ethambutol a synthetic antituberculosis bacteriostatic agent, gets absorbed rapidly and completely on oral administration, attains peak serum concentrations in 2 to 4 hours after ingestion and is excreted essentially through the kidneys, nonallergic and rarely may cause retrobulbar neuritis

ethanol (eth'a-nol) ethyl alcohol

ether (eth'er) any organic compound in which an oxygen atom links with carbon chains, used as an anaesthetic

ethics a system of moral principles or standards governing conduct

ethionamide (e-thi'on-am'id) a potent bactericidal anti-tuberculosis agent, that diffuses well in tissues and CSF. It produces most unpleasant gastrointestinal side effects, used as a reserve drug

ethmoid (eth'moyd) sieve-like

ethmoidal of or pertaining to ethmoid bone **e bone** a sieve-like spongy bone that forms the roof of the nasal fossae and part of the floor of the anterior cranial fossa. It permits the passage of olfactory nerves to the brain **e sinus** one of the three air cavities in the ethmoid bone which opens into the nasal cavity

ethmoidectomy (eth-moy-dek'to-me) excision of the ethmoidal sinuses

ethmoiditis (eth'moy-di'tis) inflammation of ethmoidal sinuses

ethnic (eth'nik) a social group sharing cultural bonds

ethology (e-thol'o-je) the biological study of behaviour

ethylene (eth'il-en) **glycol** a chemical used as an antifreeze. It is an inebriating and highly toxic substance. It is used occasionally by alcoholics. It is converted by alcohol dehydrogenase to glycolic acid

etoposide a semisynthetic chemotherapeutic agent obtained from podophyllotoxin. It inhibits nucleoside transport and mitochondral electron transport. It is active against monocytic leukaemia, lymphoma, small cell carcinoma and testicular tumour

etymology (et'i-mol'lo-je) the science of the origin and development of words

eucalyptus (u-ka-liptus) **oil** steam distilled oil from *Eucalyptus globulus* used as an expectorant and antiseptic

euchromatin (u-kro'ma-tin) nuclear chromatin that is maximally uncoiled, seen in interphase

eucrasia (u-kra'se-a) a state of health

eugenics (u-jen'iks) the study of hereditary characteristics of future generation through selective breeding

euglycaemia (u-gli'se-mea) a normal level of glucose in the blood

euglycaemic pertaining to or characterised by euglycaemia

eugonic (u-gon'ik) growing luxuriantly

eukaryon (u-kar'e-on) a highly organised nucleus bounded by a nuclear membrane

eukaryosis (u-kar'e-o-sis) the state of nucleus with a surrounding membrane and containing organelles

eukaryote (u-kar'e-ot) a true nucleus exhibiting mitosis

eukinesia (u-kin-e'se-a) normal mobility

eumenorrhoea normal menstruation

eunuch (u'nuk) a castrated person

eunuchoid (u-nu-koyd) resembling a eunuch

eunuchoidism (u-nuk-oyd-izm) a prepubertal deficiency of androgen characterised by infantile genitalia and secondary sex characters, aspermia, lack of male hair pattern, high-pitched voice, infertility, lack of libido, poor muscular development and increased long bone growth

euphoretic an agent producing euphoria

euphoria (u-for'e-a) a feeling or state intense elation

euphoric characterised by euphoria

euploid (u-ploy'd) having a balanced set or sets of chromosomes in any number

euploidy (u-ploy'de) the state of having a balanced set or sets of chromosomes in any number

eupnoea (up-ne'a) normal breathing

eustachian (u-sta'ke-an) canal *tuba auditiva*, tube that connects the middle ear cavity to the nasopharynx, 3 to 4 cm long and lined with mucous membrane, named after an Italian anatomist, Bartolomme Eustachio

eusthenuria (u-sta'nu-rea) urine of normal osmolality

euthanasia (u-tha-na'ze-a) mercy killing; painlessly putting to death persons suffering from incurable conditions or diseases direct e process of inducing death, often through the injection of a lethal drug. indirect e process of allowing a person to die by disconnecting life support systems or withholding lifesaving techniques

euthenics access to a suitable environment that enables the genes to express themselves readily

euthymic mood normal range of mood, implying absence of depressed or elevated mood

euthyroid (u-thi'royd) normally functioning thyroid

eutony harmonius; a method of achieving physical self-awareness through movement and self-observation

evacuant (e-vak'u-ant) agent to empty the bowels

evacuation (e-vak'u-a'shun) an emptying

evacuator (e-vak'u-a-tor) an instrument to remove fluid or small particles from a body cavity

evagination (e-vaj-i-na'shun) an out pouching of a layer or part

evaluation consideration of physical and mental capability of an individual

evanescent (ev'a-nes'ent) vanishing; un stable

Evans' blue a diazo dye soluble in water, used intravenously for diagnostic purpose, named after Herbert Evans, US anatomist.

evaporation change from liquid to gaseous stage

eventration (e'ven-tra'shun) protrusion of bowels from the abdomen

eversion (e-ver'zshun) a turning outward; a turning inside out

evert (e-ver't) to turn outward or to turn inside out.

evertor a muscle that turns a part outward

evil an illness

eviration (e'vi-ra'shun) 1. castration 2. *Psy* delusion in a man who thinks he has become a woman

evisceration (e-vis'er-a'shun) extrusion of the viscera or internal organs

evoked potential any stimulus-evoked response potential recorded by EEG. It varies according to intensity, modality, location and level of consciousness

evoked response a test in which the electrical activity of the brain or spinal cord in response to a specific external stimulus is measured and recorded as a tracing

evolution (evo'-lu'shun) a process of development; any time-related change in the genetic composition of a population

evulsion (e-vul'shun) extraction by fork

Ewing's tumour a cancerous bone tumour affecting children, named after James Ewing, US pathologist

exacerbation (eks-as'er-ba'shun) increase in the severity

examination general, systemic and local examination of the body which includes inspection, palpation, percussion and auscultation

exanthem (eks-an-the'm) the eruption; rash pl. exanthemata

exanthematous (eks-an'them-a-tus) pertaining to or of the nature of exanthem

exarticulation (eks'ar-tik-u-la'shun) amputation of a joint

exceration (ek'ser-a-shun) a hallowed space; the act of hollowing out

excavation (eks'ka-va'shun) 1. a hollow or depression 2. formation of a cavity.

excavator (eks'ka-va'tor) a form of scoop or gouge for surgical use

excerebration (ek'ser-e-bra'shun) removal of the brain, of dead foetus to facilitate delivery

exchange transfusion a therapeutic procedure to reduce immunotoxins in the neonate, wherein the donated blood is infused in exchange for most of an infant's circulating blood. Exchange transfusion is useful in haemolytic disease of new born and neonatal hyperbilirubinaemia

excipient (ek-sip'e-ent) a vehicle; an inert substance added to make a suitable consistency

excision (ek-si'zhun) removal; surgically cutting off

excitable responding to a stimulus

excitability sensitivity to stimulation.

excitant (ek-sit'ant) any agent that produces excitation of vital functions

excitation an act of stimulation or irritation

excited agitated purposeless motor activity, uninfluenced by external stimuli

exclamation mark hairs short irregularly thick, terminally dilated hairs with tapered proximal ends, seen in alopecia aerata

exclusion (eks-kloo'zhun) elimination; rejection; cutting off

excoriation (eks-ko-re-a'shun) a superficial wound in a body surface by deep scratching

excrement (eks'kre-ment) material passed out of the body especially faecal matter

excrescence (eks-kres'ens) any abnormal outgrowth

excreta (eks-kre-ta) waste product excreted from the body, including faeces, urine and sweat **e disposal** proper disposal of human excreta by sanitary latrines, water carriage system and sewage treatment to prevent soil pollution, water pollution, contamination of foods and propagation of flea

excretion (eks-kre'shun) the act of elimination of waste products from individual cells, tissues, organs of the body

excretory (eks'kre-to-re) of pertaining to excretion

excystation (ek-sis-ta'shun) escape from a cyst

exercise a physical or mental activity undertaken to maintain, restore or increase normal capacity **aerobic e** submaximal, rhythmic, repetitive exercise of large muscles during which the required energy is supplied by inspired oxygen. **closed- chain e.** exercise in which the distal end of the segment is fixed to a supporting surface, as the trunk and proximal segments move over the fixed point. **eccentric e** overall lengthening of the muscle due to tension and contraction to control motion against the resistance of an outside force. **e duration.** the total number of days, weeks or months during which an exercise programme is performed. **e frequency.** The number of times exercise is performed within a day or within a week. **e induced asthma** exercise can initiate or exacerbate bronchospam **e load.** the amount of weight used as resistance during an exercise. **e prescription.** individualised exercise programme involving the duration, frequency, intensity and mode of exercise. **e stress test** monitor the heart rate during vigorous exercise usually while a person walks on a exercise treadmill or rides an exercise cycle **isokinetic e.** a form of active-resistance exercise in which the speed of movement of the limb is controlled by a preset rate-limiting device. **isometric e.** a form of static exercise in which tension develops in the muscle but no mechanical work is performed. **isotonic e** a form of dynamic exercise involving concentric or eccentric muscular contractions that result in movement of a joint or body part against a constant load. **muscle-setting e.** a form of isometric exercise but not performed against any appreciable resistance, and gentle static muscle contractions are used to maintain mobility between muscle fibres and to decrease muscle spasm and pain. **open-chain e.** exercise in which a distal segment of the body moves freely in space. **pendulum e** self mobilisaition technique that uses the effects of gravity **progressive resistance e.** an approach to exercise whereby the load or resistance to the muscle is applied by some mechanical means and is quantitatively and progressively increased over time. **pumping e.** active repetitive exercise, usually of ankle or wrist, performed to maintain or improve circulation in the extremities. **resistance e.** any form of active exercise in which a dynamic or static muscular contraction is resisted by an outside force. **short-arc extension e.** active or active-resisted extension of a joint through the final degree of the range of motion, most often applied to the knee from 35 degrees flexion to full extension. **stablising e.** a form of exercise designed to develop control of proximal areas of the body in a stable, symptom-free position in response to fluctuating resistance loads.

exflagellation (eks'flaj-e-la'shun) formation of flagelliform gametes

exfoliation (eks'fo-le-a'shun) a shedding of the scales from a surface

exhalation (eks'ha-la'shun) the act of breathing out

exhale to expel from the lungs by breathing

exhaustion a state of extreme fatigue

exhibitionism exposure of the body or genitals to attract sexual interest

exhumation (eks'hu-ma'shun) removal of the dead body from the earth after burial

exocrine (eks'u-krin) secreting outwards **e gland** a gland where secretion reaches an epithelial surface either directly or through a duct

exocytosis (eks'o-si-to'sis) the discharge of particles from a cell

exodontia (eks-o-don'she-a) extraction of the teeth

exodontics (eks-o-don'tik-s) that branch of dentistry concerned with extraction of the teeth

exodous ball a rounded cluster of endometrial cells seen in vagina, 6-10 days after menstruation

exo-endophytic (eks'o-end'o-fytic) growing outward and inward from the skin surface

exoerythrocytic (ek'so-e-rith'ro-si'tik) outside the erythrocyte

exogenous (eks-oj'e-nus) growth arising from outside the body

exomphalos (eks-om'fa-lus) hernia of the abdominal viscera into the umbilical cord

exon that segment in a gene which codes for a polypeptide

exonuclease an enzyme that catalyses the hydrolysis of the nucleotides

exophthalmos (eks'of-thal'mos) abnormal protrusion of the eyeball

exophytic (eks'o-fytic) growing outward from the skin surface

exostosis (eks'os-to'sis) a bony growth projecting outward from the surface of a bone

exotic (eg-zot'ik) of foreign origin; diseases which are imported into a country in which they do not otherwise occur

exotoxin (eks'o-toks'in) a toxic substance formed by a micro-organism that is found outside the bacterial cell

exotropia (eks'o-tro'pe-a) a cross-eye in which one eye is directed outward in relation to the other eye; external squint.

expansive mood expression of one's feelings without restraint frequently over estimation of one's own significance or importance

expectorant (ek-spek'to-rant) agent promoting the coughing up of the secretions

expectoration (ek-spek'to-ra'shun) sputum; the act of coughing up and spitting

expiration (eks'pi-ra'shun) the act of breathing out; death

expiratory reserve volume (ERV) air that can be expired forcibly from the end of tidal expiration

expire to breath out; to die

exploration to examine

explosion a sudden and violet outbreak

explosive by sudden and violet outbreaks **e syndrome** *Psy* episodic outbursts of verbal abuse and physical violence in response to minor provocation, noted in organic brain disease, after cerebral trauma, psychiatric disease and metabolic dysfunctions

exponential phase phase of maximal growth, of bacteria in the culture

expose to open

exposure 1. the act of laying open 2. amount of radiation delivered over a given area

expressive dysphasia inability to produce intelligible speech despite ability to formulate it mentally

expressivity extent to which gene is manifested in a particular individual

exsanguination (ek-san'gwin-a'shun) loss of blood due to haemorrhage

exstrophy (eks'tro-fe) the turning inside out of an organ. It occurs as a developmental defect involving the bladder

extend (ek-stend) 1. to straighten 2. to move forward

extended breech breech with both knees extended and legs nearly straight

extended family a family composed of a core nuclear family unit of mother, father, children and any other blood relatives who live either in the same household or in close proximity

extender drug that prolongs action of another

extension (eks-ten'shun) a joint movement to straighten two adjoining bones

extensor that which extends **e muscle** any muscle that produces extension of a joint when it contracts

exteriorize to form a correct mental reference of the image of an object seen

external situated on the outside **e cardiac compression** application of strong pressure rhythmically over the sternum after cardiac arrest **e ligament** a strong, fibrous ligament connecting one bone to another, that lies outside the main structure of a joint **e radiation** radiation generated by machines from outside the body, used to treat cancer **e version** a gentle external rotation of the foetus from breech position to more easily deliverable cephalic position

externus a structure situated away from the centre

exteroceptor (eks'ter-o-sep'tor) a sensory nerve terminal that is stimulated by the immediate external environment

extinction disappearance of a conditioned response

extirpate (eks-tir-pa't) to pull out by the roots, to eradicate

extirpation (eks-tir-pa'shun) complete removal

extraarticular situated outside a joint

extrabronchial outside the bronchus

extracapsular extraction removal of lens of eye except posterior capsule

extracellular (eks'tra-sel'u-lar) outside a cell or cells

extracochlear implant implantation of hearing aid with electrode in middle ear usually on round window.

extracorporeal (eks'tra-kor-por'e-al) situated outside the body **e membrane oxygenation (ECMO)** a method of artificial oxygenation of blood in which a cannula in the jugular vein is connected to a small reservoir, into which blood drains by gravity: the blood is then pumped through a membrane oxygenator and heat exchanger and returned to the patient *via* the right carotid artery cannula **e shock wave lithotripsy** shock waves generated extracorporally used to disintegrate renal and biliary tract calculi

extracranial (exs'tra-kra'ne-al) outside the cranium

extract (eks-trakt) a concentrated preparation consisting of active constituents extraction preparation of an extract

extractor an instrument for removing foreign bodies

extradural (eks-tra-du'ral) situated outside the dura mater e anaesthesia injection of an anaesthetic into the space in the spinal canal outside the dura mater to cause loss of sensation in part of the body; e block e haemorrhage bleeding from meningeal vessel involved by skull fracture, characteristically there is recovery following injury, clear interval and relapse as haematoma enlarges

extrahepatic (eks'tra-he-pat'ik) outside the liver

extramedullary (eks'tra-med'u-la-re) outside the bone marrow or spinal cord

extramural (eks'tra-mu'ral) outside the wall of an organ or structure

extraneous (eks'tra-ne-us) outside and unrelated to an organism

extranuclear outside a cell nucleus

extraocular (eks'tra-ok'u-lar) outside the eye e muscle a muscle attached to the eyeball that controls eye movement and co-ordination

extrapleural outside the pleural cavity

extrapyramidal (eks'tra-pi-ram'i-dal) outside of the pyramidal tracts e lesion lead pipe or cog wheel rigidity, poverty of movement from rigidity, involuntary movements, absence of emotional movements and normal reflexes as in Parkinsonism

extrasystole (eks'tra-sis'to-le) a premature contraction of the heart

extrathoracic outside the thorax

extrauterine (eks'tra-u'ter-in) outside the uterus

extravasation (eks-trav'a-sa'shun) a discharge from a vessel into the tissues

extravascular (eks-tra-vas'ku-lar) outside a vessel

extremity a distal part lower e the lower limb including the hip, thigh, leg, ankle and foot upper e the upper limb including the shoulder, arm, forearm, wrist and hand

extrinsic (eks-trin'sik) coming from outside e allergic alveolitis a hypersensitivity reaction occurring at the peripheral gas exchanging parts of the lungs in response to repeated inhalation of antigens contained in finely particulate organic dusts of wide variety and other agents by a susceptible individual e atopic asthma commonly seen in children and young adults, due to known external allergens. There is an inborn ability to produce reaginic (IgE) antibodies in large amount very easily to substances of every day exposure in life e nonatopic asthma noted in adults and environmental factors are active in its development

extroversion (eks'tro-ver'shun) a turning inside out

extrovert a person whose interest is turned outward toward external values

extrude (eks-trud) to force out

extrusion (eks-troo'zhun) expulsion

extube (eks'tu-ba-t) to remove a tube from intubation

extubation (eks'tu-ba'shun) the removal of a previously inserted tube

exuberant (eg-zu'ber-ant) copious

exudate (eks'u-dat) material that has escaped from the blood vessels due to inflammation. The characteritics of exudate collected in the pleural cacity will have protein levels of 3 g/dl or more, ratio of pleural fluid to serum protein to be more than 0.5, pleural fluid to serum LDH more than 0.6, LDH level > 200 units/dl and a specific gravity above 1016

exudation (eks'u-da'shun) the escape of fluid from the blood vessel due to inflammatory, infectious, connective tissue or neoplastic process

exudative of or pertaining to a process of exudation e pleural effusion fluid characterised by a high protein level (fluid-to-serum ratio > 0.5), high LDH level (fluid-to-serum ratio > 0.6) and LDH level greater than 200 IU

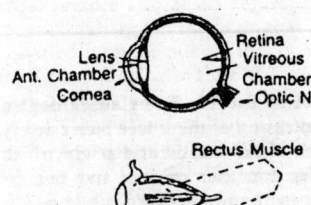

Eye Ball

eye (i) the organ of vision; oculus. It is contained in a bony cavity (orbit) embedded in the orbital fat and innervated by one of a pair of optic nerves. The eye ball consists of three layers: the inner retina containing the photo receptors – rods and cones, the middle uvea consisting of choroid, ciliary body and iris and the outer sclera and cornea. It has two cavities: smaller anterior cavity in front of the lens, which is further divided by the iris into an anterior chamber and a posterior chamber both filled with aqueous (watery) humour. There is a larger posterior chamber behind the lens containing jelly-like vitreous humour. The lens is behind the iris, held in place by the ciliary body and suspensory ligaments. The visible part of the sclera is covered by the conjunctiva, a thin membrane that continues as a lining of the eyelids. The cornea is transparent. Six extrinsic ocular muscles (superior, inferior, medial and lateral rectus muscles and the superior and inferior oblique muscles) move the eyeball in all directions **e ball** the globe of the eye **e brow** a transverse elevation at the junction of forehead and the upper eyelid covered by hairs **e ground** the fundus of the eye **e lash** hair at the edge of the eyelid **e lid** either of the two movable folds that protect the anterior surface of the eyeball **e piece** the lens of the microscope near the eye of the user, that seems to further magnify the image produced by the objective **e rolling** rhythmic eye movements which accompany rotation of the head **e worm** *Loa loa*.

F

F 1. abbreviation for Farenheit 2. chemical symbol for fluorine 3. abbreviation for frequency 4. French gauge (of size of catheters etc.) circumference in mm

f symbol for 1. respiratory frequency 2. aperture/focal length of lens

FAB classification French American British classification of acute myelogenous leukaemia

Fab fragment antigen binding, refers to either of two segments of the IgE molecule

fabella (fa-bel'la) fibrocartilaginous or bony growth in the lateral head of the gastrocnemius muscle

fabrication (fab'ri-ka'shun) a deliberate false statement

Fabry's (fa'brez) disease a genetic disorder inherited as a recessive X-linked trait due to a deficiency of the lysosomal alpha galactosidase. It results in accumulation of a glycolipid in the kidneys and other organs causing impairment in their function, named after Fabry, German physician

face (fas) front part of the head from the forehead to chin which includes the structures of the forehead, eyes, nose, mouth, cheeks and jaw. The blood supply comes from the facial, maxillary and superficial temporal branches of the external carotid arteries and the ophthalmic branch of the internal carotid artery f lift a plastic surgery to eliminate wrinkles f presentation an obstetrical presentation wherein the chin of the foetus is the point of direction

face-bow a device to measure the relationship of the maxillae to the temporomandibular joints, which is necessary for the fabrication of dental casts

facet (fas'et) a small smooth surface of a bone for articulation

facial relating to the face f angle degree of protrusion of the lower face f artery branch of external carotid artery which divides into four cervical and five facial branches f bones face has 14 bones, two each of maxilla, nasal, palatine and inferior nasal concha; zygoma and lacrimal, and one each of mandible and vomer bones f diplegia bilateral paralysis of various muscles of the face f hemiplegia paralysis of muscles of one side of the face f hemispasm bouts of facial contraction on one side f nerve seventh cranial nerve, a mixed nerve supplying all the muscles of facial expression except levator palpebrum superioris and submandibular and sublingual salivary glands, and carrying taste sensation from the anterior two-thirds of the tongue f paralysis paralysis affecting muscles of the face f spasm an involuntary contraction of the facial muscles on one side of the

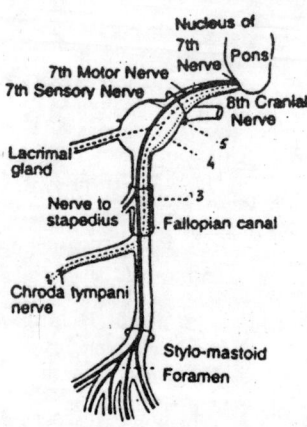

Facial nerve

face f tic repetitive spasmodic and involuntary contraction of groups of facial muscles f vein one of a pair of superficial veins draining deoxygenated blood from the superficial face

facies (fa'she-ez) 1. expression or appearance of the face 2. surface or face of any structure Hippocratic f sunken eyes and cheeks, parched dry skin, pinched nose seen in severe dehydration and wasting diseases leonine f face with flat nose, thick skin with nodules and thinning of the eyebrows mask-like f expressionless and immobile face and infrequent blinking seen in Parkinsonism Mongoloid f stupid look, epicanthic folds, slanting eyes and broad flat nose seen in Mongolism moon f round face with flushed skin, prominent cheeks, acne and hirsutism noted in Cushing's syndrome nephritic f pale puffy face, swollen eyelids noticeable more in the morning in acute glomerulonephritis and nephrotic syndrome

facilitation (fa-sil'i-ta'shun) reinforcement of an action or process

facing an inlay forming the outer surface of a tooth

faciobrachial (fa'she-o-bra'ke-al) pertaining to the face and arm

faciocervical (fa'she-o-ser-vi-kal) pertaining to the face and neck

facioplasty (fa'she-o-plas'te) plastic surgery of the face

facioscapulohumeral (fa'she-o-skap'u-lo-hu'mer-al) pertaining to the face, scapula and arm f muscular dystrophy a muscular dystrophy characterised by symmetric wasting of the skeletal muscles especially muscles of the face, the shoulder and upper arm without any sensory disturbances

faciocephalalgia (fa'she-o-sef-a-lal-je-a) neuralgia of the face and head

FACP Fellow of American College of Physicians

FACS Fellow of American College of Surgeons

factitious (fak'tish-es) self-induced; artificially produced f dermatitis a skin rash caused by the patient for secondary gain; dermatitis artifacta f disorders conditions characterised by disease symptoms caused by deliberate efforts of a person to gain attention

factor 1. a contributory cause 2. an essential element 3. a gene 4. a coagulation factor 5. physiologically active material

factor analysis stat a data reduction technique used to reduce a large number of variables to a smaller number of linear combinations of variable

facultative (fak'ul-ta-tiv) not obligatory; able to live under different environmental conditions f aerobe an organism that grows under anaerobic conditions, can develop rapidly in an aerobic environment f anaerobe an organism that grows under aerobic conditions can develop rapidly in an anaerobic environment f parasite an organism living on a host is capable of living independently

faculty 1. a normal mental attribute or sense 2. teaching staff

faecal fistula fistula between large intestine and exterior

faecal impaction the formation of a firm mass of faeces in the rectum or distal colon

faecalith (fe'ka-lith) a hard impacted mass of faeces, a faecal concretion

faecaloma (fe'kal-o-ma) a large mass of faecal material accumulated in the rectum

faeces (fe'sez) stools, excreta. It is body waste consisting of food residue, bacteria, mucus and epithelium, discharged from the bowel through the anus. faecal adj.

faeculent (fek'u-lent) vomit vomiting distinguished by faecal odour noted in late intestinal obstruction

Faget's (fazhaz') sign a constant pulse with a raising temperature as in yellow fever, described by an American physician, Jean Faget

Fahrenheit (far'en-hit) **scale** a temperature scale with the freezing point of water at 32° and the boiling point of water at 212° at sea level. It is indicated by F and devised by Daniel Fahrenheit, German physicist

failure (fal'yer) inability to function; loss of function that was existing earlier

failure to thrive failure to gain weight and even loss of weight by infants and children from conditions that interfere with normal metabolism, appetite and activity

faint 1. to feel weak and about to lose consciousness 2. syncope 3. loss of consciousness due to cerebral ischaemia

faintness lack of strength with impending loss of consciousness

falcate (fal'kat) sickle-shaped

falciform (fal-si-form) sickle-shaped or crescentic **f ligament** triangular ligament attached to the sides of sacrum and coccyx **f ligament of liver** a wide sickle-shaped reflection of the peritoneum that attaches liver to the diaphragam and serves as a boundary between right and left lobes of the liver

falciparum malaria malignant malaria; most severe form of malaria caused by protozoan *Plasmodium falciparum*

Fallopian canal facial canal in the petrous bone through which facial nerve passes

Fallopian ligament round ligament of the uterus.

Fallopian tube either of a pair of funnel-shaped ducts opening at one end into uterus and at the other end the peritoneal cavity over the ovary, named after an Italian anatomist, Gabriele Fallopio. It serves as a passage for ovum from ovary to the uterus and spermatozoa from uterus towards ovary. The tube lies in the upper border of the broad ligament. Each tube has four parts: the fimbriae, the infundibulum, the ampulla and isthmus. The fimbriae are finger-like projections from the infundibulum over the ovary. Ampulla is the widest part of the tube. An isthmus connects the ampulla to the fundus of the uterus

fallotomy (fal-oto'-me) division of the fallopian tubes

Fallot's (fal-o'z) **tetrology** a congenital heart disease characterised by ventricular septal defect, pulmonary stenosis, overriding of aorta and hypertrophy of right ventricle present with cyanosis, hypoxic spells, squatting after exertion, clubbing, needs shunt surgery, named after Etienne Fallot, French physician

Fallot's pentology rare association of atrial septal defect with Fallot's tetrology

false untrue, incorrent **f aneurysm** expansile haematoma resulting from trauma to large artery **f ankylosis** immobility of joint from an abnormal inflexibility of the parts of the body outside the joint; extracapsular ankylosis **f cyst** not lined by epithelium **f diverticulum** a protrusion of mucous membrane through a defect in the muscular layer of a hollow viscera **f joint** development of a joint at the site of former fracture **f labour** *see* labour **f negative** a test indicating an abnormality under investigation is not present when actually it is **f neuroma** a tumour that does not contain nerve elements **f passage** holes produced by unskilful bougie passage for urethral strictures **f pelvis** the part of the pelvis above the plane passing through the linea terminalis **f positive** a test indicating an abnormality under investigation is present when actually it is not **f pregnancy** a condition in which a woman believes she is pregnant when she is not **f ribs** the lowest five pairs of ribs that do not unite directly with the sternum **f vertebrae** the sacrum and the coccyx **f vocal cord** either of two thick folds of mucous membrane in the larynx separating the ventricle from the vestibule

falx a sickle-shaped structure pl. **falces f cerebelli** a fold of dura mater forming a vertical partition between the hemispheres of the cerebellum f **cerebri** a fold of dura mater lying in the longitudinal fissure separating the two cerebral hemispheres f **inguinalis** a conjoint tendon forming the origin of the transverse abdominis and internal oblique muscles f **ligamentosa** the broad ligament of the liver

familial (femi'li-yel) a characteristic condition or disease occurring in some families and it is usually but not always hereditary f **disease** follows one of the several possible inheritance patterns: autosomal dominant, autosomal recessive, x-linked recessive, x-linked dominant, polygenic, multifactorial, chromosomal, mitochondrial or non-genetic f **hypercholesterolaemia** an inherited disorder transmitted as a dominant trait, and characterised by hypercholesterolaemia, tendinous xanthomas and early evidence of atherosclerosis, especially of the coronary arteries f **Mediterranean fever** an inherited disorder presenting with fever, abdominal pain, chest pain and rash. Some may develop amyloidosis. The disease is self-limited f **megaloblastic anaemia** anaemia due to absence of intrinsic factor, with onset in infancy f **periodic paralysis** attacks of flaccid paralysis of limbs often associated with hypokalaemia f **polyposis** presence of multiple polyps in the colon and rectum inherited as an autosomal dominant condition and it exhibits high malignancy potential f **spinal muscular atrophy** progressive atrophy of the skeletal muscle from degeneration of anterior horn cells of the spinal cord

family 1. a group of individuals descended by a common ancestor 2. a divison between an order and a genus 3. a group of people living together and sharing a common attachment f **history** history about the health of other members of the family f **physician** a general practitioner; a family practice

physician f **planning** the planning and spacing of children according to the wishes of the couple f **practice** a comprehensive medical care given to the family unit

famotidine H₂ receptor blocking antihistamine used to reduce gastric acid

Fanconi's anaemia a rare congenital disorder characterised by aplastic anaemia in childhood with bony abnormalities and developmental anomalies, described by a Swiss paediatrician, Guido Fanconi

Fanconi's syndrome inborn defect of transport mechanism in the proximal renal tubule presenting with renal glycosuria, aminoaciduria, proteinuria and excessive urinary losses of phosphate, bicarbonate, potassium and water in various combinations

fang 1. a sharp pointed tooth 2. the root of a tooth.

fantasise to imagine, day dream

fantast (fan'tast) a day dreamer

fantasy (fan'ta-se') *Psy* a mechanism of creating an unusual thing or scene in the mind

farad a unit of electrical capacity, named after Michael Faraday, British physicist

faradic (fa-rad'ik) refers to induced electricity f **current** high voltage interrupted or alternating current induced in secondary coil by changes in the magnetic field produced by primary coil

faradism (far 'a-dizm) use of an interrupted current to stimulate muscles and nerves

Farber's syndrome disseminated lipogranulomatosis, named after S. Farber, US paediatrician

farinaceous (far'i-na-sh'us) 1. starchy 2. refers to the flour

farmer's lung an allergic alveolitis caused by inhalation of mouldy hay containing *Actinomyces micropolyspora* and *Themoactinomyces vulgaris*

farpoint the farthest point of vision at

which objects can be seen distinctly by the eyes

Farr's (farz) law *stat* law of regular pattern of rise and fall of epidemics, described by W. Farr, British statistician

farsightedness a refractory error wherein the parallel rays come to a focus behind the retina with accommodation completely relaxed. It allows individuals to see distant objects clearly but not near objects; hyperopia

fart flatus, passage of intestinal gas *via* the anus

fascia (fash'e-a) fibrous tissues that enclose and connect the muscles and also the body beneath the skin. pl. **fasciae deep f** fascia enclosing and binding muscles **f bulbi** a thin membranous socket that envelops the eyeball from the optic nerve to the ciliary region and allows the eyeball to move freely **superficial f** fibrous membranous covering that unites the skin with underlying tissues.

fascial (fash-e'al) pertaining to fascia **f cleft** cleavage between two contiguous fascial surfaces **f compartment** a part of the body that is walled off by fascial membranes **f space** the spaces in the hand such as middle palmar and thenar spaces where pus may accumulate

fascicle (fas'i-kal) small bundle of ovoid or spindle-cell that tends to interweave pl. fascicles

fascioplasty (fash-e-o-plas'te) plastic surgery of fascia

fasciculation (fa-sik'u-la-shun) 1. a localised uncoordinated, uncontrollable muscular twitching 2. formation of fascicles

fasciculus (fa-siku-lus) a small bundle of muscle, tendon or nerve fibres

fasciitis (fas'e-i-tis) an inflammation of the connective tissue caused by infection, injury or an auto-immune reaction

Fasciola (fa-si'o-la) a genus of flukes belonging to the class Trematodes **f hepatica** a species of flukes infesting liver; liver fluke miracidia penetrates a fresh water snail and then encysts on

Fasciola hepatica

water cress before being eaten by sheep or man

fascioliasis (fas'e-o-li'a-sis) infection with the liver fluke, *Fasciola heptica*. It presents with upper abdominal pain, fever, chills, hepatomegaly and occasionally jaundice. Eggs are demonstrable in stools. Bithionol is effective in the treatment

fasciolopsiasis (fas'e-o-lop-si'a-sis) intestinal infection due to fluke *Fasciolopsis buski* characterised by diarrhoea, abdominal pain and anorexia, and treated by praziquantel

fascioplasty (fash'e-o-plas'te) plastic surgery on the fascia

fasciotomy (fash'e-o-tome) surgical incision into an area of fascia to relieve pressure on muscles

fast 1. voluntarily not taking food 2. resistant to the effects or action of a chemical substance **acid f** bacteria not getting decolourised on treating with acid

fastidious requiring complex nutrient

fastigate pointed

fastigium (fas-tij'e-um) 1. summit 2. highest point in the course of a fever

fasting going without food

fastness the ability of bacteria to resist stains

fat 1. a substance composed of lipids or fatty acids 2. adipose tissue of the body **f boy syndrome** narcolepsy in obese males, description found in Charles Dicken's novel, Pickwick papers **f embolism** blocking of an artery in the brain by a fat embolus following a fracture of long bone **f necrosis** local breakdown of fat by liberated lipolytic enzymes

atal (fat'l) causing death

atigability (fat'iga-bil'ite) a tendency to become tired or exhausted quickly or easily

atigue (fa-tig) 1. a state of exhaustion 2. loss of ability of tissues to respond to stimuli **f fever** occurrence of fever and muscle pain after exhaustion **f fracture** any fracture resulting from excessive physical activity

atty pertaining to fat or fatty substance

atty acid a hydrocarbon in which one of the hydrogen atoms has been replaced by a carboxyl (COOH) group **essential fa** an unsaturated fatty acid that cannot be synthesised in the body and are essential to maintain health **free fa** non-esterified fatty acid which leaves the cell to be transported for use in another part of the body **omega 3 fa** fatty acid used to reduce very low density lipoproteins and chylomicrons in plasma **omega 6 fa** linoleic and arachidonic acids **saturated fa** acids with single bonds in their carbon chain. It includes palmitic and stearic acids **unsaturated fa** acids with one, two or three bonds in the carbon chain. It includes oleic, linolenic, linoleic and arachidonic acids

fauces (fo'sez) space between the mouth cavity and the oral pharynx. It is bounded by the soft palate, base of the tongue and the palatine arches

fauna (faw'na) animal life, animals characteristic of a given area or time

faveolus (fa-ve'o-lus) a depression

favism (fa'vizm) an acute haemolytic anaemia caused by ingestion of bean or inhalation of the pollen of *Viscia faba* plant and is seen in persons with an inherited deficiency of the enzyme glucose-6-phosphate dehydrogenase

favus (fa'vus) a fungal infection of the scalp by *Trichophyton schoenleino* wherein yellowish crusts occur in localised patches on the scalp

FB abbreviation for foreign body

Fc fragment a part of molecule of an antibody

FDA abbreviation for Food and Drug Administration

Fe abbreviation for iron.

fear fright, anxiety resulting from consciously recognised and realistic danger

febricula (feb'ri-cula) minor episode of fever

febrifacient (feb'-ri-fa'se-ent) causing fever

febrifuge (feb'ri-fuj) an agent that reduces body temperature; antipyretic

febrile (fe'bril) feverish **f convulsions** occurrence of convulsions with fever in the age group of six months to two to three years **f state** a condition with a rise in temperature

fecula (fek'u-la) sediment

fecundation (fe'kun-da'shun) fertilisation; impregnation

fecundity (fe-kun'di-te) fertility; ability to produce offspring

feeble-minded mentally defective who requires care but capable of most simple activities

feedback the return of information; influence of the output or result of a system on the input or stimulus **negative fb** the result of the process reverses or shuts off the stimulus **positive fb** the result of the process intensifies the stimulus

feeding giving or taking nourishment **artificial f** providing a liquid food preparation through a nasogastric tube **breast f** feeding of a infant at the breast **enteral f** feeding through a tube introduced through the mouth or nostril into the stomach **intravenous f** administration of fluids and nutrients through a vein **rectal f** introduction of fluid nutrients into the colon through rectum

feeling a conscious phase of nervous activity

feet the pedal extremities of the legs

FEF abbreviation for forced expiratory flow

fehling's (fa'lingz) **solution** a solution consisting of a mixture of copper sulphate, potassium sodium tartrate and sodium hydroxide, used to detect presence of sugar in the urine, named after Herman Fehling, a German chemist

fel bile

Feldenkrais (fel'den-kra'ise) **method.** use of movement and touch to expand body awareness and explore forgotten ways of sensing, thinking, feeling and acting to allow for more efficient and comfortable movement. Named after Israeli scientist Moshe Feldenkrais

feline (fe'lin) concerning cats

fellatio (fel-a'she-o) oral stimulation of the male genitalia

felon (fel'on) an extremely painful suppurative abscess involving the distal phalanx of a finger; whitlow

felony more severe crime

Felty's (fel'tez) **syndrome** rheumatoid arthritis in adults with splenomegaly, leukopaenia, described by an American physician, Augustus Felty

female woman, an individual of the sex that produces ova or bears young

feminism (fem'i-nizm) the possession of female secondary sexual characteristics by male

feminisation (fem'i-ni-za'shun) the development of female secondary characteristics in the male. **testicular f** an inability of the tissues to respond to testosterone produced by testicles, resulting in an apparent female in whom the genital sex is male

femoral (fem'or-al) pertaining to femur or thigh bone **f artery** artery that begins at the external iliac artery and ends behind the knee as the popleteal artery **f canal** space behind inguinal ligament between femoral vein and edge of pectineal ligament **f hernia** a protrusion of extra-peritoneal fat, peritoneum and occasionally the abdominal contents through the femoral canal; strangulation is more common **f ring** upper end of the femoral canal. It

is bounded anteriorly by the inguinal ligament, posteriorly by pectineus, medially by the concave margin of lacunar ligament and laterally by septum separating it from femoral vein **f vein** continuation of the popliteal vein upwards towards the external iliac vein **f triangle** a triangular depression on the front of upper third of the thigh immediately below the inguinal ligament bounded laterally by the sartorius, medially by the adductor longus and inguinal ligament forms the base

femur thigh bone which extends from the pelvis to the knee and is the longest and strongest bone in the skeleton

femorocoele (fem'o-ro-sel) femoral hernia

fenestra (fen-es'tra) a window-like; an aperture frequently closed by a membrane **f cochleae** the round opening leading into the cochlea, closed by secondary tympanic membrane **f ovale** f vestibuli **f rotunda** f cochleae **f vestibuli** an oval opening on the inner wall of the middle ear holding foot of stapes leading to vestibule

fenestration (fen'es-tra'shun) a surgical procedure wherein an opening is created to gain access to a cavity within an organ or a bone.

Feng shui (fen'g-sh'way) ancient Chinese art of recognising positive and negative features in the environment

fenoterol sympathomimetic bronchodilator, used as an aerosol.

Ferguson's (fer'gus-unz) **reflex** a contraction of uterus after stimulation

ferment (fer'ment) 1. to decompose 2. a substance capable of producing fermentation

fermentation (fer'men-ta'shun) an oxidative decomposition of complex substance by the action of enzyme or fements produced by bacteria, molds and yeast.

Fernandez reaction rapid erythematous response to lepromin

ferning (fer'ning) appearance of fern-like pattern in dried smear of cervical mucus

ferric (fer'ik) pertaining to or containing iron in trivalent form

FER abbreviation for forced expiratory ratio

Ferris Smith sinusectomy creation of a wide drainage tract for frontal, ethmoid and sphenoid sinuses into middle meatus by approach through medial wall of the orbit, named after Ferris Smith, US otologist

ferritin (fer'i-tin) a form in which iron is stored in the tissues of the body. It is an iron-phosphorous-protein complex

ferrotherapy (fer'o-ther'a-pe) use of iron in treating anaemia

ferrous (fer'us) pertaining to iron; a compound containing bivalent iron. The examples are ferrous fumerate, ferrous gluconate, ferrous succinate and ferrous sulphate used to treat iron deficiency anaemias

ferruginous (fer-u-ji-nus) iron containing; rust coloured **f body** the accumulation of iron on foreign material in the lung other than asbestos fibres

ferrule (fer'ul) a metallic ring applied to the end of the root or crown of a tooth to strengthen it

fertile (fer'til) capable of reproducing **f period** time of ovulation in the menstrual cycle during which fertilisation is possible

fertility (fer-til'i-te) the ability to reproduce **f drug** a hormone or hormone-related preparation used to treat infertility **f rate** live births per 1000 women between 15 and 44 years

fertilisation (fer'ti-li-za'shun) the union of male and female gametes to form a zygote from which the embryo develops **in vitro f (IVF)** technique enabling pregnancy in infertile women. Following drug-induced follicle-maturation, a sample of ova and follicular fluid is removed and mixed with the partner's sperm and incubated. The resulting zygote is introduced into the woman's uterus for implantation

festinant (fes'ti-nant) accelerating; rapid **f gait** see gait

FET abbreviation for forced expiratory time

fetal alcohol syndrome birth to alcoholic mothers of underweight infants

fetid (fe'tid) foul smelling

fetish (fe'tish) any object or idea given unreasonable or excessive attention

fetishism (fet'ish-izm) erotic stimulation following contact with non-living objects such as dress or a braid of hair

fetography x ray of foetus following intraamniotic injection of lipid-soluble contrast medium

fetology (fe-tol'o-je) the branch of medicine that is concerned with the foetus in *utero*

fetometry (fe-tom'e-tre) the measurement of the size of foetus

fetoprotein (fe'to-pro'ten) a foetal protein and it may be found in adults

fetor (fe'tor) very offensive odour **f hepaticus** musty odour due to mercaptans from excess circulating methionine encountered in hepatic coma **f oris** halitosis

fetoscope an endoscope to view the foetus in *utero*.

fetoscopy a procedure to observe foetus inside the uterus using a fetoscope

FEV₁ forced expiratory volume in first second

fever an abnormal elevation of the body temperature to above 37.7°C in a resting person; pyrexia **continuous f** temperature remains elevated for many days without showing much fluctuation as in typhoid, urinary tract infection, subacute infective endocarditis and brucellosis **drug f** prolonged fever 1-3 weeks after starting of a drug **filarial f** acute episodic adenolymphangitis in filariasis **f of unknown origin** an illness associated with prolonged fever whose diagnosis is not established after one week of hospital investigation **intermittent f** temperature rises to a variable height and touches normal level for several hours daily as in malaria, sepsis and abscess **irregular f** temperature exhibiting marked variability **jail f** epidemic louse-borne typhus **quartan f** paroxysm of intermittent fever noted on every fourth day **quotidian f** paroxysm of intermittent fever noted on every day **relapsing f** febrile state for several days alternating with variable periods of apyrexia as in Hodgkin's disease, relapsing fever, dengue fever and brucellosis **remittent f** temperature exceeding 2°C in a day without touching normal as in tuberculosis, malaria or sepsis **rose f** allergic rhinitis **saddle back f** initial fever of 2-3 days, then a remission for 2 days followed by reappearance of fever as in dengue fever **tertian f** paroxysm of intermittent fever noted every third day **undulant f** brucellosis **war f** epidemic louse-borne typhus.

Feyrter (fer'ter) **cells** APUD cells of bronchial epithelium

FFA abbreviation for free fatty acids.

FG french gauge of catheters in mm

fibre a thread-like element; an elongated thread-like structure; a slender cellulose structure **afferent f** a nerve fibre carrying sensory impulses from receptors in the periphery to CNS **circular f** collagen bundles surrounding a tooth **dietary f** the food components such as cellulose, hemicellulose, lignin and pectin that resist chemical digestion **efferent f** a nerve fibre carrying motor impulses from CNS to effector organ **motor f** axons of motor neurons innervating skeletal muscles **muscle f** a muscle cell found in striated, smooth and cardiac muscle **myelinated f** a nerve fibre whose axon or dendrite is surrounded by a myelin sheath **nerve f** a neuron **postganglionic f** the axon of a postganglionic neuron that passes from an autonomic ganglia to a vis-

ceral effector **purkinje f** any of the atypical muscle fibers lying beneath the endocardium. It is part of impulse-conducting system of the heart **unmyelinated f** a nerve fiber that lacks a myelin sheath

fiberoscope (fi'ber-skop) a flexible instrument having an inner shaft combined with light conveying thin, flexible fibres to visualise internal structures

fibril (fi'bril) a small fibre; a very small filamentous structure

fibrillation (fi'bril-a'shun) 1. involuntary recurrent inefficient contraction of muscle fibres 2. formation of fibrils **atrial f** arrhythmia wherein the atria beats rapidly, chaotically and ineffectively. Ventricles respond at irregular intervals resulting in an irregularly irregular pulse **ventricular f** arrhythmia producing rapid ineffective uncoordinated movement of ventricles, failing to produce a pulse. ECG shows chaotic, bizarre, irregular complexes

fibrin (fi'brin) an insoluble protein produced by action of thrombin on fibrinogen. It helps to plug and seal damaged blood vessels **f degradation product** substance produced when plasmin lyses either fibrin or fibrinogen

fibrinogen (fi-brin'o-jen) a plasma protein essential for blood clotting which is converted into fibrin by thrombin in presence of calcium ions

fibrinoid (fi'bri-noyd) resembling fibrin

fibrinolysis (fi'brin-ol'i-sis) a process of decomposition of fibrin

fibrinolytic (fi'brin-o-lit'ik) a drug helping to dissolve blood clot **f disorder** primary disorder very rare, may occur secondary to intravascular coagulation. Anti-fibrinolytic agents such as tranexamic acid can block excessive fibrinolysis

fibrin split products the materials produced when fibrin in a blood clot is digested by plasmin

fibroadenoma (fi'bro-ad'e-no'ma) a benign tumour composed of dense epithelial and fibroblastic tissue

fibroadipose containing fibrous and fatty tissue

fibroblast (fi'bro-blast) spindle-shaped undifferentiated cell in the connective tissue

fibroblastoma (fi'bro-blas-to'ma) a tumour derived from a fibroblast

fibrocartilage (fi'bro-kar'ti-lij) a cartilage containing thick bundles of collagenous fibres in its matrix as in the intervertebral discs

fibrochondritis (fi'bro-kon-dri'tis) inflammation of fibrocartilage

fibrochondroma (fi'bro-kon-dro'ma) a tumour of fibrous tissue and cartilage

fibrocystic (fi'bro-sis-tik) development of fibrous tissue and cystic space in a gland

fibrodysplasia (fi'bro-dis-pla'se-a) 'abnormal development of fibrous tissue

fibroid (fi'broyd) a growth of muscular and fibrous tissue

fibroma (fi'bro'ma) a benign tumour made up of muscular and fibrous tissue growing in the wall of uterus

fibromyalgia chronic pain in muscles and soft tissues surrounding joints

fibronectin (fi'bro-nek'tin) an extracellular glycoprotein that exists in a soluble form in body fluids and in an insoluble form in extracellular matrix

fibroplasia (fi'bro-pla'se-a) production of fibrous tissue as in wound healing

fibrosarcoma (fi'bro-sar-ko'ma) a sarcoma that contains connective tissue

fibroserous (fi'bro-se'rus) containing fibrous and serosal elements, as in pericardium

fibrosing alveolitis an inflammatory process of the lung with predominant involvement of the most peripheral parts of the lung in the alveolar walls. It is characterised by two histological features: an inflammatory cellular thickening of alveolar walls with marked tendency to fibrosis (mural) and the presence of a large number of large mononuclear cells presumably of alveolar origin in the alveolar spaces (desquamative)

fibrosis (fi'bro'sis) a proliferation of fibrous connective tissue **pulmonary f** the lung tissue is replaced by fibrous tissue which may be the result of inflammatory processes

fibrositis (fi'bro-si'tis) an inflammation of fibrous connective tissue

fibrothorax (fi'bro-tho'raks) adhesion of two pleural layers

fibula (fib'u-la) the lateral long thin bone of the leg extending from the knee to the ankle articulating above with the tibia and below with the tibia and talus

fictitious imaginary

field a specific area in relation to an object **f block** local anaesthesia by infiltration of an anaesthetic agent around a relevant area **f fever** a form of leptospirosis occurring in agricultural workers **high power f** the portion of an object seen through the high-magnification lens of a microscope **low power f** the portion of an object seen through the low magnification lenses of a microscope

fifth cranial nerve *see* trigeminal nerve

fifth disease erythema infectiosum; an epidemic viral febrile illness of school children and young adults presenting with a maculopapular rash and sometimes large joint arthritis

fifths estimation of amount of foetal head still above pelvic brim, 5/5 being floating and 2/5 just engaged

fifth ventricle the space separating the two layers of the *Septum pallucidum* of the brain

fight-or-flight reaction a generalised response to an emergency situation. There is intense stimulation of the sympathetic nervous system and the adrenal glands resulting in increased heart and respiratory rates, raised blood pressure and increased blood flow to muscles. This response described by

Walter Cannon, US physiologist, prepares the body to either flee or fight

figurate to represent by a figure, outline or visible change

figure 1. a body form, shape or outline 2. a number

filaria (fil-a're-a) nematode worm, examples are *Dracunculus medinensis*, *Loa loa* and *Wuchereria bancrofti* pl. **filariae**, adj **filarial**

filament a fine thread-like fibre

filariasis a disease caused by filaria or microfilaria in the tissues of the body. The condition may remain asymptomatic with circulating microfilaria, or present with acute form exhibiting lymphatic inflammation with streaky tender lymphangitis and enlarged tender lymph nodes or chronic form with lymphatic obstruction resulting in lymphoedema, hydrocoele, and elephantiasis of the limbs

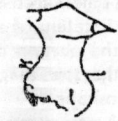

Filariasis-Scrotum

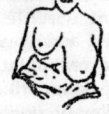

Filariasis-Breast

Filariasis

filariform thread-like

file (fil) 1. a metal device with a rough surface used for shaping bones and teeth 2. A programme, document or an image stored on a computer

filial refers to the relationship between offspring and parents

fillet (fil'et) a loop of thread, cord or tape providing traction or suspension of tissue

filling (fil'ing) 1. the material used for insertion in a prepared tooth cavity, such as amalgum 2. the operation of filling tooth cavities

film 1. a thin layer of blood or other material spread on a slide 2. a thin skin, membrane or covering 3. a thin sheet of material, usually cellulose and coated with a light-sensitive emulsion. It is used in taking photographs f **badge** a badge containing film that is sensitive to x-rays. It is used to determine the cumulative exposure to x-rays by persons working in the radiology department

filter 1. porous substance through which a liquid passes. It prevents particles larger than a particular size to pass through 2. a device for filtering liquids, light rays or radiation

filtrate (fil'trat) the fluid that has been passed through a filter **glomerular f** the fluid that passes from the blood through the glomeruli of the kidney

filtration (fil-tra'shun) the process of removing particles from a solution by allowing the liquid to pass through a membrane

filum (fi'lum) a thread-like structure **terminale** prolongation of lower end of spinal cord

fimbria (fim'bre-a) border resembling a fringe-like structure

fine needle aspiration method to aspirate material for cytological diagnosis, by inserting a hollow thin needle

finger one of the five digits of the hand f **cot** a protective covering for a finger f **nail** *see* nail f **print** an imprint made by the cutaneous ridges of the fleshy portion of the distal end of a finger f **spelling** a method of communication wherein the words are spelled out letter by letter and it is used by persons with impaired hearing f **splint** a padded strip of malleable metal used to immobilise a fractured finger f **stall** finger cot **mallet f** the terminal phalanx cannot be extended because the insertion of the extensor tendon is torn **trigger f** after closing the hand, when patient is asked to open, the ring finger remains flexed. When it is touched it snaps into line with others **webbed f** syndactylism where two or more fingers are webbed, which may involve skin, fibrous or bony region **whale f** erysipeloid cellulits of the fingers and hand due to infection from *Erysipelothrix rhusiopathiae*

FiO$_2$ fraction of inspired oxygen concentration

first aid the immediate care that is given to an injured or ill person before treatment by medically trained person

first catch urine first 15-20 ml of urine micturated

first cranial nerve *see* olfactory nerve

first degree atrioventricular block delayed atrioventricular (AV) conduction resulting in prolonged PR interval beyond 0.20 second. The diagnosis is made from the ECG. It is asymptomatic

first intention healing healing that occurs when wound edges are held or sutured together without the formation of granulation tissue

First law dictum by Hippocrates, 'above all, do no harm'-primum non nocere

first pass angiograms taken during first passage of injected material through an organ studied before occurrence of venous return

first pass effect drug effectively removed or inactivated in one passage through the liver

fish mouth small oral aperture with tight thickened skin of the face in systemic sclerosis

fish skin disease a skin disease characterised by increased horny layer and decreased secretions; ichthyosis

fish tapeworm *Diphyllobothrium latum* responsible for Vitamin B$_{12}$ deficiency due to consumption of B$_{12}$ in the gut. Praziquantel is used in the treatment

fission (fish'un) **process of splitting**
fissiparous reproducing by fission
fissure (fish'ur) groove or **a cleft on a** body surface **f-in-ano a vertical tear of** lining of anus, a painful condition with anal sphincter in spasm

fistula (fis'tu-la) an abnormal passage from an internal organ to the body surface or between two internal organs **anal f** a fistula near the anus **f-in-ano** anterior fistula communicates directly with anal canal and the posterior fistula is always horse-shoe in type entering the anal canal in the midline **arteriovenous f** a fistula between an artery and a vein **biliary f** a fistula through which bile is discharged after an operation **blind f** a fistula that is open at one end only **bronchopleural f** an abnormal communication between the pleural space and a bronchial tube **caroticocavernous f** presence of pulsatious and continuous bruit over the eyeball **cervical f** an abnormal opening into uterine cervix **faecal f** a fistula in which there is discharge of faeces through the opening **horseshoe f** a perianal fistula in which the tract goes around the rectum and communicates with the skin at one or many points **parotid f** a fistula from the parotid gland to the skin surface **pilonidal f** a fistula resulting from a pilonidal cyst **thyroglossal f** a midline fistula above thyroid gland. The tract connects the skin to a persistent embryonic thyroglossal duct **umbilical f** a fistula between the umbilicus and gut due to non-closure of the urachal duct **ureterovaginal f** a fistula between the ureter and the vagina **vesicovaginal f** a fistula between the bladder and vagina **vesicouterine f** a fistula between the bladder and the uterus

fistulectomy (fis'tu-lek'to-me) excision of a fistula

fit seizure; sudden attack of convulsion; a paroxysm; physical strength
fits convulsions, seizures

Fitz-Hugh-Curtis (fitz'hu-ker'tis) **disease** stabbing right upper quadrant pain secondary to perihepatitis caused by spread of untreated gonorrheal cervicitis into the peritoneum, named after Thomas Fitz Hugh Jr, American physician, and Arthur Curtis, American gynaecologist

five day fever trench fever

five dimensions of health major areas of health associated with strengths or limitations: physical, emotional, social, intellectual and spiritual

fixation 1. the act of holding in a rigid position 2. immobility 3. making the material adherent to the slide before staining 4. making a film-recorded image permanent

fixation point point on the retina where visual axes meet to produce clear vision

fixative (fi-k'sa-tiv) 1. a substance that makes rigid 2. a substance used to prepare microscopic slides or to preserve specimens

fixed action pattern a genetically determined behaviour pattern, which is initiated by stimuli particular to the pattern

fixed dose combination combining two or more drugs in one capsule or tablet

flaccid (flak'sid) weak; soft **f paralysis** paralysis marked by loss of muscle tone, loss of tendon reflexes, atrophy and degeneration of muscles due to lesions of lower motor neurones of the spinal cord

flagella (fla-jel'a) a long whip-like projection

flagellate 1. protozoa of class Flagellata such as Giardia, Trichomonas 2. male gamete of malarial parasite

flag sign presence of sharply demarcated alternating bands of pigmented and depigmented hair as an evidence of intermittent malnutrition in protein calorie malnutrition and rarely during treatment with methotrexate

Flagtop abbreviation for the hormones of the anterior pituitary: follicle stimulating hormone, luetinising hormone, adrenocorticotrophin, growth hormone, thyroid stimulating hormone, oxytocin, and prolactin

flail abnormal mobility **f chest** a condition of chest wall due to two or more fractures on each affected rib and it moves paradoxically in with inspiration and out during expiration **f joint** a joint exhibiting excessive mobility due to paralysis of the muscles that control it

flange (flanj) 1. a border projecting above the main structure 2. the part of an artificial denture that extends from imbedded teeth to the border of denture

flank the part of the abdomen between the ribs and the upper border of ilium

flap 1. a mass of partially detached tissue of an adjacent area 2. an uncontrolled movement **f graft** whole skin grafts including subcutaneous tissue transferable as free grafts

flapping tremor an abnormal involuntary jerky tremor of wide amplitude in hepatic precoma. It is elicited upon dorsiflexion of the pronated wrist and specially of extended fingers

flare a flush **nasal f** dilatation of the nostrils during inspiration

flashbacks intrusive memories

flask a small bottle with a narrow neck

flat affect absence of any signs of affective expression such as monotonous voice, immobile face

flat chest markedly decreased anteroposterior diameter of the chest resulting in an increased transverse diameter and chest appears like a shield

flat foot abnormal flatness of the sole and the arch of the foot

flat note impaired to dull note heard on percussion over a solid organ

flatulence (flat'u-lens) the presence of an excessive amount of air or gas in the stomach and intestine

flatus (flat'us) air or gas in the intestine that is expelled **f tube** a tube passed into the rectum to evacuate gas from the lower bowel through the anus.

This is done to relieve intestinal flatulence

flat worm a worm belonging to the phylum platyhelminthes

flavism (fla'vizm) the condition of having a yellow tinge

flavivirus (fla've-vi'rus) group B arbo viruses causing yellow fever, dengue and certain types of encephalitis

flay to strip off the skin

flea (fle) a small wingless, bilaterally compressed blood-sucking insect with a hard chitinous exoskeleton and covered with backwardly directed strong bristles, acts as a vector of bubonic plague and rickettsial disease **f index** the average number of fleas of all species per rodent. It is useful to measure the density of fleas and to evaluate the effectiveness of a spraying programme

Fleisher-Kaiser ring *see* Kaiser-Fleisher ring

flesh the soft tissues of the animal body; the muscles

flex (flek'sh) bend

flexibility the quality of bending without breaking; adaptability

flexion (flek'shun) bending

Flexner's bacillus *Shigella flexneri,* cause of severe bacillary dysentery, named after S. Flexner, US pathologist

flexor (fleks'or) a muscle that brings two bones closer together **f spasm** involuntary painful flexion of the lower extremities in presence of spinal cord lesions

flexure (flek'sher) a fold or bend

flicker the visual sensation of alternating intervals of brightness caused by rhythmic interruption of light stimuli **f epilepsy** maladjusted television sets inducing fits in some epileptics and in some otherwise normal

flight of ideas rapid progression of imperfectly connected topics

floater a body that rises in water as a result of bacterial putrefaction and gas production; extraneous tissue fragments

that can be introduced on to a histological glass slide

floaters (flo'ters) proteinaceous aggregates in the vitreous humour of the eye which drift as spots in front of the eye while reading

floating moving about **f kidney** a kidney movable from its normal position **f ribs** the 11th and 12th ribs which do not articulate with the sternum

flocculation (flok'u-la'shun) precipitation as fluffy particles

flood excessive menstrual or uterine bleeding

floor the surface that forms the lower limit of a cavity or space

floppy infant infant with poor muscular tone and/or response to stimulation of extremities caused by a variety of neuromuscular and musculoskeletal disorders

floppy valve syndrome mitral valve prolapse

flora a collection of organisms or plants in a given locality **intestinal f** bacteria present in the intestines **normal f** potentially pathogenic organisms that are harmless in the body found on the skin, oral cavity, and alimentary tract

flow 1. act of moving 2. movement with respect to time **f chart** diagram showing relationships and interventions of components of process used

flu (floo) influenza

fluctuation a physical sign to demonstrate fluid in the knee joint. The knee is kept in extension and suprapatellar pouch is squeezed with the left hand towards knee joint and kept pressed. The sides of the joint are held between the thumb and index finger of the right hand. When they are pressed firmly an impulse is felt by the left hand in presence of fluid

5 **flucytosine** an antifungal agent

fluent aphasia inability to understand the spoken word

fludrocortisone synthetic mineral corticosteroid, active orally fluid non-solid; liquid f **balance** regulation of the amount of water in the body f **diet** liquid diet f **replacement** administration of fluid to correct fluid and electrolyte deficit f **retention** failure to eliminate fluid from the body due to renal, cardiac or metabolic disorders

fluid thrill a physical sign to demonstrate fluid in the peritoneal cavity. When patient is lying down on his back, the palm is placed over the flank on one side and opposite flank is flicked with the fingers of the other hand. The patient places his hand firmly on the abdomen in the midline to dampen any impulse that may pass through the anterior abdominal wall. The fluid wave transmitted across the fluid to the other side of the flank is appreciated as a distinct impact by the palpating fingers in presence of massive ascites

fluke (flook) a parasitic worm belonging to the class trematoda phylum platyhelminthes; flatworm

fluorescein staining used to demonstrate loss of corneal epithelium. On instillation of a drop of 2% solution of fluorescein into the eye, the area devoid of epithelium takes a green stain

fluorescence (floo'o-res'ents) the light emitting property of certain substances when exposed to certain types of light radiation, usually ultraviolet light f **insitu hybridization,** FISH a molecular cytogenetic technique used as a diagnostic test in chronic myeloid leukaemia and acute promyelocytic leukaemia

fluoridation (floo'or-i-da'shun) addition of small amounts of fluoride to drinking water to reduce occurrence of cavities in the teeth

fluoride (floo'o-rid) a mineral that helps in mineralisation, development and function of bones and teeth

fluorocarbon a hydrocarbon in which some of the hydrogen atoms are replaced with fluorine

fluoroscope (floo'or-o-skop) an instrument for visual observation of the body by x-ray

fluoroscopy a method to view internal body structures or their functions by passing x-rays through the body and on to x-ray sensitive fluorescent screen

fluorosis (floo-or-o'sis) excessive ingestion of fluorine and its compounds found in water resulting in mottled, pitted enamel of tooth, chalky white discoloured teeth and osteosclerosis **dental** f excess fluoride combines with calcium to form calcium fluorapatite making the teeth to become hypoplastic and later brown discolouration **skeletal** f excess deposition in the bones causes hyperostosis and irregular new bone formation along the attachment of ligaments, muscles, joint capsules and interosseous ligaments. There can be compressive radiculomyelopathy. The bones give a structureless marble white appearance

fluorouracil pyrimidine antimetabolite, blocking DNA synthesis used in the treatment of cancer

flush 1. blush, sudden redness of the skin 2. irrigation of a cavity with water **hot** f flush accompanied with a sensation of heat, noted during menopause or neuroses **malar** f a bright flush over the malar region and cheek seen in febrile diseases and mitral stenosis

flutter 1. tremulousness 2. rapid abnormal but rhythmic contractions **atrial** f rapid atrial contraction due to intra-atrial reentry ECG a regular undulating baseline (flutter or F waves) resulting in a saw-tooth appearance. They appear at a regular rate of 250-350 min f **fibrillation** flutter waves exhibiting some irregularity **diaphragmatic** f rapid contraction of the diaphragm **ventricular** f ventricular contractions of the heart at 250 per minute

flux an excessive flow or discharge from an organ or cavity of the body fly-catcher tongue intermittent in-and-out darting of the tongue seen in tardive dyskinesia

foam stability test test for surfactant in amniotic fluid

foam test the presence of bile is recognised by shaking the freshly voided urine. The froth gives yellow colour in presence of bile pigment

foamy cells macrophages full of lipid droplets

focal emphysema dilatation of respiratory bronchioles around inhaled coal dust

focal epilepsy seizures starting in one part of the body and spreading gradually to other parts

focal nephritis segmental hyalinisation of the peripheral portions of glomerular tufts which may be associated with nephrotic syndrome

focus 1. site of convergence or divergence of rays 2. local small area of infection 3. any visible small patch of lesion

foetal (fe'tal) pertaining to foetus f monitoring the use of various techniques to check the health of a foetus f surgery an operation performed to correct defects before an infant is born

foetus (fe'tus) the developing human form in uterus from the end of the eighth week after fertilisation until birth f-in-feto rudimentary twin born as appendage attached to otherwise normal infant f papyraceous remains of death of one twin early in monovular pregnancy being flattened against membranes.

Fogarty catheter fine catheter with balloon used to pull emboli out of arteries, named after T. Fogarty, US surgeon

folate salt of folic acid

Foley's catheter a balloon-tipped rubber catheter to catheterise urinary bladder, introduced by an American urologist, F. Foley

folic (fo'lik) acid a member of vitamin B complex essential in synthesis of aminoacids and DNA and red cell maturation, whose deficiency results in megaloblastic anaemia

folie a deux communicated emotional illness between two persons

folie a trois communicated emotional illness between three persons

folinic acid an active form of folic acid

follicle a small pouch-like depression or cavity

folliculitis (fo-lik'u-li'tis) inflammation of hair follicle

fomentation (fo'men-ta'shun) a warm application

fomite (fo'mi-te) non-living material.

FNA fine needle aspiration

FNAB fine needle aspiration biopsy

font course. a particular style of type

Fontana's (fon-ta'nahz) space space at corneoscleral junction through which aqueous drains, named after A. Fontana, Italian anatomist

fontanella (fon'ta-nellah) a soft membrane covering the space at the junction of the sutures on a baby's skull

food additives chemical compounds that are intentionally or unintentionally added to our food supply

food allergy an immunologic hypersensitivity, usually acute and IgE mediated and presents with anaphylaxis, lip swelling, urticaria, rhinitis and asthma. It may be delayed as in coeliac disease presenting as malabsorption (gluten enteropathy)

food intolerance adverse reaction to food. Rarely may occur as reactions to pharmacologically active substances in the food such as caffeine (tachycardia, tremors) and tyramine (vascular headache) or as idiosyncratic reactions due to lack of enzymes such as lactase (osmotic diarrhoea after ingestion of milk) or as allergy

food poisoning occurrence of rapid onset of vomiting, profuse watery diarrhoea and abdomial pain after ingestion of preformed bacterial toxins elaborated by *Staphylococcus aureus, Clostridium perfringens* type A and *Bacillus cereus* and organic and inorganic chemicals

food supplements nutrients taken in addition to those obtained through the diet

foot the terminal portion of the lower extremity consisting of tarsus, metatarsus and the foot. pl. **feet athlete's f** a fungal infection of the foot **cleft f** extension of a cleft between digits to the metatarsal region **f drop** inability to dorsiflex or evert the foot due to damage to common peroneal nerve **flat f** flattened arch of the foot. The inner border of the sole is inclined and is worn down **f plate** the flat part of the stapes, a bone in the middle ear **f print** obtained by dusting the soles with powder and then asking the patient to walk on linoleum, useful to study the arches of the foot **f process** a cytoplasmic extension from the epithelial cell of the glomerulus; podocyte **immersion f** a condition developing from prolonged immersion in cold water. Initially there is pain followed by swelling, discolouration and numbness **march f** a spontaneous fracture of one of the metatarsal bones of the foot **trench f** degeneration of the skin of the feet due to prolonged exposure to moisture

footballer's ankle pain in front of ankle and limitation of plantar flexion with osteophytes of neck of talus

foramen (for-a'men) a natural opening

force feeding compelled feeding either against or in excess of wish of individual

forced expiratory flow (FEF) maximum rate of expiration at mid-point

forced expiratory volume (FEV) the volume of the air a person exhales with forceful expiration after maximal inspiration FEV, the forced expiratory volume in one second. The volume expired in the first second during forced vital capacity exhalation

forced expiratory time (FET) time taken with maximum effort from full inspiration to full expiration

forced vital capacity (FVC) maximum expirable, from full inspiration to full expiration

forceps (for'seps) an appliance to hold, treated both singular and plural

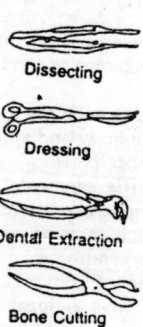

Forceps

Fordyce's (for'dis-es) **spots** sebaecous glands in buccal mucosa which appear as yellow nodules, named after J. Fordyce, US dermatologist

foregut (for'gut) the cephalic portion of embryonic alimentary tract.

foreign bodies introduction of foreign substances into the body. It may be iatrogenic as in sutures, sponges, instruments or swabs left during surgery or artificial joints, limbs and pacemakers, or accidental as in gunshot wounds. Foreign bodies may be introduced into vagina or anorectal region as a sexual deviancy

Forensic medicine branch of medical science dealing with legal aspects of health care

forequarter amputation a surgical procedure in which the upper extremity and a variable portion of the supporting shoulder girdle is amputated as in malignancy

foreskin loose fold of skin covering the tip of the penis or clitoris

forewaters the amniotic fluid between the presenting part and intrauterine membranes

form measure of regularity of shape, area

formaldehyde (for-mal'de-hid) a histologic fixative and disinfectant

formaline (for-mah-lin) saturated solution of formaldehyde

formal thought disorder *Psy* disturbance in the form of thought instead of the content of thought. There is disorder of thought process making the individual a psychotic

forme fruste (form-froost) (F) an incomplete or atypical expression of a clinical entity or pathologic condition

formication (for'mi-ka'shun) a paraesthesia wherein there is a sensation of ants running over the skin

formiminoglutamic acid (FIGLU), compound formed in the metabolism of histidine and glutamic acid which is eliminated in the urine in large amount in folic acid deficiency

formulary (for'mu-lar'e) summary listing of recommended drugs, their uses and dosage.

fornix (for'niks) an arch-shaped structure. pl. **fornices**

fortified food food that has been supplemented with essential nutrients such as iron and vitamins

forward failure decreased cardiac output and inadequate perfusion of organs

fossa (fo'sa) a depression on the surface of a bone

fossil fuel a fuel derived from decomposing fossilised organic material including oil, coal and natural gas

Foster Kennedy syndrome frontal lobe tumour presenting with optic atrophy on tumour side, papilloedema on other and anosmia, named after Foster Kennedy, British–US neurologist

Fothergill's (Foth'er-gilz) **operation** for prolapse uterus, colporrhaphy and amputation of cervix with suture together of cardinal ligaments, named after Fothergill, UK gynaecologist.

Fouchet's (foo-shaz) **test** test to detect bilirubin in the urine. A white precipitate forms on addition of 5 ml of 10% barium chloride to 10 ml urine in a test tube. It is filtered and spread over a dry filter paper. There is a play of colours varying from green to blue on additon of Fouchet's reagent (trichloracetic acid and ferric chloride) in presence of bilirubin, named after A. Fouchet, French chemist

fourchette (foor-shet') posterior commissure of labia majora

four-fold table *stat* a format of presenting data on association of two variables each having only two values, used in chi-square test

Fournier's (foor-ne-az') **gangrene** an acute inflammatory oedema of the scrotum which rapidly progresses to gangrene, described by Jean Fournier, founder of VD clinic at Paris

fourth heart sound (S4) abnormal heart sound produced by vigorous atrial contraction against ventricular resistance usually from left ventricular hypertrophy. It is low pitched sound audible immediately before the first heart sound

fovea (fo've-ah) depressed central area of retina having cones only

foveola (fo've'o-lah) most depressed, and highly sensitive part of the fovea

Foville's (fo-velz') **syndrome** paralysis of Vth and VIIth cranial nerves with contralateral hemiplegia, named after A. Foville, French psychiatrist

Fowler's (fow'lerz) **position** posture adapted by a patient wherein the head of the bed and individual's knee is elevated, described by an American surgeon, G. Fowler

fracture (frak'tur) injury to a bone wherein the continuity of the bone is broken. It is characterised by pain and tenderness, deformity in the form of swelling, shortening or angulation and loss of function, other features like abnormal mobility at the site of fracture, crepitus and loss of transmitted movements though may be present, are not sought normally. **shear** f shearing of the calcaneum into medial and lateral halves by the load of eccentrically placed talus

fragile brittle. **f X-syndrome** a sex chromosome abnormality presenting with mental retardation in males. It is associated with a 'fragile site' on the distal long arm of one x-chromosome and its inheritance is x-linked recessive

fragilitas ossium osteogenesis imperfecta. characterised by recurrent fractures of long bones and blue sclera

fragmentary disconnected , broken, incomplete

frambasia (fram-be-ze-a) yaws

Framingham heart study a study conducted by the United States Public Health Services in the town of Framingham, Massachusetts, USA since 1948 on a population of 28,000 for 20 years to determine the relation of risk factors such as blood pressure, weight, smoking and serum cholesterol to the subsequent development of cardiovascular disease

Francisella (fran'si-sel'a) a gram-negative organism causing tularaemia

FRC *see* functional residual capacity

freckle (frek'al) asymptomatic small, circular brownish macules appearing early in life on the face, hands and forearm and is due to an abnormally large amount of melanin in the epidermis

free-floating anxiety pervasive, unfocussed fear not attached to any idea

free radical one of a highly reactive family of molecules containing an unpaired electron on the outer orbital. They cause random damage to structural proteins, enzymes, macromolecules and DNA. It plays major roles in inflammation, hyperoxidation, and post-ischaemic damage. **f inactivator** any molecule re-

ducing free radical induced damage such as superoxide dismutase, glutathione, cysteine, vitamin E **f scavenger** any compound that reacts with free radicals in a biologic system and offer protection

freeze-drying method of tissue protein preservation

freezing hesitation on gait initiation seen in well developed Parkinson's disease

Frei's (friz) test skin test for lymphogranuloma inguinale described by a German dermatologist, William Frei.

Freiberg's (fri'bergz) disease osteochondritis of the heads of the second and or third metatarsal bones characterised by pain, limitation of plantar flexion and broadening of affected foot, named after Frederick Freiberg, British orthopaedic surgeon

fremitus (frem'i-tus) vibration perceptible on palpation

Freund's adjuvant a dried and pulvarised emulsion of mycobacteria used as a powerful stimulant of cellular immunity, named after Jules Freund, Hungarian-US bacteriologist

frenum a restraining structure

frenulum median fold under tongue and other similar folds.

Frey's (friz) syndrome an auriculo-temporal syndrome characterised by attacks of pain and hyperaesthesia in the auriculotemporal region, unilateral facial flushing and sweating over the cheek. The pain comes on while eating especially highly-spiced curry. It is often a sequel of an incision for suppurative parotitis, named after Lucie Frey, Polish physician.

Friedlander's (fred'len-derz) bacilli *Klebsiella pneumoniae*, described by a German pathologist, C. Friedlander

Friedman's curve a graph depicting the progress of labour, described by an American obstetrician, Friedman

Friedreich's (fred'riks) ataxia an autosomal recessive disorder characterised by progressive degeneration of dorsal root ganglia, spinocerebellar tracts, corticospinal tracts and cells of cerebellum. It develops in childhood with features of difficulty in walking, cerebellar dysarthria, ataxic weak limbs, absent deep tendon reflexes and extensor plantar response. There is loss of posterior column sensations, club foot, scoliosis and cardiac involvement

frigid (frij'id) lacking warmth of feeling; unresponsive to sexual advances

frog belly pendulous abdominal fat of children with cretinism

frog face long-standing angiofibromas of the intranasal cavities which may extend into the orbits to result in bilateral exophthalmos. It is associated with nasal congestion and a flat, croaking voice

Frohlich's (fra'liks) **syndrome** adiposogenital dystrophy, characterised by adiposity, delayed puberty, mental defect, and polydipsia, named after A. Frohlich, Austrian physician

Froin's (frow'an') **syndrome** cerebrospinal fluid having yellow colour, raised level of proteins and an absence of an increased number of cells in spinal block, named after G. Froin, German physician

frontal forehead **f bone** the bone in the front of skull that forms the forehead **f lobe** the largest part of the cerebrum that influences personality and mental activities **f sinus** an accessory nasal sinus in the frontal bone

frost-bite (frost'bit) a traumatic effect caused by freezing of body tissues from exposure to extreme cold for a long period of time. The peripheral parts of the body such as the tip of the nose, the external ears and the fingers and toes become numbed and white due to vasoconstriction

frosting finely granular salt deposits on the skin above sweat glands as in cystic fibrosis

frought freightened

frozen chest pleural or parenchymal fibrosis causing immobilisation of the chest

frozen section a rapid diagnostic procedure done on tissue obtained during operation, where the tissue is frozen, sectioned and stained with haematoxylin and eosin and examined under microscope. It helps in differentiating a benign condition from a malignant condition

frozen shoulder a painful stiff shoulder secondary to periarthritis of the shoulder joint

fructose monosaccharide obtained from honey and fruits

fructosuria presence of fructose in urine.

frusemide a thiazide loop diuretic

FSH abbreviation for follicle stimulating hormone

F test *stat* a statistical test that allows comparison of the standard deviations of two different sets of data or population

fuchsins red dyes of rosaniline group, named after L Fuchs, German botanist.

fugax transitory

fugue (fug) a state wherein an individual exhibits forgetfulness of a past event and takes a new identity

fulguration (ful'gu-ra'shun) destruction of living tissue by high frequency current

full house syndrome familial focal facial dermal dysplasia (FFFDD) an autosomal dominant condition characterised by lesion devoid of hair with finger print-like puckering of the skin, especially at the temples. It is due to alternate bands of dermal and epidermal atrophy. The condition derives its name from a card game where a full house is three cards of one value and two of another

fulminant rapid, severe illness

fumigation (fu'mi-ga'shun) 1. disinfection of room by poisonous gases 2. use of poisonous gases on fumes to destroy living organisms

Fumonisins (fu'mon'i-sins) a group of mycotoxins isolated from corn contaminated with *Fusorium moniliforme*

functional affecting the function but not the structure **f illness** an unidentified illness in which no cause has been found for the symptoms.

Functional residual capacity (FRC) the gas volume in the lungs after a normal expiration. It is measured by a gas dilution method or body plethysmography

fundal dominance normal initiation of uterine contractions in the fundus

fundus base

funduscope (fun'dus-skop) examination of the structures of the fundus of the eye by an ophthalmoscope

fungicide (fun'ji-sid) a substance that destroys fungus

fungoides bacteria that mimic true fungi. Actinomyces, Nocardia and streptomyces are some examples

fungus a parasitic plant lacking in chlorophyll. pl. **fungi f ball** a tumour-like mass of fungi. The saprophytic form of Aspergillus species may colonise a preexisting pulmonary cavity

funiculitis any abnormal inflammatory condition of a cord-like structure of the body.

funis cord-like structure

funnel chest funnel-like depression of the lower two-thirds of the sternum, behind the frontal plane of the thorax. It may extend as high as the third rib. It is usually congenital

funny bone lower end of humerus

FUO fever of unknown origin

Furrier's lung hypersensitivity pneumonitis in workers in fur industry

furrow groove

furuncle (fu'runz-k'l) a localised suppurative condition occurring in a hair follicle

furunculosis (fu-rung'ku-lo'sis) boils

fusion inhibitor an anti-HIV drug targetting the point where HIV locks to an immune cell

Fusobacterium (fu'zo-bak-te're-um) a gram-negative anaerobic rod-shaped bacteria found in the oral cavity and bowel

FVC forced vital capacity

F waves *ECG* the atrial flutter waves appear on the electrocardiogram with a 'sawtooth' pattern in leads II, III and avF and at a rate of 280-320/min; an undulation of the electromyogram that corresponds to time between the application of stimulus to the axon of the motor neuron and its return after propagation

G

γ **gamma,** third letter of Greek alphabet, symbol for microgram; immunoglobulin

G symbol for gram, gravity

G-actin a globular protein found in many cells

G cell gastrin-secreting APUD cells found mainly in stomach

GA abbreviation for General anaesthesia

Ga symbol for gallium

GABA gamma-aminobutyric acid, a major inhibiting neurotransmitter widely distributed in brain

G6PD Glucose-6-phosphate dehydrogenase

gag 1. a dental device to keep the mouth open during operative procedures of the mouth or throat 2. to retch; to prevent from talking 3. a retroviral gene that encodes a structural protein within the virus core **g reflex** elevation of the soft palate and retching which occurs on touching the posterior wall of the pharynx; a pharyngeal reflex used to test the integrity of the glossopharyngeal and vagus nerves

gain to increase in weight, strength or health

gait (gat) style of walking **ataxic g** patient walks on a broad and irregular base, keeping the feet widely apart and swinging the legs irregularly, simulating the gait of a drunken person, also called reeling gait of cerebellar ataxia **dancing g** jerky involuntary movements which exaggerate during walking and the limbs are thrown apart as in chorea **festinant g** in Parkinsonism, the patient walks with the head and body bent forwards. The hips and knees are slightly flexed. The patient walks with quick short shuffling steps giving an impression of trying to catch up with the centre of gravity **hemiplegic g** a spastic gait with abnormality involving on one side in patients with residual hemiplagia or hemiparesis. The limbs are stiff, foot plantar flexed. The leg is dragged forward in a semicircle first away from and then towards the body (circumduction) slowly **high steppage g** in polyneuropathy, poliomyelitis and peroneal muscular dystrophy the patient raises the foot to overcome the foot drop and is brought down and the toes touch the ground first **hysterical g** an irregular bizarre type of gait altering from time to time **scissor's g** in cerebral diplegia and lathyrism there is medial rotation of the legs which cross each other while walking **shuffling g** see festinant gait **spastic g** the legs are stiff and are advanced slowly on a narrow base by dragging the feet. The foot is raised from the ground by tilting the pelvis and then the leg is swung forwards. The foot makes an arc and the toes scrape the ground. This is seen in paraplegia in extension **stamping g** the patient in posterior column lesions walks by placing the feet wide apart. The feet are raised high and are brought down suddenly with the heel slamming the floor **waddling g** oscillation of the body from side to side with each step as in pseudohypertrophic muscular dystrophy, congenital dislocation of the hip, osteomalacia and advanced pregnancy

galactischia (gal'ak-tis'ke-a) suppression of milk secretion.

galacto - combining word for milk

galactagogue (gah-lak'ta-gog) agent that promotes the secretion and flow of milk

galactocele (gah-lak'to-sel) a cystic milk filled swelling in an obstructed milk duct in the breast

galactokinase (gah-lak'to-ki'nas) an enzyme that participates in the metabolism of glycogen **g deficiency** an inherited disorder of carbohydrate metabolism with deficiency or absence of galactokinase. Dietary galactose is not metabolised, causing its accumulation in the blood

galactophore (gah-lak'to-for) a milk duct.

galactorrhoea (gah-lak'to-re'ah) production of breast milk not associated with child birth or nursing. Sometimes it may be a manifestation of a pituitary gland tumour

galactosaemia (gah-lak'to-se'me-ah) a genetic disorder of galactose metabolism due to a deficiency of an enzyme galactose-l-phosphate uridyl transferase in the liver that breaks down galactose. There is intolerance to milk soon after birth, hepatosplenomegaly, cataracts and mental retardation

galactosamine (gah-lak'to-s-amine) an amino derivative of galactose

galactose (gah-lak'to-se) a monosaccharide derived from milk sugar, lactose, chiefly converted to liver glycogen

galactosidase (gah-lak'to-si'das) an enzyme that catalyses the metabolism of galactosides

galactoside (gah-lak'to-sid) a glycoside containing galactose

galactostasis (gah-lak-to'sta-sis) cessation of milk secretion

galacturia (gal'ak-tu're-ah) milky urine due to the presence of galactose

Galaganda (s) goiter *g hari* that which cures goitre

galant reflex on stroking the back along the spinal column, the hips move towards the stimulated side, in neonates. It disappears by about 4 weeks of age. Absence of reflex may indicate spinal cord lesion

galea (ga'le-ah) a helmet-shaped structure **g aponeurotica** dense vascular fibrous layer of the scalp which is loosely attached to the skull

Galeazzi's sign recognition of congenital dislocation of hip in infants. The child lying supine with the knees flexed and hips flexed at 90°, dislocation is present if one knee is higher than the other

Galenicals (gah-len'ik'lz) long standing herbal drugs, named after Greek physician, Claudius Galen

Galen's (gah-len'z) **bandage** a bandage applied to the head. It consists of a strip of cloth with each end dividied into three pieces, named after Claudius Galen, Greek physician

gall (gawl) bile, secreted by liver and stored in gall bladder, that helps in emulsification of fats and stimulation of intestines. It has no enzymes. It is discharged into the duodenum through cystic duct and common bile duct

Gallavardin's syndrome apnoea induced by exertion or emotion in individuals of coronary disease.

gall bladder (gawl'blad-er) a small pear-shaped sac under the visceral surface of the right lobe of the liver that acts as a reservoir of bile secreted by the liver. It receives bile from the liver through hepatic duct and it contracts during digestion of fats allowing the flow of the bile through the common bile duct into the duodenum **g carcinoma** a malignant condition affecting gall bladder presenting with anorexia, nausea, vomiting, weight loss, right upper abdominal pain and jaundice. The gall bladder becomes palpable and it fails to concentrate radiopaque dye **hydrops g** distension of gall bladder due to impaction of a large stone in the cystic duct with perisistant obstruction **porcelain g** long standing gall

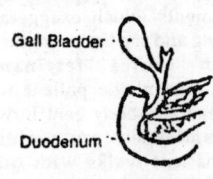

Gall Bladder

Duodenum

Gall bladder

stone disease with deposition of calcium in the fibrotic gall bladder giving an egg shell appearance on a radiograph

gallium (gal'e-um) a rare metallic element, atomic number 31 **g scan** radioscintillation imaging method using ^{67}Gallium citrate. On injection gallium binds to transferrin and any tissue that concentrates lactoferrin also concentrates gallium, used to stage lymphoms, lung cancer, hepatoma and metastases

gallop (gal'op) a cardiac auscultatory phenomenon wherein a triple or quadruple cadence of the heart sounds resembling that of a galloping horse, produced by abnormal third and fourth heart sounds.

galloping consumption diffuse tuberculous bronchopneumonia

gall stone (gawl-ston) calculus formed in the gall bladder or in a bile duct from the constituents of bile due to disturbances in cholesterol and bile pigment metabolism, infection and biliary stasis **g ileus** obstruction of ileum by a gallstone passed from cholecystoduodenal fistula

GALT *See* gut associated lymphoid tissue

Galvanic current direct current of moderate voltage, named after Italian physiologist, Luigi Galvani

Galvanic electric stimulation application of a high-voltage electric stimulation to treat muscle spasms and myofascial pain

Galvanometer (gal'vanom'eter) an instrument that measures electrical current by its effects on a needle or coil in a magnetic field as in electrocardiograph

Gambel's syndrome familial chloride-losing diarrhoea in infants, named after J. Gamble, US paediatrician

gamete (gam'et) a mature male (spermatozoon) or female (ovum) reproductive cell

gamete intrafallopian transfer (GIFT) a technique of human fertilisation for treating infertility wherein the male and female gametes are injected into the fimbrian ends of the fallopian tubes through a laparoscope

gametocide (gah-me'to-sid) an agent that destroys the gametes or gametocytes, specially the malarial parasite

gametocyte (gah-me'to-sit) a cell that produces gametes (spermatocyte or oocyte)

gametogenesis (gah-mi'to-jen'esis) formation and development of gametes

gametogony (gah-me'tog-o-ne) formation of male and female gametocytes in the life cycle of the malarial parasite, which infect the mosquito

gamgee dressing of cotton wool between two layes of a gauze

Gamma third letter of Greek alphabet, written as γ; symbol for the heavy chain of immunoglobulin G(IgG) **g aminobutyric acid** (GABA) a neurotransmitter that controls the flow of nerve impulses in the brain by blocking the release of other neurotransmitters, such as dopamine **g benzene hexachloride** a scabicide and pediculicide **g camera** a device that produces an image of the distribution of radioactive material in a patient, who has been injected with small amounts of radioactive materials **g chain disease** a variety of heavy chain disease **g globulin** (Ig) gamma fraction of protein on electrophoresis of plasma **g glutamyl transferase** an enzyme widely distributed in the body tissues. It is released into the blood when the tissue especially liver is damaged **g knife** destruction of intracranial target such as brain tumours and vascular abnormalities by ionising beams of radiation that are directed with stereotaxic precision **g rays** high-energy short wave-length radiation emitted by radioactive materials **g scan** production of image of lesions taking up radioisotope by scan of gamma ray output **g glutamyl transpeptidase** (GGTP) an enzyme that appears in the blood in disorders affecting the liver and gall bladder

gammopathy (gam-op'ah-the) abnormal increase in the level of gammaglobulin in the blood from proliferation of the lymphoid cells; paraproteinaemia **monoclonal g** paraproteinaemia, a heterogeneous group of diseases characterised by the presencé in the serum or urine of a monoclonal immunoglobin

gamogenesis (gam'o-jen'e-sis) sexual reproduction

ganciclovir (gan-si'klovir) an antiviral agent that is active against most herpes viruses but is particularly effective in the treatment of cytomegalovirus infections such as retinitis. It causes dose-related myelosuppression

Gandamala (s) scrofula

ganglion (gang'gle-on) 1. a mass of nerve cell collection situated outside the central nervous system 2. a cystic swelling developing on a tendon or an aponeurosis due to mucoid degeneration of tendinous tissue usually on the wrist. pl. **ganglia g blocker** drug that selectively blocks transmission at autonomic ganglia

gangliosides (gang'gle-o-sid'ez) complex lipids with ceramide linked to several hexoses and a sialic acid.

gangliosidosis (gan'gle-o-si-do-sis) a lipid storage disorder characterised by accumulation of gangliosides in the tissues due to a defect in the enzymes

gangrene (gang'gren) death and subsequent putrefaction of the tissues, such an occurrence is common in distal parts of lower extremities or internal organs **dry g** a condition caused by chronic occlusion of blood supply from a peripheral vascular disease that slowly progresses to severe tissue atrophy and mummification, seen in diabetes mellitus and atheroscleorisis **gas g** a condition seen in open or poorly cleaned wounds infected by Clostridia group of organisms especially *C. welchii*, *C. septicum* and *C. oedematiens* that release histolytic enzymes produce gas and crepitus may be felt **wet g**

condition caused by relatively acute vascular occlusion such as burns, crush injuries, thromboembolism and freezing. It results in liquefactive necrosis causing bleb and bullae formation with violaceous discolouration **vascular g** moist gangrene occurring in the viscera

ganja cannabis

Ganser's (gan'zeuz) **syndrome** voluntary production of severe psychological symptoms, named after Sighert Ganser, German psychiatrist

gantry (gan'tre) 1. the housing for the imaging source and detectors into which the patient is placed for computed tomography and MRI 2. place where linear accelerator and cobalt unit are housed

gap 1. an opening 2. a hiatus 3. GTPase-activating protein that acts as a growth signal in cancer **auscultatory gap** a period of silence noted sometimes while determining the systolic blood pressure by auscultation, may occur in some hypertensive patients **g junction** minute intercellular pores

GAPO syndrome a condition characterised by growth retardation, alopaecia, pseudo-anodontia (unerupted teeth) and optic atrophy

Gara (s) poison

Garbha (s) womb

Garbhapata (s) miscarriage

Garbhapatini (s) abortifacient

Garbhasaya (s) uterus

Garbhavichyuti (s) abortion

gardenhose appearance presence of tubular lumens with extensive transmural fibrosis and stenosis seen in terminal ileum in Crohn's disease and in oesophagus in progressive systemic sclerosis

garden screws screws for internal fixation of fracture of neck of femur

Gardnerella vaginalis a sexually transmitted anaerobic bacterium which is associated with vulvovaginitis, named after H. Gardner, US bacteriologist

Gardner's (Gard'nerz) **syndrome** familial polyposis of the colon in association with osseous and soft tissue tumours, described by American geneticist, Eldon Gardner

gargle mouth and throat wash wherein the fluid is allowed to accumulate in the back of the throat while agitating it by forceful expiration of air while head is tilted backwards

gargoyle cells cells that are engorged with mucopolysaccharide-laden lysosomes

gargoylism (gar'goi-izm) mucopolysaccharoidosis. Hurler's syndrome

garlic *Allium sativum* aromatic condiment rich in selenium, shown to enhance defences against systemic toxins, exhibit a non-specific anti-infective activity and inhibit platelet aggregation

Garre's (gar-az) **osteomyelitis** sclerosing nonsuppurative osteitis or osteomyelitis, named after Carl Garre, Swiss surgeon

Gartner's (gart'nerz) **duct** mesonephric duct lying adjacent to the uterus, named after Hermann Gartner, Danish surgeon.

gas one of the basic forms of matter, whose molecules move freely and swiftly. Oxygen, hydrogen, nitrogen and carbon dioxide form common important gases. Other gases are carbon monoxide, helium, sewer gas, ammonia, anaesthetic gases and the poisonous war gases **Bhopal g** *see* Bhopal gas, **blood g's** oxygen, nitrogen and carbon dioxide are found in the blood. They are found dissolved in the plasma or held in loose chemical combination with haemoglobin **g bacillus** *Clostridium perfringens* **g chromatography** separation and identification of substances by passage of gas over column of material which either absorbs or dissolves them **g distension** distension from abnormal accumulation of gas in abdominal cavity **inert g** the gas that does not react with other

substances such as helium **laughing g** nitrous oxide **marsh g** methane **nerve g** a gas that interferes with or prevents transmission of nerve impulses **nitric oxide g** administered in small quantities during mechanical ventilation **sewer g** a gas produced by decaying matter in sewage **tear g** bromoacetone that irritates the conjunctiva and produces flow of tears **toxic g** any harmful gas **vesicant g** gas causing blisters such as mustard and lewisite gases **war g** chemical substances producing poisonous gases that have irritant effects

gasometry (gas-om'e-tre) estimation of the amount of gas in a mixture

gasp to catch the breath

gasping baby syndrome condition in premature newborns consisting of severe metabolic acidosis, encephalopathy and respiratory depression with gasping following repeated administration of benzyl alcohol containing bacteriostatic solutions

gasserectomy (ga'er-ek-to-me) the excision of trigeminal (gasserian) ganglion

Gasserian ganglion trigeminal ganglion, named after G. Gasser, Austrian anatomist

gaster (gas'ter) stomach

gastralgia (gas-tral'jah) pain in the stomach

gastrectomy (gas-trek'tah-me) surgical removal of the stomach either partially or totally

gastric pertaining to stomach **g acid** digestive acid secreted by glands in the stomach **g analysis** analysis of gastric contents of the stomach for determination of amount of hydrochloric acid and for presence of blood, bile and bacteria **g carcinoma** stomach cancer, a disease of the old with features of recent onset of dyspepsia, vomiting, ulcer like pain, pain not relieved by food or antacids, easy satiety, weight loss and gastrointestinal bleeding. Majority of gastric cancers are adenocarcinomas. **g digestion** the phase of digestion that takes in the stomach. Pepsin hydrolyses proteins to peptones, and coagulates the milk **g erosion** a break in the mucosa of the stomach **g inhibitory polypeptide** a polypeptide hormone secreted by duodenum and jejunum that inhibits the motility and the secretion of gastric hydrochloric acid and pepsin **g juice** a mixture of digestive secretions (pepsin, hydrochloric acid, mucin, inorganic salts of the stomach) from stomach lining and it breaks down protein in food and destroys infectious organisms **g lavage** stomach wash. **g triangle** an anatomic region defined by the junction of systemic and common bile duct superiorly, the junction of second and third segments of the duodenum infero-laterally and the neck and body of the pancreas medially. Most gastrinomas are located in this region **g ulcer** ulceration in mucosa **benign g u** a circumscribed erosion of the mucosal layer of the stomach **chronic g u** single ulcer situated on the lesser curve within the antrum or at the junction between body and antral mucosa. It extends below to muscularis mucosa. It presents with recurrent abdominal pain sharply localised to the epigastrium, and is noted after food

gastrin (gas'trin) a polypeptide hormone secreted by the glands in the pyloric end of the stomach which stimulates the secretion of gastric acid and pepsin

gastrinoma (gas'tri-no'ma) a gastrin secreting tumour of the pancreatic islet delta cells associated with Zollinger-Ellison syndrome

gastritis (gas-trit'is) inflammation of the mucous membrane lining of the stomach **acute g** acute and sudden irritation of the gastric mucosa due to ingestion of alcohol or poisons **atrophic g** chronic gastritis with atrophied mucosa and glands **chronic g** prolonged inflammation of gastric mucosa

gastrocnemius (gas'tro-ne'me-us) the most superficial large muscle in the poste-

rior part of the leg. It flexes the knee and plantar flexes the foot

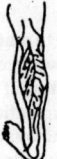

Gastrocnemius muscle

gastrocoele (gas'tro-sel) hernial protrusion of the stomach

gastrocolic (gas'tro-ko-lik) pertaining to the stomach and colon

gastrocolostomy (gas'tro-kol-os'tah-me) surgical anastomosis of the stomach to the colon

gastroduodenal (-doo-od'in-al) of or pertaining to the stomach and duodenum

gastroduodenitis (-doo-od'in-i-tis) inflammation of the stomach and duodenum

gastroduodenoscopy (-doo'od-in-os'ko-pe) endoscopic examination of the stomach and duodenum

gastroduodenostomy (gas'tro-du'o-den'os-to-me) an anastomosis of upper part of the stomach and duodenum following excision of pylorus of the stomach

gastrodynia (-din'e-ah) pain in the stomach

gastroenteric (-en'ter-ik) pertaining to the stomach and the intestine

gastroenteritis (-en'ter-it-is) inflammation of the lining of the stomach and intestine as a result of infection

gastroenteroanastomosis (-en'ter-o-ah-nas'tamo-sis) surgical anastomosis of the stomach to the small intestine

gastroenterologist (-en'ter-ol'ah-jist) a physician specialising in gastroenterology

gastroenterology (-en'ter-ol-ah-je) the study of the alimentary tract and its diseases

gastroenterostomy (-en-tros'tah-me) surgical anastomosis of the stomach to the intestine usually at the jejunum

gastroepiploic (gas'tro-ep'i-plo'ik) pertaining to stomach and greater omentum

gastroesophageal (-e-sof'a-je'al) of or pertaining to the stomach and oesophagus **g junction** the point at which the oesophagus joins the stomach that is protected by a sphincter **g reflux** a backward flow of contents of the stomach into the oesophagus as a result of incompetence of the lower oesophageal sphincter **g reflux disease** GERD backward reflux may cause oesophagitis, oesophageal ulcer, or bronchial asthma, flow of gastric contents into the oesophagus causing tissue damage which presents with heart burn and regurgitation, dysphagia, chest pain, water brash, nocturnal asthma and chronic cough

gastrogavage (-gah-vah-ze) artificial feeding through an artificial opening into the stomach

gastrograffin (-graf'in) the iodinated water soluble contrast medium

gastrointestinal (-intes'ti-nal) of or pertaining to the stomach and intestine **g bleeding** any bleeding from the gastroinstestinal tract. The common causes are peptic ulcer, oesophageal varices, carcinoma of the stomach, drugs (aspirin, NSAIDs, corticosteroids) and Mallory–Weiss syndrome **g decompression** removal of gases from intestinal tract by suction through a tube **g series** a series of barium x-ray examinations in which x-rays are taken at various intervals after a patient has swallowed a suspension of barium sulphate **g tract** alimentary tract; digestive tract, consisting of the mouth, oesophagus, stomach and intestine

gastrojejunostomy (je-joo'no-sto-me) surgical anastomosis of the stomach to the jejunum that bypasses the duodenum to prevent gastric acid from irritating a duodenal ulcer

gastrorrhagia (-ra'jah) haemorrhage from the stomach

gastroschiasis (gas-tros'ki-sis) a congenital defect with incomplete closure of the anterior abdominal wall with protrusion of the viscera

gastroscope (gas'tro-skop) an endoscope utilised to visualise the interior of the stomach

gastroscopy (gas-tros'kope) the visual inspection of the interior of the stomach by fiberoptic gastroscope inserted through the oesophagus

gastrostomy (gàs-tros'tah-me) surgical creation of an artificial opening into the stomach through the abdominal wall. **g feeding** the introduction of a nutrient solution through a tube that has been inserted into the stomach through the abdominal wall

gastrotomy (gas-trot'ah-me) incision into the stomach

gastrula (gas'troo-la) an early embryonic stage formed by the invagination of the blastula. It consists of an outer ectoderm and inner mesentoderm.

Gate theory pain does not depend on specific nerve endings but on balance and frequency of impulses reaching the spinal cord

gating 1. the opening and closing of voltage-activated channels regulated by transmembrane voltage and neurotransmitters 2. a procedure in radiology to reduce artifacts caused by involuntary movement

Gaucher's (go-shaz) **disease** a rare hereditary disorder of glucocerebroside metabolism characterised by widespread reticuloendothelial cell hyperplasia, leading to enlargement of the liver and spleen, bone damage and anaemia, described by French physician, Phillipe Gaucher

Gaussian curve *stat* normal curve of random distribution about mean, named after Friendrich Gauss, German mathematician and physicist

gauze (gawz) a light, open meshed cotton fabric used in the bandages and dressings

gavage (gah-vahzh') forced feeding through the stomach tube

gay homosexual **g bowel syndrome** a variety of infectious and non-infectious gastrointestinal symptoms in homosexuals.

gaze (gaz) to look in one direction for a period of time. **g nystagmus** jerking noted when eyes move to its limits, noted in brain stem lesion.

G-cells flask-shaped cells present in the gastric mucosa especially in the pyloric antum

G-CSF abbreviation for granulocyte colony-stimulating factor

Gee's (gez) **disease** the infantile form of coeliac disease, named after Samuel Gee, British physician

Gegenhalten (ga'gen-hal'ten) *Ger* involuntary resistance to passive movement of the extremities. It increases with the velocity of movement and continues through the full arc of motion noted in arteriosclerotic Parkinsonism

Gee-Thaysen (ge'thi'sen) **disease** the adult form of coeliac disease, named after Samuel Gee and Thorwald Thaysen, Dutch physicians

Geigel's (gi'gelz) **reflex** contraction of muscle fibres adjacent to superior portion of inguinal ligament, when the inner aspect of the upper thigh is stroked in a female. The reflex corresponds to male cremasteric reflex, named after Richard Geigel, German physician

Geiger-Muller (gi'ger-mil'er) **counter** an amplifying device that indicates the presence of ionising particles emitted by a substance, named after Hans Geiger, German physicist in England

gel (jel) a colloid that is firm in consistency **agar g** a semisolid medium prepared from the sea weed agar **aluminium hydroxide g** a white viscous suspension of aluminium hydroxide used as an antacid

gelastic epilepsy a partial seizure due to epileptic discharges in temporal lobe.

There is inappropriate laughter

gelatin (jel'a-tin) a substance obtained by partial hydrolysis of collagen

Gelineau's (zha-li-no') **tetrad** occurrence of narcolepsy, cataplexy, sleep paralysis and hypnogogic hallucinations in the same patient, named after Jean Gelineau, French neurologist

gelling stiffness following rest noted in juvenile rheumatoid arthritis

gemellipara (jem'el-lip'a-ra) one who has borne twins

gemellology (jem'el-ol'o-je) the study of twins

gemfibrozil a fabric acid derivative having potent lipid-lowering effect

gen a word termination for an agent that produces

gena (je'na) cheek

genal (ge'nil) buccal

gender the sex of an individual **g adoption** lengthy process of learning the behaviours that are traditional for one's gender **g identification** assignment of gender to a new-born on biologic basis **g identity** the sex classification of an individual where the sense of maleness or femaleness is influenced by culture **g preference** emotional and intellectual acceptance for the gender that one is **g schema** mental image of the cognitive, affective, and performance characteristics appropriate to a particular gender

gene (jen) the basic functional unit of heredity located at a definite locus on a particular chromosome. It consists of de-oxyribonucleic acid (DNA) which controls the cell function and reproduction **candidate g** a gene located in a chromosome region suspected of being involved in a disease, whose protein product suggests that it could be the disease gene in question **dominant g** a gene that expresses a trait without the assistance from its allele **g amplification** the increase in copy numbers of a gene and it is associated with

cellular oncogenes in malignancy **g diversity** a variety of immune response that an antigen is capable of evoking **g expression** transcription of a segment of DNA to mRNA and translation into a protein **g mapping** determining the relative positions of genes on a chromosome and the distance between them **g pod** the sum total of genes, with all their variations, possessed by a particular species at a particular time **g product** a polypeptide encoded by a gene **g promotion** activation of genes. It is facilitated by breaks in the ordered array of nucleosomes **g rearrangement** the shuffling of genetic material where the intervening sequences (introns) are recovered and exons are spliced together to form mRNA **g recombination** see recombinant DNA **suicide g** a strategy to make cancer cells more vulnerable to chemotherapy **g splicing** the use of micromanipulation methods to insert a portion of a gene from one species into a gene from another species enabling the altered gene to function differently **g testing** the study of genetic material to diagnose conditions caused by abnormalities of genes or chromosomes **g therapy** the introduction of normal genes into tissues expressing defective genes **g tracking** the study of DNA markers to establish the transmission pattern of a specific disease causing gene in a family **g transfer** transfer of a gene from one animal to another to repair an inherited defect in the recipient **mutant g** an altered gene that functions differently than it did before its change **recessive g** a gene that does not express itself in presence of its dominant allele. A recessive trait may be apparent in phenotype only if both alleles are recessive **sex-linked g** a gene found within the X or Y chromosomes **SRY g** sex-determining region Y gene, found at the distal end of chromosome Y and its presence dictates development of testicles while its absence results in ovarian differentiation **structural g** a gene that determines the structure of polypeptide chains by having control on the sequence of amino acids **tumour suppressor g** a gene that suppresses the growth of malignant cells **x-linked g** a gene on X chromosome for which there is no corresponding gene on Y chromosome

geneology the study of the ancestry of an individual or group.

general adaptation syndrome a defence response of the body or the psyche to injury or prolonged stress. There is an initial phase of shock followed by a phase of adaptation by utilising various defence mechanisms of the body or mind. It may lead to a stage of adjustment or exhaustion, described by Hans Selye, Austrian-Canadian endocrinologist

general anaesthesia administration of various anaesthetic agents either by inhalation or intravenous injection to cause loss of sensation and consciousness

generalise 1. to become systemic 2. to become nonspecific

General paralysis of insane (GPI) a late manifestation of syphilis seen 20 years after the infection and characterised by alteration in higher function, and dementia. It is associated with euphoric grandiose state, agitated delirium, bilateral pyramidal signs, fits and widespread tremors. There is frontal and temporal lobe atrophy

generation (jen'er'-a'shun) the act of reproducing off-spring **g time** the interval of time between receipt of infection by a host and maximal infectivity of that host

generic (jen-er'ik) 1. general 2. pertaining to a genus 3. distinctive **g drugs** non-proprietary name of the drug describing its chemical structure **g name** the nonproprietary name assigned to a drug

genesis (jen'e-sis) 1. the origin of anything 2. the act of reproducing

genetic (je-net'ik) 1. pertaining to reproduction, both or origin 2. pertaining to heredity 3. pertaining to or produced by a gene **g analysis** laboratory study of DNA to diagnose genetic disorders **g burden** the impact of pathologic changes from inherited traits or diseases **g code** genetic information carried by specific DNA molecules that determine the specific amino acids and their arrangement in the polypeptides chain of each protein synthesised by the cell **g counselling** the communication of information about disorders with a genetic component **g death** the failure of an organism to survive as a result of its genetic makeup **g disease** any inherited condition caused by a defective gene, most of which are an inborn error of metabolism **g disorder** any disease or condition that is genetically determined **g drift** tendency for variation in gene frequencies within a small population **g engineering** the manipulation of the genome of a living organism by insertion of genes or by genetic selection **g equilibrium** a condition within a population wherein the frequency of genes and genotyps does not alter from generation to generation **g fingerprint** DNA fingerprint **g heterogenicity** the presence of a variety of genetic defects which produce the same clinical disease **g linkage** existence of two genes close together on the same chromosome **g locus** the site of a gene on a pair of homologous chromosomes **g mapping** a technique to locate the site of particular genes on chromosomes **g marker** a visible mutable site on a chromosome which when mutated brings about marked changes to the host organism and on the chromosome **g predisposition** inherited tendency to develop a disease if necessary environmental factors exist **g probes** labelled fragments of DNA used in de-

tection of the presence of matching fragments in a sample of person's DNA **g recombination** the process by which blocks of homologous chromosomes exchange material by crossing over. It is seen during meiosis

geneticist (jen-et'i-sist) a person specialised in genetics

genetics (je-net'iks) 1. biological science dealing with heredity and the laws governing it 2. the genetic makeup of a particular individual, family or group **g screening** undertaking investigations to detect presence of any inherited disorder

Geneva Convention an international agreement made in 1864, whose signatory nations pledged to treat wounded persons and the army medical and nursing staff as neutrals in the battle field. It was revised and expanded in 1949. According to that the medical personnel and treatment facilities are designated as immune from attack and captured medical personnel are to be promptly repatriated

genial (je'ne-al) pertaining to the chin

genic (jen'ik) suffix meaning giving rise to; causing

genicular (je-nik'u-ler) pertaining to the knee

geniculate (je-nik'u-lat) bent **g ganglion** ganglion of facial nerve

genital (jen'i-tal) pertaining to reproductory organs or reproduction **g herpes** an infection with *Herpes simplex* acquired through sexual contact, characterised by vesicles on the genitals **g tract** organs that make up the male or female reproductive system **g ulcers genital warts g warts** warts on the genitals and anus due to human papillomavirus

genitals male and female reproductive organs, both internal and external **female g** reproductive organs of the female sex. The internal genitalia consists of two ovaries, two fallopian tubes, uterus and vagina. The external genitalia consists of vulva or pudendum that includes mons veneris, labia majora, labia minora, clitoris, fourchette, vestibule, vestibular bulb, Skene's glands, Bartholin's glands, hymen and vaginal introitus **male g** reproductive organs of male sex, consist of two testes, scrotum, two epididymis, two vas deferens, two seminal vesicles, two prostate glands, two ejaculatory ducts, urethra, two Cowper's glands and penis

genitalia (jen'i-tal'e-ah) reproductory organs

genitourinary pertaining to the genitals and the urinary organs (kidneys, ureters, urinary bladder and urethra)

genocide (jen'o-sid) the willful murder of a particular social or ethnic group

genome (je'nom) a complete set of genes in the chromosomes that give instructions for growth, development and function of the organs **human g** consist 3.2 billion base pairs. Arranged in 24 chromosomes. Humans are only 99 per cent identical; and 0.1 per cent makes them individual rather than identical clones **g map** writing out of an entire chromosome, DNA sequence, or genome

genomic imprinting affection of expression of the gene by the parental origin of chromosome

genomic library collection of cloned DNA fragments containing all genetic materials of cell line under study

genotype (jen'o-tip) the genetic constitution of an individual

gentamicin (jen'tah-mi'sin) antibiotic elaborated by Micromonospora fungi, which is effective against gram-negative and gram-positive bacteria

gentian violet a coal tar dye used as a stain in histology and also as an antibacterial and antifungal agent

genu knee **g recurvatum** hyperextension at knee joint **g valgum** knock knee **g varum** bow legs

geo -a combining word for earth

Geobiology (ge'o-bio-loji) study of an area of electromagnetics which focuses on environmental influences on the body's electromagnetic field; electromagnetic pollution

geographic distribution of disease relation between the prevalence of a disease and specific geographic-environmental conditions

geographic tongue 1. a map-like pattern noted on the tongue from breakdown of its surface cell coating in a patchy fashion 2. a chronic migrating superficial glossitis

geographic ulcer a sharply demarcated corneal ulcer with scalloped margins due to *Herpes simplex*

geophagy (geo-pha-ge) clay eating

geotrichosis (je'o-tri-ko'sis) fungal infection due to *Geotrichum candidium*

genus (je'nus) classification between family and species

GERD abbreviation for gastro-oesophageal reflux disase

Gerhardt's test ferric chloride test for acetoacetic acid in urine, named after Charles Gerhardt, French chemist

geriatrician a specialist in Geriatrics

geriatrics (jer'e-at'riks) the branch of medical science dealing with the problems of ageing and diseases of the elderly

Geriatric Society of India GSI

germ 1. a micro-organism 2. first rudiment of a developing part or organ **g layers** three primary cell layers (ectoderm, mesoderm and endoderm) in the embryo from which the organs and tissues develop **g line** inherited material that comes from the ova or sperm and is passed on to the offspring **g theory** theory stating that certain diseases are the result of pathologic microorganisms in the body

germ cells gamete or their precursors **g c aplasia** absence of spermatocytes in the testes with infertility and high FSH **g c tumours** tumours arising from malignant degeneration of the germ cell epithelium, testicular tumours and benign cystic teratomas are examples

German measles rubella, an acute exanthematous viral infection noted in children. It may occur in pregnancy to result in various developmental defects. The infection from rubella virus, a single stranded RNA virus, after an incubation period of 2-3 weeks produces an evanescent rash on the face and neck spreading downwards, accompanied by fever, malaise, sore throat, palatal enanthema and rapidly extending maculopapular rash

germicide (jer'mi-sid) agent that destroys the pathogenic micro-organisms

germinal centre the site in lymph nodes and lymphoid aggregates where normal lymphocyte transformation occurs

germination sprouting of a seed

germinoma (jer'mi-no'ma) any neoplasm with morphological features of a germ cell

gerodontics (ger'o-don-tiks) dentistry dealing with the dental problems of elderly

gerontology (je-ron-tol'o-je) scientific study of the ageing phenomenon as it affects cells and organisms

Gerota's (ga-ro'tahz) **fascia** renal or perirenal fascia, named after Dimitru Gerota, Bucharest anatomist

gestation (jes-ta'shun) period of development from fertilisation of the ovum to the birth

gestational assessment determination of the prenatal age of the foetus

gesture expression by body movement

GFR abbreviation for glomerular filtration rate

GH abbreviation for growth hormone

Ghon's focus primary pulmonary tuberculosis, named after Anton Ghon, Czech pathologist

ghost cells red blood cells having only cell membrane without any haemoglobin, seen in microscopic examination of the urine

GHRH abbreviation for growth hormone-releasing hormone

giant cell a large tissue cell **g c arteritis** a large vessel vasculitis occurring predominantly in elderly people who present with severe headache **g c carcinoma** a highly malignant tumour occurring in the lung or thyroid **g c fibroblastoma** a benign mesenchymal tumour occurring in children often located in the superficial tissues of the back and thigh **g c glioblastoma** a firm well circumscribed tumour in the brain that is highly cellular, with haemorrhage and necrosis **g c hepatitis** giant cell transformation of the liver of the newborn as a reaction to increased conjugated hyperbilirubinaemia of any aetiology **g c myocarditis** focal granulomatous necrosis with multi-nucleated giant cells in the myocardium as a virally-induced immune reaction **g c pneumonia** a fulminant respiratory disease with dyspnoea and tachycardia as a complication of measles **g c tumour** 1. a bony tumour in the weight bearing epiphysis of distal femur, proximal tibia and distal radius 2. a fibrous histiocytoma involving the flexor tendon sheath exhibiting presence of osteoclast like giant cells with hyalinisation

Giardia (je-ar'de-a) a flagellate protozoal parasite, *Giardia lamblia*, described by French biologist, Alfred Giard. It is a heart shaped single celled organism with two nucleus and four pairs of flagella. They attach to the intestinal mucosa and absorb nutrients.

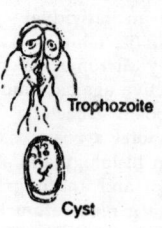

Giardia

giardiasis infestation of the small intestine by *Giardia lamblia* giving rise to diarrhoea and malabsorption. It is treated with metronidazole, tinidazole and furazolidine

Gibbon catheter narrow gauze self-retaining plastic catheter for long term urinary retention, named after N. Gibbon, UK surgeon.

gibbus a hump

Gibralter fever brucellosis.

Gibson's (gib'sunz) **murmur** a long systolic and diastolic 'machinery-like' murmur heard over the left second interspace in patent ductus arteriosus, named after Alexander Gibson, Scottish physician

giddiness dizziness

Giemsa's (gem'zas) **stain** a stain with azure dyes used to stain the blood smear to demonstrate protozoan parasites, described by German chemist, Gustav Giemsa

Gierke's (ger'kez) **disease** deficiency of glucose 6 phosphatase enzyme in the liver causing hepatomegaly, hypoglycaemia, hyperuricemia and gout, named after Edger von Gierke, German pathologist.

Giernards's disease visceroptosis. There is protrusion of lower abdomen on standing due to downward displacement of liver, spleen and kidney

GIFT 1. gamete intra-fallopian transfer, a procedure for treatment of infertility in which mature ova are removed from a woman's ovaries, combined with sperms and injected into one of the fallopian tubes of the woman 2. granulocyte immunofluorescence test

Gigabyte Gb a unit of memory capacity. One gigabyte is 1000 megabytes

Gigli's (jel'yez) **saw** flexible wire saw with handles at each end for cutting bone, named after Leonardo Gigli, Italian obstetrician

gigantism (ji'gan-tizm) increased size and stature of the body occurring before the closure of the growing ends of the bones due to hypersecretion of growth hormone

Gilbert's (zhel-barz) **disease** benign hereditary hyperbilirubinaemia and mild intermittent jaundice, described by French physician, Nicolas Gilbert

Gilchrist's disease North American blastomycosis, named after Thomas Gilchrist, US dermatologist

Gilles de la Tourette's syndrome complexities with vocalisations, often with obscene uttarances and rude gestures which may start in childhood and persist into adult life, which responds to dopaminergic receptor antagonists, named after Georges Gilles de la Tourette, French physician

Gille's test the disease of sacroiliac joint is tested while the patient is lying prone in the bed. While fixing the pelvis on the unaffected side, the affected thigh is hyperextended and the patient winces with pain if the joint is involved

ginger (jin'jer) spicy material from root of Zingiber plant, used to flavour medicines and food

gingiva (jin'ji-vah) gum, the part of the oral mucosa covering the tooth bearing border of the jaw

gingival pertaining to the gums

gingivectomy (jin'ji-vek'ta-me) surgical removal of diseased gingival tissue

gingivitis (jin'ji-vi'tis) inflammation of the gums usually caused by poor dental hygiene

ginseng Chinese herbal remedy having corticosteroid-like properties considered aphrodisiac

girdle pain painful condition due to lesions involving one or more nerve roots at the same side bilaterally

girdle a zone or belt **pelvic g** portion of lower extremities composed of 2 hip (innominate bones) bones to which the lower limbs are attached **shoulder g** portion of upper extremity composed of two clavicles and two scapulae to which the upper limbs are attached

gitter (git'er) **cell** a macrophage filled with lipoid granules from phagocytosis of damaged brain cells

glabella (glah-bel'a) the area between the eyebrows above the nasion

glabellar tap sign tapping the forehead causes repetitive blinking in Parkinsomism

glabrous (glah-brus) smooth or hairless

glacial (gla'shal) resembling ice

gladiolus (glah-di'o-lus) body of the sternum

gland an aggregation of specialised cells concerned with secretion or elimination which is not related to their own metabolism; the two main types are the endocrine glands and the exocrine glands

glanders (glan'derz) an infection caused by *Pseudomonas mallei*, it can be communicated to man from infected horses

glandular fever *see* infectious mononucleosis

glandule (glan'dul) small gland

glans (glanz) conical, acorn-shaped structure

glare temporary blurring of vision

Glasgow coma scale a quick method of grading of degree of conscious impairment in critically ill neurologically impaired patient by a numerical scale based on eyes opening, best verbal response and best motor response. Coma is indicated by a score of 7 or less

glasses 1. a transparent refractive device worn either to correct refractive errors or to protect the eyes from glare or foreign bodies **bifocal g** glasses in which the refractive power of the lower portion differs from that in the upper portion—the lower is being used to view near objects or reading and the upper to view distant objects.

glossy smooth and shiny

glaucoma (glaw-ko'mah) disease of the eye exhibiting raised intraocular pressure, causing internal damage and affecting the vision if untreated. It develops when the aqueous humour drainage is too slow to keep up with its production in anterior chamber

gleet (gl'et) a mucoid or purulent urethral discharge

glenoid (gle'no-id) a pit or a socket **g cavity** a shallow depression with which the head of the humerus articulates **g fossa** fossa of temporal bone that receives the condyle of the mandible

glia (gli'ah) neural cells having a connective tissue support, neurolgia

gliadin (gli'ah-din) a water-insoluble protein that is present in the gluten of wheat

glibenclamide oral hypoglycaemic agent of a sulphonyl group

gliclazide long-acting oral hypoglycaemic agent

gliding a smooth continuous, movement **g joint** a synovial joint in which articulation of contiguous bones allow one surface to move smoothly over an adjacent surface, as in wrist and ankle

glioblastoma (gli'o–blas-to'mah) malignant astrocytoma

glioma (glio'mah) primary tumour of the brain with glial cells, that vary widely in its degree of malignancy and rate of growth

gliomatous (gli-o-mah'tus) excess development of the neuroglia

gliosis (gli-o'sis) the proliferation of neuroglial tissue in CNS **Bergmann g** anoxic injury and death of Purkinge cells

glipizide short-acting oral hypoglycaemic agent of sulphonyl urea group and is effective when given twice daily

Glisson's (glis'enz) **capsule** the fibrous tissue sheath around the lobules of the liver that carry branches of the hepatic artery, portal vein and bile duct, named after Francis Glisson, English physician

glitter cells microscopic examination of urine revealing movement of granules in the cytoplasm of white blood cells

global complete, overall **g aphasia** combination of a grossly nonfluent aphasia and severe fluent aphasia (inability to understand the spoken word)

globi (glo'bi) encapsulated globular masses containing bacilli, especially lepra bacilli

globin (glo'bin) the protein of the haemoglobin

globular (glob'u-lar) resembling a globe or spherical

globule (glob'ul) a small spherical mass

globulin (glob'ulin) a protein found in plasma, that play important role in the formation of antibodies

globus (glo'bus) a spherical mass **g hystericus** an emotional disorder giving an uncomfortable sensation of having a lump in the throat. **g pallidus** the smaller and more medial part of the lentiform nucleus of the brain

glomectomy (glo-mek'to-me) excision of a glomus

glomerular (glo-mer'u-lar) of or pertaining to glomerulus

glomerulitis (glo-mer'u-li-tis) inflammation of a glomerulus

glomerulonephritis (glo-mer'u-lo-ne-fri-tis) (GN) a group of diseases caused by immune mechanisms in which the glomeruli are primarily involved **acute g** post-infections glomerulonephritis **chronic g** terminal stage of many forms of glomerulonephritis. The kidneys are symmetrically contracted with smooth contour. Often there is hypertension **membranoproliferative g** thickening of the glomerular basement membrane and proliferation of mesangial and endothelial cells. **mesangial proliferative g** mesangial widening and mesangial cellular proliferation similar to that seen in IgA nephropathy. It presents with features of nephrotic syndrome and runs a benign course **post infectious g** acute nephritis developing 1 to 2 weeks after a history of acute respiratory infection or in association with infected scabies noted mostly in children with sudden onset of haematuria in the form of smoky

urine, early morning puffiness of face, oliguria and hypertension. There is endocapillary proliferative glomerulonephritis. Disease is self-limiting **rapidly progressive g** a clinical syndrome in which renal function deteriorates over a period of days or weeks in a patient with glomerulonephritis. There is crescent formation, haematuria, and azotaemia. The condition may be due to antibodies to the glomerular basement membrane, or due to immune complexes or without any immunoglobulin deposition

glomerulopathy (glo-mer'ul-op'ah-the) non-inflammatory disease of the renal glomeruli

glomerulosclerosis (glo-mer'u-lo-skle-ro'sis) arteriolar nephrosclerosis wherein there is scarring as a result of damage to the glomeruli of the kidneys

glomerulus (glo-mer'u-lus) a tuft of convoluted mass of capillaries enclosed in a Browman's capsule of the kidney. This is the site of filtration which is the first step in the formation of urine

glomus (glo'mus) a small body consisting of fine arterioles communicating directly with the venules, and a rich nerve supply, the aortic body and carotid body are examples **g bodies** regulated arteriovenous anastomosis in the skin that play a role in thermoregulation **g tumour** tumour of the jugular bulb presenting with weakness of sternomastoid and trapezius

glossa (glos'ah) the tongue.

glossal (glos'al) pertaining to the tongue.

glossalgia (glos-sal'je-ah) pain in the tongue.

glossectomy (glos-sek'to-me) excision of a portion or whole of the tongue, as a treatment for cancer of tongue

glossitis (glos-it'is) inflammation of the tongue

glossodynia (glos'od-din-ea) pain in the tongue

glossolalia (glos'o-la'lea) an expression of

a revelatory message through unintelligible words

glossopharyngeal (glos'o-fer-in'je-al) of or pertaining to the tongue and pharynx. **g nerve** ninth cranial nerve **g neuralgia** severe pain in throat, tongue and ear triggered by swallowing

glottis (glot'is) larynx containing the vocal cords and the opening between them. It is the sound producing apparatus

glove a protective covering for the hand

glove and stocking region of distribution of sensory losses in neuropathies

glucagon (gloo'ka-gon) a polypeptide hormone secreted by the alpha cells of the islets of Langerhans, that stimulates the release of glucose into the blood stream

glucagonoma (gloo'ka-gon-o'mah) a glucagon secreting tumour.

glucocorticoid (gloo'ko-kor'ti-koid) corticoid hormone produced by the adrenal cortex that increases the gluconeogenesis, and suppresses inflammation

glucogenesis (gloo'ko-jen'e-sis) the formation of glucose from glycogen

glucokinase (gloo'ko-ki'nas) an enzyme found in the liver cells that in presence of ATP catalyses the conversion of glucose to glucose-6-phosphate, which is the first step in glycolysis

glucometer a battery operated device used to measure blood glucose from a few drops of blood obtained from the finger

gluconeogenesis (gloo'ko-ne'o-jen'e-sis) the synthesis of glucose from non-carbohydrate sources

glucosamine (gloo-ko'sah-min) an amino derivative of glucose

glucose (gloo'kos) a simple sugar, monosaccharide. It is the chief source of energy for living organisms

glucose-6-phosphate dehydrogenase (G6PD) the first enzyme in the hexose monophosphate from which red cells derive most of their metabolic energy. **G6PD deficiency** a genetic disorder

lacking G6PD that makes the red cells prone to damage during infections or following ingestion of certain drugs and foods

glucose tolerance test (GTT) a test of body's response to a dose of glucose after a period of fasting, used to diagnose diabetes mellitus

glucosidase (gloo'ko'si-das) an enzyme that splits glucoside

glucoside (gloo'ko-sid) a glycoside that on hydrolysis yields glucose

glucosuria (gloo'ko-su're-a) the presence of glucose in the urine

glucuronic acid carboxyl acid metabolite of glucose

glucuronide (gloo-ku'ron'id) soluble form in which many drugs are excreted and are linked to glucuronic acid in urine

glucuronyl transferases enzymes active in glucuronic acid conjugation

glue ear non-suppurative otitis media, associated with conductive deafness

GLUT glucose transport protein units, promote uptake of glucose by cells after insulin causes transfer of the GLUT from the Golgi apparatus to the cell membrane

glutamate a neurotransmitter in the brain probably participating in memory

glutamic (gloo-tam'ik) **acid** a non-essential amino acid

glutamic oxaloacetic transaminase (GOT) an enzyme that catalyses the reversible transfer of an amino group, aspartic acid

glutamic pyruvicacetic transaminase (GPT) an enzyme that catalyses the reversible transfer of alanin

glutaminase (gloo-tam'i-nas) an enzyme that catalyses the breakdown of glutamine into glutamic acid and ammonia

glutamine (gloo'ta-min) a non-essential amino acid

γ glutamyl transpeptidase GGTP an enzyme that transfers amino acids across membranes using energy of glutathione, raised in liver diseases and in metastatic cancer

glutaraldehyde (gloo-ta-ral'de-hid) 1. a sterilising agent effective against all micro-organisms 2. a primary fixative agent for electron microscopy

glutathione (gloo'ta-thi'on) a tripeptide of glycine, cystine and glutamic acid **g reductase** protect the red cells against damage due to oxidation

gluteal (gloo'te-al) relate to the buttocks

gluten (gloo'ten) the insoluble protein derived from wheat **g free diet** elimination of gluten from diet avoiding products of wheat, oats, rye or barley **g enteropathy** *see* coeliac disease

gluteus maximus the large powerful muscle in each of the buttocks that gives them their rounded shape and moves the thigh sideways and backward

glycaemia (gli-se'me-ah) presence of glucose in the blood

glycan (gli'kan) polysaccharide

glycerin (glis'er-in) trihydroxypropane used as a solvent, a preservative and as an emollient in various skin diseases. It reduces intracranial and intraocular tensions

glyceride (glis'er-id) an ester of glycerol

glycerol a constituent of many fatty substances. It is released from food during digestion and absorbed on its own or in combination with fatty acids

glyceryl trinitrate short acting vasodilator used in angina pectoris, usually under the tongue; nitroglycerin

glycine a non-essential simple aminoacid.

glycogen (gli'ko-jen) main carbohydrate reserve which is easily converted into glucose **g storage diseases** a group of familial enzyme defects affecting glycogen breakdown, usually with liver storage

glycogenesis (gli'ko-jen'e-sis) formation of glycogen from glucose

glycogenolysis (gli'ko-je-nol'i-sis) hydrolysis of glycogen to glucose

glycogenosis (gli'ko-je-no'sis) glycogen storage disease

glycolipid (gli-ko-lip'id) a compound of fatty acid with a carbohydrate containing nitrogen found in myelin sheaths

glycolysis (gli-kol'i-sis) non-mitochondrial conversion of glucose and ADP to lactate and ATP, major source of energy for voluntary and cardiac muscles

glyconeogenesis (gli'ko-ne'o-jen'i-sis) formation of glycogen from non-carbohydrate sources

glycopaenia (gli'ko-pe'ne-ah) a deficiency of sugar in an organ or tissue

glycopeptide (gli'ko-pep'tid) a compound containing sugar and aminoacids or peptides

glycoprotein (gli'ko-pro'ten) a protein-carbohydrate compound

glycoside (gli'co-si-d) any compound which on hydrolysis yields sugar and non-sugar residues.

glycosphingolipids (gli-ko-sf'ing'o-lipids) a group of carbohydrate-containing fatty acid derivatives of ceramide such as cerebrosides, gangliosides and ceramide oligosaccharides

glycosuria the abnormal presence of glucose in the urine, which usually results from diabetes mellitus

glycosylated haemoglobin haemoglobin linked to glucose non-enzymatically within circulation. It increases with glucose level and age of red cell. When it is over 10%, it indicates poor control of diabetes

glycosylation conjugation with glucose

glycyrrhiza (glis-i-ri'za) dried root of *Glycyrrhiza glabra* used as a flavouring agent; liquorice

GMP abbreviation for guanosine monophosphate

gnat (nat) minute insect belonging to the order Diptera

gnathic (na-thi'c) relating to the jaw

gnathostomiasis (nath'o-sto-mi'a-sis) visceral larva migrans, an infection of human tissues caused by the nematode parasite of dogs and cats

Gnedel's sign a system to describe the stages and planes of anaesthesia during an operative procedure, evolved by an American anaesthesiologist

gnosia (no'se-ah) ability to recognise the form and nature of a person or thing

Gn-RH abbreviation for gonadotropin-releasing hormone

goal the desired outcome of actions to alter the status or behaviour

goat's milk fever brucellosis

GOBI growth monitoring, oral rehydration, breast-feeding and immunisation-strategy to reduce infant mortality in developing countries

goblet cell mucus secreting cell in the bronchus, and intestinal tract

Goeckerman irradiation exposure to ultraviolet light for psoriasis, and vitiligo.

goitre (goit'er) enlargement of the thyroid gland visible as a swelling on the neck **colloid g** late stage of diffuse hyperplastic goitre following reduction in TSH stimulation in which there are many inactive follicles filled with colloid **diffuse g** simple goitre due to puberty, pregnancy, iodine deficiency or due to colloid goitre **endemic g** occurrence of goitre in certain geographic areas where the iodine content of food and water is deficient **exophthalmic g** goitre with exophthalmos **nodular g** presistent fluctuating TSH stimulation may lead to formation of a solitary thyroid nodule **retrosternal g** goitre arising from the lower pole of the nodular goitre **simple g** an euthyroid, nontoxic goitre which may be diffuse or nodular **toxic g** primary or secondary thyrotoxicosis. It may be diffuse or solitary and associated with excess production of the thyroid hormone

goitrogen (goy'tro-jen) anti-thyroid substance causing goitre, found naturally in cabbages

gold an yellow metallic element whose salts are tried in rheumatoid arthritis not controlled adequately by anti-inflammatory agents and radioactive iodine in treatment of certain cancers

Goldblatt hypertension hypertension produced by partial occlusion of renal artery, named after H. Goldblatt, US physiologist

golden hour the first hour following injury, term coined by Adams Cowley

Goldflam's (golt'flahmz) **disease** myasthenia gravis, named after Samuel Goldflam, Polish neurologist

gold standard a treatment procedure or action that is best available

golfer's elbow a painful inflammation on the inside of elbow from overuse of the muscles in the arm that pull back the hand and wrist

golf-hole ureter orifice of ureter in bladder appears as deep hole due to retraction of ureter

Golgi's apparatus a complex cellular organelle, described by Italian anatomist Camillo Golgi

Goltz's (golts'ez) **syndrome** focal dermal hypoplasia, a rare congenital disorder, named after Friedrich Goltz, German physician

gonad (go'nad) a sex gland, such as the testis and ovary that produces sperms or ova respectively

gonadotropic (go'nad-o-trof'ik) stimulating the gonads

gonodotropin (-trop'in) a hormone having a stimulatory effect on the gonads **g releasing hormones** hormones that stimulate the release of gonadotropic hormones

gonarthritis (gon'ar-thri'tis) inflammation of knee joint

Gondy-Gamma bodies calcium and haemosiderin deposits in the spleen, seen in setting of increased haemolysis

goniometer (go'ne-om'e-ter) instrument to measure the angles, used to quantitate joint movement

goniometry (go'ne-om'e-tre) measurement of the range of the motion in a joint

gonioscope (glone-ah-skop) an optical instrument for examining the angles of the anterior chamber of the eye

goniosynechia (go'ne-o-si-nek'e-a) adhesion of the iris to the cornea of the eye

goniotomy (go'ne-ot'ah-me) an opening for glaucoma

gonococcal (gon'o-kok'al) pertaining to or caused by gonococci

Gonococcus (go'no-kek'us) *Neisseria gonorrhoea* species causing gonorrhoea. It is gram-negative intracellular diplococcus

gonorrhoea (gon'ah-re'ah) a sexually transmitted disease predominantly affecting the lower genital tract, rectum and conjunctiva. The involvement of anterior urethra in male is associated with dysuria and purulent discharge. Involvement of lower cervical canal in women presents with vaginal discharge and dysuria. It is treated with penicillin

Goodpasture's syndrome an autoimmune disorder presenting with glomerulonephritis and pulmonary haemorrhage, described by American pathologist, Earnest Goodpasture

Goodsall's ligature method of tying off prolapsed rectal mucosa for excision, named after D. Goodsall, UK surgeon

Goodsall's line an imaginary line passing across the midpoint of the anus. The external opening of fistula-in-ano may be situated anterior or posterior to this line

Goodsall's rule the site of the internal opening of fistula-in-ano can be determined from the position of external opening. If the external opening is anterior to Goodsall's line, the fistula runs directly into the anal canal (direct type) and if the opening is located posterior to this line, the tract is curved with the internal opening in the midline posteriorly between the two sphincters in the anal canal (horse-shoe type)

goose flesh hair follicle erection

Gopalan's syndrome malnutrition with signs suggesting riboflavin deficiency with burning sensation in the extremities and hyperhidrosis, named after Indian nutrition specialist

Gordian knot compound volvulus; intertwining of crossed loops of bowel that tax the surgeon's plan of undoing it

Gordon's reflex variation of Babinski reflex where the calf muscles are compressed to determine the pyramidal tract lesions, described by American neurologist, Alfred Gordon

Gorham's (gor'hamz) disease reabsorption of whole or multiple bones and filling of residual spaces with heavily vascularised fibrous tissue, named after Lemuel Gorhom, US physician

Gorlin's equation useful to calculate the heart valve area, named after Richard Gorlin, US cardiologist

gossypol pigment of cotton seed, produces male infertility by acting on epididymis

gouge (gouj) a hollow chisel for cutting and removing bone

gourmand one who eats to excess, glutton, on who delights in luxurious food

gout an acute inflammatory response to monosodium urate monohydrate crystals formed secondary to hyperuricaemia **acute g** urate gout presenting suddenly in the night involving the first metatarsophlangeal joint of the big toe. The joint and surrounding tissues are swollen, hot, red, shiny and extremely painful. It may provoke migratory attacks affecting other joints over subsequent days **intercritical g** first attack of gout may be followed by similar episodes within one year. There is increase in frequency of attacks and number of sites involved **chronic g** tophaceous gout uncontrolled hyperuricaemia of long duration with recurrent episodes of gout. Tophi consisting of chalky white urate crystals appear as firm, nodular swellings

Gower's myopathy familial, late-onset muscular atrophy and weakness of the distal parts of the limb, named after William Gower, UK neurologist

Gower's (gou'arz) **sign** in Duchenne muscular dystrophy the patient reaches standing posture by climbing up legs due to gluteal weakness, named after Sir Wuilliam Gowers, British neurologist.

GP abbreviation for general practitioner

Gradenigo's syndrome occurrence of sixth cranial nerve palsy and unilateral headache in suppurative disease of the middle ear, named after G. Gradenigo, Italian otologist

graduate (grad'u-at) a person who has been awarded an academic degree from an University

graduated marked by a series of lines indicating degrees of measurement

Graaffian (graf'e-an) **follicle** a small sac in the ovary that encloses an ovum, described by Dutch physician, Reijnier de Graaf

graft any healthy tissue or organ taken from one part of the body or from a donor and surgically implanted in another part of the body to repair or replace damaged tissue or organ

grafting implanting any tissue or organ

Graft versus Host disease a rejection response that occurs following bone marrow transplant in the skin, gastrointestinal tract and liver when sensitised immunologically competent donor lymphocytes are transferred into an immunologically incompetent recipient tissues

Graham's law rate of diffusion of gas varies inversely as square root of its density, formulated by Thomas Graham, UK chemist.

Graham Steel (gra'am stel) **murmur** early diastolic murmur of pulmonary incompetence heard best in the second intercostal space next to the sternum, named after Graham Steel, English physician

Grainger's method palpation of abdomen by the child's own-hand. It will pull out the hand away and start crying as the point of maximum tenderness is approached. This method is useful in screaming children, who are too young to cooperate

gram a unit of weight of metric system.

Gram's (gramz) **stain** a procedure of staining bacteria with crystal violet and iodine, alcohol removes the stain from gram-negative but not from gram-positive organisms, described by Danish physician, Hans Gram

Gram-negative organisms lack teichoic acid and do not take Gram's stain that cause infections in the genitourinary and gastrointestinal tracts

Gram-positive organisms have teichoic acid on their cell wall and take Gram's stain, that cause infections on the skin and in the respiratory tract

grand mal (gran-mal) a major epilepsy exhibiting tonic-clonic seizures with loss of consciousness lasting upto 15 minutes

Granthi(s) gland

granulation (gran'u-la'shun) the process of formation of granulation tissue **g tissue** young vascular fibrous tissue developing in healing wounds and organising fibrin

granule (gran'ul) a small particle

granulocyte any cell containing granules, usually refers to the white cells such as neutrophil, eosinophil and basophil.

granuloma a small nodular chronic inflammatory swelling **g annulare** rounded skin lesion with raised edges **g inguinale** a sexually transmitted disease characterised by ulceration of the skin and subcutaneous tissue in the groin. It is caused by a small gram-negative rod-shaped organism, C. *granulomatis*

granulosa theca cell tumour ovarian tumour often secreting oestrogen with mass in the lower abdomen and precocious puberty

grasp reflex induced by stroking palm, seen in infancy and frontal lobe lesions

Grave's disease thyrotoxicosis associated with goitre and exophthalmos, described by Irish physician, Robert Graves

gravid pregnant

gravida number of pregnancies

Grawitz's (grah'vits-ez) **tumour** clear cell carcinoma of the kidney, named after Paul Grawitz, German pathologist

Gray Gy; dose of radiation that produces absorption of 1 joule of energy per kg of tissue

gray baby syndrome a toxic condition seen in neonates especially premature infants following administration of chloramphenicol. The body mechanisms are not developed to detoxify and excrete the drug and present with ashen gray cyanosis, listlessness and weakness

gray matter gray area of the brain and spinal cord where the nerve fibres are not enclosed in a myelin sheath

Green-Gordon tube endotracheal tube with cuff and carinal hook, devised by British anaesthetists.

greenhouse effect warming of the Earth's surface that is produced when solar heat becomes trapped by layers of carbon dioxide and other gases

green monkey fever *see* Marburg disease

green nail syndrome *Pseudomonas aeruginosa* infection of nail

green stick fracture an incomplete fracture wherein the bone is bent and exhibits the fracture only on the outer arc of the bend

Greenville bypass gastric bypass for obesity wherein a small part of upper end of stomach is isolated by stapling and anastomosed to Roux-en-y of jejunum, named after US city

Grenz zone a normal tumour-free space between the epithelium and a subepithelial lesion

Grey Turner's sign discolouration of abdominal wall in acute pancreatitis, named after British surgeon, Grey Turner

GRF abbreviation for growth hormone releasing factor

grid a device used in radiology department to absorb scattered radiation produced during an x-ray examination. The device contains many narrow lead strips

g iron incision for operation of simple appendicitis, division of internal and oblique muscle each in line of fibres

grief an emotional response to bereavement or loss

grinder a molar tooth

grinder's disease silicosis

grinding forceful rubbing together

gripe colicky pain especially of large bowel

grippe (F) influenza

griseofulvin an oral antibiotic used for the treatment of fungal infection

groin junction between the abdomen and thigh

groove a shallow linear hollow

gross (gro's) visible to naked eye

ground 1. foundation 2. basic substance 3. reduced to a powder **g itch** pruritic papule on the skin due to the penetration of filariform larvae of hook worm **g substance** the gel-like material containing connective tissue cells and fibres

group practice cooperative partnership of general practitioners

Group therapy a way of giving psychological help to a number of people with emotional or psychological problems at the same time

growth the progressive development or increase in the size of a living thing **g chart** a visible display of the child's physical growth and development. It is a weight-for age chart and has two reference curves. The upper curve represents the median for boys and lower for girls. The space between the two growth curves is called the 'road to health' **g hormone** a hormone secreted by anterior pituitary that regulates the cell division and protein synthesis necessary for growth **g hormone releasing factor** (GRF) a hormone from the hypothalamus that stimulates the release of growth hormone from the anterior pituitary **g monitoring** all infants should be weighed periodically at their growth charts maintained. Their longitudinal followup helps in interpreting the changes over time and to identify children at risk of malnutrition early **g rate** crude death rate is subtracted from the crude birth rate and the residual is current annual growth rate, exclusive of migration

gruel any cereal boiled in water

gryposis (gri-po'sis) abnormal curvature of any part of the body, especially nails

GTP guanosine triphosphate

GTT abbreviation for glucose tolerance test

guaicol (gwi'a-kol) methoxy phenol obtained by distillation of creosote, used as an antiseptic and germicide

guanbenz central adrenergic antagonist used as an antihypertensive agent

guanethidine antihypertensive agent which blocks release of non-adrenaline from adrenergic nerve endings

guanine (gwa-nen) purine base of nucleic acids that links with cytosine in double helix

guanosine (gwan'o-sin) the nucleoside formed from guanine and ribosome, and it is a major constituent of RNA and DNA

guard a device for protecting a part

guarding involuntary muscle spasm noted in acute peritonitis. The anterior abdominal muscles are in a state of tonic contraction giving a board-like rigidity

guar gum polysaccharide of an Indian legume, used as dietary bulking agent

gubernaculam a card-like structure that unites two structures

Gubler's (goob'lerz) **paralysis** a brainstem lesion causing paralysis of the cranial nerves on one side and of the body on the opposite side, named after Adolphe Gubler, French physician

Gudam(s) rectum

guidance counselling

guide a mechanical aid or device that helps in setting a course or directs the

movement **g line** an instructional guide indicating the course of action in a specific situation **g wire** for arteriography, a wire is introduced into artery through a needle and needle is replaced by catheter threaded over wire and wire is withdrawn

guillotine (gil'o-ten) a surgical instrument with a sliding blade **g amputation** a sharply defined loss of a portion or entire segments of extremities

guinea pig (gin'e pig) a small rodent used for experimental work

guinea worm dracunculus

guinea worm infection *see* dracunculiasis.

Guillain-Barre (ge-yan'bar-ra') **syndrome** (GBS) a neuropathy described by French neurologists Georges Guillain and Jean Barre due to an immunologic injury presenting with sudden weakness of all four limbs in a previously healthy individual. The disease is symmetrical involving proximal and distal muscles, areflexia, sensory changes, postural hypotension, and cranial nerve paralysis involving bilateral facial and bulbar muscles. CSF shows albuminocytologic dissociation with increased protein with normal cells. Nerve conduction studies show demyelination. Those who survive recover remarkably, however, many fail to reach the previous level of activity

Gull's disease atrophy of thyroid gland presenting with features of myxoedema, named after Sir William Gull, English physician

gullet throat

gum 1. a plant extract that is sticky when moist but hard or drying 2. the fleshy tissue covering the alveolar processes of the jaws

gumboil a dental abscess converted into a cyst with chronic drainage through a fistulous tract; parulis

gumma a soft gummy tumour noted in tertiary syphilis. It represents a hypersensitivity response to treponemal products. There is central caseating necrosis surrounded by epithelioid histiocytes and multinucleated giant cells

gums viscous indigestible polysaccharides of plants, component of dietary fibre

gunning splint denture without teeth used for fixation of fracture of edentulous teeth

gustation (gus-ta'shun) sense of taste

gustatory (gus'ta-tor'e) pertaining to the act or sense of taste **g hallucination** false perception of taste such as an unpleasant taste due to an uncinate seizure **g organ** taste bud

gut bowel, intestine

gut-associated lymphoid tissue (GALT) presence of gastrointestinal immune system in the mucosa and submucosa of the gastrointestinal tract. It is prominent in the tonsils, Peyer's patches and appendix

Guthrie's (guth'rez) **test** a screening test for phenylketonuria, to detect the presence of phenylalanine metabolites in the blood, named after Robert Guthrie, US microbiologist

gutta a drop. pl. **guttae**.

guttate resembling a drop

guttur (gut'ur) the throat

guttural (gut'u-ral) pertaining to throat

Guyon's (ge-yonz) **sign** ballottement of the kidney, named after Felix Guyon, French surgeon

GVH disease *see* graft versus host disease

gymnast's back pain in the back caused by exercises wherein back is arched by overstretching the muscles and ligaments

gynandrism (ji-nan'drizm) male hermophroditism

gynandroid (ji-nan'droyd) a person exhibiting sufficient hermaphrodite

sexual characters to be mistaken for a person of opposite sex

gynaeco- combining word for woman, female

gynaecoid (jin-e-koyd) resembling to female

gynaecologist (gi'ne-kol'o-jist) a specialist in gynaecology

gynaecology (gi'ne-kol'o-je) the study of the diseases peculiar to women especially those of genital tract and breasts

gynaecomastia (ji-ne-ko-mas'te-a) excess development of mammary glands in the male. It may be pubertal or due to hypogonadism, cirrhosis of the liver, lepromatous leprosy, drugs like cimetidine, digitalis, INH, spironolactone, or tumours of the adrenal gland, testes or Klinefelter's syndrome

gynandroblastoma (ji'on-and-ro-blastoma) a rare tumour of ovary with well differentiated testicular and ovarian tissue exhibiting masculanising (hirsutism, clitoral hypertrophy and deepening of voice) and/or feminising (vaginal bleeding) hormonal effects; Yin-Yang tumour

gypsum (jip'sum) a mineral containing crushed calcium sulphate hemihydrate which when calcinated becomes plaster of Paris

gyrase an enzyme first isolated from *Escherichia coli* cutting double-strand, DNA

gyrate (ji'rat) 1. convoluted or ring-shaped 2. to revolve

gyration (ji-ra'shun) a rotary movement

gyrus (ji-rus) pl. **gyri** one of the convolutions of the cerebral hemispheres of the brain. The gyri are separated by shallow grooves (sulci) or deeper groves (fissures)

H

H symbol for hydrogen, Hounsfield unit, magnetic field strength

H₁ a subtype of histamine receptors

H₂ a subtype of histamine receptors

H⁺ symbol for hydrogen ion

HaAg hepatitis A antigen

HAART abbreviation for highly active antiretroviral therapy, a combined therapy with three or more drugs for HIV infection

H antigen flagellar antigen

habena (ha-be'na) a frenum

habenula (ha-ben'ula) 1. a whiplike structure 2. a peduncle attached to the pineal body of the brain 3. a narrow band-like structure 4. a dorsomedial thalamic prominence where olfactory, visceral and somatic afferent pathways are integrated

habit an accustomed way of doing things. They are acquired by repetition, and are automatic. They can be performed only under similar circumstances **h spasm** *see* tic

habitual abortion *see* abortion

habituation an adaptive response characterised by a decreased reactivity to a repeated stimulus

habitus 1. general physical appearance 2. body build

HACEK abbreviation for *Haemophilus aphrophilus, haemophilus actinomycetemcomitans, Cardiobacterium hominis, Eikenella corrodens , Kingella kingae,* organisms that are typically associated with being fastidious or difficult for culture

haem – combining word for blood

haemachrosis (hem'a-kro'sis) abnormally bright red blood as in carbon monoxide poisoning

haemacytometer (-si'tom'-ter) an apparatus for counting blood cells

haemadsorption (-ad-sorp'shun) adher-

ence of an agent or substance on the surface of a red blood cell

haemagglutination (-a-gloo-ti-na'shun) the clumping of the red blood cells in presence of specific antibody or a microbial agent **h inhibition reaction** an immune reaction in which antigen-bearing erythrocytes are prevented from agglutinating

haemagglutinin (-a-gloo'ti-nin) an antibody that causes haemagglutination

haemagogue (-a-gog) an agent promoting the blood flow

haemal (he'mal) 1. pertaining to the blood or blood vessels 2. ventral to spinal axis in which heart is located

haemalum (hem-al.um) a mixture of haematoxylin and alum used as a nuclear stain

haemanalysis (hem'a-nal'i-sis) chemical analysis of the blood

haemangiectasis (hem'an-je-ek'ta-sis) dilatation of blood vessels

haemangion – combining form referring to blood vessels.

hemangioblast (he-man'je-o-blast) a mesodermal cell that can give rise to vascular endothelium and blood forming cells

hemangioblastoma (he-man'je-o-blasto'ma) a slow growing well circumscribed benign tumour consisting of proliferation of capillary vessel forming endothelial cells

haemangioma (he-man'je-o'ma) a developmental malformation of blood vessels in which there is intradermal or subdermal collection of dilated blood vessels. It is more common in the skin and subcutaneous tissues **capillary h** purple, or bright red lesions noted in childhood, pressure may cause disappearance of swelling or cause blanching **cavernous h** a congenital swelling containing multiple venous sinuses of varying calibre **plexiform h** a diffuse pulsatile swelling of arteries and it feels like a bag of earthworms **senile h** red papule from weakened capillary wall

haemangiomatosis (he-man′ji-o-ma-to′sis) presence of multiple haemangiomas

haemangiopericytoma (he-man′ji-o-peri-si′tom-a) a tumour of perivascular cells or pericytes occurring in the legs and retroperitoneum

haemangiosarcoma (he-man′ji-o-sar-ko′ma) a malignant tumour developing from rapidly proliferating endothelium of blood vessels

haemaphersis (hem′a-pher′sis) the removal of whole blood from a donor or a patient, followed by separation into components, retention of some components and transfusion of the recombined remaining elements to the patient.

haemarthrosis (hem′ar-thro′sis) bleeding into the joint usually from an injury which results in a swelling of the joint

haemastix dip-strip test for presence of blood in urine

haemat – combining word for blood

haematemesis (hem′at-em′e-sis) the vomiting of blood. It occurs from upper gastrointestinal haemorrhage and it may be red with clots when bleeding is profuse, or black as coffee ground, when less severe

haematencephalon (he′mat-en-sef′a-lon) cerebral haemorrhage

haematidrosis (he′mat-i-dro′sis) sweat containing blood or blood pigment

haematin (he′ma-tin) an iron-proto-porphyrin containing ferric iron

haematinic (hem′a-tin′ik) 1. pertaining to blood 2. an agent that increases the level of haemoglobin and the number of red blood cells

haematobium (he′ma-to′be-um) a protozoan parasite of blood cells

haematoblast (hem′ato-blast) a primitive undifferentiated blood cell from which erythroblasts, lymphoblasts and myeloblasts are derived

haematochezia (hem′a-to-ke′zi-a) the passage of blood in stools

haematochyluria (he′ma–to-ki-lu′re-a) presence of blood and chyle in the urine, often as a feature of filariasis

haematocoele (hem′a-to-sel) 1. a blood cyst 2. effusion of blood into a cavity. 3. effusion of blood into the tunica vaginalis testis

haematocoelia (-sel′e-a) a bleeding into the peritoneal cavity

haematocolpometra (hem′a-to-kol′po-me′tra) accumulation of blood in the uterus and vagina

haematocolpus (hem′a-to-kol′pus) accumulation of menstrual blood in the vagina due to imperforate hymen or vaginal septum

haematocrit (he-mat′o-krit) the percentage volume of red blood cells in the blood; packed cell volume **h tube** a narrow bore, thick walled short glass tube of 11 cm length with calibrations to 100 mm and has a capacity to hold 1 ml of blood

haematocyst (hem′o-to-cist) 1. bleeding into a cyst 2. a haemorrhagic cyst

haematocyturia (hem′a-to-si-tu′ria) the presence of red blood cells in the urine

haematogenesis (hem′a-to-jen′e-sis) haemopoiesis

haematogenic, haematogenous (hem′a-to-jen′ik, hem-a-toj′en-us) 1. haemopoietic 2. anything produced from blood 3. spread through blood stream

haematoid (hem′a-toy′t) resembling blood

haematoidin (hem′-a-toy′din) a golden-yellow pigment similar to bilirubin formed in tissues from haemoglobin under hypoxia

haematologist (hem′a-tol′o-jist) a physician specialised in haematology

haematology (hem′ɛ-tol′o-jey) the medical specialty concerned with the study of blood and blood forming tissues

haematolymphangioma (hem′a-to-limf′an-ji-o'ma) a benign tumour consisting of lymphatics and blood vessels

haematoma a collection of blood inside the body, caused by bleeding from an injured vessel **muscle h** occur commonly in calf and psoas muscles in haemophilia **subdural h** haematoma beneath the dura mater that produces neurologic symptoms by pressure on the brain **subungal h** a crimson, or gray brown discolouration of nail plate, frequently of the big toe

haematometra (hem'a-to-me'tra) distension of uterus with blood either as an extension of haematocolpus or from obstruction of cervix

haematomphalocoele (hem'at-om-fal'o-sel) an effusion of blood into an umbilical hernia

haematomyelia (hem'a-to-mi-e'li-a) bleeding into the spinal cord

haematomyelopore (hem'a-to-mi'il-o-por) formation of pores in the spinal cord due to haemorrhage

haematopathology (hem'a-to-pa-thol'ah-je) the division of pathology concerned with the study of diseases of the blood

haematopoiesis (hem'a-to-pou-e'sis) haemopoiesis

haemotopoietic (hem'a-to-poy-et'ik) haemopoietic

haematoporphyrin (hem'a-to-por'fi-rin) iron-free haem resulting from decomposition of haemoglobin

haematopsia haemorrhage into the eye

haematorrhachis (hem-a-tor'a-kis) bleeding within the spinal canal either intradural or extradural, but not within the cord

haematorrhoea (he'ma-to-re'a) profuse bleeding

haematosalpinx (-sal'pinks) accumulation of blood in the fallopian tube, often associated with tubal pregnancy

haematoschocoele (hem-atos'ke-o-sel) collection of blood in the scrotum

haematospermatocoele (hem'a-to-sper'ma-to-sel) a spermatocoele containing blood

haematospermia (hem'a-to-sper'me-a) semen containing blood

haematostatic (hem'a-to-stat'ik) 1. haemostatic 2. arrest of blood in a vessel

haematostaxis (hem'a-to-stak'sis) spontaneous haemorrhage due to a disorder of the blood

haematoxylin a natural dye from *Haematoxylin compechianum* used as the stain to examine tissues by light microscopy and it is used in conjunction with eosin, acting as a counterstain

haematuria (hem'a-tu're-a) passage of blood in the urine **endemic h** schistosomiasis **essential h** haematuria whose cause is undetermined **false h** passage of red coloured urine following ingestion of food or drugs containing pigment **microscopic h** presence of red blood cells in urine recognised by microscopic examination **renal h** haematuria resulting from extravasation of blood into the kidney where the urine is often smoky **urethral h** bleeding into the urethra causing passage of bright red urine at the beginning of urination **vesical h** bleeding into the urinary bladder causing haematuria

haeme (hem) an iron (ferrous) containing protoporphyrin that forms the pigmentary part of haemoglobin and it imparts red colour to haemoglobin and is responsible for its oxygen carrying capacity

haemobilia (he'mo-bil'e-a) presence of blood in the bile or bile ducts

haemobilirubin (he'mo-bil'i-ru-bin) unconjugated, lipid soluble, bilirubin, before processing in the liver

haemochorial (he'mo-ko-re'al) direct contact between chorionic villi of the placenta and maternal blood

haemochromatosis (he'mo-kro'ma-to'sis) a genetic disorder resulting in an excessive absorption and accumulation of iron in the liver, pancreas and skin. There is bronzed skin, hepatomegaly, arthritis, congestive cardiac failure, testicular atrophy and diabetes mellitus

haemoconcentration rise in the level of

red blood cell count or haematocrit due to a fall in the plasma volume

haemocyte (he'mo-sit) a blood cell

haemocytoblast (he'mo-si'to-blast) stem cell of bone marrow

haemocytometer (-si-tom'et-er) an instrument to count the blood cells

haemodiagnosis (-di'ag-no'sis) diagnosis by examination of the blood

haemodialysis (-di-al'i-sis) a dialysis carried out in renal failure, in which blood is passed through a machine and purified before being returned to the body

haemodialyser (-di'a-liz'er) a machine to undertake haemodialysis where the toxic substances are removed by exposing dialysing fluid across a semipermeable membrane

haemodilution (-di-loo'shun) fall in RBC count following bleeding and expansion of plasma volume

haemodynamics (-di-nam'iks) the study of the movement of the blood and the forces involved in circulating blood through the body

haemoflagellate (he'mo-flaj'e-lat) protozoan flagellate that are parasitic in blood which includes Leishmania and Trypanosoma species

haemofuscin (he-mo-fus'in) a brown pigment derived form haemoglobin, which imparts a reddish colour to the urine

haemoglobin (hem'o-glo'bin) an iron containing pigment in the red blood cells which carries oxygen to the tissues. Haemoglobin consists of four chains of globin, each surrounding a molecule of haeme. There are four types of normal haemoglobin in man, the embryonic, foetal (HbF) and two adult types (Hb A and Hb A2) **foetal h** the type of haemoglobin found in the normal foetus and it has the capacity to take up and give off oxygen at lower oxygen tensions **glycosylated H** HbA, or HbAic that accounts for less than 4% of total haemoglobin in blood. Its estimation is helpful in assessing chronic glycaemic control **h c disease** a

benign haemoglobinopathy causing megaloblastic anaemia in pregnancy and splenomegaly **h H disease** a condition due to failure of production of haemoglobin **h SC disease** a mild variety of sickle-cell anaemia **mean corpuscular h** (MCH) the haemoglobin content of the average red cell **muscle h** myoglobin **reduced h** haemoglobin in the red cells following release of oxygen in the tissue **sickle cell h** molecular abnormality characterised by presence of an abnormal haemoglobin Hb S which is capable of altering its structure so that red cells assume a sickle shape

haemoglobinaemia (he'mo-glo'bin-em'e-a) the presence of free haemoglobin in the blood plasma

haemoglobinolysis (-ol'i-sis) destruction of haemoglobin.

haemoglobinometer (-om'it-er) a device used for determination of haemoglobin. Erythrocytes are lysed to get intracellular haemoglobin into solution and later its conversion into acid haematin. The resulting colour is compared with permanent coloured glass standard. The method is useful to measure only oxyhaemoglobin

haemoglobinopathies (he'mo-glo'bi-nop'a-thes) genetic disorders involving globin, the protein component of haemoglobin, divided into the thalassemia syndromes such as α and β thalassemia and variant haemoglobins such as sickle cell anaemia

haemoglobinuria (-ur'e-a) the abnormal presence of haemoglobin in the urine **malarial h** Blackwater fever **march h** haemoglobinuria noted after prolonged or strenuous exercise **paroxysmal h** intermittent attacks of haemoglobinuria due to increased fragility of red cells or presence of acute haemolysis **toxic h** occurrence of haemolgobinuria from snake venom or toxic products of infection

haemogram (-gram) a detailed examination of the blood with special reference to the numbers, proportions and morphologic features of all formed elements

haemolymph (he'mo-limf) blood and lymph

haemolysin (he-mol'i-sin) a toxic substance capable of causing lysis of red blood cells and liberation of their haemoglobin

haemolysis (he-mol'i-sis) the breakdown of red blood cells. It occurs as a normal process at the end of their life span, but occasionally occurs prematurely leading to anaemia and jaundice

haemolyse (he'mo-liz) to cause liberation of haemoglobin from red cells

haemolytic (he-mo-li'e-tik) referring to lysis of red cells **h disease of newborn** a condition due to the incompatibility of foetal red cells with the maternal immune system **h jaundice** jaundice from increased destruction of red blood cells or their precursors in the marrow, causing increased bilirubin production. Jaundice is mild **h-uraemia syndrome** condition occurring in children below two years with a prodrome of bloody diarrhoea, haemolytic anaemia and thrombocytopaenia

haemopathy (he-mop'a-thi) disease of blood or haemopoietic system

haemoperfusion the perfusion of blood through activated charcoal or ion exchange resins to remove toxic substances and then returning to the patient

haemopericardium (he'mo-per'i-car'dium) blood in the pericardial sac

haemoperitoneum (-to-ne'um) blood in the peritoneal cavity

haemophagocytosis (he'mo-fag'o-si-to'sis) ingestion of red blood cells by phagocytes

haemophil (he'mo-fil) a microorganism growing in media containing blood

haemophilia (hem'o-fil'e-a) an inherited coagulation defect characterised by a permanent tendency to haemorrhages

due to a defect in the coagulation of blood **h A** a sex-linked recessive condition with a deficiency of coagulation factor VIII, noted almost exclusively in males characterised by prolonged clotting time, haemarthroses, muscle haematoma and haemorrhage after trauma **h B** Christmas disease condition clinically indistinguishable from haemophilia is due to hereditary deficiency of factor IX **h C** haemophilia due to a deficiency of factor XI **vascular h** *see* von Willebrand's disease

haemophiliac (he-mo-fil'i-ak) a person suffering from haemophilia

Haemophilus (he-mof'il-us) a small, nonmotile gram-negative bacteria that requires the growth factor (X or V or both), provided by blood. *H. aegyptius* causative agent of conjunctivitis *H. ducreyi* causative agent of chancroid *H. infulenzae* causative agent of respiratory infections and meningitis *H vaginalis* bacteria causing vaginitis

haemophobia (he-mo-fo'be-a) dislike to see bleeding or blood

haemophthalmia (he'mof-thal'mi-a) an effusion of blood into the eye

Haemophysalis (hem'afis'a-lis) a genus of ticks that include species that serve as vectors for tickborne viral diseases including Kyasanur forest disease

haemopneumopericardium (he'monu'mo-per-i-kar'di-um) accumulation of blood and air in the pericardial cavity

haemopneumothorax (-tho'raks) accumulation of blood and air in the pleural cavity

haemopoiesis (he'mo-poy-e'sis) formation and development of different types of blood cells and formed elements

haemopoietic (he'mo-poy-et'ik) related to the blood; blood forming organ

haemoprotein (he-mo-pro'ten) any protein linked with a haeme

haemopsonin (he'mop-so'nin) an antibody making red blood cell more susceptible to phagocytosis

haemoptysis (he-mop'ti-sis) coughing of

blood or blood stained sputum. It is bright red, and frothy coming from bronchial arteries **endemic h** bouts of frank haemoptysis in lung due to infection by *Paragonimus westermani* **pseudo h** expectoration of red coloured sputum in serratia infections

haemorrhage (hem'o-rij) bleeding; an escape of blood from the blood vessels. It may be dark red and continuous (venous) or bright red and flowing in spurts (arterial). Capillary bleeding is red and occurs from tissues **cerebral h** escape of blood into the cerebrum, usually in the region of the internal capsule by the rupture of the lenticulostriate artery **concealed h** internal bleeding **extradural h** an accumulation of blood between the skull and dura mater **internal h** bleeding into the area of tissue or organ that is not visible **intracranial h** bleeding into the cranium leading to the formation of a haematoma **petechial h** capillary haemorrhage into the skin or mucous membrane forming petechiae **postpartum h** haemorrhage occurring after childbirth and is more than 500 ml during the first 24 hours after delivery **primary h** bleeding occurring immediately after an injury or operation **punctate h** petechial haemorrhage **secondary h** bleeding occurring after some time following an injury or an operation **subdural h** bleeding between the dura and subarachnoid membrane

haemorrhagic (hem-o-raj'ik) relating to or characterised by haemorrhage

haemorrhagins (-ra'jins) toxins found in certain venoms and poisons that cause destruction of endothelial cells and small blood vessels

haemorrheology (he'mo-re-ol'a-ji) the study of deformation and flow properties of cellular components and plasma of the blood and the rheologic properties of the vessels with which blood comes in direct contact

haemorrhoidectomy (hem'o-royd-ek'ta-me) excision of haemorrhoids

haemorrhoids (hem'o-royd) piles; a mass of dilated, tortuous veins of the superior or inferior haemorrhoidal venous plexus at the anus **external h** varicose dilatation of a vein of inferior haemorrhoidal plexus forming a swelling on the outer side of the external sphincter and are covered by the skin of the anal canal **internal h** varicose dilatation of a vein of superior haemorrhoidal plexus at the anorectal junction and are covered by mucous membrane, and are noticeable after straining **prolapsed h** internal haemorrhoid protruding outside the anal sphincter **stangulated h** an internal haemorrhoid that has remained prolapsed for a long time by the constriction of anal sphincter, curtailing its blood supply

haemosalphinx (he'mo-sal'phinks) haematosalphinx

haemosiderin (he'mo-sid'er-in) an insoluble iron containing protein from haemoglobin following disintegration of red blood cells

haemosiderosis (-sid'er-o'sis) abnormal accumulation of haemosiderin in tissues such as liver and spleen **idiopathic pulmonary h** a condition characterised by intermittent intra alveolar and intrabronchial haemorrhage form pulmonary capillaries presenting with recurrent haemoptysis and iron deficiency anaemia

Haemosporidia (he-mo-spo-rid'e-a) a sporozoa that live in red blood cells of vertebrates and reproduce sexually in invertebrates. The genus plasmodium causing malaria is an example

haemostasis (he-mos'ta-sis) 1. the arrest of bleeding 2. the arrest of circulation in a part 3. stagnation of blood.

haemostat (he'mo-stat) 1. a small surgical clamp for constricting blood vessels and arrest flow of blood 2. an agent that controls bleeding

haemostatic (he'mo-stat'ik) 1. arresting bleeding 2. arresting the flow of blood within a blood vessel

haemostyptic (he'mo-stip'tik) an astringent that stops haemorrhage.

haemotherapy (he'mo-the'ra-pe) blood components in the treatment such as transfusion

haemothorax (-thor'aks) blood in the pleural cavity

haemotoxic (-tok'sik) 1. causing of blood poisoning 2. haemolytic

haemotoxin (-tok'sin) any substance that causes destruction of red blood cells

haemotrophic (he-mo-trof'ik), pertaining to the nutrient substances carried in the blood

haemotropic (he-mo-trop'ik) exhibiting an affinity for blood or blood cells

haemotympanum (he'mo-tim'pa-num) presence of blood in the middle ear

Hagedorn (ha'ge-dorn) **needle** a curved surgical needle with flattened sides, named after Werner Hagedorn, German surgeon

Hageman factor coagulation factor XII which initiates the intrinsic pathway of coagulation

Hailey-Hailey disease benign familial pemphigus, named after W. Hailey and E. Hailey, US dermatologists

hair a keratinised, thread-like outgrowth from the skin. A hair develops as a thin, flexible shaft of cornified cells from the hair follicle. It has a shaft and a root embedded in the follicle. The shaft consists of cuticle, cortex and medulla. The pigment found in the cortex is responsible for the colour **anagen h** actively growing hair **lanugo h** fine hair of the foetus, usually shed at birth **telogen h** nongrowing hair that is removed easily **terminal h** coarse, deeply pigmented, stiff and thick hair seen in scalp, eyebrow, chest, axilla and pubic region. Androgens are responsible for such hair **vellous h** fine, soft and downy hair of children and women

hair analysi use of hair for detection of chronic heavy metal intoxication such as arsenic, lead and mercury

hair follicle a cylindrical invagination of the epidermis in the corium layer of the skin and containing the root of a hair

half line fracture a minor fracture that appears on X ray film as a thin line between two segments of a bone

HAIR-AN syndrome abbreviation for hyperandrogenism(HA), insulin-resistance (IR) and acanthosis nigricans (AN)

hair-on end appearance a radiographic pattern seen as calcified spicules perpendicular to the bone surface seen in congenital haemolytic anaemias such as sickle cell anaemia, thalassemia, hereditary elliptosis and spherocytosis

hair pin vessels minute blood vessels that are doubled upon themselves, seen at the metaphyseal-diaphyseal junction of normal bone

hairy cell leukaemia a B cell leukaemic lymphoproliferative disorder associated with splenomegaly, pancytopaenia, recurrent infections and typical hairy cells in the blood and bone marrow. Interferon and purine analogues (deoxycoformycin chlorodeoxyadenosine) are useful in the management

hairy naevus a pigmented mole with hairs growing from it

hairy tongue *see* tongue

Hakim practitioner of herbalism

half and half nail a dull white proximal band and a distal red-brown band in the nail, seen in chronic renal insufficiency

half life time required for the amount of the drug in the body to decrease by one half during elimination **biological h l** time in which the total amount of the drug in the body after equilibrium of plasma with other physiological compartment is halved **plasma h l** time taken for the plasma concentration of the drug to fall by one-half

half normal saline a solution of 0.45% NaCl used for mucosal rehydration in respiratory therapy

halitosis (hal-i-to'sis) unpleasant breath due to oral infections and poor oral hygiene

halitus (hal'i-tus) the breath

Hallpike manoeuvre a test for the diagnosis of benign positional vertigo. A sitting patient is made to lie down with head tilted down 30° over the end of bed and then 30° to one side. The test is considered positive if a paroxysm of vertigo occurs, named after C. Hallpike, neurologist

hallucination (ha-loo-si-na'shun) *psy* false sensory perceptions not associated with real external stimuli. Hallunication indicates a psychotic disturbance only when associated with impairment in reality testing **auditory** h false perception of sound, usually voices, often associated with chronic alcohol abuse **gustatory h** false perception of taste such as unpleasant taste due to an uncinate seizure **hypnagogic h** false sensory perception occurring while falling asleep **hypnopompic h** false sensory perception occurring while awakening from sleep **Lilliputian h** false perception in which objects are seen as reduced in size **mood-congruent h** hallucination whose content is consistent with either a depressed or manic mood **mood-incongruent h** hallucination whose content is not consistent with either depressed or maniac mood **olfactory h** false perception of smell **somatic h** false sensation of things occurring in or to the body, most often visceral in origin **visual h** false perception involving sight, consisting of both formed images such as people and unformed images such as flashes of light

hallucinogen (ha-loo'si-no-jen) a drug that produces hallucinations

hallucinosis hallucinations, most often auditory that are associated with chronic alcohol abuse and occur within a clear sensorium

hallux (hal'uks) pl. **halluces** the big toe **h dolorosus** pain in the metatarsophalangeal joint of the big toe **h rigidus** a painful deformity of big toe limiting movement at the metatarsophalangeal joint **h valgus** outward displacement of the big toe **h varus** inward displacement of the big toe

halo 1. the areola especially of the nipple 2. a ring surrounding macula 3. a circle of light surrounding a shining object

halo appearance a doughnut-shaped light density within and surrounded by a rounded darker dense zones

halo naevus a pigmented melanocytic naevus surrounded by a peripheral zone of depigmentation

haloperidol (ha-lo-per'i-dol) a butyrophenon dopamine-blocking antipsychotic agent used for schizophrenia

halothane (hal'o-than) a fluorinated hydrocarbon used as a general anaesthetic

halo-vest traction a form of traction used to treat fractures of the neck in which the head is immobilised by a halo of metal mounted on a vest-like apparatus

Halsted's (hal'stedz) **operation** 1. an operation for inguinal hernia 2. a radical mastectomy for cancer of the breast, named after William Halsted, US surgeon

ham the popliteal fossa

hamartoma (ham-ar-to'ma) an error tumour consisting of components of mature tissues that are native to a site of origin. These components are arranged in an abnormal way as an island containing cartilage, fat, fibrous tissue, smooth muscle, nerve cells, epithelial tissue and foci of calcification clefts.

hamate (ham'at) hooked **h bone** the small medial bone at the ulnar side in the distal row of carpal bones

hamburger sign a CT appearance of an uncovered vertebral articular facet when the facet joint is dislocated. Normally the vertebral facet joint space looks like a hamburger.

Hamilton's (ham'il-tonz) **ruler test** a rigid ruler cannot touch simultaneously the acromion process and the lateral epicondyl of the humerus due to lateral bulging of the greater tuberosity of humerus. It is possible in dislocation of shoulder or a fracture of the neck of the scapula, named after Frank Hamilton, American Surgeon.

Hamman's (ham'anz) **disease** spontaneous mediastinal emphysema, named after Louis Hamman, US physician

hammer 1. an instrument with a head attached transversely to the handle 2. hammer-shaped bone of the middle ear, malleus **h finger** a flexion deformity of the distal interphalangeal joint of a finger caused by avulsion of the extensor tendon **h toe** the lateral deviation of the great toe that elicits callosity **percussion h** a hammer with a rubber head used to elicit reflexes

hamstring 1. any one of the three muscles on the posterior aspect of the thigh (semitendinosus, semimembranosus and biceps femoris) that flex the leg and adduct and extend the thigh 2. one of the tendons that form the medial and lateral boundaries of the popliteal fossa

Ham's test in paroxysmal nocturnal haemoglobinuria red cells lyse during one hour at 37ºC incubation with normal sera but do not lyse if complement is first removed from the sera by inactivating at 56ºC.

hamulus (ham'u-lus) any hook-shaped structure

hand the portion of the extremity attached to the wrist. It consists of carpus (wrist) with its eight bones, the metacarpus having five bones and the fingers (phalanges) with their 14 bones **ape h** median nerve injury resulting in permanent extension of the thumb **claw h** hyperextension of the metacarpo-phalangeal joints with flexion of interphalangeal joints especially of the ring and little fingers **drop h** wrist drop **obstetrician h** extension at the metacarpophalangeal and interphalangeal joints and adduction of the thumb, the position adapted by obstetrician during vaginal examination, is seen in tetany **trident h** all fingers are of similar size and diverge from one another, as in achondroplasia

hand-arm vibration syndrome a Raynaud's phenomenon-like complex due to cold induced vasospasm resulting from a prolonged use of vibrating hand-held tools

H and F haematoxylin and eosin, a stain used in histology

handedness 1. the tendency to use one hand in preference to the other **left h** sinistrality **right h** dextrality 2. a three-dimensional confrontation of a molecule, which may be left handed (laevo or L orientation) as most molecules in functioning biologic systems, or a right handed (dextro or D orientation)

hand, foot and mouth disease a coxsackie and entero virus infection characterised by painful vesicular and ulcerative lesions of the oral mucosa, tongue, hands and feet

hand-foot syndrome a crisis in sickle cell anaemia caused by sludging of red cells in vessels characterised by symmetric infarction of the small bones of the hand and foot, periosteal new bone formation, pain and swelling; sickle cell dactylitis

handicap physical and mental disability that limits the performance

Handigodu (han'di-go'du) **syndrome** a syndrome of endemic genetic epiphyseal displasia seen in Shimoga and Chikmagalur districts of Karnataka, India. Children present with dwarfism, limping, backpain, stiffness, lordosis, flexion at hips and knees and deformities of the legs. Inadequate calcium intake and consanguinity may contribute to the severity of the disease

hand mirror cell a lymphocyte with the nucleus at the mirror end and an elongated, cytoplasmic appendage mimicking a mirror's handle seen in benign or malignant haemopoietic conditions

hand piece (hand'pes) a hand instrument that holds tools used in preparing teeth for restoration and polishing

Hand-Schuller-Christian (hand-shil'er-kris'chan) **disease** multifocal eosinophilic granuloma manifesting as histiocytic granulomas of the bone, exophthalmos and diabetes insipidus. Seen in children, named after Alfred Hand Jr, US paediatrician, Arthur Schuller, Austrian neurologist and Henry Christian, US physician

hanging drop method a method for evaluating bacterial motility, where a flagellated bacterium is placed in a drop of clear physiologic solution on a cover glass (upside down) and examined by light microscopy

hang nail partially detached piece of skin at root or lateral edge of finger or toe nail

Hangman's fracture a bilateral avulsion fracture through the neural arch of the axis causing acute central spinal cord damage, seen in automobile accidents

Hanot's (a-noz) **cirrhosis** progressive biliary cirrhosis, named after Victor Hanot, French physician

Hansen's bacillus *Mycobacterium leprae*, the causative agent of leprosy, discovered by Gerhard Hansen, Norwegian physician

Hansen's disease leprosy

Hantavirus a genus of viruses belonging to Bunyaviridae family. They are trisegmented negative stranded RNA viruses that are maintained in nature in rodent reservoirs. It is responsible for haemorrhagic fever with renal syndrome and hantavirus pulmonary syndrome **h pulmonary syndrome** a febrile illness occurring in a previously healthy person characterised by unexplained adult respiratory distress syndrome or bilateral pulmonary infiltrates developing within 1 week of hospitalisation that resulted in respiratory compromise requiring supplemental oxygen or an unexplained respiratory illness resulting in death in conjunction with an autopsy examination demonstrating non-cardiogenic pulmonary oedema without an identifiable specific cause of death

H antigen histocompatibility antigen present in bacterial flagella

haploid halving half the normal number of chromosomes as in gametes, being 23 in humans

haploinsufficiency (hap'lo-in-suffi-cien-si) a situation in which the protein produced by a single copy of an otherwise normal gene is insufficient to assure normal function

haplotype a cluster of alleles that are located at the same locus of a chromosome and are usually inherited together

haptene (hap'ten) a substance that normally does not act like an antigen, but that can be combined with carrier protein and then can initiate a specific antibody response

haptics (hap'tiks) the behaviour of touching

haptoglobin (hap'to-glo'bin) a mucoprotein to which haemoglobin released from lysed red cells into plasma are bound

hard cataract nuclear cataract

hard chancre *see* Huntarian chancre

hardening 1. rendering a pathologic specimen firm 2. increased resistance to extremes of environmental temperature **h of arteries** atherosclerosis

hard exudate leakage of plasma from abnormal retinal capillaries and overlying areas of neuronal degeneration result in tiny specks to large confluent patches in diabetic retinopathy. They tend to occur particularly in the perimacular area

hard metal disease inhalation of dust containing cobalt and tungsten carbide. It may present with occupational asthma or interstitial lung disease

hardness 1. quality of water containing calcium or magnesium salts reacting with soaps to form insoluble compounds 2. X-rays of high penetration and short wavelength

hardware actual machinery of computer

hard water syndrome a clinical complex following use of hard water (contains high levels of iron, calcium and magnesium) during haemodialysis, resulting in post-dialysis nausea, vomiting, asthenia and hypertension

hard X-rays short wavelength, high frequency and highly penetrative X-rays

harelip a congenital cleft in the upper lip usually due to failure of the median nasal and maxillary processes to unite

harmony (har'mo-ne) state of working or living together smoothly

harpoon (har'poon) an instrument with a hook on one end that helps in removal of small pieces of tissue for examination

Harrison's (har'i-sunz) **groove** horizontal depression on thoracic wall and they correspond to the attachments of the diaphragm, noted at the xiphoid level in rickets described by Edwin Harrison, British physician

harsha (s) cheerfulness

Hartmann's (hart'manz) **pouch** dilatation of the neck of gall bladder, named after Robert Hartmann, German anatomist

Hartmann's solution intravenous lactated Ringer's solution for fluid and electrolyte replacement 0.31 g of sodium lactate is added to 100 ml of fluid, named after Alexi Hartmann, US paediatrician

Hartnup disease a rare hereditary disorder of renal and intestinal transport of tryptophane with clinical features resembling pellagra. The family name of the first reported case has been given to the disease

Harvard criteria criteria for irreversible coma (brain death) given by Harvard Medical School are unreceptivity and unresponsiveness, absence of movement or breathing, absent reflexes and flat electroencephalogram

harvest 1. to obtain samples or remove bacteria from a culture 2. procurement of an organ from a cadaveric or liver donor

Hashimoto's (hash'i-mo'toz) **thyroiditis** auto immune thyroiditis presenting with goitrous swelling of rubbery consistency. There is marked lymphocytic infiltration. Initially it may present with features of thyrotoxicosis, which over years may lead to hypothyroidism, named after Hakaru Hashimoto, Japanese surgeon

hashish (hash'ish) extract of the hemp plant *Cannabis sativa* which is smoked or chewed for its euphoric effects

Hassall's corpuscle a spherical body present in the medulla of the thymus. A concentrically arranged polygonal or flattened cells surround a central area of degenerated cells, named after Arthur Hassall, British physician and chemist

hasta (s) hand

haunch (hawnch) the hip and buttock

haustration (hos-tra'shun) sacculations of the colon formed by longitudinal bands that are shorter than the gut

HAV hepatitis A virus

Haverhill (ha'ver-il) **fever** febrile infection with *Streptobacillus moniliformis* transmitted to humans by rats, named after a town in Massachusetts, US, where an epidemic occurred

Haversian canal opening leading through the compact bone in a longitudinal direction and connecting with one another by transverse branches transmitting nutrient material, named after Clopton Havers, English anatomist and physician

Haversian gland a minute gland projecting from the surface of the synovial tissue into the joint space. It secretes synovial fluid

Haversian system a Haversian canal and its concentrically arranged lamellae, constituting the basic unit of the structure of compact bone

hay fever allergic rhinitis, a type I hypersensitivity reaction induced by air borne pollens giving rise to rhinitis, conjunctivitis with lacrimation and itching, nasal catarrh, sneezing and breathlessness

Hay's test test for bile salts. A pinch of sulphur when added to urine, sinks if bile salts are present. It floats in their absence, named after Mathew Hay, Scottish physician

Hawkinsinuria Excretion of unusual tyrosine metabolites in infants who present after stopping breastfeeding, vomiting, failure to thrive, acidosis and a characteristic odour like that of a swimming pool, named after Hawkinsin family which was affected by this disease

Hb haemoglobin

Hb-A normal Hb with two α and two β chains

HbA$_{1C}$ glycosylated Hb

HbCo carboxyhaemoglobin

HbF foetal haemoglobin with two α and two γ chains

HBs Ag hepatitis B surface antigen

HBV hepatitis B virus

HC human chorionic gonadotropin

HCl hydrochloric acid

HCO$_3$ chemical formula for bicarbonate ion

H$_2$CO$_3$ chemical formula for carbonic acid

HCt haematocrit

HCV hepatitis C virus

H – disease Hartnup disease

HDL high density lipoprotein

He symbol for helium

head 1. the part of the body containing the brain in the skull and organs of sight, hearing, smell and taste 2. the proximal end of a bone 3. the larger extremity of any structure or body.

head ache Cephalagia, an acute or chronic diffuse pain in various parts of the head, not confined to the area of distribution of any nerve **cluster h** a migraine variant characterised by periodic, severe unilateral periorbital pain often accompanied by unilateral lacrimation and nasal congestion. The pain is brief and occurs at a particular time of the day **coital h** a sudden, often very severe headache at the climax of sexual intercourse in middle-aged men **exertional h** brief head ache during physical exertion **postlumbar puncture h** head ache developing on removal of CSF from lumbar puncture **spinal h** frontal or occipital head ache following spinal anaesthesia **tension h** dull or tight head ache where the pain is constant and generalised. Emotional strain and anxiety are precipitating factors

head hunter curved catheter tip designed to enter carotid arteries for arteriography from femoral artery

Heaf's test six spring loaded needles penetrate a drop of tuberculin to a depth of 1-2 mm. Safe, less painful and quick method of tuberculin test. It is read 3-7 days later and graded, named after Frederick Heaf, British physician

heal (hel) 1. to cure or to restore to health 2. to cause an ulcer or wound to cicatrise and close

healer a person who heals

healing 1. the restoring to normal physical or mental condition 2. promoting the closure of wounds and ulcers **h by first intention** fibrous adhesion without suppuration or granulation tissue formation **h by second intention** union of two granulating surfaces accompanied by suppuration and delayed closure **h by third intention** slow filling of a wound or ulcer by granulations and subsequent cicatrisation

health (helth) health is a state or complete physical, mental and social well-being and not merely an absence of disease or infirmity and an ability to lead a socially and economically productive life **h care** a multitude of services rendered to individuals, families or communities by the health services or professions to promote, maintain, monitor or restore health **h development** the process of continuous progressive improvement of the health status of a population **h education** a process that informs, motivates, and helps people to adopt and maintain healthy practices and lifestyles, advocates environmental changes and conducts professional training and research **holistic h** health in terms of its physical, emotional, social, intellectual and spiritual makeup **h information system** a mechanism for the collection, processing, analysis and transmission needed for organising and operating health services and also for research and training **h insurance** insurance against some of the costs of medical, surgical and hospital care **h promotion** an activity to improve a person's or population's health by providing information about and increasing awareness of 'at risk' behaviours associated with certain diseases and to reduce such behaviours **primary h care** the first level of contact between the individual and the health system where essential health care is provided **public h** a medical speciality concerned with safeguarding and improving the health of community as a whole **secondary h care** consists essentially of curative services and is provided by district hospitals and community health centres **tertiary h care** superspecialist care by the regional/central level institutions

healthy well; free from disease; in a state of normal functioning

health centre provision of basic health services through the medium of primary health centres and subcentres for the rural and urban areas. It provides

integrated curative and preventive services

hearing power of perceiving sound **h aid** a sound-amplifying device used by the individuals with impaired hearing **impaired h** decreased ability to hear

heart (hart) cor. A hollow, muscular organ that maintains the circulation of the body by its pumping action. Two-thirds of its mass extends to the left of the midline. The wall of the heart consits of three layers – outer epicardium, the middle myocardium made of cardiac muscle and inner endocardium. The pericardium envelops the heart. There are two upper thin-walled chambers – right and left atria – separated by the interatrial septum. They receive blood from the venae cavae and pulmonary veins respectively. There are 2 lower, thick walled chambers right and left ventricles separated by interventricular septum. The left ventricle pumps blood into the aorta and right ventricle pumps

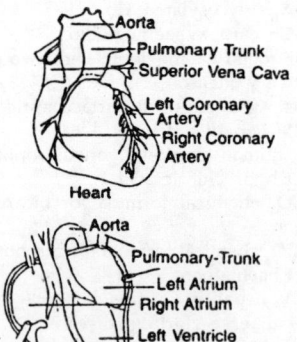

Heart Section

blood to the lungs through pulmonary artery. There are atrioventricular (mitral on left and tricuspid on right) and ventricular outflow (aortic and pulmonary) valves. The blood supply is by coronary arteries. The left main and right coronary arteries arise from the left and right coronary sinuses. The heart is innervated by both sympathetic and parasympathetic supply. The basic unit of contraction in the muscle is sarcomere **armoured h** calcium deposits in the pericardium **artificial h** a device that pumps blood like a normal left ventricle **athlete's h** hypertrophy of the heart due to prolonged physical training **beri beri h** heart disease secondary to deficiency of thiamine **fatty h** 1. fatty degeneration of the heart 2. accumulation of fat in and around heart muscle **horizontal h** rotation of electrical axis –30° **intermediate h** direction of electrical axis to +30° **irritable h** effort syndrome **left h** the left atrium and left ventricle that move blood into systemic circulation **right h** the right atrium and right ventricle that move the blood into the pulmonary circulation **semihorizontal h** direction of the electrical axis at–0° **semivertical h** direction of the electrical axis at +60° **univentricular h** double-inlet ventricle in which one ventricular chamber receives flow from both tricuspid and mitral valves, single or common ventricle **vertical h** electrical axis directed at +90° **water bottle h** chest x-ray revealing markedly enlarged cardiac silhouette with a shape of waterbottle in pericardial effusion.

heart block a defect of conduction of impulse generated at SA node to the ventricles. It may be prolonged (first degree) leading to dropped beats (second degree) or with independent ventricular rhythm (complete)

heartburn discomfort in the pit of the stomach or lower part of sternum due to acid reflux into oesophagus

heart chamber any of the four contracting regions inside the heart that regulate blood flow

heart failure *see* cardiac failure **h f cell** haemosiderin-laden macrophages found in the alveoli and it indicates occurrence of repeated bleeding

heart-lung machine an instrument that collects blood from both vena cavae, passes it through pump and oxygenator, and returns it to the femoral artery or ascending aorta. It temporarily takes over the function of the heart and lungs during heart surgery

heart rate the number of heart beats per minute

heart valve a prosthetic device to replace stenosed or 'insufficient' cardiac valve. It may be mechanical, bioprosthetic or porcine

heart worm *Dirofilaria immitis*

heat (het) a high temperature **conductive h** heat transmitted by direct contact **convective h** heat conveyed by a warm medium **h cramp** occurs in hot weather when heavy exercising muscles contract without reflex inhibition for antagonist muscles **h exhaustion** caused by salt and water loss **h illness** represents a spectrum of disorders in which the thermoregulatory mechanisms of the body remain intact **h labile** destroyed by heat **h stroke** develops due to failure of body's thermoregulatory mechanism failure. It leads to widespread cellular damage **h tetany** hyperventilation on exposure to heat leading to respiratory alkalosis manifesting as tetany **prickly h** milia rubia

heavy chain one of the two polypeptide chains forming basis of immunoglobulin molecule and determining its class **h c diseases** a family of monoclonal gammopathies or paraproteinaemias that are characterised by excess production of an immunoglobulin fragment and accompanied by lymphoproliferative disease

hebe – refers to 1. puberty 2. dull or lethargic

hebephrenia (he-be-fre'-ni-a) shallow inappropriate affect and silly regressive behaviour and mannerisms

Heberden's nodes bony swellings close to distal interphalgeal joints due to osteoarthritis. Index finger is commonly affected named after William Heberden, British physician

hebetic pertaining to youth

hebetude (heb'e-tud) stupidity

hedrocoel (hed'ro-sel) prolapse of the intestine through the anus.

heel calx h-to-knee test coordination test for skilled movements. The heel has to be kept on the opposite knee and it should be drawn along the shin towards the ankle. The procedure is done on other side. In cerebellar disease heel overshoots the knee and exhibits oscillation while it is moved down the leg. In sensory ataxia heel is lifted high and falls off many times during its downward course

height vertical measurement

Hegar's sign early diagnosis of pregnancy between the sixth and tenth weeks, when the fundus and upper part of body of uterus are enlarged and lower uterine segment is soft and empty, cervix is soft and firm. Two fingers placed in the anterior vaginal fornix appears almost to meet the fingers of the other hand pressing backwards and downwards suprapubically, named after Alfred Hegar, German gynaecologist

Heimlich (him'lik) manoeuvre a first aid technique to dislodge an inhaled object in a choking person by administering rapid upward thrusts from below the sternum, named after H.J. Heimlich, American physician

Heinz bodies clumps of precipitated oxidized haemoglobin in the cytoplasm of red cells, named after Robert Heinz, German Pathologist

HeLa cells an aneuploid epithelial cell line isolated from Henrietta (He) Lack (La) who died of anaplastic carcinoma of the uterine cervix

helical 1. relating to helix 2. coiled

helicobacter (hel'i-ko-bak'ter) a genus of motile gram-negative micro-aerophilic bacteria of the family Spirellaceae H. pylori causes gastritis and peptic ulcer

heliotrope rash lilac or violaceous discolouration of the skin of eyelids, nasal bridge and forehead in dermatomyositis

helicotrema a semilunar opening at the apex of the cochlea

heliotherapy (he'li-o-ther-api)sunbathing; therapeutic effects of the sun's rays are maximum in the early morning

helium a gaseous element, symbol He. At number 2.

helix pl. halices 1. a folded rim of cartilage forming the margin of auricle 2. a line in the shape of a coil double h helical structure as surrounded by two strands of deoxyribonucleic acid held together by hydrogen bonds, described by James Watson, US biochemist and Francis Crick, English biologist

HELLP Syndrome a syndrome noted in last trimester of pregnancy often with pregnancy-induced hypertension characterised by haemolysis, elevated liver enzymes, and low platelets

helminths (hel'minth's) worms divided into as round worms (nematodes) and flat worms (trematodes – flukes) and cestodes (tapeworms). These worms infect men when ingested or by direct penetration of the skin

helminthemesis (hel-min-them'e-sis) the vomiting or expulsion of intestinal worms through the mouth

heminthiasis (hel-min-thi'a-sis) helminths parasitising humans. Helminths are largest of human parasites

helminthic (hel-min'thik) 1. pertaining to the worms 2. pertaining to expulsion of worms

helminthoma a granulomatous nodule caused by a helminth or its products

heloma (he-lo'ma) corn; collosity

helotomy surgical treatment or corns

Helper T cells see CD4+ cells

Helsinki declaration a set of recommendations guiding physicians in biomedical research involving human subjects, adapted by the 18th World Medical Assembly in Helsinkin in 1964, which is amended later

hemaralopia (hem'er-a-lo'pe-a) day blindness

hemi – combining word for half

hemiachromatopsia (hem'e-a-kro'matop'se-a) colour blindness in one half of the visual field

hemiageusia (hem'e-a-goo'ze-a) loss of taste sensation on one side of the tongue

hemiamyosthenia (hem'e-a-mi-os-the'ne-a) diminished muscular power on one side of the body

hemianalgesia (hem'e-an'al-ge'ze-a) loss of pain sensation on one side of the body

hemianaesthesia (hem'e-an'es-the'ze-a) loss of sensation on one side of the body **crossed h** loss of sensation on one half of the face and loss of pain and temperature sense on the opposite half of the body

hemianopia (hem'e-an'o-pe-a) blindness in one half of the visual field of one or both eyes **binasal h** see binasal hemianopia **bitemporal h** see bitemporal hemianopia **heteronymous h** blindness of both nasal or both temporal halves of the visual field **homonymous h** blindness affecting the nasal half of the visual field of one eye and the temporal half of the visual field of other eye

hemiapraxia (hem'e-a-prak-se-a) inability to perform purposeful movements in the absence of motor or sensory impairment, on one half of the body

hemiataxia (hem'e-a-tak'se-a) ataxia on one half of the body

hemiathetosis (hem'e-a-th'i-to-sis) athetosis of one half of the body

hemiatrophy (hem'e-a'tro-fe) atrophy of one half of the body or of an organ

hemiaxial (hem'e-ak'se-al) any oblique angle to the long axis of the body or part

hemiballismus (hem'e-bal-liz'mus) a violent type of irregular, uncontrollable flinging movement affecting one half of the body

hemibladder (hem'e-blad'er) a developmental abnormality wherein the bladder has two separate parts each with its own ureter; a half bladder

hemiblock (hem'e-blok) failure of conduction of cardiac impulse in either of the two main divisions (anterior or posterior) of the left branch of the bundle of His

hemichorea (hem'e-kor'e-a) chorea affecting one half of the body

hemicolectomy surgical removal of a part of colon

hemicrania (hem'e-kra'ne-a) headache on one side of the scalp

hemicraniosis (hem'e-kra'ne-o'sis) hyperostosis of one side of the cranium and face

hemidesmosome site of attachment between basal surface of basal epithelial cells and the basement membrane

hemifacial (hem'e-fa'shil) pertaining to or affecting one half of the face

hemigastrectomy (hem'e-gas-trek'ta-me) surgical removal of half of the stomach

hemiglossectomy (hem'e-glos-ek'ta-me) surgical removal of one half of the tongue

hemihidrosis (hem'e-hi-dro'sis) sweating on one half of the body

hemihypalgesia (hem'e-hip'al-je'ze-a) diminished pain sensitivity on one side of the body

hemihyperaesthesia (hem'e-hi'per-es-the'zea) increased sensitiveness of one half of the body

hemihyperhidrosis (hem'e-hi'per-i-dro'sis) increased sweating on one side of the body

hemihypertrophy (hem'e-hi-per'trah-fe) increased growth on one side of the body or of a part

hemihypesthesia (hem'e-hi-pes-the'zh-ah) diminished sensitiveness on one side of the body

hemihypotonia (hem'e-hi'po-to'ne-a) decreased muscle tone on one half of the body

hemilaminectomy (hem'e-lam'i-nek'ta-me) removal of a vertebral lamina on one side only

hemilaryngectomy (hem'e-lar'in-jek'ta-me) surgical removal of one lateral half of the larynx

hemilateral (hem'e-lat'er-al) affecting one lateral half of the body.

heminephrectomy (hem'e-ne-frek'ta-me) surgical removal of one half of a kidney

hemiopia (hem'e-o'pe-a) hemianopia

hemiparesis (hem'e-pa-re'sis) weakness affecting one side of the body

hemiparetic (hem'e-pa-ret'ik) 1. pertaining to hemiparesis 2. person affected by hemiparesis

hemiplegia (hem'e-ple'je-a) paralysis of one side of the body especially of the arm and leg **hemiplegic** adj. **cerebral h** hemiplegia due to a brain lesion **crossed h** paralysis of one side of the face and opposite of the body **spastic h** hemiplegia with spasticity of the affected muscles, accompanied by exaggerated deep reflexes **spinal h** hemiplegia due to a lesion in the spinal cord

hemiptera (he-mip'ter-a) an order of insects having mouth parts adapted to piercing and sucking

hemisection (hem'i-sek'shun) division into two equal parts

hemispasm (hem'i-spazm) spasm affecting one half of the body

hemisphere (hem'is-fr) half of a spherical structure or organ **cerebellar h** either of two lobes of the cerebellum situated lateral to the vermis **cerebral h** one of the paired structures forming the bulk of the brain. **dominant h** that part of the cerebral hemisphere which is more concerned than the other in the integration of sensations and the control of voluntary functions

hemispherium (hem'is-fe're-um) either of the cerebral hemispheres

hemivertebra (hem'i-vurt'i-bra) incom-

pletely developed one side of a vertebra

hemizygosity (hem'i-zi-gos'i-te) the state of only one of a pair of alleles transmitting a specific character **hemizygois** adj.

hemizygous having only one copy of a given genetic locus

Henderson-Hasselbalch equation an equation to express dissociation constant of an acid. It states pH equals $6.1+10$ g $HCO_3^-/(PaCO_2)$. At normal pH of blood, 7.4 the ratio of HCO_3^- to $PaCO_2$ is 20 to 1, enunciated by Lawrence Henderson, US biochemist and K. Hasselbalch, Danish physician

Hepadnaviridae (hep-ad'na-vir'i-de) the hepatitis B-like viruses; a family of DNA viruses causing infection and associated with chronic disease and neoplasia

hepadnavirus (hep-ad'na-vi'rus) hepatitis B-like viruses that multiply in the nuclei of hepatocytes and induce persistent infection

hepar (he'par) the liver

heparin (hep'a-rin) naturally occurring glycosaminoglycan. It inhibits coagulation by enhancing the effect of antithrombin III in the inhibition of activated clotting factors IX, X, XI, XII and thrombin. Intravenous heparin is used for acute pulmonary embolism, acute myocardial infarction and deep vein thrombosis. It is also used while performing vascular procedures and inserting prosthetic heart valves. Bleeding is the most common complication. It has a short half life **low molecular-weight h** , LMWH fragments of unfractionated heparin produced by either chemical or enzymatic depolymerisation, used as parenteral anticoagulant for the prevention and treatment of thromboembolic diseases. **unfractionated h**, UFH a crude product derived from the intestine of pigs, used as anticoagulant for acute thromboembolic disorders. It accelerates the inactivation of thrombin and Fxa by antithrombin

heparinise (hep'a-rin-iz) to render blood incoagulable with heparin

heparinoid (hep-ari'noi-d) direct thrombin inhibitor composed of low molecular weight non-heparin glycosaminoglycan

hepatatrophia (hep'at-a-tro'fe-a) atrophy of the liver

hepatic (he-pat'ik) pertaining to the liver **h acinus** functional unit of the liver consisting of hepatocytes **h amoebiasis** *see* amoebiasis **h arterial disease** hepatic artery occlusion causing severe upper abdominal pain and high transaminase activity **h decompensation** chronic liver failure when liver functions can no longer maintain normal physiological conditions **h duct** the duct that carries bile out of the liver and it unites with the cystic duct to form the common bile duct **h encephalopathy** a neuropsychiatric syndrome caused by liver disease. Liver failure and portosystemic shunting of blood are the underlying causes. It presents with change of intellect, personality, emotions and consciousness **h failure** Liver may fail in its function acutely presenting with mental changes progressing from confusion to stupor and coma or gradually leading to ascites, oedema, hepatic encephalopathy jaundice, hypoalbuminaemia and coagulation abnormality **h flexure** the bend of colon under liver where ascending colon becomes transverse colon **h lobule** division of liver into multiple smaller units comprising a central vein, radiating sinusoids separated from each other by hepatocyte plates and peripheral portal tracts **h nodules** nodular regenerative hyperplasia giving rise to nodules in the liver **h osteodystrophy** biliary cirrhosis associated with bone pain and fractures

hepaticoduodenostomy (he-pat'i-ko-doo'o-de-nos'ta-me) surgical anastomosis of the hepatic duct to the duodenum

Henoch-Schonlein purpura a small vessel vasculitis seen in children, following an upper respiratory tract infection. There is nonthrombocytopaenic purpura over the buttocks and legs, associated with intra-abdominal pain and flitting arthritis. It is self limiting, named after Eduard Henoch, German paediatrician and Johann Schonlein, German physician

hepaticogastrostomy (-gas-tros'ta-me) surgical anastomosis of the hepatic duct to the stomach

hepaticolithotomy (-li-thot'a-me) incision of the hepatic duct for the removal of the calculi

hepatitis (hep'a-ti'tis) inflammation of the liver which results in damage to hepatocytes with subsequent cell death **acute h** acute injury to the liver from viral infections (hepatitis A, B, C, D, E viral infections, EBV, CMV, *HERPES SIMPLEX*) and drugs (rifampicin, isoniazid, chlorpromazine) **alcoholic h** alcoholic liver disease presenting with jaundice, hepatomegaly, ascites and encephalopathy. The toxic metabolites produced during conversion of acetaldehyde to acetate and immune reaction to liver cells are responsible for the condition **amoebic h** enlarged, tender liver, abscess in right lobe, fever and leucocytosis in patient with recent amoebic colotis **anicteric h** viral hepatitis without jaundice **autoimmune h** a chronic hepatitis occurring as an autoimmune disorder with presence of specific auto antibodies. It has an insidious onset with fatigue, anorexia and jaundice **chronic h** a disorder characterised by a mononuclear inflamma-

Hepatitis-B-virus

tory cell infiltrate of the portal tracts, often due to hepatitis B **hA** a self-limiting viral disease caused by hepatitis A virus, an RNA enterovirus. It spreads by faecal oral route in poor sanitation and rarely by blood. It has an incubation period of 2 weeks, presents with mild jaundice **hB** hepatitis caused by HBV, a DNA virus and only hepadnavirus causing infection in humans. It is transmitted by parenteral route; other modes of spread are through saliva, sexual intercourse, and vertically from mother to child. Humans are the only source of infection. Individuals incubating or suffering from acute hepatitis are highly infectious. It causes a severe infection and chronic infection leads to chronic liver failure. These individuals are highly infectious when markers of continuing viral replication (HBe Ag, HBV–DNA polymerase) are present **hC** an RNA containing flavivirus causing hepatitis. Humans appear to be sole source of infection and the spread is by inoculation with blood or blood products. Chronic infection with HCV may occur and is lifelong **hD** an RNA defective virus which requires HBV for replication. It can infect individuals simultaneously with HBV and cause acute severe hepatitis and it can superinfect those who are already chronic carriers of HBV and lead to progressive chronic hepatitis and cirrhosis **hE** HEV an RNA virus, spreads by faecal-oral route and found in places with poor sanitation. It is responsible for large epidemics of water-borne hepatitis. **interface h** hepatitis with invasion of inflammatory cell infiltrate into periportal parenchyma with loss of definition of the portal-peripheral interface, damage to the periportal hepatocytes and formation of hepatocyte 'rosettes' **toxic h** liver, main organ in which drugs are metabolised may get impaired in its capacity to metabolise

drugs and give rise to manifestations by hepatic damage **viral h** hepatitis caused by specific hepatitis viruses and rarely from other viruses (cytomegalovirus, EBV, HSV, yellow fever virus)

hepatisation (hep'a-ti-za'shun) transformation into a solid mass like the liver especially the consolidated lobe in pneumonia

hepat(o) combining word for liver

hepatoblastoma (hep'a-to-blas-to'ma) a malignant hepatic tumour found in infants; the tumour is single, solid, well circumscribed and contains immature histiocytes

hepatocellular carcinoma (-cel'lu-lar-kar'sin-o'ma) hepatoma; primary malignant liver tumour. Aflatoxin contamination of foods, chronic hepatitis B and C virus infection, and cirrhosis are mainly responsible factors. It presents with weakness, anorexia, weight loss, fever, a large irregular liver mass and ascites. There is marked rise in alpha-fetoprotein **fibrolemmar h** rare tumour occurring in young adults of either sexes, presents with pain due to bleeding into the tumour and later causing calcification

hepatocholangiocarcinoma (-ko-lan'je-o-kar'sin-o-ma) an uncommon tumour developing anywhere in the biliary tree. There can be intermittent jaundice, upper abdominal pain and weight loss

hepatocirrhosis (-si-ro'sis) cirrhosis of the liver

hepatocyte (hep'a-tosit) a liver cell

hepatogastric (-gas'trix) pertaining to the liver and stomach

hepatogram (-gram) 1. a radiogram of the liver 2. a tracing of the liver pulse

hepatoid (hep'a-toyd) resembling the liver

hepatojugular (hep'a-to-jug'u-lar) pertaining to the liver and jugular vein **h reflux** firm sustained pressure is exerted with hand over the right upper abdomen or elsewhere in the abdomen. In early right heart failure there is distension of the neck veins and the level of venous pulsations moves up

hepatolith (hep'a-to-lith) a calculus in the liver

hepatolithiasis (hep'a-to-lith'i-a-sis) the presence of calculi in the biliary ducts of the liver

hepatology (hep'a-tol'a-je) the scientific study of the liver and its diseases

hepatolysis (hep'a-tol'i-sis) destruction of the liver cells **hepatolytic** adj

hepatoma (hep'a-to'ma) 1. tumour of the liver 2. hepatocellular carcinoma

hepatomegaly (hep'a-to-meg'a-le) enlargement of the liver. Liver is enlarged from infections (viral hepatitis, amoebic hepatitis, malaria, kala azar, hydatid disease, tuberculosis, infectious mononucleosis), congestion (congestive heart failure, portal hypertension), early stages of cirrhosis, toxic hepatitis, heamatologic conditions (iron deficiency anaemia, reticulosis, leukaemia, multiple myeloma), metabolic (diabetes mellitus), amyloidosis, hepatoma and secondary deposits

hepatomelanosis (hep'a-to-mel'a-no-sis) deep pigmentation of the liver

hepatomphalocoele (hep'a-tom'fa-lo-sel) umbilical hernia with liver involvement in the hernial sac

hepatopexy (hep'a-to-pek'se) surgical fixation of a displaced liver

hepatopneumonic (hep'a-to-noo-mon'ik) pertaining to or communicating with liver and lungs

hepatoportal (-port-al) pertaining to the portal system of the liver

hepatopulmonary syndrome resistant hypoxaemia and intrapulmonary vascular dilatation in patients with cirrhosis

hepatorenal (-ren'al) pertaining to the liver and kidneys **h syndrome** renal dysfunction without renal pathology produced by a combination of decreased renal perfusion, hypovolaemia and

hyperaldosteronism secondary to liver disease

hepatorrhexis (hep'a-to-rek'sis) rupture of the liver.

hepatosis (hep'a-to'sis) any functional disorder of the liver

hepatosplenitis (hep'a-to-splen-it-is) inflammation of the liver and spleen

hepatosplenomegaly (-splen'o-meg'a-le) enlargement of the liver and spleen

hepatotoxin (-tok'sin) a toxic substance that destroys liver cells **hepatotoxin** adj

heptachromik (hep'ta-kro'mik) pertaining to or exhibiting seven colours

heptose (hep'tos) a sugar whose molecule contains seven carbon atoms

herald bleed an episode of bleeding often accompanied by abdominal pain that precedes a catastrophic haemorrhage as in arterial-enteric fistulas with false aneurysms

herald patch an initial lesion of pityriasis rosea that appears as a solitary, oval macule with raised border and fine, adherent scales, preceding by a week the other lesions

herb any leafy plant especially that used for remedy or as a flavouring agent

herbivorous (her-biv-a-rus) living on plants

herd an ecologic composite that includes susceptible animal species including man, vectors and environmental factors

heredity (he-red'it-e) genetic transmission of characters from parent to offspring

heredofamilial (he'red-o-fa-mil'e-al) occurrence in certain families on a hereditary basis.

heritability (her'it-a-bil'it'e) the quality of being heritable; a measure of the extent to which a phenotype is influenced by the genotype

hermaphroditism (her-maf'ro-di-tizm) presence in one individual cf both testicular and ovarian tissue

hermetic (her-met'ik) impervious to air; airtight

hernia (her'ne-a) protrusion of a portion of an organ or tissue through a normal or abnormal opening in the wall of the cavity in which it lies **hernial** adj. **abdominal h** hernia occurring through abdominal wall **Barth's h** protrusion of a loop of intestine between a persistent vitelline duct and the abdominal wall **Beclard's h** femoral hernia through the opening for saphenous vein **Bochdalek's h** congenital diaphragmatic hernia due to a defect in closure of pleuroperitoneal membrane **cerebral h** protrusion of brain through the skull **complete h** an indirect inguinal hernia in which the contents extend into the tunica vaginalis **crural h** femoral hernia **diaphragmatic h** protrusion of abdominal contents into the chest through the diaphragm **epigastric h** a protrusion of extraperitoneal fat and occasionally a small peritoneal sac through the weakness in the linea alba between the xiphoid process and the umbilicus **en glissade h** sliding hernia. The posterior wall of the hernial sac is not formed by peritoneum alone, but also by viscus such as sigmoid colon and its mesentery on the left side and caecum on the right side and the contents of the sac may be intestine or omentum **fat h** protrusion of peritoneal fat through the abdominal wall **femoral h** a protrusion of extra peritoneal fat, peritoneum and occasionally abdominal contents through the femoral canal **gastroesophageal h** hiatus hernia in which distal end of the oesophagus and part of the stomach protrude through the oesophageal hiatus of the diaphragm **hiatus h** a profusion of any structure through the oesophageal hiatus of the diaphragm. **incarcerated h** irreducible hernia **incisional h** hernia occurring through a surgical incision or scar **indirect inguinal h** common in young and it occurs in a preformed sac through the deep inguinal ring **inguinal h** com-

monest of all forms of hernia; occurs through the inguinal canal. It may be direct or indirect. Direct inguinal hernia comes out through the Hasselbach's triangle, usually bilateral and incomplete that may be shaped spherical or globular. Common in old age **interstitial h** hernial sac lies between different layers of the abdominal wall which may be intraparietal, interparietal (intermuscular) or extraparietal **paraumbilical h** painless reducible swelling around the umbilicus liable to become irreducible **reducible h** hernia in which the contents of the hernial sac can be returned back by manipulation **sciatic h** protrusion of intestine through the great sacrosciatic foramen **scrotal h** a complete inguinal hernia located in the scrotum **strangulated h** an irreducible hernia which is constricted so as to compromise the blood supply **synovial h** protrusion of a fold of synovial membrane through the *stratum fibrosum* of a joint capsule **umbilical h** herniation of abdominal contents through the centre of the abdominal scar **ventral h** hernia through the abdominal wall **vitreous h** prolapse of the vitreous into the anterior chamber

herniation (her'ne-a-'shun) abnormal protrusion of an organ or structure through a defect or natural opening found in a covering, membrane, muscle or bone

hernioplasty (her'ne-o-plas'te) surgical correction of hernia

herniorrahaphy (her'ne-or'a-fe) surgical repair of hernia, with suturing

herniotomy (her'ne-ot'a-me) a cutting operation for the repair of hernia

heroin (he'ro-in) diacetyl morphine

herpangina (her'pan-ji-na) an infectious febrile illness due to a coxsackievirus. The throat and posterior area of the mouth are covered with vesicles that rupture and ulcerate

herpes (her'pez) any inflammatory disease characterised by small vesicles in clusters caused by herpes viruses **herpetic** adj. **genital h** common sexually transmitted disease caused by herpes simplex virus (HSV) type 2. It is characterised by itchy or painful small grouped vesicles which break and produce ulcers in genital region with inguinal lymphadenopathy and fever **h encephalitis** inflammation of the brain caused by the spread of a herpes simplex virus **h febrilis** herpes simplex of the lips and nasal mucosa **h genitalis** genital herpes **h simplex** infection with the herpes simplex virus. It causes blister-like sores on the face, lips, mouth or genitals **h zoster** shingles caused by varicella-zoster virus. It involves posterior root ganglia and presents with severe continuous pain in the distribution of the affected nerve root. The lesion after 3 or 4 days becomes red and vesicles appear which dry up and leave behind small scars. The condition may be followed by neuralgia **h viruses** a group of viruses that includes herpes simplex virus, varicella-zoster virus, Epstein-Barr virus and cytomegalovirus **h whitlow** blistering of the skin on the fingers by herpes simplex viral infection

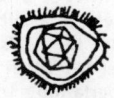

Herpes virus

herpes virus (-vi'rus) any of the group of DNA viruses which includes the causative microorganisms such as herpes simplex, herpes zoster, chickenpox Epstein-Barr virus and cytomegal o virus *H hominis* herpes simplex virus responsible for nongenital (type I) and genital (type II) infection

hersage (ar-sa'z) surgical separation of the fibres in a scarred area of a peripheral nerve

Hertz (hurts) a unit of frequency equal to one cycle per second; Hz

Herxheimer reaction *see* Jarisch–Herxheimer reaction

hesitancy (hezi-tan-si) an involuntary delay or inability in starting the urinary stream

hetacillin (het'a-sil'in) a semisynthetic penicillin which is converted in the body to ampicillin

heteraesthesia (het'er-es-the'shah) variation of cutaneous sensibility on adjoining areas

heterergic (het'er-er'jik) exhibiting different effects as in two drugs, one of which exhibits a particular effect and other does not

heterecism (her'er-e-sizm) occurrence, in parasite, of two cycles of existence, passed in two different hosts

heter (o) combining word for other; dissimilar

heteroagglutination (het'er-o-aglot'in-a-shun) agglutination of antigens of one species by agglutinins obtained by another species

heteroantibody (-an'ti-bod'e) antibody that is heterologous with respect to antigen

heteroantigen (-an'ti-jen) an antigen originating from one species producing a corresponding antibody in another species

heteroblastic (-blas'tik) developing from more than a single type of tissue

heterocellular (-sel'ul-er) composed of cells of different kinds

heterochromatin (-kro'ma-tin) 1. diversity of colour in a part normally of one colour 2. dark-appearing bands following Giemsa banding of chromosomes

heterocrine (het'er-o-krin) secreting more than one kind of material

heterocyclic (het'er-o-si'klik) having a closed chain or ring formation

heterocytotropic (-si'to-trop'ik) having an affinity for cells from different species

heterodermic (-dermic) referring a skin graft from an individual of another species

heterodont (het'er-o-don't) having teeth of different shapes

heteroduplex (het'er-o-du-pleks) hybrid DNA involving two strands which are different

heteroerotism (het'er-o-e'rah-tizm) sexual feeling directed towards another individual

heterogamety (het'er-o-gam'it-e) production of gametes of contrasting types with respect to sex chromosomes

heterogamy (het'er-og'ah-me) reproduction resulting from the union of gametes differing in their size, shape and structure. **heterogamous** adj

heterogeneous (het'er-oj'e-nus) differing in composition, quality or structure

heterogenesis (het'er-o-jen'e-sis) production of offspring unlike the parents

heterogony (het'er-og'ah-ne) heterogenesis

heterograft (het'er-o-graft) xenograft, a graft transferred from an animal of one species to one of another species

heterohaemagglutination (het'er-o-hem'a-gloot'in-a'shun) agglutination of erythrocytes of one species by a haemagglutinin derived from an individual of different species

heteroimmunity (het'er-o-i-mun'it-e) an immune state induced by immunisation with cells of an animal of another species

heterokeratoplasty (het'er-o-ker'a-to-plast'te) grafting of cornea obtained from an individual of another species

heterolalia a form of aphasia characterised by habitual substitution of inappropriate words for those intended

heterolateral contralateral

heterologous (het'er-ol-a-gus) formation of a tissue that is not normal to the part.

heterolysis (het'er-ol'i-sis) dissolution or digestion of the cells of one species by lysin of a different species

heteromeric (het'er-o-me'rik) 1. having a different chemical composition. 2. denoting spinal neurons with processes passing over to the opposite side of the cord

heterometaplasia (-met'a-pla'zhah) tissue transformation which results in the production of a tissue foreign to the part where produced

heterometropia (-me-tro'pe-a) the condition in which refraction in two eyes differs

heteromorphosis (-mor-fo'sis) development of one tissue from a tissue of another type

heteromorphous (-mor'fus) differing from the normal type

heteronomous (het'er-on'o-mus) 1. *psy* subject to another's will 2. different from the type; abnormal

heteronymous (het'er-on'i-mus) standing in opposite relations

heteroosteoplasty (het'er-o-os-te-o-plas'te) osteoplasty with bone obtained from another species

heteropathy (het-er-op'a-thi) abnormal sensitivity to stimuli

heterophagosome (-fag'o-som) an intracytoplasmic vacuole formed by phagocytosis, which gets fused with a lysosome

heterophagy (het'er-of-a-je) digestion within a cell of a substance phagocytosed from the cell's environment

heterophil (het'er-o-fil) 1. neutrophil leucocyte 2. pertaining to heterogenetic antigens and related antibody

heterophonia (het'er-o-fo'ni-a) 1. change of voice at puberty 2. any abnormality in voice sounds

heterophoria (-for'e-a) a tendency for deviation of the eyes

heterophthalmia (het'er-of-thal-me-a) a difference in the appearance of two eyes, as in colour or direction of visual axes

heteroplasia (het'er-o-pla'zhah) 1. development of cells that are not normal for the organ 2. malposition of tissue

heteroplasty (het'er-o-plas'te) tissue transplantation from one species to another; heterotransplantation

heteroploidy (-ploi-de) the state of having an abnormal number of chromosomes

heteropsia (het'er-op'se-a) unequal vision in both eyes

heteropyknosis (het'er-o-pik-no'sis) any state of variable density

heterosexual (het'er-o-sek'shu-al) 1. denoting heterosexuality 2. one who practices heterosexuality

heterosexuality (het'er-o-sek'shu-al-ite) erotic attraction or sexual behaviour between persons of the opposite sex

heterosuggestion (het'er-o-sug-jes'chun) suggestion received from another person

heterotonia (het'er-o-to'ne-a) abnormality or variation in tension

heterotopia (het'er-o-to'pe-a) 1. ectopia 2. displacement of gray matter into deep cerebral white matter

heterotransplantation (het'er-o-trans'planta'shun) transfer of a heterograft

heterotrophe (het'er-o-trof) a microorganism that obtains carbon and energy from organic compounds

heterotropia (het'er-o-tro'pe-a) strabismus

heterotypic (het'er-o-tip'i-k) pertaining to a different type

heteroxenous (het'er-o-ge'nus) requiring more than one host to complete the life cycle

heterozygosity (het'er-o-zi-gos'it-e) the state of having different allelic genes at one or more paired loci in homologous chromosomes

heterozygote an individual possessing two different alleles at the corresponding loci on a pair of homologous chromosome

hetu (s) reason

heuristics (hu-ris'tiks) direction or rules which stimulate interest from further scientific investigation. Often they are derived from common sense, personal observation or from other principles which are traditionally accepted

hexad (hek'sad) a group of six similar entities

hexadactyly (hef-sa-oak'til'e) the occurrence of six digits on one hand

hexamethonium (hek'sa-me-tho'ne-um) a ganglionic blocking agent used to reduce high blood pressure

hexobarbital (hek'so-bar'bi-tal) a short acting barbiturate sedative and hypnotic

hexokinase (hek'so-ki'nas) an enzyme that catalyses the transfer of a high energy phosphate group to a hexose

hexosamine (hek'so-so'a-men) the amine derivative of a hexose

hexosaminidase (hek'so-s-min'i-das) any of the enzymes that cleave hexosamines from ganglioside like oligosaccharides

hexose (hek'sos) a monosaccharide containing six carbon atoms in a molecule

hexuronic (hek'su-ron'ik) **acid** any uronic acid formed by oxidation of a hexose

hexyeresorcinol (hek'sil-risor'si-nol) a substituted phenol derivative used as an antiseptic

Hg chemical symbol of mercury

HGH abbreviation for human growth hormone

hiatus (hi-a'tus) a gap, cleft or opening **hiatal** adj

hibernation (hi-ber-na'shun) 1. to live in seclusion 2. to pass winter in tarpor by sharp reduction in body temperature and metabolism 3. a temporary reduction in function

hibernoma (hi'ber-no-ma) a rare benign circumscribed and symptomatic tumour consisting of brown fat that has resemblance to fat in some hibernating animals

hiccup (hik'up) spasms of the diaphragm usually due to irritation in the upper abdominal area

Hickman (hik'man) **line** a type of catheter that is surgically implanted, whose one end leads into a large vein in the chest and the other end outside the chest

hidradenitis (hi'drad-e-nits) inflammation of the sweat glands

hidradenocarcinoma (hi-drad'e-no-kar-ci-noma) carcinoma of the sweat glands

hidradenoid (hi-drad'e-noid) resembling elements of a sweat gland

hidradenoma (hi-drad-e-no'ma) a benign tumour derived from epithelial cells of sweat glands

hidr (o) combining word for sweat

hidroacanthoma (hi-dro-ak'an-tho-ma) a benign tumour of an eccrine gland

hidrocystoma (hi'dro-sis-to'ma) a retention cyst of a sweat gland

hidromeiosis obstruction of sweat glands in hot humid environments leading to decreased production of sweat

hidropoiesis (hi-dro-poi-e'sis) the formation of sweat

hidroschesis (hi-dros'kis-is) anhidrosis

hidrotic (hi-drot'ik) pertaining to or characterised by or causing sweating

high-density lipoprotein (HDL) a type of protein molecule carried in the blood that removes cholesterol from tissues and appears to protect against coronary heart disease

higher function intellectual state and mental functions

high resolution computed tomography (HRCT) a CT utilising thin collimation and image reconstruction with high-spatial frequency algorithm. HRCT lung utilises 1 to 2 mm thin slices with spacing at 1 cm intervals from the thoracic inlet to the hemidiaphragm. It is utilised to study the lungs for bronchial abnormalities, interstitial fibrosis, miliary disease or emphysema

hilum (hi'lum) pl. hila a depression or a pit on an organ. It allows entry or exit to blood vessels and nerves hilar adj. h of lung anatomic area situated between the lung laterally and the mediastinum medially, through which pass the bronchus, pulmonary vessels and are visible radiologically because of presence of surrounding aerated lung

hilus (hi'lus) pl. hili hilum

hind brain (hind'bran) the most caudal part of the brain giving rise to cerebellum, pons and medulla oblongata

hind foot (hind'foot) the back of the foot comprising the region of the talus and calcaneus

hindgut (hind'gut) the embryonic structure from which the colon is formed

hinge joint a joint in which the two bony surfaces fit tightly allowing flexion and extension as in knee or elbow joints

hip coxa area of the body lateral to and including hip joint

hippocampus (hip'o-kam-pus) a curved elevation in the floor of the inferior horn of the lateral ventricle, and is thought to be involved in memory

Hippocrates (hi-pok'rah-tez) the Greek physician who lived in island of Cos in 5th century BC, regarded as Father of Medicine. hippocratic adj

Hippocratic relating to, described by or attributed to Hippocrates h facies facial appearance in advanced case of peritonitis exhibiting sunken eyes, hollow cheeks, collapsed temples, sharp nose h nails clubbing of digits H oath an oath demanded of physician about to enter upon the practice of his profession h succussion splash splashing sound audible on shaking the chest in hydropneumothorax

hippuria (hip-u're-a) an excess amount of hippuric acid in the urine

hippuric (hip-ur'ik) acid a crystalline carboxylic acid found in the urine of some animals and man

hippus (hip'us) an abnormally exaggerated rhythmic contraction and dilatation of the pupil

Hirano (hir'a-no) body eosinophilic football-shaped inclusion seen in necrosis of the brain, part of normal ageing, but more numerous in Alzheimer's disease

hirci (hir'si) the axillary hair

hirsuitism (hir'soot'izm) abnormal growth

of hair, especially in women in a pattern that of a normal male due to an increased responsiveness of the hair follicles to the normal levels of androgenic hormones

hirudicide (hi-rood'is-id) an agent that is destructive to leeches **hirudicidal** adj

hirudin (hi'rood'in) the active principle of the buccal secretion of leeches. It prevents coagulation by acting as an antithrombin

hirudinise to render the blood non-coagulable by injection of hirudin

hirudinea (hi-rood'in-ea) a class of annelids, the leeches

hirudo (hi-roo'do) a genus of leeches *H. medicinalis* is an important example, used for drawing blood

histamine (his'ta-men) a bioactive amine stored in mast cells and basophils. It may be secreted by monocytes, neural and endocrine cells. Histamine causes smooth muscle contraction, including bronchiolar and small vessel constriction, increased vascular permeability and secretion of nasal and bronchial glands. It is a powerful stimulant of gastric secretion

histaminergic (his'ta-min-er'jic) referring to the effects of histamine at histamine receptors of target organ

histidase (his'ti-das) a liver enzyme converting histidine to urocanic acid

histidinaemia (his'ti-din-e'mea) an autosomal recessive condition characterised by a deficiency in histidase, the enzyme that converts histidine to urocanic acid in the liver and skin. Generally asymptomatic. Rarely it may have a neonatal onset with impaired speech, growth and mental retardation

histidinuria (his'ti-di-nu're-a) the presence of histidine in urine.

hist (o) combining word for tissue

histiocyte (his'te-o-sit) a resident macrophage **histiocytic** adj

histiocytoma (his'te-o-si-to'ma) a tumour containing histiocytes

histiocytosis (his'te-o-si-to'sis) an uncommon condition of undetermined aetiology presenting with involvement of flat bones and soft tissues like the lungs, skin, neurohypophysis, lymph nodes, liver and spleen, is characterised by granuloma formation with infiltration and proliferation of histiocytes **h X** a group of disorders that includes fulminant Letterer-Siwe disease of early infancy, Hand-Schuller-Christian disease of childhood, eosinophilic granuloma or Langerhans cell granulomatosis in young and middle-aged adults

histoblast (his'to-blast) a tissue cell

histochemistry (his'to-kem'is-tre) the study of chemistry of the cells and tissues

histoclinical (-klin'i-kl) combining histologic abnormality with clinical features

histocompatibility (-kom'pat'i-bil'it-e) the state of being histocompatible **h antigen** one of the multiple antigens found in all nucleated cells in the body capable of identifying the cell as 'self' and they determine the compatibility of tissue for transformation

histocompatible capable of being accepted and remaining functional

histodifferentiation (-dif'er-en'she-a'shun) the morphologic appearance of tissue characteristics during development

histogenesis (-jen'is-is) the formation and development of tissues from the undifferentiated cells of the germ layers of the embryo

histogenous (his'to-j'in-is) formed by the tissues

histogram (his'to-gram) a pictorial diagram of a frequency distribution and are represented by vertical bars or rectangles

histoid (his'toid) resembling in structure one of the tissues in the body

histokinesis (his'to-ki-ne'sis) movement in the tissues of the body

histology (his-tol'a-je) 1. the study of microscopic structure of organ tissues 2. the science dealing with the microscopic study of cells and tissues. **histologic** adj

histolysis (his-tol'i-sis) breakdown of living tissue

histone (his'ton) one of simple proteins that contains a high proportion of basic aminoacids

histopathologist a medically qualified person who interprets histologic slides prepared from diseased tissues

histopathology (his'to-pa'tho-lo-je) the study of diseases affecting the tissue cells

histophysiology (his'to-fiz'e-ol'a-je) microscopic study of tissues in relation to their functions

Histoplasma (his'to-plas'ma) a genus of fungi *H. capsulatum* the causative agent of histoplasmosis. It exists in mycelial form in nature and in yeast phase in the human body temperature

histoplasmoma (-plas-mo-mah) an infectious granuloma caused by *Histoplasma capsulatum* develops around a healed primary focus. There is a calcified central core surrounded by concentric layers of fibrous tissue

histoplasmosis (-plaz-mo'sis) the infection from *H. capsulatum* is acquired from the moist soil often contaminated by bird droppings in the river basins in temperate zones, especially in central United States. It presents as primary infection, or acute or chronic histoplasmosis **acute h** presents with cough, chest pain, fever, lassitude, multiple, soft pneumonic infiltrates in the lung leave behind multiple calcification **chronic h** associated with tissue necrosis and cavity formation. Amphotericin B is used in treatment **disseminated h** noted when histoplasmosis develops as an opportunistic infection

histothrombin (-throm'bin) a thrombin derived from connective tissue

histotomy (his-tot'ah-me) dissection of the tissues; microtomy

histotoxic (his'to-tok'sik) any substance that is poisonous to the tissues

histotrophic (his'to-trof'ik) favouring the formation of tissues

histotropic (-trop'ik) attracted toward tissues.

histrionism (his'tre-o-nizm) exaggerated facial expressions, speech or body movements.

hita(s) wholesome, favourable, useful

HIV abbreviation for human immunodeficiency virus

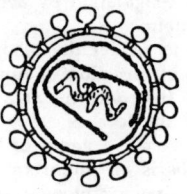

HIV

hives (hivz) urticaria, an itchy raised rash on the skin surrounded by inflammation, that results from an allergic reaction

HLA abbreviation for human leucocytic antigen

H_2O symbol for water

hoarse having a rough, harsh quality of voice

Hodgkin's disease a lymphoma of B cell origin. It may involve single lymph node region or extralymphatic site (stage 1), two or more lymph node regions or an extra-lymphatic site and lymph node regions on same side above or below diaphragm (stage 2), lymph nodes of both sides of diaphragm with or without localised extralymphatic involvement or involvement of spleen or both (stage 3) and diffuse involvement of one or more extralymphatic tissues (stage 4). Histologically, it is characterised by large malignant lymphoid cells. There is painless, rubbery lymphadenopathy or mediastinal masses. The spread is contiguous. Treatment includes radiotherapy, chemotherapy or both, named after Thomas Hodgkin, British physician

Holdswath test palpation of spinous processes and presence of a gap in the interspinous space is indicative of unstable fracture due to a tear in the interspinous ligament

holandric (hol-an'drik) 1. inherited exclusively through the male descent 2. designing genes located on the non-homologous portion of the Y-chromosome

Hoffmann's sign an abnormal reflex elicited by sudden, forceful flicking of the nail of the middle finger, resulting in flexion of the thumb and of the middle and distal phalanges of one of the other fingers. It indicates pyramidal lesion above the level of C_7 segment of the spinal cord, described by Johann Hoffmann, German neurologist

holagogue (hol'a-gog) a drastic remedy

holism (hol'izm) man as a functioning whole. **holistic** adj

hol (o) a prefix meaning whole; entire

holoacardius (hol'o-akar'-de-us) a separate, grossly defective monozygotic twin foetus. It appears like a shapeless, non- formed mass with absent heart

holoarthritis (-arth-ri'-tis) a form of arthritis affecting all joints

holoblastic (ho'lo-blas'tik) pertaining to an ovum dividing completely

holocrine (-krin) secretion of the gland wherein the entire secretory cell containing secretory products is cast off as of sebaceous glands

holodiastolic (-di'a-stol'ik) pertaining to the entire diastole

holoendemic (-en-dem'ik) affecting every person in a particular region

holoenzyme (en'zim) a substance formed by a mixture of a coenzyme and an apoenzyme that gives full catalytic activity

holography (hol-og'ra-fe) a method of production of three-dimensional images with ultrasound equipment

hologynic (hol-og'in'ik) inheritance exclusively through the maternal line

holoprosencephaly (hol'o-pro-sen-sepha'li)

a birth defect where the forebrain does not separate properly into two halves during early foetal life

holorachischisis (hol-o-ra-kis'ki-sis) fissure of the entire spinal cord

holosystolic (hol'o-sis-tol'ic) pansystolic, occupying whole of the systole

Holter monitor a device to record ECG tracing or a portable tape recorder while the patient carries normal activities, devised by Normann Holter, US biophysicist

Holt Oram syndrome an autosomal disorder characterised by anomalies of the upper limbs and heart abnormalities like ASD or VSD, named after Mary Holt and Samuel Oram, British physicians

homaluria (hom'a-lu're-a) production and excretion of urine at a normal rate

homans' sign calf pain on forced dorsiflexion of the ankle with knee extended in deep vein thrombosis, named after John Homans, US surgeon

homatropine (ho-mat'ro-pen) a weak anticholinergic agent used as a mydriatic

homaxial (ho-mak'se-il) having axes of the same length

home care a health service provided in the patient's place of residence

home page the introductory page of a Web site. It contains links toother pages in the site

homeoplasia (ho'me-o-pla'zhah) formation of new tissue like that normal to the part

homeostasis (-sta'sis) a relative constancy in the internal environment of the body maintained by a variety of active processes in the body

homeothermy (ho'me-o-ther'me) maintenance of a constant body temperature despite changes in the envrionmental temperature

homergic (hom-er'jik) having same effect, pertains to drugs possessing similar effect.

homicide (hom'isi'd) the killing of an

human being by another human, usually intentional.

homo the genus of primates *h. sapiens* species of man

homocarnosine (ho'mo-kar'no-sin) a dipeptide consisting of aminobutyric acid and histidine, found in brain tissue

homocysteine (-sis'te-en) a sulphur containing amino acid produced by demethylation of methionine

homocystine (-sis'ten) a homologue of cystine formed from two molecules of homocysteine. It acts as a source of sulphur in the body

homocystinuria (-sis'tin-u're-a) a genetic disorder characterised by an abnormal presence of homocystine in the blood and urine and causes bony deformities

homocytotropic (-sit'o-trop'ik) having an affinity for cells of the same species

homodromous (ho-mod'ra-mus) moving in the same direction

homoeopathy (ho'me-op'a-the) a system of therapeutics based on the theory that 'like cures like', founded by Samuel Hahnemann, German physician. He believed that administration of a large amount of a particular drug may cause symptoms of a disease and moderate dosage may reduce those symptoms

homoeopathist a physician who practises homoeopathy

homoeotherapy (ho'me-o-ther-a-pe) treatment of disease with a substance similar to the causative agent of the disease.

homogametic (ho'mo-ga-met'ik) a tissue made unifom in quality by grinding cells

homogenesis (-jen'isis) reproduction by the same process in succeeding generations

homogenise (ho'moj'in-iz) to render homogeneous

homogentisic (ho'mo-jen-tis'ik) **acid** alkapton; an intermediate in tyrosine metabolism

homograft (ho'mo-graft) *see* allograft, a tissue or organ transplanted from one individual to another of same species

homolateral (ho'mo-lat'eral) pertaining to the same side of the body; ipsilateral

homologous (ho-mol'a-gus) corresponding or alike in certain characteristics

homologue (hom'a-log) a member of homologous pair

homolysin (ho'mol'i-sin) a sensitising haemolytic antibody formed as a result of stimulation by an antigen derived from an animal of the same species

homonomous (ho-mon'om-us) referring the parts having similar form and structure arranged in a series as the digits

homonymous (ho-mon'in-mus) having the same sound or name **h hemianopia** blindness in the right or left halves of the visual fields of both eyes

homophil (ho'mo-fil) referring to an antibody that reacts only with the specific antigen that induced its formation

homoplastic (-plas'tik) similar in form and structure

homorganic (hom'or-gan'ik) produced by the same organs

homosapiens (ho'mo-sa'pe-ans) genus and species indentifying humans

homosexual (ho'mo-sex'shoo-il) 1. sexually attracted by persons of the same sex

homosexuality sexual attraction to members of the same sex

homotropic (-trop'ik) referring to or occurring at the same place or part of the body

homotype (ho'mo-tip) any part or organ of the same structure or function as another

homovanilic (ho'mo-va-nil'ik) **acid** a phenol substance in the urine that arises as a degradation product of tyrosine, dopa and hydroxy tyramine

homozygosis (-zigo'sis) the formation of a zygote by the union of gametes that have one or more identical alleles

homozygote an individual possessing identical alleles at the corresponding loci on a part of homologous chromosomes

homozygous possessing two identical forms of gene that controls a specific inherited trait

honeycombing the end stages of interstitial lung diseases in which coarse reticulations surround air spaces greater than 5 mm in diameter

honeymoon cystitis urinary tract infection in woman that is associated with sexual intercourse

hook a curved instrument for traction or holding

hookworm a nematode parasite in the intestine and *Ankylostoma duodenale* (old world h) and *Necator americanus* (New world h) are two important species causing ankylostomiasis

hoose (hooz) a bronchopulmonary disease by nematodes in cattle, sheep and swine

Hoover's (hoo'verz) sign unilateral lag in motion of one side of the chest due to pleurisy or pleural effusion, elicited by comparing the displacement from the midline during a deep inspiration of the examiner's hands, each placed lightly over one hemithorax, with thumbs touching beneath the xiphoid process at the start of breath, named after Charles Hoover, US physician

hordeolum (hor-de'o-lum) stye. painful swelling from inflammed hair follicles at the margin of eyelid **h externa** inflammation of the sebaceous gland of an eyelash **h interna** acute purulent infection of meibonian gland

horizon (hah-ri'zin) a specific development stages of an embryo from fertilisation to the end of foetal stage

horizontal 1. parallel to the plane of the horizon 2. a transverse plane of the body that is at right angles to vertical axis of the body

hormion (hor'me-on) point of union of

the sphenoid bone with the posterior border of vomer

hormonal pertaining to hormones **h implant** an implant placed under the skin that slowly releases a dose of synthetic hormone **h antagonist** a drug that blocks the action of a particular organ

hormone (hor'mon) a chemical substance that is produced in the body by an organ or cells of an organ and released directly into the blood stream. It has a specific regulatory action on the activity of a certain organ **adrenocortical h's** hormones secreted by adrenal cortex. The major ones being glucocorticoids, mineralocorticoids, and androgens **adrenocorticotropic h** ACTH corticotropin, hormone of anterior lobe of pituitary that stimulates the growth and functional activity of the adrenal cortex **androgenic h** masculinising hormone **anterior pituitary h** one of the several hormones secreted by the anterior lobe of the pituitary such as growth hormone, TSH, ACTH, FSH, ICSH, LH, prolactin and MSH **antidiruretic hormone** ADH, a peptide hormone produced by the hypothalamus and stored in posterior pituitary. It increases reabsorption of water by kidneys; vasopression **chorionic gonadotropic h** chorionic gonadotropin, **corpus luteum h** progesterone secreted by corpus luteum **cortical h** adrenocortical hormones **corticotropin-releasing h** (CRH), a neuropeptide from hypothalamus that stimulates the anterior pituitary to release ACTH **ectopic h** hormonal substances released from a neoplasm or cells outside the usual source of hormones **follicle-stimulating h** (FSH), a gonadotropic hormone of anterior pituitary that stimulates growth and maturation of graafian follicles in the ovary, and stimulates the epithelium of seminiferous tubules in the testis for spermatogenesis **follicle stimulating h** releasing h (FSH-RH), a factor secreted by hypothalamus to promote release of FSH gonadotropic h gonadotropin gonadotropin-releasing h (GHRH) a hypothalamic hormone that stimulates anterior pituitary to release gonadotropins such as FSH and LH growth h (GH), somatotropin; a secretion of anterior pituitary that stimulates growth by directly influencing protein, carbohydrate and fat metabolism. growth h-releasing h (GH-RH), a substance elaborated by hypothalamus stimulating the release of growth hormone from anterior pituitary interstitial cell stimulating h (ICSH), luteinising hormone lactogenic h prolactin luteinising h (LH), a gonadotropic hormone of the anterior pituitary that stimulates ripening of the follicles and secretion of progesterone by them, their rupture to release the ova and conversion of the ruptured follicle into the corpus luteum luteinising h-releasing h (LH-RH), a hormone from the hypothalamus that stimulates anterior pituitary to release FSH and LH luteotropic h (LTH), an anterior pituitary hormone that maintains the function of the corpus luteum. melanocyte stimulating h (MSH), a peptide hormone secreted by the intermediate lobe of the pituitary that causes melanin formation and deposition in the body tissues and bring about darkening of skin neuro hypophysical h's posterior pituitary hormones ovarian h one of the hormones secreted by the ovary, as an oestrogen parathyroid h a polypeptide hormone of the parathyroid gland which influences calcium and phosphorous metabolism placental h's substances secreted by the placenta such as chorionic gonadotropin, relaxin and other substances posterior pituitary h substances such as vasopressin and oxytocin released from posterior pituitary progestational h progesterone sex h's steroid hormones possessing oes-

trogenic (female) or androgenic (male) activity. somatotropic h (STH), somatotropin or growth hormone steroid h's hormones possessing cyclopentanoperhydrophenanthrene ring in their molecules thyroid h's thyroxin, triidothyronine and calcitonin thyroid stimulating h (TSH), thyrotropin thyrotropin releasing h (TRH), hormone from the hypothalamus that stimulates anterior pituitary to release thyrotropin

hormonogen (hor'mon-o-jen) prohormone

horn cornu; 1. a cutaneous outgrowth as a pointed projection 2. any horn shaped structure

Horner's syndrome a syndrome characterised by ptosis, meiosis, enophthalmos and anhidrosis over one side of the face due to paralysis of the cervical sympathetic nerve trunk, named after Johann Horner, Swiss ophthalmologist

horny layer the epidermis or non-sensitive outer skin layer which protects the true skin or dermis

horopter (hor-op'ter) the sum of all points, the images of which for a given distance fall on corresponding retinal points

horror (hor'er) terror; intense fear

horsepox (hors'poks) a mild variety of small pox affecting horses

hospice (hos'pis) a hospital or a part of a hospital devoted for the care of dying patients.

hospital (hos'pit'l) an institution for the care of the patients flying h air borne fully equipped hospital established in 1996, a charitable humanitarian organisation teaching h hospital in which undergraduate and postgraduate medical students receive clinical experience

hospitalisation (hos'pit'l-iz-a'shun) admission in a hospital as a patient for diagnosis and treatment

host the organism in or on which a parasite lives obtaining its nourishment from the host definitive h the host in which the parasite develops the adult or sexually mature stage **intermediate h a** host in which there is no development of the parasite, however its presence is required as an essential link to complete the life cycle of the parasite **reservoir h** a potential source of human reinfection, that sustains the parasite or agent when it is not infecting man

hot flush reddening of the face, neck and chest, accompanied by a sensation of warmth and often followed by sweating

Hounsfield numbers expression of density of tissue in computerised tomographic scanning, named after Godfrey Hounsfield who first developed CT

housefly fly belonging to the order Diptera *Musca domestica* responsible for transmission of infections of faecal-oral route

housedust the mixed dust which accumulates in the air of dwellings. The mite Dermatophagoides that lives on human skin scales forms important element in the house dust and cause allergic reactions in some persons

housemaid's knee swelling of prepatellar bursa situated over the lower half of the patella and in the upper half of the *ligamentum patellae*

Howel-Jolly bodies presence of spherical granules in the erythrocytes in the slides of stained blood smear, and are thought to be nuclear particles, seen in asplenia following splenectomy and haemolytic anaemia, named after William Howell, US physiologist and Justin Jolly, French histologist

HP abbreviation for house physician

HPV abbreviation for human papilloma virus

HRCT abbreviation for high resolution computed tomography

Hrdayam (s) heart

Hrdroga (s) disease of the heart

HSV abbreviation for herpes simplex virus

HTLV abbreviation for human T-cell leukaemia/lymphoma virus

hum (hum) a continuous roaring murmur **venous h** heard on auscultation over the internal jugular vein on the right side above the clavicle and turning the neck up and away from area of auscultation. It becomes less prominent on relieving venous obstruction. It is heard in hyperdynamic circulatory states. It may be heard over the umbilicus with large portal anastomotic veins

human chorionic gonadotropin a hormone produced by the anterior pituitary that stimulates normal body growth and development

human ehrlichiosis a tick-borne zoonosis acquired by human by outdoor activity. *E. chaffeensis* and granulocytic ehrlichiosis sp. produce fever, chills, headache, myalgia and malaise initially and later diarrhoea, abdominal pain, cough, dyspnoea and maculopapular rash. It is treated by tetracycline or doxycycline

Human genome a complete list in order, of the chemical letters that make up the DNA in human cells **h g project** an international research project to map each human gene and to completely sequence human DNA

human growth hormone a chemical messenger produced by the anterior pituitary that stimulates normal body growth and development

human immunodeficiency virus (HIV), a Lentivirinae subfamily of retrovirus having an RNA genome. The viral enzyme reverse transcriptase has the property of transcribing a DNA copy of the RNA genome following viral penetration of the host cell. The DNA copy randomly integrates into host cell genome and it is used as a template to transcribe new RNA viral copies. HIV occurs in two types: HIV1 and HIV2. HIV infects CD4 + helper T lymphocytes and cause attrition of the CD4 cell population resulting in gradual and increasing failure of immune function

human leucocyte antigens one of the important types of histocompatibility antigens studied to determine tissue compatibility between donors and recipients for transplants. These antigens are also associated with specific diseases

human T-cell lymphotropic virus a virus resembling HIV, infects T lymphocytes and is associated with adult T-cell leukaemia and T-cell lymphomas

humectant (hu-mek'tant) a preparation intended to preserve moisture in the skin

humeral relating to the humerus

humerus (hu'mer-us) see table of Bones

humor (hu'mer) pl. **humors** 1. one of the elemental body fluids such as blood, bile and phlegm 2. a clear fluid with hyaline substance **aqueous h** the watery fluid that fills the anterior and posterior chambers of the eye **vitreous h** the fluid component of the vitreous

humoral relating to a humor

hump a rounded eminence **dowager's h** dorsal kyphosis

humpback (hu'mp'bak) kyphosis

hunchback (hunch'back) 1. kyphosis 2. a person with kyphosis

hunger (hung'er) 1. a desire or need for food 2. strong desire or craving for food

Huntarian chancre hard chancre, a single round painless ulcer on the genitalia. It has a characteristic indurated base which feels like a button. It is seen in first stage of syphilis after three weeks of infection at the site of entry of treponemas, named after John Hunter, Scottish anatomist and surgeon

Hunter's syndrome a genetic disorder causing dwarfism and mental retardation, named after Charles Hunter, Canadian physician

Huntington's chorea an inherited disorder of CNS with onset in middle age exhibiting degeneration of cerebral cortex and basal ganglia. It is characterised by chorea, progressive dementia, named after George Huntington, US physician

Hurler's syndrome a genetic disorder that causes severe mental retardation, named after Gertrad Hurler, German paediatrician

hurry sickness increased time dependence

hyalin (hi'a-lin) a clear, eosinophilic, homogeneous substance

hyaline (hi-a-lin) a glossy, homogeneous, translucent appearance **h cartilage** smooth, semi-transparent cartilage **h cast** transparent, pale and homogeneous casts seen in chronic nephritis **h membrane disease** respiratory distress syndrome of the newborn characterised by loss of alveolar stability leading to progressive atelectasis of the affected lung presenting as respiratory distress at or shortly after birth

hyalinisation formation of hyalin

hyalinosis (hi-a-lin-o'sis) hyaline degeneration

hyalitis (hi'a-lit'is) inflammation of vitreous humour. The inflammatory changes extend into the vitreous from adjacent structures

hyal (o) combining word for glassy

hyalogen (hi-al'o-jen) substances related to mucoids which on hydrolysis yield sugars, and they are found in cartilage, vitreous humour and hydatid cyst

hyalohyphomycosis (hila'lo-hi'fo-mi-ki'sis) any opportunistic infection by mycellial fungi that possess colourless walls

hyaloid (hi'a-lo-id) **canal** remnant of a channel in the centre of vitreous humour that carried an artery during the eyes' development in the foetus

hyalomere (hi'a-lo-mer) the clear periphery of a blood platelet

hyalomma (hi'a-lom'a) a genus of large ixodid ticks that parasitise domestic and wild animals

hyalomucoid (hi'a-lo-mu'koid) mucoid found in vitreous humour

hyalonyxis (-nik'sis) surgical puncture of vitreous humour

hyalophagia (-fa'jah) the eating of glass

hyaloplasm (hi'a-lo-plazm) the protoplasmic fluid of cell

hyaloserositis (hi'a-lo-ser'o-sit'is) inflammation of a serous membrane with a fibrous exudate that eventually gets hyalinised. It gives a relatively thick, glistening white coating

hyalosis (hi'a-lo'sis) degenerative changes in vitreous humour

hyalosome (hi-a-lo-sum) a oval or round structure within a cell nucleus that stains faintly

hyaluronate (hi'a-loo'ro-nat) an ester of hyaluronic acid

hyaluronic (hi-a-loo'ro-nik) **acid** a mucopolysaccharide forming a gelatinous substance in the tissue spaces and an intercellular cement substance throughout the body

hyaluronidases (hi'a-loo-ron'i-das-us) any of the three enzymes (hyaluronoglucosaminidase, hyaluronoglucoronidase and hyaluronate lyase) that hydrolyse hyaluronic acid

hybrid (hi'brid) an animal or plant produced from two different species

hybridisation (hi'brid-ii-za'shun) 1. the pairing of complementary DNA or RNA 2. identification of single strand nucleic acid by linking it with labelled complementary strand of same or nearly same constitution

hybridoma (hi'brid'o-ma) a 'tumour' cell line originating from two cells that are interdependent upon one another's metabolic machinery, created by fusing a normal mouse cell line producing a large amount of antibody against an antigen of interest, with an immortal myeloma cell line

hydatid (hi'da-tid) 1. hydatid cyst 2. any cyst like structure **h cyst** a cyst in the liver or lung containing the larva of *Echinococcus granulosus*

hydatidiform (hi'da-tid'i-form) having a form or appearance of a hydatid **h mole** an intrauterine mass of grape-like enlarged chorionic villi. Such a degeneration from the proliferation of the trophoblast results in rapid growth of the uterus compared to the duration of gestation

hydatidosis (hi-da-ti-do'sis) hydatid disease with presence of hydatid cysts

hydatidostomy (hi'da-ti-dos'ta-me) surgical evacuation of a hydatid cyst

hydrogogue (hi'dra-gog) producing a discharge of watery fluid, refers to cathartics that retain fluid in the intestine and help in the removal of oedema fluid

hydralazine (hi-dral'a-zin) a peripheral vasodilator used as an antihypertensive

hydramnios presence of excess amount of amniotic fluid in uterus during pregnancy

hydranencephaly (hi'dran-en-sef'a-le) absence of the cerebral hemispheres resulting in an internal hydrocephalus

hydrargyria (hi'drar-jir'e-a) mercury poisoning

hydrargyrum (hi-drahr'ji-rum) mercury

hydrarthrosis (hi-drar-thro'sis) collection of serous fluid in the joint cavity

hydratase (hi'dra-tas) enzyme catalysing hydration

hydrate (hi'drat) a compound crystallising with one or more molecules of water

hydration (hi-dra'shun) 1. addition of water 2. taking in of water to correct a deficit

hydraulics (hi-draw'liks) the science of mechanics of liquids

hydroa (hid-ro'a) any bullous eruption

hydroblepharon (hi-dro-ble'ph-e-ron) swelling of the eyelid

hydrocalycosis (hi-dro-kali'i-ko'sis) dilatation of the renal calyx due to an obstruction of the infundibulum

hydrocarbon (hi'dro-kar'bon) a compound containing only hydrogen and carbon

hydrocoele (hi'dro-sel) a collection of serous fluid in a sacculated cavity, as in the tunica vaginalis testis

hydrocoelectomy (-lek'to-mi) excision of a hydrocoele

hydrocephalic (-se-fal'ik) relating to hydrocephalus

hydrocephalus (-sef'a-lus) distension of the cerebral ventricles by increased cerebrospinal fluid. It may be due to decreased absorption from congenital malformations, obliteration of aqueduct, haemorrhage, infection, neoplasms and trauma. Rarely it can be due to an increased production of CSF. The brain becomes oedematous and the gyri flatten

hydrochloric (-klor'ik) **acid** (HCl), a strong acid that is a major component of gastric juice

hydrochloride (-klor'id) a salt of hydrochloric acid

hydrochlorothiazide (-klor'o-thi-a-zid) an oral thiazide diuretic and antihypertensive

hydrocholecystis (-ko'le-sis'tis) effusion of serous fluid into the gall bladder

hydrocholeresis (-ko'le-re'sis) promotion of flow of watery bile

hydrocirsocoele(-sir'so-sel) hydrocoele complicated with varicocoele

hydrocodone (-ko'don) a semisynthetic derivative of codeine possessing analgesic properties

hydrocolloid (-kol'oid) a colloid system where water is the dispersion medium

hydrocortisone(kor'ti-son) one of two main glucocorticoids secreted by adrenal cortex

hydrocyanic (-si-an'ik) **acid** hydrogen cyanide, a colourless liquid poison

hydrocyst (hi'dro-sist) a cyst containing watery fluid

hydrocytosis familial haemolytic anaemia with swollen red cells due to a membrane defect and water inflow

hydrodelineation (-de-lin'e-a'shun) injection of fluid between the layers of the nucleus of lens to delineate the nuclear zones during cataract surgery

hydrodissection (-di-sek'shun) injection of fluid into the capsule of the lens for dissection during cataract surgery

hydroencephalocoele (-en-sef'a-lo-sel) congenital herniation of meninges to exterior with sac containing brain with ventricular space

hydroflumethiazide (-floo'me-thi'a-zid) a thiazide diuretic

hydrogen (hi'dro-jen) gaseous element, atomic number 1, symbol H

hydrogenase (hi'dro-jen-as) an enzyme that catalyses reduction by molecular hydrogen

hydrokinetic (hi'dro-ki-net'ik) referring to the motion of fluids and the forces giving rise to such motion

hydrolase (hi'dro-las) hydrolysing enzyme that cleaves substrates by addition of H_2O.

hydrolyase (hi'dro-li'as) an enzyme removing H and OH as water, forming new double bonds within the affected molecule

hydrolysate (hi-drol'i-sat) a solution containing the products of a hydrolysis

hydrolysis (hi-drol'i-sis) a chemical process enabling the cleavage of compound into two or more simpler compounds, with addition of H and OH parts of a water molecule on either side of the chemical bond cleaved

hydroma (hi-dro'ma) hygroma

hydromeningocoele (hi'dro-mening'gosel) a sac formed by protrusion of the meninges containing cerebrospinal fluid

hydrometer (hi-drom'it-er) an instrument to determine the specific gravity of a fluid

hydrometrocolpos (hi'dro-me'tro-kol'pos) a collection of watery fluid in the uterus and vagina

hydrometry (hi-drom'i-tre) measurement of specific gravity with a hydrometer

hydromicrocephaly (hi'dro-mi'kro-sef'a-le) abnormally small head with an increased amount of cerebrospinal fluid

hydromyelia (-mi-el'e-a) fluid in the central canal of the spinal cord

hydromyelomeningocoele (-mi'e-lo-mening'go-sel) projection of meningeal sac containing spinal cord tissue and cerebrospinal fluid through a spinal defect

hydromyoma (-mi-o'ma) a leiomyoma

containing cyst-like foci of proteinaceous fluid

hydronephrosis (hi-dro'ne-fro'sis) dilatation of the pelvis and calices of one or both kidneys due to obstruction of the ureter to the flow of urine and leads to atrophy of renal parenchyma

hydropericarditis (hi-dro-per'i-kar-dit'is) collection of serous fluid in the pericardium

hydroperitoneum (-per'it-o-ne'im) ascites

hydrophilic (-fil'ik) attracting or associating with water molecules, a property possessed by ions

hydrophobia (-fo'be-a) fear of water, *see* rabies

hydrophobic (-fo'bik) 1. tendency to repel water 2. relating to or suffering from hydrophobia

hydrophthalmos (hi'drof'thal'mos) distension of the eye ball due to accumulation of fluid within it as in infantile glaucoma

hydropic (hi-drop'ik) pertaining to oedema; oedematous

hydropneumatosis (hi'dro-noo'ma-to'sis) presence of liquid and gas in the tissues

hydropneumogony (-noo-mo'go-ne) injection of air into a joint to determine the amount of effusion

hydropneumoperitoneum (-noo-mo-per'it-o-ne'um) a collection of fluid and gas in the peritoneal cavity

hydropneumothorax (-thor'aks) a collection of fluid and gas in the pleural cavity

hydrops (hi'drops) oedema; distension with fluid **h foetalis** intrauterine death of foetus with oedema and anaemia due to severe rhesus incompatibility

hydrorrhoea (-re'a) a profuse discharge of water fluid

hydrosol (hi'dro-sawl) the fluid state of a colloid solution

hydrostatic (hi'dro-stat'ik) pertaining to the pressure of fluids or to their properties when in equilibrium

hydrotaxis (-tak'sis) movement of cells or organisms in relation to water

hydrotherapy (hi-dro-ther'a-pe) the use of water to treat muscle and joint disorders

hydrothorax (-thor'aks) a collection of serous fluid in the pleural cavity

hydrotropism (-tro'pizɪn) the property in growing organisms to move towards or away from moisture

hydrotubation (hi'dro-too-ba'shun) injection of liquid medication or saline solution through the cervix into the uterine cavity and fallopian tubes for dilatation and medication of the tubes

hydroureter (-ur-et'er) distension of the ureter with urine or watery fluid due to obstruction

hydroxide (hi-drok'sid) any compound containing a hydroxyl group

hydroxy – prefix referring to addition or substitution of the –OH group to or in a compound

hydroxyamphetamine (hi-drok'se-am-fet'a-men) a sympathomimetic amine which is a nasal decongestant and a mydriatic

hydroxyapatite (-ap'a-tit) a natural mineral substance which resembles the lattice of bones and teeth, used in chromatography of nucleic acids

hydroxybutyrate (-bu'ti-rat) a salt of hydroxybutyric acid

hydroxybutyric (-bu-tir'ik) **acid** any of the hydroxy derivatives of butyric acid, such as beta hydroxy-butyric acid, a ketone body

hydroxy chloroquine (-klor'o-kwin) an antimalarial and antiinflammatory preparation used in malaria and rheumatoid arthritis

hydroxy corticosteroid (-kor'ti-ko-ster'oid) 17 OHCS steroid hormones formed in the adrenal gland by the action of 17 hydoxylase. The urinary excretion of 17 OHCS reflect the functional status of adrenal gland. The rates of catabolism of 17 OHCS are increased in pregnancy, Cushing's disease, obesity and pancreatitis, and decreased in Addison's disease and hypopituitarism

hydroxyprolinaemia (-pro'li-ne'mea) a disorder from a deficiency of hydroxyproline oxidase causing a raised level of hydroxyproline in blood and urine and mental retardation

hydroxyproline (hi-drok'se-pro'len) a hydroxylated proline found in high concentrations in collagen. It plays an important role in cross-linking collagen

5 hydroxytryptamine (-trip'ta-men) serotonin

hydroxyurea (-u-re'a) an orally active cytotoxic agent used in refractory cases of chronic myeloid leukaemia

hydruria (hi-droor'e-a) excretion of urine of low specific gravity or low osmolality

hygiene (hi'jen) the science concerned with promotion and preservation of health

hygienist (hi-jen'ist) a person technically trained in the principles of healthful living or as an assistant to a professionally qualified person such as dental hygienist, industrial hygienist

hygroma (hi-gro'ma) cavernous lymphangioma especially of neck

hygrometry (hi-grom'e-tre) measurement of moisture content in atmosphere

hygroscopic (hi'gro-skop'ik) capable of absorbing and retaining water

hymen (hi'men) a thin, membranous ring surrounding the opening to vagina which gets torn during first sexual intercourse or by use of tampon

hymenolepiasis (hi-me-no-lep-i'a-sis) infestation with hymenolepis

Hymenolepis (hi'me-nol'e-pis) a genus of tapeworm *H. nana*, the dwarf tapeworm of 2.5 cm length capable completing its life cycle in a single host

hymenology (hi'men-ol'a-je) the branch of science concerned with the study of membranes of the body

Hymenoptera (hi'men-op'ter-a) an order of insects having two pairs of well developed membranous wings, that includes ants, bees and wasps

hyoepiglotic (hi'o-ep'i-glot'ik) pertaining to the hyoid bone and the epiglottis

hyoglossal (-glos'l) pertaining to the hyoid bone and the tongue or to the hyoglossus muscle

hyoid (hi'oid) shaped like Greek letter upsilon **h bone** *see* table of bones. **h fracture** fracture of hyoid bone indicating throttling

hyoscine (hi'o-sin) scopalamine

hyoscyamine (hi'o-si'a-men) an anticholinergic alkaloid from Hyoscyamus and other solanaceous plants

hypalgesia (hi'pal-je'ze-a) decreased pain sensation. **hypalgesic** adj

hypamnios (hip-am'ne-os) deficiency of amniotic fluid

hyparterial (hip'ar-ter'e-il) beneath an artery

hypaxial (hi-pak'se-al) ventral to the long axis of the body

hyper – combining word meaning excessive or abnormally increased

hyperacidity (hi'per-as'idi-te) an increased production of gastric acid by the stomach, a feature of duodenal ulcer and indigestion

hyperactivity (-ak-tiv'ite) overactivity being restless, aggressive and destructive activity; hyperkinesis

hyperacusis (-a-koo'sis) sounds heard with unusual loudness in paralysis of the stapedius muscle as it affects dampening influence on the stapes

hyperadenosis (-ad'in-o'sis) enlargement of glands

hyperadiposis (-ad'i-po'sis) an extreme degree of fatness

hyperadrenalism (-a-dren'a-lizm) Cushing's syndrome

hyperadrenocorticism(-a-dren'o-kort'i-sizm) an increased secretion of adrenocortical hormones, usually cortisol

hyperalgesia (-al-je'ze-a) markedly increased pain sense. **hyperalgesic** adj

hyperalimentation (-al'i-men-ta'shun) providing nutrients in excess amount needed by the body to patients who are not able to take food by mouth or who are grossly under-nourished

hyperalphalipoproteinaemia (-al'fah-a-lip′o-pro′te-ne′me-a) abnormally high levels of high density lipoproteins in the serum

hyperammonaemia (-am′o-ne′me-a) an excess amount of ammonia in circulating blood

hyperaphia (-a′fe-a) tactile hyperaesthetic **hyperaphic** adj

hyperazotaemia (-az′o-tem′e-a) an abnormally increased amount of non-protein nitrogenous substance, especially urea, in the circulating blood

hyperbaric (-barik) 1. referring to atmospheric pressure greater than 1. 2. solution more dense than the diluent or medium **h oxygen** therapy exposing a person to oxygen at higher than normal atmosphere to increase oxygen supply in the tissues. It is indicated in decompression sickness, carbon monoxide poisoning, gas gangrene and arterial gas embolism

hyperbarism (-bar′izm) disturbances in the body from the atmospheric pressure greater than 1 atmosphere

hyperbetalipoproteinaemia (-bat′ah-lip′o-pro′te-ne′me-a) familial disorder of feed-back control of lipoprotein level, where homozygotes demonstrate skin and tendon xanthomas in childhood and ischaemic heart disease during young age and heterozygotes demonstrate an increased incidence of ischaemic heart disease

hyperbilirubinaemia (-bil′i-roo′bi-ne′me-a) an increased concentration of bilirubin in the blood which leads to jaundice

hypercalcaemia (-kal-sem′e-a) an abnormally high level of calcium in the blood

hypercapnia (-kap′ne-a) an abnormally increased amount of carbon dioxide in the circulating blood

hypercarbia (-kar′be-a) hypercapnia

hypercarotenaemia (-kar′o-te-ne′me-a) an increased level of carotene in the blood which may colour the skin yellow

hypercatabolism an accelerated breakdown of tissue proteins following major trauma, sepsis or surgery

hypercatharsis (-ka-thar′sis) excessive purgation

hypercellularity (-sel′ul-ar′ite) abnormal increase in the number of cells in any part, as in bone marrow

hyperchloraemia (-klor-em′e-a) markedly increased amount of chloride ions in the circulating blood

hyperchlorhydria (-klor-hi′dre-a) presence of an increased amount of hydrochloric acid in the stomach

hypercholesterolaemia (-kol-es′ter-ol′e-me-a) an abnormally high levels of cholesterol in the blood

hyperchromatism (-kro′ma-tizm) 1. excessive pigmentation 2. increased amount of chromatin in cell nuclei 3. increased staining capacity of the nuclei

hyperchromia (-kro′me-a) markedly increased colour index of the blood

hyperchylia (-kil′e-a) increased secretion of gastric juice

hyperchylomicronaemia (-ki′lomi′kro-ne′me-a) a familial disorder of lipid metabolism

hypercortism (-kort′i-zm) an increased production of adrenal cortical hormones in the body

hypercryaesthesia (-kri′s-the′zhzh) excessive sensitivity to cold

hypercupraemia (-ku-pre′me-a) an excess of copper in the blood

hypercythaemia (-si-them′e-a) presence of an abnormally increased number of red blood cells in the circulating blood

hypercytosis (-si-to′sis) abnormally increased number of cells, in the circulating blood or tissues, especially white blood cells

hyperdynamia (-di-na′me-a) hyperkinesis exhibiting muscular restlessness **hyperdynamic** adj

hyperechema (-e-kem′a) auditory exaggeration

hyperemesis (-em′i-sis) excessive vomiting **hyperemetic** adj **h gravidarum** a feature of early pregnancy characterised by vomiting of marked severity in the first trimester

hyperaemia (-e'me-a) presence of an increased amount of blood in a part or organ

hypereosinophil (-e'o-sin'o-fil) **syndrome** a peripheral and bone marrow eosinophilia with infiltration of many organs such as heart, skin, muscle, lungs, CNS and intestine with mature eosinophils

hyperequilibrium (-e'kwi-lib're-um) an increased tendency to have vertigo while making even slight movements

hyperexophoria (-ek'so-for'e-a) a tendency of one eye to deviate upward and outward

hyperextension injury an injury caused by straightening of a joint beyond its normal limits

hyperferraemia (-fe-rem-e-a) raised level of iron in the serum

hyperfibrinogenaemia (-fi-brin'o-je-ne'me-a) raised level of fibrinogen in the blood

hyperfiltration (-fil-tra'shun) an elevated glomerular filtration rate

hyperfractionation (-frak'shun-a'shun) a radiation treatment schedule in which there is reduction in dose per exposure to minimise the side effects

hypergalactia (-ga-lak'she-a) excessive secretion of milk

hypergalactosis (-gal'ak-to'sis) excessive secretion of milk

hypergammaglobulinaemia (-gam'a-glob'u-lin-e'me-a) an increased amount of gamma globulins in the plasma

hypergenesis (-jen'e-sis) excessive development of parts or organs of the body

hypergeusia (-goo'ze-a) abnormal acuteness of sense of taste

hyperglucagonaemia (-gloo'ka-gon-e'me-a) markedly raised levels of glucagon in the blood.

hyperglycaemia (gli-se'mea) an abnormally high level of glucose in the blood

hyperglycinemia (-gli-se'ne-mea) an autosomal recessive disorder with glycine accumulation due to a defect in the catabolic pathway. There is marked CNS depression, seizures and atonia

hyperglycaemic (-gli-sem'ik) 1. pertaining to or causing hyperglycaemia 2. an agent raising the level of glucose in the blood **h hyperosmolar, non ketotic coma** (HHNK) profound hyperglycaemia, hyperosmolarity and severe dehydration in the absence of significant ketosis. Fluid replacement is the main stay of therapy

hyperglyceridaemia (-glos'er-i-de'me-a) raised levels of glycerides in the plasma, usually within chylomicrons and it is normal or transiently increased following a fatty meal but abnormal if the condition persists

hyperglycerolaemia (-glis'er-ol-e'me-a) increased levels of glycerol due to a deficiency of an enzyme catalysing its phosphorylation

hyperglycogenolysis (-gli'ko-jin-ol'i-sis) increased glycogenolysis

hyperglycorrhachia (-gli'ko-ra'ke-a) excessive amounts of sugar in the cerebrospinal fluid

hypergonadism (-go'nad-izm) excess secretion of gonadal hormones leading to precocious puberty

hyperhidrosis (-hi-dro'sis) increased sweating

hyperhydration (-hi-dra'shun) over-hydration; excess water content of the body

hyperimmune (-i-mun) presence of an increased amount of specific antibodies in the serum

hyperimmunoglobulinaemia (-im'un-o-glob'u-lin'em'e-a) markedly raised levels of immunoglobulins in the serum

hyperinsulinism (in'sul-in-izm) an increased secretion of insulin by the islets of Langerhans resulting in hypoglycaemia

hyperirritability (-ir'it-ab-bil'it-e) increased response to a stimulus

hyperisotonic (-i'so-ton'ik) hypertonic; a solution containing more than 0.45% salt

hyperkalaemia (-kal-em'e-a) raised level of potassium ions in the circulating blood.

hyperkeratinisation (-ker'a-tin'i-za'shun) hypertrophy of the horny layers of the epidermis especially of the palms and soles

hyperkeratosis (-ker'a-to'sis) 1. hypertrophy of the horny layer of epidermis 2. hypertrophy of the cornea

hyperketonaemia (-ke'to-ne'me-a) increased amount of ketones in the blood

hyperkinaemia (-ki-ne'me-a) increased rate of circulation

hyperkinesia (-ki'ne-zha) excessive activity or motor function

hyperkinesis (hi'per-ki-ne'sis) excessive, purposeless motor activity

hyperlactation (-lak-ta'shun) continuation of lactation beyond the normal period

hyperlipaemia (-li-pe'me-a) an excess amount of lipids in the blood

hyperlipidaemia (-lip'i-de'me-a) increased amount of circulating fatty acids, triglycerides and cholesterol. It develops as a complex interaction between genetic predisposition and dietary indiscretion

hyperlipoproteinaemia (-lip'o-pro'te-ne'me-a) an increase in the level of lipoprotein in the blood

hyperlithuria (-li-thur'e-a) excretion of an increased amount of uric acid in the urine

hyperlucency (-loo'sen-se) increased radiolucency

hyperlysinaemia (-li'si-ne'me-a) an autosomal recessive condition of childhood characterised by an increase in lysine or its metobolites

hypermagnesemia (-mag'ne-se-me-a) markedly increased level of magnesium in blood

hypermastia (-mas'te-a) excessively large mammary glands

hypermenorrhoea (-men'or-e'a) menorrhagia; excessively profuse or prolonged menstruation

hypermetabolism (-me-tab'o-lizm) an increased rate of metabolism

hypermetria (-me'tre-a) an ataxia exhibiting over reaching a desired object or goal

hypermetropia (-me-tro'pe-a) long-sightedness which needs convex lenses for correction

hypermorph (hi-per-morf) a person with long limbs, consequently making his standing height greater than sitting height

hypermotility (hi'per-mo-til'it-e) an abnormally increased motility

hypermyotrophy (-mi-a'tro-fe) muscular hypertrophy

hypernatraemia (-na-tre'me-a) markedly increased plasma concentration of sodium ions

hypernephroma (-ne-fro'ma) adenocarcinoma of the kidney presenting with painless, profuse, intermittent haematuria

hypernutrition (-noo-trish'un) overfeeding and its associated ill-effects

hyperopia (hi'per-o'pe-a) hypermetropia; far-sightedness

hyperorchidism (-or'kid-izm) increased size or functioning of the testes

hyperorexia (-o-rek'se-a) bulimia

hyperorthocytosis (-or'tho-si-to'sis) increase in the number of white blood cells in which the relative percentages of different types of cells are within the normal range

hyperosmolality (-oz'mol-al'it-e) increased concentration of a solution and is expressed as osmols of solute per kg of serum water

hyperosmolarity (-oz'mol-ar'it-e) increased osmotic concentration of a solution and is expressed as osmols of solute per litre of solution

hyperostosis (-os'to'sis) a proliferation of a bony matrix

hyperoxaluria (-ok'sa-lu're-a) markedly increased amount of oxalic acid or oxalates in the urine hyperoxia (-ok'se-a) 1. an excess amount of oxygen in tissues or organs 2. an increased tension of oxygen than normal that is produced while breathing air or oxygen at pressures greater than 1 atmosphere

hyperparathyroidism (-par'a-thi'roid-izm) a condition associated with an autonomous secretion of parathyroid hormone by a single parathyroid adenoma (primary) or by hyperplasia secondary to chronic renal failure (secondary) or adenoma formation by continuous stimulation of parathyroid (tertiary). Primary hyperparathyroidism is associated with features of hypercalcaemia that include polyuria and polydipsia, renal colic, lethargy, anorexia, dyspepsia, paptic ulceration, constipation, depression and drowsiness. There is osteitis fibrosis from increased bone resorption with fibrous replacement

hyperpathia increased pain sensation to stronger pin pricks in an area that has decreased sensation to milder pricks

hyperperistalsis (-per'i-stal'sis) increased peristalsis allowing rapid passage of food through the stomach and intestine

hyperphalangism (-fal'an-jizm) presence of a supernumerary phalanx in a finger or toe

hyperphenylalaninaemia (-fen'il-al'a-nine'me-a) a group of congenital enzymopathies characterised by accumulation of phenylalanins and related metabolites and a deficiency of tyrosine. Phenylketonuria is the common example of the disorder

hyperphonesis (-fon-e'sis) increase in sound audibility

hyperphoria (-for'e-a) upward deviation of the visual axis of one eye

hyperphosphatesmia (-fos'fa-ta-se'me-a) a rare condition with a benign increase in the intestinal isoenzyme of alkaline phosphatase

hyperphosphaturia (-fos'fa-tu're-a) increased excretion of phosphates in the urine

hyperpigmentation (-pig'men-ta'shun) excessive pigmentation in a tissue or part

hyperpituitarism (-pi-tu'it-er-izm) increased production of hormones of anterior pituitary, especially somatotropin and it leads to gigantism or acromegaly

hyperplasia (-pla'zhah) overgrowth in numbers of tissue cells

hyperplasmia (-plaz'me-a) an abnormal increase in the number of cells resulting in an increase in the size of an organ

hyperploidy (hi'per-ploid-e) a condition of having one or more chromosomes in addition to the normal number

hyperpnoea (hi'perp-ne'a) deeper and more rapid breathing than normal

hyperpolarization (hi'per-pol'er-iz-a'shun) an increase in polarisation of membranes, or nerves or muscle cells

hyperponesis (-po-ne'sis) increased activity within the motor system

hyperposia (-po'ze-a) markedly increased intake of fluids in a relatively short period of time

hyperpotassaemia (-pot'a-se'me-a) hyperkalaemia

hyperprebetalipoproteinaemia (-pre-ba'ta-lip'o-pro'te-ne'me-a) increased concentration of pre-beta lipoproteins in the blood

hyperprolinaemia (-pro'li-ne'me-a) a condition characterised by a defect in amino acid metabolism. There may be a defect of proline oxidase producing pyrroline carboxylate from proline and is associated with renal tube defects without mental defects (type I) or a defect of delta pyrroline 5 carboxylic acid dehydrogenase with variable mental retardation and renal tube defects (type II)

hyperprosexia (-pro-sek'se-a) preoccupation with one idea

hyperproteosis (-prot'e-o'sis) a condition resulting from an excess amount of protein in the diet

hyperpyrexia (-pi-rek'se-a) extremely high fever with a temperature above 41°C

hyperreactive (-re-ak'tiv) exhibiting greater than normal response to stimuli

hyperreflexia (-re-flek'se-a) markedly exaggerated deep tendon reflexes

hyperreninaemia (-re'ni-ne'me-a) increased levels of renin in the blood that can lead to hypertension and aldosteronism

hyperresonance (-rez'on-ans) increased resonance on percussion of the chest

hypersalivation (-sal'i-va-shun) excessive salivation

hypersecretion (-se-kre'shun) excessive secretion

hypersensitivity (-sen'si-tiv'it-e) 1. abnormal sensitivity to any stimulus exhibiting an excessive response 2. a state of altered reactivity in which body exhibits an exaggerated immune response to a foreign agent or allergen **delayed h** a hypersensitivity reaction by immunocompetent T-lymphocytes (cell mediated immunity) developing several hours after injection of·an antigen in the skin of a sensitive person **immediate h** a constitutional predisposition of underlying immune dysfunction or both in the atopic individuals for the occurrence of an immediate anaphylactic reaction when exposed to common environmental allergens

hypersomnia (-som'ne-a) excessive sleeping.

hypersomnolence (-som'no-lens) a condition in which one sleeps for an excessively long duration

hypersplenism (-splen'izm) enlargement of spleen. The condition is associated with pancytopaenia and hyperplasia of the marrow precursor cells. Splenectomy improves the condition **congestive h** due to stasis of blood flow, mostly secondary to cirrhosis of the liver

hypersthenia (-sthen'e-a) an excessive strength or tension of part or all of the body

hyperteleorism (-te'lor-izm) an excess separation of paired organs such as the eyes or breast rarely

hypertension (ten'shun) persistent high blood pressure. It is a quantitative deviation from the normal **accelerated h** complicates hypertension of any aetiology. There is accelerated microvascular damage with necrosis in the walls of small arteries and arterioles and intravascular thrombosis. The blood pressure is very high and there is rapidly progressive end-organ damage **borderline h** the arterial blood pressure being within normal range sometimes and in hypertensive range sometimes **essential h** hypertension without any specific underlying cause **idiopathic intracranial h** development of raised intracranial pressure without a space occupying lesion, ventricular dilatation or impaired consciousness. Presents with headache, transient diplopia and visual abnormalities **malignant h** accelerated hypertension **ocular h** persistently elevated intraocular pressure in the absence of any other signs of glaucoma **portal h** prolonged elevation of the portal venous pressure and is due to extrahepatic (sepsis) and intrahepatic parenchymal (cirrhosis) diseases. The clinical features are due to portal venous congestion and collateral vessel formation. Splenomegaly is constant **pregnancy induced h** hypertension complicating pregnancy with proteinuria and oedema **primary h** essential hypertension **pulmonary h** markedly increased pressure in pulmonary circulation. There is marked narrowing of pulmonary vascular bed from anatomic or vasomotor mechanisms **renal h** hypertension produced by renal diseases **renovascular h** hypertension due to diminished blood flow to the kidney from renal artery stenosis **secondary h** hypertension as a consequence of a specific disease or abnormality leading to sodium retention and/or peripheral vasoconstriction **venous h** incompetent valves in deep leg veins resulting in retrograde blood flow to superficial system causing a rise in capillary hydrostatic pressure **whitecoat h** recording of blood pressure by a doctor causing unrepresentative surge in blood pressure and it has been ascribed to anxiety

hypertensive (-ten'siv) 1. marked by increased blood pressure 2. an individual with abnormally high blood pressure

hyperthecosis (-the-ko'sis) hyperplasia of *theca interna* of a maturing ovarian follicle. It may be associated with hirsutism and amenorrhoea

hyperthelia (-thel'e-a) presence of supernumerary nipples on the breast or elsewhere

hyperthermalgesia (-therm'al-je-ze-a) extreme sensitivity to heat

hyperthermia (therm'e-a) a body temperature of greater than 42°C. It is associated with peripheral vasodilatation, tachycardia, hypoxia, hyperkalemia and cardiac failure **malignant h** a hyper-metabolic myopathic syndrome that is chemically or stress induced, presenting by abrupt rise in temperature, vigorous muscular contractions, metabolic and respiratory acidosis, and ventricular arrhythmias, especially noted when inducing anaesthesia

hyperthymia (-thi'me-a) 1. increased excitability 2. excessive emotionalism

hyperthymism (-thi'mizm) increased activity of thymus gland

hyperthyroidism (-thi'ro-id-ozm) a clinical syndrome resulting from exposure of the body tissues to excess circulating levels of free thyroid hormones. The condition is due to Grave's disease, multinodular goitre or autonomously functioning solitary thyroid nodules. The condition develops insidiously and involves almost every system of the body. There is diffuse or nodular goitre, weight loss despite increased appetite, anorexia, palpitations, nervousness, irritability, muscle weakness, heat intolerance, fatigue, exophthalmos, lid retraction, amenorrhoea, loss of libido and tremor

hypertonia (-ton'e-a) increased tension of muscles or arteries

hypertonic (-ton'ik) 1. spastic; increased degree of tension 2. having an increased osmotic pressure than a reference solution

hypertonicity (-to-nis'it-e) 1. increased osmotic pressure of body fluids 2. hypertonia

hypertrichosis (-tri-ko'sis) generalised distribution of coarse hairs and is not restricted to the male pattern

hypertriglyceridaemia (-tri-glis'er-i-de'me-a) an increased concentration of triglycerides in the blood

hypertrophy (hi-per'tro-fe) an increase in the size of an organ that causes an increase in the size of its constituent cells

hypertropia (hi'per-tro-pe-a) strabismus in which there is an upward deviation of the visual axis of an eye

hypertrophic cardiomyopathy *see* cardiomyopathy

hypertrophic osteoarthropathy a clinical condition exhibiting clubbed digits, periosteitis of the ends of long bones, arthritis and pain and is classically associated with lung cancer and rarely in pachydermoperiostosis

hyperuricaemia (-u'ri-se'me-a) increased blood level of uric acid noted in renal failure, and disorders of purine metabolism such as gout

hyperventilation (-ven-til-a'shun) tachydyspnoea noted in neurotics with anxiety attacks leading to respiratory alkalosis, tightness in the chest, dizziness, numbness of hands and feet, and tetany. Rebreathing air in a paper bag facilitates to increase CO_2

hyperviscosity (-vis-kos'it'e) marked increase in plasma viscosity, commonly seen in Waldenstrom syndrome due to massive increase in circulating IgM, less commonly in IgG and IgA plasma cell dyscrasias

hypervitaminosis (-vit′a-min-o′sis) a condition caused by an excessive intake of vitamins especially vitamins A and D

hypervolaemia (-vol-em′e-a) plethora; an abnormally increased volume of blood

hypesthesia (hi-per-the′zhah) decreased sensitivity to stimulation

hypha (hi′fah) pl. hyphae a branching tubular cell seen during the growth of filamentous fungi

hyphedonia (hip′he-do′ne-a) an abnormally lessened degree of pleasure

hyphema (hi-fe′ma) injury to the iris resulting in bleeding into the anterior chamber

hyphidrosis (hip′hi-dro′sis) decreased sweating

hyphomycetes (hi′fo-mi-set′ez) the molds; the mycelial fungi

hypnogogue (hip′na-gog) an agent that induces sleep

hypnalgia (hip-nal′ja) pain during the sleep

hypnoanalysis (hip′no-a-nal′i-sis) psychoan-alysis employing hypnosis as an adjunctive technique

hypnodontics (-don′tiks) use of hypnosis and controlled suggestion in dental practice

hypnogenic (-jen′ik) relating to induction of sleep or of hypnotic state

hypnoid (hip′noid) resembling hypnosis

hypnolepsy (hip′no-lep′se) narcolepsy

hypnology (hip′nol′a-je) study of sleep or of hypnotism

hypnosis (hip-no′sis) a state of suspended consciousness characterised by a heightened suggestibility

hypnotic (hip-not′ik) 1. something, usually a drug, that induces sleep. Therapeutically it is a central nervous system depressant 2. relating to hypnotism

hypnotise (-tiz) to induct into hypnosis

hypnotism (hip′no-tizm) the process of inducing hypnosis

hyp (o) combining word for beneath, under, deficient

hypoactivity decreased activity or retardation, hypokinesis

hypoacusis (hi′po-a-ku′sis) impaired hearing

hypoadrenalism (-a-dre′nal-izm) reduced adrenocortical function

hypoadrenocorticism (a-dren′o-kort′is-izm) diminished secretion or the effect of the adrenal cortical hormones.

hypoalbuminosis (-al-bu′min-o′sis) abnormally low level of albumin

hypoalimentation (-al′i-men-ta′shun) insufficient nutrition

hypoalphalipoproteinaemia (-al-fah-lip′o-opro′te-ne′me-a) deficiency of high density (alpha) lipoproteins in the blood

hypobaric (-bar′ik) pertaining to pressure of ambient gases less than 1 atmosphere

hypobarism (-bar′izm) condition resulting from decreasing barometric pressure on the body without hypoxia

hypobaropathy (-bar-op′a-the) sickness produced by reduced barometric pressure

hypobetalipoproteianemia an autosomal dominant condition due to decreased LDL, low level of serum cholesterol and acanthocytosis

hypoblast (hi′po-blast) endoderm

hypocalcaemia (hi′po-kal-se′me-a) an abnormally low levels of calcium in the circulating blood

hypocapnia (-kap′ne-a) markedly decreased tension of carbon dioxide in the circulating blood

hypocarbia (kar′be-a) hypocapnia

hypochloraemia (-klor-em′e-a) markedly decreased level of chloride ions in circulating blood

hypochlorhydria (klor-hi′dre-a) markedly decreased amount of hydrochloric acid in the stomach

hypochlorite (-klorit) bleach

hypochlorisation (-klor′i-za′shun) decreased amount of sodium chloride in the diet

hypocholesteraemia (-kol-es′ter-em′e-a) markedly decreased amounts of cholesterol in the circulating blood

hypocholesterolaemia (-kol-es′ter-ol-e′me-a) hypocholesteraemia

hypochondria (-kon'dre-a) 1. exaggerated concern over one's health that is not based on real organic pathology, but rather on unrealistic interpretation of physical signs or sensations as abnormal 2. plural of hypochondrium.

hypochondriac (-kon'dre-ak) a person obscessed with real or imaginary disease in himself

hypochondriasis (-kon-dri-a-sis) a person exhibiting persistent and irrational fear that he or she is ill despite medical reassurance to the contrary

hypochondrium (hi-po-kon'dre-um) the area on either side of the abdomen covered by the costal cartilages, lateral to the epigastrium

hypochondroplasia (hi'po-kon'dro-pla'zea) an autosomal dominant condition characterised by short stature, short limbs and caudal syringomyelia

hypochromasia (-kro-ma'zhah) hypochromia, where the red blood cells have decreased amount of haemoglobin

hypochromatism (-kro'mat-iam) 1. the condition of being hypochromatic 2. hypochromia

hypochromatosis (-kro'ma-to'sis) gradual disappearance of the cell nucleus

hypochromia (-kro'me-a) 1. hypochromasia 2. a condition of anaemia wherein the percentage of haemoglobin in the red blood cells is less than the normal range

hypocomplementaemia (-kom'ple-mente'me-a) a disorder of the blood in which one or another component of complement is deficient or decreased in amount

hypocorticism (-kort'is-izm) adrenocortical insufficiency

hypocyclosis (-si-klo'sis) deficient accommodation of the eyes

hypocythaemia (-si-them'e-a) markedly reduced numbers of red and white cells and platelets in the circulating blood, as in aplastic anaemia

hypoderma (-derm'a) the larvae belonging to genus of botflies causing cutaneous larva migrans

hypodermiasis (-der-mi'a-sis) a creeping eruption of the skin from the larva of hypoderma

hypodermic (-derm'ik) subcutaneous **h needle** a hollow needle attached to a syringe that is used to inject medication under the skin, into a muscle or directly to blood vessel

hypodermis (-derm'is) subcutaneous tissue

hypodermoclysis (-der-mok'li-sis) subcutaneous injection of a saline or other solution

hypodipsia (-dip'se-a) markely decreased thirst

hypodontia (-don'shi-a) 1. oligodontia 2. congenital absence of teeth

hypodynaemia (-di-nam'e-a) decreased muscular power

hypoeccrisia (-e-kris'e-a) reduced excretion of waste matter

hypoechoic (-e-ko'ik) tissues or structures, in ultrasonography reflecting few of the ultrasonic waves directed at them

hypoergia (-er'ja) hyposensitiveness

hypoesophoria (-es'o-for'e-a) downward and inward deviation of the eyeball

hypoesthesia (-es-the'zhah) markedly decreased sensitivity particularly to touch

hypoexophoria (ek'so-for'e-a) outward and downward deviation of the eyeball

hypoferraemia (-fe-rem'e-a) decreased amount of iron in the circulating blood

hypofertility (-fer-til'it-e) decreased capacity to produce

hypofibrinogenaemia (-fi-brin'o-j'in-em'e-a) markedly decreased amount of fibrinogen in the circulating blood plasma

hypogalactia (-ga-lak'she-a) decreased amount of milk secretion

hypogammaglobulinaemia (-gam'a-glob'u-lin-em'e-a) decreased production of immunoglobulins which may be congenital with B cell defects or acquired as in chronic lymphocytic leukaemia

hypoganglionosis (-gang'gle-on-o'sis) a decrease in the number of ganglionic nerve cells

hypogastrium (-gas'tre-um) pubic region; the lower middle area of the abdomen below the umbilicus

hypogenesis (-jen'i-sis) underdevelopment of parts or organs of the body

hypogenitalism (-jen'i-tl'izm) partial or complete failure of maturation of the genitalia, commonly due to hypogonadism

hypogeusia (-goo'ze-a) a decrease in taste sensation

hypoglucagonaemia (-gloo'ka-gon'e-me-a) markedly decreased levels of glucagon in the blood

hypoglycaemia (-gli-sem'e-a) a decrease in circulating glucose and occurs as a symptom **fasting h** caused by hypopituitarism, Addison's disease, adrenogenital syndrome, islet cell tumours, retroperitoneal sarcoma, hepatic disease, ectopic insulin production and glycogen storage disease **postprandial h** noted in postgastrectomy, oral hypoglycaemic agents, insulin, alcohol, aspirin or idiopathic

hypoglycaemic (-gli-sem'ik) pertaining to or characterised by hypoglycaemia **h drugs** drugs that lower glucose levels in the blood in patients with type 2 diabetes, and their action depends upon a supply of endogenous insulin such as sulphonylureas and biguanides. Thiazolidinediones act by insulin enhancement and alpha-glucosidase, by delaying carbohydrate digestion and absorption of glucose

hypoglycorrhachia (-gli-ko-ra'-ke-a) decrease in the amount of sugar in the cerebrospinal fluid

hypogonadism (-gon'ad-izm) a clinical disorder characterised by decreased or absent phenotypic expression of a person's sexual genotype. It may be primary due to lack of end-organ response to FSH or LH produced normally by pituitary or secondary to defective hypothalamic or pituitary hormonal activity

hypogonadotropic (-gon'a-do-top'ik)

implies inadequate secretion of gonadotropins and the resultant condition

hypohidrosis (-hi-dro'sis) decreased sweat production **acquired h** noted in Sjogren's syndrome, systemic sclerosis, psoriasis, pemphigus vulgaris, anticholinergics, hypothyroidism, diabetes insipidus, heat stroke, dehydration, peripheral neuropathies **inherited h** noted in ichthyosis, hereditary anhidrotic ectodermal dysplasia

hypokalaemic (-ka-lem'ik) hypopotassaemia; abnormally decreased level of potassium ions in the circulating blood

hypokinesia (-ki-ne'zhah) slow movement

hypolactasia (-lak-ta-zhah) deficient amount of lactase in the intestine

hypoleydigism (-lid'ig-izm) decreased secretion of androgens by the cells of Leydig

hypolipidaemic (-lip'id-em-ik) decreased lipid concentration in the blood

hypolipoproteinaemia a group of conditions exhibiting decreased lipoproteins. It may be congenital or acquired secondary to malabsorption, anaemia and hyperthyroidism

hypomagnesaemia (-mag'nes'em'e-a) decreased concentration of magnesium in circulating blood plasma

hypomania (-man'e-a) mild excitement with a moderate alteration in behaviour

hypomenorrhoea (-men'o-re-ah) a decreased flow or a shortened duration of menstruation

hypomere (hi'po-mer) 1. the ventrolateral part of myotome that forms the body wall muscle innervated by an anterior ramus of the spinal nerve 2. the lateral mesoderm giving rise to the lining of the body cavities

hypometria (hi'po-me'tre-a) an ataxia characterised by under reaching of an object or goal

hypomnesia (hi'pom-ne'sia) impaired memory

hypomorph (hipo-morf) a person having

disproportionately short legs compared to the length of the trunk

hypomyxia (hi'po-mik'se-a) diminished secretion of mucus

hyponatraemia (-na-trem'e-a) an abnormally low concentration of sodium ions in the circulating blood

hyponeocytosis (-ne'o-si-to'sis) a 'shift to the left' where leucopaenia is associated with the presence of young and immature leucocytes in the peripheral blood

hyponoia (-noi'a) sluggish mental activity

hyponychium (-nik'e-um) the epithelium of the nail bed particularly in the posterior part of the lanula

hypoorthocytosis (-or'tho-sito'sis) leucopaenia in which the relative numbers of different types of white blood cells are within the normal range

hypoparathyroidism (-par'a-thi'roid-izm) parathyroid insufficiency due to diminution or absence of secretion of parathormones **pseudo h** condition with normal or reduced parathormone secretion but lack of target tissue response to the hormone associated with congenital malformations **pseudopseudo h** normal levels of PTH, calcium and phosphorus, with congenital abnormalities of pseudo- hypoparathyroidism

hypoperfusion (-per-fu'zhun) decreased flow of blood through an organ

hypopharynx (-fa'rinks) upper airway between the base of the tongue and larynx

hypophonesis (-fo-ne'sis) diminished intensity of the sound

hypophonia (-fo'ne-a) decreased voice from incoordination of vocal muscles including weakness of respiratory muscles

hypophoria (-for'e-a) downward deviation of the visual axis of one eye compared with the other eye

hypophosphatasia (-fos-fa-ta-zhah) a congenital rickets-like metabolic disease exhibiting low serum alkaline phosphatase and clinical manifestations in infants with premature loss of deciduous teeth, growth retardation, increased fractures, and in adults with early loss of permanent teeth, osteoporosis, fractures and pseudofractures

hypophosphataemia (-fos'fah-te'me-a) markedly decreased concentration of phosphates in the circulating blood

hypophrenia (-fre'ne-a) mental deficiency

hypophysectomy (hi-pof'i-sek'ta-me) surgical removal of the pituitary gland

hypophyseoportal (hi'po-fiz'o-por'tl) pertaining to the portal system of the pituitary gland in which hypothalamic venules connect with the capillaries of anterior pituitary

hypophysioprivic (fiz'e-o-priv'ik) deficient hormonal secretion from pituitary gland

hypophysis (hi-pof'i-sis) pea-sized conductor of endocrine orchestra present in the sella turcica and is separated into an anterior lobe containing cells producing ACTH, FSH, GH (growth hormone or somatotropin), LH and TSH, intermediate lobe producing MSH and posterior lobe (neurohypophysis) which under the influence of hypothalamus produces antidiuretic hormone (vasopressin) and oxytocin

hypopiesis (hi'po-pi-e'sis) hypotension

hypopituitarism (-pi-tuit-ar-izm) a condition due to diminished activity of the anterior lobe of the pituitary with inadequate secretion of one or more anterior pituitary hormones

hypoplasia (-pla-zhah) failure of an organ or tissue to develop fully

hypopnoea (hi-pop'ne-a) significant decrease, not absence of airflow for at least 10 seconds

hypoporosis (hi'po-por-o'sis) deficient callus formation at the site of bone fracture

hypopotassaemia (-po'ta-se'me-a) hypokalaemia

hypoprosody (-pros'o-de) decreased variation in stress, pitch and rhythm of speech

hypopselaphesia (hi'pop-sel'a-fe'zhah) blunted touch sensation

hypoptyalism (-ti-a-lizm) decreased salivation

hypopyon (hi-po'pe-on) presence of pus in the anterior chamber of the eye, resulting from corneal ulceration and uveitis

hyposalivation (hi'po-sali'i-va'shun) decreased salivation; hypoptyalism

hyposecretion (-se-kre'shun) decreased secretion, as by a gland

hyposensitive (-sen'sit-iv) decreased ability to respond

hyposomatotropism (hi'po-so'mat-o-tro'pizm) decreased secretion of pituitary growth hormone

hyposmia (hi-poz'me-a) diminished sense of smell

hypospadius (-spa'de-is) a developmental defect in which urethra opens on the undersurface of the penis

hypostasis (hi-pos'ta-sis) collection of fluid or blood in dependent parts

hypostatic (hi-po-stat'ik) resulting from a dependent position

hyposthenia (hi-pos-the'ne-a) weakness

hyposthenuria inability to concentrate urine

hypoteleorism (-tel'er-izm) abnormal closeness of the eyes

hypotension (-ten'shun) an abnormally low blood pressure that reduces blood flow to the brain causing dizziness and fainting

hypotensive (-ten'siv) 1. characterised by low blood pressure 2. an agent causing a reduction in blood pressure

hypothalamic-pituitary axis a group of feedback systems that coordinate the activity of hypothalamus and pituitary. The hypothalamus synthesises releasing hormones that act on the pituitary which in turn evokes end-organ responses from adrenal gland, thyroid, gonads and breast, and has also growth hormone-somatotroph axis

hypothalamus (-thal'a-mus) a portion of diencephalon of the brain forming the floor and part of the ventral wall of the third ventricle. It lies beneath the thalamus. It controls some metabolic activities, regulate body temperature and secretion of releasing and inhibiting hormones acting on pituitary gland. It integrates the activity of autonomic nervous system

hypothenar (-the'na-r) the fleshy mass at the ulnar side of the palm

hypothermia a dangerous fall in body temperature to below normal level (35°C or less), it causes drowsiness, and reduced breathing and heart rates and may lead to unconsciousness and death

hypothesis (hi-poth'e-sis) 1. a statement derived from a theory that predicts the relationship among variables 2. an assumption advanced as a basis for reasoning or argument **null h** hypothesis that observed differences or variation in scores can be attributed to random sources

hypothymia (hi'po-thi'me-a) depression of spirits

hypothymism (-thi'mizm) insufficient synthesis and release of thyroid hormones

hypothyroidism (-thi'roid'izm) a condition due to deficient secretion by thyroid. It develops insidiously manifesting in tiredness, somnolence, weight gain, cold intolerance, hoarseness, bradycardia, dry skin, non-pitting oedema or myxoedema, menorrhagia, constipation, delayed relaxation of tendon reflexes, depression and psychosis **congenital h** thyroid agenesis **drug induced h** administration of lithium and iodine causing hypothyroidism **goitrous h** hypothyroid-state from Hashimoto's thyroiditis, iodine deficiency and genetically determined defect in thyroid hormone secretion **postablative h** disorder of thyroid following I^{131} therapy for Grave's disease. There is low levels of thyroid hormones associated with raised TSH **spontaneous atrophic h** an organ specific autoimmune disorder with fibrosis and atrophy of thyroid **subclinical h** asymptomatic state with low levels of thyroid hormones but with raised serum TSH

hypotonia (ton'e-a) 1. a condition of diminished tone or tension 2. relaxation of arteries 3. diminished muscular tonicity.

hypotonic (-ton'ik) having a lesser concentration of solute than another solution hence exerting less osmotic pressure than that solution

hypotrichosis (-tri-ko'sis) a less than normal amount of hair on the scalp and/or body

hypotrophy (hi-po-tra-fe) atrophy

hypotropia (hi'po-tro'pe-a) downward deviation of the visual axis of one eye

hypotympanotomy (-tim'pa-not'a-me) surgical incision into the lower tympanic cavity

hypotympanum (-tim'pa-num) the lower part of the tympanic cavity

hypouricaemia (-ur'is-em'e-a) decreased blood concentration of uric acid

hypoventilation (-ven'ti-la'shun) reduced ventilation resulting in an increase in arterial carbon dioxide tension and decrease in arterial oxygen tension

hypovolaemia (vo-lem'e-a) an abnormally low circulating blood volume

hypovolia (-vol'e-a) diminished water content or volume of a given compartment

hypoxaemia (hi'pok-sem'e-a) a decrease in PaO_2 below normal expected value. It may develop in presence of normal or lowered arterial carbon dioxide tension. An inadequate gas exchange due to ventilation-perfusion inequality, increased right-to-left intrapulmonary shunting of blood, impaired diffusion and hypoventilation result in hypoxaemia

hypoxia (hi-pok'se-a) an inadequate level of oxygen in the tissues, blood or air

hypsokinesis (hi$_1$ so-ki-ne'sis) a tendency to sway or fall backward when standing seen in Parkinson's disease

hysterectomy (his'ter-ek'ta-me) surgical removal of the uterus **abdominal h** excision of the uterus through the abdominal wall **caesarean h** caesarean section followed by removal of the uterus **radical h** removal of ovaries, fallopian tubes, lymph nodes and lymph channels with uterus and cervix **total h** removal of uterus and cervix

hysteresis (his'te-re'sis) a phenomenon in which values or data point in a cyclical fashion or periodic proceses occur along a different route in one direction as the other.

hystereurysis (-u're-sis) dilatation of the lower segment and cervical canal of the uterus

hysteria (his-ter'e-a) the conversion of mental or emotional illness into physical symptoms such as blindness, paralysis

hysterical (his-ter'ikal) relating to or suffering from hysteria **h anaesthesia** loss of sensory modalities resulting from emotional conflicts **h dyspnoea** a frequent cause of dyspnoea without any systemic cause, where dyspnoea is evident at rest **h fits** occur in emotionally charged situation in presence of onlookers and do not occur when patient is alone. Consciousness is not lost during fits. The movements are bizarre **h neurosis** a psychogenic loss or disorder of function manifested either as conversion reaction (sensory or motor) or as a dissociative reaction (psychic symptoms) **h personality** emotionally labile, dramatising, defensive, and demanding, tendency to be untruthful **h trans** the twilight state or stupor. Patient gets detached from reality and may also be immobile and immersed in his own self

hysterics (his-te'riks) an emotional expression accompanied often by crying, laughing and screaming

hyster (o) combining word for uterus, hysteria

hysterocoele (his'ter-o-sel) 1. an abdominal hernia containing part or all of the uterus 2. protrusion of uterine contents into weakened area of uterine wall

hysterocleisis (his'ter-o-kli'sis) operative closure of the uterus

hysteroepilepsy (-ep'il-ep'se) hysterical convulsions

hysterography (his'ter-og'ra-fe) a radiographic picture of a uterus made after the injection of a contrast medium into the uterine cavity

hysteroid (his'ter-oid) resembling or simulating hysteria

hysterolith (his'ter-o-lith) uterine calculus

hysterolysis (his'ter-ol'i-sis) severing of adhesions between the uterus and the surrounding structure

hysteromyoma (his'ter-o-mi-o-ma) a myoma or leiomyoma or fibromyoma of the uterus

hysteromyotomy (-mi-ot'a-me) incision into the uterine muscle for removal of an uterine fibroid

hysteropexy (his'ter-o-pek'se) surgical fixation of a misplaced or abnormally moveable uterus

hysteroptosis (his'ter-op-to'sis) prolapse of the uterus

hysterorrhaphy (his'ter-or-ah-fe) surgical repair of uterus

hysterorrhexis (his'ter-o-rek'sis) rupture of the uterus

hysterosalpingectomy (-sal'pin-jek-ta-me) surgical removal of the uterus and one or both fallopian tubes

hysterosalpingogram (-sal'ping-go-gram) an X-ray film of the uterus and fallopian tubes using gas or a radiopaque substance introduced through the cervix

hysterosalpingography (-sal'ping-gog'ra-fe) an X-ray examination of the uterus and fallopian tubes used to investigate infertility

hysterosalpingoophorectomy (-sal'ping-go-o'of-o-rek'ta-me) surgical removal of one or both ovaries and fallopian tubes along with the uterus

hysterosalpingostomy (-sal'ping'gos'ta-me) an operation to restore the patency of a fallopian tube

hysteroscope (his'ter-o-skop) a viewing instrument for examination of the cervix and the interior of the uterus

hysteroscopy (his'ter-o-sko-py) direct visualisation of the cervix and the uterus through a hysteroscope

hysterospasm (-spazm) a spasmodic contraction of the uterus

hysterotomy (his'ter-otao-me) a miniature caesarean section, wherein the incision of uterus is made either transabdominally or vaginally to remove produts of conception

hysterotrachelorrhaphy (his'ter-o-tra-kel-or'a-fe) surgical repair of a lacerated cervix uteri

hysterotrachelotomy (-tra'kel-ot'a-me) incision of the cervix uteri

hysterotubography (-too-bog'ra-fe) hysterosalpingography

Hz abbreviation of hertz

HZV abbreviation for herps zoster virus

I

I chemical symbol for the element iodine, inspired gas

I¹³¹ symbol for radioactive iodine, atomic weight 131

ia suffix indicating condition, especially abnormal

I and O abbreviation for intake and output

IAP Indian Academy of Paediatrics

–iasis suffix indicating condition, especially pathologic

–iatric (ia'trik) suffix pertaining to medicine or to a physician

iatro a combining word for relating to a physician or to medicine

iatrogenesis (i'at-ro-jen-i-sis) new situation created from treatment

iatrogenic (ia'trojen'ik) physician-produced **i disease** any disease or disorder that has resulted in a patient from effects of treatment by a physician or a surgeon

iatrology (i'a-trol'o-je) medical science

I band an isotropic band of striated muscle fibre that appears dark in polarised light but light when stained

IBD abbreviation for inflammatory bowel disease

IBS abbreviation for irritable bowel syndrome

ibid (ib'id) *ibidem* in the same book, chapter or page

iccha(s) intention

ibuprofen a low-risk non-steroidal anti-inflammatory drug

IC abbreviation for inspiratory capacity

IC 50/ IC90 the inhibitory concentration of a drug needed to inhibit viral replication by either 50% or 90%

ice (is) a solid form of water produced by freezing **i bag** a watertight bag enabling to keep ice cubes, also called ice pack, used to cool an area **i box** an insulated cabinet with a partition for ice **iceberg** (is'burg) more subclinical than clinical cases and what comes to the notice is only the tip of the iceberg **i cold** cold as ice **i water** water chilled with ice.

ice-cream headache a migraine headache triggered by oropharyngeal irritation due to cold foods

ICD abbreviation for International Classification of Diseases

ICDS Integrated Child Development Service Programme. A scheme sponsored by Government of India to improve the physical, mental and social development of pre-school children, to improve the capacity of mothers to look after the health and nutritional status of their children and to reduce the maternal, the infant and the pre-school child morbidity and mortality. Now the programme is known as Integrated Mother and Child Development Service

ichor (i'kor) thin, fetid discharge from an ulcer or wound

ichthyosis (ik'theo'sis) hypertrophy of horny layer characterised by thick, dry, scaly skin resembling fish skin. **ichthyotic** adj. **bullous i** epidermolytic hyperkeratosis with bullous lesions and hyperkeratosis in infants **i congenita**, a severe variant of lamellar ichthyosis exhibiting thick sheet of hyperkeratosis **i hystrix** bilateral symmetric epidermal naevus arranged in a geometrical pattern **i vulgaris** presence of brownish angulated scales over the body, especially on the front of the legs, inherited as an autosomal dominant character **lamellar i** presence of diffuse erythema and scaling in flexural aspects of cubital and popliteal fossae, inherited as an autosomal recessive character **X-linked i** transmitted by a recessive gene which manifests in males, though resembles autosomal dominant ichthyosis

ICSH interstitial cell stimulating hormone, produced by the anterior lobe of pituitary gland

ictal (ik'tal) pertaining to a sudden attack such as an epileptic seizure

icteric (ikter'ik) affected with jaundice; jaundiced

ictero (ik-ter'o) pertaining to jaundice.

icterogenic (ik'ter-o-jen'ik) causing jaundice

icterus (ik'ter'us) jaundice **i gravis neonatorum,** erythroblastosis foetalis a haemolytic jaundice of the newborn baby with incompatibility between mother's serum and red blood cells of infant **i index** comparison of blood serum in intensity of colour with that of potassium dichromate. Normally it is 3–5. In presence of jaundice the index shows a rise to 15 or more **i neonatorum** jaundice noted in infants between second and fifth days of life

icthyol a product of tar, a 10 percent ointment is applied in diseases associated with erythemas and scaling or fissures

ictus (ik'tus) a seizure, stroke, sudden attack or a fit noted at birth

ICU abbreviation for intensive care unit

ICCU abbreviation for intensive coronary care unit

ID abbreviation for infectious disease

id *psy* selfish and supremely egocentric

-id 1. a rash occurring in a region away from the main lesion of the disease 2. obscure, inaccessible part of personality

IDDM insulin-dependent diabetes mellitus. *see* diabetes mellitus

idea (ide'a) a concept; a mental image; any thought

ideational apraxia the inability to execute a sequence of movements in an orderly fashion

ide eruption allergic vesicular reaction on the sides of fingers and palms from which no fungus can be isolated though

develops as a complication of dermatophytosis, stasis dermatitis and eczema

idem the same as previously mentioned

identical (iden'itkel) exactly the same or similar **i twin** one of a pair of twins of the same sex resembling one another closely who have developed from a single fertilised ovum

identification (iden'tefeka'shen) the act of identifying

identify (iden'tefi') to recognise or verify the identity

identity (iden'ti'te) the condition of being oneself

ideokinetic apraxia the dissociation of an idea and the motor act

idiocy (ide-o-se) severe mental retardation

ideogram (id'e-o-gram) the graphic representation of chromosome complement of a cell

ideoglossia (id'e-o-glos'e-a) an inability to articulate properly

idiopathic (idie-o-path'ik) of undetermined origin **i hypertrophic subaortic stenosis** *see* hypertrophic cardiomyopathy **i midline destructive disease** a midline granuloma of undetermined aetiology characterised by local destruction of the upper respiratory tract and acute and chronic inflammation with variable necrosis **i pulmonary fibrosis** appears as a fibrosing lesion in the alveolar walls. It is chracterised by dyspnoea, small stiff lungs and hypoxaemia **i pulmonary haemosiderosis** recurrent haemoptysis and iron deficiency due to intrapulmonary haemorrhage **i scoliosis** an abnormal condition characterised by a lateral curvature of the spine. **i thrombocytopaenic purpura** (ITP), occurrence of ecchymotic haemorrhage secondary to viral infection or vaccination in children (acute) or widespread haemorrhage, bruisability and transient thrombocytopaenia in adults (chronic)

idiosome (id'e-o-some) ultimate element of living matter

idiosyncrasy (id'e-o-sin'kra-se) 1. a habit or quality peculiar to any person 2. an abnormal susceptibility to some drug or protein peculiar to a person

idiot person with gross mental retardation

idioventricular (id'e-o-ven-trik'u-lar) relating to the cardiac ventricle alone when dissociated from the atrium

Ig immunoglobulin. **IgA** immuno-globulin A, **IgD** immunoglobulin D, **IgE** immunoglobulin E, **IgG** immunoglobulin G, **IgM** immunoglobulin M

IGF-1 insulin-like growth factor

IGF – BP–3 iGF binding protein–3

ignis fire; cautery

ileal (il'e-al) pertaining to the ileum **i conduit** an irreversible obstruction of the urinary tract, ureters may be anastomosed to an isolated loop of ileum opening on the abdominal wall **i bypass operation** a surgical procedure where the distal one-third of the small intestine is bypassed and bowel continuity is restored by an end-to-end ileocaecostomy, performed in extreme obesity or high serum cholesterol **i resection** surgical removal of ileum as in Crohn's disease. It leads to vitamin B_{12} and bile salt malabsorption resulting in diarrhoea

ileitis (il'ei'tis) inflammation of the ileum **regional i** a non-specific, chronic, inflammatory, granulomatous lesion involving terminal ileum. *See* Crohn's disease

ileo (il'e-o) relation to the ileum

ileocaecal (il'e-o-se'kal) relating to the ileum and caecum. **i valve** sphincter that helps to close the ileum where it opens into the ascending colon

ileocolic (il'e-o-kol'ik) pertaining to the ileum and caeum

ileocolitis (il'e-o-ko-li'tis) inflammation of ileum and colon

ileocolostomy (il'e-o-ko-los'to-me) anastomosis between the ileum and colon

ileocystoplasty (il'e-o-sist'o-plas'te) surgical procedure connecting a portion of ileum to the urinary bladder so as to increase the size of the bladder

ileoileostomy(il'eo-li'eo-s'to-me) surgical creation of an opening between two parts of the ileum

ileorectal (il'e-o-rek'tal) pertaining to the ileum and rectum

ileostomy (il'e-os'to-me) an operation to bring ileum through an incision in the abdominal wall and formed into an artificial outlet to allow discharge of faeces into a bag attached to the skin

ileum (il'e-um) the longest and narrowest distal part of the small intestine connecting jejunum to the caecum

ileus (il'e-us) impairment of the forward flow of the intestinal contents which is either paralytic secondary to electrolyte abnormalities, surgery, peritoneal irritation or mesenteric artery accidents or obstructive due to adhesive bands, foreign bodies, intussusception or tumours. **paralytic i** omnious silence of abdomen without normal intermittent gushings and gurglings

iliac (il'e-ac) pertaining to the ileum **i artery** either of two large arteries that carry blood to the pelvic region and lower limbs; common iliac artery. It has an outer branch – external iliac artery that becomes femoral artery and an internal iliac artery conducting blood to gluteal region **i crest** upper free margin of the ileum **i fossa** one of the concavities of the iliac bones of the pelvis **i region** inguinal region on either side of the hypogastrium **i spine** one of the four spines of the ileum such as anterior and posterior superior spines and anterior and posterior inferior spines

ilio-relation to ilium or flank

ilium (il'e-um) the broad upper part of the hip bone; one of the bones of each half of the pelvis. It forms part of the acetabulum and provides attachment to several muscles.

Ilizarow technique a technique devised by a Russian surgeon Ilizarow for the treatment of non-union or malunion deformity, chronic osteomyelitis or limb length discrepancy. It consists of external rings and thin wires. The wire is passed through the bones on both sides of fracture which after tensioning are fixed to the ring fixator. Bone lengthening can be achieved by corticotomy

ill (il) sick, diseased, not healthy

illness (il'nis) sickness, condition of ill health ailment

illumination (il-lu-min-a'shun) lighting up of a part for examination or an object under microscope

illusion (il'lu-shun) misperceptions or misinterpretations of real external stimuli. **illusory** adj. **optical i** a visual impression that is inaccurate

illusive (il'lu-siv) deceptive, misleading

IM abbreviation for intramuscular

IMA abbreviation for Indian Medical Association

image (im'aj) a picture of an object or person, a mental representation, appearance **i intensifier** device to increase the brightness of an image produced by x-ray **mirror i** an image of an object reflected in a mirror, in which right and left are reversed

imagery (im-ij-re) imagination

imagination (im'aj-i-na'shun) formation of mental images of things, persons or situations different from those previously known.

imaging creation of images, pictures or shadows of the structures inside the body by using magnetic fields, sound waves, or radiation often combined with computers

imago (i-ma'go) 1. sexually mature adult stage of an insect 2. a memory developed during childhood that has been clouded by imagination and idealism

imbalance (im-bal'ens) without equality between two; faulty muscular or glandular co-ordination

imbecile (im'be-sil) mentally defective person, above the level of idiocy; mental retardation

imbecility a state of mental retardation; feebleness of mind

imbedding to fix into a surrounding tissue; implantation referring to the human blastocyte attaching to the endometrium of the uterus

imbibe (im'bi-b) to consume, to drink to soak, or to absorb

imbibition (im'bi-bish'un) the absorption of a liquid

imbrication (im'bri-ka'shun) overlapping.

imipenem a beta-lactam broad spectrum antibiotic active on aerobic and anaerobic, gram-positive and gram-negative organisms. It is partially inactivated by a renal enzyme, hence given along with an inhibitor of that enzyme, called cilastatin

imipramine (i-mip'ra-men) a tricyclic antidepressant drug

immature (im'ma-chur) not fully developed

immediate occurring without delay, instant

immedicable (i-med'i-ka-b'l) incurable

immersion (im-er'shun) placing a body under water or other fluid **i lens** a special lens with oil placed between the lens and the object being visualised to produce a higher magnification **i oil** an oil with a refractive index of 1.52 that allows high power magnification for light microscopy

immiscible (i-mis'i-bl) not mixing

immobilisation making part immovable

immobilise to fix so as to be immovable

immotile cilia syndrome defects in the ultrastructure of the cilia and of the sperm may affect their motility and function. The cilia lose their orientation and are unable to beat in a coherent way. The sperm tails stand straight and stiff without exhibiting any motility. Clinical manifestations include sinopulmonary infections with bronchiectasis, Kartagener's syndrome, situs inversus, middle ear infections and infertility

immune (im-un') resistant to a disease due to the development of antibodies **i body** antibody **i complexes** circulating aggregates of antibody and antigen, whose deposition in the tissues such as blood vessel walls cause inflammation and tissue damage **i deficiency** decreased effectiveness of the immune system. It is encountered in people who are malnourished, infected with HIV or undergoing chemotherapy for treatment of cancer **i globulin** a sterile solution of globulins containing different antibodies normally found in human blood, used in passive immunisation of non-immune persons exposed to diseases **i reaction** antigenic response to a specific antibody **i reconstitution** improvement of the function of the immune system **i response** reaction of the body to foreign substances **i serum** a serum containing naturally or artificially produced antibodies **i system** a collection of body cell substances and structures that work to protect the body from disease-causing organisms and from the development of cancer.

immunity 1. a state of resistance to a disease through the defense activities of the immune system 2. protection from a disease **active i** resistance to infection that is acquired as a result of previous infection with a disease-causing organism or following vaccination **adaptive i** an immune system where distinct antigens generate specific responses and different lymphocytes recognise antigens. Reexposure to antigen induces more rapid and effective response **cell mediated i** (CMI), antibacterial activity induced and expressed by T-lymphocytes **humoral i** immunity mediated by antibodies found in the plasma or lymph, synthesised by B lymphocytes **innate i** natural immunity where cellular and mediator events provide effective protection **passive i** injection of antibodies to provide temporary protection against a disease-causing organism

immunisation the process of inducing immunity as a preventive measure against specific infectious diseases. **i schedule** (*see* **table 4**)

immunoadsorbent any material such as gel or inert solid used to adsorb or purify antibodies from a solution

immunoassay (im'u-no-as'sa) laboratory methods to measure antibodies and antigens in a person's blood or tissue to diagnose infectious diseases

immunoblast lymphoblast **i test** *see* Western blot test

immunocompetence (im'u-no-kom'petens) the ability of the body to develop an immune response

immunocompromised condition of not possessing a normal immune system

immunodeficiency (im'u-no-de-fish'en-se) a deficiency in immune response **i diseases** may be primary affecting one or more components of the immune system such as B cells, T cells, macrophages, NK cells and complement and exhibits an increased susceptibility to infection or chronic due to drugs, irradiation or HIV infection

immunodiagnosis (im'u-no-di'ag-no'sis) diagnosis based on demonstration of antibodies to antigens

immunodiffusion (im'u-no-di-fu'-zhun) the diffusion of antigen and antibody from different regions

immunoelectrophoresis (im'u-no-e-lek'-tro-fo-re-sis) a method of electrophoresis and double diffusion to recognise the proteins based on their electrophoretic mobility and antigenic specificities

immunoenhancement the process of increasing the level of immune response

immunofluorescence (im'u-no-floo'o-re's-ens) determination of the site of antigen or antibody in the tissue by fluorescence

immunogen (i-mu-no-jen) any substance capable of eliciting an immune response

immunogenetics (im'u-no-je-net'iks) study

Table 4: Immunisation schedule

The following is the National Immunisation schedule

Age	Vaccine	Symbol	Dose	Route of administration
1. For infants				
0–3 days	BCG		0.1 ml	I.D.
	OPV	OPVO	0.1 ml (2 drops)	Oral
	OPV	OPVI		
6 weeks	DPT	DPT 1	0.5 ml	IM
10 weeks	OPV	OPV II		
	DPT	DPT II		
14 weeks	OPV	OPV III		
	DPT	DPT III		
9–12 months	Measles		0.5 ml	SC
2. For preschool children	DPT	DPT Booster		
	OPV	OPV Booster		
6 years	DT	DT Booster		
3. For older children	TT	TT	0.5 ml	IM
10 years		Booster		
16 years	TT	TT Booster		
4. For pregnant women				
16-22 weeks	TT	TT I		
34-36 weeks	TT	TT II		

Table 5: Immunoglobulins

IgA	constitutes 20% of total immunoglobulins. Gut mucosa and lamina propria of the respiratory tract are major sites of IgA production. Secretory IgA provides local immunity
IgD	useful in the maturation and regulation of B-lymphocytes
IgE	produced in the lining of the respiratory and intestinal tracts, needed for immediate hypersensitivity reactions
IgG	constitutes 70% of total immunoglobulins and is distributed equally between the blood and extracelluar fluid. It protects against infectious agents and participates in immunologic reactions. It is the only immunoglobulin transported across the placenta and provides passively acquired immunity to the newborn. There are four subclasses of IgG as IgG1, IgG2, IgG3 and IgG4
IgM	earliest immunoglobulin to be synthesised by the foetus. An intravascular macromolecule stimulating complement activity

of genetic factors influencing the immune response

immunogenic (im'-o-no-jen'ik) inducing immunity

immunogenicity (im'u-no-je-nis'i-te) the degree to which a protein is capable of evoking an immune response and production of specific antibody

immunoglobulin (im'-u-no'-glob'o-lin) a protein produced following exposure to an antigen possessing the activity of an antibody. They are the effector products of B cells in response to an antigen. There are five types of immunoglobulins - IgA, IgD, IgE, IgG and IgM (*see* table 5)

immunoglobulinopathy gammopathy

immunologic (im'u-no-loj'ik) pertaining to immunology **i tolerance** limitations on the responsiveness of lymphocytes to self-antigens

immunologist (im'-u-no-lo-jist) a person specialised in immunology

immunology (im'u-nol'o-je) the study of the molecular and cellular biology of antigen recognition and of immune reactions

immunomodulation manipulation of the immune system with non-specific biological modifiers such as lymphokines or specific molecules produced against a patient's self-cells

immunopathology (im'u-no-pa-tho'lo-je) branch of science dealing with immune reactions and disease

immunophenotyping typing of cells with immunological markers such as monoclonal antibodies

immunoprecipitation (im'u-no-pre'-sip-ta'-shun) precipitation resulting from antigen antibody reaction

immuno proliferative small intestinal disease (IPSID), diffuse affection of the small intestine especially proximally by a dense lymphoplasmacytic infiltrate and present with malabsorption, anorexia and fever in young adults; alpha heavy chain disease

immunoprophylaxis prevention of disease by using vaccines or antisera

immunoprotein gammaglobulin

immunoreaction (i-mu'no-re-ak'shun) the reaction between an antigen and its antibody

immunosenecence weakened immune system with advancing age

immunosorbent antigen adsorbing homologous antibody from a mixture

immunostimulant (i-mu'no-stim'u-lant) a substance increasing the efficiency of the immune system

immunosuppressant (i-mu'no-su-pre-sant) a substance decreasing the immune response

immunosuppression (i-mu'-no-su-presh'un) prevention of activation of an excessive or inappropriate immune response by drugs such as corticosteroids, cyclophosphamide, methotrexate or cyclosporine

immunosurveillance (im'u-no-ser-va'lens) monitoring the function of immune system

immunotherapy (im'u-no'-ther'a-pe) 1. passive immunisation by preformed antibodies to build up a person's immunity to which he or she is allergic 2. use of body's immune system to counteract side effect of therapy especially cancer chemotherapy

impacted wedged in; **i fracture** a break in a bone in which the fragmented bony ends are forced into one another making it difficult to set **i tooth** tooth confined in its socket as to be incapable of normal eruption

impaction (im-pak'shun) wedged into a part

impair (im'par) to weaken, to cause to worse,

impairment any loss or abnormality of a structure or function

impalpable (im-pal'pa-bl) not felt; not palpable; incapable of being perceived by touch

impassive (im-pas'iv) without emotion, apathetic, showing no feeling

impedance (im-pe'dans) resistance **i audiometry** a test to find out whether hearing loss is due to damage to the middle ear i **plethysmography** a technique for detection of blood vessel occlusion

impede (im-ped) to hinder, to limit or obstruct

impediment (im'pe'de-ment) an obstruction, that which hinders

imperative involuntary; obligatory

imperforate (im-per'fo-rat) not open i **anus** malformed opening at the anus which needs surgical correction i **hymen** a hymen without an opening

impermeable (im-per'me-a-b'l) not allowing passage; impervious

impetiginisation (im'pe-tij'i-ni-za'shun) the development of impetigo upon an area which was seat of some other skin disorder

impetigo (im-pe-ti'go) a highly contagious skin infection showing confluent vesicles, pustules which rapture and exhibit bright yellow crusts i **contagiosa** a highly contagious form of impetigo affecting the most superficial layers of epidermis, occurs commonly on the face of children **bullous** i diffusely, scattered, tense bullae filled with clear fluid occurring in children **Bockhart's** i superficial folliculitis, infection at the opening of the hair follicles on legs and thighs presents with pustules, named after Max Bockhart, German physician

impetuous (im-pech'us) hasty, impulsive, rash

impetus (im'pi-tus) driving energy, momentum, impulse, stimulus

impinge to trespass, intrude

implant (im'plant) to graft or to insert a natural or artificial material into a body surgically

implantation (im'plan-ta'shun) process of grafting or insertion i **dermoid** painless, soft cyst in the pulps of the fingers probably due to continued proliferation of a fragment of epidermis that is driven beneath the dermis

impotence (im'-po-ten's) inability to achieve or maintain a penile erection, adequate for the successful completion of intercourse, terminating in ejaculation

impotent (im'po-tent) 1. sterile 2. unable to copulate

impoverish (im-pov'or-ish) to make poor, to exhaust

impregnate (im-preg'-nat) to fertilise an ovum to make pregnant

impregnation (in'preg-na'shun) fertilisation of an ovum

impressior 1. a depression in a surface 2. an effect produced upon the mind 3. the imprint of all or part of the dental arch or teeth using appropriate dental materials

imprint a mark made by pressure; a depression in a surface

imprinting differential effects of maternally and paternally derived DNA; a specialised form of learning occurring early in life and often influencing behaviour later in life

impulse (in'puls) an act of driving outward with sudden force **cardiac** i heartbeat felt at the cardiac apex **excitatory** i impulse stimulating the activity **inhibitory** i impulse dampening the activity **nerve** i an electrical change transmitted along the membrane of a nerve **proprioceptive** i an afferent nerve impulse arising from stimuli originating in joints, muscles, tendons or other sensory endings

impulsion idea to do something

IMV intermittent mandatory ventilation *see* ventilation

Inaba a serotype of *Vibrio cholera*

inanimate without life

inaction (in-ak'shun) failure of response to a stimulus

inactivation rendering inactive

inadequacy (in-ade'-kwa-se) insufficiency; incompetence

inanimate not alive; lifeless

inanition (in'a-nish'un) marked weight loss and weakness

inapparent not noticeable

inarticulate not jointed; not articulate; lack of ability to express; inability to use articulate speech

inaudible incapable of being heard

inborn formed during intrauterine life; innate or inherent

inbreeding a mating of closely related individuals

INC Indian Nursing Council

incarcerated hernia herniation of a loop of intestine into a mesothelial sac that cannot return to its original position without surgery

incarceration unnatural retention of a part

inception 1. beginning 2. ingestion 3. intrussusception.

incest (in'sest) sexual intercourse or activity between close blood relatives

incidence (in'si'dans) the frequency of occurrence of any event or condition over a period of time; the number of new cases of a disease in a specified period, usually per year **i rate** the incidence rate per 1000 persons in a population is the number of new cases that occur within a defined unit of time, divided by the persons exposed or at a risk during the same unit, multipled by 1000

incidentaloma an incidentally-discovered tumour mass detected by imaging procedures or other modality

incineration (in-sin'er-a'shun) the act of burning

incinerator a furnace to burn the solid wastes

incipient (in-sip'e-ent) coming into existence

incisal (in-si'zal) cutting

incise (in-siz) to cut

incision (in-sizh'un) a cut or a wound produced by a sharp instrument

incisor (in-si'zor) that which cuts **i teeth** one of the four anterior teeth in each jaw at the front of the mouth used for cutting through food

incisura (in-si-su'ra) a notch as in bone

incitant (in-sit-ant) stimulus that sets off a reaction, disease or incident

incite to stimulate

inclusion an act of enclosing **i body** a particle of foreign (virus or lead) or metabolically inactive materials (Mellory body) within the cytoplasm or nucleus of a cell **i blennorrhoea** inclusion conjunctivitis **i body myositis** an idiopathic myositis causing atrophy and weakness of quadriceps **i conjunctivitis** inflammation of the conjunctiva

i criteria the condition in which a person must meet to join a clinical trial **dental i** a tooth unable to erupt due to excessive surrounding tissue

incoagulability (in'ko-ag'ula-bil'i-te) not coagulable

incoherence (in'ko-her'ens) inability to express coherently

incoherent (in'ko-he'rent) not understandable, without logical connection; disjointed

incompatibility quality of not being suitable for mixing

incompatible not compatible; pertaining to biologic substances which interfere with one another physiologically; pertaining to drugs which interfere with one another physiologically

incompetence insufficiency or inadequate ability to function **aortic i** regurgitation of blood through the aortic valve **mitral i** leaky mitral valve allowing regurgitation of blood from left ventricle to left atrium **pulmonary i** inability of pulmonary valve to close permitting regurgitation of blood to right ventricle **tricuspid i** leaky valve allowing blood to flow backward into right atrium

incomplete not complete **i fracture** a fracture wherein the bone is broken partially across **i miscarriage** a miscarriage in which not all of the foetal and placental tissue has been expelled from the uterus

incomprehensible unintelligible, not understandable

incontinence inability to control the passing of natural discharges or evacuations as urine or faeces **faecal i** an involuntary passage of faces can develop following obstetric trauma, severe diarrhoea, anorectal diseases or cauda equina lesions of urine when urinary retention progresses to a point at which bladder can no longer expand and pressure within the bladder exceeds outlet pressure noted in outflow tract obstruction or neurologic abnormalities **stress i** laxity of pelvic floor musculature causing urine leak in women **urinary i** an involuntary loss of urine in large amounts, may be transient or persistent **retention and overflow i** incontinence

incoordination (in'ko-or'-di-na'shun) inability to produce a coordinated action; lack of coordination

incretins gastrointestinal hormones secreted in response to oral administration of nutrients such as gastrin-inhibiting polypeptide

incubate to place in an optimal condition for development

incubation (in'ku-ba'shun) 1. the process of incubating period; the period lapsing between entry of a pathogen and appearance of the clinical features 2. development of pathogens

incubator 1. an apparatus in which media inoculated with microorganisms are cultivated in appropriate temperature 2. enclosed crib where oxygen, temperature and humidity are regulated to take care of prematurely born infants

incudal (ing'ku-dal) relating to the incus

incudectomy (ing'ku-dek'to-me) surgical removal of all the parts of incus

incudomalleal (ing'ku-do-mal'e-al) pertaining to the incus and malleus in the middle ear

incudostapedial (ing'ku-do-sta-pe'de-al) pertaining to the incus and stapes in the middle ear

incurable not capable of being cured

incus (in'kus) the middle one of a chain

of small bones in the middle ear which conduct vibrations from the tympanic membrane to the inner ear; anvil

indentation a notch, pit or depression

independent variable *stat* a variable studied in relation to an outcome or dependent

index (in'deks) 1. an indicator 2. the forefinger 3. the ratio of the measurement of a given substance with that of a fixed standard 4. a sequential arrangement of material; gives an idea of how many are affected, and how many are having different grades of the disease. pl. **indices cardiac i** the cardiac output of blood **cephalic i** skull breadth multiplied by 100 and divided by the length of the skull **i card** small card used for recording information and usually filled in an index **i case** the first disease as contrasted with the appearance of subsequent cases **i cells** densely hyperchromatic cells seen in small cell carcinoma of the lung **i finger** forefinger **pelvic i** the ratio of pelvic conjugate and transverse diameters. **thoracic i** the ratio of the thoracic anteroposterior diameter to the transverse diameter

indeterminate indefinite, uncertain

inebriant (in-e'bre-ant) an intoxicant

Index Medicus a publication of the National Library of Medicine that lists the articles published in the journals of biomedical and health sources

India ink a black pigment consisting of lamp black mixed with glue **i cells** densly hyperchromatic cells seen in small carcinoma of the lung **i preparation** an even smear is made on a slide by placing a loopful of culture and loopful of India ink. Organisms do not take up the stain. A depot is formed around the cells. Colourless cells appear against dark background. **I spot nuclei** nuclei that have dark homogeneous chromatin and a smooth contour seen occasionally in keratinising epidermoid carcinoma

Indian childhood cirrhosis a fatal familal disease of early childhood onset, first described in middle class Hindu families of rural india. It is characterised by fever, anorexia, hepataomegaly, fulminant cirrhosis and hepatic failure, excessive dietary copper intake appears to be the cause and discontinuation of use of copper cookware has reduced its incidence

Indian cobra a highly venomous cobra, *Naja naja* found in India and it has makings resembling a pair of spectacles on the back of the foot

Indian multipurpose food vegetable blend consisting of 25% roasted Bengal gram flour and 75% groundnut cake, fortified with minerals and vitamins

indication (in'dika-shun) a sign or situation that indicates the proper treatment of a disease

indifferent 1. not responsive to normal stimuli 2. cells that have not differentiated

indigenous (in-dij'en-us) orginating in and characterising a particular region, native

indigestible (in-di-jest'ti-bl) not digestible; not easily digested

indigestion common disorder producing nausea, belching, gas bloating, heart burn and abdominal cramps brought on by eating

indigo a blue dye

indirect laryngoscopy a method of examining the larynx with a mirror

indisposition a mild illness or disorder

indistinct not distinct, not clearly distinguishable

indriya(s) faculties in the body *antar i* mind, consciousness, ego and memory

indole (in'dol) the product of bacterial decomposition of tryptophans. It is partially responsible for faecal odour

indoleacetic (in'dol'ase'tik) **acid** a major terminal metabolite of tryptophan

indolent (in'do-lent) lazy, causing little or no pain

indomethacin (in'do-meth-a-sin) an antiinflammatory analgesic and antipyretic agent

Indomoeba butschilli a non-pathogenic amoebae

induce (in-dus) to move by persuasion or influence

induction (in-duk'shun) initiation **i chemotherapy** drug treatment given as a primary treatment for those presenting with an advanced cancer **i of labour** use of drugs to initiate the process of child birth

indurate (in'du-rat) to make hard

induration (in'du-ra'shun) 1. the process of hardening 2. the hardened area of a tissue

indwell to possess; to inhabit

indwelling inside the body such as catheter, drainage tube or other device remaining inside the body

inebriation (in-e'bre-a'shun) the condition of being drunk, state of intoxication

inelastic not elastic, lacking flexibility

inert (in-ert) having no action.

inertia (in-er'she-a) inactivity; sluggishness **uterine i** absence or weakness of uterine contractions of labour

infancy early period of life of an infant; early childhood

infant a young child; baby. **i mortality rate**

$$\frac{\text{number of deaths under 1 year} \times 1000}{\text{number of live births}}$$

infanticide (in-fan'ti-sid) the act of killing of viable conceptus that is older than 20 gestational weeks

infantile (in'fan'til) pertaining to an infant. **i paralysis** poliomyelitis **i glaucoma** buphthalmos, enlargement of the whole eye in infant **i pyloric stenosis** presence of visible peristalsis from left to right where the infant vomits the water that is imbibed

infantilism (in-fan'til-izm) a condition wherein the characters of childhood persist into adult life

infarct an area of necrosis due to a deficient blood supply

infarction the formation of an infarct

myocardial i an infarction in the cardiac muscle due to coronary occlusion.
pulmonary i infarction due to pulmonary embolism
Infatuation a shallow, intense attraction to another person
infect to affect with disease-producing organisms
infection (in-fek'shun) the invasion of the body by microorganisms that reproduce and multiply causing disease **acute i** an infection that occurs suddenly **airborne i** an infection caused by inhalation of microorganisms in the air **apical i** an infection located at the apex of the lung or at the tip of the root of a tooth **blood-borne i** an infection transmitted through contact with blood **chronic i** an infection having a prolonged course **cross i** the transfer of an infection from one patient to another in the hospital **droplet i** an infection acquired by inhalation of a microorganism in the air especially one added to the air by coughing or sneezing **endogenous i** reactivation of a quiescent primary lesion as in tuberculosis **exogenous i** infection acquired from outside from an active case **local i** infection confined to the site of entry **nosocomial i** an infection acquired during hospitalisation **opportunistic i** any infection that results during immunocompromised conditions **pyogenic i** an infection resulting from pus-forming organism **secondary i** infection made possible by a primary infection that lowers host's resistance **subacute i** an infection intermediate between acute and chronic **subclinical i** an infection without presenting symptoms **systemic i** an infection in which the infecting agent is found throughout the body
infectious (in-fek'shus) capable of being communicated by infection **i disease** any communicable disease **i mononucleosis** glandular fever. An acute infectious condition caused by

Epstein-Barr virus. It principally occurs in teenagers and young adults. The virus infects and replicates in B lymphocytes. It is characterised by exudative tonsillitis, petechial rash on palate, lymphadenopathy, splenomegaly and maculopapular rash. There is atypical lymphocytosis and treated symptomatically
infective (in-fek'tiv) capable of producing infection. **i arthritis** disease of joints resulting from the invasion of bacteria. **i endocarditis** microbial infection of a heart valve, the endocardium or blood vessel or a congenital anomaly. The causative organism is usually a bacteria often *Streptococcus viridans, S. faecalis, Staphylococcus aureus* and rarely a rickettsia, chlamydia or fungus. **acute** presents as a severe febrile illness with prominent and changing heart murmurs and petechiae. Embolic events are common. *Staphylococcus aureus* is a common cause. **i hepatitis** inflammation of the liver due to hepatitis virus (A,B,C,D, E) EBV, CMV, herpes simplex, which results in damage to hepatocytes. It presents with nausea, anorexia, fatigue, jaundice and hepatomegaly **i parotitis** *see* mumps **Post-operative i endocarditis** affects the valve ring and presents with unexplained fever in a patient who has undergone heart valve surgery. **subacute i endocanditis** presents with persistent fever in a patient known to have congenital or valvular heart disease. It is associated with clubbing, splinter haemorrhages under finger or toe nails, painful tender swellings at the finger tip (Osler's nodes), splenomegaly, petechial rash, changing murmurs and microscopic haematuria. Vegetations are demonstrated by echocardiography. Benzyl penicillin and other antibiotics are to be given
infecund (in-fe-kun'd) barren
infer to derive by reasoning

inference the act of inferring

inferential statistics methods used for drawing general conclusions about probabilities on the basis of a sample

inferior (in-fe're-or) located below a point of reference **i vena cava** large vein draining deoxygenated blood to the heart from parts of the body below the diaphragm. It is formed by the junction of two common iliac veins at the right of L5 vertebra and ascend along the vertebral column ultimately to open into the right atrium

infertile not fertile, sterile

infertility sterility; the inability of a couple of reproductive age to produce offspring, inspite of having regular unprotected sexual intercourse

infestation presence of animal parasite such as lice or mites on the skin or hair or worms inside the body

infibulation (in-fib-u-la'shun) the process of fastening as in joining of the lips of the wound

infiltrate (in-fil'trat) to penetrate a tissue to filter into; to permeate

infiltration (in'fil-tra'shun) growth of tissue or cells which are not normal or in amounts in excess of the normal **cellular i** an infiltration of blood cells into tissues; invasion of malignant cells into adjacent tissue **fatty i** a deposit of fat in the tissues

infirm feeble or weak

infirmary a hospital for care of sick

infirmity feeble state; physical weakness; ailment

inflammation a bodily response to injury, infection or destruction characterised by heat, redness, pain, swelling and disturbed function referred to as *calor, rubor, dolor, tumour* and *functio laesa* respectively

inflammatory pertaining to or marked by inflammation **i bowel disease** genetic or environmental factors causing an infiltration of the intestinal wall with acute and chronic inflammatory cells as in ulcerative colitis and Crohn's

disease; IBD **i carcinoma** invasion of dermal lymphatics with malignant cells mostly of breast origin **i oncotaxis** the attraction of malignant cells to the sites of tissue trauma **i response** occurs from a complex interplay of different mediator cascades such as complement, cytokines, chemokines, inflammatory cells found in circulating blood such as neutrophils, eosinophils, and monocytes and the tissue cells

inflate to distend; to swell

inflation (in-fla'shun) the distension of a part by air, gas or liquid

influenza (in'floo-en'za) flu; an acute infection of the respiratory tract by influenza virus A and B characterised by sudden onset of fever, headache, malaise, myalgias and arthralgias with dry cough and nasal discharge. Influenza C virus causes upper respiratory tract infection. The virus is transmitted in respiratory secretions. Treatment is symptomatic. Amantadine and rimantadine can shorten illness if given early in cases of influenza A. Inactivated influenza vaccine offers protection against influenza A and B

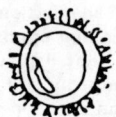

Influenza virus

influx an inflow

informed consent 1. an agreement to participate in a clinical trial, or to take part in a test, after full written or verbal explanation of the trial including the risks and benefits of participation 2. permission to surgical or diagnostic procedure after getting a thorough explanation of the procedure and the risks involved

infra below i clavicular below the clavicle i costal below the ribs i diaphragmatic below the diaphragm i mammary below the mammary gland i nuclear peripheral to a nucleus i orbital beneath the orbit i patellar bursitis painful swelling adjacent to insertion of the patellar tendon into tibial tubercle i red the part of the invisible spectrum that is contiguous to the red end of the visible spectrum i scapular beneath the shoulder blade i sonic sound wave frequency lower than those normally heard i spinous beneath the scapular spine i umbilical below the umbilicus

infrequent occurring rarely

infundibulum (in'fun-dib'u-lum) structure having a funnel-shaped passage

infuse to instill

infusion (in-fu'zh'un) the introduction of a fluid, drug or nutrient into a blood vessel or body cavity i pump an apparatus designed to inject measured amounts of a drug over a period of time

ingestant (in-jes'tant) a substance taken by oral route

ingestion the act of taking any substance into the body through the mouth

ingrain to fix deeply and freely

ingravescent gradually increasing in severity

ingredient (in-gre'de-ent) any part of a compound or a mixture

ingress act of entering

ingrowth an inward growth

inguinal (ing'gwi-nal) pertaining to the groin i hernia protrusion of part of the intestines into the muscles of the groin i axillary veins superficial venous communications between the axilla and femoral triangle. They may get dilated on one side if there is pressure on the common or external iliac vein of that side or both sides if there is inferior vena caval obstruction i canal a narrow passage in the lower part of the abdominal wall, extending from the internal (abdominal) ring to the

external (subcutaneous) inguinal ring. Its length is 4 cm, in men it transmits spermatic cord and ilioinguinal nerve and in women the round ligament of the uterus and the ilioinguinal nerve. It forms a channel for descent of indirect inguinal hernia i region the iliac region on either side of pubes i triangle bounded by deep epigastric vessels, Poupart's ligament, and outer border of rectus sheath, described by Hesselbach, a German surgeon also called Hesselbach's triangle

INH isonicotinic acid hydrazide.

inhabit to live in

inhalant a substance that can be taken into the respiratory tract

inhalation (in'ha-la'shun) the act of drawing air or other substances into the lungs

inhale (in-hal) to breathe in

inhaler a device to administer a drug in powder or vapour form by inhalation dry powder i (DPI) a breath actuated device which permits inhalation of medication in powder form metered dose i (MDI) drug either dissolved or suspended in a liquid propellant mixture of chlorofluorocarbons and surfactant in a sealed canister, aerosol is released on actuation

inheritance (in-her'i-tans) the acquisition of characters from the parents to children through the influence of genes

inhibin (in-hib'in) a peptide hormone released by the testicular Sertoli cells that inhibits FSH, also produced by the ovarian granulosa cells in response to FSH

inhibit to arrest

inhibition (in'hi-bish'un) arrest a process.

inhibitor a substance interfering with the process

ingrown grown inwardly i toe nail one or both edges of the nail of big toe pressing into the adjacent skin resulting in infection and inflammation

inimical unfriendly, unfavourable as in climate

inion (in'e-on) the most prominent point of the external occipital protuberance

initiate to begin, to introduce

initiation *mol* the first step in the synthesis of polypeptide chain. It requires the formation of a ribosome-mRNA-initiator tRNA complex

injectable capable of being injected

injection (in-jek'shun) the act of introduction of a drug, liquid or vaccine into the tissue or vasculature or an organ from a syringe through a needle **intralesional i** injection of a large dose of a drug in a small volume of vehicle, directly in a place where it is required to act, example corticosteroids **intramuscular** injection into the muscles in the anterior thigh, deltoid or buttocks **intraosseous i** injection of an anaesthetic directly into the cancellous bone of the alveolar process adjacent to the tooth **intraperitoneal i** injection into the peritoneal cavity **intrapleural i** injection into the pleural cavity **intravenous i** injection into a vein **subcutaneous i** injection beneath the skin

injector a device for making injections

injury trauma or damage to some parts of the body

inlay (in'la) a solid filling made to the precise shape of a cavity of a tooth and cemented into it

inlet a passage leading to a cavity

innate genetically determined behaviour patterns **i releasing mechanism** sensory mechanism selectively responsive to specific external stimuli and responsible for triggering the stereotyped motor response

innervation (in'rt-va'shun) nerve supply to a part

innocent (in'o-sent) **murmur** any cardiac murmur that occurs in a normal person

innocuous (i-nok'u-us) innocent

innominate (i-nom'i-nat) nameless such as hip bone, brachiocephalic artery and brachiocephalic trunk

inoculate (in-ok'u-lat) to communicate a disease by inserting the causative agent to introduce vaccine or immune serum.

inoculation (in-ok'u-la'shun) introduction of infective agent, vaccine, serum into the tissues

inoculum (in-ok'u-lum) a substance introduced by inoculation

inocyte (in'o-sit) fibroblast

inoperable unsuitable for surgery

inorganic not pertaining to living organisms

inosculation (in-os'ku-la'shun) anastomosis

inositol (in-os'i-tol) a member of vitamin B complex.

inotropic (in'o-trop'ik) affecting the force of muscular contractions **i agent** agent that maintains tissue perfusion. They are sympathetic catecholamines such as dopamine and dobutamine

inpatient a patient who is hospitalised

inquest a legal inquiry into the manner of a death

insane (in-san) mentally deranged

insanity mental derangement with unreliability of behaviour with concomitant danger to himself and other

insatiable (in-sa'she-a-bl) incapable of being satisfied

inscription (in-skrip'shun) the body of prescription giving the names of the drug

insect organism belonging to class Insecta of the phylum arthropoda, flies, mosquitoes, lice, fleas, ticks, spiders, bees, hornets and wasps are some examples

insecticide (in-sek'ti-sid) a preparation causing destruction of insects

insemination (in-sem'in-a'shun) deposition of semen into the vagina or cervix

insensible not perceptible

insert (in'surt) to put or set in , to introduce or cause to be introduced into the body of something

insertion 1. the movable attachment of the distal end of the muscle 2. placement or implantation 3. *mol* the interposition of one or more nucleotides in a chain of DNA or RNA

insidious (in-sid'e-us) gradual

insight *psy* ability of the patient to understand the true cause and meaning of a situation **impaired i** diminished ability to understand the objective reality of situation **intellectual i** understanding of the objective reality of a set of circumstances, without the ability to apply the understanding in any useful way to master the situation **true i** understanding of the objective reality of situation coupled with the motivation and emotional impetus to master the situation

in situ (in si'tu) (L) in place, confined to the site of origin **in situ hybridisation** hybridisation of a DNA probe to a metaphase chromosome spread or a tissue section on a slide

insoluble (in-sol'u-bl) incapable of being dissolved

insomnia inability in getting sleep or remaining asleep

inspection visual examination of the external surface of the body

inspiration (in'spir-a'shun) inhalation, drawing air into the lungs

inspiratory (in-spir'a-ter-e) pertaining to inspiration. **i capacity** the maximum amount of air a person can breath in after a resting expiration **i reserve volume** (IRV) the volume of air that can be inspired by maximum voluntary effort starting from resting and inspiratory position

inspissation (in-spi-sa'shun) the process of rendering the material dry or thick

instillation (in'stil-a'shun) administration of a liquid drop by drop

instinct (in'stingkt) a developmental process resulting in species typical behaviour

instruction 1. a direction or command 2. the act of teaching 3. furnishing information

instrument (in'stroo-ment) 1. a mechanical device 2. a special equipment for accomplishing specific tasks

insufficiency (in'su-fish'en-se) the condition being not adequate for a given purpose

insufflation the act of blowing gas or powder into a body cavity

insufflator (in'su-fla-tor) an instrument used to perform insufflation

insula (in'su-la) 1. island 2. a triangular area of cerebral cortex lying in the floor of lateral fissure

insulation protection of a body or substance with nonconducting medium

insulin a protein hormone produced by the beta cells of the islets of Langerhans in the pancreas. It is essential to the body's use of glucose as an energy source. It lowers blood glucose by suppressing hepatic glucose production and stimulating peripheral uptake mainly in skeletal muscle and fat

insulin-dependent diabetes mellitus (IDDM), diabetes beginning in childhood requiring regular injections of insulin. *see* Diabetes

insulin-like growth factor (IGF) IGF-1 a polypeptide hormone structurally similar to proinsulin which is synthesised in the liver and fibroblasts. IGF-2 a protein structurally homologous to IGF-1 that may be produced by tumours

insulin kinase an enzyme that activates insulin

insulin lipodystrophy the loss of local fat deposits in diabetes patients as a complication of repeated insulin injections

insulin pen a device with the size and shape of a pen to administer insulin. It is a syringe containing prefilled insulin cartridge with a very fine needle

insulin preparations they are rapid acting (regular and semilente), intermediate acting (NPH-isophane and lente), long acting (ultra lente and protamine zinc insulin– PZI). The purified porcine and human insulins are actrapid, insulatard, mixtard and huminsulin

insulin pump an implantable device that delivers insulin at low levels at a regulated rate

insulin-regulatable glucose transporter (IGRT), a protein expressed in muscle and fat that migrates from the cytoplasm to plasma membrane in response to insulin. It results in increased intracellular transport of glucose

insulin resistance a condition exhibiting suboptimal response to physiological levels of insulin. It may be due to increased circulating glucogan or a relative insulin receptor deficiency where plasma insulin is high relative to glucose

insulin shock administration of excess insulin causes profound hypoglycaemia to that required for normal brain function

insulin tolerance test a test of body's ability to utilise insulin. The blood glucose is measured periodically following administration of insulin. The blood glucose falls in thirty minutes and returns to normal after 90 minutes. The fall in glucose in patients with hypoglycaemia is lower and is slower to return to normal

insulinoma (in'su-lin-o'ma) a tumour of the beta cells of the islets of Langerhans that secretes excessive amounts of insulin. It causes a marked fall in the amount of glucose in the blood which can lead to collapse and coma

insulitis infiltration of the islets of pancreas with mononuclear cells in type I diabetes

insult any stressful stimulus which results in morbidity when it occurs in a background of preexisting compromised condition

intake (in-tak) that which is taken in especially food and liquids

integrase (in-te'graze) an enzyme that the virus uses to insert the genetic material into that of an infected cell

integration (in'te-gra'shun) bringing together of various parts or functions so as to perform in harmony

integrin the receptor on cell surfaces that links proteins and chemical mediators

to increase cell to cell communication

integument (in-teg'u-ment) a covering, the skin.

intellect thinking; mild; conscious brain function

intellectual property rights patents, copyrights and trademarks

intelligence the ability to understand; ability to think and comprehend **i quotient** *see* quotient

intensity a state of increased force or energy

intensive care unit (ICU), a special unit in the hospital for patients who because of their illness, injury or surgery require continuous monitoring of their condition by specially trained staff

intention (in-ten'shun) 1. a natural process of healing 2. purpose **first i** healing without granulation **second i** healing by adhesion of two granulated surfaces. **third i** healing of an ulcer or cavity by filling with granulation tissue and cicatrization

inter - prefix meaning between

intercellular between the cells

intercellular adhesion molecule–1 (ICAM-1), production of a protein ligand induced by gamma-interferon required for neutrophils to migrate into inflamed tissue

interclavicular between the clavicles

interferon (in-ter-fer'on) biologic substances elaborated by the viral infected host cells and they inhibit subsequent viral replication **interferon alpha and beta** produced by leucocytes and fibroblasts **interferon gamma** produced by T cells, NK cells and fibroblasts

interleukins protein substances that regulate immune responses. They are produced by several different cell types rapidly (Table 6)

intercostal between the ribs

interlobar between the lobes

interlocking a rare complication of vaginal delivery of twins where the first twin presents in breech and descends locking his head above the head of the second twin

intermediate-density lipoprotein (IDL), a plasma lipoprotein formed by VLDL hydrolysis with lipoprotein lipase. It transports cholesterol from the intestine to the liver

intermittent (inter-mit'ent) suspending activity at intervals **i claudication** an intermittent cramp-like pain occurring in the extremity during exercises and relieved by rest. It occurs due to accumulation of P substance in occlusive vascular diseases **i limping** a patient with endarteritis is unable to meet the demand of blood supply of the muscles on walking and the muscles go into cramp and patient limps intermittently

intern (in'tern) a fresh medical graduate receiving training in the hospital by rotation in different disciplines over 12 months before being eligible to receive licence to practice medicine

internal within the body; within; inward **i capsule** a fan-like mass of white fibres in the brain between the lentiform nucleus and caudate nucleus and thalamus. It consists of an anterior limb, a genu and a posterior limb carrying the afferent and efferent fibres of the cerebral cortex **i fixation** method to hold together the fragments of a fractured bone with pins, wires, screws, nails and plates **i injury** any wound or damage to the viscera **i malleolus** the round process of tibia forming the internal surface of the ankle joint **i medicine** the branch of medicine concerned with the study of pathophysiology, diagnosis and management of disorders of internal organs **i os** the internal opening of cervical canal **i rotation** the turning of a limb inward the midline of the body **i secretion** secretions in which substances pass directly from a gland into the blood stream **i version** a procedure that attempts to convert a difficult foetal presentation to a vaginally deliverable situation

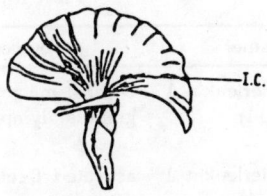

Brain : internal capsule.

International classification of diseases ICD a system of disease classification which is regularly updated by WHO

international system of units SI, an internationally standard system of units. It is measured as metre (length), kilogram (mass), second (time), ampere (electric current), kelvin (temperature), candela (luminous intensity) and mole (amount of a substance)

international unit IU, an internationally-sanctioned unit of measurement for a naturally occurring substance such as hormone, enzyme or vitamin

Internet (in'ter-net) A worldwide network of computers linked together via telephone and cable lines. An access to internet allows one to retrieve information from millions of sources

internist a physician specialised in internal medicine

internship (in'tern-ship) the period an intern undergoes training in a hospital or health centre

internuncial (in'ter-nun'she-al) centre of communication between the nerve cells

interosseal situated between the bones

interosseus pl. **interossei.** situated between bones such as muscles, ligaments or vessels

interosseal muscles muscles of the hands and feet, intergrity of the muscles is tested by card test, wherein the patient keeps the fingers straight and a piece of stiff paper is inserted into an interdigital cleft and the patient is asked to grip the paper between the

Table 6 : Interleukins and their function

Name	Sources	Functions
Interleukin 1 (IL-1)	B cells, macrophages, large granular lymphocytes	activation of lymphocytes and macrophages, increased leucocyte-endothelial adhesion, fever
Interleukin 2 (IL-2)	activated T-cells	activation of T-cell cytotoxic responses
Interleukin 3 (IL-3)	T-cells	colony stimulation factors, stimulation of production of pleuripotent stem cells
Interleukin 4 (IL-4)	activated T-cells, mast cells	proliferation and differentiation of B and T-cells, IgE isotype switching
Interleukin 5 (IL-5)	T-cells, mast cells	B cells and haemopoietic cell growth and differentiation of eosinophils
Interleukin 6 (IL-6)	monocytes, fibroblasts, transformed T-cells	growth and differentiation of B, T and haemopoietic cells
Interleukin 7 (IL-7)	bone marrow stromal cells	growth and differentiating factor for B and T cells
Interleukin 8 (IL-8)	many cell types on induction with IL-1, TNF lipopolysaccharides, infective agents	chemotactic activating factor for neutrophils, T-cells and eosinophils
Interleukin 9 (IL-9)	T-helper cells	mast cell activation
Interleukin 10 (IL-10)	T-cells, macrophages, monocytes, T-cells, keratinocytes	potent immunosuppressant, inhibits cytokine synthesis, enhances B-cell growth
Interleukin 11 (IL-11)	bone marrow stromal cells	inflammatory mediator, growth factor for megakaryocyte colonies
Interleukin 12 (IL-12)	macrophages, B-cell	production on interferon gamma, activates NK cells
Interleukin 13 (IL-13)	T-cells	growth of B-cells, IgE isotype switching
Interleukin 14 (IL-14)	T-lymphocytes	stimulates proliferation of B-cells
Interleukin 15 (IL-15)	macrophages, other cell types	growth of T-cells

fingers. When the paper is pulled the clasping fingers offer resistance and when the grip is feeble the paper just slides out of the cleft

interparietal (in'ter-pa-ri'e-tal) 1. between the walls 2. between the parietal bones or lobes

interpersonal concerning the relations between persons

interphalangeal (in'ter-fa-lan'je-al) situated between two contiguous phalanges

interrogation history taking, to elicit the symptoms of the patient

interphase 1. a stage of cell division during which there is replication of DNA 2. the area or zone where two phases of a substance (a gas and liquid) come in contact with each other

interpolation 1. the study and analysis of a radiograph and the integration of the findings with the clinical picture 2. *psy* the deeper analysis of the statements made by the patient

interscapular situated between the scapulae.

intersection the site where one structure crosses over another

intersegmental (in'ter-seg-men'tal) between segments

intersex (in'ter-seks) an individual exhibiting features of both sexes in varying degrees.

interspace the space between two similar parts.

interstitial (in'ter-stist'al) in the interspaces of a tissue **anterior i nerve** it is tested by asking the patient to flex the terminal joint of the thumb when it is held at the metacarpophalangeal joint in order that no movement occurs at that place. **i deletion** loss of DNA or part of a chromosome which does not occupy a terminal position **i keratitis** occurrence of blindness **i lung disease** disease of lungs characterised by inflammation and disruption of gas exchanging parts of the lung affecting diffusion capacity **posterior i nerve** supplies external digitorum, which is

tested by asking the patient to resist the attempt to flex the extended fingers **tertiary i orchitis** rounded, densely hard 'billiard ball' like testis in its scrotal covering as in syphilis

intertrigo (in'ter-tri-go) dermatitis occurring on opposed surfaces of the skin **acute i** a painful deep fissure in a fold of skin with inflammatory changes in surrounding skin commonly the retroauricular fold or the interdigital areas **candidial i** areas of erythema, itching and burning in a fold of skin as in groins, interdigital spaces of toes or fingers, under breast, caused by candida **i haemorrhage** bleeding from internal organs presents with increasing pallor, increasing pulse-rate and there may be restlessness and air hunger

interview the process of getting information from a person by asking questions and recording the answers

intertrochanteric (in'ter-tro'kan-ter-ik) between the greater and lesser trochanter of the femur

interval a space or time between two objects or periods

intervention (in'ter-ven'shun) action taken to modify an effect

interventricular between the ventricles

intervertebral between two adjacent vertebrae

intestinal pertaining to the intestine

intestine (in-tes'tin) the largest portion of digestive system extending from the pyloric opening of the stomach to the anus; bowel; gut. It is divided into the small intestine and large intestine **large i** large intestine extends from the ileocaecal junction to the anus and is of 1.5 m in length. The mucosa has no villi but contains mucous secreting glands. It absorbs water, minerals and vitamins and eliminates undigested material during defecation. It consists of caecum, vermiform appendix, ascending colon, transverse colon and descending colon, sigmoid colon, rectum, anal canal and anus **small i** small intestine consists of duodenum, jejunum and ileum. Duodenum receives chyme from the stomach through pyloric orifice and by common bile duct, bile from the liver and gall bladder and pancreatic juice from pancreas. Ileum opens into the caecum and ileocaecal valve prevents regurgitation of intestinal contents. The wall of intestine contains circular folds of mucosa and submucosa containing villi and microvilli which provide surface area for absorption of products of digestion

intima (in'ti-ma) an innermost layer of an artery containing continuous layer of endothelial cells

intolerance an inability to endure or an incapacity to bear pain; effects of a drug

intorsion (in-tor'shun) rotation of the eyeball inwards towards the nose

in toto entirely, wholly, altogether

intoxicant (in-toks'i-kant) an agent that produces intoxication

intoxication the state of being intoxicated by a drug, or alcoholic beverage **water i** excessive retention of water from excess ingestion of water, administration of hypotonic solutions, or oxytocin or increased secretion of ADH. It is characterised by abdominal cramps, dizziness, lethargy, convulsions and coma

intra-abdominal within the abdomen

intra-arterial within the artery

intra-articular (in'tra-ar-tik'u-lar) within a joint

intrabronchial (in'tra-brong'ke-al) within a bronchus

intracapsular within a capsule **i extraction** surgical technique for cataract removal wherein the nucleus, cortex and capsule are removed together

intracardiac with the heart

intracath an inflexible needle surrounded by a catheter which is inserted into a vein

intracellular (in'tra-sel'u-lar) within the cell

intracerebellar (in'tra-ser'e-bel'ar) within the cerebellum

intracerebral (in'tra-ser'e-bral) within the cerebrum

intracranial within the cranium or skull

intractable (in'trak'ta-b'l) unresponsive to treatment

intradermal (in'tra-dermal) within the skin

intraepithelial neoplasia an *in situ* carcinoma that is confined to an epithelium

intralobar (in'tra-lo'bar) within a lobe

intramedullary (in'tra-med-u-lar'e) 1. within the medulla oblongata 2. within the spinal cord 3. within the bone marrow cavity

intramural within the walls of a hollow organ or cavity

intramuscular inside or into a muscle

intranasal within the nasal cavity

intraocular within the eyeball

intraoperative (in'tra-op'er-a'tiv) occurring during operation

intraorbital within the orbit

intrapartal the period from the onset of labour to its termination

intrapartum (in'tra-par-tum) occurrence during childbirth

intrapelvic (intra-pel'vik) within the pelvis

intraperitoneal within the peritoneal cavity

intrapleural within the pleural cavity

intrascrotal (in'tr-skro'tal) within the scrotum

intraspinal within the spinal cord

intrathecal (in'tra-the'kal) within the spinal canal

intrathoracic (in'tra-tho-ras-ik) within the thorax

intratracheal (in'tra-trak-e-al) introduced into the trachea

intrauterine (in'tra-u'ter-in) within the uterus **i contraceptive device** (IUCD), a device with a small, flexible plastic frame. It often has copper wire or copper sleeves on it. It is inserted into a woman's uterus through her vagina. It has one or two strings or threads tied to them, which hang through the opening of the cervix into the vagina. It works chiefly by preventing sperm and ova from meeting. It is very effective and does not interfere with sex. Hormone-releasing IUDs release small amount of progesterone or levonorgestrel **i device** (IUD) **i growth retardation** a decreased rate of foetal growth may occur as a result of any condition that interfer with the blood supply to the placenta or general health and nutritional status of the mother

intravasation (in-trav'a-za'shun) entry of extraneous material into the blood vessel through traumatic or pathologic conditions

intravenous (in-tra-ve'nus) inside a vein.

intravesicle (in'tra-ves'i-kal) within the urinary bladder

intrinsic located in or originating from a tissue or organ **i asthma** a variety of asthma where an extrinsic allergen can't be identified as the cause, and asthmatic attacks are not mediated through IgE **i factor** a vitamin B_{12} binding glycoprotein secreted by the gastric parietal cell

introflexion (in'tro-flek'shun) a bending inwards

introitus (in-tro'i-tus) an opening or entrance into a canal or cavity as the vagina

introjection *psy* identification of the self with another person or object

intromission (in'tro-mish-un) insertion of one part into another, as insertion of the penis into the vagina

intron segment of DNA which is transcribed but does not contain coding information for a polypeptide; intervening sequence

introversion (in'tro-ver'shun) the turning outside in of an organ

introvert individual having his interest toward himself

intubation (in tu-ba'shun) the introduction of a tube into any hollow organ **endotracheal i** insertion of an

endotracheal tube through the mouth or nose into the trachea to maintain the airway **nasogastric i** *see* nasogastric intubation

intubator a device for controlling, directing and placing an intubation tube within the trachea or blood vessel

intuition knowing something without going through a rational process of thinking

intumescence 1. a swelling 2. the process of enlarging

intussusception (in'tu-su-sep'shun) one part of the intestine telescoping into the lumen of adjoining part. It is felt as a hard swelling as the wave of peristalsis begins often in the right hypochondrium. It may be associated with a red-current jelly exudate from the rectum

inulase (in'u-las) an enzyme that converts inulin to levulose

inulin a vegetable homopolysaccharide of D-fructose used to measure renal clearance

inunction (in-ungk'shun) the act of applying an ointment with friction

in utero (in-u'ter-o) (L) within the uterus

in vacuo (in vak'u-o) (L) within a cavity from which air has been removed

invaginate (in-vajiin-at) to infold a part of a structure within another part

invagination the infolding of one part within another **i test** a little finger when inserted into the inguinal canal if finds it empty in presence of a lump, the swelling can't be inguinal hernia

invalid disabled

invasion attack, enter

invasive 1. a medical procedure in which body tissues are penetrated by an instrument 2. a cancer exhibiting a tendency to spread beyond its site of origin

invasiveness ability to enter and to spread

inventory any list of items

inversion (in-ver'shun) a turning inside-out

invert (in-vert) 1. homosexual 2. to turn inside out or upside down

invertase (in-ver'tas) enzyme that converts a disaccharide into a monosaccharide

invertebrate species of animals not possessing a backbone

inverted comma sign a radiologic abnormality in a plain chest film of variation of the azygos lobe which is invested with its own pleural membrane in the medial aspect of the right upper lobe

invertor (in-ver'tor) a muscle that rotates a part inwards

investing ensheathing with a coating or a suitable material

investment a covering or sheath

inveterate chronic

in vitro (in-ve'tro) (L) within a test tube or in an artificial environment **i fertilisation** (IVF), a method of treating infertility. An ova is removed from a woman, and fertilised in the laboratory with sperm and reinserted into her uterus or a fallopian tube **i fertilisation and embryo transfer.** IVF-ET fertilisation in the laboratory of an ovum taken from the woman with subsequent return of the developing embryo into the woman's uterus

in vivo (in-ve'vo) (L) occurring within the living body

involuntary occurring without conscious control

involute to return to normal size after enlargement

involution (in'vo-lu'shun) turning inward; a retrograde process; reduction in size

iodamoeba (Ii-da-me'ba) a genus of amoeba found in the intestinal tract

iodide (io-did) a compound of iodine containing another element as potassium iodide **i mumps** bilateral parotid enlargement after administration of iodine

iodine (i'o-din) an essential micronutrient, mostly present in the thyroid gland in the form of thyroglobulin. It is essential to form thyroid hormone. It is found in sea foods and iodised salts. Its de-

ficiency results in goitre or cretinism. Radioisotopes of iodine are useful in radioisotope scanning and in palliative treatment of cancer of thyroid

ion an atom or a group of atoms carrying positive (cation) or negative (anion) electric charge **i channels** voltage activated proteins that control the permeability of cells to specific ions such as sodium, potassium, calcium and chlorides by opening or closing in response to differences in potentials across the plasma membrane

ionisation the dissociation of substance in solution into ions

ionising radiation radiation used in therapy to destroy malignant tumours and in x-ray imaging. It may cause genetic or cellular damage

iontophoresis (i-on'to-fo-re'sis) 1. the introduction of ions of soluble salts into the tissues by electric current 2. the process of electric current passing through a salt solution causing migration of positive ion to the negative pole and the negative ion to the positive pole

IOP abbreviation of intraocular pressure

IP abbreviation for incubation period

iopanic acid a radiopaque dye used in cholecystography

ipecac (ip'e-kak) the dried root of ipecacuanha, source of emetine

IPPB abbreviation for intermittent positive-pressure breathing

IPPV abbreviation for intermittent positive- pressure ventilation

ipratropium bromide an anticholinergic administered by inhalation, used in COPD

ipsilateral (ip'si-lat'er-al) situated on the same side

IQ intelligence quotient, a measure of a person's intelligence. It is based on the results of special tests

iridectasis (ir'id-ek-ta'sis) dilatation of the iris or pupil

iridectome (ir'i-dek'tom) an instrument for cutting the iris in iridectomy

iridectomy surgical removal of a part or all of the iris of the eye

iridocyclitis inflammation of the iris and of the ciliary body

iridodilator the dilator muscle of the pupil

iridodonesis (ir'id-o-do-ne'sis) abnormal tremulousness of the iris on movements of the eye

iridokeratitis (ir'id-o-ker'a-ti'tis) inflammation of the iris and cornea

iridology (i'rid'i-o-logi) a technique of diagnosis of a person's state of health by studying the appearance of the iris

iridomalacia (ir'id-o-ma-la'she-a) softening of the iris

iridoplegia (ir'id-o-ple'je-a) paralysis of the sphincter of the iris

iridoptosis (ir'i-dop-to'sis) prolapse of the iris

iridotomy (ir-i-dot'o-me) incision of the iris

iris 1. the circular pigmented membrane suspended between the lens and the cornea with pupil at the centre. It separates anterior chambers of the eyeball. By contraction it regulates the amount of light that enters the eye. **irides** the godess of the rainbow in Greek mythology for whom the iris of the eye is named. **i bombe** bulging of iris forward by pressure of the aqueous humour **i lesions** ring-shaped papules with a central purpuric punctum and a peripheral rim of dusky erythema, as in erythema multiforme

iritis inflammation of the iris which can impair vision. It is characterised by pain, photophobia, lacrimation and diminution of vision. Iris is swollen, dull and muddy. Pupil is contracted and irregular.

iron (i'ern) a mineral essential for the production of haemoglobin and enzymes. Iron is used as a haematinic in the form of its salts and complexes such as ferrous sulphate, ferrous gluconate, ferrous fumarate and iron-dextran. Red meat, liver, egg yolk, green leafy vegetables, dry fruits and jaggery are good sources of iron **i deficiency anaemia** a microcytic hypochromic anaemia caused by poor dietary intake, poor bioavailability of iron from cereal-based diets, increased requirements and blood loss

irradiate (i-ra'de-at) to treat with ionising radiation

irradiation 1. treatment by ionising radiation 2. spreading in all directions from a centre

irrational contrary to what is reasonable or logical

irreducible (ir're-du'si-bl) not capable of being reduced as a fracture or hernia

irrigation cleansing an area by flushing it with a stream of water or other fluid **bladder i** washing out of bladder with water or other fluids, often normal saline **colonic i** flushing of the colon with water.

IRV abbreviation for inspiratory reserve volume

irritability 1. excitability 2. excessive response to a stimulus

irritable bowel syndrome (IBS), a functional bowel disorder in which abdominal pain is associated with defecation or a change in bowel habit

irritation 1. a reaction to that which is irritating 2. a normal response to stimulus of a nerve or muscle

ischaemia (is-ke'me-a) deficiency of blood supply to an organ or tissue **myocardial i** an imbalance between myocardial oxygen supply and demand leading to angina pectoris and if untreated to myocardial infarction

ischemic colitis colicky abdominal pain with nausea, tenesmus, fever and bloody diarrhoea resulting from atherosclerosis of the mesenteric arteries supplying the intestine

ischaemic (is'ke-mik) **heart disease** myocardial impairment due to imbalance between coronary blood flow and myocardial requirements. Atherosclerotic coronary artery disease forms the most common cause. Angina pectoris occurs when the vessel is critically narrowed so as to compromise the blood supply to the myocardium during period of stress. Unstable angina is noted when there is spasm over a fixed obstruction or when platelet aggregates occur or in presence of increased sympathetic flow resulting in increased myocardial oxygen consumption. Myocardial infarction occurs when a vessel gets totally occluded

ischaemic reperfusion injury tissue damage following restoration of blood flow in an organ with oxygen deprivation

ischial (us'ke-al) pertaining to ischium

ischiorectal (is'ke-o-rek'tal) pertaining to the ischium and rectum **i abscess** presents with redness and swelling between the anal margin and the ischial tuberosity

ischium (is'ke-um) the inferior dorsal part of the innominate (hip) bone

ischuria retention or suppression of urine

Ishihara's (ish'i-ha'rahz) **test** a test for colour vision using round dots of varying sizes and colours, introduced by a Japanese ophthalmologist, Shinoby Ishihara

island a structure detached from surrounding tissue or characterised by different structure

islet (i'let) a tiny isolated mass of one kind of tissue within another type

islets of Langerhans groups of cells located inside the pancreas that secrete the hormone insulin and glucagon, named after Paul Langerhans, German pathologist

isoagglutination (i'so-a-gloo'ti-na'shun) agglutination of red blood cells by agglutinins from blood of another member of same species

isocoria (i'so-ko're-a) pupils of equal size

isoetharine (i-so-eth'a-ren) beta-2 adrenergic agonist used as a bronchodilator

isoenzyme (i'so-en'zim) a protein catalyst found in different tissues; isozyme

isolate to separate from others

isolation the process of isolating; separation of a patient from other people to prevent him or her from infecting them or from being infected by them

isomer (i'so-mer) chemical substances that have the same molecular formula but different chemical and physical properties due to a different arrangement of the atoms in the molecule

isometric exercise active exercise that strengthens the muscle by applying pressure against resistance

isoniazid (INH), isonicotinic acid hydrazide. A powerful bactericidal agent acting on rapidly dividing extracellular tubercle bacilli, by interfering with the essential enzymes concerned in the terminal steps of the oxidative sequence of susceptible strains of tubercle bacilli. It is absorbed rapidly on oral administration, achieving a peak serum level in 1-2 hours and gets distributed to all organs, metabolised by acetylation in the liver. There is no cross-resistance between INH and other anti-tuberculosis drugs. It is a most widely used drug in the treatment of all types and severity of tuberculosis.

isoproterenol (i'so-pro'to-re-nol) a beta-adrenergic agonist used as a bronchodilator

isoprenaline (i'so-pre'na-lin) a potent, non-selective ß-adrenergic agonist with a very low affinity to a - adrenergic receptors. Used in emergencies to stimulate heart rate in patients with bradycardia or heart block

isospora (i'so-spo-ra) a sporozoan parasite. *I. belli* agent producing acut diarrhoea

isosthenuria (i'sos-then-u're-a) the excretion of urine with the same osmolality as that of plasma despite variations in fluid intake

isothermia (i'so-ther-mea) having same temperature

isotonic (i'so-ton'ik) 1. a solution having same tonicity 2. maintenance of a constant amount of resistance during muscular contraction

isotope (i'so-top) a chemical element possessing the same number of protons and atomic number while differing in the number of neutrons and the atomic mass.

issue (ish'u) 1. offspring 2. a discharge of pus or blood

isthmitis (is-mi'tis) an inflammation of the throat and fauces

isthmus (is'mus) a narrow connection between two larger parts

Italian millet *Setaria italica*, a cereal grain 100 gm supplies 12 gm protein and 378 Kcal energy

itch 1. pruritus 2. scabies **barber's i** tinea barbae **dhobie i** tinea cruris **ground i** a local irritation by penetration of the skin of the foot by hookworm larvae **swimmer's i** dematitis following swimming in water containing larval form of schistosomes

itching an unpleasant cutaneous sensation caused by scratching the skin; pruritis.

itch mite an extremely small, globular arthropod just visible to the naked eye. The female parasite, *Sarcoptes scabei*, is the example

ITP abbreviation for idiopathic thrombocytopaenic purpura

IUCD abbreviation for intrauterine contraceptive device

IUD abbreviation for intrauterine device

IUGR intrauterine foetal growth restriction, failure of foetus to fulfill with programmed growth potential

IV abbreviation for intravenous

Ivermark's (iver-mar-kz) **syndrome** histologic features of congenital hepatic fibrosis in addition to pancreatic cystic and dysplastic changes named after Bjorn Ivermark, Swedish Pathologist

ivermectin an antibiotic useful in the treatment of human filarial infections from *Wuchereria bancrofti*, *Brugia malayi*, and *Onchocerea valvulus*

IVF abbreviation for *in vitro* fertilisation

ivory vertebrae osteosclerosis of vertebrae seen in osteoblastic metastases from adenocarcinoma of prostate

IVP abbreviation for intravenous pyelogram

ixodes (iks-o'dez) a genus of ticks of the family Ixoididae

Ixodidae (iks-od'i-de) a family of ticks which transmit disease in domestic animals and humans, such as Kyasanur forest disease, Rocky mountain spotted fever, Lyme disease, ehrlichiosis and relapsing fever

J

J symbol for joule, unit of energy of work

jaagsiekte (jahg-sek'te) a fatal viral pulmonary adenomatosis of sheep. A Dutch term meaning 'to go quickly in sickness'

jab a sudden thrust or stab

jabber talk in what seems to be a rapid and confused manner

Jaboulay's (zha'boo-laz) operation amputation of the thigh and removal of hip bone, named after a French surgeon, Mathieu Jaboulay

Jaccoud's (zhah-kooz') arthritis recurrent episodes of rheumatic fever with joint abnormalities especially metacarpophalangeal joints, named after French physician, Sigismond Jaccoud

Jaccoud's fever fever associated with slow and irregular pulse noted in adults suffering from tuberculous meningitis, named after a French physician, Sigismond Jaccoud

Jaccoud's sign prominence of the aorta in the suprasternal region

jacket (jak'it) 1. a protective covering of plaster applied especially on the upper part of the body to immobilise the spine 2. an artificial crown composed of acrylic resin Minerva j plaster cast applied to the trunk and head with spaces cut out for the face area and the ears, named after Roman Goddess of wisdom plaster of Paris j a casing of plaster of Paris enveloping the body, used to correct deformities straight j a jacket-like device to restrain the limbs

Jack (jak) used as a familiar name

jack in the box a box with a figure in it that springs up when the lid is opened

jack-knife pocket knife j position lying on the back with shoulders elevated, legs fixed on thighs and the thighs at right angles to the trunk j spasms infantile epilepsy making the body bent sharply at waist

jack screw (jak'skroo) a device containing a screw in a threaded socket, useful in orthodontics to expand the dental arch and move individual teeth, and also to position bone fragments properly after a fracture

Jackson (jak'sun) crib a removable orthodontic appliance retained in position by crib-shaped wires, named after Victor Hugo Jackson, an American dentist

Jacksonian (jak-so'ne-an) epilepsy, named after John Hunglings Jackson, British neurologist, characterised by unilateral clonic movements that begin in one group of muscles and spread gradually to adjacent group reflecting the march of the epileptic activity (e.g. mouth, thumb, great toe) through the motor cortex. The attacks may vary in duration from a few seconds to several hours

Jackson's law the nerve functions that have developed at the end are the earliest to go in a paralysis, framed by John Hunglings Jackson

Jackson's (jak'sunz) membrane a thin sheet of peritoneum passing in front of ascending colon to the lateral part of posterior abdominal wall, named after Jabez Jackson, U.S. surgeon

Jackson's rule after an epileptic attack the simple nervous processes are recovered earlier than the complex ones formulated by John Hunglings Jackson

Jackson's safety triangle sign a triangular space bound below by the lower end of the thyroid cartilage with sides by sternomastoid muscles and apex in the suprasternal notch. Chevaliar Jackson, an American laryngologist, described that the trachea may be safely incised in this region

Jackson's syndrome paralysis of the tenth, eleventh and twelfth cranial nerves of the same side due to vascular lesion in the medulla, named after John Hughlings Jackson, British neurologist

Jacobaeus (yah'ko-ba'us) **operation** removal of pleural adhesions by thoracoscopy and cauterisation, formulated by a Swedish surgeon, Hans Jacobaeus

Jacobine (ja'ko-bin) poisonous alkaloid from plant *Senecio jacobea*, may cause necrosis of the liver

Jacobson's (ja'kub-sunz) **nerve** tympanic nerve, named after a Danish anatomist, Ludwig Jacobson

Jacobson's organ vomeronasal organ present in most mammals but rudimentary in man. It responds to odours in the same way as olfactory receptors, named after Ludwig Jacobson, Danish anatomist

Jacob's (zhah-kobz') **membrane** layers of rods and cones in retina described by Arthur Jacob, Irish ophthalmologist

Jacob's syndrome conjunctivitis, angular stomatitis and scrotal dermatitis due to riboflavin deficiency, described by E.C. Jacob, US physician

Jacquemier's (zhak-me-az) **sign** blue or purple colour of vaginal mucosa sometimes noted after fourth week of pregnancy, described by Jean Jacquemier, a French obstetrician

jactitation (jak'ti-ta-shun) rhythmic rolling, tossing from side to side seen in acute illness

jaculate to throw

Jaeger's (ya'gerz) **test types** use of letters of seven different sizes imprinted on a card to test near vision, named after an Austrian ophthalmologist, Eduard Jaeger

Jaffe's (zhah-faz') **reaction** serum creatinine assay which is based on the red colour of the creatinine complex with alkaline picrate, named after Max Jaffe, German chemist

jag a notch

jaggery (jag'er-i) coarse sugar prepared from sugarcane. 100 gms gives 383 Kcal, energy and 11.4 mg iron

Jaipur foot a cheap light weight water resistant below knee prosthetic device, devised by P.K. Sethi, Jaipur. Rajasthan, that is functional and cosmetically acceptable. The person can walk, climb and squat without any difficulty

Jail bars sign an x-ray of the chest demonstrating dense osteosclerosis of the ribs in the form of horizontal bands simulating the bars of a prison window. It may be encountered in osteopetrosis, sickle cell anaemia and myeloid metaplasia

jail fever louse-borne typhus fever

Jakob Creutzfeldt (jak'ob-kroits'felt) **disease** a rare slow virus encephalopathy with partial degeneration of the pyramidal and extra pyramidal systems, named after two German psychiatrists, Alfons Jakob and Hans Creutzfeldt

jal (s) water *Jeevan j* oral rehydration solution.

jala (s) network

jalap (jal'ap) cathartic from *Ipomoea*

jalauka (s) acquatic blood sucking worm

jalaukya (s) leech. *j. vidhi* application of leeches

jalodara (s) ascites

Jamaican hepatic phlebitis veno-occlusive disease of liver

Jamaican neuropathy tropical spastic paraparesis with sensory ataxia, optic atrophy and nerve deafness

Jamaican vomiting sickness violent vomiting, prostration, convulsions and hypoglycaemia caused by hypoglycin A present in 'bush tea' made from unripe ackee fruit

Jamais vu (zham' a-voo) psychomotor epilepsy with a mental reaction of false feeling of unfamiliarity with a real situation one has experienced

James fibres accessory bundle connecting the atrium with the lower part of AV node or to His bundle. It is a pathway for conduction of cardiac impulses so that they bypass the atrioventricular node. It allows preexcitation of ventricle with resultant tachycardia, described by US physician, T.N. James

Jamshedi's needle instrument to perform trephine biopsy of the bone marrow

Janeway's (jan'waz) **lesion** small, flat erythematous non-tender macules on the thenar and hypothenar eminences in subacute infective endocarditis, described by Edward Janeway, US physician

jangali vaidya (s) tribal physician

jangama (s) motile

janiceps (jan'i-seps) a monster with one head and two faces on its anterior and posterior aspects

Janma(s) birth

Jansen's (yan'senz) **test** inability to cross the legs with a point above the ankle resting on the opposite knee and is seen in osteoarthritis of the hip, named after Murk Jansen, Danish orthopaedic surgeon

Janet's (zhah-naz') **test** a test to differentiate organic anaesthesia from functional anaesthesia, named after Pierre Janet, French physician

Japanese encephalitis JE, an arbo-virus disease spread by bites of infected culicine mosquitoes. Pigs are important sources of infection. Children are more susceptible. It is characterised by abrupt onset of fever, headache, convulsions, altered sensorium, muscular rigidity, drowsiness to deep coma and neurologic deficits. The condition may last from a few days to 2 weeks or longer. The CSF is under raised pressure. The protein and cells are raised. There is no specific treatment

Japanese summer house HP a hypersensitivity pneumonia suspected to be due to house dust or bird droppings containing *Trichosporon cutaneum*

Jaques (zhah-kvez) **catheter** ordinary soft rubber urethral catheter, named after British engineer, Jacques

jar 1. a wide mouthed glass, plastic or earthenware container 2. a sudden movement

jargon (jar'gun) 1. a vocabulary peculiar to a specific profession 2. unintelligible speech **j aphasia** a speech defect wherein several words run into one

and nonsense words repeated with various intonations

Jarish-Herxheimer (yah'rish-herks'him-er) **reaction** profound fall in temperature, shock and cardiac failure within a few hours following administration of drug and it is due to liberation of antigens from killed organisms, named after Austrian and German dermatologists, Adolf Jarisch and Rarl Herxheimer respectively

Jarotzky's (yar-ot'skez) **treatment** dietary therapy for peptic ulcer consisting of eggs, milk, bread and butter, formulated by Alexander Jarotzky, Moscow physician

Jarvell (jar'wel) **syndrome** congenital long QT syndrome

Jarvik-7 an artificial heart, designed by Robert Jarvik, U.S. physician for use in humans. It requires air processor to drive the ventricles

Jarvis' snare a snare for removal of growths in the nasal cavities, named after William Jarvis, US laryngologist

jasper opaque crystalline quartz

jatajanya (s) congenital

Jatane operation anastomosis of the aorta and pulmonary arteries

jatara (s) stomach

jataragni stomach fire, a figurative expression for the heat in the organ which digests food

Jatropha crucas, seeds of *Jangli arandi* containing an acrid oil, which on swallowing causes burning in the throat, vomiting, thirst and depression

jaundice (jawn-dis) yellowish discolouration of the conjunctiva, sclera, mucosa under the tongue and skin due to deposition of bile pigments from haemolytic, hepatocellular or obstructive disorders of hepatobiliary system, and occurs as a symptom **acholuric j** elevated unconjugated bilirubin that is not excreted by the kidney **cholestatic j** jaundice from biliary obstruction with passage of very dark urine and clay coloured stools **drug induced j** chemical compounds and drugs causing liver damage due to either direct hepatotoxicity or by poison. Hypersensitivity may cause hepatic damage **haemolytic j** excess red cell breakdown causing jaundice from excess unconjugated bilirubin **hepatocellular j** jaundice due to hepatocellular injury, dysfunction, inflammation or destruction **leptospiral j** jaundice present with leptospirosis **mechanical j** obstructive jaundice **nonhaemolytic j** jaundice caused by an abnormality in the metabolism of bilirubin resulting in excessive accumulation of unconjugated bilirubin **j of new born** icterus neonatorum **obstructive j** jaundice from biliary obstruction **physiologic j** mild icterus neonatorum lasting the first few days of life

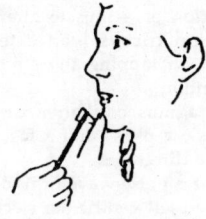

Jaw jerk

jaw bony framework in the face bearing teeth, divided as upper and lower jaw (maxilla and mandible) **dislocation of j** traumatic or spontaneous displacement of the mandible **j bone** a bone of either jaw **j breaker** words hard to pronounce **j drop** bilateral paralysis of the muscles of mastication resulting in failure to elevate the lower jaw **j jerk** reflex elicited by tapping chin with a rubber while mouth is half open and the jaw muscles relaxed. Normally there is no response. An upward jerk closing the jaw occurs in the lesions of upper motor neuron above the level of the pons governing the motor activity of the trigeminal nerve **j thrust** a manoeuvre that manually displaces the jaw to establish an airway during resuscitation **j winking phenomenon** unilateral ptosis wherein lid is lifted following voluntary movements of the lower jaw due to faulty innervation of *levator palpebrae*; Marcus Gunn's syndrome **j wiring** wiring the jaws temporarily to prevent eating and allow liquid feeds only to reduce weight **lumpy j** actinomycosis

J chain a polypeptide allowing polymerisation of immunoglobulins

JC virus a polyoma virus named after the index patient responsible for progressive multifocal leucoencephalopathy in immunocompromised hosts

jecor (je'kur) liver.

Jeddah (jed'ah) **ulcer** cutaneous leishmaniasis named after a city in Saudi Arabia

Jefferson's fracture burst fracture of the ring of the atlas vertebrae, often noted in diving accidents, and is asymptomatic, named after Sir Geoffrey Jafferson, English neurosurgeon

Jeffries probe *Mol* DNA finger printing probe specially useful in paternity testing

Jehovah's witness patients sign a special consent absolving the doctors from problems arising from failure to transfuse blood or blood products

jejunal (je-ju-nal) pertaining to the jejunum

jejunectomy (jejoo-nek-ta-me) excision of jejunum

jejunitis (jejoo-nitis) inflammation of the jejunum

jejunoileal (je-joo'no-il'e-al) concerning the jejunum and ileum **j bypass** anastomosis of approximately 18 cm of jejunum to the terminal 18 cm of ileum

jejunocolostomy (je-joon'o-col'os-tah-me) operative establishment of an anastomosis between the jejunum and the colon

jejunojejunostomy (jejoon-'o-jejoon'os'tah-me) anastomosis between two portions of the jejunum

jejunostomy (jejoo-nos'tah-me) formation of an artificial opening through the abdominal wall into the jejunum **j feeding** administration of liquid foods through a hollow tube inserted into the jejunum through the abdominal wall

jejunum (je-joon'um) empty; the middle portion of small intestine between duodenum and ileum. It is about 2.4 m long forming about two-fifths of the small intestine adj. **jejunal**

Jekyll-and Hyde-syndrome a syndrome seen in elderly who cyclically improve with hospitalization and undergo mental and physical deterioration while at home

Jello sign undulation of the scrotum that occurs with foetal limb movements. It helps in determination of infant's sex by ultrasonography

jelly (jel'e) a translucent soft elastic material containing gelatin and pectin **contraceptive j** a non-greasy jelly used in the vagina as a contraceptive agent **j fish** venomous marine animal **pertroleum j** petrolatum **Whorton's j** the intracellular substance of the umbilical cord

Jendrassik's (yen-dra'siks) **manoeuvre** procedure to enhance the knee jerk wherein the patient hooks his hands together by flexed fingers and tries to pull them apart vigorously, named after Erno Jendrassik, Hungarian physician

Jenner's (jen'erz) **stain** eosin methylene blue stain evolved by Louis Jenner, British physician

Jennerisation (jen'er-i-za'shun) production of immunity to a disease by inoculation of an attenuated virus producing the disease, named after English physiciar, Edward Jenner

Jensen's (yen'senz) **classification** a classification of bacteria based on their nutritive characteristics, named after Orla Jensen, Danish physiologist

jentigo a histologic finding consisting of a combined junctional naevus and simple lentigo

jerk (jurk) a sudden reflex, involuntary muscular movement **ankle j** contraction of calf muscles on tapping the stretched Achilles tendon **biceps j** a reflex contraction, of the biceps brachii on tapping the thumb of the evaluator, placed over the insertion of the tendon at the head of the radius in the cubital fossa **jaw j** a movement that occurs on tapping the mandible when the jaw is half open **knee j** the extension of the leg due to contraction of quadriceps femoris on striking the patellar tendon when the knee is flexed **supinator j** flexion of the elbow and the finger flexion on striking the styloid process of the radius **tendon j** the contraction of a muscle after tapping its tendon **triceps j** an extension of forearm on tapping the stretched triceps tendon

jerky nystagmus oscillation of the eyes with a slow phase and a fast phase in opposite directions

jerky pulse a pulse waveform found with shortened left ventricular ejection as in severe mitral regurgitation, hypertrophic obstructive cardiomyopathy and in heart failure

Jervell-Longe Nielsen syndrome deafness with cardiac dysrhythmias, long QT interval and enlarged T-wave, named after Jervell and Longe Nielsen, US physicians

jessur (jes'ur) Russell's viper, Bengali name

jesuit a member of a Roman catholic religious order

jet humidifier a humidifier that increases the surface area for exposure of water to gas by breaking the water into small aerosol droplets

jet lag an acute shift in the circadian rhythm, caused by travelling across multiple time zones resulting in excess day time sleepiness, insomnia, alterations in mood and performance efficiency

Jet lesion development of vegetation when a regurgitant jet of turbulent blood flow strikes the endocardium, causing fibrosis and roughening of the endocardial wall as in infective endocarditis

jet nebulizer a humidifier that converts a source of liquid into a fine mist of aerosol particles

jet phenomenon a narrow column of barium gushing past the stenosis due to an oesophageal web

jet ventilation intermittent blowing of high velocity stream of humidified gas into the endotracheal tube at rapid frequencies, entraining additional fresh gas during insufflation

Jeune's (ju'nz) **syndrome** asphyxiating thoracic dystrophy with a small thorax, pulmonary hypoplasia, polydactyly, biliary dysgenesis and may have a component of renal dysplasia, named after Mathis Jeune, French paediatrician

Jewett (joo'et) **nail** a nail for internal fixation of a trochanteric fracture, named after Eugene Jewett, U.S. surgeon.

jhin jhinia (jin jin'e-ah) tingling sensation in the sole of feet accompanied by trembling

jiggers infestation with jigger flea, *Tunga penetrans*

jiggle to move to and fro or up and down with short, quick jerks

jignasa (s) inquiry

jigsaw puzzle cells bizarre erythrocytes of variable size and shape simulating pieces of a jigsaw puzzle. Such poikilocytes may be due to mechanical damage as in severe hereditary spherocytosis

jigsaw puzzle tumour cylindroma of the skin, histologically exhibiting cell islands consisting of central light staining cells with large nuclei and peripheral palisade of cells with small dark nuclei

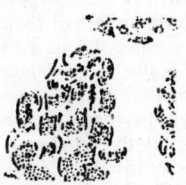

Jigsaw puzzle tumour

jihva (s) tongue

jirna (s) senile; digest

jitatma (s) restrained in mind.

jitters (jit'erz) nervousness; an uneasy nervous feeling

jiva (s) life; principle of life; personal soul

jivan (s) organisation of the physical body, mind, sensory faculties and soul

jivitam (s) life

J-junction *ECG* the junction of QRS and the ST segment in the electrocardiogram

jnana (s) conscious

jnanendriya (s) sense organs – visual, auditory, gustatory, olfactory and touch

Jo-1 a clinical complex related to the production of antibodies against the Jo-1 antigen which is associated with polymyositis

Job's (jobz) **horn probe** instrument for ENT examination

Job syndrome recurrent infections of the skin due to impaired defense, associated with high levels of serum IgE and defective neutrophil and monocyte, chemotaxis named after a Biblical character.

Jacosta (jo-kas'ta) **complex** sexual attraction of mother towards her son after Jocasta of Greek mythology, who was mother of Oedipus

jocund (jok'und) cheerful, merry, pleasant.

jocose merry, humorous

jod iodine

jod Basedow (i'od-bas'e-do) **phenomenon**

development of acute hyperthyroidism as an adverse effect of iodine supplementation especially in a hyperplastic endemic goitre, named after German physician, Carl von Basedow

Joffroy's (zhof-rwhaz) **sign** absence of wrinkling of the forehead when the eyes are suddenly turned upwards while the head is bent down. It may be seen in thyrotoxicosis, described by Alexis Joffroy, French physician

jog to run at a steady slow pace.

jogger's heel an irritation of the fibrous and fatty tissue covering the heel. It is encountered in joggers in whom the heel strikes the surface first

jogging running at a slow pace, usually over a long period as part of physical exercise

Johne's (yo'nez) **disease** enteritis in cattle from *M. paratuberculosis* named after Heinrich Johne, German pathologist

Johnson's (john'sonz) **method** a technique to fill root canals in dentistry with plastic material

Johnson's test a method to demonstrate protein in the urine sample wherein a white coagulum appears on pouring a strong solution of trinitrophenol, described by George Johnson, English physician

joint an articulation, a place of junction where two or more bones come in contact. A joint is formed of fibrous connective tissue and cartilage; a cigarette made from dried marijuana (*Cannabis sativa*) leaves (substance abuse) **ball and socket j** a joint in which the round end of one bone fits into the cavity of another enabling movement freely in almost all directions as in hip and shoulder joints **flail j** an unusually mobile joint **hinge j** notably in elbows and knees, swing back and forth like doors on hinges **gliding j** joints permitting a gliding motion as vertebral joints and finger joints **j capsule** sac-like structure enclosing the ends of bone **j cavity** articular space enclosed

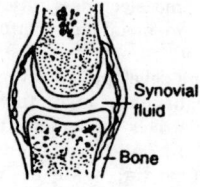

Joint

by the synovial membrane and articular cartilage **j crepitus** when a joint is moved with one hand while the other hand is laid, upon the joint fine crepitus may be appreciated in subacute and chronic affections of the joint and coarse crepitus in osteoarthritis **j fracture** a fracture of the articular surfaces of the bony structures of a joint **j mice** loose bodies composed of fibrous tissue covered by cartilage within the joints as in osteoarthritis **j protection** technique to minimise stress on joints and avoidance of weight bearing **j replacement** arthroplasty where one (partial) or both (total) sides of the deformed joint surfaces are replaced with prosthesis **j sense** sense of passive movement. The patient is asked for the direction of the movement of the joint as soon as he appreciates. It is lost in posterior column disorders **j space** radiologic appearance produced by separation of bones by articular cartilages **saddle j** each of the bones is concave in one direction, convex in the other and allow movement at right angles to each other, as in wrist and thumb **simple j** joint in which only two bones articulate **spheroidal j** a synovial joint in which a spheroidal surface of one joint (ball) moves within the concavity of (socket) the other bone **suture j** inflexible joints in adult skull **synovial j** union of the bony surfaces being surrounded by an articular capsule enclosing a cavity lined by synovial membrane **temporomandibular j** a bicondylar joint formed by the head of the mandible and the mandibular fossa, and the articular tubercle of the temporal bone **uniaxial j** one which permits movements in one axis only

Jolle's (yol'ez) **test** demonstration of colours in urine in presence of bile pigments, test devised by Adolf Jolles, Austrian chemist

Jolly's (zho-lez') **reaction** absence of response to faradic stimulation in a muscle, named after Friedrich Jolly, German neurologist

Jones' criteria major and minor manifestations of acute rheumatic fever, described by T. D. Jones, US physician. The major manifestations are polyarthritis, carditis, chorea, subcutaneous nodules and erythema marginatum. The minor manifestations include fever, arthralgia, previous rheumatic fever or known rheumatic heart disease, raised levels of ESR or C-reactive protein, leucocytosis, first degree or second degree AV block. Presence of two major or one major and two minor criteria establishes the diagnosis of rheumatic fever

Jones' (jonz) **position** acute flexion of the forearm for treatment of fracture of the internal condyle of the humerus, named after Sir Robert Jones, English surgeon

Jones' nasal splint a splint for fracture of nasal bones, named after John Jones, American surgeon

Jones' test fluorescein instilled into conjunctiva reaches nasopharynx if lacrimal passage is patent

Jorgensen technique a method of intravenous sedation, introduced by Jorgensen of United States by injection of pentobarbitone supplemented by a mixture of pethidine and hyoscine. The technique though safe requires long induction and recovery times

Joseph complex intense sibling rivalry

Joseph disease striatonigral degeneration and degeneration of dentate nucleus of cerebellum with features of Parkinsonism, named after Joseph, an Azorean family affected by the disease

joule (jool) unit of work or energy-named after English physicist, James Joule

Jourdain's (zhoor-daz') **disease** suppurative inflammation of the gums, named after Anselme Jourdain, French surgeon

journal club a medical education programme where a group meets once a week or month to discuss, analyse and review a limited number of articles from major medical journals

jowl lower part of the face flesh hanging from the chin

J-point *ECG* a point on ECG indicating end of S wave, and beginning of normally flat ST segment

J-pouch a faecal reservoir formed surgically by folding the distal end of the ileum in an ileoanal anastomosis, preserving anal sphincter

J-receptors juxta pulmonary capillary receptors located close to pulmonary capillaries within the interstitium of the alveolar walls, described by A.S. Paintal of India, which behave as interstitial stretch receptors and are stimulated by distortion of the interstitial space, as with interstitial oedema or fibrosis, and mediate the rapid shallow breathing encountered in those conditions

J-reflex stimulation of J receptors produces the pulmonary chemoreflex, a triad of apnoea, bradycardia and hypotension

J segment *Mol* part of DNA sequence of Ig heavy and light chains

Judd method a technique in radiology for positioning a patient while taking an x-ray of the atlas and odontoid process

judgement ability to assess a situation correctly and act appropriately within that situation **critical j** ability to assess, discern, and choose among different options in a situation **automatic j** reflex performance of an action **impaired j** diminished ability to understand a situation correctly and to act appropriately

Judkin's coronary arteriography coronary catheterization by inserting the catheter *via* femoral artery, named after Judkin, US radiologist

jugal (joo'gl) 1. connecting 2. pertaining to cheek **j bone** zygomatic bone

jugate (joo-ga'te) locked together

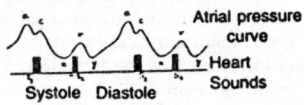

Jugular venous pulse

jugular (jug'u-lar) pertaining to neck **j bulb** slight dilatation of internal jugular vein emerging from skull **j foramen** opening formed by jugular notches of the temporal and occipital bones **j fossa** depression in petrosal part of the temporal bone **j ganglion** nodes of vagus and glossopharyngeal nerve in the jugular foramen **j process** projection of occipital bone towards the temporal bone **j pulse** a pulsation in the jugular vein **j veins** external, draining blood from exterior of the cranium and the deep parts of the face; and internal draining blood from the brain and superficial parts of the face and neck **j venous pressure** vertical distance above sternal angle at which jugular veins collapse. It is measured from the sternal angle when the patient is propped up at 45° angle. The vertical distance between the top of the oscillating venous column to the sternal angle is recorded in cm H_2O **j venous pulse** three positive (a,c,v) and two negative waves (x,y) in the neck veins. The oscillating top of the distended proximal portion of the internal jugular veins represents volumetric changes which faithfully reflect the

right atrial pressure at all stages of the cardiac cycle

jugular glomus (jug'u-larglo'mus) an ovoid structure of 0.5 mm size situated in the adventitia of the superior bulb of internal jugular vein. It consists of two or more masses related to IXth or Xth cranial nerve, and may form tumours

jugulation (jug-u-la'shun) the sudden arrest of disease by therapy

jugulum (jug'u-lum) neck, throat

jugum (ju'gum) a depression or ridge connecting two structures

jugum sphenoidale (joo'gum sphe'no-i-da'le) smooth area on the superior surface of the body of sphenoid bone

juice (joos) any fluid from animal or plant tissue **gastric j** the secretion of the gastric glands **intestinal j** the secretion of glands in the intestinal lining **pancreatic j** the enzyme containing secretion of the exocrine part of the pancreas

jujube lozenges of gelatin, flavoured and sweetened

julab purgative

julep (joo'lep) a sweet liquid drink in which other nauseous medicine is taken

jump to move from one Web page to another

jumper syndrome blunt trauma from jumping or falling from heights and is associated with multiple fractures

jumping (jump'ing) the skipping of several steps in a series **j gene** *Mol* a unit of genetic information found in a DNA segment that can move from one position in the genome to another

junction (junk, shun) the place of meeting or coming together **dentinocemental j** the line of meeting of the dentin and cementum on the root of a tooth **dentino enamel j** the plane of meeting between dentin and enamel on the crown of a tooth **gap j** a narrow portion of the intercellular space containing channels linking adjacent cells and allowing passage of ions **gastro-oesophageal j** the site of transition from the stratified squamous epithelium of the oesophagus to the simple columnar epithelium of the cardia of the stomach **ileocaecal j** the junction of the ileum and caecum, located in the right lower abdomen **mucocutaneous j** the site of transition between skin and mucous membrane **myoneural j** neuromuscular junction **neuromuscular j** the site of opposition between a nerve fibre and the motor end plate of the skeletal muscle which it innervates **sclerocorneal j** the line of union of the sclera and cornea **tight j** an intercellular junction at which adjacent plasma membranes are joined tightly together

junctional (junk'shun-al) pertaining to a junction **j rhythm** heart beat arising in or near AV node which is slow and regular **j naevus** a mole which can become highly malignant **j tachyarrhythmia** rhythm due to re-entry within the AV node generally without any structural heart disease with normal QRS complexes at a rate of 140-220 beats per minute

junctura (junk-too'rah) 1. a site of union between different structures 2. suture of bones

Jung's (yoong) **method** analytic psychology, named after Carl Jung, Swiss psychiatrist

Jungling's (yeng'lingz) **disease** sarcoidosis, named after German surgeon, Otto Jungling

Junin virus infection acute febrile illness characterised by haemorrhagic manifestations, marked myalgia and shock found particularly in workers harvesting corn; Argentine haemorrhagic fever

juniper (joo'niper) the dried ripe fruit of *Juniperus communis* which possesses diuretic property

junk DNA *Mol* repetitive DNA sequences that serve no known function

junk food food containing lot of fat and sugar and hardly any roughage

jurisprudence (joor'is-pro'dens) the scientific study or application of the principles of law and justice

juscul broth, soup

jute (jut) strong, coarse fibres of tropical shrub, *Corchorus capsularis*

juvantia (joo-van'she-ah) adjuvant and palliative medicines or appliances

juvenile (joo'venil) young or immature **j aponeurotic fibroma** a benign tumour of fibrous tissue of the hand and wrist in children or adolescents **j arthritis** chronic polyarthritis seen in childhood **j cell** the early developmental form of white blood cells **j delinquency** habit of indulging in antisocial or criminal acts by older children **j diabetes** insulin-dependent diabetes mellitus **j glaucoma** raised intraocular tension in an young individual due to development of structural defects restricting the outflow of fluid **j myoclonic epilepsy** a seizure disorder seen in adolescence, affecting the flexor muscles of the head, neck and shoulders, the attacks occur as clonic-tonic-clonic seizures upon awakening **j nephronopthisis** an autosomal recessive condition causing renal failure in childhood **j polycystic kidney disease** a recessively inherited disorder with multiple cysts in kidney with hepatic fibrosis and cysts which leads to renal and/or hepatic failure early **j periodontitis** periodontitis affecting adolescents, characterised by an early loss of alveolar bone surrounding permanent teeth **j polyposis** multiple benign colonic polyps present with bleeding **j rheumatoid arthritis** arthritis developing in persons less than 16 years; juvenile chronic arthritis **j spinal muscular atrophy** progressive degeneration of anterior horn cells leading to skeletal muscle wasting and it begins in childhood **j xanthogranuloma** a skin disorder with yellow, or brown papules or nodules on the extensor surfaces of the arms and legs, and the lesions are noted in infancy or early childhood and disappear later

juxta (juks'tah) near to or adjoining **j articular** near a joint **j epiphyseal** (juks'ta-ep-i-fiz-i-al) adjoining an epiphysis **j glomerular** (juks'tah-glo-mer,ul-er) adjacent to a glomerulus **j glomerular apparatus** granular cells in the wall of afferent arteriole before its entry into glomerulus, which secrete renin and possibly erythropoietin **j phrenic peak** a triangular opacity with its base on the hemidiaphragm near the highest point of the dome, a radiographic sign of atelectasis **j position** (juks'ta-pah-zish'un) placing close together or side by side **j spinal** near the spinal column

jvara (s) fever *jirna j* chronic fever *jvarahara* antipyretic

JVP jugular venous pulse, jugular venous pressure

J-wave *ECG* appearance of a wave in hypothermia at the junction of the QRS complex with the ST segment in ECG. It disappears on rewarming the patient.

K

k symbol for potassium

k symbol for kilo

Kahn (kan) test 1. a serologic precipitin test for syphilis, devised by American bacteriologist, Reuben Kahn 2. a three dimensional projective test to assess psychosexual development, devised by American psychiatrist, Theodore Kahn

kakamukha (s) crow-shaped surgical instrument.

kakke disease *see* **Beri beri.**

kala (s) extremely minute anatomical structures; time, season *k janya* disease due to seasonal changes

Kala-bala-pravrtta (s) diseases having their origin in time such as seasonal changes

kala azar (ka'la-az'ar) (H) Black disease, visceral leishmaniasis, an infectious disease caused by *Leishmania donovani*. It is carried by sand flies (phlebotomous). They multiply in the cells of reticuloendothelial system, and cause irregular fever, anaemia and hepatosplenomegaly. It is prevalent in Bihar and West Bengal, India. Also called Dumdum fever. It is treated with sodium stibogluconate and meglumine antimoniate (pentavalent antimonials), pentamidine methanosulphate and amphotericin B

kalaemia presence of potassium in the blood.

kalakrta (s) passage of time.

kaliopaenia (ka'le-o-pe'ne-a) hypokalaemia

kalium potassium

kaliuresis (ka'le-u-re'sis) potassium excretion in the urine

kalka (s) paste

kallidin (kal'i-din) a kinin liberated by the action of kallikrein or a plasma globulin; bradykinin

kallikrein (kal'i-krei'n) a group of enzymes that help in conversion of kininogen to a vasodilator substance, bradykinin

kallikrein-kinin system endogenous vasopeptides that maintain blood pressure. Kallikrein stimulates renin release and kinin production. Kinins are potent vasodilators and natriuretics

kallikreinogen (kal'I-kri-nah-jen) the inactive precursor of kallikrein

Kallmann's syndrome a condition characterised by absence of the sense of smell due to agenesis of the olfactory bulbs and by secondary hypogonadism; named after Franz Kallmann, American psychiatrist

kaluresis (kal'u-re'sis) increased urinary excretion of potassium.

kama (ka'ma) (s) erotic desire

kamale (s) jaundice.

Kamino body an eosinophilic inclusion found in the epidermis

kanamycin (kan'ah-mi-sin) antibiotic from *Streptomyces kanamyceticus* effective against aerobic, gram-negative bacteria and some gram-positive bacteria including mycobacteria

Kanavel's (kan-a'velz) **sign** point of maximal tenderness in suppurative tenosynovitis, described by Allen Kanavel, US surgeon

Kandahar sore cutaneous leishmaniasis, named after city in Afghanistan

kandara (s) tendon responsible for movements

kandu (s) itching

Kane surgery any surgical procedure performed by the surgeon on himself, named after O'Neill Kane, who operated upon himself for an inguinal hernia, appendicitis and amputation of a finger

Kangri cancer development of heat-induced squamous cell carcinoma due to wearing kangri basket made of *cinar*

wood on abdomen to keep the body warm, seen in Kashmir

kanka mukha (s) heron faced surgical instrument

K antigen antigens present on the surface of gram-negative bacteria such as Klebsiella species and *Escherichia coli*

kaolin (ka'o-lin) hydrated aluminium silicate acting as an adsorbent

kaolinosis (ka'o-lin-o'sis) pneumoconiosis caused by the inhalation of clay dust, kaolin

Kapha (s) 1. one of the three *doshas* in the body and it is composed principally of water and has inertia in its general orientation. It is viscous, cold, white, smooth, heavy and compact. It is aggravated by day time sleep, laziness, inactivity and certain foods; phlegm *k. prakrti* a person with *kapha* constitution, tender and clear complexion, pleasing appearance, well formed muscular body, firm mind, slow in action 2. phlem, sputum, expectoration

kappa the tenth letter of the Greek alphabet, a light chain immunoglobulin

kappa chain one of the two light chain immunoglobulins

Kaposi's (kap'o-se') **sarcoma** a multifocal malignant neoplasm of reticuloendothelial cells involving skin, described by Austrian dermatologist, Moritz Kaposi. An opportunistic neoplasm often associated with AIDS

karana (s) causal

karaya (kar'aya) (H) a bulk cathartic

Karelian (ker'i-lean) **fever** a culicine mosquito -borne Sindbis viral infection seen in Egypt, characterised by malaise, fever, myalgia, arthralgia, tendonitis and vesicular rash

karma (s) action directed towards therapy

karmendriya (s) organs of action such as hands, feet, speech, anus and genital organs

karna (s) ear *k. purana* filling the ear

Karnofsky (kar'nof-ski) **scale** a scale of objective criteria for the quality of life, used in patients with incapacitating disease named after David Karnofsky, American oncologist

Kartagener's (kar-tag'-enerz) **syndrome** an immotile cilia syndrome, described by Swiss physician, Manes Kartagener, presenting with dextrocardia, bronchiectasis, sinusitis and sterility

kary(o) – combining word for nucleus of a cell

karyoclasis (kar-e-ok'la-sis) fragmentation of a cell nucleus

karyocyte a nucleated, immature normoblast

karyogamy (kar'e-og'ah-me) union of nuclei of cells as in fertilisation

karyogenesis (kar'e-o-jen'e-sis) formation of a cell nucleus

karyokinesis (kar'e-o-ki-nesis) division of the nucleus into two equal parts in the early stages of cell division, mitosis. **karyokinetic,** adj

karyolymph (kar'e-o-limf) the liquid portion of the nucleus of a cell

karyolysis (kar'e-ol'i-sis) the dissolution of the nucleus of a cell, **karyolytic,** adj

karyon (kar-e-on) the nucleus of a cell

karyophage (kar'e-o-faj) phagocytosis of the nucleus of the cell

karyoplasm (kar'e-o-plasm) nucleoplasm, the substance of the nucleus of a cell

karyopyknosis (kar'e-o-pik-no'sis) shrinkage of a cell nucleus with condensation of the chromatin

karyorrhexis (kar-e-o-rek'sis) rupture of the cell nucleus resulting in disintegration and extrusion of chromatin. **karyorrhectic,** adj

karyosome (kar'e-o-som') condensed irregular clumps of chromatin dispersed in the chromatin network of a cell

karyotin (kar'eo'tin) nuclear material; chromatin

karyotype (kar-e-o-tip) the chromosomal constitution of the cell nucleus

karyotyping chromosome analysis

Kasabach-Merritt syndrome a rapidly enlarging haemangioma and thrombocytopaenia noted during early infancy, described by Haig Kasabach, US paediatrician and Merrit, US physician

kasaghna (s) cough suppressant

kashaya (s) 1. decoction 2. astringent flavour

kashta sadhya (s) with difficulty.

kata (s) extremely minute anatomical structures

Katayama fever acute systemic schistosomiasis due to *Schistosoma japanicum* and *S. mansoni* presenting with serum sickness-like disease. The condition was first reported from Katayama river valley in Japan

kathina (s) hard

katolysis (kah-tol'i-sis) incomplete breakdown of complex chemical substances into simpler compounds, as in digestion

katu (s) pungent

Kaumara(s) pertaining to children   **k bhrtya** paediatrics, care of children

Kava intoxicating drink made from the roots of a shrub

Kawasaki disease mucocutaneous lymph node syndrome of undetermined aetiology affecting children under age 5 years. It presents with high fever, rash, conjunctivitis and cervical lymph node enlargement. It was first described by Japanese paediatrician, Tomsaku Kawasaki. There is a high incidence of coronary artery aneurysms, occlusions and myocardial infarction. Treatment includes aspirin in large doses and supportive care

kaya (s) body *k chikista* one of the eight branches of Indian medicine dealing with physical and mental diseases of the adult. *k sadhana* to make the body efficient.

Kayser-Fleisher (ki'zer-fli'sher) **ring** a gray- green to red-gold pigmented ring at the outer margin of cornea, described by German ophthalmologists Bernard Kayser and Bruno Fleisher. It is seen in Wilson's disease and pseudosclerosis

Kcal kilocalorie

K cell killer cell; Kulchitsky cell

Kco carbon monoxide gas transfer coefficient

kD kilodalton

Kearn's syndrome external ophthalmoplegia, pigmentary degeneration and cardiomyopathy

Kearns-Sayre (ke'arnz-sa're) **syndrome** a single large mitochondrial deletion presenting with progressive external ophthalmoplegia, retinitis pigmentosa, heart block, hearing loss, short stature, ataxia, peripheral neuropathy and delayed secondary sexual characters, named after Thomas Kearns, US ophthalmologist and George Sayre, US Pathologist

Kegel exercises specific exercises to strengthen the pelvic-vaginal muscles to control stress incontinence in women, and to strengthen the pelvic floor, and are named after Arnold Kegel, a gynaecologist who devised them first

Kehr's (karz) **sign** patient with haemoperitoneum when lies flat on the back with foot of bed raised, the liquid blood gravitates towards the under-surface of the diaphragm causing referred pain in one or other shoulder, described by Hans Kehr, Berlin surgeon

Keith's (keths) **node** sinoatrial node of the heart, named after Sir Arthur Keith, British anatomist

Keith-Wagener-Barker classification a classification of degree of hypertension and arteriosclerosis based on retinal changes; constriction of retinal arterioles (grade I); constriction and sclerosis of retinal arterioles (grade II); cotton-wool exudates and haemorrhages in the background of grade II hypertensive retinopathy (grade III), and papilloedema (grade IV), named after Norman Keith, Canadian-US physician, Henry Wagener, US Physician and N.W. Barker, US Physician.

Kell blood group one of the human blood groups showing presence of red cell antigens (k gene) that react with antibodies (anti-k) and cause haemolytic disease, named after a patient in whom the antibodies were first discovered, named after propositus first observed

Kellgren's (kel'grinz) **syndrome** erosive

osteoarthritis, described by Swedish physician, Henry Kellgren

Kellogg Speed's test method to test the integrity of the anterior horn of the medial semilunar cartilage, described by US surgeon, Kellogg Speed

Kelly clamp a curved haemostat forcep without teeth, devised by American gynaecologist, Howard Kelly, to grasp vessels in gynaecological procedures

Kelly-Paterson syndrome iron deficiency anaemia associated with dysphagia, named after Joseph Kelly, US otolaryngologist and Donald Paterson, laryngologist from Wales; also referred as Plummer Vinson syndrome

Kelly plication surgical plication of bladder-neck and urethra for stress incontinence of urine, named after Howard Kelly, US surgeon

keloid (ke'loyd) a progressively enlarging firm, elevated scar with irregular margins at the site of a wound or burn of skin due to overgrowth of collagen. Its surgical removal is often followed by recurrence

keloplasty operative removal of a scar or keloid

kelotomy (kelot'o-me) herniotomy

Kempner (kemp'ner) **diet** rigid salt restricted diet providing 2000 calories, used in the treatment of hypertension, consisting of rice, fruits and sugar, formulated by Walter Kempner, US physician.

ken(o) empty

kennel place where dogs are cared during quarantine

Kenny treatment physical therapy for poliomyelitis, suggested by sister Elizabeth Kenny, an Australian nurse

kenophobia (ken'o-fo-be'a) fear of empty spaces

Kent's bundle an accessory conducting pathway between atria and ventricles, described by English physiologist, Albert Kent

Kent's test estimation of general intelligence by a test consisting of ten oral questions

Kenya tick bite fever an infection from *Rickettsia conorii* characterised by fever, headache, myalgia, eschar and regional lymphadenopathy: Mediterranean spotted fever

Keogh coefficient ratio of diffusion capacity/alveolar ventilation

Kerandel's (ker'and'elz) **sign** avoid closing doors in Gambian sleeping sickness, named after Jean Francois Kerandel, Fvench Physician in Africa.

kerasin (ker'a-sin) a cerebroside found in brain tissue

keratalgia (ker'ah-tal'je-a) pain in the cornea

keratectasia (ker'atek-ta'she-a) protrusion of a thin scarred cornea

keratectomy (ker'ah-tek'to me) excision of a portion of the cornea

keratic (ker-at'ik) horny

keratin (ker'a-tin) a scleroprotein consisting of sulphur that is a major component of epidermis, hair, nails, horny tissues and the organic matrix of the enamel of the teeth

keratinase (-as) a proteolytic enzyme that catalyses the cleavage of keratin

keratinocyte (ker-at'in-o-sit) the epidermal cell that synthesises keratin

keratinisation process of development of/ or conversion into keratin.

keratinise (ker'-atin-iz) to become hard or horny

keratinous (ke-rat'inos) composed of keratin; horny

keratitis (ker'ah-tit'is) inflammation of the cornea

keratoacanthoma (ker'ah-to-ak'an-tho'ma) rapidly evolving tumour of the skin composed of keratinising squamous cells originating from the pilosebaceous follicles. It may resolve spontaneously

keratocentesis (ker'ah-to-sen-te'sis) puncture of the cornea.

keratocoele (ker'ah-to-sel) hernial protrusion of Decemet's membrane of the cornea.

keratoconjunctivitis (ker'a-to-kon-junk'-ti-vi'tis) inflammation of the cornea and the conjunctiva **k sicca** dryness of cornea due to a deficiency of lacrimal secretion seen in Sjogren's syndrome, vitamin A deficiency and trachoma

keratoconus (ker'o-toko'nos) conical protrusion of the central part of the cornea

keratocyte (ker'ah-to-sit) an erythrocyte with one or two notches or horns. Such a phenomenon may occur when the red cells are squeezed through strands of intravascular fibrin as in DIC

keratoderma (ker'ah-to-der'mah) 1. hypertrophy of the horny layer of the skin 2. a horny skin 3. hyperkeratosis **diffuse k** hyperkeratosis of entire surface of the palms and soles **k blennorhoea** thickened scaly lesions of the soles of the feet in Reiter's disease **localised k** hyperkeratosis in localised areas **punctate k** hyperkeratosis in small punctate areas

keratogenous (ker'ah-toj'i-nus) giving rise to a growth of horny material

keratoglobus (ker'ah-to-glo'bus) megalocornea

keratoid (ker'a toid') producing horny substance

keratohelcosis (-hel-ko'sis) ulceration of the cornea

keratoleukoma (-loo-ko'ma) a white corneal opacity

keratolysis (ker'ah-tol'i-sis) loosening of or separation of the horny layer of the epidermis

keratolytic (ker'ah-to-lit'ik) drug causing peeling and softening of the outer layer of the skin, examples being salicylic acid, resorcin, urea, sodium hydroxide and potassium hydroxide

keratoma (ker'ah-to-mah) a callus or callosity

keratomalacia (ker'ah-to-mah-la'she-a) softening and necrosis of the cornea with absence of inflammation noted in vitamin A deficiency

keratome (ker'ah-tom) a knife to incise cornea

keratometer (ker'ah-tom'itar) an instrument used for measurement of the curvature of the anterior surface of the cornea

keratometry (ker'ah-tomi-tre) measurement of the anterior curvature of the cornea by a keratometer

keratomileusis (ker'ah-to-mi-loo'sis) keratoplasty wherein a portion of the patient's cornea is removed and shaped to the desired curvature and sutured back

keratomycosis (-mi-ko'sis) fungal infection of the cornea

keratopathy (ker'ah-top'ah-the), a noninflammatory disorder of the cornea

keratophakia (ker'ah-to-fa'ke-a) keratoplasty wherein a portion of donor's cornea is shaped to a desired curvature

keratoplasty (ker'ah-to-plas'te) corneal grafting

keratorrhexis (ker'ah-to-rek'sis) rupture of the cornea

keratoscleritis (ker'a-to-skler-i-tis) inflammation of cornea and sclera

keratoscope (ker'ah-to-skop') an instrument for determination of the symmetry of the curvature of cornea

keratoscopy (ker'ah-tos'kah-pe) inspection of the cornea

keratose (ker'a-tos) horny

keratosis (ker'ah-to-sis) horny growth

keratotome (ker-at'o-tom) a knife to incise cornea.

keratotomy (ker'ah-tot'ah-me) corneal incision

keratotorus (ker'ah-to-tor'us) a vault-like protrusion of the cornea

kerion (ker'e-on) an inflammatory condition that has produced a boggy swelling on the scalp. It is caused by a superficial fungal infection, common example being *Trichophyton mentagrophytes* or *T. verrucosum*

Kerly lines thickened interlobular connective tissue septa or distended interlobular lymphatics as water-density lines less than 1 mm thick visible radiologically in the region of costophrenic angles (B lines) and in the region of hilum (A lines), described by British radiologist, Peter Kerly, seen in congestive heart failure

kernel (kur'nel) the soft edible part in the shell of a nut

kernicterus (ker-nik'ter-us) a grave form of *icterus neonatorum* presenting with severe neurologic symptoms with high levels of circulating bilirubin in newborn

Kernig's (ker'nigz) sign sign of meningitis, described by Russian physician, Vladimir Kernig, wherein there is an inability to extend the leg completely with thigh flexed upon the abdomen

kerosene a flammable liquid fuel distilled from petroleum

Kerr incision a low transverse incision made in the noncontractile portion of the uterus, pioneered by Kerr for Caesarean section

kesaridhal Lathyrus sativa pulse rich in protein (28%) and carbohydrate (57%)

Keshan disease selenium deficiency in water resulting in dilated cardiomyopathy and increased platelet aggregation, first noted in Keshan province of China

ketamine hydrochloride a non-barbiturate rapidly acting general anaesthetic

keto (ke'to) acid a carboxylic acid containing carbonyl group

ketoacidosis (ke'to-a-si-do'sis) metabolic acidosis due to accumulation of ketone bodies in the blood noted in poorly controlled diabetes mellitus from incomplete metabolism of lipids

ketoaciduria (ke'to-as'id-ur'e-a) the presence of keto acid in the urine

ketoaminoacidaemia (ke'to-ah-me'no-aside-me-a) maple syrup urine disease

ketoconazole a broad spectrum synthetic antifungal agent, used in the treatment of histoplasmosis, coccidioidomycosis and blastomycosis

ketogenesis (ke'to-jen'e-sis) the production of ketone bodies in the body

ketolysis (ke'tol'i-sis) the breaking down of ketones

ketone bodies acetone, acetoacetic acid and beta hydroxy butyric acid, that are intermediate organic molecules in the metabolism of the fatty acids. They appear to be a physiological defence in starvation, in diabetes mellitus and in defective carbohydrate metabolism

ketonaemia (ke 'to'ne'mea) an excess of ketone bodies in the blood

ketone (ke'ton) an organic compound containing a carbonyl group

ketonuria (ke'to-nu're-a) presence of ketone bodies in the urine; ketosuria

ketoprofen a non-steroidal anti-inflammatory substance with analgesic and antipyretic properties

ketorolac a non-opioid anti-inflammatory agent with analgesic equivalence of morphine

ketosis (ke-to'sis) an abnormal accumulation of ketone bodies in the blood and tissues due to an inadequate utilisation of carbohydrates

17 ketosteroid (ke'to-ster'oid) any of the adrenal cortical hormones having ketone groups on functional carbon atoms at position 17

ketotifen a prophylactic orally active agent used in extrinsic bronchial asthma. It possesses antihistaminic and cromolyn-like properties. It inhibits eosinophil activation and accumulation and diminishes development of airway hypersensitivity

key (ke) means of understanding or solving k hole sign trapping of radiocontrast barium in the mucosa of duodenal bulb which disappears with peristalsis k hole surgery minimally invasive surgery k note address a speech presenting important issues, principles and policies k sign hyperaesthesia where patient avoids locking door, in Gambian sleeping sickness

khaini cancer a squamous cell carcinoma of oral cavity in men keeping lime and tobacco in lower gingivolabial fornix, seen in Uttar Pradesh and Bihar States, India

khanija (s) mineral; metal

khanda-paka (s) confections, medicated syrups

kheer a milk product, 100 ml giving 176 Kcal energy. It contains 6.9 gm protein

khellin active alkaloid of *Ammi visnaga* which acts on tissue mast cell and stabilises its cell membrane used as prophylactic in asthma in the form of cromolyn sodium

khova (kho-a) a milk product 100 gm supplying 400 Kcal energy and 14 (buffalo milk) and 20 (cow's milk) grams of protein

kick chart a record of foetal movements maintained by a woman during later stages of pregnancy

KID syndrome a triology of symptoms-keratitis, ichthyosis and deafness

Kidd blood group the red cell antigen (Jk gene) that reacts with the antibodies (anti-Jk), named after the patient in whom the antibodies were first found

kg kilogram

kHz kilohertz

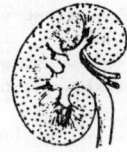

Kidney

kidney (kid'ne) either of a pair of bean shaped organs in the lumbar region that filters the blood and excretes water, solute and waste products of metabolism. The upper level of the kidneys is opposite 12th thoracic vertebra and the lower level opposite the 3rd lumbar vertebra. The right kidney is slightly at a lower level than the left. Each kidney is about 11 cm long, 6 cm wide and 2.5 cm thick. **abdominal k** an ectopic kidney situated above the iliac crest with its hilum at second lumbar vertebra **amyloid k** renal amyloidosis **artificial k** a haemodialyser: an extra-corporeal machine through which blood circulates and gets rid of the substances that are normally excreted in the urine **cake k** a bizarre shaped, irregularly lobed kidney **cement k** calcified contracted scarred kidney as in healed tuberculosis of the kidney **cicatricial k** a shrivelled, irregularly scarred kidney due to pyelonephritis **contracted k** a scarred, granular, atrophic kidney **fatty k** kidney with fatty degeneration **flea-bitten k** kidney exhibiting petechiae on its surface **floating k** hypermobile kidney **fused k** fusion of renal anlagen resulting in a single anamolous kidney **Goldblatt k** kidney with obstruction to its blood flow resulting in hypertension **horse-shoe k** an anomalous kidney from fusion of the corresponding poles of renal analgen **hypermobile k** freely mobile kidney **lumbar k** an ectopic kidney situated opposite sacral premontory in the iliac fossa **k machine** artificial kidney **k stone** renal calculus **pelvis k** ectopic kidney situated opposite the sacrum and below the aortic bifurcation

Kielland (ke'land) **forceps** a forceps used to turn the head of the foetus from an occipitoposterior or occipitotransverse position to an occipitoanterior position. It was devised by a Norwegian obstetrician, Christien Kielland

Kienbock'atrophy acute atrophy of bone seen in inflammatory conditions of the extremity, described by Robert Kienbock, Austrian physician

kieselguhr silica, diatomaceous earth

Kiesselbach's (ke'sel-boks) **area** an area anterior to the nasal septum consisting of a rich network of veins which may be the site of epistaxis, named after Wilhelm Kiesselbach, German laryngologist

kila-baddha-samdamsa (s) gripping instrument

Kilian's (kil'e-anz) **pelvis** pelvis affected by osteomalacia, named after Hermann Kilian, German gynaecologist

Kilian's dehescence weak area in the posterior wall of pharynx where pharyngeal diverticula are common, named after Gustar Kilian, German laryngologist

killed vaccine a vaccine containing dead but antigenically active bacteria or virus which are capable of producing protective antibodies without causing disease e.g. DPT vaccine

killer (K) cell a large granular lymphocyte that can lyse target cells coated with specific antibody. They are of two types – the natural killer (NK) cells and the killer (K) cells

kilo - one thousand (10^3), a unit of measurement, K.

kilobase unit of one thousand nucleotides on a single RNA or DNA strand; Kb

kilobyte Kb a unit of memory capacity/A single kilobyte is equivalent to 1000 bytes

kilocalorie (kil'o-kal'o-re) the amount of energy required to raise the temperature of 1 kilogram of water by 1° C; a unit of heat equal to 1000 calories (Kcal)

kilodalton (kil'o-dawl-ton) a unit of protein mass, being 1000 daltons (KD or KDa)

kilogram (kil'o-gram) 1000 grams (kg).

kilohertz (kil'o-hurts) 1000 (10^3) hertz (kHz)

kilometre (kil'o-me'tre) 1000 metres (km)

kilovolt (kil-ah-volt) 1000 volts (kV)

Kimmelstiel-Wilson syndrome diabetic glomerulosclerosis presenting with albuminuria, oedema and hypertension, described by Paul Kimmelstiel, German physician and Clifford Wilson, British physician

kinanaesthesia (kin'an-es-the'za) loss of power of appreciation of movement

kinase (ki'nas) a phosphorylase subclass of transferase enzyme that catalyses the transfer of a high energy phosphates from a donor molecule

kine- movement

kineplasty (kin'e-plas'te) making use of the stump of an amputated extremity to produce motion of the prosthesis

kinesalgia (kin'e-sal'je-a) pain caused by movement

kinescope (-skop) an instrument to ascertain ocular refraction

kinesi (o) combining word for movement

kinesia (ki-ne'zha) motion sickness

kinesiatrics (ki-ne'se-at-riks) treatment involving active and passive movements

kinesimeter (kin'e-sim-e-ter) an instrument to measure movements quantitatively

kinesiology (ki-ne'se-ol'ah-je) scientific study of muscular movements of body parts

kinesioneurosis (ki-ne'se-o-noo-ro'sis) a neurologic disorder with motor disturbances

kinesis (ki-ne'sis) 1. movement 2. stimulus-induced motion which responds to the intensity of the stimulus

kinesitherapy (ki-ne'si-ther'ah-pe) utilisation of movements or exercise as therapy

kinesthesia (kin'es-the'zhah) 1. appreciation of position, weight, tension and movement 2. sense of movement. **kinesthetic**, adj

kinesthesis (-sis) kinesthesia

kinetic (ki-net'ik) pertaining to body motion.

kinetics (kinet'iks) the forces acting on the body during movement and the interactions of sequence of movements

kinetocardiogram (ki-ne'to-kahr'de-o-gram) the graphic record obtained by kinetocardiography

kinetocardiography (-kar'de-og'rah-fe) the graphic recording of slow vibrations of the arterier chest wall over the cardiac region. The vibrations represent the absolute motion at a given point of the chest

kinetochore (ki-ne't ah-kor) a specialised region of chromosome overlying the centromere, which is critical in mitosis

kinetogenic (ki-ne'to-jenik) producing movement

kinetoplast (ki-net'o-plast) a rod-shaped structure found in parasitic flagellates near the base of the flagellum

kinetosis (ki-ne-to'sis) any disorder due to unaccustomed movements

kinetosome a structure within the cilia of a cell, about 1 cm size

kingdom (king'dum) one of the categories of classification of natural objects such as animal, plant, mineral and single-celled organisms

King-Armstrong units units of phosphatase, named after Canadian and UK biochemists

King syndrome a malignant hyperthermia characterised by facial dysmorphia, pectus carinatum, delayed motor development and cryptorchidism, named after J.O. King, Australian Physician

King's evil scrofula; tuberculous lymphadenopathy supposed to be cured by the royal touch

Kingella (king'ella) a genus of non-motile, gram-negative, facultative anaerobic rod

kinin (ki'nin) vasoactive endogenous polypeptide inducing smooth muscle contraction

kininase II (-as) an enzyme that catalyses the cleavage of dipeptides from oligopeptides. Angiotensin-converting enzyme is an example which converts angiotensin I to angiotensin II

kink (kingk) a twist or curl

kininogen (ki'nin'o-jen) an α_2-globulin of plasma that is precursor of kinins

kinesia paradoxa ability to run or walk fast for a few seconds by a patient with Parkinsonism

kinky hair disease an X-linked recessive disorder with defective copper metabolism presenting with failure to thrive, seizures, hypothermia, short, poorly pigmented hair with twisted and broken shafts, infections and seborrheic dermatitis

kinocilium (ki'no-sil'e-um) a motile, protoplasmic filament on the cell

Kinsbourne syndrome myoclonic encephalopathy of childhood

kinship (kin'ship) a group of individuals who are descent from a common ancestor; family relationship

Kinyoun method a staining technique similar to the Ziehl-Neelsen procedure to demonstrate Mycobacteria, instead of hot stain, a higher concentration of basic funchsin, alcohol and phenol are used and the slide is not heated

kionectomy (ki'o'nek'to'me) uvulectomy

kiotomy (ki'not'eme) uvulotomy

kiraunophobia a morbid fear of thunder and lightning storms

Kirkland knife a surgical knife with a heart-shaped blade, sharp on all edges, used for a gingivectomy incision, devised by Olin Kirkland, US dentist

Kirschner (kursh'ner) **wire** a steel wire used to transfix the fractured bones, devised by German surgeon, Martin Kirschner

kissing disease infectious mononucleosis

kissing ulcer 1. an ulcer occurring on opposing surfaces or parts as in opposing side of vulva due to autoinoculation by *Haemophilus ducreii* 2. pair of duodenal ulcers facing each other on the anterior and posterior walls

kitta (s) undigested or indigestible food residue or waste products to be expelled

Klebsiella (kleb'se-el'a) a genus of gram-negative bacteria that appear as small, plump rods with rounded ends, named after German bacteriologist Theodore Klebs. It includes *K. pneumoniae* responsible for necrotising pneumonia K **pneumonia** rapidly progressive pneumonia with necrotic lesions; it presents with high fever, chills, chest pain, cough with jelly-like blood stained sputum, dyspnoea and prostration. There is volume expansion of the involved lobe and abscess cavities, treated with aminoglycosides

Klebs-Loeffler (klebz'lef'ler) **bacillus** *Corynebacterium diphtheriae*, named after German bacteriologists Theodor Klebs and Friederich Loeffler

Kledahara(s) that which removes fatigue

kledana (s) moistening.

kleptomania (klep'to-ma'ne-a) an abnormal uncontrollable desire to steal things

kleptomaniac (klep'to-ma'ne-ak) a person exhibiting kleptomania

Klima needle short bevelled, wide bore needle with a stylet fitted with an adjustable guard, used in bone marrow aspiration

Klinefelter's (klin'fel-terz) **syndrome** a condition described by American physician Harry Klinefelter characterised by small testes, azoospermia, gynaecomastia, excess elimination of urinary gonadotropins and subnormal intelligence

Kline test a flocculation test for syphilis, named after Benjamin Kline, an American pathologist

Kline-Levin (klin'lev'in) **syndrome** psychosis of unknown aetiology characterised by periodic somnolence, excessive eating and hyperactivity, described by German psychiatrist William Kline and American neurologist, Max Levin

Klippel-Feil (kli-ipel'fil) **syndrome** reduction in the number of cervical vertebrae or the fusion of multiple hemivertebrae into one piece resulting in shortness of the neck, low hair line and limitation of neck movements and facial asymmetry. It is named after Maurice Klippel and Andre Feil, French physicians

Klippel-Trenaunay-Weber syndrome a macular vascular nexus in combination with bony and soft tissue hypertrophy and venous varicosities

Klumpke's (kloomp'kez) **paralysis** paralysis of intrinsic muscles of the hand which results in a claw hand. It is the result of an injury of the eighth cervical and first thoracic nerve roots as a result of forceful abduction of the shoulder mostly occurring during breech presentation with arms above the head, described by Madame Augusta Klumpke, French neurologist. It can occur in later life due to dislocation of the shoulder joint or violent upward pull on the arm or during anaesthesia at operation

Kluver-Bucy (klu'ver-buk'i) **syndrome** bilateral loss of anterior temporal lobes characterised by memory deficit, hypersexuality, excessive exploratory behaviour, emotional placidity, hyperoration and agnosis, named after Heinrich Kluver, US Psychologist and neurologist, and Paul Bacy, US neurologist

km kilometre

kneading (ned'ing) a form of massage; making firm paste by working with hand

knee (ne) genu; a complex hinge joint that connects the thigh with the leg and is formed by the distal end of femur, proximal end of tibia and patella **knee cap** patella **housemaid's k** inflammation of the bursa anterior to the patella in persons who kneel frequently **knock** (nok) **k** genu valgum; a deformity of the thigh or leg or both, in which the knees are abnormally close together **k jerk** patellar jerk, reflex extension of the leg caused by contraction of the quadriceps following a sharp tap on the patellar tendon **k joint** a hinged joint with the articulation between the femur, tibia and patella **k replacement** the surgical insertion of a hinged prosthesis

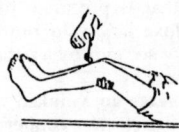

Knee jerk

kneeled chest pectus carinatum

Knock-down effect pyrethrum, an insecticide is a nerve poison that kills arthropods within a matter of seconds

knock out inactivation of specific genes

knol-khol green leafy vegetable *Brassica oleracea*, 100 g supplies 740 mg calcium and 50 mg phosphorus

knot (not) 1. an intertwining of the ends or parts of threads, sutures or strips of clothing 2. a knob-like protuberance

knob 1. small lump, round swelling on surface 2. a specialised red cell membrane enabling red cells infected with *Plasmodium falciparum* to adhere to the vascular epithelium

knuckle (nuk'l) the dorsal aspect of any interphalangeal or metacarpophalangeal joint **k pad** symmetrical erythematous papules over the dorsal surface of finger joints in gout

knuckling (nuk'ling) upward and forward displacement of the *fetlock* joint of a horse.

Koch's (koks) **bacillus** *Mycobacterium tuberculosis*, named after Robert Koch, German bacteriologist

Koch's (koks) **phenomenon** altered reaction in guinea pig previously infected with tubercle bacilli with the latter's reinoculation

Koch's postulates the prerequisites, described by German bacteriologist, Robert Koch, necessary to establish a given micro-organism to be the causative agent of a given disease: 1) demonstration of micro-organism 2) isolation and culture in a laboratory media 3) reproduction of the disease in an experimental animal following inoculation of such a culture and 4) demonstration of micro-organism from the diseased experimental animal

Kocher-Debre-Semelaigne syndrome (Ko'ker-de-bra'se-ma-len'ye) a rare childhood disorder of hypothyroidism associated with muscular enlargement named after Emil Kochar, Robert Debre and Georges Semelaigne, French Paedistricians.

Kocher manoeuvre a method of reducing dislocation of shoulder

Kocher's (ko'kerz) **forceps** forceps having notched jaws interlocking teeth and curved or straight powerful handles, devised by Swiss surgeon, Emil Kocher

Kocher sign a sign of hyperthyroidism wherein the eyelid retracts faster than the eyeball while the patient looks up thus exposing the sclera above the cornea

Kocher's test slight compression on the lateral lobes of thyroid in goitre produces stridor due to pressure on trachea, described by Emil Kocher, Swiss surgeon

Koch-Weeks (kok-weks) *bacillus Haemophilus influenzae*, named after Robert Koch and John Weeks, US ophthalmologists

Kocks, pouch surgically created urinary bladder utilising a segment of ileum, named after Joseph Kocks, German surgeon

Koebner's (kob'ner) **phenomenon** development of isomorphic lesions at the site of injury in cases of psoriasis, lichen planus, and verruca planus, described by Polish dermatologist, Heinrich Koebner

Koerber-Salus-Elschnig syndrome the sylvian aqueduct syndrome with vertical gaze palsy and pupillary abnormalities named after Hermann Koerber, German ophthalmologist, Robert Salus and Anton Elschnig, Austrian ophthalmologist

Koffler's tear drop a tear drop-shaped radio-opaque outline immediately superolateral to the obturator foramen in innominate bone

Kohler's bone disease 1. osteochondrosis of the navicular bone in children 2. thickening of the shaft of second metatarsal bone named after Alban Kohler, German physician

Kohn's (konz) **pores** interalveolar pores, named after Hans Kohn, German pathologist

koil (o) combining word for concave or hollow

koilocytes (koi'lo-sit'z) large cells with clear nuclear membranes with inconspicuous nucleoli

koilocystosis (koi'lo-sito'sis) presence of koilocytes that are vacuolated with clear cytoplasm and hypochromatic nucleus seen in condyloma acuminata

koilonychia (koi'lo-nik'e-a) dystrophy of

the nails which are abnormally thin and concave from side to side with edges turned up. Such spoon nails are seen in iron deficiency anaemia

koilosternia (koi'losturn'e-a) funnel chest

kolypeptic (ko'le-peptik) hindering digestion

koviocortex granular type of cerebral cortex containing densely packed stellate cells

Kopan's (ko'penz) **needle** a long biopsy needle to locate position of a breast tumour

Koplick spots small bright red spots with a minute white speck in the centre, on buccal and lingual mucosa, noted in measles before the appearance of rash, described by American paediatrician, Henry Koplick

Korean haemorrhagic fever hartavirus haemorrhagic fever with renal syndrome

Koronion (ko-ro'ne-on) apex of the coronoid process of the mandible

Korotkoff's sounds sounds heard over brachial artery during auscultatory determination of blood pressure, described by Nickoloi Korotkoff, a Russian physician. On slow deflation of inflated pneumatic arm cuff, tapping sounds are heard synchronous with systolic blood pressure. On further deflation, the sounds become louder and then become muffled and disappear, which corresponds to diastolic blood pressure

Korsakow's syndrome memory loss of recent events due to lesions in limbic system

Korsokoff's syndrome psychosis, described by Sergei Korsokoff, Russian neurologist. There is amnesia in chronic alcoholics due to deficiency of vitamin B1.

koshtha (s) cavity

KPa kilopascal

Krabbe's disease galactosylceramide lipoidosis; a familial form of leucoencephalopathy noted in infants

with deficiency of beta galactosidase, named after Knud Krabbe, Danish neurologist. It is characterised by progresive psychomotor deterioration

krait (krit) one of the several extremely venomous elapid snakes. It shows white bands on the body. Dorsal scales on the body are hexagonal. Head and the sides of the lower jaw are covered with large shields

K-ras gene one of the three proto-oncogenes

kraurosis (kraw-ro'sis) a dried, shrivelled condition. **k vulvae** dryness, itching and atrophy of external genitalia in aged women

Krause's corpuscles tiny cylindrical or oval sensory end organs, described by German anatomist, Wilhelm Krause

Krause's membrane transverse line bisecting I bands of skeletal muscle, also called as Z band

Krebs (krebz) **citric acid cycle** a sequence of enzymatic reaction involving metabolism of carbon chains of sugars, fatty acids and amino acids to yield carbon dioxide, water and high energy phosphate bonds, described by German-English biochemist Hans Krebs

kre(o) **krept**(o) crypt(o)

kriyaghnah (s) normal therapeutic procedures.

kriya-kala(s) the onset of disease as a result of the vitiation of the *doshas*; developmental stages in the course of disease

krodha (s) anger

Krogh coefficient ratio of diffusing capacity to alveolar ventilation, described by August and Marie Krogh

Kronig's isthmus a band of resonance corresponding to the apex of the lung, bounded medially by neck laterally by structures of shoulder, anteriorly by clavicle and posteriorly by trapezius muscle. It is normally resonant becomes dull in apical fibrosis

Krukenberg's (kroo'ken-bergz) **tumour** a neoplasm of the ovary developing as a metastasis of stomach cancer, named after Friedrich Krukenberg, German pathologist

krypton (krip'ten) Kr. Noble gas Krypton 81^m radioactive gas used to evaluate regional ventilation.

kshara(s) caustic

kshaya (s) wasting; tuberculosis

kshira (s) milk *k-paka* decoction in milk.

KUB a plain x-ray picture of the abdomen giving information about kidneys, ureters and bladder

Kuf's disease amaurotic familial idiocy, named after H. Kufs, German psychiatrist

Kugelberg-Welander disease a hereditary juvenile form of muscular atrophy due to loss of anterior horn cells of the spinal cord, described by a Swedish neurologists, Eric Kugelberg and Lisa Welander. There is involvement of the proximal muscles of all four limbs, and runs a benign course.

Kultner's (kul't-nerz) **tumour** chronic sclerosing sialadenitis occurring in submandibular gland and it is not a tumour

kumarabhrtya (s) Paediatrics

Kultschitsky cell argentaffin cell, described by Nicolai Kultschitsky, a Russian histologist **K carcinoma** pulmonary neuroendocrine tumour

kumkum a red powder applied to the forehead by Hindu women

Kummell's (kim'elz) **disease** a compression fracture of the vertebrae presenting with pain, intercostal neuralgia, kyphosis and weakness of legs, named after Hermann Kummell, German surgeon

kuncha (s) brush.

Kuntscher (koon'cher) **nail** a stainless steel nail used to fix the fractured ends of the long bones, named after Gerhard Kuntscher, German surgeon

Kupffer's cells large stellate or pyramidal intensely phagocytic reticuloendothelial cells lining the sinusoids of the liver, named after a German anatomist, Karl von Kupffer

Kuru (koo'roo) a fatal neurologic prion disease transmitted by subhuman primates in certain Melanesian tribes in New Guinea which in their language means to shiver from fever or cold. It presents with cerebellar ataxia, tremors, dysarthria progressing to complete motor paralysis and death

kusa-patram (s) instrument used for extraction of fluids

Kussmaul's disease periarteritis nodosa

Kussmaul's respiration air hunger characterised by a deep, very rapid sighing respirations seen in metabolic acidosis, described by French physician, Adolf Kussmaul

Kussmaul's sign a paradoxical rise in venous pressure with distension of jugular veins during inspiration, seen in constrictive pericarditis, or mediastinal tumour.

kusta (s) leprosy

kV kilovolt

kvatha (s) decoction; *Kashaya*, where one part of the drug or drugs is mixed with four, eight or sixteen parts of water and the whole is boiled down in an open vessel until one quarter of water remains

Kveim reaction appearance of noncaseating granuloma 4 weeks after injection of an antigen obtained from a lymph node of a patient with sarcoidosis, a diagnostic skin test for sarcoidosis described by Norwegian physician, Morton Kveim

kVp kilo volts peak

kwashiorkor (kwahsh'e-or'kor) a protein-energy malnutrition seen in infants and young children after weaning from breast. It is characterised by oedema, pigmentary changes in skin and hair, impaired growth and development and abdominal distension. First recognised in Ghana (earlier Congo) by British paediatrician Cicely Williams which in Ga language means displaced child

Kyasanur forest disease Monkey disease, an arbovirus disease, transmitted by soft wood tick, *Haemophysalis spinigera*, maintained by monkeys in the forest areas of Shimoga, Udipi, Uttara Kannada, districts, Karnataka, India, characterised by fever, headache, muscular aches, back ache, orbital pain, prostration and occasionally haemorrhagic manifestations. The treatment is symptomatic

kymatism (ki'mah-tizm) myokymia

kymograph an instrument to record undulations of an artery

kynurenic (kin'u-ren'ik) **acid** an aromatic compound produced from tryptophan catabolism and excreted in the urine in disorders of tryptophan catabolism

kynurenine (kin'-u-re'nen) an intermediate amino acid in tryptophan catabolism

Kyphoplasty (ki'poh-plasti) repair of the vertebral deformity caused by a collapsing spine

kyphos (ki'fos) the hump of the spine in kyphosis

kyphoscoliosis (ki'fo-sko'le-o'sis) backward and lateral curvature of the spine

kyphosis (ki'fo'sis) an abnormally increased convex curvature of the thoracic spine, hunchback. **kyphotic,** adj

kyrtorhachic (kir'to-rak'ik) posterior concavity of the lumbar vertebral curvatue

L

L a description prefix for an optically active organic compound; litre; levorotatory

L1-5 first to fifth lumbar nerve, first to fifth lumbar vertebra

l symbol for length, litre

LA abbreviation for left atrium

lab abbreviation for laboratory

label 1. a marker 2. a substance having a special affinity for an organ, tissue, cell or organism in which it may get deposited and fixed

la belle indifference *Psy* bland and indifferent to their defect as in hysterical patients

labetalol (lah-bet'ah-lol) beta-adrenergic blocking antihypertensive agent, useful in the treatment of all grades of hypertension and pheochromocytoma

labia (la'be-a) lips, fold of skin at the opening of the mouth or vagina **l majora** the two folds of skin and adipose tissue lying on either side of the vaginal opening that form the lateral borders of the vulva **l minora** the two thin folds that lie inside the vagina and between labia majora and hymen

labial (la'be-al) pertaining to the lips **l bar** a connector installed labial or buccal to the dental arch **l glands** small mucous or serous glands in the lips **l notch** a depression in the denture border

labile (la-bil) unstable; unsteady **l affect** *Psy* rapid and abrupt changes in emotional feeling, tone, unrelated to external stimuli **l hypertension** wide swings in blood pressure as an accentuation of normal variability

lability (la'bil'i-te) the state of being unstable **emotional l** *Psy* excessive emotional reaction associated with frequent changes in emotions and mood

labio - combining word for lip

labiocervical (la'be-o-ser'vi-kal) relating to the buccal surface of the neck of an anterior tooth

labiochorea (la'be-o-ko're-a) a chronic spasm of the lips as in chorea

labiodental (la'be-o-den'tal) relating to the lips and teeth

labioglossolaryngeal (la'be-o-glos'o-lar-in'je-al) relating to the lips, tongue and larynx

labioglossopharyngeal (la'be-o-glos'o-far-in'je-al) relating to the lips, tongue and pharynx

labiograph (la'be-o-graf) an instrument to record the movement of the lips while speaking

labiomental (la'be-o-men'tal) relating to the lower lips and the chin

labionasal (la'be-o-na'zal) pertaining to upper lips and the nose

labiopalatine (la-be-o-pal'a-tin) relating to the lips and the palate

labioplasty (la'be-o-plas'te) plastic operation on a lip

labiotenaculum (la'be-o-ten-ak'u-lum) an instrument to hold the lips during an operation

labioversion (la'be-o-ver'zhun) labial displacement of a tooth from the line of occlusion

labium (la'be-um) a lip with a fleshy border. pl. **labia**

laboratory (lab'ra-tor'e) a building or a room equipped for scientific experimentation, research, testing or studies of materials, fluids or tissues obtained from patients **l diagnosis** a diagnosis arrived at after study of secretions, excretions, blood or biopsy specimen through chemical, microscopic and bacteriologic means

labour the physiological process of expulsion of the products of conception from the uterus *via* the cervix and vagina to the outside world **active l** regular uterine contractions with increasing dilatation of the cervix and descent of the presenting part **arrested l** failure of the labour to progress through the normal stages **complicated l** labour occurring in association of an abnormality such as haemorrhage or inertia **dry l** premature rupture of the membranes leading to drainage of most of the amniotic fluid and then occurrence of labour **false l** occurrence of uterine contractions which are not accompanied by effacement or dilatation of the cervix. **induced l** administration of oxytocin to stimulate uterine contractions **instrumental l** application of forceps to complete the labour **l pain** painful uterine contractions at term **missed l** labour in which true labour pains stop as in dead foetus or extra uterine pregnancy **normal l** progressive dilatation of the cervix with descent of presenting part **obstructed l** obstruction to the foetal passage through the birth canal from foetal malposition, malpresentation and cephalopelvic disproportion **precipitate l** labour of less than three hours in duration in a primigravida **preterm l** premature labour wherein labour begins between 20 and 37 (i.e <37 weeks) weeks of gestation **prolonged l** abnormally slow progress of labour which may last 20 hours or more **spontaneous l** labour taking place without any mechanical or operative interference

labrocyte (lab'ro'sit) a mast cell

labrum (la'brum) an edge; rim; lip; liplike structure

labyrinth (lab-i-rinth) 1. any group of inter-connecting membranous cavities, cells or canals separated from the bony labyrinth by the perilymph both of which lie within the petrous portion of the temporal bone 2. internal ear comprising the semicircular canals, vestibule and cochlea

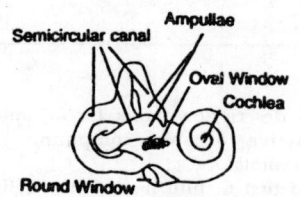

Membranous labriynth

labyrinthectomy (lab-i-rin-thek'to-me) surgical removal of the labyrinth of the ear

labyrinthitis (lab-i-rin-thi'tis) inflammation of the three interconnecting fluid-filled chambers in the internal ear; otitis interna. The condition causes sudden vertigo typically precipitated or aggravated by movement, lasting minutes or hours. Nausea and vomiting are associated symptoms

labyrinthotomy (lab-i-rin-that'o-me) incision into the labyrinth of the ear

lac (lak) milk, milky fluid

lacerate (las'er-at) to tear into irregular segments

lacerated (las'er-at-ed) torn with a ragged edge

laceration (las'er-a-shun) a torn, jagged wound

laceratus (la-ser'tus) the muscular part of the arm

Lachman test a test to determine the integrity of the anterior cruciate ligament of the knee. The examiner standing on the side to be examined, grasps the tibia at the level of tibial tuberosity while stabilising the femur with the other hand. The patient is asked to relax the leg while the exminer is holding the knee fixed at 30° pulls forward on the knee. The test is considered positive when there is an excess motion.

lacquer crack appearance optic fundus exhibiting branching clefts in the lamina vitrea with choroidal atrophy, seen in progressive myopia

lacrimal (lak'rim-al) relating to tears **l. apparatus** a system of glands and ducts that produces tears and drains away from the inner corners of the eyes to the back of the nose

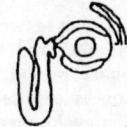

Lacrimal apparatus

lacrimation (lak'rim-a-shun) the secretion and discharge of excessive amount of tears

lacrimator (lak'rim-a-ter) a substance irritating the eyes and producing tears

lacrimatory (lak'ri-ma-to're) causing lacrimation

lacrimotome (lak'ri-mo-tom) a cutting instrument used for incision of the lacrimal sac or duct

lacrimotomy (lak'rim-ot'o-me) incision of the lacrimal duct or sac

lactacidosis (lak-ta-sid-o-sis) acidosis due to increased lactic acid; lactic acidosis

lactaciduria (lakt-a-sid-u're-a) presence of lactic acid in the urine

lactalbumin (lak'tal-bu'min) an albumin found in milk. It is found in higher concentration in human milk than in cow's milk

b.lactamase (ba-ta-lak'ta-mas) enzyme which alters the β-lactam ring of penicillins and cephalosporins β**-resistant antibiotics,** antibiotics exhibiting resistance to the action of β-lactamase, hence effective against microorganisms producing β-lactamase

lactase (lak'tass) enzyme converting lactose into dextrose and galactose, found in intestinal juice **l deficiency** an inherited disorder with an inability to digest milk, sugar, lactose due to a deficiency of the enzyme, lactase on the intestinal brush borders

lactate (lak'tat) 1. any salt derived from lactic acid 2. to secrete milk

lactation (lak-ta'shun) the production and secretion of milk after childbirth; period of suckling **l suppression** suppression of milk production by high levels of oestrogen in the blood

lactator female who is producing breast milk

lacteal (lak'te-al) 1. a lymphatic vessel carrying chyle from the intestine. 2. pertaining to milk

lactic (lak'tik) **acid** a glycolytic product by the action of the lactic acid bacillus, on milk or milk sugar; a weak acid produced during anaerobic exercise **l dehydrogenase,** LDH, an enzyme catalysing the oxidation of lactate to pyruvate, also called lactate dehydrogenase. It is found in humans in several molecular forms called isoenzymes and any damage to the tissues is associatd with release of an isoenzyme of LDH into the blood

lactiferous (lak'tif'er-us) producing milk

lactifuge (lak'ti-fuj) causing the arrest of the secretion of milk

lactigenous (lak-tij'en-us) producing milk

lactobacillus (lak-to-ba-sil'us) gram-positive, non-motile, rod-shaped bacteria capable of production of lactic acid from carbohydrates and cause souring of milk **l. acidofilus** an organism capable of producing lactic acid by fermenting the sugars in the milk. It is found in milk and in the faeces of bottle-fed infants. **L. bulgaricus** a bacillus found in fermented milk **L. casei** a bacillus found in milk and cheese

lactoferrin a nonspecific protein found in milk and neutrophil granules that combines with iron in the blood

lactogen (lak' to-jen) an agent stimulating milk production

lactoglobulin (lak'to-glob'u-lin) a protein found in the milk

lactometer (lak'tome-ter) a device to determine the specific gravity of milk

lactose milk sugar, a disaccharide sugar

present in milk and milk products which on hydrolysis yields glucose and galactose l **intolerance** a lactase deficiency causing an inability to digest lactose. The individual complains of bloating, nausea, diarrhoea and abdominal cramps following intake of milk

lactosuria (lak-to-su′rea) excretion of lactose in the urine which occur during pregnancy and lactation

lactulose a synthetic disaccharide that is not hydrolysed or absorbed in humans. It is metabolised by bacteria in the colon

lacuna (la-ku′na) a gap, space, pit or cavity. pl. **lacunae** adj. **lacunar lacunar cell** an enlarged Reed-Strenberg cell variant of 40-50 millimicrons which has a polylobated nucleus and lacy chromatin surrounded by a rim of clear cytoplasm and is seen in clear lacunae thought to be artefact of formalin fixation, occurs in Hodgkin's disease and nasopharyngeal carcinoma l **infarcts** multiple small cerebral infarcts whose resolution leaves behind lacunae l **skull** shallow depressions in the skull with smooth contour, seen radiologically over frontoparietal region in conditions of meningocoele complicated by hydrocephalus l **state** multiple lacunae in the basal ganglia which may lead to dementia or a lacunar syndrome l **syndrome** motor weakness, dysarthria or ataxia due to lacunae in the cerebral hemisphere

lacus (la′kus) a small collection of fluid

LAD left anterial descending artery, a branch of left coronary artery

Laddergram a schematic method for analysis of complex arrhythmias in which a ECG rhythm strip is divided into atrial (A) line, atrio-ventricular junction (AV) line and ventricular (V) line

ladder pattern stepped pattern of parallel loops of distended small intestine suggestive of obstruction of the small intestine and it indicates a late diagnosis

Lafora-body disease myoclonic epilepsy and dementia, skin biopsy shows Lafora bodies, acid - Schiff-positive inclusions consisting of polyglucosans, named after Gonzalo Lafora, Spanish physician

lag the period of time between the application of stimulus and the resulting reaction l **phase** period between the time a person is exposed to a toxic inhalent and development of pulmonary oedema

laghu (s) light, lightness

lagophthalmos (lag′of-thal′mos) an incomplete closure of the eyelids over the eyeball

la grippe (la-grip′) influenza

Lahey method palpation of thyroid gland from the front, in which to palpate right lobe, thyroid gland is pushed from left to the right to make it more prominent for palpation with the other hand and *vice versa*, named after Frank Lahey, US surgeon

lake a small cavity of fluid

laky plasma or serum giving a bright red appearance due to presence of haemoglobin released from destroyed red blood cells

laliatry (lal-i′a-tre) the study and treatment of speech disorders

lalling stammering wherein the speech is almost unintelligible

lalopathy (la-lop′a-the) any disorder of speech

laloplegia (lal-o-ple′je-a) paralysis of the muscles concerned in the mechanism of speech

lAM leucocyte adhesion molecule

Lamaze (la-maz) **method** a method of preparation for uncomplicated vaginal delivery which includes relaxation, physical conditioning and breathing exercises, devised by Fernand Lamaze, French obstetrician

lambda (lam′da) junction of the sagittal and lamdoid sutures at the site of posterior fontanella; a symbol for immunoglobulin light chain **l waves** sharp or sawtooth waves over the occipital areas in a normal EEG, and are evoked by visually scanning an object or a picture

lambdoid (lam'doyd) resembling the Greek alphabet lambda

Lambert-Eaton syndrome a myasthenia characterised by muscle weakness, hyporeflexia and autonomic dysfunction frequently associated with small cell carcinoma of the lung, described by Edward Lambert, US physiologist and Lee Eaton, US physician

lame disabled in one or more limbs often of the leg or foot affecting normal movement

Lambl's excrescences small fibrin vegetations overlying sites of endothelial damage on flow side of cardiac valves

Lamblia (lam'ble-a) Giardia, named after Bohemian physician Vilem Lambl

lambliasis (lam-bli'a-sis) giardiasis

lamella (la-mal'a) a thin layer, thin plate or scale; disc of gelatin

lamellar (la-mel'ar) arranged in thin plate or scales **l body** concentrically layered, fingerprint like, osmiophilic material obtained form membranes and organelles, seen by electron microscopy in skin and lungs

lameness limping

lamin a fibrous protein

lamina (lam'i-na) a thin, flat plate or layer or membrane. pl. **laminae**

laminagram (lam'i-na-gram) a radiogram of a selected section of the body taken by a laminagraph

laminagraph (lam'i-nag-raf) a radiographic technique to give details of a specific region of the body

laminagraphy (lam'i-nag'ra-fe) tomography

laminar flow smooth movement of gas particles along lines parallel to the walls of the tube

lamination (lam'in-a'shun) layer-like arrangement

laminectomy (lam-i-nek'to-me) surgical removal of the entire lamina of a vertebra as a treatment of herniation of intervertebral disc

laminotomy (lam'i-not'o-me) a division of one of the vertebral laminae

lamp a device to produce and apply light, heat, radiation and different forms of radiant energy to treat diseases **infrared l** a lamp that develops a high temperature, emitting infrared rays **slit l** a lamp emitting intense light through a slit and used for examination of eyes **ultraviolet l** a lamp producing ultraviolet light

lamprophonia (lam'pro-fo'ne-a) a clear voice

lanatoside (lan-at'o-sid) a glycoside obtained from the leaves of *Digitalis lanata*

lanceolate shaped like a lance

lancet (lan'set) a surgical knife having a small, sharply pointed double edged blade

lancinating (lan'si-nat'ing) sharply cutting or tearing

Landau reflex an infantile reflex wherein there is flexion of the body when head is passively flexed forward in a prone position. It appears by third month and is absent in children with cerebral palsy, named after William Landau, US neurologist

landmark a reference point in a skeletal or soft tissue structure and it is used to take measurement and to describe the location of anatomical structures

Landolfi's sign change in the size of the pupil synchronous with the cardiac cycle, seen an aortic incompetence

Landouzy-Dejerine (lan-du -ze'de'zhe-ren) **dystrophy** a slowly progressive dystrophy involving the facio-scapulo-humeral muscles, described by Louis Landouzy and Joseph Dejerine French physician It is noted in 10-40 years of age as an autosomal dominant disease

Landsteiner's (lan'sti-nerz) **classification** a classification of blood into A, B, AB and O groups based on the presence of antigens on the erythrocytes, named after Carl Landsteiner, physician, who worked in Vienna and New York

Langerhans' cell a macrophage that presents antigen to lymphocytes in the upper dermis which sends dendritic processes, named after Paul Langerhans, German pathologist.

Langerhans' cell granuloma eosinophilic granuloma, histocytosis X. Presents with a combination of cavitary lung disease, intraphagocytic cytoplasmic inclusions (X bodies, Birbeck bodies) and recurrent pneumothorax.

Langerhans' islets endocrine cells distributed in irregular groups in the pancreas, described by a German pathologist Paul Langerhans. There are three types of cells - alpha cells secreting glucogon, beta cells secreting insulin and delta cells secreting somatostatin

Langer's (lang'erz) **lines** natural cleavage lines in the body giving structural orientation of the fibrous tissue of the skin. They are visible prominently as palmar creases. Incisions are made during an operation, parallel to them which enables to make smaller postoperative scar than those made at right angles to the lines, described by Carl Langer, Austrian anatomist

Lange's (lang'ez) **test** a test for diagnosis of neurosyphilis by the degree of gold precipitation of colloidal gold solution and cerebrospinal fluid named after Carl Lange, German Physician

Langhans' giant cell a giant cell composed of fused epithelioid cells. A large number of nuclei are arranged like garland surrounding cytoplasm. These cells are diagnostic of tuberculosis when accompanied by caseation, described by T. Langhans, Swiss pathologist

languor (lang'ger) lassitude; lack of vigour; exhaustion

lanolin (lan'o-lin) a water-adsorbable ointment base prepared from wool of sheep

lanugo (la-nu'go) hair; fine, soft downy hair that covers a foetus and is shed before birth

LAO left anterior oblique

laparo loin; abdomen

laparocoele (lap'a-ro-sel) an abdominal hernia

laparoscope (lap'a-ro-skop) peritoneoscope with a tiny camera at its tip to visualise internal organs in the abdominal cavity

laparoscopy (lap-ar-os'ko-pe) examination of the interior of the abdominal cavity using a laparoscope. The laparoscope is inserted through a small incision in the abdomen and the image is displayed on TV-screen

laparotomy (lap-ar-ot'o-me) surgical incision to open up the abdomen

Laplace's law the wall tension (T) is a function of the ventricular pressure (P) and the size of the chamber (radius = r), formulated by 18th century mathematician Laplace

$$T = \frac{PT}{r}$$

laptop a portable computer

larva immature form of an insect or a worm during the developmental stage. pl. **larvae l migrans** an infestation with larvae that move through the skin or intestine

larvicidal destructive to larvae

larvicide an agent that kills larvae

laryngeal (lar-in'je-al) relating to the larynx **l obstruction** obstruction to the entry of air from oedema of glottis resulting in harsh respiration

laryngectomee (lar'in-jek'to-me) a person whose larynx has been removed

laryngectomy (lar'in-jek'to-me) surgical removal of the larynx either partially or totally

laryngismus (lar'in-jis'mus) spasm of the larynx

laryngitis (lar-in-ji'tis) inflammation of the mucosa lining larynx that causes hoarseness

laryngocoele (lar-in'go-sel) a narrow-necked pouch having connection with the larynx and the condition is suspected if a swelling of the neck appears when the patient blows his nose

laryngoedema a swelling of the larynx caused by an allergic reaction

laryngologist (lar'in-gol'o-jist) a specialist in laryngology

laryngology (lar'in-gol'o-je) medical speciality dealing with the diseases of the throat, pharynx, larynx and tracheobronchial tree

laryngometry (lar-in'gom'e-tre) measurement of the larynx

laryngoparalysis (lar-in'go-par-ali-sis) paralysis of the muscles of the larynx

laryngopharyngeal (lar-in'go-far-in'je-al) relating to larynx and pharynx

laryngopharyngeus (la-ring'go-fa-rin-je-us) muscle constricting the inferior pharynx

laryngopharyngitis (lar-in'go-far-in-ji'tis) inflammation of the larynx and pharynx

laryngoplasty (lar-in'go-plas'te) surgical repair of the larynx

laryngophony (lar-in-gof'o-ne) voice sounds heard on auscultating, the pharynx

laryngophthisis (lar'ing-gof'thi-sis) tuberculosis of the larynx

laryngoplegia (lar-ingo-ple'je-a) paralysis of the laryngeal muscles

laryngoscope (lar-in'go-skop) an illuminated endoscope to examine the interior of the larynx

laryngoscopic (lar'in-go-skop'ik) pertaining to observations of the interior of the larynx with the help of a small long-handled mirror

laryngoscopy (lar'in-gos'ko-pe) visual examination of the larynx with a laryngoscope

laryngospasm (lar-in'go-spazm) spasm of the laryngeal muscles

laryngostenosis (lar-ing'go-ste-no'sis) narrowing of the larynx

laryngostomy (lar-in-gos'to-me) establishment of a permanent opening through the neck into the larynx

laryngotomy (lar-in-got'o-me) surgical incision of the larynx.

laryngotracheal (la-ring'go-tra'ke-al) relating to larynx and trachea

laryngotracheitis (la-ring'go-tra-ke-i'tis) inflammation of the larynx and trachea

laryngotracheobronchitis (la-ring'go-tra'ke-o-brong-ki'tis) inflammation involving the larynx, trachea and bronchi

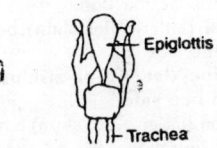

Larynx

larynx (lar'inks) a musculocartilaginous structure concerned with voice production located between the pharynx and the trachea at the level of 3rd and 6th cervical vertebrae and comprises a number of articulated cartilages surrounding the upper end of the trachea and lined with ciliated mucous membrane; voice box containing vocal cords.

Lasegue's (la-segz') **sign** aggravation of pain in the back and leg in sciatica while raising the heel from the bed with knee straight, described by French physician Ernest Lasegue

laser (la'zer) light amplification by stimulated emission of radiation; a device that transfers a narrow beam of visible light into an extremely intense monochromatic small beam of radiation with high energies which is able to cut and dissolve tissue

Lassa fever a highly contagious fatal acute febrile disorder caused by an arena virus first reported in Lassa city in Nigeria. It is characterised by fever, headache, prostration and severe pharyngitis. There is lymphadenopathy, vomiting, diarrhoea, a maculopapular rash and mucosal bleeding. Treatment is symptomatic

lassitude (las'i-tud) weariness; weakness; exhaustion

latency (la'ten-se) a period of inactivity between the time of stimulus and the movement of response

latent not manifest; inactive; dormant

lateral (lat'er-al) pertaining to a side; away from the midline; situated on one side

lateralis (lat'er-a'lis) located away from the midline of the body

lateroflexion (lat'er-o-flek'shun) bending toward one side

lateroposition (lat'er-o-po-zish'un) displaced to one side

lateropulsion (lat'er-o-pul'shun) tendency to fall to one side

lateroversion (lat'er-o-va'shun) a turning to one side

latex fixation test a serologic test using antigen-coated latex particles for agglutination

lathyrism (lath'ir-izm) a spastic paraplegia developing from consumption of kesari dal, *Lathyrus sativus*. The disease affects men more frequently and more severely. It passes through non-stick, one-stick, two-stick and crawler stages. There is spasticity, a 'scissor type' of gait and weakness

latissimus (la-tis'i-mus) a broad or large structure such as a muscle

latitude a range of exposure that would produce a technically proper radiograph

latrine (la-tren) a toilet **sanitary l** nonservice type of latrine wherein excreta does not contaminate the ground or pollute the soil, and is not accessible to flies, rodents or animals and does not create a nuisance **trench l** latrines suitable for camps and temporary use

LATS long-acting thyroid stimulator

lattice (lat'is) a network formed by a structure intertwined at right angles with each other

latus (la'tus) flank; broad; side

laudanum (law'dan-um) a tincture containing opium

laugh (laf) sound produced by laughing.

laughing death uncontrollable compulsive laughter encountered at terminal stages of *Kuru*

laughing disease pseudobulbar palsy

laughing gas an anaesthetic gas, nitrous oxide

laughter (laf'ter) inarticulate sounds produced as an expression of emotion, usually happiness

Laurence-Moon-Biedl syndrome (la'rensmoon'be'del) a hereditary disorder characterised by girdle-type obesity, hypogonadism, retinitis pigmentosa, polydactyly, mental retardation and skull defects, described by English ophthalmologist John Laurence, American ophthalmologist Robert Moon and Czechoslovakian physician Arthur Biedl

lavage (la-vazh) the washing out of a hollow cavity **gastric l** washing out of the stomach using a stomach wash tube

lavana (s) salt

law 1. a statement that holds true uniformly 2. body of rules, regulations and legal opinions of conduct and action that are legally binding

lax (laks) 1. loose 2. without tension

laxative (lak'sa-tiv) an agent that stimulates evacuation of soft, formed stools.

laya (s) dissolution; mental inactivity

layer (la'er) a thin sheet-like structure of uniform thickness

lazy leucocyte syndrome an immunodeficiency disease of children with defective neutrophil chemotaxis after appropriate stimuli, and deficient random mobility of neutrophils leading to recurrent pyogenic infections

LBBB left bundle branch block

LD lethal dose

LDH lactate dehydrogenase; lactic acid dehydrogenase

LDL low-density lipoprotein.

L-Dopa, levo dopa l-3,4 dihydroxyphenyl alanine useful in the treatment of Parkinsonism

LE lupus erythematosus

lead (led) plumbum, a metal; the conductor connected to the electrocardiograph; insulates wires that connect a patient to a monitoring device **l line** a blue line consisting of a series of grey-black dots situated about a mm from the free margin of the gums in patients who work with lead

lean (len) emaciated

Leber's optic atrophy hereditary bilateral atrophy of the optic nerves resulting in rapid loss of vision in young adult males, named after German ophthalmologist Theodor Leber

LE cell lupus erythematosus cell. A mature polymorphonuclear leucocyte that contains the phagocytosed nucleus of another cell.

lecithin (les'ith-in) a phospholipid. It is part of a cell membrane, also found in blood and egg yolk

lecithinase (les'i-thin-as) a phospholipase that catalyses the decomposition of lecithin

leech (letch) a blood-sucking water worm It is parasitic on humans and other animals. The worms are source of hirudin; an anticoagulant substance

leeching application of a leech for withdrawal of the blood

leg the lower limb between the knee and ankle, often the term is applied to whole of the lower limb. pl. **legs bow l's** outward bowing of the legs with separation of the knees widely; genu varum

legal pertaining or according to law

Legg's (legz) **disease** osteochondritis of the epiphysis of the head of the femur, named after Arthur Legg, US surgeon

Legg-Perthes disease epiphyseal aseptic necrosis of the head of the femur, described by US surgeon, Arthur Legg, and German surgeon Georg Perthes

Legionella a genus of gram-negative rod-shaped bacteria **l pneumophila** bacteria that is responsible for Legionnaire's disease

Legionellosis; legionnaire's disease; a disease caused by *Legionella pneumophila*. It is a multisystem disorder affecting the lungs, kidney, alimentary tract and central nervous system. It presents with fever, chills, cough, dyspnoea and prostration. There can be vomiting, abdominal pain, diarrhoea, headache and mental confusion. It is treated with erythromycin. Rifampicin is added in severely ill patients

legume (le'gum) pulse

leha (s) thickened extract for licking, got from boiling the decoction down to a thick consistency

Leigh's disease a leucodystrophy manifesting in the first year of life with loss of head control, hypotonia and crying. It is followed by irregular, external ophthalmoplegia and dysphagia

Leiner's (li'nerz) **disease** exfoliative dermatitis, named after Karl Leiner, Austrian paediatrician

leiodermia (li'o-der'me-a) smooth and glossy skin

leiomyofibroma (li'o-mi'o-fi-bro'ma) a benign tumour composed of smooth muscle and fibrous tissue

leiomyoma (li'o-mio'ma) a benign tumour of smooth muscle containing a relatively small amount of fibrous tissue

leiomyosarcoma (li'o-mi'o-sar-ko'ma) a malignant tumour of smooth muscle

Leishman-Donovan bodies small round or oval bodies found in the reticuloendothelial cells in a patient suffering from kala azar, described by an English army surgeon William Leishman and Irish Physician Charles Donovan while working in Chennai, India

Leishmania (lesh-ma'ne-a) a protozoan flagellate spread by bite of female sandfly responsible for leishmaniasis

leishmaniasis (lesh-ma-ni'-a-sis) infection from protozoa leishmania presenting in three different forms as visceral (kala azar), cutaneous and mucocutaneous leishmaniasis. Disease manifestations depend on the species of parasite, geographical region and immune status of the patient. The disease is transmitted by biting of sand flies **cutaneous l** single or multiple painless papular-ulcerative lesions on the skin which leave an atrophic, depigmented scar on healing. Delhi boil or Bagdad sore is an example. When a large number of parasites spread throughout the skin the condition becomes diffuse **mucocutaneous l** destructive lesions involving nasal and oropharyngeal region may occur following recovery from cutaneous ulcer and is seen in Latin America **visceral l** *see* kala azar

lema (le'ma) the dried secretion of the tarsal gland that collects in the inner canthus of the eye

lemniscus (lem-nis'kus) a band or bundle of sensory nerve fibres in the medulla and pons

lemon fruit of citrus lemon containing citric acid and is rich in ascorbic acid

lemon sign an abnormally-shaped foetal head and flattening of frontal bones seen in antenatal ultrasonographic examination during second trimester, and it implies open spina bifida

length the measurement of the distance between two points

lens (lenz) a transparent biconvex body lying in the internal compartment of the eye that adjusts focus; a transparent refracting medium usually of glass which converges or scatters light rays

lentectomy (len-tek'to-me) removal of the lens of the eye

lenticulostriate (len-tik'u-lo-stri'at) relating to the lenticular nucleus and the corpus striatum

lenticonus (len'ti-ko'nus) a conical projection of the lens

lenticular resembling a lens; having a shape of a lentil

lenticulothalamic (len'tik-u-lo-thal-amik) relating to the lenticular nucleus and the thalamus

lenticulus an intraocular lens of inert plastic material

lentiform (lent'i-form) lens-shaped

lentigines (len-ti-jin-ez) flat, brown spot on ageing skin of the back of the hands due to accumulation to lipofuscin

lentigo (len-ti'go) a brown macule with a regular border on the skin due to excess deposition lipofuscin and is brought on by sun exposure; a freckle

lepa (s) external application

leontiasis (le'on-ti-a-sis) The lion-like appearance of the face in some cases of advanced lepromatous leprosy

Leopald's (le'o-pal'dz) **manoeuvre** use of four steps in palpating the uterus to determine the position and presentation of the foetus, described by Christian Leopald, a German physician

leper (lep'er) a person suffering from leprosy

lepidic (le-pid'ik) concerning scales

lepidosis (lep'i-do'sis) any scaly eruption

leprologist (lep-rol'o-jist) a specialist in leprology

Leprology (lep'rol'o-je) the study of leprosy and its management

leproma (lep-ro'ma) a granulomatous nodule caused by *Mycobacterium leprae*

lepromatous (lep'ro'ma-tus) referring to leproma

lepromin (lep'ro-min) an extract of tissue infected with *Mycobacterium leprae* used in skin tests to determine tissue resistance in leprosy

leprosarium a hospital for patients suffering from leprosy

leprosy (lep'ro-se) Hansen's disease, a chronic granulomatous infectious disease caused by *Mycobacterium leprae*, the organisms were demonstrated by Hansen, a Norwegian physician **borderline l** patients showing features closer to either lepromatous or tuberculoid leprosy. There can also be features lying midway between the two **indeterminate l** early lesion of leprosy appearing as a hypopigmented macule **lepromatous l** occurs in individuals with low resistance. It is a highly bacillary disseminated disease. The lesions are bilaterally symmetrical, ill-defined, hypopigmented macules or diffusely infiltrated plaques **tuberculoid l** a high resistance form of the disease with individual exhibiting high degree of immunity. The lesions are well defined, anaesthetic, and hidrotic and alopaecic. The superficial nerves are thickened and tender

lepti frail; thin; delicate

leptin (lep'tin) a hormone produced by adipose tissue, that acts at the level of the hypothalamus to suppress appetite

leptocephalus (lep'to-se-fa'l-us) an abnormally vertically elongated narrow skull

leptochromatic (lep'to-kro'mat'ik) a fine chromatin network

leptocyte (lep to-sit) an unusually thin, flat red blood cell with a central rounded area of pigmentation like a "bull's eye" surrounded by a clear zone and a pigmented rim, often referred as `target' or 'Mexican hat' cell

leptocytosis (lep'to-si-to'sis) presence of leptocytes in the blood

leptodactyly (lep'to-dak'ti-le) abnormally slender fingers

leptomeninges (lep'to-men-in-jes) soft thin membranous covering of brain and spinal cord, the piamater and arachnoid mater

leptomeningitis (lep'to-men-in-ji'tis) inflammation of the leptomeninges

leptomona (lep'to-mo'na) a parasitic flagellate

leptonema (lep'to-ne'ma) the early stage of prophase in meiosis

leptophonia (lep'to-fo'ne-a) feeble voice

Leptospira (lep-to-spi'ra) a thin, spiral and hook-ended bacteria belonging to the family Treponemataceae. It has 240 serotypes and 23 serovars

leptospirosis (lep'to-spi-ro'sis) infection with species of *Leptospira interrogenes* that is acquired by domestic and wild animal hosts especially rodents. The illne s is biphasic with initial leptospiraemia and later immune phase. Initially there is frontal headache, muscular pains, fever and chills. Then there is involvement of one organ system giving rise to any of the conditions such as hepatitis, nephritis, atypical pneumonia, influenza or gastroenteritis. The condition responds to penicillin or doxycycline

leptotene (lep'to-ten) the early stage of prophase of cell division where the chromosomes become visible.

leptotrichia (lep'to-tri-ki-a) a gram-negative bacteria found in the oral cavity

Leriche's (le-resh'ez) **syndrome** aorto-iliac occlusive disease. Obstruction of terminal aorta, absence of pulsation in femoral arteries, pallor, cold and claudication in lower limbs, described by French Surgeon, Rene Leriche

lesbian (les'be-an) referring to homosexuality between females

lesbianism sexual desire of women toward those of their own sex

Lesch-Nyhan syndrome a hereditary disease of purine metabolism affecting males characterised by mental retardation, aggressive behaviour, impaired renal function, described by American paediatricians Michael Lesch and William Nyhan

lesion (le'zhun) a circumscribed area of pathologically altered tissue. Primary lesions are in the form of macules, papules, vesicles, pustules, blebs, bullae, chancres, tubercles, wheals and tumours. Secondary lesions are the result of primary lesions and consist of crusts, excoriations, fissures, scales, scars, pigmentations and ulcers

lethal deadly; fatal **l agranulocytosis** an autosomal recessive condition seen in infants characterised by profound neutropaenia and recurrent pyogenic infections **l dose** a dose of toxin that is lethal within a specified period **l gene** a mutant gene is lethal when it is autosomal dominant in a homozygous state. **l midline granuloma** a clinical syndrome consisting of a destructive lesion of upper respiratoy tract

lethality ability to cause death

lethargic (le-thar'jik) affected with lethargy, drowsy, dull, inactive

lethargy (leth'ar-je) drowsiness; indifference

lethologica (leth-o-loj'i-ka) the temporary inability to remember a word, name or intended action

Letterer-Siwe (let'er-er-si'we) **disease** a non-lipid reticuloendotheliosis of early childhood, described by German physician Erich Letterer and Swedish physician August Siwe

leucine (loo'sin) an essential amino acid, essential for normal growth and metabolism

leucoblast (loo'ko-blast) an immature granular leucocyte

leucocyte (loo'ko-sit) a white blood cell or corpuscle, WBC

leucoblastosis (loo'ko-blast'o-sis) abnormal proliferation of immature leucocytes

leucocidin (loo'ko-ci-din) a heat labile bacterial toxic substance destroying the white blood cells

leucocoria (loo'ko-co-ria) white or abnormal pupillary reflex noted in retinoblastoma, congenital cataract and retrolental fibroplasia

leucocytosis (loo'ko-si-to'sis) an abnormally large number of circulating white blood cells

leucoderma (loo-ko-der'ma) local or total absence of pigmentation in the skin

leucodystrophy (loo'ko-dis'tro-fe) degeneration of the white matter of the brain

leucoencephalitis (loo'ko-en-sef-a-li'tis) inflammation of the white matter of the brain

leucoencephalopathy disease affecting the white matter of the brain

leucoerythroblastosis (loo'ko-e-rith'ro-blasto'sis) anaemia occurring from space-occupying lesions in the bone marrow. There are immature erythroid-myeloid cells in the circulation

leucoma (loo-ko'ma) a dense white corneal opacity

leuconychia (loo'ko-nik'e-a) unusually white nails

leucopaenia (loo'ko-pe'ne-a) a condition with diminished number of circulating white blood cells

leucopedesis (loo'ko-pe-de'sis) the passage of leucocytes through the walls of the blood vessels

leucopheresis a process by which the white blood cells are separated from withdrawn blood

leucoplakia (loo'ko-pla'ke-a) white thickened firmly attached patches on the mucous membrane, considered as precancerous condition

leucopoiesis (loo'ko-poy-e'sis) the production of leucocytes

leucorrhoea (loo'ko-re-a) a white viscid malodourous discharge from the vagina or cervical canal. It may be accompanied by intense pruritus

leucotaxis (loo'ko-taks'is) cytotaxis of leucocytes

leucotomy (loo'kot'o-me) incision into the white matter of the frontal lobe of the brain

leukaemia (loo-ke'me-a) a form of cancer characterised by disorganised proliferation of abnormal leucocytes **acute l** disorder of primitive stem cells which proliferate showing little or no differentiation. There are two main varieties, myeloid and lymphoid. The symptoms are due to bone morrow failure from replacement of normal haemopoietic tissue by leukaemic blast cells. It is characterised by anaemia, infection, mouth ulceration, gingival overgrowth, skin lesions, shock and bleeding. There may be bone pain, joint pain, tonsillar enlargement and splenomegaly. There is presence of blast cells. The treatment is to induce remission with cytotoxic drugs. Bone marrow transplantation may be necessary in some cases **chronic basophilic l** resembles CGL. There is gross increase in basophils **chronic granulocytic l (CGL),** a malignant disease of myeloid stem cells noted in middle age and it passes through three stages — benign responsive; accelerated unresponsive and a terminal phase resembling acute leukaemia. Majority show presence of Philadelphia chromosome. The condition is of insidious onset with weakness and weight loss and symptoms of anaemia. There is massive splenomegaly. The white cell counts are markedly raised. There is neutrophilia with immature forms like bands, metamyelocytes, and myelocytes. Benign phase responds to busulphan or hydroxyurea **chronic lymphatic l (CLL),** a progressive proliferation of lymphocytes (usually B cells) with infiltration of the bone marrow causing a peripheral blood lymphocytosis, seen in elderly patients. Often the condition is asymptomatic. There is lymph node enlargement, splenomegaly, anaemia and thrombocytopaenia. There is marked lymphocytosis and blood film shows disintegrated lymphocytes. Many patients survive for many years without treatment **chronic monocytic l** a blood picture of CGL with marked increase in the number of monocytes **hairy cell l** a variant of CLL rare and males are more frequently affected. Leucocyte count may be normal or high. There is massive splenomegaly. There is presence of hairy cells having features of B lymphocytes and monocytes. The cytoplasm exhibits a number of villi giving a hairy appearance. Corticosteroids and splenectomy are advised **promyelocytic l** a rare variant of CLL, seen in males above 60 years of age, associated with gross splenomegaly and very high white cell count. Lymphadenopathy is rare. Peripheral blood shows large lymphocytes with a prominent nucleolus. Its prognosis is poor.

leukaemic (loo-ke-m'ik) pertaining to leukaemia

leukaemid (loo-ke'mid) any non-specific skin eruptions frequently associated with leukaemia

leukaemoid (loo-ke'moyd) leucocytosis with clinical features resembling leukaemia **l reaction** leucocytosis in the circulating blood simulating leukaemia

leuko combining word for white

leukoblast (loo'ko-blast) an immature white blood cell

leukoplakia (loo'ko-pla'ke-a) raised white patch on the mucous membrane which has the potentiality to develop into cancer

leukosarcoma (loo'ko-sar-ko'ma) a type of malignant lymphoma with circulation of a large number of immature cells of lymphocytic series

leukotrichia (loo'ko-trik'e-a) white hairs

leukotrienes biologically active products of arachidonic acid metabolism which act as mediators of inflammation and allergic reactions

levator (le-va'tor) a muscle or an instrument to raise a part **l ani** a broad muscle forming the floor of the pelvis **l palpebrae superioris** a muscle that elevates the upper eyelid

LeVeen shunt a shunt from the peritoneal cavity to the venous circulation to control ascites, devised by Harry LeVeen, U.S. surgeon

Levin's (le-vinz) **tube** a plastic catheter which is introduced through the nose and extends through the stomach into the duodenum to remove intestinal liquids and gas during, and following intestinal surgery, named after American physician Abraham Levin

levo - combining word for left

levocardia (le'vo-kar'de-a) normal position of heart in presence of *situs inversus* of the viscera

levodopa active form of dopa used in the treatment of Parkinsonism.

levoduction (le'vo-duk'shun) a rotation of one or both eyes to the left

levorotation (le'vo-ro-ta'shun) a turning to the left

levoversion a turning toward the left

levulinic acid an acid produced on addition of dilute hydrochloric acid on certain sugars

levulose fruit sugar, fructose

lewdness a homosexual behaviour making obscene telephone calls

Lewis blood group antigen of red blood cells specified by Lewis that react with the antibodies designated anti Le after a patient in whose blood the antibodies were discovered, named after English propositus who first reported

lewisite (lu'i-sit) a toxic gas used in warfare to disable and kill.

Lewy bodies neuronal cells with pigmented inclusion bodies, which may be seen in the brain in substantia nigra and locus ceruleus in Parkinsonism, named after Frederic Lewy, German neurologist

Leydig's cells interstitial cells of the testis that secrete testosterone, named after German anatomist, Franz Leydig

LH luteinizing hormone

Lhermittes' (lar'mits) **sign** a sensation like an electric shock coursing down the spine when neck is flexed, described by Jacques Lhermittes, French neurologist. The aetiology may be cervical cord trauma or tumour, cervical spondylosis or multiple sclerosis

LH-RH luteinizing hormone-releasing hormone

libido (li-bi'do) sexual desire or drive

Libman-Sacks (lib'man-saks') **disease** nonbacterial verrucous endocarditis associated with SLE, described by Emanuel Libman and Benjamin Sacks, US physicians

lice plural of louse

lichen (li'ken) discrete shiny, itchy papular skin lesions resembling lichens growing on rocks l **planus** pruritic purple polygonal papules

lichenification (li-ken'i-fi-ka'shun) leathery induration and thickening of the skin

Lichtheim's (likt'himz) **syndrome** subacute combined degeneration of the spinal cord associated with pernicious anaemia, named after German physician, Ludwig Lichtheim

lichenoid resembling lichen

Lichtenberg (lai'ten-burg) **figures** arbores-cent fern-like markings due to cutaneous injuries from lightening strike, named after Christoph Lichtenberg, a German Physicist

lie the relation which the long axis of the foetus bears to that of the mother

lien (li'en) spleen

lienal (li'e'nal) splenic

lienitis inflammed spleen

life support measures the care provided to a person in a moribund state in an intensive care unit to maintain the patient in a stable condition

life style the way people live, includes personality traits, living habits, nutrition, physical exercise, use of alcohol, drugs and smoking and behavioural pattern

life table a statistical record which reflects the course of mortality in a population

life threatening illness a morbid condition in which the likelihood of death is high unless the course of disease is interrupted

ligament (lig'a-ment) a tough slightly elastic band of fibrous tissue that binds together the bony ends in a joint

ligamentopexy (lig'a-men'to-pek-si) fixation of the uterus by shortening the round ligament

ligand (li'gand) an organic molecule attached to a tracer element

ligation (li-ga'shun) the process of tying of a structure

Ligat's sign marked hyperaesthesia as a sign of early appendicitis, described by English surgeon, Ligat. It consists of picking up between the fingers and thumb a portion of the skin and subcutaneous tissue and lifting it from the abdominal musculature. The facial expression of pain is looked at

ligature (lig'a-chur) any material, a thread or wire used in surgery to tie off blood vessels around a structure

light chain a subunit of an immunoglobulin **l c disease** multiple myeloma producing only monoclonal light chain proteins

lightening an abrupt sensation of relief from the weight felt by the mother in later weeks of pregnancy due to the descent of foetal head into the pelvic cavity

lightning foot burning feet, described by Gopalan, nutrition specialist from India characterised by intense burning pain of the feet with hyperaesthesia due to a deficiency of vitamins and protein

lightning mark an arborescent charring of skin from high voltage electricity that may be seen in persons dying of electrocution

lightning pains sudden, sharp, painful crisis, may be idiopathic or precipitated by cold, a classic symptom of tabes dorsalis

light reflex reaction to light is dependent on the reflex arc with afferent fibres in the optic nerve, oculomotor nerve nuclei and efferent fibres in the oculomotor nerve

ligneous thyroiditis Riedel's disease, stony hard goitre producing tracheal compression early in the course of the disease and is noted in young adults of both sexes

lignocaine a local anaesthetic of moderate potency and duration, but of good penetrating power and rapid onset of action; xylocaine

limb (lim) an extremity; a segment of any jointed structure

limbic (lim'bik) **system** a part of the brain which controls emotions and instincts

limbus (lim'bus) an edge or border of a part

lime calcium oxide; citrus fruit

limen (li'men) entrance; threshold

liminal (lim'i-nal) pertaining to a threshold.

limping Walking with abnormal, jerky movements may arise from painful lesion, deformity, shortening or paralytic condition of the lower limb, trunk or abdomen

linctus (link'tus) a confection containing a medical preparation taken by licking

Lindau-von Hippel disease a hereditary disorder characterised by angioma of retina and cerebellum, and sometimes of spinal cord and viscera, after Arvid Lindau and Eugen-von Hippel, German ophthalmologists

linea (lin'e-a) a line or strip distinguished from the adjacent tissues by its colour or texture

linear (lin'e-ar) resembling a line **l regression** a generic term for statistical methods that are used to 'fit' a straight line to scattered data points of paired values. **l staining** a pattern of immune deposition that are described as continuous, smooth, thin, delicate and ribbon like **l transformation** the mathematical conversion of an equation into one providing data that can be plotted in a straight line

line diagram diagram to show the trends of events with the passage of time such as birth and death rates

line of demarcation a separating line at the junction of dead and living tissues, which is well marked in senile gangrene

lingua (ling'gwa) tongue

lingual (ling'gual) relating to the tongue **l thyroid** ectopic thyroid as a round swelling at the back of the tongue which may produce dysphagia, dyspnoea and heaemorrhage

Linguantula a blood sucking arthropod, tongue worm

linguantuliasis human infection by the third stage larvae of linguantula which presents with pain, itching and irritation in the throat with dyspnoea, dysphagia and vomiting

linguiform (ling'gwi-form) tongue-shaped

linguine (lin'gui-ne) **sign** a breast magnetic resonance imaging, characterised by fine, curvilinear low-signal-intensity strands within the gel of breast implants that have ruptured

lingula (ling'gu-la) a tongue-shaped structure

liniment an oily medicated liquid preparation for external application on the skin as a counter-irritant or anodyne

linitis (lin-i-tis) inflammation of the gastric tissue l **plastica** a diffuse fibrosis and rigid thickening of the wall of stomach encountered in a variant of gastric carcinoma

linkage presence of two or more genes sufficiently close to each other on the same chromosome to be passed on together from a parent to a child; chemical covalent bond l **disequilibrium** the tendency for some genes at a locus to be found with certain genes at another locus on the same chromosome with frequencies greater than would be expected by chance alone l **map** a genetic map based on the coinheritance of allele combinations across multiple polymorphic loci l **number** the number of times two strands of DNA cross through each other; winding number l **study** a study that identifies the chromosome responsible for a disease

linoleic acid an essential 18-carbon fatty acid with 2 unsaturated bonds obtained from vegetable oils

linolenic acid an essential 18-carbon fatty acid with 3 unsaturated bonds derived from either plants or animals

lint (lint) an absorbent surgical dressing material

LIP lymphocytic interstitial pneumonia

lip a muscular fold with an outer mucosa l **stripping** excision and advancement of the buccal mucosa

lipaemia (li-pe'me-a) increased amount of lipids in the circulating blood

lipase (li'pas) an enzyme secreted by pancreas that breaks down fat l **deficiency** decreased secretion of lipase by pancreas resulting in fats to pass through the intestine without being digested. It results in stools that are bulky, greasy and foul smelling

lipectomy (li'pek'to-me) surgical removal of fatty tissue

lipoedema chronic swelling of lower limb by fat and fluid

lipids (lip'ids) a group of fatty substances insoluble in water; they are stored in the body and used for energy

lipidosis disorder of metabolism that results in excessive accumulation of lipids in brain, liver, spleen or other parts of the body. It includes hereditary disorders such as Gaucher's disease, Tay-Sachs disease and Niemann-Pick disease. Usually they occur as recessive disorders in Jews. It presents with dementia, epilepsy and blindness

lipoatrophy (lip'o-a-tro'fe) atrophy of subcutaneous fat

lipoblast (lip'o-blast) an embryonic fat cell.

lipocoele (lip'o'sel) presence of fatty tissue in a hernial sac

lipochondrodystrophy (lip'o-kon-dro'dis' tro-fe) a connective tissue disorder, Hurler's syndrome

lipochrome (lip'o-krom) a generic term for any natural, fat-soluble pigment including lipofuscin, carotenes and lycopenes

lipocrit an apparatus used to separate and analyse the amount of lipid in blood or other body fluid

lipocyte (lip'o-sit) a fat storing cell in the liver

lipodystrophy (lip'o-dis'tro-fe) absence of subcutaneous fat associated with systemic abnormality

lipofibroma (lip'o-fi-bro'ma) a benign tumour of fibrous tissue with a large number of adipose cells

lipofuscin (lip'o-fus'sin) a yellow to brown pigmented lipid degradation product after destruction of mitochondria or mitochondrial polyunsaturated lipid membrane; lysosomal digestion pigment accumulates with age in the muscle, heart, liver, nerve cells and in lysosomes

lipogenesis (lip'o-jen'e-sis) production of fat

lipogranuloma (lip'o-gran-u-lo'ma) a granulomatous condition in association with deposits of lipid substance in tissues

lipoid (lip'oyd) fat like l pneumonia a pneumonitis following inhalation of oil into the lungs. Liquid paraffin or nasal instillation of mineral oil may be inhaled by elderly people with neurologic disturbances. The malnourished young children may inhale milk or codliver oil

lipoidosis (lip'oy-do'sis) a disorder of metabolism wherein there is excessive accumulation of some lipids in the body

lipolysis (lip-ol'i-sis) hydrolysis of fat

lipoma (li-po'ma) a benign tumour of fatty tissue in the subcutaneous tissue, which. is soft, mobile and slow growing. Most lipomas fluctuate as fat is fluid at body temperature

lipomatosis (li-po'ma-to'sis) abnormal deposits of fat in the tissues; adiposis l dolorosa a disorder of women with multiple localised masses of adipose tissue accompanied by local pain at the sites of accumulation

lipomeria (li-po'me're-a) the congenital absence of a limb or other part

lipopaenia (li-po'pe'ne-a) a deficiency of lipids in the body

lipophage (li'po-fag) a cell that ingests fat

lipophil (lip'o-fil) a substance possessing hydrophobic properties

lipophilic (lip'o-fil-ik) capable of absorbing lipids

lipopolysaccharide (lip'o-pol'e-sak'a-rid) a compound formed by lipids and carbohydrates

lipoproteins a family of lipid-carrying, water soluble proteins including chylomicrons, high -, intermediate-, low-and very-low density lipoproteins that are responsible for the transport of cholesterol and cholesterol esters, phospholipids and triglycerides throughout the circulation

liposarcoma (lip'o-sar-ko'ma) a malignant condition consisting of lipoblasts or fatty tissue

liposis (li-po'sis) fatty infiltration

liposome (lip'o-som) synthetic spherical vesicle with a lipid bilayer. It functions as artificial membrane systems to deliver DNA etc. into cells, and as a drug delivery system of toxic drugs

liposuction a cosmetic surgery in which localised areas of fat are removed from subcutaneous tissue through a metal cannula with side holes connected to a high pressure vacuum

lipotrophy (li-pot'ro-fe) increase in body fat

lipoxygenase (li-poks'i-je-nas) an enzyme that catalyses oxidation of unsaturated fatty acids

Lippes (li'pez) **loop**, an intrauterine contraceptive device, devised by Jacob Lippes, US obstetrician

lipping (lip'ing) formation of a lip-like structure at the articular end of a bone

lipuria (li-pu're-a) excretion of lipids in the urine

liquefacient (lik'we-fa'shent) making liquid

liquefaction (lik'owe-fak-shun) change from a solid to a liquid form

liquor (lik'er) liquid l **folliculi** clear fluid containing cavities surrounding the ripening Graafian follicle

Lisch (li'sh) **nodules** pigmented iris hamartomas seen in patients with type 1 neurofibromatosis, named after Karl Lisch, Austrian ophthalmologist

lissencephaly smooth brain without gyrae

Listeria a genus of gram-negative bacteria, named after Baron Lister, founder of modern antiseptic surgery, a Scottish surgeon.

listeriosis (lis-ter'e-o'sis) an infection contracted by eating undercooked meat that has been contaminated by *Listeria monocytogenes*

lithectasy (li'th-ek'ta-se) urethral extraction of a vesical calculus

lithiasis (lith-i-a-sis) formation of calculi

lithodialysis (lith'o-di-al'i-sis) fragmentation of calculi

lithogogue causing dislodgement or expulsion of a stone

lithotome (lith'o-tom) a knife to perform lithotomy

lithotomy (lith'ot'o-me) surgical removal of stone **l position** the position assumed by the patient lying supine with the hips and knees flexed and the thighs abducted and rotated externally for vaginal examination

lithotripsy (lith'o-trip'se) the crushing of a calculus by concentrated ultrasonic shock waves. It is a non-surgical, non-invasive method to dissolve renal and biliary tract calculi

lithotriptor (lith'o-trip'tor) a machine used for lithotripsy

lithotrite (lith'o-trit) an instrument used to crush a calculus

Litten's sign absence of normal peeling movements of the diaphragm on the thoracic cage named after Moritz Litten, German Physician

Little's disease cerebral spastic paralysis or diplegia, described by William Little, British physician

Littre's hernia hernia of Meckel's diverticulum named after Alexis Littre, French surgeon

Littritis (lit-tri'tis) inflammation of the urethral glands, named after French surgeon, Alexis Littre

live birth complete expulsion or extraction from its mother of a product of conception which after such separation, breathes or shows other evidence of life

live vaccine vaccine prepared from live, attenuated organisms such as BCG, measles, oral polio. These organisms have lost their capacity to produce full blown disease but retain their immunogenicity

livedo (li-e'do) a discoloured area on the skin due to passive congestion

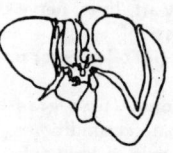

Liver-Inferior view

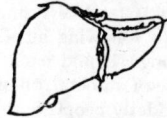

Liver-Front views

liver (liv'er) the largest gland of the body lying in the right upper abdomen, containing a large number of minute lobules performing many functions essential to life **cirrhosis of l** a chronic generalised liver disease resulting from necrosis and regeneration of liver cells. It is characterised by liver cell dysfunction, increased hepatic fibrosis and nodular degeneration **l abscess** it may be pyogenic or amoebic **l cancer** primary, derived from hepatocytes known as hepatoma **l fluke** a flatworm which on infecting liver causes jaundice **l tongue** blue-red tongue with engorged capillaries seen in advanced cirrhosis

livid (liv'id) discoloured

Loa loa (lo'a lo'a) a filarial nematode, named after a term used in Angola, West Africa, causative agent of loiasis; eyeworm

lobar (lo'bar) pertaining to a lobe

lobate (lo'bat) divided into lobes; lobe-shaped

lobe (lob) a well demarcated subdivision in any organ or gland

lobectomy (lo-bek'to-me) surgical removal of a lobe

lobotomy (lo'bo-tomi) a surgical procedure to treat psychiatric disorders where the nerves connecting the hypothalamus to the prefrontal cortex are severed by introducing surgical instruments into the frontal lobe of the brain

Lobstein's (lob'stinz) **disease** osteogenesis imperfecta, named after Johann Lobstein, German surgeon

lobular (lob'u-lar) pertaining to a lobule

lobule (lob'ul) a small lobe or subdivision of a lobe

local (lo'kal) restricted to one area

localization (lo-kal-i-za'-shun) determination of the place of any process or lesion

lochia (lo'ke-a) the vaginal discharge noted during the first three to four weeks following childbirth. It contains mucus, blood and tissue debris

lochiometra (lo'ke-o-me'tra) distension of the uterus with retained lochia

lock and key model A biochemical model that assumes an enzyme and substrate have a rigid interaction with each other, where a substance fits in a key-like fashion to its lock. The enzyme turning on the reaction

locked-in syndrome a condition of flaccid tetraplegia with facial paresis and complete incapacity to express voluntary response due to bilateral interruption of the corticobulbar and corticospinal tracts at the level of the pons

lock jaw painful spasm of the masseter muscles with stiffness of the jaw noted in tetanus

locomotor (lo'ko-mo'tor) pertaining to the movement of the body

loculation (lo'ku-la'shun) a space formed between surfaces of organs or membrane

loculi (lok'u-li) plural of loculus.

loculus (lok'u-lus) a small space or cavity

locus (lo'kus) a site in the body or site of a gene on a chromosome

lod abbreviation of the $\log_{10}$ of the odd's favouring linkage **l score** statistical test to determine whether a set of linkage data are linked or not linked

LOD score a statistical estimate of whether 2 loci are likely to lie near each other on a chromosome

Loffler's syndrome a benign disorder of pulmonary eosinophilia, cough and transient opacity in the lung, named after Swiss physician, Wilhelm Loffler

log abbreviation of logarithm

logagnosia (log'ag-no-se-a) aphasia.

logarithm a scale of measurement, often used while describing viral load. A one log change refers to a ten-fold change such as from 100 to 10; A two-log change refers to a hundredfold change such as from 1000 to 10

logging on the process of accessing computers or files using a password or other instructions

log-on to identify yourself and gain access to a computer

logopaedics (log'o-pe'di-ks) the science concerned with the study and treatment of speech defects

logoplaegia (log-o-ple'je-a) paralysis of the organs of speech

logospasm (log'o-spazm) the spasmodic utterance of words

loiasis (lo-i'sis) infection with nematodes of the genus *Loa loa*

loin (loyn) the part of the back on either side of the spine between the thorax and pelvis

lomustine a nitrosurea anticancer drug

longissimus (lon-jis'i-mus) longest

longitudinal (lon'ji-tu-di-nal) parallel to the long axis of the body

longus (long'gus) a long structure

looking at the ceiling test the patient with degenerative changes in the cervical intervertebral discs will complain of discomfort either in the base of the neck, or interscapular region when he or she is asked to look at the ceiling and maintain the neck in extension for a minute

loop a turn or a curve

loose body something felt 'moving about in the joint' often called mouse, in osteoarthritis

loosening of associations *Psy* flow of thought in which ideas shift from one subject to another in a completely unrelated way

Looser's zone a radiologic abnormally showing linear zones of decalcification which tend to be symmetric and extend perpendicular to the cortex, named after Emil Looser, Swiss Surgeon

lordosis (lor-do'sis) abnormal increase in the anterior curvature; saddle back

lotion (lo'shun) a liquid medicated suspension for external application to the body

Louis angle sternal angle, a transverse ridge in upper sternum corresponding to second rib, named after Antoine Louis, French surgeon, who designed guillotine

Louis-Bar (loo-we'bar) **syndrome** ataxiatelangiectasia, described by Denise Louis-Bar, European physician

loupe (loop) a convex lens to magnify light upon an object

louse an ectoparasitic insect infesting mammals. pl. **lice**

lower motor neuron (LMN) the motor cells of the cranial nuclei of the brain stem and the anterior horn cells of spinal cord **LMN lesion** loss of all movements, flaccidity, wasting followed by contracture, loss of tendon reflexes and unaltered superficial reflexes

Lowe's (loz) **disease** oculocerebrorenal syndrome, described by Charles Lowe, U.S. paediatrician

Lown-Ganong-Levine Syndrome an electrocardiographic abnormality with a short PR interval and normal QRS complex giving rise to paroxysmal supraventricular tachycardia, named after Bernard Lown, US cardiologist, William Ganong, US physiologist and Samuel Levine, Polish-US Cardiologist

lozenge (loz'enj) a small disc-shaped body containing a drug

lubb (lub) a syllable representing the first heart sound

lucid (lu'sid) clear **l interval** a window period preceding the loss of consciousness and coma that occurs in subdural and epidural haematomas

lucidity (lu-sid'i-te) clarity

lucio phenomenon severe type 2 reaction caused by vasculitis occurring in lucio leprosy, characterised by erythematous macules which become ulcerated, later heal with atropic scarring

Ludwig's (lud'vigz) **angina** diffuse purulent inflammation around the submaxillary glands due to streptococcal infection, named after Wilhelm von Ludwig, German surgeon

lues syphilis

luetic (lu-et'ik) syphilitic

Lugol's (lu'golz) **solution** a strong iodine solution named after Jean Lugol, French physician

lumbago (lum-ba'go) pain in the lumbar region.

lumbar (lum'bar) pertaining to the loin **l plexus** an interlacing network of nerves located on either side of the spine in the low back **l puncture** insertion of a hollow needle into the lower part of the spinal canal to withdraw cerebrospinal fluid or to inject drugs, anaesthetic agents or radiographic substances **l spine** the part of the spine situated between the lowest pair of ribs and the top of pelvis; it consists of five lumbar vertebrae

lumbarization (lum'bar-i-za'shun) a condition wherein the first segment of the sacrum is not fused with the second segment of the sacrum and remains as a separate vertebra

lumbar root lesions characterised by low back pain. The lesions of L3-4 root have pain in anterior thigh, L5 root lesion in lateral thigh and lesions of sacral 1-2 segments have pain in posterior thigh

lumbosacral pertaining to the loin and groin

lumbrical (lum'bri-kal) a muscle in the hand; of the earthworms

lumbricide (lum'bri-sid) an agent that kills intestinal worms.

lumbricoid (lum'bri-kyod) resembling the earthworm

lumbricus (lum-bri'kus) the ascaris

lumbus loin

lumen (lu'men) channel within a tubular structure

luminous (loo'mi-nus) emitting light

lumpectomy segmental mastectomy

lunacy (lu'na-se) insanity

lunar pertaining to the moon

lunate moon-shaped especially a half moon; crescentic

lunatic (lu'na-tik) a mentally deranged individual

lung either of the organs of respiration situated on either side of the heart within the thoracic cavity. The right lung has three lobes (upper, middle and lower) and the left two lobes (upper and lower). The lungs have double arterial supply from pulmonary and bronchial arteries and double venous drainage. They provide a surface for transfer of gases through which blood gets rid of CO_2 and absorbs oxygen. The aim of the lungs is to achieve normal oxygenation (arterialisation) of the mixed venous blood perfusing the pulmonary capillaries l **abscess** a localised collection of pus in the parenchyma of the lung as a result of tissue necrosis and suppuration from a pyogenic infection l **agenesis** a rare congenital abnormality exhibiting failure of development of the primitive lung bud l **aplasia** a total absence of the lung and bronchi **budgeriger** l people exposed to droppings of Turkey pigeon are sensitised to avian serum proteins result in extrinsic allergic alveolitis **cheese worker's** l exposure to mouldy cheese resulting in extrinsic allergic alveolitis **coffee worker's** l coffee bean dust acting as a sensitising agent to cause extrinsic allergic alveolitis **honeycomb** l an endresult of many diverse interstitial lung diseases presenting radiologically with a pattern of coarse reticular interstitial areas of increased opacity with intervening cystic spaces, and pathologi-

cally cystic spaces with walls consisting of a variable amounts of fibrous tissue l **collapse** shrinkage of lung volume either from the obstruction of a lobar bronchus or from presence of air or fluid in the pleural space **lung compliance** a measure of the distensibility of the lungs (C_L). It measures the ease with which the lung volume is changed and is expressed in litres per cm H_2O l **rupture** expansion of the air in the lungs on ascent in divers, leading to its entry into the pleural space and the mediastinum l **scars** scars in the lung from a previous infection that acts as a weak point for action of environmental carcinogens l **tumours** see bronchogenic carcinoma l **volume** consists of four basic subdivisions as tidal volume, inspiratory reserve volume, expiratory reserve volume and residual volume. The former three are dynamic lung volumes. The lungs do not become totally airless at the end of each expiration and it can't be expelled (residual volume) **mushroom picker's** l inhalation of mouldy mushroom compost dust resulting in extrinsic allergic alveolitis **pigeon fancier's** l people exposed to pigeon droppings are sensitised to avian serum proteins to result in extrinsic allergic alveolitis

lungworm the trematode, *Paragonimus westermani.*

lunula (lu'nu-la) a small crescentic area

lupus (lu'pus) a chronic inflammation of connective tissue with skin lesions; wolf.

luteal pertaining to corpus luteum

lutein (lu'tein) a yellow pigment

luteinization (lu'te-in-i-za'shun) the process of transformation of the ovarian follicle into corpus luteum following ovulation

luteinizing hormone (LH) secretion of anterior pituitary and corpus luteum is formed by its influence. Ovulation requires a sudden surge of LH

luteinizing hormone releasing hormone (LMRH). The main effect of gonadotrophin-releasing hormone is on the release of luteinising hormone

Lutembacher's (loo'tem-bak'erz) **syndrome** mitral stenosis associated with atrial septal defect, described by Rene Lutembacher, French physician

luxation (luks-a'shun) dislocation

luxuary perfusion syndrome an overall increase in cerebral blood flow in excess of metabolic demands noted in brain lactic acidosis

lycopene (li'ko-pen) the red carotinoid pigment especially found in tomato

Lyell's syndrome toxic epidermal necrolysis; acute bullous lesion caused by epidermal separation, frequently at mucocutaneous junctions, named after Allan Lyell, British dermatologist

lying in puerperal

Lyme disease a multi-system disease by a bacterial *(Borrelia burgodorfi)* infection transmitted by tick bites initially described at old Lyme, Connecticut, USA

lymph (limf) a transparent, slightly yellowish fluid circulating in the lymphatics. It plays an important part in the immune system and in the absorption of fats from the intestine **l node** a small gland that lies along the course of a vessel in the lymphatic system. It filters lymph and acts as a barrier to the spread of infection

lymphadenectasis (lim-fad'e-nek'ta-sis) enlargement of a lymph node

lymphadenectomy (lim-fad'e-nek'to-me) excision of the lymph node

lymphadenitis (lim-fad'en-i'tis) inflammation of one or more lymph nodes

lymphadenoid goitre Hashimoto's disease; a rubbery hard, fixed enlargement of the whole of thyroid gland with evidence of myxoedema

lymphadenopathy (lim-fad'e-nop'a-the) disease of the lymph nodes

lymphadenosis (lim-fad'e-no'sis) hypertrophy of the lymphoid tissue

lymphangial (lim-fan'je-al) pertaining to a lymphatic vessel

lymphangiectasis (lim-fan'je-ek'ta-sis) dila-

tation of the lymphatic vessel

lymphangiogram (lim-fan'je-o-gram) a roentgenogram of the lymphatic vessels

lymphangiography (lim-fan'je-og'ra-fe) roentgenography of the lymphatic vessels following injection of contrast medium

lymphangioleiomyomatosis (LAM) a rare pulmonary disorder characterised by an abnormal proliferation of smooth muscle-like cells that can lead to obstruction of airways, lymphatics and blood vessels. It affects primarily young women of child-bearing age

lymphangioma (lim-fan'je-o'ma) a tumour composed of newly formed lymphatic vessels

lymphangitis (lim'fan-ji'tis) inflammation of a lymphatic vessel or vessels

lymphatic (lim-fat'ik) pertaining to lymph or lymph vessel

lymph node any of the accumulations of lymphoid tissue in the course of lymphatic vessels

lymphoblast (lim'fo-blast) the immature precursor of the mature lymphocyte

lymphoblastosis (lim'fo-blas-to-sis) excess number of lymphoblasts in the blood

lymphocyte (lim-fo-sit) a mononuclear leucocyte with a deeply staining nucleus containing dense chromatin and a pale-blue staining cytoplasm. It is divided into B and T lymphocytes responsible of humoral and cellular immunity respectively

lymphocytic (lim-fo-sit'ic) pertaining to the lymphocyte **l leukaemia** an uncontrolled proliferation and accumulation of mature B lymphocytes. The symptoms result from bone marrow failure

lymphocytopaenia (lim-fo-sit'o-pe'-ne-a) a decreased number of lymphocytes in the blood.

lymphoedema (limf-e-de'ma) chronic oedema of the extremities due to accumulation of interstitial fluid due to stasis of lymph **primary l** due to congenital defect such as aplasia or hypoplasia of subcutaneous lymphatic vessels or due to incompetence and dilatation of lymphatics and noted in middle aged adults as a painless swelling **secondary l** occurs due to nonlymphatic conditions producing obstruction to normal lymphatics

lymphocytopoiesis (lim'fo-sit'-o-poy-e'sis) the development of lymphocyte

lymphocytosis (lim'fo-si-to-sis) increase in the number of normal lymphocytes in the blood

lymphogranuloma (lim'fo-gran'u-lo'ma) condition with granulomas or granuloma-like lesions **l inguinale** a sexually transmitted disease caused by *Chlamydia trachomatis* affecting lymph nodes in inguinogenital region. Also called tropical bubo **l venereum** (LGV), responds to tetracyclines and aspiration not incision of buboes

lymphography (lim-fog' ra-fe) roentgenography of the lymphatic vessels and lymph nodes following injection of contrast medium in a lymphatic vessel

lymphoid (lim'foyd) pertaining to lymph or lymphatic system **l tissue** a tissue rich in lymphocytes that is found in lymph nodes and in the spleen

lymphokine (lim'fo-kin) mediator released by sensitised lymphocyte

lymphoma (lim-fo'ma) any neoplastic condition of the lymphoid tissue. It consists of Hodgkin's disease, non-Hodgkin's lymphoma and T-cell lymphoma

lymphomatoid granulomatosis a systemic disorder characterised by granulomatous vasculitis affecting the lungs, kidneys, skin and central nervous system. It is treated by immuno-suppressive therapy

lymphomatosis (lim'fo-ma-to'sis) the development of multiple lymphomas in different parts of the body

lymphopaenia (lim-fo-pe'ne-a) decrease in number of lymphocytes in the blood

lymphopoiesis (lim'fo-poy-e'sis) the development of lymphatic tissue

lymphorrhagin profuse exudation of lymph from the vesicles formed on the lymph scrotum

lymph scrotum filarial condition presenting as dilatation and tortuosity of the cutaneous lymphatics of the scrotum. It may be associated with gross rugosity of scrotal skin

lymph varix dilatation and tortuosity of the cutaneous lymphatics, noted in the scrotum

Lynch (li'n-ch) **syndrome** hereditary nonpolyposis colorectal syndrome

lyonisation (lion'isa-shun) all but one X-chromosome are inactivated randomly early in development

lyophil (li'o-fil) a substance that readily goes into solution

lyophilisation (li-of'i-li-za'shun) the production of a stable biologic substance by rapid freezing and dehydration of the frozen product under high vacuum; freeze-drying

lyse (liz) to cause disintegration

lysergic acid diethylamide, (LSD), synthetic hallucinogen obtained from ergot alkaloids that produces mood elevations, sensory distortion and depersonalisation and there can be panic attacks

lysin (li'sin) an antibody which can cause dissolution of cells

lysine (li'sen) an amino acid

lysis (li'sis) dissolution by enzymes

lysosome (li'so-som) a minute membrane bound cytoplasmic organelle present in the cells that contains a variety of digestive enzymes

lysozyme (li'so-zim) a hydrolytic enzyme which hydrolyses mucopolysaccharides and mucoproteins, found in tears, milk, saliva, serum and neutrophils and acts as an antibacterial enzyme

lyssa (lis'sa) madness : rabies

M

M symbol for mega (10⁶), molar concentration, mitosis

m metre, minim, mean of a sample, messenger, molar concentration; mass

MAC *Mycobacterium avium* complex

MacCallum's plaques maplike thickening of the endocardium over myocardial lesion in acute rheumatic fever, named after William Maccallum, Canadian-US Pathologist

macerate (mas'er-at) to soften by soaking in water

maceration (mass-er-a'shun) process of softening a solid by steeping in a fluid

machinary murmur a harsh, rasping continuous murmur of patent ductus arteriosus heard in the left second intercostal space near the sternum. The murmur begins shortly after the first sound reaches a maximum at the end of systole and wanes in late diastole. It is accompanied by a thrill or buzz

machine any mechanical device or instrument

macies (ma'she-ez) wasting, atrophy

macrencephaly (mak-ren'sef'a-le) abnormally large size of the brain

macr(o) combining word for large or long

macroaggregated albumin used as a carrier for radio-isotopes for angiographic imaging

macroamylase a salivary type of plasma amylase that circulates complexed to various high-molecular weight plasma proteins

macrobrachia (mak'ro-bra'ke-a) abnormal size or length of arm

macrocardius (mak'ro-kar'de-us) person with an abnormally large heart caused by congenital heart disease

macrocephaly (mak-ro-sef'a-le) abnormal large and globular head, seen in hydrocephalus, acromegaly, osteitis deformans, gorgoylism or as a congenital condition

macrocheilia (mak'ro-ki'le-a) abnormal size of the lip

macrocheria (mak-ro-ki're-a) large hands

macrocnemia (mak'rok-ne'me-a) abnormally large legs

macrocornea (mak-ro-kor'ne-a) abnormal size of the cornea

macrocyst (mak'ro-sist) a large cyst

macrocyte abnormally large erythrocyte with increased haemoglobin and decreased life span seen in haemolytic anaemia, massive bleeding, hyperthyroidism and erythroblastosis foetalis

macrocytic (mak'ro-sit'ik) pertaining to cells larger than normal **m anaemia** an impaired erythropoiesis and presence of large red blood cells in the blood, often a result of folic acid or vitamin B_{12} deficiency

macrocytosis (mak'ro-si-to'sis) condition in which erythrocytes are larger than normal; macrocythaemia

macrodontia (mak'ro-don'she-a) abnormal increase in size of the teeth

macrogamete (mak'ro-gam'et) a large immobile zygote formed by conjugation of female gamete with the microgamete (male). It is encountered in the plasmodium life cycle that occurs in human

macrogametocyte (mak'ro-ga-me'to-sit) a large immobile reproductive cell developing from the merozoite of certain protozoa

macrogenitosomia (mak'ro-jen'i-to-so'me-a) abnormal size of genitalia due to excess androgens

macroglia (mak-rog'le-a) astrocyte

macroglobulin (mak'ro-glob'u-lin) any large serum protein. Its level in the blood is increased in multiple myeloma, collagen disorders, cirrhosis of the liver and amyloidosis

macroglobulinaemia (mak'ro-glob'u-lin-e'me-a) presence of macroglobulins in the blood, which causes increased viscosity of the blood, *see* Waldenstrom's macroglobulinaemia

macroglossia (mak'ro-glos'e-a) markedly enlarged tongue seen in acromegaly, cretinism, myxoedema, primary amyloidosis, mangolism, haemangioma or lymphangioma

macrognathia (mak-ro-na'the-a) abnormal size of the jaw

macrography (mak-rog'va-fe) writing with large letters

macrogyria (mk-ro'ga-y-re-a) excessively large size of convolutions of cerebral hemispheres

macrolabia (mak-ro-la'be-a) abnormal size of lip

macrolide (ma'kro-lid) antibiotic, any of a group of broad-spectrum antibiotics e.g. erythromycin, clarithromycin, azithromycin and spiramycin which contain a lactone ring and inhibit protein synthesis in target bacteria

macromania (mak'ro-ma'ne-a) a delusion of possessing extremely large body parts or surroundings; megalomania

macromastia (mak-ro-mas'te-a) abnormally large breasts

macromelia (-mel'e-a) excessive size of an organ or part especially limbs

macromelus (mak-rom'e-lus) an individual with abnormally large extremities

macromolecule (mak'ro-mol'e-kul) a large molecule such as protein, polysaccharide or polymer

macronodular cirrhosis coarsely nodular 'hob-nail' liver of portal cirrhosis

macronucleoli (mak'ro-ni'kle-o-le) enlarged nucleoli seen in certain malignancies such as carcinoma of the kidney, breast and thyroid, malignant melanoma and Hodgkin's disease. They are also seen in tissue repair

macronucleus (mak'ro-nu'kle-us) a nucleus occupying most of the cell

macronutrients minerals needed in relatively high amounts

macronychia (mak'ro-nik'e-a) abnormal length of the finger nails

macrophage (mak'ro-faj) cells of reticuloendothelial system possessing the ability to phagocytose bacteria and other foreign particles. They are monocytes comprising 3-5% of circulating leucocytes, tissue-bound macrophages located in the alveoli (dust cells), central nervous system (microglial cell), liver (Kupffer cells, lymph nodes), peritoneum and skin (Langerhans cells) and histiocytes found in connective tissues **alveolar m** multipotent cells normally petrolling the interior of alveoli which recognise and destroy bacteria as the foreign organic particles **fixed m** a nonmotile macrophage **foamy m** macrophages that stain positive with periodic acid-Schiff reagent and infiltrate small intestinal mucosa in Whipple's disease **free m** a wandering or amoeboid macrophage **m activating factor** MAF, a lymphokine that stimulates alteration in the appearance and activities of the macrophage cells so that they can kill some microbes **m chemotactic factor** any cytokine that functions in tandem with macrophages mediating migration **m migration inhibiting factor** a substance that prevents the migration of macrophages in culture

macrophallus (mak'ro-fal'us) abnormally large penis

macrophthalmia (mak'rof-thal'me-a) abnormally large eye ball

macroplasia (mak'ro-pla'ze-a) abnormally large size of a tissue or part

macropodia (mak'ro-po'de-a) abnormally large feet

macropsia (mak-rop'se-a) condition wherein the objects look larger than they actually are

macrorhinia (mak-ro-rin'e-a) abnormally large nose

macroscelia (mak-ro-se'le-a) abnormally large legs

macroscopic (mak-ro-skop'ik) large enough to be seen by the naked eye

macroscopy (mak-ros'ko-pe) examination of an object with naked eye

macrosis (ma-kro'sis) increase in size

macrosomia (mak-ro-so'me-a) abnormally large body

macrostomia (mak-ro-sto'me-a) excessively large mouth

macrotia (mak'ro'she-a) abnormally large ears

macrotome (mak'ro-tom) an instrument for cutting large anatomical sections

macula (mak'u-la) 1. a small spot 2. a coloured area **m densa** a specialised region in the distal renal tubule at which point specialised cells converge and macula densa is part of the juxtaglomerular apparatus **m lutea** yellowish area of retina centred on *fovea centralis*

macular (mak'u-lar) relating to or having macules **m degeneration** a disorder of blood vessel in which the central part of the retina in the eye deteriorates causing partial loss of vision **m rash** skin eruptions in which the lesions are flat

macule (mak'ul) circumscribed area of variable size on the skin with an alteration in colour and without any elevation as in leucoderma, mole, purpura, erythema, or leprosy

maculopapular (mak'u-lo-pap'u-lar) an eruption consisting of both macules and papules

maculopathy (mak'u-lop'a-the) pathologic changes affecting the macula of the eye.

mad irrational, insane

mad cow disease bovine spongiform encephalopathy

madarosis (mad-a-ro'sis) loss of eyebrows or eyelashes

Madelung's disease generalised symmetrical deposits of fatty tissue on the upper part of the posterior part of the thorax, shoulders and neck, named after Otto Madelung, German surgeon

Madhura (s) sweet

Madura foot a chronic fungal disease of deep soft tissues and bones, most commonly of the limbs, named after the city Madurai, Tamil Nadu

Maduromycosis (mad-u'ro-mi-ko'sis) It is caused by two groups of organisms Eumycetes (*Madura mycetomatis*, *Madurella grisea*) and aerobic Actinomycetes (*Actinomadura madurae*). They produce a chronic granuloma with a fibrous stroma and cyst-like space, which contain grains of colonies of matted organisms. Those caused by Actinomycetes can be treated by rifampicin or streptomycin and dapsone or co-trimoxazole

MAF abbreviation for macrophage activating factor

Magendie's (ma-jen'dez) **foramen** the median of the three openings in the roof of the 4th ventricle and it connects the ventricle with the subarachnoid space, named after Francois Magendie, French physiologist

Magenblase syndrome *Ger* accumulation of swallowed air in the stomach that leads to fullness of stomach after food. Radiologically there will be a large gastric bubble

magenstrasse *Ger* the pliable, linear rugal folds along the lesser curvature of the stomach from cardia to pylorus

megenta bodies red-to-purple perinuclear inclusions seen by Romanovsky stain in breast carcinoma

magenta tongue a deeply red-to-purple, smooth tongue seen in riboflavin deficiecy

maggot larve of an insect especially of flies. They are parasitic and thrive in necrotic tissues

magic bullet any agent that would act with specificity of an antibody and have the lethal potential of a toxin

magnesia (mag-ne'ze-a) magnesium oxide MgO **milk of m** magnesium oxde and water used as an aperient

magnesium a white mineral substance found in soft tissue, muscles, bone and body fluids. Magnesium is widely distributed in foods, especially whole grains, fruits and vegetables. It activates enzymes that catalyse reactions between phosphate ions and ATP. Its deficiency may be associated with tetany, weakness and mental depression **m carbonate** a white odourless powder, on oral administration it neutralises acid in the stomach **m chloride** useful in treatment of electrolyte disturbances and in dialysis solution. **m citrate** used as a purgative **m hydroxide** milk of magnesia used as a laxative and antacid **m oxide** white powder used as an antacid and laxative **m sulphate** epsom salt used as a cathartic, anticonvulsant and topically as an anti-inflammatory agent **m trisilicate** used as an antacid

magnet (mag'net) any body possessing the property of attracting iron **magnetic** adj.

magnetic field the region around any magnet in which its effects can be detected

magnetic resonance MR the absorption or emission of electromagnetic energy by nuclei in a static magnetic field after excitation by a suitable resonance fequency magnetic field

magnetic resonance imaging MRI the creation of images by the phenomenon of magnetic resonance which is a function of the distribution of hydrogen nuclei (protons) in the body. The MR image is a computerised interpretation of the physical interaction of unpaired protons with electromagnetic radiation in the presence of a magnetic field

magnetotherapy (mag-ne-to-ther'a-pe) application of magnets in the treatment of diseases

magnification (mag-ni-fi-ka'shun) 1. a process of increasing the size of an object as under microscope 2.*Psy* cognitive distortion in which the effects of one's behaviour are magnified

magnum great; large

mahakushtha (s) leprosy

maharoga (s) major disease

MAI *Mycobacterium avium intracellulare*

maim (mam) to disable

main (man) hand **m d'accoucheur** *Fr* hand with fingers straight but bent of metacarpophalangeal joint as in tetany **m en griffe** *Fr* claw hand **m en trident** *Fr* a short broad hand with a fore shortened middle finger resulting in equal length of all digits, seen in achondroplasia

maintenance dose the amount of drug required to keep a desired mean steady-state concentration in the tissues

Majja(s) bone marrow

major affective disorder any of a group psychotic disorders characterised by severe and inappropriate emotional responses, by prolonged and persistent disturbances of mood, and other symptoms either of depression or maniac states.

major basic protein protein found in eosinophilic granules that causes bronchial epithelial damage and is related to asthma.

major histocompatibility complex MHC a set of polymorphic genes on chromosome 6 that code for the antigens that determine tissue and blood comptibility. They are referred as human leucocyte antigens (HLA) in humans

major surgery any surgical procedure requiring general anaesthesia or respiratory assistance

mal a disorder or illness.

Mal de mer L sea sickness

mala (ma'lo) 1. the cheek 2. the cheek bone. **malar** adj.

mala (s) waste product

malabsorption (mal'absorp'shun) impaired absorption of nutrients from gastrointestinal tract **m syndrome** a complex of symptoms resulting from disorders in the intestinal absorption of nutrients characterised by abdominal distension, borborygmi, cramps, weight loss, undigested food in the stools, or bulky, pale and offensive stools, lethargy and malaise and deficiencies of specific vitamins, trace elements and minerals

malacia (ma-la'she-a) abnormal softening of tissues or an organ

malacoplakia (mal'a-ko-pla'ke-a) presence of soft patches in the mucous membrane of a hollow organ especially in urogenital tract

maladie (mal'a-de) **de Roger** *Fr* congenital interventricular septal defect, named after Henry Roger, French physician

maladjusted poorly adjusted

malady (mal'a-de) a disease or illness

malaise (ma-laz) uneasiness; indisposition

malalignment (mal'a-lin-ment) improper alignment of structures, such as teeth or parts of a fractured bone

malaria (ma-la're-a) a tropical disease caused by the presence of sporozoa plasmodium, species of protozoa and transmitted to humans by the bite of an infected female mosquito of the genus *Anopheles* that previously sucked the blood from a person with malaria. It mainly affects the hepatocytes and red blood cells and presents with fever and splenomegaly. Four species of plasmodium, *Plasmodium vivax, P falciparum, P. ovale* and *P. malariae* have man as their vertebrate host in their life cycle. The sporozoites injected by mosquito are transported to the liver by circulating blood, where they undergo a sexual maturation and become schizonts and later merozoites. The infected hepatocytes rupture after 8-14 days and release merozoites into circulation, and infect the red blood cells, where further asexual cycles of multiplication occurs producing schizonts. Rupture of schizont releases more merozoites into the blood and causes fever whose periodicity depends on the species of plasmodium. *P. vivax* and *P. ovale* may persist in liver cells as dormant forms (hypnozoites), capable of developing into merozoites months or years later. *P. falciparum* and *P. malariae* have no exoerythrocytic

phase. However recrudescences of fever occurs from multiplication of parasites in the red cells which have not been eliminated by therapy or immune processes **acute m** commonest presentation of malaria due to *P. vivax* and *P. falciparum*. It is characterised by abrupt onset of chills necessitating to cover the body with blankets (cold phase). There is uncontrollable shivering (rigors). It is followed by fever, headache, and flushing (hot phase). The fever remits in 3-8 hours with profuse sweating (wet phase). The paroxysms coincides with haemolysis **cerebral m** falciparum malaria in which brain is affected due to tendency of parasites to agglutinate in the capillaries and is manifested either by confusion or coma, usually without localising signs **chronic m** persistent hepatic infection by *P. vivax* resulting in progressive splenomegaly **falciparum m** malaria caused by *P. falciparum*. It invades red cells of all ages and haemolysis is more severe. The condition is more dangerous than other forms of malaria. The fever has no particular pattern. Liver and spleen are enlarged and anaemia develops rapidly **quartan m** malaria of short duration caused by *P. malariae* where sporulation occurs every 72 hours and bouts of fever every third day **quotidian m** Malaria produced by *P. vivax* with classical bouts of fever on alternate days **tertian m** malaria in which sporulation occurs at 48 hours interval. Benign tertian malaria is caused by *P. vivax* and malignant tertian malaria by *P. falciparum* **vivax m** most common form of malaria produced by *P. vivax*. It is characterised by frequent recurrences

malaricidal (ma-la're-a-si'dal) possessing the property of killing malaria parasite

Malassezia (mal'a-se'ze-a) *furfur* a genus of fungus causing tinea versicolor, named after Louis Malassez, French physiologist

malathion (mal′a-thi′on) an organo-phosphorous insecticide

male 1. an individual of male sex 2. denotes sex to which those belong have organs for production of spermatozoa 3. masculine **genetic m** an individual with normal male karyotype including one X and one Y chromosome **m erectile disorder** inability to attain or maintain adequate erection of penis until completion of sexual activity

Malecot catheter a self-retaining rubber catheter-named after A. Malecot, French surgeon

malemission (mal′e-mish-un) failure of semen to be ejaculated during coitus

maleruption (mal-e-rup′shun) incorrect eruption of teeth

malformation (mal-for-ma′shun) deformity; abnormal shape or structure

malfunction (mal′funk′shun) defective function

malic acid hydroxysuccinic acid

malice (mal′a′s) desire to harm someone or show ill-will

malignancy a neoplasm or a cancerous tumour, that is life threatening, not confined to the site of origin but by spreading by invasion or metastases

malignant (ma-lig′nant) 1. condition resisting treatment especially of cancerous growth 2. virulent. **m hyperpyrexia** a familial tendency to develop severe form of hyperpyrexia during the use of muscle relaxants or general anaesthesia with succinylcholine or halothane **m hypertension** a severe form of hypertension that progresses rapidly accompanied by widespread fibrinoid necrosis. It has a poor prognosis **m melanoma** see melanoma **m mimics** lesions that either grossly or microscopically mimic malignancy **m narcissism** *Psy* personality disorder characterised by marked narcissistic and antisocial traits **m neoplasm** a tumour that tends to invade and metastasise

malingerer (ma-ling′ger-er) one who pre-tends to be ill to elicit sympathy

malleable (mal′e-a-bl) possessing a property of being shaped by pressure

malleolus (mal-e′o-lus) pl. **malleoli** the bony protuberances on either side of the ankle joint **lateral m** protuberance in lower end of the fibula **medial m** protuberance in lower end of the tibia

mallet a hammer-like tool **m finger** flexion deformity of terminal phalanx due to avulsion or rupture of extensor tendon **m fracture** avulsion fracture of the dorsal base of the distal phalanx **m toe** fixed flexion deformity of distal interphalangeal joint of lesser toes

malleus (mal′e-us) largest auditory ossicle in the middle ear that connects tympanus to incus

Mallary (mal′ore) **bodies** an eosinophilic cytoplasmic inclusion in liver cells, may be seen in acute alcoholic liver injury, named after Frank Mallory, US pathologist

Mallory-Weiss syndrome tear of mucosa of the lower end of oesophagus or gastroesophageal junction during severe vomiting especially in alcoholics, causing haemorrhage, named after Kenneth Mallory, US pathologist and Soma Weiss US physician

Malmstom's cup cup for obstetric vacuum extraction, named after T. Malmstom, Scandinavian obstetrician

malnutrition (mal′nu-tri′shun) any disorder of nutrition caused by a deficiency of proper food substances. It may also be due to deficient breakdown, assimilation or utilisation of the food

malocclusion (mal′okloo′zhun) malposition and imperfect contact of the teeth in upper and lower jaw, causing a poor bite

malonaldehyde a metabolic product of prostaglandin that is raised in Vitamin E deficiency

Malpighian (mal-pig′e-an) **body** 1. renal corpuscle consisting of a glomerulus enclosed in Bowman's capsule 2. periarticular lymphoid nodule in the spleen, named after Marcello Malpighi, Italian anatomist

Malpighian layer inner layer of epidermis that is a live cell segment consisting of basal cells and prickle cells

malposition (mal-po-zi'shun) abnormal position of the parts of the body or of foetal presenting part in relation to the maternal pelvis

malpractice professional misconduct or unreasonable lack of skill in the performance of a professional act

malrotation (mal'ro-ta-shun) failure of normal rotation of viscera during embryogenesis

MALT mucosa-associated lymphoid tissue, extranodal aggregates of lymphoid tissue in the bronchus (BALT), gut (GALT), skin (SALT), breast and uterine cervix. It acts as an immune defence that is in close contact with exogenous antigens

malt germinated grain, usually barley, used in manufacture of beer **m sugar** maltose

Malta fever Brucellosis, named after Malta island

maltase (mawl'tas) an enzyme that converts maltose by hydrolysis to glucose

MALToma low grade lymphoma in the stomach closely associated with *Helicobacter pylori* infection

malturned abnormally turned

malt worker's lung an extrinsic allergic alveolitis due to hypersensitivity to spores from *Aspergillus clavatus* and *A. fumigatus* in mouldy hay and barley

malunion union of fragments of fractured bone in a faulty position to affect function

mamillary (mam'iler'e) **body** either of the two small round masses of gray matter in the hypothalamus

mamillated (mam'il-la-ted) having protuberances like a nipple

mamilliplasty (ma-mil-i-plas'te) plastic operation on a nipple

mamillitis (mam'il-i'tis) inflammation of a nipple

mamma (mam'a) pl. **mammae** breast

mammal (mam'al) an animal class, mammalia characterised by having breasts.

mammary (mam'ere) pertaining to or resembling the mammary gland **m gland** a milk secreting glandular structure situated in female on either side of the chest over the anterolateral area between the third and sixth ribs. Glandular tissue forms a radius of lobes containing alveoli, each lobe contains ducts for passage of milk from the alveoli to the nipple. The central part of the breast contains glandular tissue and the periphery consists of adipose tissue **m souffle** an innocent systolic or continuous murmur of arterial origin during late pregnancy. It is unaffected by Valsalva manoeuvre

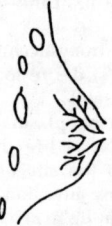

Mammary gland

mammectomy mastectomy

mammogram (mam'o-gram) an x-ray film of the soft tissues of the breast

mammography (mam-og'ra-fe) radiography of the mammary gland

mammoplasty plastic reshaping of the breasts, performed to reduce or lift enlarged or sagging breasts; to enlarge small breasts or to reconstruct a breast with a plastic prosthesis, after removal of a tumour

mammose (mam'os) 1. having very large breasts 2. shaped like a breast

mammothermography a diagnostic procedure in which thermography is used for examining the breast to detect abnormal growths

mammotropin (ma-met′ro-pin) prolactin

mamsa (s) flesh; muscle

man 1. member of the human species 2. human race 3 male member of the species.

mandagni (s) indigestion

manas (s) the mind

manasa (s) mind; mental

mancinism (man′sin-izm) state of being left handed

mandelic acid a urinary antiseptic

mandible (mon′di-b′i) a large bone constituting lower jaw. It consists of a curved body and two perpendicular rami that join the body at almost right angles. The superior border contains sockets for 16 lower teeth

mandibular pertaining to or of mandible **m arch** the first visceral arch from which the mandible develops **m canal** a passage extending from the mandibular foramen on medial surface of the ramus of the mandible to the mental foramen, that contains mandibular blood vessels and a portion of the mandibular branch of trigeminal nerve **m notch** a depression in the inferior border of the mandible where external facial muscles cross the lower border of the mandible **m process** 1. the upper alveolar part of the mandible 2. the projection of the ramus of the mandible bearing the condyle **m reflex** *see* jaw jerk **m sling** the connection between the mandible and maxilla by the masseter and pterygoid muscles at the angle of the mandible

mandibulofacial relating to the mandible and face

mandibulooculofacial relating to the mandible and the orbital part of the face

mandibulopharyngeal relating to the mandible and pharynx

mandril (man′drel). 1. a staff to which a tool is attached and used for rotation 2. a handle that holds in dentistry, a disk, stone or cup used for grinding, smoothing or finishing

mandrin a stylet or a stiff wire inserted in the lumen of a soft catheter

manganese (man′ga-nez) a metallic element, atomic number 25, found in many foods and tissues. Daily requirement is 2-3 mg. Its deficiency is rare **m poisoning** extrapyramidal manifestations may develop in workers exposed to manganese regularly

mania *Psy* a hyperkinetic psychiatric reaction **m episode** a persistently elevated, expansive or irritable mood, increased energy, decreased sleep, distractability, impaired judgement, grandiosity and flight of ideas

maniac (ma′ne-ak) person afflicted by mania

maniacal (ma-ni′a-kl) 1. relating to or characterised by mania 2. afflicted with mania

maniac-depressive (man′ik-de-pres′iv) alternating between attacks of mania and depression

manifest to reveal

manifestation the demonstration of the presence of a sign or symptom in association with a disease

manikin (man′i-kin) a model of human body or its parts used to teach anatomy and nursing procedures

man-in-the-barrel syndrome a type of reverse paraplegia with severe weakness of upper extremity without weakness of lower extremity may occur in comatose patients who survive an episode of severe hypotension

manipulation (ma-nip′u-la′shun) 1. any manual precedure 2. a joint mobilisation technique 3. a method of realigning a fractured bone 4. influencing another person

mannerism a peculiar mode of movement, action or speech

mannitol (man′i-tol) hexahydric alcohol obtained by reduction of fructose, used as an osmotic diuretic and to measure glomerular filtration

mannose (man′os) an aldohexose from plant source

mannoside (man'o-sid) a glycoside of mannose

mannosidosis (man'os-i-do'sis) a lysosomal storage disease due to congenital deficiency of mannosidase and is associated with mental retardation, kyphosis, enlarged tongue, vacuolated lymphocytes and accumulation of mannose in the tissues

manoeuvre (men-oo'ver) 1. a skillful manipulation or procedure **Bracnt m** delivery of a foetus in breech position by which foetal head is expelled spontaneously **Heimlich m** *see* Heimlich maneuvre **key-in-lock m** a method by which obstetrical forceps are used to rotate the foetal head **Mauriceau- Smellie m** method adopted to deliver the aftercoming head in breech presentation **Muller's m** inspiratory effort with a closed glottis at the end of expiration **Munro Kerr m** a method to determine the presence of disproportion between the foetal head and the maternal pelvis. **Pajot m** a method of forceps extraction of the foetal head **Pinard's m** a method of bringing down the foot in breech extraction **Prague m** a method for delivery of the foetus in breech position when the foetal occiput is posterior **Scanzoni's m** forceps rotation and traction in a spinal course with reapplication of forceps for delivery **Sellick's m** application of pressure to the cricoid cartilage to prevent regurgitation during endotracheal intubation in the anaesthesised patient **Toynbee m** pinching the nostrils and swallowing to determine the patency of auditory tube **Valsalva's m** 1. forced expiratory effort with closed nose and mouth to inflate the eustachian tubes and middle ears 2. forced expiratory effort against a closed glottis to increase intrathoracic pressure. It impedes venous return to the right atrium

manometer (man-om'et-er) an instrument for determining liquid or gaseous pressure. The measurement is expressed in millimetres of either mercury or water, or in torr

manometry (-e-tre) measurement of pressure of gases or liquids by means of manometer

Mansonia (man-so'ne-a) a genus of culicine mosquitoes that are vectors of *Wuchereria bancrofti* and *Brugia malayi*, named after Patrick Manson, British physician

mantha (s) emulsion

mantle 1. a covering 2. cerebral cortex **m port** a radiotherapy field that covers the axillary, mediastinal, hilar, cervical, supra- and infraclavicular lymph nodes, especially used to treat multiple contiguous lymphoid regions affected by Hodgkin's disease

Mantoux (man-tu') **test** an intradermal injection of 0.1 ml of purified protein derivative on flexor surface of forearm and measuring appearance of induration between 48 and 72 hours. An induration of 10 mm diameter is considered positive. It indicates person has been infected with *Mycobacterium tuberculosis*, named after Charles Mantoux, French physician

manual (man'u-al) 1. pertaining to the hands 2. performed by or with hands

manubrium (ma-noo'bre-um) a handlelike structure **m mallei** process of malleus that is attached to the middle layer of tympanic membrane, and tensor tympani muscle is attached to it **m sterni** the upper segment of the sternum articulating with the clavicle and the first two pairs of costal cartilages

manusha (s) man

MAO abbreviation for 1. monoamine oxidase 2. maximum acid output

map a two-dimensional graphic representation of arrangement in space **gene m** a graphic representation of linear arrangement of genes indicating the relationship of genes to each other on a chromosome

maple bark stripper's lung an extrinsic allergic alveolitis due to hypersensitivity to spores from *Cryptostroma corticale*

maple syrup urine disease MSUD branched chain ketoaciduria. A rare inborn error of metabolism due to decreased branched chain-ketoacid dehydrogenase complex activity resulting in accumulation of branched chain aminoacids (valine, leucine and isoleucine). It has a neonatal onset, with dyspnoea, spasticity, mental and growth retardation, feeding difficulties and convulsions. It is treated by excessive administration of thiamine

mapping location of the genes on a chromosome

marana (s) death

marantic endocarditis a non-bacterial endocarditis with sterile vegetations on either side of valve leaflets composed of fibrin and clot

marasmus (mar-az'mus) a state of severe malnutrition, due to decreased ingestion of protein and calories resulting from an inadequate diet, improper feeding habits or metabolic disturbances. It is characterised by failure to thrive, emaciation, weight loss, loss of skin turgor and subcutaneous atrophy. The children are listless, and wizened. There is muscular atrophy, hypotonia and hypothermia

marble bone disease osteopetrosis, an autosomal recessive condition of early onset with failure to thrive, bone fragility and multiple fractures and bony over growth of cranial foramina resulting in proptosis, blindness, deafness and hydrocephalus, and osseous replacement of marrow spaces

Marburg virus disease a viral haemorrhagic fever due to direct contact with infected monkey tissues. It presents with headache, fever, myalgia, rash and haemorrhage, first recognised in Marburg, Germany

marc (mark) the residue remaining after percolation of a drug.

march (mar'ch) the spread of electrical activity through the motor cortex **m fracture** a metatarsal stress fracture **m haemoglobinuria** haemolysis due to repeated trauma that impacts on red cells that pass through small vessels overlying the bones of the hands and feet in long distance marching, or marathon running **m in place** repetitive movements of the legs when standing as in tardive dyskinesia

Marche a petit pasi *Fr* patients with multiple small-vessel cerebrovascular disease walking with small steps with instability. There is no variable pace and freezing

Marchiafava-Micheli (mar'ke-a-fa'va-me-ka'le) **syndrome** a rare haemolytic anaemia associated with paroxysmal nocturnal haemoglobinuria, named after Ettore Marchiafava, Italian pathologist and Ferdinando Micheli, Italian physician

Marcus Gunn (mar'kus-gun) **pupil** a pupil of the eye that shows constriction more to an indirect than direct light, described by Robert Marcus Gunn, British ophthalmologist

Marcus Gunn syndrome a congenital disorder in which the ptosis disappears on opening the mouth or on moving the jaw to one side; jaw winking phenomenon

marfanoid (mar'fan-oid) having characteristics of Marfan's syndrome.

Marfan's (mar-fahnz) **syndrome** an autosomal dominant heritable disorder of connective tissue characterised by musculoskeletal, ocular and cardiovascular abnormalities. The affected persons are tall with long slender limbs; the lower segment (pubis to sole) length is greater than the upper segment (pubis to vertex) and arm span exceeds height. The muscles are underdeveloped and hypotonic. The fingers are long, tapering and spidery, there is upward bilateral dislocation of lens and diffuse dilatation of ascending aorta, described by Bernard-Jean Marfan, French physician

margin an edge or border of a structure **marginal** adj. **gingival m** the border of the gingiva surrounding a tooth

margination (mar'ji-na'shun) adhesion of leucocytes to the walls of blood vessels at the site of injury in the initial stages of inflammation

marginoplasty (mar-jin'o-plas'te) plastic surgery of a border, as of an eyelid

margo (mar'go) margin

Marie-Bamberger (ma-re'-bahm'ber-ger) **syndrome** hypertrophic pulmonary osteoarthropathy, named after Pierre Marie, French neurologist and Eugen Bamberger, Austrian physician

Marie's ataxia, hereditary cerebellar ataxia from bilateral cortical atrophy of the cerebellum, named after Pierre Marie, French neurologist

Marie-Strumpell (ma-re'strim'pel) **disease** ankylosing spondylitis, named after Pierre Marie, French neurologist and Adolf von Strumpell, Leipzig physican

Marie-Tooth (ma-re'tooth) **disease** peroneal muscular dystrophy, named after Pierre Marie, French neurologist and Howard Tooth, English physician

Marion's sign an enlarged prostate projecting into the bladder that brings the edge of internal urethral meatus and ureteric orifice into one cystoscopic field, named after Jean Baptiste Camille Georges Marion, French surgeon

Marion's syndrome Bladder-neck obstruction in women due to enlarged periurethral glands, described by Georges. Marion

Marjolin's (mar'zho-lanz) **ulcer** malignant growth arising at the edge of a chronic ulcer, named after Jean Nicolas Marjolin, French surgeon

mark a spot, scar, or naevus visible on the surface of the body **birth m** a circumscribed blemish or spot on the skin **portwine m** naevus flammeus **strawberry m** naevus vascularis

marker 1. an identifying characteristic 2. a device used to mark something **genetic m** an identifiable physical location on a chromosome **tumour m** a biochemical substance indicative of presence of neoplasm

marketing advertising, detailing

marma (s) energy point

marrow (mar'o) the soft tissue filling the cavities of bones **m aspiration** procuring a specimen of bone marrow for examination using a special aspirating needle. It is obtained from the upper portion of the sternum or the iliac crest **red m** marrow found in spongy bones and is concerned with the production of different blood cells **spinal m** the spinal cord **yellow m** marrow found in medullary cavities of the long bones. It is made up of fat cells and connective tissue

marsupialisation (mar-su'pe-al-i-za'shun) process of conversion of a closed cavity into an open pouch by incising it and suturing the edges of the abdominal wound

marsupium (mar-su'pe-um) 1. scrotum 2. a pouch that serves to hold the young of marsupials such as kangaroos

masculation (mas-ku-la'shun) development of male secondary sexual characteristics

masculine (mas-ku-lin) 1. pertaining to male sex 2. possessing male characteristics

masculinisation (mas'kul-in-i-za'shun) 1.the normal development of male sex characters at puberty 2. abnormal development of male secondary sex characters in the female and it may be due to testosterone producing tumours or intake of testosterone or anabolic steroids; virilisation

maser (ma'zer) a device that produces intense, small nondivergent radiation beam

mask 1. to cover or conceal 2. immobile apperance of the face 3. an appliance for shading or protecting 4. to diminish sound by the presence of another sound of different frequency 5. to cover metal parts of dental prosthesis by an opaque material **aerosol m·a** mask used for administration of a nebuliser, humidity or oxygen **BLB m** *see* BLB mask **m area** central area of face where boils may drain to the cavernous sinus **Mary Catheral mask** MC mask oxygen mask for delivery of high concentrations of oxygen **m of pregnancy** hyperpigmented macules in the facial and neck skin seen in pregnancy and in oral contraceptive use **m phenomenon** evanescent punctate macules on the face and neck following prolonged retching and violent coughing **venturi m** oxygen flowing at a high velocity in the form of a jet through a narrow orifice to the base of the mask creates a negative pressure entraining atmospheric air through the perforations in the face piece and there is no rebreathing

masked concealed

masochism (mas'o-kizm) a perversion in which infliction of pain gives sexual gratification to the recipient, named after Leopald Masoch, Austrian novelist

masochist (mas'o-kist) a person who derives pleasure from masochism

mass 1. a collection of cohering particles or components 2. a cohesive mixture to be made into pills 3. that characteristic of matter giving it the property of inertia **m reflex** multiple muscle and visceral responses in cord section after stimulus below the level of lesion

massage systematic pressure, stroking and kneeding of the body **cardiac m** manual compression of the heart to restore heart beat in cardiac arrest. It is done by applying intermittent pressure over the sternum (closed cardiac massage) or through an incision in the chest wall (open cardiac massage) to reinstate and maintain circulation **carotid sinus m** firm rotatory pressure applied to one side of the neck over the carotid sinus to cause vagal stimu-

lation to terminate tachycardia **electrovibratory m** massage by an electric vibrator

masseter (mas-se'ter) *see* table of muscles

masseur (ma-soor) 1. a man who performs massages 2. an instrument for massaging

masseuse (ma-sooz) a woman who performs massages

massive (mas'siv) huge; a large mass; bulky **m transfusion** an infusion within a 24-hour period of a blood volume that approaches or exceeds the recipient's own collected blood volume

mastadenitis (mast-ad-e-ni-tis) inflammation of a mammary gland

mastadenoma (mast'a-de-no'ma) a tumour of the breast

mastalgia (mast-al'je-a) pain in the breast

mastatrophy (mast-at'ro-fe) atrophy of the breast

mast cell a type of cell that stains metachromatically due to its high proteoglycan content and electron dense granules and plays a role in the immune system and in allergic reactions. It releases mediators of inflammation in response to the presence of allergens **m stabilisers** drugs that prevent the release of mediators of inflammation from the mast cells such as disodium cromoglycate and nedocromil sodium

mastectomy (mas-tek'to-me) surgical removal of all or part of the breast as treatment of breast cancer **modified radical m** total mastectomy with removal of axillary lymph nodes, subcutaneous fat and involved skin but leaving the pectoral muscles intact **radical m** removal of breast, skin, pectoral muscle, subcutaneous fat and axillary lymph nodes **simple m** removal of breast, nipple, areola and the involved overlying skin

Master two-step test a standard exercise test to evaluate cardiac function. The patient repeatedly walks up and down 2 steps of 22.5 cm high while monitoring the electrocardiogram, devised by Arthus Master, US physician

mastheleosis (mas'thel-o'sis) ulceration of the breast

mastication (mas'ti-ka'shun) the process of chewing food. It helps in breaking of food and mixing with saliva in the mouth **masticatory** adj.

mastigophora (mas'ti-gof'o-ra) a division of protozoa characterised by one or more flagella, includes giardia and trypanosomes

mastitis (mas-ti'tis) inflammation of the breast

mastocarcinoma (mast'o-kar-sin-o'ma) carcinoma of the breast

mastocyte (mas'to-sit) a mast cell

mastocytosis (mas'to-si-to'sis) an aggregation of mast cells in the tissues. The condition may be restricted to the skin in the form of urticaria pigmentosa or systemic involving bone marrow, lymph nodes and abdominal organs

mastodynia (mast-o-din'e-a) pain in the breast

mastography roentgenography of the breasts

mastoid (mas'toyd) 1. shaped like a breast 2. mastoid process of temporal bone 3. pertaining to the mastoid process **mastoidal** adj

mastoidale (mas-toy-da'le) the tip of the mastoid process

mastoidalgia (mas-toyd-al'je-a) pain in the mastoid region

mastoidectomy (mas-to-id'ek-to-me) excision of mastoid cells

mastoidocentesis (mas-toid'e-o-sen-te-'sis) paracentesis of mastoid cells

mastoiditis (mas-toyd-it'is) inflammation of the air cells of mastoid process

mastoidotomy (ma-toyd-ot'o-me) incision into the mastoid process

mastomenia (mas-to-me'ne-a) vicarious menstruation from the breast

mastooccipital (mas'to-ok-sip'i-tal) relating to the mastoid process and occipital bone

mastopathy (mas-to-pa-the) any disease of the mammary gland

mastopexy (mas'to-peks-e) surgical fixation of a pendulous breast

mastoptosis (mas'to-to-sis) pendulous breasts

mastorrhagia (mas-ter-a'je-a) bleeding from the breast

mastoscirrhus (mas-to-skir'us) hardening of the breast

mastosquamous (mas-to-skwa'mus) relating to the mastoid process and the squamous portion of temporal bone

masturbate (mas'ter-bat) to practice masturbation

masturbation (mas'ter-ba'shun) stimulation of genitals to induce orgasm by some means other than intercourse.

matching (mach'ing) 1. comparison to make selection of objects, controls or persons with indentical characteristics 2. a method of measuring tissue compatibility between individuals 3. being indentical **group m** assigning cases to sub-categories based on their characteristics **m. of blood** a technique of determining the immunologic and genetic characteristics of the patient's blood. It facilitates to make selection of appropriate blood for transfusion **cross m** a technique of determining the compatibility of the blood of a donor and that of a recipient before transfusion.

mater (ma'tur) the trilaminal membranous covering of the brain and spinal cord **arachnoid m** a membrane that bridges hemispheric sulci. It offers connective tissue support to the blood vessels communicating with pia mater **dura m** a tough fibrous membrane intimately attached to the inner aspect of the cranial bones. It covers the bra'n, cranial nerves, and spinal cord **pia m** the inner most layer of loose connective tissue and is a continuation of the arachnoid membrane of the blood vessels

materia (ma-ter'e-a) material or substance **base m** the basic ingredient of a denture such as polymers or metal im-

pression m any material used to make an impression of teeth **m alba** white cheese- like deposit along gum line about the necks of teeth **m medica** pharmacology

maternal 1. relating to the mother 2. from a mother **m death** death of a woman on account of, aggravated by or resulting in the course of management of pregnancy, childbirth or puerperium **m deprivation syndrome** premature loss or absence of mother leading to emotional, physical and nutritional neglect of an infant or a child **m mortality rate** maternal deaths at a place during a calendar year divided by the number of live births at the same place and year, multiplied with 1000 or 100,000

maternity (ma-tunr'it-e) 1. motherhood 2. the obstetrics department of a hospital

mating (mat'ing) pairing of individuals of opposite sexes especially for reproduction **assortive m** the mating of individuals having similar qualities and constitution **random m** the mating of individuals without regard to any similarity between them

matricide killing of one's mother

matrilineal (ma'tri-lin'e-al) concerning descent through the female line

matrix (ma'triks) 1. the basic substance from which a structure develops 2. the intracellular substance of a tissue 3. a mold for casting amalgums in dental restoration 4. a form for casting **bone m** the intercellular substance of bone **extracellular m** any substance produced by cells and excreted into the extracellular space within the tissue **m unguis** nail bed

matt dull surface seen on culture plates of bacteria that do not produce capsules as Enterobacteriaceae species

matter (mat'er) 1. substance such as gas, liquid or solid 2. anything that occupies space 3. pus **gray m** gray portions of the central nervous system which includes cerebral cortex, basal ganglia

and nuclei of the brain and H-shaped gray columns of the spinal cord. It is composed of cell bodies of the neurones **white m** white substance of the brain and spinal cord consisting mainlynerve fibres

matting enlargement and cohesion of lymph nodes as in tuberculosis

maturate (mat'u-rat) 1. to ripen 2. to mature 3. to suppurate

maturation (mat'u-ra'shun) 1. the process of becoming mature or ripe as a graafian follicle 2. attainment of emotional and intellectual maturity 3. a process of cell division during which the number of chromosomes in the germ cells are reduced to one half 4. suppuration 5. attaining menarche 6. the completion of mineralisation pattern **m index** squamous cell index to evaluate female oestrogen status

maturational arrest 1. presence of immature nucleus in a relatively mature cytoplasm as in megaloblastic anaemia due to a deficiency of vitamin B_{12} and/ or folic acid 2. failure of testes to produce spermatozoa despite normal multiplication of earlier stages

mature (ma-tur) fully developed or ripened

maturity 1. fully developed 2. time when an individual becomes capable of reproducing **m onset diabetes** non-insulin dependent diabetes mellitus

matutinal (ma-tu'tinal) occurring in the morning

Maurer's (mos'erz) **dots** coarse stippling of red cells in falciparum malaria, named after Georg Maurer, German physician who worked in Sumatra

maxilla (mak-sil-ah) the bone of the upper jaw *see* Table of bones **maxillary** adj

maxillary sinus *see* sinus

maxillitis (maks'il-i'tus) inflammation of the maxilla

maxillodental (mak-sil'o-den'tal) pertaining to the maxilla and the teeth it supports

maxillofacial (mak-sil'o-fa'shal) pertaining to the maxilla and face **m syndrome** facial abnormalities due to improper ossification of the foetal cartilages in the facial area

maxillojugal (mak-sil'o-ju'gal) pertaining to the maxilla and zygomatic bone

maxillomandibular (mak-sil'o-man-dib'ular) pertaining to the upper and lower jaws

maxillopalatine (mak-sil'o-pal'a-tin) pertaining to the maxilla and palatine bone

maxillotomy (mak-sil'o-to-me) surgical section of the maxilla to facilitate its movements

maximal aerobic power the maximal volume of oxygen consumed per unit of time

maximal heart rate reserve the difference between the resting heart rate and the maximal heart rate

maximum (mak'si-mum) pl. **maxima** 1. the greatest quantity or effect 2. largest or utmost 3. height of a disease **maximal** adj. **m breathing capacity** MBC the maximum volume of air that can be breathed in and out of the lungs in one minute **m dose** the largest dose that is safe to administer **m permissible dose** the highest dose of radiation allowed to a person exposed over a period of one year

Mayaro virus a mosquito-borne virus causing epidemic of acute polyarthritis in Brazil and Bolivia

Mayo's (ma'oz) **operation** devised by William Mayo and Charles Mayo, US surgeons. 1. excision of head of metatarsal bone for hallux valgus 2. excision of pyloric end of the stomach and construction of gastrojejunostomy 3. operation for radical cure of umbilical hernia 4. subcutaneous removal of varicose vein

maza (maz'ah) the placenta

Mazdaznan (maz'daz-nan) a way of life derived mainly from Zarathustrian teaching which recommends lactovegetarian diet and naturopathic remedies for illness

maze (maz) a complicated system of intersecting paths used in intelligence tests

mazopexy (mas'zo-pex'se) mastopexy

mazoplasia a mammary dysplasia with fibrosis and ductal desquamation

MBBS Bachelor of Medicine and Bachelor of Surgery

MBC maximum breathing capacity.

MBP major basic protein

MC millicurie

m chain one of the two proteins required to form a tetramer of lactic dehydrogenase

m component a narrow peak noted on serum protein electrophoresis and is considered as an evidence of a monoclonal proliferation of mature B cells producing IgG, and IgM.

McArdle's disease a rare disorder of muscle metabolism with an abnormal accumulation of glycogen in muscle tissue due to a deficiency of myophosphorylase and the condition is characterised by muscle pain on exercise, named after Brian McArdle, British paediatrician

McBurney's incision an abdominal incision for appendectomy. The incision is made parallel to the path of external oblique muscle, devised by Charles McBurney, US surgeon

McBurney's point a point situated at the juction of lateral one third and medial two thirds of the right spinoumbilical line, denoting the site in appendicitis

McCune-Albright syndrome polyostotic fibrous dysplasia with café-au-lait spots and endocrinopathy, named after Donovan McCune, US Paediatrician, and Fuller Albright, US physician

mcg microgram

MCH mean corpuscular haemoglobin refers to the average haemoglobin content of an erythrocyte

Mch Master of Surgery

MCHC mean corpuscular haemoglobin

_concentration, refers to the average haemoglobin concentration in erythrocytes

MCTD abbreviation for mixed connective tissue disease

MCV mean corpuscular volume that is a calculated value for the average volume of peripheral red blood cells

MD Doctor of Medicine

MDR abbreviation for multiple drug resistance

MEA abbreviation for multiple endocrine adenomatosis

meal (mel) a portion of food eaten at a particular or fixed time to satisfy the appetite

mean (men) an average *stat* a numerical value intermediate between two extremes

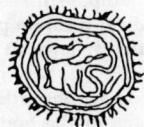

Measles virus

measles (me'zle) a paramyxoma virus in-

fection commonly noted in childhood. It spreads by droplet infection and begins as a catarrhal stage with fever, running nose, red watery eyes followed by cough, photophobia and Koplik's spots. After third day a red macular or maculopapular rash develops. It is noted initially at the back of the ears and at the junction of the forehead and the hair. Within a short period the whole skin is invaded by the rash, giving bloachy appearance. Fever settles when the rash begin to fade and desquamate. The condition may have complications such as postviral encephalitis, bronchopneumonia, corneal ulceration and weight loss. Live attenuated measles vaccine gives protection **black m** a severe form of measles with dark eruptions due to bleeding into the skin **German m** rubella

measly (me'zle) pork infested by cysticerci

measure (me'zhur) 1. the dimentions, capacity or quantity of anything 2. to determine the length, area, volume and mass of the materials (Table 6A).

Table 6A: Measures

Length

Millimetre	Centimetre	Decimetre	Metre	Decametre	Hectometre	Kilometre
1	0.1					
10	1.0					
100	10	1				
1000	100	10	1			
10^4	1000	100	10	1		
10^5	10^4	1000	100	10	1	
10^6	10^5	10^4	1000	100	10	1
10^7	10^6	10^5	10^4	1000	100	10
10^9	10^8	10^7	10^6	10^5	10^4	1000

Volume (fluid)

Millilitre	Centilitre	Decilitre	Litre
1			
10	1		
100	10	1	
1000	100	10	1

measurement use of certain prefixes for international system (SI) units

meat the flesh of animals

meatoscopy (me-a-tos'ko-pe) instrumental examination of a meatus, as of urethra

meatotomy (me-a-tot'o-me) incision of urethral meatus to enlarge the opening

meatus (me-a'tus) an opening or passage **meatal** adj. **acoustic m** either of two passages in the ear, external from external ear to tympanic membrane, and internal on the posterior surface of the petrous portion of temporal bone through which cochlear and vestibular nerves pass **m nasi** one of the four portions of the nasal cavity (common, inferior, superior and middle) on either side of the septum **urinary m** external opening of the urethra

mebendazole (me-ben'do-zol) a broad spectrum anthelmintic

mecamylamine (mek'a-mil'a-min) a ganglion-blocking antihypertensive

mechanical (me-kan'i-kal) 1. performed by means of an instrument 2. automatic **m restraint** a device applied to an individaul to restrict free movement **m ventilation** mechanically-assisted respiration in which inspiration is driven at a preset frequency or triggered by the patient. Though expiration is passive the intra-alveolar pressure may be raised by positive end-expiratory pressure (PEEP). It is indicated when measures fail to secure clinical improvement from respiratory failure and blood gases worsen and the patient shows signs of fatigue with rapid shallow breathing or reduced ventilatory volume and force

mechanics (me-kan'iks) the science of force and matter

mechanism (mek'a-nizm) 1. response to a stimulus 2. response pattern to achieve a result 3. a machine or machine-like structure 4. details of a process

mechanoreceptor (mek'a-no-re-sep'tor) a receptor that is excited by mechanical pressures

mechanotherapy (mak'an-o-ther'a-pe) use of different mechanical apparatus to perform passive movements

Meckel's (mek'elz) **diverticulum** a blind pouch sometimes found in lower portions of ileum. It represents the persistent proximal end of the yolk stalk.

It is a favoured site for carcinoids, named after Johann Meckel the younger, German anatomist

meclizine (mek'li-zen) an antithistamine useful for control of nausea and vomiting of motion sickness

meconium (me-ko'ne-um) 1. the thick, sticky greenish black faecal material consisting of salts, amniotic fluid, mucus, bile and epithelial cells passed by newborn infant in the first 24 hours 2. opium **m aspiration syndrome** the aspiration of meconium by the newborn prior to delivery **m ileus** ileus due to impacted meconium in the intestines, characteristic of cystic fibrosis

medas (s) fat; adipose tissue

media (me'ode-a) **medium** pl. 1. the middle or muscular layer of an artery or vein

mediad (me'de-ad) towards the median line or plane of the body

medial 1. pertaining to the middle 2. situated in or towards the midline

medialis (me'de-a'lis) close to the midline of the body

median (me'de-an) 1. middle 2. *stat* a number obtained by arranging the given series in order of magnitude and taking the middle number **m nerve** *see* table of nerves **m plane** a vertical plane through the head and trunk dividing the body into right and left halves

mediastinal (me'de-as'ti-nal) pertaining to the mediastinum **m crunch** a substernal crepitant sound audible in mediastinal emphysema

mediastinitis (me'de-as'ti-ni'tis) inflammation of the tissues of mediastinum

mediastinography (me'de-as'ti-nog'rafe) radiography of the mediastinum

mediastinopericarditis (me'de-as'ti-noper'i-kar-di'tis) inflammation of the pericardium and mediastinum

mediastinoscopy (me'de-as'ti-nos'ko-pe) examination of the mediastinum by means of an endoscope through an incision in the neck

mediastinotomy (me'de-as'ti-not'o-me) surgical incision of the mediastinum

mediastinum 1. (me'de-as-ti'num) pl. **mediastina** a median septum between two parts of an organ 2. structure lying centrally within the chest spanning the region vertically from the thoracic inlet to the diaphragmatic hiatus, transversely between the parietal pleura, and coronally between the sternum and vertebral column. It contains all soft-tissue thoracic organs except the two lungs. It is divided empirically as anterior (posterior surface of sternum, the pericardium posteriorly and the visceral pleurae laterally), middle (includes the thoracic inlet superiorly and extends from the pericardium anteriorly to the anterior surface posteriorly) and posterior (bounded by middle compartment anteriorly and the costophrenic angles laterally) compartments **mediastinal** adj **m testis** the thickened portion of *tunica albugenia* on posterior surface of testis

mediate (me'de-at) 1.indirect; accomplished by an intervening medium 2. between two sides or parts **m percussion** indirect percussion used over the chest; digito-digital percussion

mediation (me'd-a'shun) the action of a mediating agent

mediator (me'de-a'tor) that which mediates, such as a chemical, nerve, cellular substance or a person

medicable (med'i-ka-bl) treatable; curable

medical (med'i-kal) 1. pertaining to medical science 2. requiring treatment by medicines as distinct from surgical treatment **m ethics** moral dilemmas affecting broad medical decisions **m examiner** a physician qualified and trained to undertake physical examination of a person or to the task of investigation of the cause of death **m failure** a patient not responding to a non-interventional method of treatment

m grand rounds a medical education programme undertaken in a teaching hospital where the clinical case is presented and discussed **m history** a detailed record of present illness, and past illness **m informatics** application of information technology to various aspects of medical knowledge, practice and management **m jurisprudence** application of the principles of law to the practice of medicine **m preparation** a preparation of medical substance **m record** a written documentation of information regarding the patient's clinical history, physical findings, diagnostic tests and treatment **m specialty** different branches of medical sciences providing specialised patient care **m staff** licensed qualified medical persons **m team** a group of physicians and health care workers responsible for the patients' care while in hospital or in emergency

medicament a medicine or remedy

medicamentosa (med'i-ka-men-to-sa) pertaining to the drug

medicare (med'i-kar) a programme of health care covered by the health insurance plans

medicate (med'i-kat) to treat disease with drugs

medication (med'i-ka'shun) 1. the administration of remedies 2. impregnation with medicine 3. a medicament

medicinal (me-di'sin-al) 1. pertaining to a medicine 2. possessing healing qualities

medicine (med'i-sin) 1. any drug or remedy 2. the art and science of prevention of diseases, promotion of health and curing diseases 3. the study and treatment of diseases affecting internal organs 4. treatment of disease by medicines **adolescent m** the branch of medicine dealing with the treatment of youth **aerospace m** branch of medicine concerned with the problems involved in aviation **alternative m** the diagnosis and management of medical conditions by use of generally not accepted scientific disciplines such as ayurveda, homoeopathy, naturopathy, holistic method, siddha, unani, yoga etc. **clinical m** 1. study and practice of medicine in the clinical setting at the bed side 2. the curriculum in a medical college after study of preclinical subjects **Cnidean m** anti-Hipppocratic School of Medicine at Cnidus in Asia Minor which regarded disease as originating within the organism itself **community m** medical science concerned with the population, with emphasis on preventive medicine **complementary m** therapies which are not considered as orthodox that can be used along conventional medicine **emergency m** the medical specialty dealing with acutely ill or injured who require an immediate attention and treatment **empirical m** treatment born of actual experience **environmental m** branch of medicine dealing with the effects of the environment on humans **essential m** those that satisfy the priority health care needs of the population. They are selected with due regard to public health relevance, evidence on efficacy and safety, and comparative cost **experimental m** the study of diseases by experimentation upon animals or by clinical research **family m** medical speciality concerned with providing medical care to all members of the family **foetal m** the medical speciality concerned with the study, development, care and treatment of the foetus **folk m** treatment of diseases by home remedy and measures based upon experience and knowledge passed from generation to generation **forensic m** medical jurisprudence **group m** practice of medicine by a group of physicians representing various specialities who are associated together in providing total care of the patient **holistic m** a comprehensive total health care of the patient affecting physical, mental, social and spiritual aspects **industrial m** specialty concerned with the diseases peculiar to the work environment **internal m** branch of medicine concerned with diagnosis and medical treatment of internal organs of the body **legal m** forensic medicine **nuclear m** the branch of medicine concerned with the use of radionuclides in the diagnosis and treatment of disease **occupational m** industrial medicine **patent m** a drug or remedy that is protected by patent and is available without a prescription **perinatal m** the specialty concerned with care of the mother, foetus during pregnancy, labour and delivery **physical m** physiatry; treatment of disease by mechanical devices or the physical agents such as heat, cold, light, electricity or manipulation **preclinical m** the first year of training in a medical college **preventive m** medical science concerned with the prevention of diseases and promotion of health **proprietary m** a remedy where formula and mode of manufacture are the property of the producer **psychosomatic m** branch of medicine that is concerned with mind-body interrelationship in diseases or abnormal states **rehabilitation m** branch of medicine concerned with the restoration of form and function following an injury or illness **socialised m** the control of medical practice by a governmental agency **sports m** the branch of medicine concerned with physiology, pathology and psychology as applied to the individuals who participate in sports and to the injuries sustained by athletes and sportsmen **tropical m** medical science dealing with the diseases occurring in tropics and subtropics especially diseases of parasitic origin **veterinary m** the branch of medical science concerned with the diseases and health of animals

Medicine sans Frontiers (MSF) Doctors

without borders. The world's largest independent medical relief organisation that provides short- and long-term medical aid to war zones, sites of natural disasters and refugee camps in the form of emergency care, immunisation services, food, hygiene, education and training, got Nobel Peace Prize 1999 for the outstanding humanitarian work

medico combining word for medical.

medicochirurgical (med'I-ko-ki-rur'ji-kal) concerning to both medicine and surgery

medicolegal (med'i-ko-le'gal) relating to medical jurisprudence

medicosocial (med'i-ko-so'shil) concerning both medical and social aspects

medio combining word for middle.

mediocarpal (me'de-o-kar'pal) pertaining to the central part of carpus

mediolateral (me'de-o-lat'er-al) relating to the midline and one side

medionecrosis (-ne-kro'sis) necrosis of the tunica media of a blood vessel

mediotarsal (-tar'sal) relating to the middle of the tarsus

meditation the art of meditating, deep thought or serious contemplation **transcendental m** practice of meditation where the person tries to relax by sitting quietly for regular periods while chanting a prayer

Mediterranean fever a familial disease characterised by repetitive episodes of high fever, peritonitis, pleuritis and inflammatory arthritis, oral colchicine acts as a prophylactic and prevents the development of amyloidosis

medium (med'e-um) pl. **media** 1. a means 2. anything through which an action is performed 3. substance used for cultivation of microorganisms 4. substance through which impulses are transmitted 5. the liquid holding a substance in solution or suspension **clearing m** a substance that makes histologic specimens transparent **contrast m** a radio- opaque substance such as barium used in radiography to permit visualisation of internal organs **culture m** a liquid or solid matrix with nutrient substance on which microorganisms are cultivated, such as agar, broths or gelatin **differential m** media that allow visualization of metabolic differences between groups or species of bacteria **dispersion m** a liquid in which colloid is dispersed **enriched m** a growth media that contains added growth factors such as blood, vitamins, and yeast extracts **nutrient m** a medium to which nutrient substances have been added **refracting m** the transparent tissues and fluid through which light rays pass and get refracted and focussed on retina **separating m** a substance applied to the surface of an impression or mold to prevent interaction of materials and to allow their separation after casting, in dentistry **transport m** a culture medium used to transport specimens for bacteriologic examination, as alkaline-peptone water to transport stool or vomitus in suspected cases of cholera

medius (me'de-us) middle, situated in the mid-position

MEDLARS Medical literature analysis and retrieval system, a computerized system of databases and data banks of biomedial literature, available from US National Library of Medicine

MEDLINE MEDLARS-on-line. The computer-accessible bibliographic data base that links telephone lines to the MEDLARS data bases

medorrhoea (me-dur-re'a) gleet or gleet on genitals

medo-vrddhi (s) obesity

medroxyprogesterone (med-rok'se-pro-jes'ter-on) a long acting progestational agent

medulla (me-dul'a) 1. the marrow 2. innermost portion of an organ **medullary** adj **adrenal m** inner portion of the adrenal gland, that consists of cells displaying a chromaffin reaction and it secretes adrenaline and non-adrenaline m of bone bone marrow m of hair shaft central axis of some hairs m of kidneys renal pyramid m oblongata the lowest sub division of brain stem, continuous with the pons above and the spinal cord below. It regulates all the vital functions such as heart rate, respiration, blood pressure, swallowing etc. m ossium bone marrow. The tissue that fills the cavities of bone, having a stroma of reticular fibres and fat (yellow bone marrow) or developmental stages of erythrocytes, leucocytes and megakaryocytes (red bone marrow) m of ovary central portion of the ovary m renis the renal pyramid composed chiefly of collecting ducts, loops of Henle and vasa recta spinal m spinal cord m of thymus the central portion of each lobule of thymus containing reticular cells

medullated (med'u-lat'ed) 1. myelinated 2. having a medulla or marrow

medullectomy (med'u-lek'to-me) excision of any medullary substance

medulloarthritis (med-ul'o-ar-thri'tis) inflammation of cancellous articular ends of a long bone

medulloblast (med-ul'-o-blast) a cell of neural tube that may develop into either a nerve cell or neuroglial cell

medulloblastoma (med-ul'o-blas-to'ma) a tumour of childhood affecting the cerebellar vermis. A highly cellular tumour, presenting with a short history of headache, vomiting and truncal ataxia

medulloepithelioma (med'ul-o-ep'i-thel-e-ma) a rare neuroepithelial tumour in the brain or retina

Mees' lines transverse white lines above the lunula of the finger nails following exposure to arsenic, named after R. Mees, Dutch scientist.

mefloquin an ar 'imalarial agent acting on blood trophozoites and gametocytes. It acts more slowly than chloroquine or quinine. It is also used as a chemoprophylactic in chloroquine-resistant P. falciparum malaria

mega 1. combining word for large, oversize 2. indicates a unit of measurement of 1 million

megabacterium a large-sized bacteria.

megabladder (meg'a-blad'er) abnormal enlargement of the urinary bladder

megabyte MB. A unit of memory capacity. A single megabyte is 1000 kilobytes

megacalycosis (meg'a-kal'i-ko'sis) nonobstructive dilatation of the renal calices

megacolon (meg'a-ko'lon) extreme dilatation of the colon and refractory constipation. It may be congenital or develop later in life acquired m colonic enlargement as a result of voluntary withholding of stools or chronic constipation and prolonged abuse of stimulant laxatives congenital m a congenital aganglionosis of large intestine, with failure of relaxation of internal anal sphincter. Constipation, abdominal distension and vomiting develop immediately after birth. see Hirschsprung's disease toxic m marked dilatation of the colon as a complication of ulcerative colitis

megadose a dose of vitamin administered in a larger dose than recommended

megadactyly (meg-a-dak'ti-li) large fingers

megaoesophagus (meg'a-e-sof'a-gus) enlargement of lower portion of oesophagus, usually associated with achalasia or occur as a late complication of Chaga's disease

megahertz (meg-a-hartz) one million (10^6) hertz (cycles per second); MHz

megakaryoblast (meg-a-kar'i-o-blast) precursor of a megakaryocyte

megakaryocyte (meg-a-kar'i-o-sit) a large cell with a multilobed nucleus found in the bone marrow that gives rise to blood platelets

megakaryocytosis (meg'a-kar'e-o-si-to'sis) presence of increased number of megakaryocytes in the bone marrow or in the blood

megalencephaly (meg'al-en-sef'a-le) an abnormally large head; megacephaly

megalo combining word for great or large

megaloblast (meg'a-lo-blast) an erythroid precursor with an enlarged nucleus related to Vitamin B_{12} and/or folic acid deficiency which causes a change in the nuclear cytoplasm maturation

megaloblastic anaemia anaemia produced by vitamin B_{12} or folic acid deficiency

megalocephalic (meg-a-lo-sef-al'ik) relating to or characterised by a large head

megalocephaly (meg-a-lo-sef-a'le) megacephaly

megalocheiria (meg'a-lo-ki're-a) markedly large hands

megalocornea (meg'a-lo-kor'ne-a) an unusually large cornea

megalocyte (meg'a-lo-sit) markedly enlarged erythrocyte

megalocytic anaemia megaloblastic anaemia

megalodactyly (meg'a-lo-dak'ti-le) markedly increased size of the fingers or toes

megalodontia (meg'a-lo-don'she-a) a condition associated with abnormally large teeth

megalomania (meg'a-lo-ma'ne-a) over-evaluation of one's importance

megalonychosis (meg'a-lo'ni-ko'sis) hypertrophy of nails

megalophthalmus (meg'a-lof-thal'mus) abnormal enlargement of the eyes

megalopodia (meg'a-lo-po'de-a) abnormally large feet

megaloscope (meg'a-lo-skop) a large magnifying lens

megaloureter (me'a-lo-u-re'ter) markedly dilated ureter

megamitochondria markedly enlarged mitochondria seen in the liver, associated with alcoholic liver disease

megarectum a faeces-filled dilated rectum resulting in constipation

-megaly combining word for an enlargement of specific organ or body part.

megavitamin therapy administering of excess doses of water soluble vitamins

megavolt (meg'a-vot) one million, 10^6 volts.

meglitinide pancreatic beta cell stimulator

meglumin N-methyl glucamine combined with iodinated acids in contrast media to increase its viscosity and to reduce toxicity

meglumine(meg'lu-men) an antimony preparation used in the treatment of leishmaniasis

Meibomian (mi-bo' me-an) **cyst** a retention cyst of a tarsal gland occurring in either lid and it moves with the eye lid, named after Heinrich Meibom, German anatomist

Meibomian glands row of large sebaceous glands within the upper lid discharging to lid margin

meibomitis (me-bo'mi-tis) inflammation of the Meibomian glands

Meigs' syndrome ascites and hydrothorax associated with ovarian fibroma or other pelvic tumour, named after Joseph Meigs, US gynaecologist

meiosis (mi-o'sis) reduction cell division that produces ova or sperm, each of which contain half the genes of the original cell

Meissner's (mis'nerz) **corpuscle** medium-sized encapsulated touch corpuscles of dermal papillae of finger tips, palms and soles, named after Georg Meissner, German anatomist

Meissner's plexus autonomic nerve plexus found in the submucosa of the gut from the cardia downwards that acts as a sensory side of peristaltic control

mela 1. a religious fair 2. a congregation of people in connection with a festival

melagra (mel-a'gra) muscular pain in the arms or legs

melalgia (mel-al'je-a) pain in the limbs

melancholia (mel-an-ko'le-a) *Psy* psychotic depression with an uninterested affect and lack of interest in activities that normally cause pleasure more common in women and is accompanied by helplessness, suicidal ideation or attempts

melancholy (mel-an-ko'le) a state of depression occurring temporarily as in mourning the loss of a loved one

melanin (mel'a-nin) a complex polymer synthesised from DOPA and bound to a carrier protein by melanocytes. It gives skin, eyes and hair their colour

melanoblast (mel'an-o-blast) precursor cell of melanocyte

melanoblastoma (mel'a-no-blas'to-ma) melanoma

melanocyte (mal'an-o-sit) melanin producing cell of neural crest origin found in basal layer of epidermis and hair matrix m stimulating hormone a polypeptide hormone secreted in the middle lobe of hypophysis, that stimulates dispersion of melanocytes in the skin and their production of melanin

melanocytic naevus pigmented naevus in the dermis containing inactive melanocytes

melanoderma (mel'an-o-der'ma) presence of an abnormally increased amount of melanin in the skin

melanodermatitis (mel'a-no-der'ma-ti'tis) increased deposition of melanin in an area of dermatitis

melanoepithelioma (mel'an-o-epi'-the-le-o'ma) melanin containing malignant epithelioma

melanogen (me-lon'o-jen) melanin-related compound that is excreted in the urine of patients with advanced malignant melanoma

melanogenesis (mel'an-o-jen'e-sis) the production of melanin

melanoglossia (-glo'se-a) black hairy tongue

melanoleukoderma (mel'an-o-lu'ko-der'ma) a mottled appearance of the skin

melanoma (mel'a-no'ma) tumour of melanocytes acral m large macular lentiginous pigmented area on the palms and soles lentigo maligna m melanoma on exposed skin in elderly

nodular m melanoma develop on a pigmented nodule and has poor prognosis malignant m a malignant tumour arising from melanocytes located in the epidermis, dermis or mucosal epithelium or from naevus cells. The growth is asymmetrical with irregular border, colour and elevation. It may spread to regional lymph nodes or produce distant disease

melanonychia (mel'a-no-nik'e-a) blackening of the nails by melanin pigmentation

melanophage (mel-a-no-phage) a macrophage that has ingested melanin

melanophore (mel'an-o-for) a cell containing melanin pigment

melanophoroma blue naevus with collections of pigmented melanocytes in dermis

melanoplakia (mel'an-o-pla'ke-a) the development of pigmented patches on the buccal mucosa and the tongue

melanosarcoma (mel'a-no-sar-ko'ma) melanin containing sarcoma

melanosis (mel'an-o'sis) 1. a condition with abnormal dark brown or brown-black pigmentation of tissues and organs 2. disorder from widespread metastases of melanoma m coli segmental or global darkening of the colonic mucosa associated with chronic constipation due to prolonged abuse of laxatives containing anthraquinone

melanosome (mel'a-no-sum) pigmentary granules within the melanocytes

melanotroph (-trof) a pituitary cell that produces melanocyte-stimulating hormone

melanuria (mel'an-ur'e-a) darkening of urine on standing due to presence of melanin precursor, seen in extensive metastases from melanoma

MELAS mitochondrial encephalopathy with lactic acidosis and stroke-like episodes due to an adenine-to-guanine substitution in the gene affecting mitochondrial transcription

melasma (me-laz'ma) chloasma

melatonin (mel'a-to'nin) a hormone produced by the pineal gland in response to light

malena (me-le'na) the passage of dark coloured stools from upper gastrointestinal bleeding

Meleney's ulcer symbiotic action of microaerophilic streptococci and haemolytic streptococci and staphylococci acting as causative agent in producing an acute spreading painful ulcer and a gangrene of the postoperative wound of a perforated viscus and following of drainage of empyema thoracis

melioidosis (mel'e-oi-do'sis) an infection caused by *Burkholderia pseudomallei* a saprophyte found in soil and water. Infection is through abrasions characterised by fever, prostration, pneumonia, hepatosplenomegaly and multiple abscess. Ceftazidine and tetracyclines are useful

melituria passage of any sugar such as glucose, fructose, maltose, or pentose in the urine

Melkerson's syndrome recurrent facial palsy, swelling of lips and congenital furrowing of tongue, named after E. Melkerson, Scandinavian physician

meli, melli- combining word for sugars, sweetness.

melon seed bodies soft small free bodies found in joint cavities in various inflammations

meloplasty (mel'o-plas-te) plastic surgery of the cheek

melphalan (mel'fa-lan) alkylating cytotoxic agent used in myelomatosis

membra (mem-bra) plural of membrane

membrana (mem-bra'na) membrane **m flaccida** upper loose segment of ear drum **m reuniens** fibrous link of skin to dura in spina bifida occulta

membrane (mem'bran) a thin layer or sheet of tissue that covers a part, lines a cavity or divides a cavity or connects two structures **m bone** bone formed from fibrous tissue without intervention of cartilage **m potential** electrical potential due to the differences of ions on either side of a semipermeable membrane. **m transport** active translocation of proteins from the site of production in the cell to the sites of storage or to the cell membrane for later release. **serous m** a connective tissue sheet lubricated with slippery serum

membranes amnion; extraembryonic parts of conceptus

membranocartilagenous (mem'bra-no-kart'il-aj'i-nus) 1. partly membranous and partly cartilagenous 2. developed in both membrane and cartilage

membranoid (mem'bra-noid) membrane like

membranolysis (mem'bran-ol'i-sis) disruption of a cell membrane

membranoproliferative glomerulonephritis thickening of the glomerular basement membrane and proliferation of mesangial and endothelial cells, in a progressive renal lesion

membrum (mem'brum) pl. **membra** a limb or extremity

membranous resembling mucosa involving epithelial layer **m pharyngitis** Vincent's angina **m urethra** a thin walled 1 cm canal between the urethral sphincter and prostate

memory (mem'a-re) 1. recollection of that which was once experienced or learnt 2. mental information system consisting of encoding, storage and retrieval 3. a computer's capacity for storing information **long term m** memory process that is permanently retained for future retrieval **short term m** memory process in which the stimuli that have been recognised are stored for a brief period **m cells** lymphocytes already primed by exposure to antigen

MEN multiple endocrine neoplasia. A group of autosomal dominant diseases characterised by hyperplasia or neoplasia of more than one endocrine gland, many of which are members of APUD system

menacme (me-nak'me) the period between menarche and menopause

menadiol (men'a-di'ol) synthetic analogue of vitamin K

menadione (men'a-di'on) vitamin K_2 compound exhibiting vitamin K activity, and is synthesised by the intestinal flora

menarche (me-nar'ke) onset or beginning of menstruation

Mendelian 1. of or pertaining to Gregor Mendel 2. referring to the laws of heredity enunciated by Gregor Mendel

Mendel's law 1. different forms of one character remain distinct without blending in crosses (of segregation) 2. forms of any one character behave independently of those of any other character (of recombination), formulated by Gregor Mendel, Austrian monk and naturalist

Mendelson's syndrome acute lung injury from aspiration of acid gastric contents especially from general anaesthesia, during labour, named after Curtis Mendelson, US obstetrician

Menetrier's disease giant hypertrophic gastritis, wherein there is a diffuse thickening of the gastric mucosa by excessive proliferation of epithelial cells of stomach mucosa, without damage to glandular elements, named after Pierre Menetrier, French physician

Menghini needle an aspiration needle for liver biopsy available in lengths of 4 cm and 7 cm and has varying internal diameter. It has a blunt nail inside preventing the suction of the biopsy material into the syringe and hence its fragmentation. The tip of the needle is oblique with an effective cu..ing edge, named after G. Menghini, Italian physician

Meniere's disease labyrinthine vertigo. The condition is characterised by tinnitus, distorted hearing and paroxysmal attacks of vertigo, preceded by a sense of fullness in the ear, named after Prosper Meniere, French physician

meningeal pertaining to meninges m carcinomatosis diffuse infiltration of meninges by malignant tissue presenting with seizure, headache, cranial nerve palsies and disturbances of mentation

meninges (men-in-jez) 1. membranes 2. the three membranes enclosing the brain and spinal cord, comprising the dura mater, the arachnoid and pia mater

meningioma (me-nin'je-o'ma) a fibroblastic tumour of the meninges seen in adults. It grows slowly and occurs most commonly in the cortical dura. It offers best prospects for complete removal by surgery

meningism (men'in-jizm) meningitis-like symptoms without inflammation of the meninges

meningismus meningeal irritation without any objective signs

meningitis (men'in-ji'tis) acute infection of meninges presenting with features of fever, headache, stiffness of neck and irritability of meninges **bacterial m** develops secondary to a bacteraemic illness or from direct spread from an adjacent focus of infection in the ear, sinus or skull fracture. *Neisseria meningitidis, Haemophilus influenzae* and *Streptococcus pneumoniae* are common causes. CSF is cloudy due to presence of neutrophils **fungal m** a recognised complication of HIV infection **tuberculous m** may develop after a primary infection in childhood or as part of miliary tuberculosis. CSF demonstrates a fine clot (cobweb) on standing, with a rise in protein and a marked fall in glucose. There is increased number of leucocytes **viral m** a benign and self-limiting illness. Headache is more severe than meningism. CSF shows excess leucocytes with normal proteins and glucose

mening (o) combining word for meninges, membrane.

meningocoele (me-ning'ga-sel) protrusion of meninges through spina bifida

meningococcaemia (me-nin'gokok-sem'e-a) a disease caused by *Neisseria meningitidis* in the blood. It has a sudden onset with fever, chills, myalgia, headache, petechiae and severe prostration

meningococcus (me-ning'go-kok'us) pl. **meningococci** a bacterium of the genus *Neisseria meningitidis*, a non-motile, gram-negative diplococcus, often found in the nasopharynx of asymptomatic carriers that may cause septicemia, cerebrospinal fever and meningitis

meningocyte (me-ning'go-sit) a mesenchymal epithelial cell of the subarachnoid space

meningoencephalitis (me-ning'go-en-sef'a-lit'is) inflammation of meninges and brain

meningoencephalocoele (-en-sef'a-lo-sel) protusion of the meninges and brain through a congenital defect in the skull

meningoencephalopathy (-en-sef'a-lop'a-the) disease affecting meninges and brain

meningogenic (-jen'ik) arising in the meninges

meningomalacia (-ma-la'she-a) softening of a membrane

meningomyelitis (-mi'e-li'tis) inflammation of the spinal cord and meninges

meningomyelocoele (-mi'le-lo'sel) protrusion of the spinal cord or the cauda equina along with meninges through spina bifida. The cord and nerves appear as dark shadows in the brilliantly translucent swelling during transillumination test

meningomyeloradiculitis (-mi'e-lo-ra-dik'u-li'tis) inflammation of the meninges, spinal cord and roots of the spinal nerves

meningo-osteophlebitis (-os'te-o-fli'bit'is) inflammation of the veins of the periosteum

meningopathy (me'in-gop'a-the) any disease affecting the meninges

meningoradicular (me-nin'gora-dik'ul-er) pertaining to the meninges and the nerve roots

meningorrhagia (-ra'je-a) haemorrhage from the meninges

meningosis (me'ing-go'sis) membranous union of bones, as in the skull of newborn

meningovascular (me-ning'go-vas'ku-lar) pertaining to the blood vessels in the meninges or the meninges and blood vessels

meninx (me'ninks) singular of meninges

meniscitis (men'i-sit'is) inflammation of a meniscus of the knee joint

meniscocyte (me-nis'ko-sit) a sickle cell

meniscocytosis (me-nis'ko-si-to'sis) sickle cell anaemia

meniscosynovial (-sin-o-ve-il) pertaining to a meniscus and the synovial membrane

meniscus (me-nis'kus) 1. curved edge of liquid-solid line of contact 2. concavo-convex lens 3. a crescent-shaped structure as of cartilage of knee **m sign** *radiol*1. a semilunar radiolucency peripheral to a pulmonary mass lesion, seen in hydatid cyst, aspergilloma 2. a large semilunar hypodense zone in ulcerated gastric adenocarcinoma

men (o) combining word for menstruation

menolipsis (men'a-lip'sis) decreased menstruation noted at any age from any cause

menometrorrhagia (-me'tra-ra'je-a) excessive uterine bleeding at and between menstrual periods

menopause (men'a-pawz) the cessation of menstrual activity which occurs between ages of 45 and 50, characterised by menstrual irregularity, hot flushes, irritability, increased weight, osteoporosis and atrophy of female tissues

menorrhagia (men'ar-a'jea) excessive or prolonged menstrual bleeding

menorrhalgia (men'ar-al'jea) dysmenorrhoea

menoschesis (me-nos'ke-sis) suppression of menstruation

menostasis (men'o-sta'sis) amenorrhoea

menostaxis (men'a-stak'sis) a prolonged menstrual period

menoxenia (men'ok-e'nea) abnormal menstruation

menses(men'sez) the monthly flow of menstrual bood from the uterus

menstrual extraction suction extraction of an early conceptus (upto 8 weeks of gestation)

menstrual regulation suction evacuation of the uterus at a very early stage of pregnancy

menstruation (men'stro-a'shun) cyclic endometrial shedding and discharge of bloody fluid from the uterus , and it occurs at approximately 4-week intervals. **anovulatory m** menstruation without the discharge of ovum **retained m** haematocolpus **retrograde m** backward flow of menstrual blood through the fallopian tubes **vicarious m** periodic bleeding occurring from any surface other than uterine mucous membrane.

menstrum (men'str-um) 1. a solvent medium 2. menstrual fluid

mensuration (men'ser-a'shun) the act of measurement

mental (ment'l) 1. pertaining to the mind 2. pertaining to the chin **m age** *psy* the level of the mental ability of a person as determined by an intelligent test in relation to chronological age of an average person at this level **m deficiency** lowered mental capacity **m disorder** significant behavioural or psychological syndrome associated with distress or disability, not just an expected response to a particular event **m retardation** impaired intellectual functioning and adaptive behaviour

mentalis *see* table of muscles

menthol (men'thol) an alcohol from different mint oils used as a flavouring agent and as an antipruritic

mentoanterior face presentation in labour with chin anterior

mentoplasty (men'to-plas'te) plastic surgery of the deformities of chin whereby its shape or size is altered

mentoposterior face presentation in labour with chin posterior

mentum (men'tum) chin

mepacrine 4-aminoquinoline antimalarial, also used in tapeworm infestation

meperidine (me-per'i-den) a narcotic analgesic

mephenteramine (me-fen'tar-men) an adrenergic vasopressor agent used as a nasal decongestant, and to maintain blood pressure

mephenytoin (me-fen'i-to'in) an anticonvulsant agent

mephitic (me-fit'ik) emitting foul odour; poisonous; noxious

mephobarbital (mef'o-bar'bi-tal) a long acting barbiturate

MEq abbreviation for milliequivalent

meralgia (me-ral'je-a) pain in the thigh **m parasthetica** a sensory neuropathy resulting from compression of the lateral femoral cutaneous nerve at the level of inguinal ligament or in the fascia lata and it is characterised by pain and parasthesia involving lateral and occasionally anterior proximal thigh unilaterally

M:E ratio the ratio of maturing myeloid cells to erythroid cells within the bone marrow, normally it is 3-4:1

mercaptan (mer-kap'tan) thioalcohol, a substance in which the oxygen of an alcohol has been replaced by a thiol (-SH) group

mercaptopurine (mer'kap'to-pur'en) a purine antimetabolite used in acute leukaemia

mercurial (mer-kur'e-il) 1. pertaining to mercury 2. a mercurial preparation

mercuric (mer-kur'ik) pertaining to mercury as a bivalent element

mercurous (mer-kur-us) pertaining to mercury as a monovalent element

mercury (mer'kur-e) a heavy , silver white metallic element, atomic no. 80, symbol Hg, fluid at ordinary temperatures used in barometers, thermometers, pesticides, dental fillings and pharmaceutical preparations

meridian (me-rid'e-an) a line encircling a globular body at right angles to its equator and touching both poles

Merkel cell tactile receptor cell in deeper layers of epidermis, named after Friedrich Merkel, German anatomist

meroblastic (mer'a-blas'tik) pertaining to or characterising an ovum that contains a large amount of yolk. The cleavage is restricted only to a part of the cytoplasm

merocrine (mer'a-krin) a secretion in which the secreting cell remains intact while producing and discharging the secretory product

merogenesis (mer'o-jen'i-sis) reproduction by segmentation

merogony(me-rog'a-ne) 1. an incomplete development of an ovum which has been disorganised 2. schizogony seen in sporozoan protozoa, in which the nucleus divides several times before the cytoplasm divides. The dividing cell (schizont) breaks up to form daughter cells (merozoites)

meromyosin (mer'o-mi'a-sin) a subunit of myosin, which may be heavy (H) or light (L)

meropia (me-ro'pe-a) partial blindness

merorachischisis (me'ro-ra-kis'ki-sis) fissure of a portion of spinal cord

merotomy (me-rot'a-me) fissure of part of the spinal cord

merozoite (mer'a-zo-it) a motile, pre- and extra-erythrocytic form of plasmodial parasites, resulting from the asexual division of plasmodia in the liver or erythrocytes which either infect other erythrocytes or spontaneously develop into sexual forms

MERRF myoclonus epilepsy with ragged red fibres. A mitochondrial myopathy exhibiting myoclonus epilepsy, ataxia, presence of ragged red muscle fibres on staining by Gomori trichrome and increased mitochondria demonstrable by electron microscopy

merycism (mer'i-sizm) rumination

mesangial (mes-an'ji-al) referring to the mesangium m ring annular deposition of C3, C4 and properidin in the glomerular mesangium in membranoproliferative glomerulonephritis

mesangiocapillary (mes-an'je-o-kap'il-er'e) pertaining to or affecting the mesangium and associated capillaries

mesangium (mes-an'je-um) a framework containing basement-membrane like material giving support to the centre of renal glomerulus, between capillaries

mesatipellic (mes-at'i-pel'ik) an individual with a pelvic index between 90 and 95

mesaxon (mes-ak'son) the plasma membrane of the neurolemma surrounding a nerve axon

mesectoderm (me-sek'to-derm) that part of the masenchyme derived from ectoderm

mesencephalon (mes'en-sef'a-lon) the mid- brain

mesencephalotomy (mes'en-sef'a-lot'a-me) sectioning of any structure in the midbrain, especially the spinothalamic tracts for relief of unbearable pain

mesenchyma (me'seng'ki-ma) an aggregation of mesenchymal cells

mesenchyme (me'senz'kim) mesenchyma

mesenchymoma (mes'en-ki-mo'ma) any benign or malignant tumour containing two or more mesenchymal elements and fibroblasts

mesenteriopexy (mes'en-ter'e-o-pek'se) surgical fixation of a torn mesentery

mesenteric relating to the mesentery m adenitis inflammation of mesenteric lymph nodes, often in respiratory infection m artery syndrome obstruction of duodenum by angulation of origin of mesenteric artery m thrombosis embolic obstruction of superior mesenteric artery resulting in infarction of small intestine

mesenteriplication (-mes'en-ter'i-pli-ka'shun) shortening of the mesentery by taking tucks in it surgically

mesenterium (mes'en-ter'e-um) mesentery

mesenteron (mes-en'ter-on) midgut

mesentery (mes'en-to're) the peritoneal fold that encircles the small intestine and connects it to the posterior abdominal wall **mesenteric** adj

mesiad (me'ze-ad) toward the midline or centre

mesial (me'ze-il) nearer the centre of dental arch

mesiobuccal(me'ze-o-buk'l) pertaining to or formed by the buccal surface of a tooth

mesioclusion (-kloo'zhun) malocclusion in which mandible articulates with maxilla in a position mesial to normal

mesiodens (me'ze-o-dens) a supernumerary tooth in the maxilla between the central incisor teeth

mesion (me'ze-on) division of the body into right and left symmetrical halves

mesioversion(me'ze-o-ver'zhun) malposition of a tooth in a posterior direction following the curvature of the dental arch

mesmerism a system of therapeutics from which hypnotism and therapeutic suggestions have been developed, named after Franz Mesmer, Austrian physician

mesmerison (mes'mer-izon) hypnotism

mes (o) combining word for middle.

mesoappendix (mes'o-a-pen'diks) the peritoneal fold connecting the appendix to the ileum

mesobilirubinogen (-bil'i-roo-bin'a-jen) a reduced form of bilirubin, formed in the intestine; sterocobilin forms on its oxidation

mesoblast (mes'o-blast) initial stage of mesoderm

mesoblastema (mes'o-blas-tem'a) cells constituting the early undifferentiated mesoderm

mesocardia (-kar'de-a) situation of the heart in the middle of the thorax

mesocardium (-kar'de-um) an embryonic mesentery giving support to the heart, and connecting it to the foregut and the central body wall

mesocolon (mes'o-ko'lon) the peritoneal process attaching the colon to the posterior abdominal wall

mesocolopexy (mes'o-kol'o-pek'se) surgical fixation of colon

mesocoloplication (-kol'o-pli-ka'shun) an operation to shorten the mesocolon to correct undue mobility and ptosis

mesocord (mes'o-kord) an umbilical cord adhering to the placenta

mesocortex (mes'o-kor'teks) the cortex of cingulate gyrus

mesoderm (mes'o-derm) an embryonal tissue layer that gives rise to muscle, cartilage, bone and subcutaneous tissue, cardiovascular system, urogenital system except urinary bladder, serous membranes, spleen and adrenal glands

mesodiastolic (mes'o-di'a-stal'ik) pertaining to the middle of diastole

mesoduodenum (-doo'o-de'num) the mesenteric fold connecting the duodenum to the abdominal wall

mesoepididymis (-ep'i-did'i-mis) a fold of tunica vaginalis that sometimes connects the epididymis and testis

mesogastrium (-gas'tre-um) primitive mesentery enclosing the stomach. Greater omentum develops from it

mesogluteus (-gloot'e-us) gluteus medius muscle

mesoileum (-il'e-um) the mesentery of the ileum

mesomere (mes'o-mer) a blastomere

mesometrium (mes'o-me-tre-um) the broad ligament of the uterus below the mesosalpinx

mesomorph (mez'o-morf) a body build characterised by predominance of tissues derived from mesoderm and the individual is stocky and muscular

meson (mes'on) particle of mass intermediate between electron and proton, that may be charged positive, negative or neutral

mesonephroma (mes'o-ne-fro'ma) a rare malignant neoplasm of the ovary with tubular pattern and focal proliferation of epithelial cells

mesonephros (-nef'ros) the second stage in renal development which appears as an oblong mass along with the embryonal gonads and disappears with foetal maturation

mesophile (mes'o-fil) a microorganism with an optimum temperature between 25°C and 40°C, but growing between 10°C and 45°C.

mesophlebitis (mes'o-fle-bit'is) inflammation of the middle coat of a vein

mesophryon (mes'of're-on) the glabella

mesopulmonum (mes'o-pul-mon'um) embryonic mesentery of the lung

mesorchium (mes-or'ke-um) a fold of tunica vaginalis testis between the testis and epididymis

mesorectum (mes'o-rek'tum) the peritoneal covering of the rectum, which covers its upper part only

mesosalpinx (mes'o-sal'pinks) the part of the broad ligament covering the fallopian tube

mesosigmoid (-sig'moid) mesentery of sigmoid flexure attaching it to the posterior abdominal wall

mesosigmoidopexy (-sig-moid'a-pek'se) surgical fixation of the mesosigmoid

mesosome (mes'o-som) an invagination of the bacterial cell membrane

mesosternum (mes'o-stern'um) middle part of the sternum

mesotendineum (-ten-din'e-um) synovial sheath of a tendon connecting the lining of tendon sheath to the fibrous sheath covering the tendon

mesothelioma (mez'o-the'le-o-ma) a neoplasm of serosal surfaces. Exposure to asbestos can lead to pleural, or peritoneal mesothelioma after a long latent period **peritoneal m** presents as a diffuse abdominal mass due to omental infiltration and with ascites.

pleural m diffuse malignant tumour spreading along pleural surface. It encases the lungs and invades tissues. There is accumulation of large amounts of haemorrhagic pleural fluid

mesothelium (-thel'e-um) a single layer of flattened cells forming an epithelial lining of serous cavities

mesotympanum (-tim'pa-num) the portion of the middle ear medial to the tympanic membrane

mesovarium (-var'e-um) a short peritoneal fold connecting the anterior border of the ovary with the posterior layer of the broad ligament of the uterus

messenger (mes'en-jer) an information carrier **mRNA** the transcript of a structural gene carrying genetic information to the site of protein synthesis in ribosomes

mestranol (mes'tra-nol) synthetic oestrogen used in oral contraceptive

MET metabolic equivalent

meta change, after, beyond

metaanalysis (met'a-a-nal'i-sis) an analytical discipline that critically reviews and combines the results of multiple studies and apply statistical methodology to arrive at an unbiased conclusion

metabasis (me-tab'a-sis) a change in the clinical manifestations or alteration in the course of a disease

metabiosis (met'a-bi-o'sis) dependence of one organism upon another

metabolic relating to metabolism **m acidosis** an acid base disturbance developing from an increased acid production or accumulation of non-volatile acids or from loss of bicarbonates. There is an increase in hydrogen ion concentration and a fall in pH **m alkalosis** an acid base disturbance caused by an increase in plasma bicarbonate concentration. The condition is initiated by marked loss of acid other than H_2CO_3 from the stomach or the kidney. The plasma chloride level is low (hypochloraemic). There is fall in hydrogen ion concentration **basal m**

measurement of metabolism under basal conditions and it is expressed as a percentage of normal **m rate** in a steady state the amount of oxygen taken by the lungs exactly equals the amount utilised by the tissues and the amount of carbon dioxide eliminated by the lungs equals that formed in the tissues. The amount of oxygen consumed varies with the surface area of the body. It is around 250 ml per minute

metabolism (me-tab'o-lizm) the process of transforming food stuffs into tissue elements and into energy for use in the growth, repair and general function of the body **m equivalent,** MET. The amount of oxygen required per minute under quiet resting conditions, equal to 3.5 ml of oxygen consumed per kilogram of body weight per minute

metabolite (-lit) any product of metabolism

metacarpal (met'a-kar'pal) 1. pertaining to the metacarpus 2. a bone of metacarpus

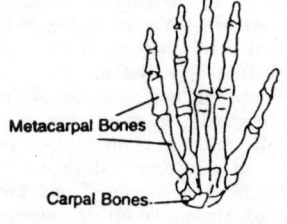

Metacarpal Bones

Carpal Bones

metacarpus (-kar'pus) the part of the hand between the wrist and fingers. It is formed by five metacarpal bones that extend from the carpus to the phalanges

metacentric (-sen'trik) location of centromere toward middle in a chromosome

metacercaria (-ser-ka're-a) the encysted state in the life cycle of a trematode,

which occurs in the intermediate host, a species of fresh water snail

metachromasia (-kro-ma'zhah) the property of a tissue that enables it to stain differently from the colours used in the dye

metachrosis (-kro'sis) alteration of colour in animals

metacone (met'a-kon) the distobuccal cusp of an upper molar tooth

metaconid (met'a-kon'id) the mesiolingual cusp of a lower molar tooth

metagenesis (-jen'e-sis) alteration of generations

megagonimus (-gon'i-mus) a genus of flukes that encyst on fish, and may infest man

metalodobenzylguanidine (-a'lo-do-ben'zil-gwa-ne-din) a noradrenaline analogue labelled with radioactive iodine, used in the imaging study of adrenal medulla

metal (met'l) an element possessing a peculiar lustre, malleability, fusibility, and conductivity for heat and electricity and capable of getting ionised positively in solution. **metallic** adj **m fume fever** an influenza-like illness due to occupational exposure to copper dust or fumes

metaloenzyme (me-tal'o-en'zim) an enzyme that contains a metal ion on the aminoacid side chains such as cytochromes

metaloporphyrin (me-tal'o-por'fi-rin) a combination of a metal with porphyrin as in haeme

metaloprotein (-pro'ten) a combination of metal ion with protein, such as haemoglobin

metallurgy (met'al-urj-e) 1. the science of separating metals from their ores 2. the technique of making and compounding alloys

metamere (met'a-mer) one of a series of homologous body segments

metamorphopsia (met'a-mor-fo'p-sea) distorted vision due to macular affections such as macular scar or oedema metamorphosis (met'a-mor'fah-sis) transformation wherein there is a change in form, structure and function

metamyelocyte (-mi'l-o-sit) a maturing granulocyte between a myelocyte and a polymorphonuclear neutrophil, are confined to bone marrow. The nucleus is reniform with coarsely clumped chromatin

metanephrine (-nef'rin) a metabolite of epinephrine that is normally excreted in the urine

metanephros (-nef'ros) the embryonic precursor of the adult kidney. It arises from mesonephric ducts

metaphase (met'a-faz) a stage in mitosis, wherein there is loss of nuclear membrane, with aggregation of chromosomes on equatorial plane and formation of nuclear spindle

metaphysis (me-taf'i-sis) the zone of growth between the epiphysis and diaphysis during development of a bone.

metaplasia (met'a-pla-zhah) the conversion of one type of adult cells into another, especially those of the epithelium.

metaplasm (met'a-plazm) inactive materials found in protoplasm such as yolk

metapneumonic (met'a-noo-mon'ik) following pneumonia

metaproterenol (-pro-ter'e-nol) orciprenaline

metapsychology (-si-kol'a-je) an attempt to describe what lies beyond the laws of psychology, such as the relation between the body and mind

metaraminol (-ram'i-nol) a sympathomimetic agent with potent vasopressor action

metarubricyte (-roo'bri-sit) the last cell type in the development of red blood cell prior to extrusion of the nucleus

metastasectomy (me-tas'ta-sek'ta-me) surgical removal of one or more metastatic deposits

metastasis (me-tas'ta-sis) pl. metastases 1. distal spread of a malignant cell either through blood or lymphatic vessel or along a serosal membrane. It develops a secondary focus of malignancy 2. transportation of microorganisms from one part of the body to another through the blood stream or lymph 3. the shifting of the manifestation of a disease from one part of the body to another

metatarsal (met'a-tar'sil) 1. pertaining to the metatarsus 2. a bone of metatarsus m dome a rounded support under middle of forefoot to relieve metatarsalgia

metatarsalgia (-tar-sal'je-a) pain in the forefoot, symptom due to any abnormality of foot resulting in faulty distribution of weight

metatarsus (-tar'sus) the part of the foot between the instep and the toes, consists of five metatarsal bones extending from the tarsus to the phalanges

metathalamus (-thal'a-mus) the most caudal part of the thalamus composed of the medial and lateral geniculate bodies

metathesis (me-tath'e-sis) transfer of a pathologic product from one place to another so as to decrease its effect

metatrophic (met'a-trof'ik) ability to obtain nourishment from different sources

metazoa (met'a-o-zoa) multicellular animal organisms in which the cells are differentiated and form tissues

metazoon (-zo'on) multicellular animal organism

metencephalon (met'en-sef'a-lon) the anterior of two major subdivisions of the rhombencephalon consisting of pons and cerebellum

metaenkaphaline endorphin 5-peptide

mateorism (met'e-a-rizm) tympanitis

meteorotropism (met'e-o-ra'tra-pizm) response to influence by meteorological factors such as climate and weather

metformin a biguanide oral hypoglycaemic agent

methacrylate (meth-ak'ri-lat) an ester of methacrylic acid or the acrylic resin formed upon its polymerisation, used in dentures, contact lenses and as glue in prosthetic joints

methacycline (meth'a-si-klen) a semisynthetic tetracycline derivative

methadone (meth'a-don) a synthetic, relatively long-acting oral opiate

methaemalbumin (met'hem-al-bu'min) haem attached to plasma albumin, noted after a major intravascular haemolysis

methaemoglobin (met-he'mo-glo'bin) (MetHb) a type of haemoglobin in which iron is oxidised from the ferrous to ferric state and it cannot carry oxygen. It is found in traces in the blood normally

methaemoglobinaemia (met-he mo-globin'e-mi-a) presence of methaemoglobin in the circulating blood

methaemoglobinuria (met-he'mo-glo-bin-u'ri-a) presence of methaemoglobin in the urine

methenamine (meth-en'a-men) an antibacterial agent used in urinary tract infections

methamphatamine (met'am-fet'a-men) a methyl derivative of amphetamine, a CNS stimulant

methandrostenolone (meth-an-dro'sten'o-lon) an anabolic steroid possessing androgenic effects

methane (meth'an) (CH_4) an odourless combustible gas produced by the decomposition of organic matter

methanol (meth'a-nol) a highly toxic polar alcohol used as an industrial solvent, often abused as an inebrient. It gets metabolised to formaldehyde and formate causing metabolic acidosis and damage to the optic nerve and blindness. Ethanol is used to reduce methanol metabolites and toxic effects

methantheline (me-than'the-len) a quaternary ammonium anticholinergic

methapyrilene (meth'a-pir'i-len) an antihistaminic agent with sedative action

metharbital (me-thar'bi-tal) an anticonvulsant agent used to control epileptic seizures

methdilazine (meth-di'la-zen) an antipruritic antihistaminic

methicillin (meth'i-sil'in) a semisynthetic penicillinase-resistant penicillin

methimazole (meth-im'a-zol) antithyroid agent that inhibits synthesis of thyroid

methionine (me-thi'o-nen) a sulphur-containing essential amino acid

method (meth'od) the mode or manner of events of a process or procedure

methadology (meth'ed-ol'a-je) the system of principles of procedures employed in scientific study

methotrexate (meth'o-trek-sat) a folic acid antimetabolite used in choriocarcinoma and in combination with other agents for lymphoproliferative malignancy

methoxsalen (me-thek'sa-len) an acrylic acid compound that is capable of inducing melanin production on exposure of skin to ultraviolet light, used in the treatment of vitiligo and psoriasis

methoxyphenamine (me-thok'si-fen'a-men) sympathomimetic bronchodilator

methsuximide (meth-suk'si-mid) an anticonvulsant used in the treatment of epilepsy

methyl (meth'il) the radical $-CH_3$ **m alcohol** CH_4O, solvent and antifreeze

methylate (meth'i-lat) 1. a compound of methyl alcohol and a base 2. to add methyl group, CH_3 to a chemical compound

methylcellulose (meth'il-sel'u-los) hydrophilic colloid, used as bulk-makiŋ ʒ purgative and to adjust osmatic effects of lotions

methylcobalamine (-ko-bal'a-min) a metabolically active cobalamine synthesised by vitamin B_{12}

methyldopa (-do'pa) a centrally acting antihypertensive, inhibits DOPA-decarboxylase

methylene (meth'i-len) **blue** a thiazine dye. Used as an indicator for theoxidation-reduction reaction and as an agent to reduce methaemoglobin. It is used in Wright-Giemsa stain and as a counter-stain

methylene dioxyamphetamine (-di-ok'se-am-fet'a-men) an analogue of amphetamine

methylmalonic (meth'il-ma-lon'ik) **acid** a carboxylic acid intermediate in the metabolism of fatty acid

methylmalonic acidaemia (-as-de'me-a) 1. presence of excess methylmelonic acid in the blood 2. an inherited metabolic disorder caused by an inability to convert methylmelonic acid to succinic acid, and characterised by metabolic acidosis, hyperglycinaemia, hyperglycinuria, failure to grow and mental retardation

methylmalonic aciduria (-as'i-du're-a) an excess amount of methylmalonic acid in the urine, a feature of methylmalonic acidaemia

methylphenidate (meth'il-fen'i-date) an agent used to control attention deficit/hyper-activity disorder

methylprednisolone (-pred-nis'a-lon) a synthetic glucocorticosteroid

methyltestosterone (-tes-tos'ter-on) a methyl derivative of testosterone

methyltransferase (-trans'fer-as) any enzyme transferring methyl groups from one compound to another

methysergide (meth'i-sur'jid) lysergic acid derivative, 5 HT antagonist used for prevention of migraine. Prolonged use is associated with retroperitoneal fibrosis

metmyoglobin (met-mi'a-glo'bin) myoglobin in which the ferrous ion of the haeme is oxidised to ferric ion

metoclopramide (met'o-clo-pr'a-mide) a prokinetic agent used as an antiemetic

metolazone (me'tel'a-zon) a thiazide diuretic

metopic (me-top'ik) pertaining to the forehead

metopion (me-to'pe-on) glabella

metoprolol (met'a-pro'lol) adrenergic beta-blocker used in hypertension and arrhythmias

metoxenous (me-tok'se-nus) having more than one host, refers to parasite passing different states of its existence in different animal hosts

metra (me'tra) the uterus

metratonia (me'tra-te'ne-a) atony of the uterus

metratrophia (-tro'fe-a) atrophy of the uterus

metre (me'ter) 1. measure of length 2. measuring instrument

metrectopia (me'trek-to'pe-a) displacement of the uterus

metreurynter (me'troo-rin'ter) an inflatable bag to dilate the cervix

metric (me'trik) quantitative; relating to measurement

metritis (me-trit'is) inflammation of the uterus

metrizamide (me-triz'a-mid) a contrast medium, used in radiography. It is a substituted amide of metrizoic acid and is less hyperosmolar. It is used for myelography and for enhancing CT images

metrizoate a water-soluble triiodobenzene radiographic contrast medium used for angiography and urography

metr (o) combining word for uterus

metrocoele (me'tro'sel) hernia of the uterus

metrocolpocoele (-kol'pa-sel) protrusion of uterus into the vagina, pushing the vaginal wall downwards

metrocystosis (-sis-to'sis) formation of cysts in uterus

metrocyte (me'tro-sit) a mother cell

metrofibroma a fibroma of the uterus

metrodynia (me'tro-din'e-a) pain in the uterus

metroleukorrhoea (-loo'ka-re'a) a discharge from the uterus of white or yellowish fluid containing mucus and pus

metromalacia (-ma-la'she-a) softening of the uterus

metronidazole (-ni'da-zol) a nitro-imidazole derivative having high activity against anaerobic bacteria and intestinal protozoa. It is effective against *Trichomonas vaginalis, Giardia lamblia* and *Entamoeba histolytica* and is active against infections caused by anaerobic bacteria, specially *B. fragilis*

metroparalysis (-pa-ral'i-sis) paralysis of the uterus during or immediately following childbirth

metropathia haemorrhagica cystic glandular hyperplasia of endometrium resulting in abnormal, excessive uterine bleeding

metropathy (me-trop'a-the) any disease of the uterus

metroperitonitis (me'tro-per'i-ton-it'is) inflammation of uterus involving the peritoneum

metrophlebitis (-fle-bit'is) inflammation of uterine veins following childbirth

metroptosis (me'trop-to'sis) prolapse of the uterus

metrorrhagia (me'tro-ra'je-a) irregular uterine bleeding superimposed on normal cycle

metrorrhoea (-re'a) a discharge from the uterus

metrosalpingography (-sal'ping-gog'ra-fe) hysterosalpingography

metrostaxis (-stak'sis) continuous bleeding from uterus in small amounts

metrostenosis (-sto-no'sis) a narrowing of the uterine cavity

-metry combining word for measurement

metyrapone (me-ter'a-pon) inhibitor β-hydroxylase, the final enzyme in corticosteroid synthesis used for evaluation of the hypothalamus-pituitary-adrenal axis

mexiletine (mek'si-le-ten) cardiac anti-arrhythmic agent used in ventricular tachycardia and fibrillation

Meyer-Betz syndrome paroxysmal idiopathic myoglobinuria with muscle necrosis, named after Friedrich Meyer Betz, German physician

meziocillin (mez'io-sil'in) synthetic broad-spectrum penicillin

Mg chemical symbol magnesium.

mcg microgram

MHC mg milligram abbreviation for major histocompatibility antigen

MHz megahertz, frequency of million per second

MI abbreviation for myocardial infarction; mitral incompetence.

MIC abbreviation for minimum inhibitory concentration; methyl isocyanate

mica (mi'ka) a mineral composed of various rock forming minerals and occur in thin, sparkling scales

micaceous (my'kase-us) scales, particularly those of psoriasis, that peel off like sheets of mica

mication (mi-ka'shun) a quick movement, such as winking

miconazole (mi-kon'a-zol) imidazole antifungal agent, topical for cutaneous candidiasis and intravenous for systemic candidiasis and intrathecal for cryptococcal meningitis

micr (o) combining word for very small; units of measurement to designate an amount 10^{-6} (one millionth) the size of the unit to which it is joined; apparatus for study of small objects

micracoustic (mi'kra-koo'stik) 1. pertaining to faint sounds 2. a process of magnification of very faint sounds

micrencephaly (mi'kren-sef'a-le) abnormally small brain

microabscess (mi'kro-ab'ses) a focal aggregate of neutrophils

microadenoma (mi'kro-ad'e-no'ma) a pituitary adenoma of less than 1 cm in diameter

microaerophilic (-a'ero-fil'ik) a bacterium requiring oxygen only as a terminal electron acceptor. They grow poorly at ambient oxygen levels and in anaerobic conditions

microaggregate (-ag're-gat) clumps of leucocytes, platelets and fibrin that may cause intravascular sludging

microalbuminuria (-al-bu-min-u're-a) passage of a small amount of albumin in the urine. The amount may be 30-300 mg/24 hours. It is an important indicator of risk of developing overt diabetic nephropathy

microanalysis (-a-nal'i-sis) an analytical examination of minute quantities of material

microanatomist (-a-nat'o-mist) histologist

microanatomy (-a-nat'a-me) histology

microaneurysm (-an'ur-izm) focal dilatation of capillaries occurring at arteriolocapillary junctions, or at retinal capillaries

microangiopathy (-an'je-op'a-the) any defect of very small blood vessels, usually capillaries, common in diabetes mellitus

microarray technology a new method of studying how large number of genes interact with each other and how a cell's regulatory networks control vast number of genes simultaneously

microbe (mi'krob) a microorganism including bacteria, spirochaetes, rickettsiae and virus

microbicide (mi-kro'bi-sid) an agent destructive to microbes

microbiology (mi'kro-bi-ol'a-je) the science concerned with the study of microscopic and ultramicroscopic organisms

microbiophotometer (-bi'o-fo-tom'it-er) an instrument for measuring the growth of bacterial culture by turbidity of the medium

microbiota (-bi-ot'a) the microorganisms of a region

microblast (mi'kro-blast) a small nucleated red blood cell

microblepharia (mi'kro-ble-far'e-a) a developmental abnormality wherein the eyelids have an abnormally small vertical dimension

microbody (mi'kro-bod'e) an organelle occurring in animal and plant cells containing membrane-bound granular cytoplasmic particles and enzymes

microcardia (-kar'de-a) abnormally small heart

microcephaly (-sef'a-le) abnormally small brain

microcheilia (-ki'le-a) abnormally small lips

microcheiria (-ki're-a) abnormally small hands

microchemistry (-kem'is-tre) branch of chemistry concerned with analysis of minute quantities of chemical substances

microcirculation (-sur'kul'-a'shun) blood circulation in arterioles, capillaries and venules

Micrococcaceae (-kok-a'se-e) a family of bacteria of the order Eubacteriales, containing gram-positive spherical cells, that may be saprophytic, parasitic or pathogenic

micrococcus (-kok'us) pl. **micrococci** a genus of bacteria belonging to the family of Micrococcaceae, that are gram-positive spherical cells. They occur in irregular masses, and are saprophytic or parasitic, such as *M. luteus*

microcomputer (-com'pu-ter) a computer that uses a microprocessor for its central processing unit and control circuitry

microcoria (-kor'e-a) congenital contraction of the pupil

microcornea (-kor'ne-a) an abnormally small cornea

microcurie (mi'kro-ku're) a measure of radium emanation, one millionth of a curie

microcyte (-sit) a small non-nucleated red blood cell

microcytotoxicity (mi'kro-si'to-tok-sis-it-e) extremely minute quantities of substance damaging the cells

microdeletion syndrome deletion of contiguous genes from small sections of chromosome material resulting in dysmorphic syndromes associated with retardation

microdetermination (-de-tur'mi-na'shun) chemical analysis of extremely small quantities of substance

microdiskectomy (-dis-kek'ta-me) surgical removal of a herniated intervert-ebral disc using an operating microscope

microdissection (-di-sek'shun) dissection of tissues under magnification

microdontia (-don'shi-a) markedly small dentition to the build of the body

microenvironment (-in-vi'ron-ment) the environment at the microscopic or cellular level

microerythrocyte (-e-rith'ro-sit) microcyte

microfarad (-far'ad) a microunit of electrical capacity; one millionth of a farad

microfauna (-faw'na) the microscopic animal organisms in a specific region

microfilament (-fil'a-mint) actin fibres of 5 mm diameter found in cytoplasm of cells forming a cytoskeletal lattice work

microfilaria (-fi-la're-a) larvae of nematodes of the family Filarioidea. They are 170-320 microns long that migrate in blood or skin. The life cycle is completed when mosquitoes take up microfilariae while feeding on humans. Microfilariae appear in the blood at night and can be seen moving in a wet blood film

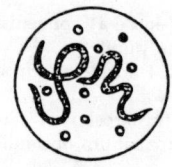

Microfilaria

microflora (-flor'a) a community of microorganisms in one environment

microfold cell an intestinal mucosal cell overlying Peyer's patches that has microfolds allowing entry of lymphocytes to approach intestinal lumen

microfracture (mi'kro-frak'cher) a minute incomplete break or discontinuity in a bone

microgamete (mi'kro-gam'et) the smaller (male) of the two motile conjugating gametes in sexual cycle of plasmodium

microgametocyte (-ga-met'a-sit) the mother cell producing microgametes

microglia (mi-krog'le-a) specialised form of macrophages in CNS

microgliocyte (mi-krog'le-o-sit) an embryonic cell of microglia

microglossia abnormally small tongue

microglobulin (mi'kro-glob'ul-in) a polypeptide expressed on the surface of antigen presenting cells

micrognathia (-nath'e-a) abnormally small jaws, especially mandible

microgonioscope (-go'ne-o-skop) an instrument for measurement of minute angles, used in the study of glaucoma

microgram (mi'kro-gram) one millionth of a gram

micrograph (-graf) 1. an instrument for magnifying and recording minute movements 2. photograph of an object or specimen as seen through a microscope

micrographia (mi'kro-graf'e-a) minute handwriting

microgyria (-ji're-a) shrinkage of convolutions from localised brain atrophy

microgyrus (-ji'rus) a small, malformed convolution of the brain

microinfarct (-in'farkt) very small infarct due to obstruction to the blood flow in arterioles or capillaries

microinjector (-n'jek'ter) an instrument for injection of very small amounts of drugs

microinvasion (-in-va'zhun) invasion of tissue immediately adjacent to a carcinoma *in situ*

microiontophoresis delivery of minute quantities of drugs by passage of electric currents through capillary tubes containing appropriate solutions

microlitre (mi'kro-let'er) one-millionth of a litre

microlithiasis (mi'kro-li-thi'a-sis) the formation, presence or discharge of minute concretions

micromanipulator (-ma-nip'ul-at-or) a microscope used in microdissection, microinjection and other activities

micromelia (-me'li-a) disproportionately small limbs

micromere (mi'kro-mer) a blastomere of small size

micrometastasis (mi'kro-me-tas'ta-sis) metastasis in which the secondary deposits are too small to be detected

micrometre (mi-krom'e-ter) 1. thousandth of millimetre (m.) 2. a lens that is accurately marked for measuring microscopic forms

micromethod (-meth'od) any chemical or physical procedure dealing with exceedingly small quantities of material

micromyelia (-mi-el'e-a) abnormally short spinal cord

micromyeloblast (-mi'e-lo-blast) a small myeloblast

micron (mi'kron) micrometer

microneedle (mi'kro-ne'dl) extremely minute needle used in microdissection

microneurosurgery (-noor'o-sur'je-re) a highly specialised surgery on minute vessels and structures of the nervous system undertaken under high magnification

micronodular presence of minute nodules

micronucleus (noo'kle-us) 1. small nucleus in a large cell 2. the smaller of the two nuclei in ciliates

micronutrients minerals needed in relatively small amounts

microorganism (-or'ga-nizm) a microscopic organism

micropathology (-pa-thol'a-je) microscopic study of the changes in the tissues and organs brought about by disease process

microperfusion (-per-fu'zhun) perfusion of a minute quantity of a substance

microphage (mi'kro-faj) polymorphonuclear leucocyte

microphakia (mi'kro-fa'ke-a) a congenital abnormality in which the lenses of the eye are small and spherical, often subjected to subluxation

microphallus (-fal'us) abnormally small penis

microphone (mi'kra-fun) a device picking and converting sound energy into an electronic signal, which is then transmitted

microphonic (mi'kro-fon'ik) 1. helping to amplify the sound 2. cochlear membrane

microphotograph (-fot'a-graf) a minue photograph of any object.

microphthalmos (mi'kro-thal'mos) abnormally small eye ball(s)

micropinocytosis (mi'kro-pi'no-si-to'sis) formation of small vesicles in the cytoplasm on taking up into the cell of macromolecules by invagination of the plasma membrane and then pinched off

micropipette (-pi-pet) an extremely small pipette used to measure small quantities of liquids

microplethysmography (-pleth'is-mog'ra-fe) a technique of measurement of minute alterations in the volume of a part as a result of blood flow into or out of it

micropodia (-po'dea) abnormally small feet

Micropolyspora faeni fungus of mouldy hay, causative agent of farmer's lung

microprobe (mi'kro-prob) a very small probe used in microsurgery

microprocessor the hardware component of a microcomputer containing the central arithmetic unit, a logic board and the associated circuitry fitting on one or several silicon chips

micropsia (mi-krop'se-a) subjective perception of objects as smaller than they actually are

micropyle (mi'kro-pil) the opening in the ovum of some animals, for entry of spermatozoon

microradiography (mi'kro-ra'de-og'ra-fe) technique of radiography of minute objects

microrefractometer (-re-frak·tom'it-er) a refractometer used for the study of blood cells

microrespirometer (-res'pi-rom'it-er) an instrument to measure the use of oxygen by small particles of isolated tissues

microsatellite repetitive structures of short sequences of DNA, used as genetic markers to track inheritance in families

microscope (mi'kro-skop) an instrument that gives an enlarged image of an object that is not visible to the naked eye **binocular m** microscope having two eye pieces, **compound m** microscope having two or more lenses **dark field m** a variant of light microscopy in which light is directed at an oblique angle and the specimen appears bright in a dark background, useful to observe spirochaetes **electron m** a beam of electrons pass through the specimen providing a magnified image of an object on a fluorescent screen **fluorescent m** a variant of light microscopy in which light is projected onto the specimen by halogen-quartz, mercury or xenon lamps and reemitted at another wavelength **operative m** microsurgery **phase-contrast m** technique used to observe living cells **simple m** microscope consisting of a single magnifying lens **slit lamp m** a low power light microscopy which has an attachment for examination of cornea

microscopy (mi-kros'ka-pe) study of minute objects by a microscope

microsecond (mi'kro-sek'ond) one millionth of a second

microshock (-shok) direct application of a low level electric current to the myocardial tissue in ventricular fibrillation

microshunt arteriovenous shunt at capillary level

microsome (mi'kra-som) smallest sized lipoprotein-rich cytoplasmic bodies, chiefly ribosomes

microspherocyte (-sfer'a-sit) small rounded erythrocytes seen in excess blood loss, burns, pernicious anaemia and myelofibrosis

microspherocytosis (-sfer'o-si-to'sis) presence of small and more globular red cells in the blood in haemolytic anaemia

microsphygmia (-sfig'me-a) a pulse that is difficult to be felt

microsplenia (-sple'ne-a) abnormal smallness of spleen

microsporon (mi-kros'po-ron) a genus of fungi causing dermatophytosis

microsporum (-um) a fungus often involved in superficial mycoses

microsurgery (mi'kro-sur'je-re) surgery utilising operating microscope

microsyringe (-si-ring) hypodermic syringe that can deliver an accurately measured minute quantities of fluid

microtia (mi'kra-she-a) abnormally small external ear

microtome (mi'kra-tom) an instrument used to cut histological sections. The metal blades cut paraffin embedded tissues for high power microscopy and diamond blades cut plastic-embedded tissues for electron microscopy

microtubule (mi'kro-too'bul) structural component of cytoplasm containing tubulin protein subunits; constituent of mitotic spindles

microvasculature (-vas'kul-a-chor) the system of minute terminal capillaries

microvillus (-vil'us) finger-like cell processes without showing complex structure of cilia. They are constructed of complex plasma membrane folds surrounding an actin microfilament core and form striated border of small intestinal mucosa to increase their cell surface area

microvolt (mi'kro-vot) one millionth of a volt; symbol mV

microwave (-wav) a wave on the electromagnetic spectrum

microzoon (mi'kro-zo'on) a microscopic organism

micrurgy (mi'krur-je) surgical procedures on minute structures under a microscope

micturate (mik'cher-at) urinate

micutrition passing of urine

midbrain (mid'bran) upper segmer᠎ brain stem consisting of colli᠎ tegmentum and cerebral peduncle᠎

middiastolic middle of diastole **m murmur** low pitched rumbling diastolic murmur, especially of mitral stenosis

midget (mij'it) a person who is undersized, but possessing normally developed organs

midgut (mid'gut) 1. the central portion of the digestive tract, the small intestine 2. the portion of embryonic gut between the foregut and hindgut

midlife period between 45 and 65 years of age **m crisis** period of emotional upheaval encountered among some midlife persons

midpalmar space a deep space situated deep to the flexor tendons and superficial to the medial three metacarpals and the intervening interossei and is separated from thenar space by a septum attached to the third metacarpal bone posteriorly and fascia on undersurface of flexor tendons anteriorly

midriff (-rif) the region between the breast and waistline

midsystolic murmur a midsystolic ejection murmur heard in aortic or pulmonary stenosis

midwife (-wif) a person who practises midwifery

midwifery (-wif'ri) science dealing with care of women antepartally, intrapartally and postpartally

migraine (mi'gran) paroxysmal headache, vomiting and focal usually visual, neurological events. The attack begins with malaise and irritability followed by a severe throbbing hemicranial headache, photophobia and vomiting. The aetiology is unknown and there is a genetic predisposition with a great female preponderance **m equivalents** a condition where the visual, sensory, motor or psychic disturbances characteristic of migraine is not followed by headache

migranous neuralgia a migraine variant with periodic unilateral periorbital pain, conjunctival injection, unilateral lacrimation and nasal congestion often in middle-aged males

migration (mi-gra'shun) 1. passing from place to place, of diseases or of symptoms 2. diapedesis 3. movement of a tooth or teeth from normal position 4. movement of molecules during electrophoresis **m inhibiting factor** (MIF) a lymphokine localising the macrophages

milia tiny white spots on the face especially around the nose during first three or four weeks of life due to temporary blocking sebaceous glands

Mikulicz's syndrome painless progressive non-suppurative enlargement of the lacrimal glands and salivary glands, named after Johannes Mikulicz, Breslau surgeon

milestones developmental landmarks to assess the child development e.g. holds head erect 3 months, sits without support 6–8 months, crawling 9–10 months, stands with support 10–11 months, walks with wide base 12–14 months, walks with narrow base 18–21 months

miliaria (mil'ar'e-a) an eruption of minute vesicles and papules due to retention of sweat at the mouths of sweat follicles **m rubra** prickly heat, papular lesions seen in persons exposed to hot environment especially in high humidity. They occur due to blockage of sweat glands by the prickle cell layer of epidermis

miliary (mil'e-ar'e) 1. like scattered millet seeds 2. characterised by lesions resembling millet seeds **m tuberculosis** presence of widespread lesions of tuberculosis occurring after a haematogenous dissemination of tubercle bacilli. It occurs in individuals who have inadequate cell-mediated immunity

milieu environment **m interieure** *Fr* environment presented to the body cells by body fluids

milium (mil'e-um) tiny keratin-filled cyst lying superficially within the skin, usually of face in the newborn

milk 1. an opaque white liquid secreted by the mammary glands of female mammals serving for nourishment of their young 2. any whitish milky fluid 3. a pharmacopeial preparation containing a suspension of insoluble drugs in a water medium

milk alkali syndrome a condition which occurs after prolonged use of absorbable antacids over years along with large amounts of milk. It leads to hypercalcaemia, metastatic calcification and renal failure

milking (milk'ing) removal of contents of a tubular structure by pressing the fingers along it

Milkman's lines pseudofractures of bone seen in X-ray of bones, are linear zones of decalcification that tend to be symmetrical and extend perpendicular to the cortex, named after Louis Milkman, US roentgenologist

milkpox variola minor

Millard-Gubler syndrome paralysis of the lateral rectus with or without a lower motor neuron facial palsy and contralateral pyramidal tract signs due to a lesion in the pons, named after Auguste Millard and Adolphe Gubler, French physicians

Miller-Abbott tube long double-lumen tube with balloon tip for small bowel intubation, named after US physicians, Grier Miller and William Abbott

milli (m) prefix used in metric system to signify one thousandth (10^{-3})

milliampere (mil'e-am'per) one thousandth of an ampere

millicurie (mil'i-kur'e) (mCi) one thousandth (10^{-3}) curie

milliequivalent (mil'e-e-kwiv'a-lint) (MEq) one thousandth (10^{-3}) of a chemical equivalent

milligram (mil'i-gram) (mg) one thousandth (10^{-3}) of a gram

millilitre (-let'er) (ml) one thousandth (10^{-3}) of a litre

millimetre (-met'er) (mm) one thousandth (10^{-3}) of a metre

millimicron (mil'i-mi-kron) one thousandth (10^{-3}) of a micron; nanometre.

millimole (mil'i-mal) (mmol) one thousandth of a mole

milliosmole (mil'e-oz'mol) one thousandth (10^{-3}) of an osmole

millisecond (mili'ske'and) (ms, msec) one thousandth (10^{-3}) of a second

millivolt (mili-vot) (mv) one thousandth of a volt

Millwaukee brace brace for scoliosis applying pressure to pelvis, occiput and chin

mill wheel murmur a loud churning sound over the right ventricle and pulmonary artery, heard in air embolism

milphosis (mil'fo-sis) the falling of eyelashes

Milroy's oedema nonpitting oedema due to congenital lymphatic deficiency, named after William Milroy, US physician

mimesis (mi-me'sis) 1. simple, imitative motor activity of childhood 2. hysterical simulation of an organic disease

mimetic of similarity; similar effect produced by agents of different kind

min abbreviation for minute, minim, minimum

Minamata disease cerebral cortical atrophy due to methyl mercury poisoning, that occurred in Japan bay

mind 1. the organ or seat of consciousness, memory and reasoning 2. all mental processes and psychic activity

mineral (min'er-al) a metallic substance found in nature; many minerals are essential for human and animal nutrition

mineralocorticoid (min'er-al-o-kor'ti koid) an adrenocortical hormone that influences sodium and potassium metabolism

miniature radiography photofluorography, method of case finding undertaken in the antituberculosis campaign

minilaparotomy (min'i-lap'a-rot'a-me) a small incision to enter abdominal cav-

/ity to undertake an operative procedure

minim (min'im) a unit of capacity such as liquid measure, equivalent of 0.0616 ml

minimal lesion nephropathy common cause of nephrotic syndrome in children, which is immunologically mediated, follows infections and responds to immunosuppressants

minimum inhibitory concentration MIC; identifying amount of antimicrobial agent required to inhibit the growth or multiplication of a bacterial isolate

minipill low-dose progesterone oral contraceptive

miniplate (min'e-plat) a small bone plate

minocycline (mi-no-si'klen) a semisynthetic antibiotic of tetracycline group

minor smaller; lesser

minoxidil (mi-nok'si-dil) a directly acting vasodilatory antihypertensive agent

minute (mi-noot) extremely small **m volume** volume of air breathed in one second

miocardia (mi-a-kor'de-a) systole

miosis (mi-o'sis) 1. contraction of the pupil 2. the period of decline of disease

miotic (mi-ot'ik) 1. pertaining to, characterised by or producing miosis 2. an agent producing miosis

miracidium (mi'ra-sid'e-um) free-swimming larva of schistosome, hatched in water to infect snails

mire (mer) a test object in ophthalmometry, by means of the images of which the amount of astigmatism is calculated

mirror (mir'or) a polished surface that reflects light to give images of objects in front of it **dental m** an instrument to view occlusal and distal surfaces of teeth **head m** a circular mirror strapped to the head of the examiner. It is used to reflect light into a cavity especially in the examination of nose, pharynx and larynx **mouth m** dental mirror

mirror movement simultaneous, contralateral, involuntary identical movement that accompany voluntary movements.

misanthropy (mis-an'thra-pe) hatred of people

miscarriage (mis'kor-ij) loss of products of conception from the uterus before the foetus is viable

miscegenation (mis'i-ji-na'shun) inbreeding of individuals of different races

miscible (mis'i-b'l) capable of being mixed

misdiagnosis wrong diagnosis

misogamy (mi-sog'a-me) aversion to marriage

misogyny (mi-soj'i-ne) aversion to women

misuse inappropriate use of legal drugs intended to be medications

mita(s) moderate

Mitchell's method treatment of piles by injecting 5% phenol, named after Mitchell, US surgeon

mite (mit) a minute arthropod of the order Acarina that can act as a vector or intermediate host of pathogenic agents, or may cause dermatitis or tissue damage

mithramycin (mith-ra-mi'sin) a cytotoxic antibiotic from Streptomyces, used in teratoma and in hypercalcaemia occurring in malignancy

mithridatism (mith'ri-dat'izm) acquired immunity against the action of poison produced by administering it in small and gradually increasing doses, name derived from Mithridates, King of Poritus who practised such a method

miticide (mit'i-sid) an agent destructive to mites

mitochondria (mi'to-kon'dre-a) an organelle of the cell cytoplasm which is the main source of energy to the cell. It contains cytochrome enzymes. It has a smooth outercoat and an inner membrane arranged in the form of tubules or folds

mitochondrial myopathy a disorder of muscle with abnormal structure, size, form and number of mitochondria in the muscle

mitogen (mi'to-jen) a substance that induces mitosis especially in T cells

mitomycin (mi'to-mi'sin) an anti-tumor antibiotic from streptomyces

mitosis (mi-to'sis) somatic cell division; process in which chromosomes duplicate and segregate during cell division

mitral (mi'tril) 1. relating to mitral or bicuspid valve 2. shaped like a bishop's miter **m apparatus** mitral annulus, the cusps, chordae and papillary muscles functioning in coordination with left atrial and left ventricular muscles. The anterolateral and posterolateral groups of papillary muscles support the corresponding halves of the anterior (aortic) and posterior (mural) cusps **m incompetence** occurs due to dilatation of the mitral annulus, shrivelling of the cusps, alteration in the chordae, prolapse of the cusps, shortening of the cusps and rupture of chordae **m murmurs** *see* murmurs **m stenosis** commonest valvular lesion of rheumatic heart disease due to thickening of mitral cusps, fusion of valve commissures and shortening and fusion of chordae tendinae causing obstruction to the flow of blood across the mitral valve in diastole **m valve prolapse** (MVP) Barlow's syndrome, floppy valve syndrome, an abnormal displacement of one or both mitral leaflets into the left atrial cavity during systole. Presents with chest pain and a mid-systolic click **m valvulotomy** an operative procedure disrupting the fibrous union of the two cusps at either commissures

mitralization (mi'tril-i-za'shun) straightening of the left border of the heart due to prominent left atrium and the pulmonary conus, an x-ray chest finding in mitral stenosis

Mitsuda reaction a skin test to detect delayed hypersensitivity in leprosy, subcutaneous injection of lepromin (Dharmendra antigen) giving a second reaction with induration 3-4 weeks after injection, named after Kensuke Mitsuda, Japanese physician

mixed astigmatism long-sighted in one meridian and short-sighted in other **mixed connective tissued disease** a condition wherein the features of scleroderma, SLE and polymyositis overlap

mixed parotid tumour a pleomorphic salivary gland tumour

mixture (miks'cher) 1. a liquid preparation holding an insoluble medicine 2. combining together of two or more substances without a chemical union, each retaining its physical characteristics

µl Microlitre

MLC medicolegal case

MLD abbreviation for minimum lethal dose

mL ml, millilitre

mm millimetre

m-mode an ultrasound presentation of the changes in echoes. The depth of echo-producing interfaces is displayed along one axis and time is displayed along with second axis, recording motion of interfaces toward and away from the transducer

MMFR 1. maximal mid-expiratory flow rate 2. mean mid-expiratory flow rate

MMR mass miniature radiography.

MMWR morbidity and mortality weekly report, a journal brought out by the Centers for Disease Control in Atlanta, Georgia. It provides information on epidemiology of communicable diseases

Mn chemical symbol, manganese

mnemonic (ne'mon-ik) pertaining to memory named after Mnemosyae, Greek Goddess of memory

MO abbreviation for medical officer

Mo chemical symbol, molybdenum

MOAb monoclonal antibody

mobilisation (mo'bi-li-za'shun) making movable 1. restoration of movement in a joint 2. excitation of a physiologic activity.

Mobiluncus (mo'bi-lung'kus) a genus of gram-negative anaerobic bacteria responsible for bacterial vaginosis.

Mobitz type I block *ECG* second degree heart block where PR interval increases progressively till a QRS is totally missed. Clinically the pulse exhibits a regular irregularity

Mobitz type II block *ECG* second degree heart block that is a very serious arrhythmia, it is mostly due to a block in His-Purkinje system. The PR interval of conducted beats is fixed; but some of the P waves fail to be conducted to the ventricles and are not followed by QRS. The P waves outnumber the QRS complexes

modality (mo-dal'i-te) 1. method of procedure 2. any form of therapeutic intervention 3. different forms of sensation

mode (mod) 1. *stat* in a set of measurements, that value which appears most frequently 2. different approaches in the mechanical ventilation

modem hardware that converts electronic signals from a computer into sound signals that can be transmitted by phone. The data can be reconverted by another modem into the original electronic data

modification (mod'i-fi-ka'shun) the process of altering the form or characteristics of an object

modifier (mod'i-fi'er) an agent that changes the form or features of an object or substance **biologic response m** a substance such as interferon produced in the body may stimulate immune system

modiolus (mo-di'o-lus) conical bony axis of cochlea.

modulation (mod'u-la'shun) regulation of the rate at which a specific gene is transcribed

modus operandi L mode of operating or living

MODY maturity-onset diabetes of the young, an autosomal dominant variant of NIDDM, and the responsible gene is located on the long arm of chromosome 20

Moebius sign failure of convergence of the eyes when the patient is asked to look at the finger brought in front, a sign in thyrotoxicosis, named after Paul Moebius, German neurologist

MOF multi-organ failures

MOH medical officer of health

moiety (moi'it-e) one of the two or more parts into which something can be divided

mol mole

molal (mo'lal) refers to one mole of solute dissolved in 1000 grams of solvent

molality a fraction of a solution that is expressed in moles of solute per kilogram of solvent

molar (mo'lar) 1. grinding 2. relating to a mass 3. molar tooth 4. relating to hydatidiform mole 5. denoting specific quantity **m tooth** a tooth having a crown with four to five cusps on the grinding surface, attached to lower jaw with a bifid root and upper jaw with three conical roots. They are three in permanent dentition situated on either side behind premolars. Their number is two in deciduous dentition and are situated on either side behind the canines

molarity (mo-lar'it-e) the amount of substance of a solution that is expressed in moles of solute per liter of solution (mol/L)

mold fungi which produce spores; mould

molding (mold'ing) 1. changes that the foetal skull undergoes to accommodate itself into the birth canal

mole (mol) 1. a pigmented benign or malignant lesion 2. an intrauterine mass formed by degeneration of the partly developed products of conception **hydatidiform m** a vesicular mass resulting from proliferation of trophoblast with degeneration and avascularity of the chorionic villi

molecular relating to molecules **m biology** study of biology at the molecular level, involving DNA, RNA and proteins **m disease** any condition that is traceable to a defect in the gene encoding one, or a limited number of molecules such as sickle cell anaemia

molecule (mol'e-kul) the smallest quantity into which a substance may be divided without loss of its characteristics

molimen (mo-li'men) a laborious effort made for the performance of a normal function

mollities (mo-lish'e-ez) soft consistency

molluscum (mo-lus'kum) any of small round superficial skin lumps **m bodies** intracytoplasmic inclusion bodies seen within the epithelial cells of molluscum contagiosum **m contagiosum** a viral disease caused by a DNA pox virus, the largest virus affecting the human beings. The virus gets implanted on the skin by contact with other infected persons. It presents with pearly white or pink smooth surfaced papules of 2-10 mm size over any part of the body in diffusely scattered clusters **m fibrosum** soft pink skin nodule of neurofibromatosis

mol wt molecular weight.

molybdenum (mo-lib'di-num) metal atomic no. 42 found in bones, liver and kidney and is a component of xanthine oxidase

monaesthetic (mon'es-thet'ik) pertaining to or affecting a single sense or sensation

monad (mon'ad) 1. unit 2. single protozoon

monarthritis (mon'ar-thrit'is) inflammation of a single joint

monarticular (-ar-tik'u-ler) pertaining to a single joint

monaster (mon-as'ter) the single star figure at the end of prophase in mitosis

monathetosis (-ath'i-to'sis) athetosis of one limb

Monckeberg's sclerosis medial calcifica-

tion of larger arteries described by J. Monckeberg, German pathologist

monday fever chest tightness and wheeze after the weekend break in a cotton mill worker, who later develops byssinosis

Monge's disease chronic mountain sickness in long term residents' at high altitude having polycythaemia and pulmonary hypertension, named after Carlos Monge, Peruvian pathologist

mongolism (mong'go-lizm) Down's syndrome; trisomy 21

monilethrix (mo-nil'e-thriks) a congenital abnormality of hairs which are beaded and fragile

monilia (mo-nil'e-a) candida

monilial (-al) pertaining to or caused by monilia

moniliform (mo-nil'I-form) beaded

monitor (mon'it-er) 1. to check constantly on a specific condition 2. a device that records specified data for a given series of events

monitor (mon'it-or) the viewing screen showing computer's files

mon (o) combining word for one, single, combined with one atom

monoamide (mon'o-am'id) a molecule containing one amide group

monoamine (mon'o-a-men) a molecule containing one amine **m oxidase** (MAO) enzyme that converts methylamine groups to aldehydes **m oxidase inhibitor** drugs inhibiting action of monoamine oxidase used as antidepressants

monoaminergic (-am'in-er'jik) neurones or nerve fibres that transmit nerve impulses by medium of catecholamines

monoamniotic (-am'ne-ot'ik) having or developing within a single amniotic cavity, such as monozygotic twins

monobactum (-bak'tam) antibiotics produced by bacteria with b-lactam ring (possessed by penicillin)

monobasic (-ba'sik) an acid with one replaceable hydrogen atom monoblast (mon'o-blast) an immature cell that develops into a monocyte

monoblepsia (mon'o-blep'se-a) a condition in which the vision is better when one eye is used

monochorea (-kor-e'a) chorea affecting only one limb or head

monochorionic (-kor'e-on'ik) relating to or having one chorionic sac, as in monoovular twins

monochromatic (-kro-mat'ik) 1. having only one colour 2. staining with one dye at a time

monochromatism (-kro'ma-tizm) 1. state of having or exhibiting only one colour. 2. complete colour blindness

monochromatophil (-kro-mat'a-fol) 1. cell taking only one stain 2. stainable with only one kind of stain

monoclonal (-klon'al) forming single clone, especially of myeloma cells and their products m antibody a highly specific antibody formed by fusing an immortal cell from mouse myeloma to a cell producing an antibody against a desired antigen m gammopathy increased production of single gammaglobulin from clone of plasma cells as in myelomatosis m immunoglobulin a protein produced by clonally-expanded immunoglobulin-producing cells as in multiple myeloma, chronic lymphocytic leukaemia and Waldenstrom's disease

monocular (mon-ok'ul-er) 1. relating to or having only one eye 2. having only one eye piece, as in microscope

monocyte (man'o-sit) large mononuclear leucocyte of blood

monocytopaenia (mon'o-sito-pe'ne-a) diminution in the number of monocytes in the peripheral blood

monocytosis increase in the number of monocytes in the blood seen in chronic infections, monocytic leukaemia and Crohn's disease

monodermoma (-der-mo'ma) a tumour composed of tissues from a single germ layer

monoecious (mon-e'shus) presence of male and female sex organs in the same individual

monogamous (mon'o-ga-mus) paired relationship with one partner

monoiodotyrosine (-i-o'-do-ti'ro-sen) an amino acid intermediate in the synthesis of thyroxine and triiodothyronine

monokine (mon'o-kin) soluble chemical meditor released by the monocytes and macrophages during the immune response

monolocular (mon'o-lok'u-lar) having one cavity or compartment, as a cyst

monomania (-ma'ne-a) preoccupation with a single object

monomer (mon'o-mer) one unit substance from which polymer is formed

monomeric (mon'o-mer'ik) 1. consisting of or affecting a single part 2. a hereditary disease or characteristic controlled by genes at a single locus

monomolecular (-mo-lek'ul-er) referring to a single molecule

monomorphic (-mor'fik) unchangeable in form or shape

mononeuritis (-noo-ri'tis) inflammation of a single nerve

mononeuropathy (-noo-rep'a-the) disease of a single nerve m multiplex simultaneous or sequential involvement of non-contiguous nerve trunks

mononuclear (-noo'kle-ar) having only one nucleus, such as a monocyte or lymphocyte

mononucleosis (-noo'kle-o'sis) presence of increased number of mononuclear leucocytes in the peripheral blood, especially forms that are not normal infectious m glandular fever; an acute infectious disease caused by Epstein-Barr virus occurs in young adults. The virus infects and replicates primarily in B lymphocytes. It presents with malaise, tiredness, headache, anorexia and fever. There is lymphadenopathy, splenomegaly, exudative tonsillitis and rash

mononucleotide (-noo'kle-a-tid) a product of hydrolysis of nucleic acid containing phosphoric acid with a glucoside or pentoside

monophasia (-fa'zhah) inability to speak other than a single word or sentence

monophyletic (mon'o-fi-let'ik) having a single source of origin

monoplegia (-ple'jah) paralysis of only one limb **monoplegic** adj

monorchidism (mon-or'kid'izm) a condition in which there is one descended testis, other may be undescended or absent

monosaccharide (mon'o-sak'a-rid) a simple sugar that cannot be further hydrolysed

monosodium glutamate a flavour-enhancing amino acid that functions as an excitatory neurotransmitter

monosomy (mon'o-so'me) presence of one chromosome only of a pair

monospasm (mon'o-spazm) spasm affecting one muscle or a group of muscles

monospecific (mon'o-spe-sif'ik) having an effect only on a particular type of cell or tissue or reacting with a single antigen

Monosporium (-spor'e-um) a genus of fungi including *M. apiospermum*, a causative agent of maduromycosis

monostotic (mon'o-sto-tik) affecting a single bone

monostratal (-strat'l) composed of or pertaining to a single layer

monosynaptic (-si-nap'tik) a simple reflex involving one motor and one sensory neuron with one synapse

monotherapy (-ther'a-pe) treatment of a disorder by a single agent

monothermia (-ther'me-a) maintenance of even body temperature throughout the day

monotocous (mo-not'a-kis) giving birth to one offspring at a time

monounsaturated (mon'o-un-sach'er-at'ed) a chemical compound having one double or triple bond

monovalent (-va'lent) 1. possessing the combining power of a single hydro-

gen atom 2. capability of combining with either one specific antigen or antibody

monoxenic (-zen'ik) associated with a single known species of micro-organism

monoxenous (mon-ok'sin-is) requiring one host to complete the life cycle

monoxide (mon-ok'sid) any oxide having only one atom of oxygen

monozygotic (mon'o-zi-got'ik) arising from one zygote especially of identical twins **m twins** genetically identical twins formed by the division into two at an early stage in the development of an embryo derived from a single fertilised ovum

mons a prominence **m pubis, m veneris** the prominence caused by a pad of fatty tissue over the symphysis pubis in female

monster (mon'ster) foetus or infant with gross deformities, generally incompatible with survival

Montgomery's glands large sebaceous glands without hairs in areola of nipple, named after William Montgomery, Irish obstetrician

monticulus (mon-tik'u-lus) a small eminence

mood a pervasive and sustained emotion, subjectively experienced in the form of depression, elation or anger **dysphoric m** an unpleasant mood **elevated m** air of confidence and enjoyment **ethymic m** normal range of mood without depression or elation **expansive m** expression of one's feelings without restraint **irritable m** easily annoyed and provoked to anger **m swings** oscillations between periods of euphoria and depression

moon face rounded swollen facies of adrenocorticosteroid excess

Mooren's ulcer chronic painful superficial ulcer of cornea in elderly, named after A. Mooren, German ophthalmologist

moot debatable, disputable

MOPP a four-drug combination consisting of nitrogen mustard, vincristine, procarbazine and prednisone used to treat stage III Hodgkin's disease, myelosuppression and increased infections occur as complications

Moraxella (mo-rak'sel'a) a genus of gram-negative coccobacillus that are parasitic on the mucous membrane of man and animals *M. lacunata* causes conjunctivitis

morbid (mor'bid) 1. diseased or pathologic 2. *Psy* abnormal or deviant

morbidity (mor-bid'it-e) 1. prevalence of the disease in a community 2. a diseased state

morbilli (mor-bil'I) measles

morbilli: form (mor-bil'i-form) measles-like; resembling of the eruptions of measles

morbillivirus (-vi'rus) genus of paramyxoviruses, including measles

morbus (mor'bus) disease

morcellation (mor'sil-a'shun) removal of small fragments in succession

mordant (mord'ant) a substance that fixes a stain or dye

morgue (morg) mortuary; a building where dead bodies are kept for identification or until claimed for burial or for autopsy

moribund (mor'i-bund) in a dying state

morning the beginning of day; the dawn **m after pill** a high dose oestrogen given in the early post-ovulatory period to prevent implantation of a potentially fertilised egg following unprotected intercourse **m dip** increased airway obstruction in the early morning in some asthmatics **m sickness** pregnancy-related nausea, often accompanied by vomiting on getting up in the morning, noted in the first 2–12 weeks of gestation

moron mentally subnormal

Moro reflex a neonatal reflex that disappears by three to four months of age. It is elicited by holding the baby at an angle of 45° with the horizontal and the head is allowed to suddenly fall back for a short distance. There is abduction and extension of the arms followed by adduction of the arms, named after Ernst Moro, German paediatrician

-morph combining word for shape

morphea (mor'fe'a) localised scleroderma

morphine (mor'fen) an opium alkaloid with powerful analgesic properties

morphogen (mor'fa-jen) a substance that triggers the growth, proliferation and differentiation of cells and tissues

morphogenesis (mor'fo-jen'is-is) differentiation of cells and tissues in early embryonic stage

morphology (mor-fol'a-je) the study of the structure of animals or plants

morphometry quantitative morphology.

morphosis (mor-fo'sis) mode of development of a part

Morquio's disease familial dwarfism due to defective growth of cartilage named after Louis Morquio, French paediatrician

morrhuate (mor'u-at) agent used as injection in the treatment of varicose veins

mors (murs) death

morsus (mor'sus) bite

mortal (mort'l) 1. destined to die 2. pertaining to causing death

mortality (mor-tal'it-e) 1. the state of being mortal 2. death rate **foetal m** the number of foetal deaths per 1000 live births per year **infant m** the number of deaths of children less than one year per 1000 live births per year **maternal m** the number of deaths of women during child bearing per 1,00,000 births **neonatal m** the number of deaths of infants less than 28 days per 1000 live births per year

mortar (mort'er) a vessel with rounded interior in which crude drugs are beaten, crushed and ground with a pestle

mort d'amour death due to coitally induced cardiac overload, and in any person with underlying cardiac disease

mortification (mort'i-ti-ka'shun) gangrene; necrosis

mortuary (mor'chu-a-re) morgue

morula (mor'ul-a) earliest embryo as a solid clump of cells from first division occurring in fallopian tube

mosaicism (ma-za'i-sizm) a condition in which an individual has two or more cell lines of different genetic or chromosomal constitution

mosm milliosmole

mosquito (mos-ke'to) a blood sucking dipterous insect of the family Culicidae which includes Aedes, Anopheles, Culex and Haemogogus and they act as vectors of many diseases including malaria, filariasis, dengue, viral encephalitis and yellow fever

motherboard the circuit board which houses computer's central processing unit

motilin (mo-til'in) a polypeptide hormone secreted by enterochromaffin cells of the duodenum and jejunum. It increases gut motility and stimulates pepsin secretion

motility (mo-til'ite) the ability to move spontaneously

motion sickness a clinical manifestation occurring in response to real or apparent motion to which a person is not adapted and presents with nausea, pallor, sweating and vomiting

motoneuron (mot'o-noor'on) motor neuron. It carries impulses to muscle to stimulate its contraction or to gland to stimulate its secretion

motor (mot'er) 1. producing motion 2. nerve structure by which impulses are generated and transmitted **m neuron disease** a group of chronic neurologic disorders that selectively affect with varying combination the anterior horn cells of the spinal cord and lower brainstem

M unit group of muscle fibres related to one anterior horn cell

mottling (mot'ling) 1. an area of skin with macular lesions of different col-

ours 2. minute, discrete radiologic shadows in chest roentgenogram

moulage (moo-lazh) 1. smooth contour of the small intestine with loss of mucosal folds seen in radiocontrast studies in sprue 2. a technique of casting from negative impressions, employed in reproduction of anatomical and pathological specimens

mouldy hay disease farmer's lung.

mounding (mound'ing) myxoedema

mount 1. to prepare a specimen or slide for microscopic study 2. a support on which something may be fixed 3. to climb on for purpose of copulation

mountain sickness sudden exposure to altitude above 2500 m may lead to hyperventilation, tachycardia, palpitation and headache resulting from lowered oxygen tension. In susceptible individuals untoward symptoms follow after 6 to 7 hours of ascent, in pulmonary (cough, dyspnoea, chest pain), cerebral (headache, giddiness, irritability, insomnia, convulsions) or hypoxic (muscle cramps, anorexia) forms

mouse (mous) 1. a small rodent of the genus *Mus* 2. a small piece of tissue that become separated in a body cavity or joint.

mouth 1. oral cavity, within the cheeks, containing the tongue, teeth, hard and soft palate and communicating with the pharynx 2. the opening, usually external of a cavity or canal **m stick** a device for use by persons who have no functioning hands **m wash** a pleasant preparation to rinse the mouth, but having no medicinal value **trench m** necrotising ulcerative gingivitis

movement (moov'mint) 1. the act of motion of the entire body or its parts 2. defecation.

mover (moo'ver) that which produces movement

moxalactum (mok'sa-lak'tam) a semisynthetic antibiotic having a broad spectrum of activity

moya moya disease an arteritis of unknown aetiology involving large intracranial arteries. The lenticulostriate arteries give rise to many collaterals giving a puff of smoke appearance in angiography. It affects young adults; often there is bilateral stroke

moxibustion a variant form of acupuncture that uses heat

MPH Master of public health

MPO myeloperoxidase

MR mitral regurgitation

mR milliroentgen

MRC Medical Research Council

MRCP Member of Royal College of Physicians

MRCS Member of Royal College of Surgeons

MRI Magnetic resonance imaging.

mRNA messenger RNA

mrdu (s) soft

MS 1. Master of Surgery 2. Mitral stenosis 3. Medical superintendent 4. Multiple sclerosis

MSc Master of Science

MSH melanocyte-stimulating hormone

MSOF multisystem organ failure

mtDNA mitochondrial DNA

MTX methotrexate

muciferous (mu-sif'er-us) secreting mucus

mucigen (mu'si-jen) a glycoprotein substance found in mucous cell, which on extrusion, is converted into mucin

mucilage (-lij) a watery solution of gummy substance used as a vehicle or demulcent

mucin (mu-sin) a secretion containing mucopolysaccharides, such as that from mucous glands and it is also found in the ground substance of connective tissue **mucinoid** adj

mucinosis (mu'si-no'sis) presence of excessive amounts of mucin in the skin

mucinous (mu's-nis) 1. mucoid 2. relating to or containing mucin **m cystadenoma** large ovarian cyst with mucinous contents

mucins mucopolysaccharides and mucoproteins

mucinuria (mu'sin-ur'e-a) presence of mucin in the urine.

muc(o) combining word for mucus; pertaining to a mucous membrane

mucociliary (mu'ko-sil'e-ar-e) pertaining to ciliated mucosa

mucocoele (mu'ko-sel) mucin containing cyst

mucocutaneous lymph node syndrome *see* Kawasaki syndrome

mucoenteritis (-en'ter-i'tis) inflammation of intestinal mucosa

mucoepidermoid (-ep'i-der'moid) squamous and mucin secreting epithelium

mucogingival (-jin'ji-val) pertaining to the oral mucosa and gingiva

mucoid (mu'koid) 1. mucinoid 2. pertaining to or relating to or resembling mucus

mucolipidoses (mu'ko-lip'i-do'ses) rare enzyme defects with storage of complex mucolipids

mucoperichondrium (-pe're-kon'dre-um) perichondrium having a mucosal surface as in nasal septum

mucoperiosteum (-os'te-um) mucosa and underlying periosteum firmly bound into a single layer

mucopolysaccharide (-sak'a-rid) 1. a group of polysaccharides containing hexosamine, including glycosaminoglycans and neutral polysaccharides 2. glycosaminoglycan

mucopolysaccharoidosis (-sak'a-ri-do'sis) a group of diseases caused by an accumulation of mucopolysaccharides (glycosaminoglycans) due to an enzyme deficiency characterised by developmental delay, mental retardation, skeletal anomalies, coarse facial features and hepatosplenomegaly

mucoprotein (-pro'ten) a protein-polysaccharide complex **Tamm-Horsfall m** a matrix of urinary casts derived from the ascending loop of Henle named, after Igor Tamm, Russian born US virologist and Frank Horsfall, US physician

mucopurulent (-pu'roo-lent) containing both mucus and pus

mucopus (mu'ko-pus) mucus blended with pus

mucor (mu'kor) a genus of fungi found in dead or decaying matter, belong to the family of Mucoraceae, and may cause mucormycosis

mucormycosis (-mi-ko'sis) infection with certain species of Mucor, Rhizopus and Absidia, common saprophytic fungi which can cause an opportunistic infection in the lung

mucosa (mu-ko'sa) mucous membrane

mucous (mu'kus) 1. mucous membrane 2. mucus

mucoviscidosis (mu'ko-vis'i-do-sis) cystic fibrosis

mucus (mu'kis) a clear viscid fluid that is produced by mucous membrane. It consists of mucopolysaccharides, enzymes, IgA and other proteins, desquamated epithelial cells and in organic salts.

mula (s) root

Mullarian ducts paramesonephric ducts from which in female the fallopian tubes, uterus and part of vagina develop; and in male appendix, testis and prostatic utricle, named after Johannes Muller, German physician

mullebria (mu'le-eb're-a) the female genitalia

multi- combining word for many.

multifactorial diseases diseases which result from an intervention of environmental factors with multiple genes at different loci

multifid (mul'ti-fida) divided into many segments or clefts

multiform (-form) polymorphic with many forms or shapes

multigravida (mul'ti-grav'i-da) a pregnant woman who has been pregnant one or more times previously

multiinfection (mul'te-in-fek'shun) mixed infection with two or more pathogens developing at the same time

multimedia (mul-ti-med'ia) any combination of different types of media such as text, pictures, sound and video

mutimeric having many segments or parts.

multipara (mul-tip'a-ra) a woman who has given birth at least two times to viable foetuses, whether alive or dead

multiparity (mul'ti-par'it-e) the condition of being a multipara

multiple sclerosis (MS) disorder of CNS white matter with preservation of axons compared with loss of myelin. It presents with multiplicity of lesions with sclerotic appearance that are scattered throughout CNS. Relapses and remissions are common. It presents with muscle weakness, ocular disturbance, gait ataxia, parasthesia, dysarthria and mental disturbances

multipuncture test tuberculin test carried out with an instrument which carries a small plate with fixed short steel needles. On release of a spring the 6 needles puncture the skin to a depth of 2 mm

multivalent (-val'int) 1. having a combining power of more than one atom of hydrogen 2. active against several strains of an organism 3. efficacious in more than one direction

mummification (mum'i-fi-ka'shun) 1. dry gangrene 2. drying and shrivelling of a body as a dead and retained foetus

mumps an inflammatory disease caused by a paramyxovirus infection leading to acute painful inflammation of the parotid and occasionally other salivary glands. orchitis, oophoritis, pancreatitis, meningitis and encephalitis may occur as complications

Munchausen (men-chow'zen) syndrome repeated freigning of major disorders to obtain hospital admissions, name derived from Baron Karl Munchausen, a fictional character

mural (mur'l) pertaining to a wall of an organ or a body cavity m thrombus thrombus attached to wall of a large blood vessel or heart chamber.

muramidase (mu-ram'i-das) lysozyme.

murchchha (s) fainting, loss of consciousness

murine (mur'en) pertaining to rodents

murmur (mur'mur) vibrations heard due to a turbulent blood flow with an increase in its velocity at or near a valve or of an abnormal communication within the heart. They are audible on auscultation of the heart, or blood vessels **aortic diastolic m** failure of cusps of aortic valves coming in apposition during the diastole resulting in a high pitched soft blowing murmur **aortic systolic m** an ejection systolic murmur heard in aortic stenosis, dilatation of the ascending aorta, and in hyperkinetic circulatory states apical diastolic m a diastolic filling murmur at the apex **Austin-Flint m** a diastolic rumble at the apex in severe aortic incompetence **cardiac m** a murmur produced within the heart **cardiopulmonary m** an innocent murmur synchronous with the heart beat, that disappears when the breath is held **Carey Coomb's m** a shortlived diastolic murmur at the apex in mitral valvulitis due to acute rheumatic fever **continuous m** murmur heard continuously during systole and diastole due to continuous flow of blood through an abnormal communication from a region of high pressure to low pressure with a large pressure gradient between the two regions **crescendo m** a murmur increasing in its intensity due to atrial systole facilitating increased blood flow across the stenotic valve from left atrium to the left ventricle **diastolic m** a murmur heard during diastole **Duroziez m** systolic and diastolic murmur audible on compression of femoral artery in aortic incompetence **ejection m** murmur produced by the forward flow of blood across the right or left ventricular outflow tract. Murmur is mid-systolic, medium pitched with intensity ascending and descending in a diamond-shaped configuration **flint m** Austin-Flint murmur **flow m** increased velocity and volume of blood flow across a normal mitral valve producing short mid-diastolic rumble at the apex. **Gibson's m** a machinery murmur audible over left second and third intercostal space near the sternum in patent ductus arteriosus **Graham Steell's m** an early diastolic murmur in the second left intercostal space next to sternum heard in pulmonary incompetence **haemic m** faint systolic murmur over the pulmonary area and to a lesser extent over the apex in severe anaemia **innocent m** functional murmur **inorganic m** functional murmur **late systolic m** heard at the apex in mild mitral incompetence due to an unusual distortion of the mitral valve leaflet, chordae tendinae or papillary muscles. **machinery m** Gibson's murmur **mitral diastolic m** narrowing of the orifice of the mitral valve causing a low pitched, rumbling mid-distolic murmur **mitral systolic m** a soft blowing pansystolic murmur at the apex, that is conducted towards the axilla due mitral valve incompetence **obstructive m** a murmur produced as a result of a forward flow of blood across a stenosed region **organic m** murmur when arises from the damaged heart **pansystolic m** a murmur begins with the first heart sound and continues through to the second heart sound. The intensity of the murmur is uniform **presystolic m** atrial systolic ejection murmur **pulmonary diastolic m** Graham Steell's murmur **pulmonary systolic m** an early-to-mid systolic murmur of PDA or tricuspid stenosis audible at the apex due to transmission of the murmur **tricuspid regurgitant m** a pansystolic murmur heard over tricuspid area that tends to get louder on inspiration **tricuspid stenotic m** a low pitched presystolic scratchy murmur audible near the lower end of sternum and it has a crescendo-decrescendo character

Murphy's sign a method to elicit tenderness of the gall bladder. It is performed with the patient lying down or sitting, the examiner's thumb or fingers are hooked under the right costal margin at the lateral border of the rectus, simultaneously the patient takes a deep breath so that the gall bladder descends to strike the examining fingers. The patient winces with pain and there will be catch in the breath in case of an inflamed gall bladder, named after John Murphy, US surgeon

Mus a genus of rodents including mice and rats

Musca (mus'ka) a genus of flies belonging to the order Diptera *M domestica* common house fly which may serve as a vector of various causative agents of typhoid, bacillary dysentery, cholera, trachoma, and its larva may cause myiasis.

muscarine (-ren) a highly toxic alkaloids from various mushrooms **m receptors** cholinergic receptors mostly of parasympathetic nervous system stimulated by muscarine

muscarinic (mus'ka-rin'ik) pertaining to cholinergic effects of muscarine on parasympathetic

muscle (mus'l) tissue composed of contractile cells or fibres that causes movement of an organ or part of the body. They are classified as skeletal, cardiac or smooth muscles, *see* Table of Muscles. **m spindle** small voluntary muscle fibres covered by sensory nerve endings

muscle phosphorylase (fos-for'l-las) a muscle isoenzyme of glycogen phosphorylase and its deficiency results in glycogen storage disease, type V

muscular cirrhosis of the lung pulmonary muscular hyperplasia, a variant of diffuse fibrosing alveolitis presenting with honeycombing radiologically

muscularis (mus'ku-la'ris) relating to muscle coat of a hollow organ or tubular structure **m mucosa** unstriated muscular tissue layer of mucous membrane

musculature (mus'kul-a-char) the arrangement of muscles in the body or its parts.

musculoaponeurotic (mus'kul-o-ap'-o-noor-ot'ik) pertaining to a muscle and its aponeurosis

musculoskeletal (-skel'e-t'l) referring to the framework of the body including muscles and skeleton

musculus (mus'ku-lus) pl. **musculi** muscle

mushroom worker's lung extrinsic allergic alveolitis produced by inhalation of mushroom compost

Musset's (mu'saz) **sign** repetitive head nodding synchronous with ventricular contractions of the heart in free aortic regurgitation, named after Louis de Musset, French poet

mustard (mus'trad) yellow powder of mustard seed of genus *Brassica* used as a counterirritant, emetic, stimulant and condiment **nitrogen m** an alkylating agent used in the treatment of malignancy

mutagen (mu'ta-jen) an agent that causes genetic mutations

mutagenesis (mu'ta-jen'e-sis) the induction of genetic mutation

mutagenic (mut'a-genik) capable of promoting genetic alterations in cells

mutagenicity (-je-nis'it-e) having power to cause mutation

mutant (mut'nt) 1. an organism that has undergone genetic mutation 2. produced by mutation

mutase (mu'tas) an enzyme that catalyses the intramolecular shifting of a chemical group from one position to another

mutation (mu-te'shun) an alteration in genetic material. It could be a single base change (point mutation) or more extensive losses of DNA (deletion) **nonsense m** a single DNA base change resulting in a premature stop codon There is gene mutation that ends the gene rathen than continuing with the sequence of base pairs **point m** a genetic change involving a single base pair

Table 7: Muscles

Name	Origin	Insertion	Nerve supply	Action
Abductor hallucis	medial tubercle of calcaneum and plantar fascia	base of proximal phalanx of great toe on medial side	medial plantar	abduction and flexion of great toe
Abductor digiti minimi of little finger	pisiform bone	base of proximal phalanx of little finger on its medial side	ulnar	abduction of little finger
Abductor digiti minimi of little toe	tubercles of calcaneum and plantar fascia	base of proximal phalanx of little toe on its lateral side	lateral plantar	abduction of little toe
Abductor pollicis longus	posterior surface of radius-ulna and interosseous membrane	1st metacarpal bone and trapezium	posterior interosseus	abduction and extension of thumb
Abductor pollicis brevis	scaphoid, trapezium and flexor retinaculum	base of proximal phalanx of thumb	median nerve	abduction of thumb
Adductor magnus	ramus of pubis, ischium and ischial tuberosity	linea aspera of femur and adductor tubercle	obturator and sciatic	adduction and extension of thigh
Adductor hallucis	2,3,4 metatarsals and plantar ligaments	proximal phalanx of great toe	lateral plantar	adduction and flexion of great toe
Adductor longus	body of pubis	linea aspera of femur	obturator	adduction, medial rotation and flexion of thigh
Adductor brevis	pubis-body and ramus	linea aspera of femur in its upper part	obturator	adductor, medial rotator and flexor of thigh
Adductor pollicis	oblique head from 2nd metacarpal, capitate and trapezium. Transverse head from 3rd metacarpal	proximal phalanx of the thumb on its medial side		adduction and opposition of thumb

Name	Origin	Insertion	Nerve supply	Action
Anconeus	posterior aspect of lateral epicondyl of humerus	posterior surface of ulna and olecranon process	radial	extension of forearm
Arrectores piloreum	from skin deep surface	root of hair follicles	sympathetic	raising hair
Articularis genu	Anterior surface of lower part of femur	capsule of the knee joint	femoral nerve	raising of capsule of knee joint
Aryepiglotticus	Apex of arytenoid cartilage	lateral margin of epiglottis	recurrent laryngeal nerve	closure of inlet of larynx
Arytenoideus obliques	muscular process of arytenoid cartilage	apex of opposite arytenoid cartilage	recurrent laryngeal nerve	narrowing of laryngeal inlet
Arytenoideus transversus	posterior surface of arytenoid cartilage	posterior surface of opposite arytenoid cartilage	recurrent laryngeal nerve	adduction of vocal cords
Auricularis anterior, oblique posterior and superior	temporal fascia and mastoid process	cartilage of pinna	branches of facial nerve	movement of auricle
Biceps brachii	supraglenoid tubercle of scapula and corocoid process	tuberosity of radius and bicipital aponeurosis	musculo-cutaneous	flexion of arm and supination of forearm
Biceps femoris	ischial tuberosity and linea aspera	head of fibula, lateral condyle of tibia	tibial	flexor and lateral rotator of leg, extensor of thigh
Brachialis	anterior surface of humerus	coronoid process of ulna	musculo-cutaneous	flexor of forearm
Brachioradialis	lateral supra-condylar ridge of humerus	lower end of radius on its lateral side	radial	flexor of forearm and supinator of semipronated forearm
Buccinator	mandible, maxilla and pterygo-mandibular raphe	fibers merge with orbicularis oris muscle of mouth	facial	blowing, retraction of angle of mouth

Name	Origin	Insertion	Nerve supply	Action
Bulbocavernosus	perineal membrane and median raphe	fascia of penis or clitoris	pudendal nerve	sphincter of urethra in male and of vagina in female
Chondroglossus	lesser horn and body of hyoid bone	merges with muscles of tongue	hypoglossal	retraction and depression of tongue
Ciliaris	corneoscleral junction	choroid and ciliary processes	short ciliary	increases convexity of lens
Coccygeus	ischial spine	sacrum and coccyx on its side	sacral 3rd and 4th nerve	raises coccyx, supports pelvic viscera, movement of tail in animals
Constrictor of pharynx-inferior	cricoid and thyoid cartilages	median raphe on the posterior wall of pharynx	glossopharyngeal plexus, recurrent laryngeal nerve	constriction of pharynx
Constrictor of pharynx-middle	horns of hyoid bone and lower part of stylohyoid ligament	median raphe on the posterior wall of pharynx	pharyngeal plexus of Xth and IXth nerves	constrictor of pharynx
Constrictor of pharynx-superior	pterygoid plate, pterygomandibular raphe, mandible	median raphe on the posterior pharyngeal wall	pharyngeal plexus of Xth and IXth nerve	constrictor of pharynx
Coracobrachialis	coracoid process of scapula	shaft of humerus on its medial surface	musculocutaneous	flexor and adductor of arm
Corrugator supercilii	superciliary arch	skin under eyebrow	facial	pulling of eyebrow medially and downwards
Cremaster	from internal oblique near its insertion	pubic tubercle	genital branch of genitofemoral	draws the testes upwards
Cricoarytenoideus lateral	cricoid cartilage on its lateral surface	muscular process of arytenoid cartilage	recurrent laryngeal	adduction of vocal cords

Name	Origin	Insertion	Nerve supply	Action
Cricoarytenoideus posterior	lamina of cricoid cartilage on its posterior surface	muscular process of arytenoid cartilage	recurrent laryngeal	abductor of vocal cords
Cricothyoid	arch of cricoid cartilage	lamina and inferior horn of thyroid cartilage	superior laryngeal nerve-external branch	tension of vocal cords
Deltoid	acromion, clavicle and spine of scapula	deltoid tuberosity of humerus	axillary nerve	abductor, flexor and extensor (posterior fibres) of arm
Depressor anguli oris	mandible	angle of mouth	facial	pulls down angle of mouth
Depressor labii inferioris	lower border of mandible anteriorly	fibers merge with orbicularis muscle of mouth	facial	depressor of lower lip
Depressor septi nasi	incisive fossa of maxilla	ala and septum of nose	facial	depressor of ala of nose and constrictor of nostrils
Detrussor	smooth muscle of the urinary bladder wall, arranged in longitudinal and circular layer			contraction of bladder for expulsion of urine
Diaphragm	in front of bodies of upper lumbar vertebrae, lateral arcuate ligaments, inner surface of lower costal cartilage and ribs and xiphoid process	central tendon of diaphragm	motor by phrenic, sensory by intercostal nerves	increase in volume of thoracic cavity
Digastric	anterior belly from diagastric fossa on mandible, posterior belly from mastoid notch on temporal bone	two belly from intermediate tendon above hyoid bone	anterior belly by mylohyoid branch of inferior alveolar, posterior belly by branch from facial	depression of lower jaw and elevation of hyoid bone
Dilator pupillae	radial fibres originating from sphincter of pupil	ciliary margin	sympathetic	dilates the pupil

Name	Origin	Insertion	Nerve supply	Action
Erector spinae	sacrum, spines of lumbar and lower thoracic vertebrae, iliac crest	fibres terminate as iliocostalis, longissimus and spinalis	thoracic and lumbar spinal nerves	extension, lateral bending and rotation of vertebral column
Extensor digitorum	lateral epicondyle of humerus	exterior expansion of digits	posterior interosseous, branch of radial nerve	exterior of wrist and phalanges
Extensor hallucis longus	anterior surface of fibula and interosseous membrane	distal phalanx of great toe near its base	deep peroneal	extensor of ankle and great toe
Extensor indicis	posterior surface of ulna and interosseous membrane	extensor expansion of index finger	posterior interosseous branch of radial nerve	extensor of index finger
Extensor digiti minimi	lateral epicondyle of humerus	extensor expansion of little finger	deep branch of radial	extensor of little finger
Extensor pollicis longus	posterior surface of ulna and interosseous membrane	distal phalanx of thumb on its posterior surface	posterior interosseous branch of radial nerve	extensor and adductor of thumb
Extensor pollicis brevis	posterior surface of radius	proximal phalanx of thumb on its posterior surface	posterior interosseous nerve	extensor of thumb
Extensor digitorum longus	lateral condyle of tibia, anterior surface of fibula and interosseous membrane	extensor expansion of toes	deep peroneal nerve	extensor of toes
Extensor digitorum brevis	upper surface of calcaneum	joins extensor tendon of 4 medial toes	deep peroneal nerve	extensor of toes
Extensor carpi radialis longus	lateral supracondylar ridge of humerus	base of IInd metacarpal bone on its dorsal aspect	radial nerve	extension and abduction of wrist
Extensor carpi radials brevis	lateral epicondyle of humerus	bases of 2nd and 3rd metacarpal bone on its dorsal aspect	deep branch of radial nerve	extension and abduction of wrist joint

Name	Origin	Insertion	Nerve supply	Action
Extensor carpi ulnaris	lateral epicondyle of humerus and posterior border of ulna	base of 5th metacarpal bone	deep branch of radial nerve	extensor and abductor of wrist
Flexor digitorum profundus	shaft of ulna and coronoid process interosseous membrane	distal phalanges of fingers near its bases	ulnar nerve and anterior interosseus branch of median nerve	flexor of distal phalanges
Flexor digitorum superficialis	medial epicondyle of humerus, coronoid process of ulna and anterior border of radius	on the two sides of middle phalanges of fingers	median nerve	flexor of middle phalanges
Flexor hallucis longus	posterior surface of fibula	distal phalanx of great toe near its base	tibial nerve	flexor of great toe
Flexor digiti minimi brevis	hook of hamate and transverse carpal ligament	proximal phalanx of little finger on its medial side	ulnar nerve	flexor of little finger
Flexor digiti minimi of foot	peroneal sheath	proximal phalanx of little toe on its lateral surface	lateral plantar	flexor of little toe
Flexor pollicis longus	medial epicondyle of humerus, coronoid process of ulna and anterior surface of radius	distal phalanx of thumb near its base	anterior interosseous branch of median nerve	flexor of thumb
Flexor pollicis brevis	flexor retinaculum, trapezium	proximal phalanx of thumb on its lateral side	median and ulnar	flexor of thumb
Flexor digitorum longus of foot	posterior surface of tibia	distal phalanges of toe	tibial nerve	flexor of toes and foot
Flexor digitorum brevis of foot	tuberosity of calcaneum and plantar fascia	middle phalanges of toes	medial plantar	flexor of toes
Flexor carpi radialis	medial epicondyle of humerus	bases of IInd and IIIrd metacarpal bones	median	flexion and abduction of wrist

Name	Origin	Insertion	Nerve supply	Action
Flexor carpi ulnaris	medial epicondyle of humerus, olecranon process of ulna and posterior border of ulna	pisiform, hook of hamate and base of Vth meta-carpal bone	ulnar nerve	flexor and adductor of wrist joint
Gastrocnemius	two heads medial head from popliteal suface of femur, medial condyle upper part, cap-sule of knee joint; lateral head from lateral condyle of femur and capsule of knee joint	joins the tendon of soleus muscle to form tendo calcaneus	tibial nerve	plantar flexor of foot and flexor of knee joint
Gemellus inferior	tuberosity of ischium	joins tendon of obturator inter-nus	nerve to quad-ratus femoris	lateral rotator of thigh
Gemellus superior	ischial spine	joins tendon of obturator inter-nus	nerve to obtu-rator internus	lateral rotator of thigh
Genioglossus	superior genial tubercle on mandible	hyoid bone and tongue	hypoglossal	depression and protrusion of tongue
Geniohyoid	inferior genial tubercle of mandible	hyoid bone	1st cervical through hypo-glossal nerve	elevation of hyoid bone
Gluteus maximus	dorsal surface of ilium, sacrum, coccyx, sacro-tuberous ligament and fascia	glutetal tubero-sity of femur and iliotibial tract	inferior gluteal nerve	extensor, ab-ductor and lateral rotator of thigh
Gluteus medius	dorsal surface of ilium between anterior and posterior gluteal lines.	greater troch-anter of femur	superior gluteal nerve	abductor and medial rotator of thigh, stabli-ses the pelvis while walking

Name	Origin	Insertion	Nerve supply	Action
Gluteur minimus	dorsal surface of ilium between anterior and inferior gluteal lines	greater trochanter of femur	superior gluteal nerve	abductor and medial rotator of thigh
Gracilis	body and inferior ramus of pubis	upper part of medial surface of tibia	obturator nerve	adductor of thigh and flexor of knee
Hyoglossus	body and greater cornua of hyoid bone	between intrinsic muscles of tongue	hypoglossal nerve	depression and retraction of tongue
Iliacus	iliac fossa, ala of sacrum	lesser trochanter of femur	femoral nerve	flexor of thigh and trunk
Iliococcygeus	fascia on obturator internus	coccyx and anococcygeal raphe	nerve to levator ani	part of pelvic diaphragm, supports the viscera
Iliocostalis	lateral part of erector spinae muscle, divided into lumbar, thoracic and cervical part			
Iliocostalis cervicis	3rd, 4th, 5th, 6th ribs near their angles	transverse process of 4th, 5th and 6th cervical vertebrae	cervical nerves	extensor of cervical vertebrae
Iliocostalis lumborum	iliac crest	lower 6-7 ribs near their angles	thoracic and lumbar nerves	exterior of lumbar spine
Iliocostalis thoracis	angles of lower 6 ribs	angles of upper ribs and 7th cervical vertebra	thoracic nerves	extensor of thoracic vertebrae
Iliopsoas	iliacus and psoas muscle together called as iliopsoas			
Incisive labi inferior and superior	incisive fossa of mandible and maxilla	angle of mouth	facial	narrowing of vestibula of mouth
Infraspinatus	infraspinous fossa of scapula	greater tubercle of humerus	suprascapular nerve	lateral rotator of arm elevator
Intercostalis external	inferior borders of ribs	superior border of rib below	intercostal nerves	of rib during inspiration

Name	Origin	Insertion	Nerve supply	Action
Intercostalis internal	inferior border of ribs and costal cartilages	superior border of ribs and costal cartilages below	intercostal nerves	act on ribs in expiration
Interossei dorsal of foot	sides of adjacent metatarsal bones	proximal phalanges of 2nd, 3rd and 4th toes	lateral plantar nerve	flexor and abductor of toes
Interossei palmaris	sides of 1st, 2nd 4th and 5th metacarpal bones	extensor tendons of 1st 2nd, 3rd and 4th fingers	ulnar	adduction, flexion of proximal mal and extension of middle and distal phalanges
Intercrossei plantaris	medial side of 3rd, 4th and 5th toes	medial side of bases of proximal phalanges of 3rd, 4th and 5th toes	lateral plantar nerve	flexion and adduction of toes
Interspinalis cervicis, thoracis, and lumborum	part of errector spinalis muscle, extending between spinous processes of adjacent vertebrae		spinal nerve	lateral bending of vertebral column
Intertransversalis	part of erector spinalis muscle extending between transverse processes of adjacent vertebrae		spinal nerve	lateral bending of vertebral column
Ischiocavernosus	ramus of ischium	crus of penis or clitoris	pudendal nerve	maintain erection of penis or clitoris
Latissimus dorsi	spines of lower thoracic, lumbar and sacral vertebrae thoracolumbar fascia, iliac crest, lower ribs and inferior angle of scapula	bicipital groove of humerus	thoracodorsal nerve	adduction, extension and medial rotation of arm
Levator anguli oris	canine fossa of maxilla	fibres merge with orbicularis oris muscle	facial nerve	elevation of angle of mouth
Levator ani	posterior surface of púbis, obturator fascia	coccyx around prostate in male as puboprostalis, vagina in female as pubovaginalis and around rectum— as puborectalis	3rd and 4th sacral nerves	supports pelvic viscera

Name	Origin	Insertion	Nerve supply	Action
Levator costareum	transverse processes of 7th cervical and thoracic vertebrae except of 12th thoracic	medial to the angle of rib below	intercostal nerves	elevation of ribs
Levator glandulae thyroideae	isthmus or pyramidal process of thyroid gland	body of hyoid bone	superior laryngeal nerve	not significant, muscle fibres developed around remnants of thyroglossal duct
Levator labii superioris	zygomatic bone at the lower margin of orbit	fibres merge with muscles of upper lip	facial nerve	raises upper lip
Levator labii superioris alaeque nasi	frontal process of maxilla	skin and cartilage of ala of nose and upper lip	branch of facial nerve	dilates nostrils and raises upper lip
Levator palpabrae superioris	orbital surface of sphenoid bone near the apex of orbit, above optic foramen	skin and superior tarsal plate	oculomotor nerve	elevation of upper eye lid
Levator palati	undersurfaces of petrous part of temporal bone and cartilagenous part of auditory tube	aponeurosis of soft palate	pharyngeal plexus	elevation of soft palate
Levator prostatae	fibres of pubococcygeus inserted into prostate		sacral nerves and branch from pudendal nerve	supports and compresses prostate
Levator scapulae	transverse processes of upper 4 cervical vertebrae	medial border of scapula above spinous process	3rd and 4th cervical nerve	elevation of scapula
Longus capitis	transverse processes of 3rd, 4th, 5th and 6th cervical vertebrae	part of occipital bone	basilar cervical nerves	flexor of head
Longus colli	muscle has 3 parts, superior oblique, inferior oblique and vertical part			

Name	Origin	Insertion	Nerve supply	Action
Superior oblique	transverse processes of 3rd to 5th cervical vertebrae	tubercle on anterior arch of atlas vertebrae	anterior cervical nerve	flexion of neck
Inferior oblique	from bodies of 1st to 3rd thoracic vertebrae	transverse processes of 5th and 6th cervical vertebrae	anterior cervical nerve	flexion of neck
Vertical part	from bodies of 3 lower cervical and 3 upper thoracic vertebrae	bodies of 2nd and 4th cervical vertebrae	anterior cervical nerve	flexion of neck
Longissimus capiti	transverse processes of upper 4 thoracic vertebrae and articular processes of lower 4 cervical vertebrae	mastoid process of temporal bone	cervical nerves	exterior and rotator of head
Longissimus cervicis	transverse processes of upper 4 thoracic vertebrae	transverse processes of 2nd to 6th cervical vertebrae	lower cervical and upper thoracic nerves	extensor of neck
Longissimus thoracis	transverse and articular processes of lumbar vertebrae and fascia	transverse processes of thoracic vertebrae and lower ribs	lumbar and thoracic nerves	extensor of thoracic vertebrae
Lumbricals of foot	from tendons of flexor digitorum longus	base of proximal phalanges of 4 lateral toes	medial and lateral plantar	flexor of metatarsophalangeal joint and extensor of distal phalanges
Lumbricals of hand	from tendons of flexor digitorum profundus	extensor tendons of 4 lateral fingers	median and ulnar	flexor of metacarpophalangeal joint, and extensor of middle and distal phalanges
Masseter	zygomatic process of maxilla, lower border and deep surface of zygomatic arch	angle of the mandible and upper half of lateral surface of ramus of mandible	nerve to masseter, a branch of mandibular division of trigeminal nerve	elevator of lower jaw

Name	Origin	Insertion	Nerve supply	Action
Multifidus	dorsal surface of sacrum, sacroiliac ligament, mamillary processes of lumbar vertebrae, transverse processes of thoracic vertebrae and articular processes of cervical vertebrae	spines of the vertebrae above	spinal nerves	extensor and rotator of vertebral column
Mylohyoid	from mylohyoid line of mandible	body of hyoid bone and median raphe	mylohyoid branch of inferior alveolar nerve	elevation of hyoid bone
Nasalis	maxilla	ala of the nose, aponeurosis with muscle of opposite side	facial	widening of nostrils, depressor of nasal cartilage
Oblique capitis inferior	spinous process of axis	transverse process of atlas	spinal nerves	rotator of atlas
Oblique capitis superior	transverse process of atlas	occipital bone	spinal nerves	extensor of head, also bends head laterally
Oblique external of abdomen	lower 8 ribs near costal cartilages	iliac crest and linea alba of rectal sheath	lower thoracic	flexor and rotator of vertebral column and supports abdominal viscera
Oblique inferior of eye	orbital surface of maxilla	sclera—posteriorly and inferiorly	oculomotor	upward and outward movement of eyeball with abduction
Oblique internal of abdomen	iliac crest and fascia	lower 4 costal cartilages, linea alba, forms conjoint tendon to attach to pubis	lower thoracic	flexor and rotator of vertebral column and support abdominal viscera
Oblique superior of eye	orbital surface of lesser wing of sphenoid above optic foramen	sclera—superiorly and anteriorly	trochlear nerve	downward and outward movement of eyeball with abduction

Name	Origin	Insertion	Nerve supply	Action
Obturator externus	pubis, ischial rami and obturator membrane	trochanteric fossa of femur	obturator nerve	lateral rotator of thigh
Obturator internus	inner margins of obturator foramen and obturator membrane	greater trochanter of femur	lumbar 5th and sacral first and second nerves	lateral rotator of thigh
Occipitofrontalis	lateral half of highest nuchal line on occipital bone and occipital aponeurosis	skin of eyebrows and aponeurosis	branches of facial nerve	draws scalp backward and raises eyebrows
Omohyoid	superior border of scapula	body of hyoid bone	ansa cervicalis upper cervical nerves	depressor of hyoid bone
Opponens digits minimi of hand	hook of hamate bone	fifth metacarpal bone—anterior aspect	ulnar nerve branch	abductor, flexor and rotator of 5th metacarpal
Opponens pollicis	flexor retinaculum and tubercle of trapezium	first metacarpal on its lateral side	branch of median nerve	flexion and opposing movement of thumb
Orbicularis oculi three parts—orbital, palpebral and lacrimal	medial margin of orbit, frontal process of maxilla; medial palpebral ligament and posterior lacrimal crest	medial palpebral ligament; orbital tubercle of zygomatic bone and lateral palpebral raphe	branch from facial nerve	closure of eyelid and compression of lacrimal sac
Orbicularis oris	encircling muscle fibres around mouth having labial part and marginal part	raphe at the angles of mouth	branch of facial nerve	sphincter of mouth, protrudes lips
Orbitalis	margins of inferior orbital fissure	fascia covering inferior orbital fissure	sympathetic nerves	protrudes eye in animals
Palatoglossus	undersurface of palatine aponeurosis	side of the tongue	pharyngeal plexus	elevation of tongue and constriction of oropharyngeal isthmus

Name	Origin	Insertion	Nerve supply	Action
Palatopharyngeus	posterior border of hard palate and palatine aponeurosis	posterior border of thyoid cartilage and merges with side wall of pharynx	pharyngeal plexus	constrictor of pharynx
Palmaris longus	medial epicondyle of humerus	flexor retinaculum and palmar aponeurosis	median nerve	tensor of palmar aponeurosis
Palmaris brevis	from palmar aponeurosis distal border	skin on medial side of hand	branch of ulnar nerve	deepening hollow of palm
Papillary muscles	walls of ventricles of heart	atrioventricular valve cusps by chordae tendeneae		prevents eversion of atrioventricular cusps
Pectineus	pectineal line of pubis	pectineal line of femur	branches of femoral and obturator nerve	flexion and adduction of thigh
Pectoralis major	front of clavicle, sternum and upper 6 costal cartilages	lateral lip of bicipital groove of humerus	lateral and medial pectoral nerves	adduction, flexion and medial rotation of arm
Pectoralis minor	from second, third, fourth and fifth ribs	coracoid process of scapula	medial and lateral pectoral nerves	raises upper ribs in forced inspiration, draws shoulder forward and downward
Peroneus longus	lateral condyle of tibia, head and lateral surface of fibula	medial cruciform and 1st metatarsal bone	superficial peroneal nerve	plantar flexor, abductor and everter of foot
Pterygoid lateral	infratemporal surface of greater wing of sphenoid and infratemporal crest, lateral surface of lateral pterygoid plate	neck of mandible and capsule of temporomandibular joint	mandibular nerve	depressor and protrusion of lower jaw helps in chewing

Name	Origin	Insertion	Nerve supply	Action
Pterygoid medial	maxillary tuberosity, medial surface of lateral pterygoid plate	ramus and angle of mandible on its medial side	mandibular nerve	elevation and protrusion of lower jaw
Pubococcygeus	posterior surface of pubis, part of levator ani	anococcygeal ligament and lateral side of coccyx	third and fourth sacral nerves	supports pelvic viscera as part of pelvic diaphragm
Puboprostaticus	anterior surface of prostate	posterior surface of pubis, part of levator ani	third and fourth sacral and autonomic supply for smooth muscle fibres component	supports and compresses prostate gland
Puborectalis	posterior surface of pubis, part of levator ani	fibres of two sides form a sling around ano-rectal junction	third and fourth sacral	supports pelvic viscera
Pubovaginalis	posterior surface of pubis, part of levator ani	neck of urinary bladder	sacral and pudendal nerves	helps to control micturition
Pyloric sphincter	circular smooth muscle fibres around pyloric canal	forming a thick muscular layer	autonomic nerves	sphincteric control of pyloroduodenal junction tion
Pyramidalis	body of the pubis	linea alba	twelfth thoracic nerve	tensor of linea alba
Quadratus femoris	ischial tuberosity	quadrate tubercle of femur and intertrochanteric crest	fourth and fifth lumbar and first sacral nerve	adduction and lateral rotation of thigh
Quadratus lumborum	iliac crest and fascia	transverse process of lumbar vertebrae and twelfth rib	twelfth thoracic and first and second lumbar nerves	flexion of trunk laterally
Quadratus plantae	calcaneum and plantar fascia	joins tendon of flexor digitorum longus of sole	lateral plantar nerves	flexion of toes

Name	Origin	Insertion	Nerve supply	Action
Quadriceps femoris	consisting of four muscles—one rectus femoris and 3 vasti-lateralis, medialis and inter-medialis. Vasti muscles taking origin from shaft of the femur and rectus femoris from hip bone by two heads	forms a common tendon that surrounds the patella and is attached to tuberosity of tibia	femoral nerve	extensor of leg
Rectus abdominis	pubic crest	xiphoid process, fifth, sixth and seventh costal cartilages	lower thoracic nerves	flexion of vertebrae in lumbar region and forms part of abdominal wall to support viscera
Rectus inferior	common tendinous ring in the orbit	sclera on the inferior surface of eyeball	oculomotor nerve	rotation of eyeball downwards and medially and adduction
Rectus lateralis	common tendinous ring in the orbit	sclera on the lateral surface of eyeball	abducent nerve	abduction of eyeball
Rectus medialis	common tendinous ring in the orbit	sclera on the medial surface of eyeball	oculomotor nerve	adduction of eyeball
Rectus superioris	common tendinous ring in the orbit	sclera on the superior surface of eyeball	oculomotor nerve	rotation of eyeball upwards and medially and adduction
Rector capitis anterior	lateral mass of atlas	basilar part of occipital bone	first and second cervical nerves	flexion of head
Rectus capitis lateralis	transverse process of atlas	jugular process of occipital bone	first and second cervical nerves	flexion and lateral bending of head
Rectus capitis posterior major	spine of axis vertebra	occipital bone	suboccipital and greater occipital nerve	extension of head

Name	Origin	Insertion	Nerve supply	Action
Rectus capitis posterior minor	posterior tubercle of atlas	occipital bone	suboccipital and greater occipital nerve	extension of head
Rectus femoris	anterior inferior iliac spine and area above acetabulum	joins vasti tendon to attach on tuberosity of tibia	femoral nerve	extension of leg, flexion of thigh
Rhomboideus major	spines of 2nd to 5th thoracic vertebrae	medial border of scapula	dorsal scapular nerve	retraction of scapula
Rhomboideus minor	spine of 7th cervical, 1st thoracic vertebrae and ligamentum nuchae	medial border of scapula near root of spinous process	dorsal scapular nerve	retraction of scapula
Risorius	masseteric fascia	skin at angle of mouth	buccal branch of facial nerve	draws angle of the mouth laterally
Rotators	deep muscle fibres attached between spines and transverse process of vertebrae		spinal nerves	extension and rotation of vertebral column
Sacrospinalis	*see* erector spinae			
Salpingo-pharyngeus	cartilage of auditory tube	fibres merge with palato-pharyngeus	pharyngeal plexus	pulls pharyngeal wall upwards
Sartorius	anterior superior iliac spine	upper part of medial surface of tibia	femoral nerve	flexion of thigh and leg abduction and lateral rotation of thigh
Scalenus anterior	transverse process of 3rd to 6th cervical vertebrae	scalane tubercle of first rib	2nd to 7th cervical nerves	elevation of first rib, flexion of cervical vertebrae
Scalenus medius	transverse process of first to seventh cervical vertebrae	superior surface of first rib	2nd to 7th cervical nerves	elevation of first rib, flexion of cervical vertebrae

Name	Origin	Insertion	Nerve supply	Action
Scalenus posterior	transverse processes of fourth to sixth cervical vertebrae	second rib	2nd to 7th cervical nerves	elevation of first rib, flexion of cervical vertebrae
Semimembranosus	ischial tuberosity	medial condyle of tibia	sciatic nerve	flexion of leg, extension of thigh
Semispinalis capitis	transverse process of upper thoracic and lower cervical vertebrae	occipital bone	suboccipital, greater occipital and cervical nerves	extension of head
Semispinalis cervicis	transverse processes of upper thoracic vertebrae	spines of lower cervical and upper thoracic vertebrae	spinal nerves	extension and rotation of vertebrae
Semispinalis thoracis	transverse processes of lower thoracic vertebrae	spines of lower cervical and upper thoracic vertebrae	spinal nerves	extension and rotation of vertebrae
Semitendinosus	ischial tuberosity	upper part of medial surface of tibia	sciatic nerve	flexion and medial rotation of leg, extension of thigh
Serratus anterior	first to eighth ribs anterolaterally	medial border of scapula	long thoracic nerve	protraction and rotation of scapula during abduction
Serratus posterior inferior	spines of lower thoracic and upper lumbar vertebrae	lower four ribs posteriorly	ninth to twelfth thoracic nerves	helps to pull ribs downwards during expiration
Serratus posterior superior	spines of upper thoracic vertebrae and ligamentum nuchae	second to fifth ribs posteriorly	upper four thoracic nerves	elevation of ribs during inspiration
Soleus	soleal line of tibia, fibula and tendinous arch	calcaneum along with gastrocnemius by a common tendon	tibial nerve	plantal flexion of foot
Sphincter ani externus 3 parts—subcutaneous, superficial and deep	anococcygeal raphe, coccyx	perineal body	inferior rectal and fourth sacral perineal branch	sphincter of the anal canal

Name	Origin	Insertion	Nerve supply	Action
Sphincter ani internus	ring of circular muscle fibres at the lower end of rectum		autonomic nerves	sphincteric control at ano-rectal junction
Sphincter Oddi	circular smooth muscle fibers at the opening of bile duct within the wall of duodenum			
Sphincter pupillae	circular fibres of	iris	parasympathetic nerves through ciliary ganglion	constriction of the pupil
Sphincter urethrae	inferior ramus of pubis	fibres surround urethra on perineal membrane	perineal branch	compresses membranous urethra
Spinalis capitis	spines of lower cervical and upper thoracic vertebrae	occipital bone	spinal nerve branch	extension of head
Spinalis cervicis	spines of seventh cervical vertebrae	spine of axis vertebra	cervical nerve branch	extension of vertebral column
Spinalis thoracis	spines of lower thoracic and upper lumbar vertebrae	spines of upper thoracic vertebrae	spinal nerve branches	extension of vertebral column
Splenius capitis	spines of seventh cervical and upper thoracic vertebrae, ligamentum nuchae	mastoid part of temporal bone, occipital bone	cervical nerves	extension and rotation of head
Splenius cervicis	spines of upper thoracic vertebrae	transverse processes of upper cervical vertebrae	cervical nerves	extension and rotation of head and neck
Stapedius	within pyramid of tympanic cavity	neck of stapes	facial nerve branch	reducing movements of stapes
Sterno-cleidomastoid	manubrium of sternum and medial third of clavicle	mastoid process of temporal bone and superior nuchal line of occipital bone	accessory nerve and branches from cervical plexus	flexion of neck, rotation of head to opposite side

Name	Origin	Insertion	Nerve supply	Action
Sternocostalis	posterior surface of sternum and xiphoid process	second to sixth costal cartilage	intercostal nerves	helps in respiratory movements of chest
Sternohyoid	manubrium of sternum	body of hyoid bone	ansa cervicalis	depression of hyoid bone
Sternothyroid	manubrium of sternum	lamina of thyoid cartilage	ansa cervicalis	downward pulling of thyroid cartilage
Styloglossus	styloid process	margin of tongue	hypoglossal nerve	elevation and retraction of tongue
Stylohyoid	styloid process	body of hyoid bone	facial nerve	drawing hyoid bone upwards and backwards
Stylopharyngeus	styloid process	thyroid cartilage and lateral pharyngeal wall	glossopharyngeal nerve	elevation of pharyngeal wall
Subclavius	superior surface of first rib and its cartilage	inferior surface of clavicle	nerve to subclavius from upper trunk of brachial plexus	depression of clavicle
Subcostals	inferior border of ribs	superior border of two or three ribs below	intercostal nerves	elevation of ribs on inspiration
Subscapularis	subscapular fossa of scapula	lesser tubercle of humerus	subscapular nerve	medial rotation of humerus
Supinator	lateral epicondyle of humerus	upper part of shaft of radius bone	deep branch of radial nerve	supination of forearm
Supraspinatus	supraspinous fossa of scapula	greater tubercle of humerus	suprascapular nerve	abduction of arm
Suspensory muscle of duodenum	smooth and skeletal muscle fibres from left crus of diaphragm	merges with muscular coat of duodenum at duodenojejunal junction	autonomic and phrenic	supports duodenojejunal junction
Tarsal-inferior	fibres from inferior rectus of eye ball	tarsal plate of lower eye lid	sympathetic	depression of lower eye lid

Name	Origin	Insertion	Nerve supply	Action
Tarsal-superior	fibres from levator palpabrae superioris of upper eye lid	tarsal plate of upper eye lid	sympathetic	elevation of upper eye lid
Temporalis	temporal fossa and fascia	coronoid process and anterior ramus of mandible	mandibular nerve	elevation of upper eye lid
Tensor fascia lata	iliac crest	iliotibial tract	superior gluteal nerve	flexion and medial rotation of thigh
Tensor palati	scaphoid fossa and spine of sphenoid bone	aponeurosis of soft palate	mandibular nerve	tensor of soft palate
Tensor tympani	cartilage of auditory tube	handle of malleus	mandibular nerve	tensor of tympanic membrane
Teres major	inferior part of lateral border of scapula	medial lip of intertubercular sulcus of humerus	lower subscapular nerve	adduction, extension and medial rotation of arm
Teres minor	lateral border of scapula	lower part of greater tubercle of humerus	axillary nerve	lateral rotation of arm
Thyro-arytenoideus	inner surface of thyoid cartilage lamina	muscular process of arytenoid cartilage	recurrent laryngeal nerve	relaxation of vocal folds
Thyro-epiglotticus	lamina of thyoid cartilage	margins of epiglottis	recurrent laryngeal nerve	sphincter of laryngeal inlet
Thyrohyoid	lamina of thyoid cartilage	greater horn of hyoid bone	aura cervicalis	elevation of larynx
Tibialis anterior	lateral condyle and surface of tibia, interosseous membrane	medial cuneiform and base of first metatarsal bone	deep peroneal	dorsiflexion and inversion of foot
Tibialis posterior	tibia, fibula and interosseous membrane	bases of 2nd to fourth metatarsal bones and tarsal bones except talus	tibial nerve	plantar flexion and inversion of foot
Trachealis	smooth muscle fibre, transversely arranged to fill up the gap of the back of each tracheal cartilage		autonomic nerves	reduction of diameter of tracheal passage

Name	Origin	Insertion	Nerve supply	Action
Transversus abdominis	iliac crest, thoraco-lumbar fascia and lower six costal cartilages	linea alba through rectus sheath	lower thoracic spinal nerves	compression of abdominal cavity
Transversus auricularis	cranial surface of auricle	circumference of auricle	posterior auricular branch of facial	retraction of helix
Transversus perinei—deep	ramus of the ischium	perineal body	perineal branches	fixation of perineal body contributes to form urogenital diaphragm
Transverse perinei—superficialis	ramus of ischium	perineal body	perineal nerves	fixation of perineal body, contributes to form urogenital diaphragm
Transversus linguae	median septum of tongue	dorsum and margins of tongue	hypoglossal nerve	changing shape of tongue helping mastication and swallowing
Trapezius	occipital bone, ligamentum nuchae, spines of seventh cervical and all thoracic vertebrae	lateral third of clavicle, acromion and upper border of crest of scapula	accessory nerve and branches from cervical plexus	elevation and retraction of shoulder, helps in abduction of arm by rotating scapula with serratus anterior
Triceps brachii	infraglenoid tubercle of scapula, posterior surface of humerus above and below radial groove	olecranon process of ulna	radial nerve	extension of forearm, weak adduction of arm
Uvulae-muscularis	aponeurosis of soft palate, posterior nasal spine	uvula	pharyngeal plexus	raises uvula

Name	Origin	Insertion	Nerve supply	Action
Vastus inter-medius	anterior and lateral surface of femur	patella, forms quadriceps tendon to attach on tibial tuberosity	femoral nerve	extension of leg
Vastus lateralis	lateral surface of femur	patella, forms quadriceps tendon to attach on tibial tuberosity	femoral nerve	extension of leg
Vastus medialis	medial surface of femur	patella, forms quadriceps tendon to attach on tibial tuberosity	femoral nerve	extension of leg
Verticalis linguae	fascia on dorsal surface of tongue	fascia on sides and ventral surface of tongue	hypoglossal nerve	flattening of tongue, helps in mastication and swallowing
Vocalis	thyoid laminae near its angle on inner side	vocal process of arytenoid cartilage	recurrent laryngeal nerve	variation in tension of vocal folds
Zygomaticus major	zygomatic bone	angle of mouth	facial nerve	draws angle of mouth upwards and backwards
Zygomaticus minor	zygomatic bone	fibres merge with orbicular muscle of mouth and levator labii superioris	facial nerve	draw upper lip upwards and laterally

mute (mut) 1. unable or unwilling to speak 2. one who is unable to speak

mutilation (mut'i-la'shun) 1. disfigurement or injury or removal or destruction of a part of the body 2. a condition so resulting

mutism (mut'izm) inability to speak **akinetic m** a situation of being immobile or silent with loss of emotional feeling due to lesions of the upper brain stem **elective m** inability to speak due to hysteria

mutra (s) urine

mutragatha (s) obstruction to urination

mV millivolt

μV microvolt

MVA modified vaccinia virus that replicates in bird cell lines

MVP mitral valve prolapse.

MVV maximum voluntary ventilation

my(o) combining word for muscle

myalgia (mi-al'je-a) pain in a muscle

myasthenia (mi'as-the'ne-a) weakness and easy fatigability of muscles **m gravis a**

defect at neuro-muscular junction, wherein the antibodies against acetylcholine receptors do not permit acetylcholine to combine with the receptors, thus blocking the chemical transmission. The thymus gland acts as a source of antigen directing humoral and cellular immune responses. There is easy fatigability of muscles, worsened on exertion and the disability is relieved by rest. Diplopia, ptosis, ophthalmoplegia, dysphagia and dysphonia occur due to involvement of muscles supplied by cranial nerves

myasthenic relating to myasthenia **m crisis** serious complication of myasthenia gravis with rapid development of muscle weakness which results in respiratory paralysis and is due to inadequate drugs **m reactions** a clinical picture closely resembling myasthenia gravis may develop as a paraneoplastic phenomenon, however, ocular muscles are unaffected

myotonia (mi-a-to'ne-a) deficiency or loss of muscle tone

myotonic dystrophy myotonia, cataract, ptosis, frontal baldness and gonadal atrophy caused by expansion of a trinucleotide repeat of chromosome 19

myatrophy (mi-at'ro-fe) atrophy of a muscle .

mycelium (mi-se'le-um) mass of interlaced hyphae (fungus) or of filamentous bacteria (actinomycetes)

mycete (mi-set) a fungus

mycetoma (mi-se-to'ma) a chronic granulomatous inflammation caused by several species of fungi or actinomycetes

Myc (o) combining word for fungus.

mycobacterium (-bak-ter'e-um) a genus of aerobic non-motile, gram-positive acid fast bacteria, belonging to the family Mycobacteriaceae. It consists of parasitic and saprophytic species pl. **mycobacteria** *M. avium*, complex causes a chronic pulmonary disease resembling tuberculosis *M. balnei*, *M. marinum* causes swimming pool granuloma *M. bovis* causative agent of tuberculosis in cattle, transmitted to man through milk *M. kansasii* a photochromogen produces a chronic pulmonary disease resembling tuberculosis *M. leprae* an obligate parasitic species which causes leprosy. *M. marinum* a species causing swimming pool granuloma *M. scrofulaceum* a scotochromogen causes cervical lymphadenitis exclusively in children *M tuberculosis* the tubercle bacillus, the cause of tuberculosis in man, most commonly of the lungs **non tuberculous m** (NTM) ubiquously distributed in the environment and can cause disease similar to tuberculosis, also called atypical mycobacteria, anonymous mycobacteria, or mycobacteria other than *M. tuberculosis*

mycodermatitis (-der'ma-ti'tis) candidiasis

mycologist (mi-kol'o-jist) a person specialised in mycology

mycology (mi-kol'o-je) the science concerned with the study of fungi

mycomyringitis (mi'ko-mir'in-jit'is) fungal disease of tympanic membrane

mycoplasma (-plaz'ma) an incomplete intracellular and extracellular infectious particle that causes pneumonia and genitourinary infection

Mycoplasmal pneumonia pneumonia caused by *Mycoplasma pneumoniae* common in adolescents and young adults, develops insidiously with headache, low grade fever, chills, arthralgia, myalgia, skin rash, anorexia followed by sore throat and cough. Sensitive to macrolides and tetracycline.

mycosis (mi-ko'sis) fungal infection **deep m** fungal infection involving subcutaneous tissue and organs **m fungoides** cutaneous T cell lymphoma **subcutaneous m** subcutaneous fungal infection such as sporotrichosis, chromomycosis, phycomycosis and rhinosporidosis **superficial m** fungal infection limited to the dead keratinised tissue of the skin wherein the cellular response of the host is minimal and it includes superficial mycoses and dermatophytoses **systemic m** fungal infection affecting various systems of the body.

mycotic (mi-kot'ik) of fungi **m aneurysm** ulceration or degeneration of the wall of an artery due to local inflammation from an infected embolus lodging within the vessel results in formation of a small aneurysm. Severe haemorrhage results from rupture of a mycotic aneurysm

mycotoxicosis (mi-ko-tok-si-ko'sis) toxicity due to ingestion of substances produced by certain moulds on particular food stuffs or ingestion of fungi themselves

mycotoxin (-tok'sin) a fungal toxin.

mydriasis (mi'dri-a'sis) dilatation of pupil

mydriatic (mi'dre-at'ik) 1. of mydriasis 2. drug causing dilatation of pupil

myectomy (mi-ek'ta-me) excision of a muscle

myectopia (mi'ek-to'pe-a) dislocation of a muscle.

myelapoplexy (mi'il-ap'a-plek'se) haematomyelia

myelatrophy (-at'ra-fe) atrophy of the spinal cord

myelencephalon (-en-sef'a-lon) medulla oblongata

myelin (mi'e-lin) a complex lipid material of axon sheath. It is rich in cerebrosides and phosphatidyl ethanolamine

myelinisation (mi'e-lin'i-za'shun) formation of a myelin sheath around a nerve fibre

myelinolysis (mi'e-lin-ol'i-sis)dissolution of the myelin sheaths of nerve fibres

myelinotoxic (mi'e-lin'o-tok'sik) having a damaging effect on myelin sheath

myelitis (mi'e-li'tis) inflammatory lesions of the spinal cord encompassing diverse pathological processes which may be infective or noninfective **acute necrotic m** a necrotising myelitis affecting the white matter of the cord,

characterised by acute onset of paraplegia or quadriplegia with sensory deficit and sphincter paralysis **ascending m** symptoms of spinal syndrome ascending progressively **transverse m** transverse and complete spinal syndrome with flaccid paralysis, sensory loss below the lesion, presence of a zone of increased sensation between the area of sensory loss and the area of normal sensation, and involvement of bladder

myel (o) combining word for marrow, spinal cord

myeloablation (mi'e-lo-ab-la'shun) severe myelosuppression

myeloblast (mi'e-lo-blast) earliest recognisable granulocyte precursor. It has basophilic cytoplasm without granules

myeloblastaemia (mi'e-lo-blas-tem'e-a) the presence of myeloblasts in the blood

myeloblastoma (-blas-to'ma) a nodular collection of myeloblasts

myelocoele (mi'e-lo-cel) protrusion of the spinal cord through a defect in the vertebral column

myelocyst (-sist) a benign cyst developing from a rudimentary medullary canal in CNS

myelocystocoele (mi-e-lo-sis'to-sel) myelomeningocoele

myelocystomeningocoele (-sis'to-mening'go-sel) combined myelocystocoele and meningocoele

myelocyte (mi'e-lo-sit) granulocyte precursor in the bone marrow. It has a round nucleus with numerous granules in the cytoplasm

myelocytoma (-si-to'ma) a nodular, dense collection of myelocytes

myelocytosis (mi'e-lo-si-to'sis) occurrence of abnormally large numbers of myelocytes in the blood, tissues, or both

myelodysplasia (mi'e-lo-dis'pla-zhah) a developmental anomaly with an incomplete fusion of neural tube in the embryo; a non-progressive condition associated with spina bifida

myelodysplastic syndromes (MDS) a group of clonal proliferative disorders of bone marrow characterised by cytopaenias of one or more cell lines in the peripheral blood and dysha-emopoietic changes in the bone marrow. They evolve into acute non-lymphoid leukaemia

myencephalitis (-en-sef'xa-lit-is) inflammation of the spinal cord and brain

myelofibrosis (-fi-bro'sis) replacement of bone marrow by fibrous tissue. There is extramedullary haemopoiesis with massive splenomegaly

myelogenesis (-jen'e-sis) development of bone marrow

myelogenous (mi'e-log'i-nus) produced in the bone marrow

myelogone (mi'e-lo-gon) an immature white blood cell of myeloid series having a relatively large, finely reticulated nucleus with pale nucleoli and scanty cytoplasm

myelography (mi'e-log'ra-fe) X-ray to demonstrate spinal subarachnoid space, taken after introduction of contrast agent into the theca and positioning the patient to allow the dye to pass up or down

myeloid (mi'e-loid) 1. pertaining to or derived from bone marrow 2. spinal cord 3. pertaining to certain features of myelocytic forms in the bone marrow **m leukaemia** a disorder of unrestrained and excessive proliferation of haematopoietic tissue showing full range of granulocyte precursors from myeloblasts to mature neutrophils in

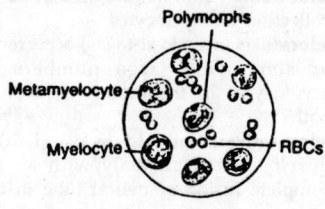

Myeloid leukaemia

the peripheral blood. It is associated with extramedullary haemopoiesis with active marrow tissue **m metaplasia** spleen and liver with a leucoerythroblastic blood picture

myeloidosis (mi'e-loi-do'sis) hyperplasia of myeloid tissue

myelolipoma (mi'e-lo-li-po'ma) nodules containing accumulations of cells derived from localised proliferation of reticuloendothelial tissue of the adrenal gland and adipose tissue

myeloma (mi'e-lo-ma) a tumour composed of cells derived from haemopoietic tissue of bone marrow **multiple m** a malignant proliferation of plasma cells. The plasma cells produce an immunoglobulin of a single heavy and light chain. The malignant plasma cells are present in the bone marrow and a small number in the peripheral blood. It causes bone erosion, pathological fracture, renal damage, increased blood viscosity, and impaired immune function

myelomalacia (mi'e-lo-ma-la'she-a) softening of the spinal cord

myelomatosis (-ma-to'sis) multiple myeloma

myelomeningitis (-men'in-ji'tis) meningomyelitis

myelomeningocoele (-me-ning'go-sel) hernial protrusion of the spinal cord and its meninges through a defect in the vertebral column

myelomere (mi'e-lo-mer) any segment of the embryonic spinal cord

myelopathy (mi'e-lop'a-the) 1. disease affecting the spinal cord 2. a disease of myelopoietic tissues

myeloperoxidase (mi'e-lo-per-ok'si-das) enzyme of myeloid cells producing free halogens from halides. Its deficiency prevents cell adhesion and migration of phagocytes

myelopetal (mi'e-lop-i-t'l) moving toward the spinal cord

myelophthisis (mi'e-lo-thi'sis) 1. atrophy of the spinal cord 2. replacement of haemopoietic tissue in the bone marrow by fibrous tissue or metastatic carcinoma

myeloplast (mi'e-lo-plast) any of the premature forms of the leucocyte series of cells in the bone marrow

myelopoiesis (mi'e-lo-poi-e'sis) myeloblast undergoing several divisions, simultaneously maturing into five sequential cells such as promyelocyte, myelocyte, metamyelocyte, band (stab) form and neutrophil

myeloproliferative (-pro-lif'er-a-tiv) pertaining to or characterised by unusual proliferation of myelopoietic tissue

myeloradiculitis (-ra-dik'ul-it'is) inflammation of the spinal cord and nerve roots

myeloradiculodysplasia (-ra-dik'u-lo-displa'zhah) congenital maldevelopment of the spinal cord and spinal nerve roots

myelorrhagia (-ra'jah) haematomyelia

myelosarcoma (-sar-ko'ma) a malignant tumour derived from bone marrow or one of its cellular elements

myelosclerosis (-skle-ro'sis) 1. myelofibrosis 2. obliteration of marrow cavity 3. sclerosis of the spinal cord.

myelosis (mi'e-losis) 1. abnormal proliferation of bone marrow 2. abnormal proliferation of medullary tissue in the spinal cord

myelospongium (mi'e-lo-spon'je-um) a network developing into neuroglia

myelosuppressive (-su-pres'iv) 1. inhibiting bone marrow activity 2. an agent exhibiting such properties

myelotoxic (my-uh'low'tock'sik) damage to the bone marrow

myenteron (mi-en'ter-on) the muscular coat of the intestine

myesthesia (mi'es-the'zhah) muscle sense; sensation appreciated during muscular contraction

myiasis invasion of tissues or body cavities by the maggots (larvae) of dipterous flies

myoarchitectonic (mi'o-ar'ki-tek'ton'ik) pertaining to the structural arrangement of muscle or muscle fibres

myoatrophy (-a'tra-fe) muscular atrophy

myoblast (mi'o-blast) a primitive muscle cell

myoblastoma (mi'o-blas-to'ma) a tumour of immature muscle cells

myocardial pertaining to the myocardium or disease affecting the myocardium **m cell** myocyte of 100 m long, each cell branches and interdigitates with adjacent cells **m contraction** basic unit of contraction is the sarcomere, which is aligned to those of adjacent myofibrils. During contraction there is shortening of sarcomere, and contraction is initiated in presence of calcium ions **m infarction** myocardial damage, due to the formation of occlusive thrombus at the site of rupture of an atheromatous plaque in a coronary artery. It presents with pain, breathlessness, anxiety, nausea, vomiting, collapse or syncope **m ischaemia** disease of coronary artery presenting with angina, myocardial infarction, heart failure, arrhythmia or sudden death **m stunning** viable myocardium surrounding a fresh infarct may contract poorly for a few days

myocardiopathy (-kar'de-op'a-the) cardiomyopathy

myocarditis (-kar-di'tis) an acute inflammatory condition that may complicate a wide variety of infections, mostly from viruses. It may present with inappropriate tachycardia or fulminant heart failure. Some forms may lead to chronic low grade myocarditis or dilated cardiomyopathy

myocardium (-kar'de-um) the middle and thickest layer of the heart wall composed of cardiac muscle

myocardosis (-kar-do'sis) any degenerative disorder of the heart

myoclonic seizure sudden, brief bilaterally synchronous muscle contraction without loss of consciousness

myoclonus (mi-ok'lo-nus) a brief involuntary random muscle contraction occurring either with rest. in response to sensory stimuli or with voluntary movements

myocoele (mi'o-sel) protrusion of a muscle through a rent in its ruptured sheath

myocutaneous flap skin and underlying muscle with its blood supply used for plastic repair

myocyte (-sit) a muscle cell

myocytolysis (mi'o-si-tol'i-sis) disintegration of muscle fibres

myodystonia (-dis-to'ne-a) a disorder of muscular tone characterised by slow relaxation interrupted by a succession of slight contractions following an electrical stimulation of a muscle

myodystrophy (-dis-tro-fe) muscular dystrophy

myoidema (-e'de-ma) myotatic irritability: a transitory localised swelling on light tap, due to the contraction of the unduly irritable muscles in conditions associated with cachexia

myoepithelioma (-ep'i-el'e-o'ma) a benign tumour of myoepithelial cells

myoepithelium (-ep'i-the'le-um) contractile cells forming outer layer of secretory epithelium, as of breast, salivary and sweat glands

myofascial (-fash'e-al) pertaining to or involving the fascia surrounding muscle tissue

myofasciitis (-fa-sit'is) inflammation of a muscle and its fascia

myofibre (mi'o-fi'ber) muscle fibre

myofibril (mi'o-fi'ril) one of the slender, longitudinal fibrils occurring in a skeletal or cardiac muscle fibre

myofibroblast (-fi-bro-blast) contractile fibroblasts that help in contraction of healing wounds

myofibroma (-fi-bro'ma) a benign tumour composed of fibrous connective tissue and muscle cells

myofibrositis (-fi'bro-sit'is) inflammation of the fibrous sheath enveloping the muscle fibres

myofilament (-fil'a-ment) ultramicroscopic thick and thin threads making up myofibrils in striated muscles

myogenesis (-jen'i-sis) formation of muscle fibres

myogenous (mi-og'in-is) myogenetic

myoglobin (mi'o-glo'bin) haemoglobin in the muscle having one haem per globin unit instead of four

myoglobulin (mi'o-glob'ul-in) globulin found in muscle tissue

myograph (mi'o-graf) an instrument by which tracings are made of muscle contractions

myography (mi-og'ra-fe) the recording of muscular contractions by the myograph

myoid (mi'oid) resembling muscle

myokinase (mi'o-ki'nas) an enzyme in the muscle that catalyses the synthesis of adenosine triphosphate

myokinesis (-ki-ne'sis) 1. muscular activity 2. displacement of muscle fibres by surgery

myokymia (-ki-me-a) irregular twitching of muscle fibres

myolipoma (-li-po'ma) a benign tumour of muscle with variable number of fat cells

myology (mi-ol'a-je) the branch of science concerned with the study of the muscles and their parts

myolysis (mi-'ol'i-sis) dissolution of muscle tissue

myoma (mi-o-ma) a benign tumour of muscle tissue

myomalacia cordis softening of infarcted myocardium

myomatosis (mi-o'ma-to'sis) the development of multiple myomas

myomectomy (mi'o-mek-ta-me) surgical removal of a myoma, specifically of a uterine myoma

myomelanosis (-mel'a-no'sis) abnormal dark pigmentation of muscle tissue

myomere (mi'o-mer) a muscular segment

myometer (mi-om'it-er) an instrument for measurement of the extent of muscular contraction

myometritis (mi'o-me-trit'is) inflammation of the muscular wall of the uterus

myometrium (-me'tre-um) the muscular wall of the uterus

myoneme (mi'o-nem) a muscle fibre

myoneural (mi'o-noor'al) pertaining to the synapse of the motor neuron with striated muscle fibres

myopalmus (-pal'mus) muscle twitching

myoparalysis (-pa-ra'i-sis) muscular paralysis

myoparesis (-pa-re'sis) muscle paresis

myopathy (mi-op-a-the) any abnormality of the muscular tissue especially involving the skeletal muscle **carcinomatous m** Eaton-Lambert syndrome **centronuclear m** slowly progressive generalised muscle weakness and atrophy beginning in childhood. The nuclei of most muscle fibres are found near the centre of the fibre **congenital m** an inherited disorder, central core disease with its gene being located on chromosome 19, associated with structural changes in muscle fibres, floppy at birth or early childhood, generally non-progressive, weakness more prominent in proximal muscles **distal m** myopathy affecting predominantly distal portions of the limbs, has an autosomal dominant inheritance **myotubular m** centronuclear myopathy **nemaline m** myopathy with dystrophic facial features and skeletal deformities, deteriorates rapidly **ocular m** begins in early childhood with bilateral symmetrical ptosis and progressive external ophthalmoplegia **proximal myotonic m** autosomal dominant condition with proximal muscle weakness, cataract and myotonia **thyrotoxic m** generalised muscle weakness with predilection to girdle muscles in thyrotoxicosis

myopericarditis (mi'o-per'i-kar-di'tis) inflammation of the muscular wall of the heart and the pericardium

myophosphorylase (mi'o-fos-for'i-las) muscle isoenzyme of glycogen phosphorylase whose deficiency results in glycogen storage disease V

myopia (mi-o'pe-a) short sight in which parallel rays entering the eye focus in front of the retina **myopic** adj. **curvature m** myopia due to excessive corneal curvature **index m** myopia due to abnormal refractivity of the media of the eye **malignant m** progressive myopia leading to retinal detachment and blindness **progressive m** myopia increasing during adult life

myopic (mi-op'ik) pertaining to myopia **m crescent** pale area round the optic disc developing in pathological myopia

myoplasm (mi-o-plazm) the contractile part of muscle cell

myoplasty (-plas'te) plastic surgery of muscle tissue

myorrhexis (-rek'sis) tearing of a muscle

myosarcoma (-sar-ko'ma) a malignant tumour derived from muscle tissue

myosclerosis (-skle-ro'sis) hardening of a muscle

myosin (mi'u-sin) fibrous protein of skeletal and heart muscle

myositis (mi'o-sit'is) inflammation of a muscle **epidemic m** epidemic pleurodynia **m fibrosa** induration of a muscle through an interstitial growth of fibrous tissue **inclusion body m** a progressive inflammatory myopathy affecting muscles of pelvis and lower limbs **multiple m** polymyositis **m ossificans** myositis accompanied by calcium deposits in the muscle **m purulenta** suppurative myositis with abscesses **traumatic m** myositis due to injury **Trichinous m** myositis due to the presence of *Trichinella spiralis*

myospasm (mi'o-spazm) spasmodic muscular contraction

myotactic (mi'o-tak-tik) pertaining to muscle sense

myotasis (mi-ot'a-sis) stretching of a muscle

myotenositis (mi'o-ten'o-si'tis) inflammation of a muscle and tendon

myotome (mi'o-tom) 1. a knife used for cutting muscles 2. that part of an embryonic somite that gives rise to striated muscle 3. all muscles derived from one somite and innervated from a single spinal segment

myotonia (mi′o-to-ne-a) delayed relaxation after contraction **m congenita** an inherited condition begining in early childhood characterised by difficulty in getting up and walking, difficulty in relaxing a grip, and generalised muscular hypertrophy. There is reduced chloride membrane conductance and reduced number of chloride channels

myotonoid (mi-ot′o-noid) a muscle reaction showing a slow contraction and relaxation

myotonus (-nus) a tonic spasm of muscle.

myotrophic (mi′o-tro′fik) pertaining to myotrophy

myotrophy (mi-ot′ra-fe) nutrition of a muscle

myotube (mi′otoo′b) a developing skeletal muscle fibre with a tubular appearance

myringa (mi-ring′ga) the tympanic membrane

myringectomy (-mir′in-jek′ta-me) excision of the tympanic membrane

myringitis (mir′in-jit′is) inflammation of tympanic membrane

myring (o) combining word for tympanic membrane

myringomycosis (mi-ring′go-mi-ko′sis) fungal disease of tympanic membrane

myringoplasty replacement of eardrum with temporal fascia

myristic (mii-ris′tik) **acid** straight chain-saturated 14 carbon fatty acid

mysophilia (mi′so-fil′i-a) an increased attraction towards excretions

mysophobia (-fo′be-a) morbid fear of contamination and filth

myxadenitis (miks′ad-e-ni′tis) inflammation of mucous gland

myxoedema (mik′se-de′ma) primary hypothyroidism in juveniles and adults, it has an insidious onset, slowing of

activities, lethargy, somnolence, constipation, gain in weight, increased sensitivity to cold, accumulation of fluid and adipose tissue, lustreless thick, dry skin with scanty hair, husky voice, and non- pitting oedema **m coma** untreated cases of myxoedema leading to somnolence, stupor and coma **m madness** psychiatric disturbance in myxoedema **pretibial m** localised myxoedematous deposits in front of the leg in hyperthyroidism

Myx (o) combining word for mucus; mucin.

myxochondroma (mik′so-kon-dro′ma) a chondroma in which the stroma has resemblance to primitive mesenchymal cell

myxofibroma (-fi-bro′ma) a benign fibrous connective tissue tumour which contains primitive mesenchymal tissue

myxofibrosarcoma (-fi′bro-sar-ko′ma) a fibrosarcoma containing primitive mesenchymal tissue

myxoid (mik′soid) resembling mucus

myxolipoma (mik′so-li′po′ma) a lipoma containing elements of myxomatous degeneration

myxoma (mik-so′ma) a slow growing soft, lobulated tumour occurring in subcutaneous tissue, spinal cord, urinary bladder, bones and heart

myxomatosis (mik′so-ma-to′sis) 1. mucoid degeneration 2. multiple myxomas

myxorrhoea (mik′so-re′a) excessive flow of mucous

myxosarcoma (-sar-ko′ma) a sarcoma containing tissue having resemblance to primitive mesenchymal tissue

myxovirus (mik′so-virus) RNA viruses having affinity to mucous surfaces. Includes influenza viruses A, B and C and para influenza and respiratory syncytial virus that cause the respiratory infections

MZ monozygotic

N

N Chemical symbol for nitrogen, normal solution symbol for population size

n – nano, 10⁹; symbol for normal, refractory index, sample size

Na chemical symbol for sodium (natrium)

nabhi (s) naval

nabothian (nabo'the'-en) **cyst** a cyst formed in a nebothian gland of uterine cervix. It appears pearly white and firm and has no adverse effects

nabothian gland one of many small, mucus-secreting glands of uterine cervix, named after Martin Naboth, German physician

NACO National AIDS control organization

NAD abbreviation for no appreciable disease

nadi (s) pulse channel in the body along which life-force flows *n pariksha* examination of pulse *n yantra* tubular instrument

nadir (na'der) the lowest point

nadolol (nad'e-lol) a beta-adrenergic blocking agent, used in treatment of hypertension and angina pectoris

Naegele's obliquity the sagittal suture nearer the promontory than the symphysis when the vertex engages in the pelvic brim; anterior asynclitism

Naegele's (na'ge-lez) **rule** estimation of the day of onset of labour by counting back 90 days from the day of beginning of last menstrual period and adding seven days to that date, rule formulated by Franz Naegele, German obstetrician

Naegleria free-living soil amoebae that may produce primary amoebic meningoencephalitis. The organisms are carried in the nose and the throat of asymptomatic carriers

naevus (ne'vus) mole, birthmark, a circumscribed area of hyperpigmentation angioma of skin. pl. **naevi. bathing trunk n** pigmented naevus consisting of large nodules on the trunk **compound n** presence of a naevus at the dermo-epidermal junction and in the dermis **dermal n** naevus located in the dermis **halo n** presence of a halo of depigmented skin around a pigmented lesion **junctional n** naevus located at dermo-epidermal junction **epidermal n** a congenital malformation characterised by papillated or digitated epidermal proliferations accompanied by hyperkeratotosis **n flaromeus** a flat capillary haemangioma that is present at birth and that varies in colour from pale red to deep reddish purple seen commonly on the occiput **intradermal n** a lesion composed of nests, cords and strands of melanocytes of a naevus within the dermis wholly **melanocytic n** pigmented naevus located on any site of the body and remain unchanged throughout life, used as an identification mark **n achromaticus** a single large irregular depigmented area limited to a single nerve segment **n anaemicus** an irregular area of hypopigmentation present at birth which remains unchanged throughout life. The cutaneous capillaries exhibit an abnormally exaggerated tendency for vasoconstriction **n of lto** naevus in supraclavicular, deltoid or scapular regions **n of Ota** dermal naevus in the territory of ophthalmic and/or maxillary divisions of trigeminal nerve unilaterally. **n verruosus** excessive proliferation of the epidermal cells that present as asymptomatic hyper-keratotic verrucous areas unilaterally

nafcillin penicillinase–resistant synthetic penicillin, used in infections from penicillinase producing streptococci

Naffziger's method method of examination for exophthalmos while standing behind a seated patient the head is tilted backwards while holding the head the eyeballs are observed with the plane of vision being that of the superciliary ridges, named after Howard Naffziger, US surgeon

nail (nal) an epidermal plate with keratin covering the sensitive tips of the fingers and toes; a slender metallic rod used in operation to fasten pieces of broken bone pl. **nails brittle n** weakening of nail edges with splitting and softening often due to effects of solvents, detergents and soaps **Hippocratic n** *see* clubbed digits **ingrown n** growth of the nail edge into the soft tissue, a result of improper pairing of the nails or pressure on a nail edge from improperly fitted footwear **n bed** the portion of the tip of a finger or toe covered by the root and body of the nail **n biting** a neurotic condition wherein the edges of the nails are bitten **n fold** a fold of skin supporting the nail at its base **n groove** a shallow depression between the nail bed and the nail wall **n- patella syndrome** an autosomal dominant disease involving structures of mesodermal and ectodermal origin and presenting with defective nails of thumb and great toe, flexion contraction of multiple joints, defective or absent patellae, lordosis, renal abnormalities, exostosis of ileum and pigmentary anomalies of iris, cataract, microcornea and ptosis; hereditary osteo-onychodysplasia, **n plate** the hard portion of the dorsum of the fingers and thumb **Smith-Peterson n** a three-fanged nail to fix the fractures of the neck of the femur devised by Marius Smith Paterson, US orthopaedic surgeon **spoon n** koilonychia, a nail with depressed centre and elevated lateral edges seen in iron deficiency anaemia

nailing (nal'ing) operative procedure to fix a fracture t bone by a nail

naïve 1. never receiving treatment before 2. not having any previous exposure

naja (nah'jah) cobra *Naja naja*, a common cobra of India

naked granuloma hard tubercle with Langhans giant cells and mononuclear cells without necrosis as in sarcoidosis and granuloma annulare

naked nuclei elongated, cytoplasm poor cells with hyperchromatic nuclei as in ovarian endometriosis; cells with friable nuclei and scant or absent cytoplasm as in small cell carcinoma

nakha (s) nail

nalidixic (nal-i-diks'ic) **acid** a quinolone preparation active against bacterial urinary tract infections

nalika (s) tube

nalorphine (nal'or-fen) a morphine antagonist

naloxone (nal-oks'on) an antagonist of morphine and other narcotics

name (nam) word by which a person, animal, place or thing is known or called

NANB non A, non B type hepatitis

nandrolone (nan'dro-lon) an anabolic androgenic steroid

nanism (na'nizm) dwarfism

nano division by 10^9, dwarf

nanocephalous (na'no-sef'a-lus) microcephalus

nanocephaly (na'no-sef 'a-le) microcephaly

nanogram (na'no-gram) a unit of mass that is one billionth (10^{-9}) of a gram

nanomelia (na'no-me'le-a) a developmental abnormality showing abnormal smallness of the limbs

nanophthalmos (na'n-of-thal-mos) very small eyes

nanous (na'nus) dwarf

nap a short sleep

NAP neutrophil alkaline phosphatase

nape (nap) the back of the neck

naphazoline (naf-az'o-len) a vasoconstrictor used as a topical nasal decongestant and as a mydriatic.

naphthalene a crystal formed from 2 benzene rings, used for mothballs and insecticide

naphthaline a carcinogen found in tobacco smoke

napkin a small towel **n rash** irritant contact dermatitis

naproxen a non-steroid anti-inflammatory drug

narcissism (nar'si-sizm) sexual attraction towards self

narcoanalysis (nar'ko-a-nal'li-sis) encouraging the patient to talk about their experiences following induction of light anaesthesia by IV, babiturate

narcolepsy (nar'ko-lep'se) a sudden collapse into sleep at irregular intervals during daytime whose cause is undertermined

narcosis (nar-ko'sis) depression of neuronal excitability causing stupor/ or sleep **carbon dioxide na** clinical picture of lethargy, drowsiness, flapping tremors, altered consciousness due to sudden increase in arterial carbon dioxide tension

narcotic (nar-kot'ik) a substance capable of inducing stupor and insensibility **n addict** a person who has become dependent on narcotics **n analgesics** pain killing drugs used in the treatment of pain. They diminish perception of pain by combining with pain receptors on brain cells and block transmission of pain signals **n antagonist** a drug used in the treatment of narcotic-induced respiratory depression, such as nalorphine and naloxone **n poisoning** poisoning by narcotics which cause depression, decreased heart rate and respiration, sleep and coma

naris (na'ris) nostril; anterior opening of nose on either side of the nasal cavity, pl. **nares**

narrate (na-rat) to give an account of or to tell

narration act of telling

narrowing decreasing in the diameter of a space or a vessel

nasal (na'zal) relating to the nose **n bleeding** epistaxis **n bone** either of two small bones forming the arch of the nose **n**

cannula low flow oxygen delivery system which protrude 1 cm into both nares and are held in position by a head strap **n catheter** low flow oxygen delivery device which is of rubber or polyvinylchloride catheter inserted to a level just below the soft palate **n CPAP** application of continuous positive airway pressure to nose through tightly fitting mask to prevent airway collapse **n cartilage** any of the cartilages forming the framework of the external nose **n cavity** one of a pair of cavities that open on the face through the pear-shaped anterior nasal aperture and communicate with the pharynx **n cycle** alternating congestion and decongestion of the nasal airway **n discharge** discharge from the nose. It may be thin, watery (coryza), mucopurulent or purulent (infections) or blood stained **n flaring** outward movement of nostrils with each inspiration indicative of increased work of breathing **n obstruction** obstruction to nasal passage from atresia, adenoids, foreign body, polyp deviated nasal septum or growths **n packing** the filling of nasal cavities with aseptic gauze **n prongs** low flow oxygen delivery devices that are simple and comfortable to the patient, though FiO_2 can't be well controlled **n polyp** chronic inflammatory pedunculated growth of nasal mucosa **n septum** central cartilage partition inside the nose **n sinus** any one of the numerous cavities in various bones of the skull. It is lined with ciliated mucous membrane continuous with that of the nasal cavity. The nasal sinuses consist of frontal sinuses, ethmoidal air cells, sphenoidal sinuses and maxillary sinus **n speculum** bivalved instrument to examine the nasal vestibule **n swab** a specimen of mucus taken from the nose with a sterile cotton tipped stick called a swab **n voice** change in tone of voice due to diseases of nose and nasopharynx

nasalis (nazal'is) one of the three muscles of the nose divided into a transverse part and an alar part

nascent (nas'ent) just beginning to exist; just born **n oxygen** oxygen that has just been liberated from a chemical compound

nasion (na'ze-on) 1. a point on the skull which corresponds to middle of the nasofronta! suture 2. the depression at the roof of the nose

naso – a combining word for - relating to the nose.

nasoantral (na'zo-an'tral) relating to the nose and maxillary (antrum) sinus

nasoendoscopy rigid or flexible endoscope to visualise areas of nose which are inaccessible for direct visualisation

nasofrontal (na'zo-fro'n-tal) relating to nasal and frontal bones

nasogastric (na'zo-gas'trick) connection of the nose down the oesophagus into the stomach **n feeding** introduction of liquid nutrients directly into the stomach *via* a nasogastric tube **n intubation** placement of a nasogastric tube through the nose into the stomach to relieve gastric distension, to instil medication, food or fluids or to obtain a specimen for gastric analysis, and as a post-operative procedure **n suction** the removal by suction of solids, fluids or gases from the gastro-intestinal tract through a nasogastric tube **n tube** a narrow plastic or rubber tube that is passed through the nose down oesophagus and into the stomach to introduce fluids into or remove secretions from the stomach

nasolabial (na'zo-la'beal) relating to the nose and the upper lip **n reflex** a sudden backward movement of the head, arching of the back and extension and stretching of the limbs that occur in infants in response to a light touch to the tip of the nose and the reflex disappears by the age of 5 months

nasolacrimal (na'zo-lak'ri-mal) relating to the nasal cavity and lacrimal appara-

tus **n duct** a channel that carries tears from the lacrimal sac to the nasal cavity **n groove** a groove on the nasal surface of the upper jaw, which is the site of the nasolacrimal duct **n reflex** reflex secretion of tears produced by stimulation of nasal mucosa by irritating substances

nasology (na'zo-l'o-je) study of nose and its diseases

nasomental reflex a reflex elicited by tapping the side of the nose. There is contraction of mentalis muscle with elevation of the lower lip and wrinkling of the skin of the chin

nasopharyngeal (na'zo-fah-rin'je-al) relating to the nose or nasal cavity and the pharynx **n angiofibroma** a benign tumour of the nasopharynx, noted in puberty presenting with nasal and eustachian tube obstruction, adenoidal speech and dysphagia **n cancer** a malignant condition of nasopharynx which may present with nasal obstruction, otitis media, hearing loss, bony destruction of the skull and lymphadenopathy

nasopharyngitis (na'zo-far-in-ji'tis) inflammation of the nasopharynx

nasopharyngoscope an electrically-lighted instrument for examining the throat and larynx

nasopharynx (na'zo-far'inks) the part of the pharynx above the soft palate which opens above into the nasal cavity; back of the throat

nasopharyngolaryngoscopy instrumentation to get the view of the larynx and laryngopharynx and to demonstrate the lesions

nasopharyngoscopy use of rigid or flexible nasopharyngoscope to visualise lesions of nasopharynx and to obtain biopsy for diagnosis

nasoscope (na'zo-skop) an electrically lighted instrument to inspect the nasal cavity

nasosinusitis (na'zo-si'nu-si'tis) inflammation of the nasal cavities and of the accessory sinuses

Nasse's law refers to X-linked inheritance wherein only males are affected by condition transmitted by females, described by Nasse, German physician

nasus (na'sus) nose

nasya karma (s) errhine therapy, treatment by nasal insufflation

natal (na'tal) relating to birth; relating to the buttocks **n teeth** teeth in some neonates in the position of central incisors in the lower jaw or there can be early eruption of deciduous teeth

natality (na'tal'i-te) the birth rate in any community

nates (na'tez) the buttocks; breech; upper two corpora quadrigemina.

native (na'tiv) inborn, innate; normal to a location

National Academy of Medical Sciences NAMS a multidisciplinary body catering to highest talent of the country in various disciplines of medicine

National Board of Examination NBE an autonomous body conducting postgraduate and higher examinations in various disciplines of medical sciences of high and uniform standard at the national level. Successful candidates are awarded 'Diplomate of National Board'

National Health Policy policy of Government of India enunciated in 1983 stressing preventive, promotive, public health and rehabilitation of aspects of health care

National Health Programmes Government of India has undertaken several measures to improve the health of the people through various health programmes such as National malaria eradication programme, National filaria control programme, National leprosy eradication programme, National tuberculosis programme, Diarrhoeal disease control programme, Acute respiratory disease control programme, Guineaworm eradication programme, Japanese encephalitis control programme, iodine deficiency disorders programme, Kala-azar control programme, STD control programme, National programme for control of blindness, National cancer control programme, National mental health programme, National diabetes control programme, Child survival and safe motherhood programme, Universal immunisation programme, National family welfare programme, National water supply and sanitation programme, Minimum needs programme, 20-point programme and AIDS control programme

National Institutes of Health NIH the major federal agency supporting medical research in the US, located in Bethesda, Maryland

natraemia (nah'tre'me-a) presence of sodium in the circulating blood

natrium (na'tre-um) sodium

natriuresis (na'tre-u-re'sis) increased urinary elimination of sodium

natriuretic (na'tre-u-ret'ik) agent increasing urinary elimination of sodium

natural (nat'u-ral) true to life **n antibody** an antibody present in the circulation without known previous exposure to the antigen such as antibodies to the ABO group **n carcinogen** a substance that is normally present in foods which may be carcinogenic **n childbirth** techniques to facilitate a woman to give birth with a minimum medical intervention **n dentition** the entire array of natural teeth in the dental arch **n immunity** an innate and permanent form of immunity to a specific disease **n killer cells**, NK cells, large granular lymphocytes with a high cytoplasmic: nuclear ratio and an intrinsic non-antibody mediated ability to kill various cells **n selection** the genotypes best adapted to their environment have a tendency to survive; Darwinism

nature innate dispositoin

naturopath (na'tur-o-path) a practitioner of natural healing who utilises natural methods such as diet, air, sun and water to treat diseases.

naturopathy (na'tur-op'ah-the) a system of healing that espouses the philosophy that disease is the result of violation of natural laws of living

Naughton test treadmill test of cardiac function, to assess effort tolerance

nauli (s) an exercise in yoga for cleansing the bowel

nausea (naw'se-a) an unpleasant sensation of impending desire to vomit. It is usually associated with salivation, inhibition of gastric peristalsis and rise in the tone of the duodenum and proximal jejunum

nauseant (naw'se-ant) an agent causing nausea

navel (na'vel) umbilicus; a small depression in the middle of abdomen

navicular (nah-vik'u-lar) boat-shaped **n bone** scaphoid bones in the carpus and tarsus **n fossa** terminal dilatation of male urethra within glans **n cells** glycogen-rich squamous cells seen in the papanicolaou-stained cytological preparations of the vagina and cervix, seen in great numbers in pregnancy and early menopause **n pads** tarsal supports for flat feet

NBE National Board of Examination; nonbacterial endocarditis

Nd chemical symbol for neodymium

Nd-YAG laser neodymium-yttrium, aluminium garnet laser, a photocoagulation unit used in control of gastrointestinal bleeding

near death experience the subjective observations of individuals who have either close to clinical death or who may have recovered after having been declared dead

near drowning a situation in which the person has survived exposure to circumstances that usually cause drowning

nearsighted able to see the objects clearly when held close to the eyes; myopic

nearthrosis (ne'ar-thro'sis) a new joint following total joint replacement; an abnormal articulation developing after a non-united fracture

nebula (neb'u-lah) a faint corneal opacity; cloudiness in urine

nebulous indistinct

nebulisation (neb'ul-i-za'shun) production of particles such as a spray or mist from liquid

nebuliser (neb'u-liz'er) a device which makes liquid medication into an extremely fine mist or aerosol, which is administered through a face mask **ultrasonic n** an aerosol produced by vibrating ultrasonic transducer under water

Necator (ne-ka'tor) hookworm; cold murderer *N. americanus* a new world nematode that resembles *Ankylostoma duodenale*, but shorter and slender

necatoriasis (ne-ka'tor-i-asis) hookworm disease caused by *Necator americanus*

neck (nek) constricted structure of the body between the head and shoulders; the region between the crown and the root of tooth **bull n** marked swelling of the neck due to massive lymphadenopathy or subcutaneous emphysema **n dissection** surgical removal of the cervical lymph nodes. It is undertaken to prevent the spread of malignant tumours of the head and neck **n movements** from a neutral position with head erect and chin drawn in, right and left rotation, flexion, extension and lateral bending movements are possible **n of femur** the portion of the femur between the hand and the greater and lesser trochanters **n pulsations** pulsations in the neck, arterial or venous **n rigidity** an inability to flex and turn the neck as in meningitis, tetanus and disorders of cervical vertebrae **n stiffness** resistance to the movement of the neck by spasm in the extensor muscles of the neck due to meningeal irritation or diseases of cervical spine **n veins** jugular veins which communicate directly with the right atrium

neck face syndrome a transient clinical manifestation showing oropharyngeal spasms, dysarthria, tachycardia and hypertension following commencement of chlorpromazine therapy

necro – a combining word for death

necrobiosis (nek-ro-bi-o'sis) gradual degeneration of cells or tissues **n lipoidica** reddish-yellow shiny plaques on shins, with atrophy and telangiectasia, often associated with diabetes mellitus

necrobiotic nodule least common pulmonary manifestations of rheumatoid arthritis. It is characterised by a central area of fibrinoid necrosis surrounded by a zone of chronic inflammatory cells and a variable number of fibroblasts. Symptoms occur when the nodule undergoes liquefaction and forms a cavity or get infected

necklace (nek'las) an encircling band around the neck **Casal's n** an area of hyperpigmentation around the neck in pellagra **n of venus** rash around the neck with hyperpigmentation in secondary syphilis **n pattern** annular distribution of lesions seen in AIDS-related Kaposi sarcoma

necrectomy (nek-rek'to-me) surgical removal of any necrosed tissue

necrocytosis (nek'ro-si-to'sis) abnormal death of cells

necrologist (nek'ro-lo-gist) one who compiles a list of people who have died

necrology (ne-karol'o-je) study of the causes of death; mortality statistics

necrolysis (ne-krol'i-sis) necrosis and separation of tissue

necrophilia (nek'ro-fil'e-a) a morbid liking to be in company of dead bodies; an impulse to have sexual contact with a dead body

necropsy (nek'rop-se) autopsy.

necrose (nek'ros) to undergo necrosis

necrosis (ne-kro'sis) death of cells, tissue or organ within living body **anaemic n** necrosis following deficient blood supply **aseptic n** occurring without infection **caseous n** necrosis with cheesy material **central n** necrosis occurring only in the central part **coagulation n** occurrence of coagulation in necrotic

area due to lack of blood supply **colliquative n** necrosis caused by liquefaction of tissues **fat n** necrosis in fatty tissue **fibrinoid n** not a true necrosis, but a homogeneous, granular eosinophilic material seen in necrotising vasculitis **liquefactive necrosis** necrosis that occurs during abscess formation caused by enzymatic degradation **pathergic n** dissolution of tissue without apparent cause as in Wegener's granulomatosis. **putrefactive n** necrosis by bacterial decomposition

necrotic (ne-kro'tic) relating to death of a portion of tissue

necrotising (nek'roti-zing) causing the death of tissues **n enterocolitis** a disease of premature infants affecting the terminal ileum characterised by abdominal distension, vomiting, gangrene, sepsis and perforation, less common in breast-fed children **n vasculitis** an inflammatory condition of blood vessels characterised by necrosis, fibrosis and proliferation of the inner layer of the vessel wall

nedocromil an anti-inflammatory agent that inhibits immediate and late broncho-constriction provoked by inhaled allergen or by exercise when administered 10 to 15 minutes prior to provocation

needle (ne'd'l) a slender, sharply pointed instrument used for suturing, ligaturing or puncturing **n aspiration** removal of material from a clinically or radiologically identified mass by aspirating it through a hollow needle attached to a syringe **n biopsy** removal of a piece of tissue for examination by cutting it out with a wide-bore hollow needle **n holder** a surgical forceps to hold and pass a suturing needle through tissue **needle-stick injury** accidental puncture by the needle

nef a human immunodeficiency virus gene that encodes the regulatory protein *nef*.

negative (neg'a-tiv) 1. numerical value less than zero 2. an absence or not present **n anxiety** *psy* an emotional state in which anxiety prevents a normal functioning **n feedback** a decrease in function in response to a stimulus **n identity** the assumption of a person that is at odds with the accepted values of the society **n pressure** less than ambient atmospheric pressure **n reinforces** *psy* a stimulus that when presented immediately after a behaviour decreases the probability of its recurrence **n relationship** an inverse relationship between two variables **n sign** minus sign (–) used in subtraction and to indicate a lack **n study** investigation in which only negative results are obtained **n symptom** in the process of a disorder certain symptoms may not be present in the patient, but still their absence is to be recorded

negativism (neg'ath-tiv-izm) performing opposite of what is asked

neglect (neg-lek't) to treat carelessly; failure to provide minimal physical and emotional care

negligence (neg'li-jens) the failure to exercise ordinary, reasonable, usual or expected care, resulting in harm or injury to patients; carelessness

Negri (na'gre) **bodies** inclusion bodies in the cytoplasm of nerve cells in rabies, named after Adelchi Negri, Italian pathologist. They are seen in large numbers in the hippocampal gyrus, Purkinje cells of the cerebellum and the pyramidal cells

Neisseria (nis-se're-a) gram-negative cocci occurring in pairs with the adjacent sides flattened named after Albert Neisser, Polish dermatologist **N. gonorrhoeae,** gonococcus gram-negative, non-motile, diplococcus which appear as flattened pairs within the cytoplasm of neutrophils. **n meningitidis** meningococcus non-motile, gram-negative diplococcus frequently found in the nasopharynx

NEJM abbreviation for New England Journal of Medicine

Nelaton (na-la-ton) **line** when a line is drawn from the anterior superior iliac spine to the ischial tuberosity when a patient lies on his side with hip semiflexed; it normally passes across the tip of greater trochanter. If there is shortening in the head or neck of the femur or dislocation upwards of the head the top of trochanter will be above this line, described by Auguste Nelaton, Paris surgeon

Nelson's syndrome bilateral adrenalectomy may be followed after a few years by enlargement of the pituitary, pressure effects on optic chiasma and raised intracranial pressure and increased pigmentation, named after Donald Nelson, US physician

nema – a prefix meaning pertaining to a thread

-nema a suffix meaning pertaining to a thread-like stage in the development of chromosomes

nemathelminthes (nem'ah-thel-min'thez) nematode worms

nemathelminthiasis (nem'ah-thel'minthi'ah-sis) infestation by nematodes

nematocide (nemat'i-sid) agent that kills nematodes

nematode (nem'ah-tod) parasitic worms such as intestinal and filarial round worms

nematology (nem'a-tol'o-je) the division of parasitology that deals with the study of nematodes

neo- a prefix meaning 'new'

neocerebellum (ne'o-ser'e-bel'um) the large lateral portion of the cerebellar hemisphere; little brain

neocortex (ne'o-kor'teks) most recent evolution of cerebral cortex except hippocampus and incus

neodymium (ne'o-dim'e-um) Nd, one of the rare earth elements, atomic weight 144.

neogenesis (ne'o-jen'e-sis) regeneration, as of tissue

neolalism (ne'o-lal'izm) coining new words that are meaningless

neolithic (ne'o-li'thik) of the new stone age

neologism new words created by the patient often combining syllabus of other words

neomembrane a thin sheet of reactive fibrous tissue overlying a chronic subdural haematoma

neomycin (ne'o-mi'sin) aminoglycoside antibiotic used topically and for gut sterilisation

neonatal (ne'o-na'tal) newborn, period from birth to first 28 days of life **n convulsion** twitching of a limb and fluttering of the eyelids and not an obvious major fit as the neurones are not mature **n death** the death of a liveborn infant during the first 28 days after birth **n hepatitis** diseases affecting the newborn hepatic parenchyma associated with raised levels of conjugated hyperbilirubinaemia **n intensive care unit** a ward providing intensive medical care to the infants with a 24-hour availabiltiy of trained medical personnel, monitoring devices, continuous assessment of vital functions, equipment for resuscitation, respiratory therapy, drugs and full laboratory coverage **n mortality** infant death during the first 28 days after live birth, expressed as the number of such deaths for 1000 live births in a specific region in a given time **n myasthenia** swallowing difficulty and generalised hypotonia in the first few weeks following birth in infants born to mothers with myasthenia **n ophthalmia** inflammation of the eye in a newborn from an infection acquired during the birth process

neonate (ne'o-nat) a neonatal infant; a new-born child from birth upto four weeks of age

neonatologist (ne'o-na-tol'o-jist) a specialist in neonatology

neonatology (ne'o-na-tol'o-je) the medical speciality concerned with the study, care and treatment of disorders of the neonate

neopathy (ne-op'a-the) a new disease

neophilism (ne'o-fil-izm) abnormal love of new persons, things and scenes

neophobia (ne'o-fo'bi-a) dread of novelty

neoplasia (ne'o-pla'ze-a) the pathologic process resulting in the formation and growth of a neoplasm

neoplasm (ne'o-plazm) a tumour; an abnormal growth serving no function **benign n** a localised growth that does not spread by metastases or infiltration **malignant n** tumour that infiltrates and spreads by metastasis

neoplasty (ne'o-plas-te) surgical restoration of parts

neoplastic (ne'o-plas'tik) pertaining to neoplasia or containing a neoplasm

neostigmine (ne'o-stig'min) a cholinergic agent to improve muscle function in myasthenia gravis

neostriatum (ne'o-stri-a'tum) the caudate nucleus and putamen

neovascularisation capillary ingrowth and endothelial proliferation

nephelopia (nefe-lo'pe-a) cloudy vision

nephralgia (ne'fral'je-a) renal pain

nephrectasia (nef'rek-ta'ze-a) dilatation of the pelvis of the kidney

nephrectomy (ne-frek'to-me) surgical removal of the kidney

nephritic syndrome haematuria, oliguria and hypertension

-nephric (nef'rik) a suffix meaning pertaining to the kidney; nephritic

nephritic (nef'tik) pertaining to an inflammation of the kidney

nephritis (ne-fri'tis) inflammation of the kidneys

nephritogenic (ne-frit'o-jen'ik) causing nephritis

nephro- prefex referring to the kidney

nephroblastoma (nef'ro-blas-to'ma) Wilm's tumour, rapidly growing tumour of the kidney that occurs in children

nephrocalcinosis (nef'ro-kal'si-no'sis) diffusely scattered calcification in the kidneys

nephrogenic (nef'ro-jen'ik) capable of giving rise to renal tissue; originating in the kidney **n ascites** accumulation of fluid in the peritoneal cavity of patients undergoing haemodialysis for renal failure **n diabetes insipidus** condition in which the renal tubules are unresponsive to ADH and presents with polyuria and polydipsia

nephrogram (nef'ro-gram) radiograph of the kidney following intravenous injection of a radiopaque substance.

nephrography (ne-frog'ra-fe) radiography of the kidneys obtained after intravenous injection of contrast medium

nephroid (nef'roid) resembling a kidney

nephrolith (nef'ro-lith) a renal calculus

nephrolithiasis (nef'ro-li-thi'a-sis) the presence of calculi in the kidneys or the urinary passages. It is characterised by the combination of renal colic with haematuria, presence of stones in the urine or radiologic visualisation of the stone

nephrolithotomy (nef'ro-li-thot'o-me) incision into the kidney to remove a stone

nephrology (ne-frol'-je) the branch of medical science concerned with renal disorders

nephroma (ne-fro'ma) a tumour arising from the renal tissue

nephromegaly (nef'romeg'a-le) hypertrophy of one or both kidneys

nephron (nef'ron) the microscopic functional unit of the kidney consisting of the renal corpuscle (a glomerulus enclosed within Bowman's capsule) and the tubule (proximal convoluted tubule, loop of Henle and distal convoluted tubule) that filter waste products from the blood and regulate the excretion of salts and water in the urine. Each kidney has one million nephrons

nephropathy (ne-frop'a-the) any disease of the kidney **diabetic n** a major com-

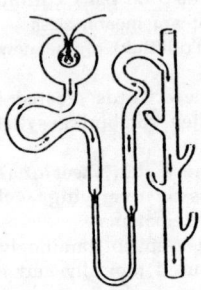

Nephron

plication of diabetes, that leads to end-stage renal failure. It is caused by diabetic microvascular disease. There is glomerulosclerosis with basement membrane thickening and increased mesangial matrix **IgA n** a form of glomerulonephritis occurring in young adult males. There is mesangial cell proliferation and presents with recurrent haematuria and renal failure

nephropexy (nef'ro-pek'se) surgical fixation of a floating kidney

nephroptosis (nef'rop-to'sis) prolapse of the kidney

nephropyosis (nef'ro-pi-o'sis) suppuration of the kidney

nephrorrhapy an operation that fixes a floating kidney in place

nephrosclerosis (nef'ro-skle'ro-sis) scarred contracted kidney, commonly seen in arteriosclerotic kidneys

nephrosis (ne-fro'sis) nephrotic syndrome wherein there is a non-inflammatory derangement of glomerular function characterised by an increased glomerular leak with loss of albumin

nephrostomy (ne-fros'to-me) introduction of a small tube into the kidney to drain urine to the abdominal surface bypassing the ureter; the procedure is done to facilitate healing of the ureter after surgery

nephrotic (ne-frot'ik) **syndrome** a condition characterised by hypoalbuminaemia, hyperlipidaemia, oedema and hypercoagulability resulting from increased glomerular permeability to protein leading to massive proteinuria (3.5 g in 24 h)

nephrotomy (ne-frot'o-me) surgical incision of the kidney

nephrotoxic (nef'ro-tok'sik) toxic to the kidney

nephrotoxin (nef'ro-tok'sin) a toxin with specific destructive properties for the kidneys

nephroureterectomy (nef'ro-u're-ter-ek'to-me) surgical removal of a kidney and its urreter

nephroureterolithiasis (nef'ro-u're-ter-o-lithi'asis) the presence of calculi in the kidneys and ureters

nerve (nerv) a whitish cord consisting of fibres held together by a connective tissue that transmits electrochemical messages back and forth between the brain and spinal cord and other parts of the body (*see* Table 8) **afferent n** a nerve that conducts sensory impulses from receptors to the central nervous system **efferent n** a nerve that conducts motor impulses from CNS to the effector organs and tissues **mixed n** nerve containing both sensory and motor fibres **n block** injection of a narcotic into or around a nerve to produce loss of sensation in a part of the body supplied by that nerve **n cell** the basic unit of the nervous system that detects sensory information and transmits it from one part of the body to another **n compression** pressure on a nerve to cause its damage and muscle weakness **n conduction studies** non-invasive method to assess a nerve's ability to carry an impulse. It provides information on latency periods and conduction velocities **n ending** the termination of a nerve fibre in a peripheral structure. **n entrapment** mononeuropathy characterised by nerve damage and muscle weakness or atrophy. Repeated compression of peripheral nerve trunks are vulnerable to entrapment as in carpal tunnel syndrome **n excitability** the readiness of a nerve cell to respond to a stimulus **n fibre** axon of a neuron which may be myelinated or unmyelinated **n impulse** the electrochemical process involved in neural transmission **n plexus** an interwoven network of nerves such as brachial or lumbar plexus **n sheath** coverings for nerve fibre

Table 8 Nerves

Accessory n	eleventh cranial nerve has two roots - cranial and spinal arising from a nucleus in the floor of fourth ventricle along glossopharynegeal and vagus nerves and the upper portion of the spinal cord. The cranial branch emerging from the medulla joins the vagus nerve contributing sensory innervation to the palate, pharynx and larynx. The spinal accessory supplies upper part of the trapezius and sternomastoid muscle
'Abducent n	sixth cranial nerve arises from the nucleus situated in the floor of the fourth ventricle at the level of pons, and emerges between the pons and medulla, runs through cavernous sinus and enters orbit to supply lateral rectus, has a very long intracranial course, making it vulnerable to the effects of pressure

Alveloar - superior	originates from maxillary nerve by anterior, middle and posterior branches, supplies upper jaw, teeth and maxillary sinus
Alveolar - inferior	branch from mandibular nerve, supplies teeth and gums of lower jaw, skin of chin and lower lip, motor to myelohyoid and anterior belly of digastric, branches are inferior dental, mental, gingival and muscular
Anococcygeal	originates from coccygeal plexus, supplies sacro-coccygeal joint, coccyx and skin over coccyx
Auditory n	eighth cranial nerve. **Vestibulocochlear n** has two divisions-cochlear concerned with hearing and vestibular with equlibrium. The auditory fibres arise from the cochlear (spiral) ganglion having receptors in spiral organ of cochlea terminate in the dorsal and ventral nuclei situated in the pons. The vestibular fibres arising from vestibular ganglion having receptors in the semicircular canals, ventricle and saccule, terminate in a group of nuclei in the pons and medulla. The secondary auditory tracts after partial decussation end in the inferior colliculi and the medial geniculate bodies. The fibres arising from them pass through internal capsule to the cortical centre for hearing in the first and second temporosphenoid convolusions of the brain. The vestibular fibres are connected with the cerebellum
Auricular - great	origin from cervical plexus, supplies parotid gland, mastoid process and pinna
Auriculotemporal	branch of mandibular nerve, supplies parotid gland, skin of temporal region and tympanic membrane, external acoustic meatus and pinna
Axillary	C5, 6 from posterior cord of brachial plexus, muscular and cutaneous branches supply deltoid and teres minor muscle and skin over back of arm
Buccal	sensory branch from mandibular nerve, supplies skin and mucous membrane of cheek, gums, molar and premolar teeth
Cardiac - superior, middle and inferior cervical	originates from superior cervical, middle cervical and cervicothoracic ganglion, carries sympathetic supply and pain afferents from heart

Cardiac - thoracic	originates from thoracic 2 to 5 sympathetic ganglias supplies heart through plexus formation
Carotid - external and internal	origin from superior cervical ganglion, supplies cranial blood vessels and glands *via* plexuses
Cervical	origin from cervical segments of spinal cord. 8 pairs, upper cervical branches from cervical plexus, lower branches contribute in the formation of brachial plexus
Cervical - transverse	origin from cervical plexus, supplies skin of side and front of neck by its superior and inferior branches.
Ciliary - long	branch of nasociliary nerve of ophthalmic division of trigeminal nerve, supplies dilator pupillae and cornea
Ciliary - short	originates from ciliary ganglion by 10-12 branches, carries sympathetic, parasympathetic and sensory fibres to smooth muscles and eye ball coverings
Cranial n.	There are 12 pairs of cranial nerves and they are classified into three categories depending on their function as sensory, motor and mixed **motor n** oculomotor, trochlear, abducent, and hypoglossal **mixed n** trigeminal, facial, glossopharyngeal, vagus and spinal accessory **sensory n** olfactory, optic and auditory. The cranial nerves have been numbered serially by Roman numerals
Cutaneous nerve of arm	superior lateral, inferior lateral, medial and posterior branches from axillary, radial and medial cord of brachial plexus supplying skin on the medial, lateral and posterior aspects of arm
Cutaneous nerves of forearm	lateral, medial and posterior branches of musculocutaneous nerve, medial cord of brachial plexus and radial nerve respectively supply corresponding areas of fore arm for general sensation
Cutaneous nerves of calf	lateral and medial branches of common fibular and tibial nerve supplies lateral and posterior aspects of leg.
Cutaneous nerves of thigh	Lateral - arises from lumbar plexus. Supplies front and lateral side of thigh and calf
Cutaneous nerves of thigh	posterior - arises from sacral plexus. Supplies skin of buttock, genitalia and back of thigh and calf
Dorsal nerve of clitoris	a branch from pudendal nerve, supplies deep trans-

verse muscle of perineum, sphincter urethrae muscle, skin, prepuce and glans of clitoris

Dorsal nerve of penis — a branch from pudendal nerve, supplies deep transverse muscle of perineum, sphincter urethrae muscle, skin, prepuce and glans of penis

Dorsal scapular — branch of brachial plexus, motor supply of rhomboid and levator scapulae muscle

Ethmoidal nerves — anterior and posterior – branches from nasociliary of ophthalmic nerve supplies upper part of nasal septum, nasal cavity, ethmoidal and sphenoidal air sinuses, skin of the nose

Facial n — seventh cranial nerve. The motor fibres take their origin from the nucleus situated in the lower part of the pons lateral to that of the abducent nerve, and emerge at pontomedullary junction. It enters the internal auditory meatus along auditory nerve and reach geniculate ganglion. The nerve pursues its course in the facial canal close to middle ear emerges through the stylomastoid foramen and divides into many branches to supply all the muscles of facial expression except levator palpabrae. It gives branch to platysma and stapedius muscle

the secretomotor fibres in the greater superficial petrosal nerve supply lacrimal, submandibular, and sublingual salivary glands

the taste sensation from the anterior two thirds of the tongue is carried by the lingual nerve and the taste fibres leave and go in the chorda tympani which join the facial nerve and reach geniculate ganglion. The axons from the ganglia pass along the facial nerve (nervous intermedius) and reach medulla and terminate in the tractus solitarius. Sensations from the skin of external auditory meatus and part of pinna are also carried by sensory part of the facial nerve

Femoral — originates form lumbar plexus, supplies skin of the thigh and leg, hip and knee joints and muscles of front of thigh by its muscular, articular and cutaneous branches

Frontal — branch of ophthalmic division of trigeminal nerve, divides into supratrochlear and supraorbital nerve for sensory innervation of forehead and scalp

Genitofemoral — origin from lumbar plexus, divides into genital and femoral branches to supply cremaster muscle and skin of scrotum or labium majus and thigh

Glossopharyngeal n	ninth cranial nerve. Takes its origin in an elongated nucleus in the medulla in the floor of fourth ventricle and emerges by several roots along the lateral aspect of the medulla and leave the skull through the jugular foramen along accessory nerve. The nerve innervates stylopharyngeus muscle and middle constrictor of the pharynx. The sensory fibres carry sensation from the upper part of the pharynx and taste as well as somatic sensations from the posterior third of tongue, through tympanic, pharyngeal, tonsillar and lingual branches
Gluteal - inferior	origin from sacral plexus, supplies gluteus maximus muscle
Gluteal - superior	origin from sacral plexus, supplies gluteus medius, gluteus minimus, tensor fascia lata and hip joint.
Gliohypogastric	origin from lumbar plexus (L_1) supplies skin above pelvis and lateral side of buttock by its lateral and anterior branches, may supply pyramidalis muscle also
Glioinguinal	origin from lumbar plexus (L_1) passes through inguinal canal to supply skin of scrotum, labia-majora and thigh by its anterior scrotal or labial branches
Infraorbital	continuation of maxillary division of trigeminal, branches are middle and anterior superior alveolar, inferior palpebral, internal and external nasal and labial to supply upper incisor, premolars, skin and conjunctiva of lower eye lid, nose, part of septum, skin of upper lip and mucous membrane of mouth
Infratrochlear	branch of nasociliary from ophthalmic supplies skin of root of nose, lower eye lid, conjunctiva and lacrimal duct
Intercostobrachial	formed by second and third intercostal nerves, supplies skin on posterior and medial aspects of arm
Intermedius of facial	parasympathetic and special sensory root of facial supplying lacrimal, palatine, submandibular and sublingual glands and anterior 2/3rd of tongue through greater petrosal and chorda tympani branches
Interosseous of forearm - anterior	branch of median nerve, supplies flexor pollicis longus, flexor digitorum profoundus, pronator quadratus muscles and wrist and intercarpal joints
Interosseous of forearm - posterior	branch of radial nerve, supplies abductor pollicis longus, extensors of thumb and index finger, wrist and intercarpal joints

Interosseous of leg	branch of tibial nerve, supplies interosseous membrane and inferior tibiofibular joint
Lacrimal	branch of ophthalmic division of trigeminal, supplies lacrimal gland, conjunctiva and skin of upper eye lid
Laryngeal – external	motor branch of superior laryngeal nerve to supply cricothyroid and inferior constrictor muscle
Laryngeal – internal	sensory branch of superior laryngeal nerve to supply mucosa of epiglottis, base of tongue and larynx
Laryngeal - recurrent	branch of vagus nerve, supplies intrinsic muscles of larynx by its inferior branch and mucosa of trachea and oesophagus, contributes in formation of cardiac plexus
Laryngeal – superior	origin from inferior ganglion of vagus, supplies cricothyroid muscle, inferior constrictor, mucous membrane of posterior part of tongue and larynx by its external and internal branches
Lingual	sensory branch of mandibular nerve, supplies anterior 2/3 of tongue and adjacent areas of mouth and gums
Lumbar	origin from lumbar segments of spinal cord, 5 pairs, ventral branches of these nerves contributes in formation of lumbo-sacral plexus
Mandibular	*see* trigeminal n
Masseteric	branch of mandibular nerve, supplies masseter muscle
Maxillary	*see* trigeminal n
Median	origin from lateral and medial cord of brachial plexus (C_6-T_1) supplies skin of hand, flexor muscles of front of forearm, short muscles of the thumb and elbow joint
Mental	continuation of inferior alveolar nerve supplies skin of chin and lower lip
Musculocutaneous	origin from lateral cord of brachial plexus (C_5-C_7) supplies coracobrachialis, biceps brachialis, skin of forearm and elbow joint
Nasociliary	branch of ophthalmic division of trigeminal nerve supplies ethmoidal air sinuses by ethmoidal branches and skin of upper eyelid by infratrochlear branch gives long ciliary branch to supply sclera of eye ball and a communicating branch to ciliary ganglion
Nasopalatine	parasympathetic and sensory branch from pterygopalatine ganglion, supplies mucosa and glands of nasal septum and anterior part of hard palate

Obturator	origin from lumbar plexus (L_3-L_4) supplies adductor muscles, gracilis, skin of medial side of thigh and hip joint
Obturator - accessory	origin from lumbar (L_3 and L_4) supplies pectineus muscle and hip joint
Obturator - internal	origin from ventral branches of L_5-S_2 supplies gemellus superior and obturator internus muscle
Occipital - greater	origin from dorsal branch of cervical second, supplies semispinalis capitis and skin of head posteriorly
Occipital - lesser	origin from cervical plexus, sensory supply to skin of medial surface of pinna and adjacent area of head
Occipital - third	arises from dorsal branch of cervical third, supplies skin of back of neck and head
Oculomotor n	third cranial nerve. Takes origin from a series of nuclei in the mid-brain. The nuclei in the front (Edinger-Westphal nucleus) supply parasympathetic innervation to the ciliary muscles and iris and nuclei behind are concerned with innervation to the extraocular muscles. The nerve passes through cavernous sinus, enters the orbit divides into superior, medial and inferior rectus, inferior oblique and levator palpebrae
Ophthalmic	*see* trigeminal nerve
Olfactory n	first cranial nerve, nerve of smell, arises from the sensory cells in the olfactory epithelium located in the upper part of the nasal fossa, consists of 15-20 bundles, pass through cribriform plate of ethmoid, ends in olfactory bulb. The fibres forming the olfactory tract emerge from the olfactory bulb and reach the uncus of hippocampal gyrus (olfactory area) in the cerebral cortex
Optic n	second cranial nerve, nerve of vision. The fibres originate in the retina and pass behind as optic nerve. The nerves of both sides meet at optic chiasma. There is partial decussation and the fibres from the temporal half of the same side and nasal half of the retina of the opposite side emerge as optic tract and terminate in the internal geniculate body. The optic radiation arising from the lateral geniculate body passes through the posterior limb of the internal capsule on either side to reach visual cortex in occipital lobe
Palatine - greater	origin from pterygopalatine ganglion supplies palate

Palatine - lesser	origin from pterygopalatine ganglion, supplies soft palate and tonsil
Perineal	branch of pudendal nerve, supplies bulbospongiosus, ischiocavernosus, bulb of penis, sphincter ani externus, levator ani, superficial transverse perinei and skin of scrotum and labia majora
Petrosal - deep	sympathetic nerve from internal carotid plexus, forms nerve of pterygoid canal with greater petrosal to supply lacrimal, nasal and palatine glands through branches from pterygo-palatine ganglion
Petrosal - greater	branch from geniculate ganglia, joins deep petrosal to form nerve of pterygoid canal, parasympathetic and sensory supply to lacrimal, nasal, palatine glands and nasopharynx through branches from pterygopalatine ganglion
Petrosal - lesser	origin from tympanic plexus, carrying fibres of glossopharyngeal nerve supply parotid gland through auriculotemporal nerve, having parasympathetic post-ganglionic fibres in otic ganglion
Phrenic	origin from cervical plexus (C4-5) supplies diaphragm, pleura, pericardium, peritoneum and a communicating branch to sympathetic plexus
Phrenic - accessory	separate origin and course from cervical fifth, enter the thorax and joins phrenic nerve
Plantar - lateral	origin as terminal branch of tibial nerve, passing through layers of sole muscles supplies intrinsic muscles of sole and gives cutaneous branches to skin of lateral half of sole and fourth and fifth toes
Plantar - medial	origin as larger terminal branch of tibial nerve, supplies intrinsic muscles of the sole of the medial side and cutaneous supply to skin of medial half of sole and first to fourth toe
n of pterygoid canal	formed by union of deep petrosal and greater petrosal nerve carrying sympathetic and parasympathetic fibres, joins pterygopalatine ganglion
Pudendal	origin from sacral plexus (S2-4) supplies muscles, skin and erectile tissue of perineum by its branches inferior rectal, and perineal and dorsal nerve of penis and clitoris
Radial	origin from posterior cord of brachial plexus supplies extensor muscles at the back of the arm and forearm, joints and skin of back of arm, forearm and hand

Rectal - inferior	origin as a branch of pudendal nerve supplies sphincter ani exterior muscle, lower part of anal canal and skin around anus
Sacral	five pairs of sacral nerves arising from sacral segments of spinal cord, contributes in the formation of sacral plexus (S1-4)
Saphenous	termination of femoral nerve supplies skin on medial side of leg and foot, forms subsartorial plexus and supplies knee joint
Sciatic	origin from sacral plexus (L4-S3) divides into common peroneal and tibial nerve
Splanchnic	greater - origin from thoracic sympathetic chain and ganglia (T5-10), ends in coeliac ganglion
	lesser - from sympathetic chain or thoracic ganglion (T9-10) joins coeliac plexus and communicates with renal and superior mesenteric plexuses
	lowest - from last ganglion of sympathetic trunk joins aorticorenal and other plexus. Lumbar from lumbar ganglia, joins coeliac, mesenteric and superior hypogastric plexus. Pelvic - origin from sacral plexus (S3-4) joins inferior hypogastirc plexus and supplies pelvic viscera
	sacral - from sacral part of sympathetic chain, supplies pelvic viscera and blood vessels
Subcostal	ventral branch of spinal nerve T12 supplies transversalis, oblique, rectus abdominis and skin of lower abdomen and lateral part of gluteal region
Suboccipital	origin as dorsal branch of C1 supplies muscles of suboccipital triangle and semispinalis capitis
Subscapular	origin from posterior cord of brachial plexus (C5), two nerves-upper and lower-supplies subscapularis and teres major muscles
Supraclavicular	medial, intermediate and lateral, originate from cervical plexus (C3-4), supplies skin of shoulder, pectoral and deltoid region
Supraorbital	terminal branch of frontal nerve, supplies skin of upper eyelid, forehead, scalp and mucosa of frontal sinus
Suprascapular	origin from upper trunk of brachial plexus supplies supraspinatus, infraspinatus muscles and also to shoulder joint and acromioclavicular joint
Supratrochlear	terminal branch of frontal nerve, supplies skin of forehead and upper eyelid

Sural	formed by union of medial sural and a communicating branch from common peroneal, supplies skin of the back of leg, lateral side of foot and heel
Temporal - deep	branch of mandibular supplies temporal muscle
Thoracic - long	origin from ventral branches of T5-7 of brachial plexus, supplies serratus anterior muscle
Thoracodorsal	origin from posterior cord of brachial plexus (C7-8) supplies latissimus dorsi muscle
Tibial	continuation of sciatic nerve in lower part of thigh, supplies semimembranosus, semitendinosus, biceps, abductor magnus and muscles of calf and sole and toes. Also supplies joints and skin of back of leg, sole and toes
Trigeminal n	fifth cranial nerve. Has a long sensory nucleus extending from the pons to the upper cervical portion of the spinal cord and a small motor nucleus in the pons near the floor of the fourth ventricle. The sensory part has three divisions - ophthalmic, maxillary and mandibular - and carry the sensations from the face, teeth, mouth and nasal cavity and its motor part is related to mandibular division and it innervates the muscles of mastication (pterygoids, masseter, temporalis, tensor tympani and tensor palati)
	Mandibular branch carries sensations from the lower part of the face, the lower lip, ear, tongue and lower teeth. Maxillary branch carries sensations from the cheek, upper lip, lower eyelid and its conjunctiva, side of the nose, mucous membrane of the nose, upper teeth, upper part of the pharynx and tonsils. Ophthalmic branch carries sensations from the upper eyelid and its medial part of the conjunctiva, nose upto the tip, forehead and anterior part of the scalp.
	The sensations carried through the sensory divisions reach the Gasserian (trigeminal) ganglion. The sensory root originating from the ganglion terminates in the brain stem
Tympanic	origin from inferior ganglion of glossopharyngeal, contributes in the formation of tympanic plexus, supply mucous membrane of tympanic cavity, auditory tube and mastoid air cells
Trochlear n	fourth cranial nerve. Arises in the midbrain caudal to the nucleus of oculomotor nerve. The nerve fibres decussate unlike other cranial nerves before it emerges near the roof of the fourth ventricle. It supplies superior oblique muscle of the eye ball

Ulnar	origin form medial cord of brachial plexus (C8-T1) supplies flexor muscles on the front of arm and short muscles of the hand. Also carries sensory fibres from skin of the joint and medial part of hand and 11/2 fingers on medial side
Vagus	tenth cranial nerve arises from the nucleus in medulla in the floor of fourth ventricle and emerges by several rootlets from the lateral side of the medulla and passes through jugular foramen, continues in the neck, thorax and abdomen. It carries sensations from the pharynx and larynx. Motor fibres innervate muscles of the soft palate, pharynx and larynx. The parasympathetic branches supply to the thoracic and abdominal viscera. Branches are superior and recurrent laryngeal, meningeal, auricular, pharyngeal, cardiac and other visceral plexus
Vestibular	part of VIIIth cranial nerve, fibres arise form vestibular ganglion, receptors in semicircular canals, ventricle and saccule of internal ear concerned with sense of equilibration
Vertibulocochlear	see auditory nerve
Vidian	formed by union of deep petrosal and greater petrosal nerve, carries sympathetic and parasympathetic fibres to nasal mucous membrane
Zygomatic	origin as a branch from maxillary nerve, communicates with lacrimal nerve, sensory for skin of temple and adjacent part of face

nervous excited or agitated; relating to a nerve or the nerves **n breakdown** any mental disorder disrupting normal functioning **n system** the extensive, intricate network of structures that activates, co-ordinates and controls the functions of the body. It consists of central nervous system comprising the brain and the spinal cord, and the peripheral nervous system

nervousness a condition of unrest and of irritability

nesidioblastosis the admixture of islets of Langerhans with pancreatic ducts; ductulo-insulin complexes

nest a small mass of cells resembling a bird's nest

nested nails a pair of nails placed side by side in the medullary canal of long bones

net a nest-like structure of interlocking fibres

net reproduction rate of one NRR replacement of a mother by just one living daughter within her reproductive period

netilmycin aminoglycoside active on organisms resistant to gentamicin

nettle rash an urticarial eruption following stinging nettle, a common weed

network 1. an interconnected group or system 2. (network) the connection of two or more computers and printers. It is used to share resources such as documents, programs, and pointers

Neufeld nail an orthopaedic nail with V-shaped tip and shank used to fix an inter-trochanteric fracture, named after Alonzo Neufeld, US surgeon

neuro- relating to the nervous system

neural (nu'ral) relating to nerve cells or its processes **n crest** the dorsal region of the embryonic nervous system that gives rise to the sensory and autonomic nervous systems and melanocytes **n tube** tube in the back of an embryo that develops into the spinal cord and brain **n tube defects** failure of normal development of the spinal cord or brain in an embryo resulting in birth defects such as spina bifida and anencephaly

neuralgia (nu-ral'je-a) severe pain in the course or distribution of a nerve due to irritation or damage to a nerve **glossopharyngeal n** recurrent, paroxysmal intense pain originating in the tonsillar fossa and may radiate to the ear on the same side **occipital n** paroxysmal pain in the occipital, suboccipital and posterior parietal areas on one side due to spontaneous irritation of the greater occipital nerve **postherpetic n** severe burning pain may occur following herpes zoster and persist for a long time **post-traumatic n** occurrence of persistent pain and sensory changes following trauma to a peripheral nerve **temporomandibular n** recurrent unilateral, severe pain originating in one temporomandibular joint and spreading either into the face or into the temporal muscle **trigeminal n** recurrent paroxysmal, brief episodes of intense pain over one side of the face confined to one of the three divisions of trigeminal nerve

neuraminidases (nur'a-min'i-dases) enzymes removing one sialic acid from polysaccharides

neurapraxis (nu'rah-prak'sis) injury to a nerve causing temporary interruption of conduction

neurasthenia (nu'ras-the'ne-a) fatigue accompanying depression; nervous debility

neurectoderm (nu'rek'to-derm) tissues derived from neural tube and neural crest

neurectomy (nu-rek'to-me) excision of a segment of a nerve

neuraxis (nu-rak'sis) brain stem and spinal cord together; cerebrospinal axis

neurilemma (nu'ri-lem'ma) sheath of schwann, the external sheath of a nerve fibre

neurilemmoma (nu'ri-lem-mo-ma) schwannoma, benign encapsulated tumour from cells structurally identical to schwann cells, neurinoma.

neurinoma (nu'ri-no'ma) a tumour of the nerve sheath

neuritis (nu-ri'tis) inflammation of a nerve

neuro - a combining word for nerve or pertaining to nerves

neuroablation the destruction of nerve tissue

neuroanatomy (nu'ro-a-nat'o-me) the anatomy of the nervous system

neuroanaesthesia (nu'r-on'as-the'zhah) anaesthesia for neurosurgery.

neuroarthropathy (nu'ro-ar-throp'a-the) disease of joint combined with disease of CNS

neurobiology (nu'ro-bi-ol'o-je) the biology of the nervous system

neuroblast (nu'ro-blast) an embryonic nerve cell that develops into a neuron

neuroblastoma (nu'ro-blas-to'ma) a malignant tumour with neuroblasts that usually originates in the adrenal medulla. It may also originate in any part of the sympathetic nervous system

neurocanal (nu'ro-ka-nal) the central canal of the spinal cord

neurocheck a brief neurologic assessment.

neurocirculatory (nu'ro-sur'ku-la-to're) pertaining to circulation and the nervous system **n asthenia** a psychosomatic disorder exhibiting irregularities in nervous system and cardiovascular system, often result from or associated with psychologic stress

neurocoele (nu'ro-sel) a system of cavities in the CNS. It consists of ventricles of brain and the central canal of the spinal cord which originated from the neural tube

neurocranium (nu'ro-kra'ne-um) the part of the skull enclosing the brain

neurocrine (nu'ro-krin) a chemical transmitter; an endocrine influence on nerves or *vice versa*

neurocutaneous syndromes diseases affecting the brain, skin, eyes and other systems as in neurofibromatosis, tuberous sclerosis, Von Hipple-Lindau disease, Sturge-Weber syndromes and ataxia-telangiectasia.

neurocysticercosis neurological parasitosis by larvae of *Taenia solium*. It presents with focal or secondary generalised seizure. There may be single small enhancing lesion on the CT scan

neurocyte (nu'ro-sit) nerve cell

neurocytolysis (nu'ro-si-to'ly-sis) destruction of nerve cell

neurodermatitis (nu-ro-der'ma-ti'tis) a chronic indurated and thickened skin lesion often associated with emotional stress

neurodiagnosis (nu'ro-di-ag-no'sis) diagnosis of nervous disorders

neuroectoderm (nu'ro-ek'todurm) the part of the embryonic ectoderm that gives rise to the central and peripheral nervous system

neuroendocrine cells pulmonary endocrine cells situated in contact with the basement membrane throughout different regions of extra- and intrapulmonary airways. Some of the cells reach the lumen with their microvillus projections. The cells contain electron dense membrane bound vesicles in water clear cytoplasm. The vesicles are capable of amine precursor uptake and decarboxylation. Hence considered as APUD cells; Kulchitsky or Feyrter cells

neuroendocrine tumours growth with malignant potential that secrete one or more hormones with neuroendocrine properties. They are derived from embryonic neural crest cells, also called APUD tumours. carcinoids, insulinoma, VIPoma, somatostatinoma, glucagonoma and Zollinger-Ellison syndrome are some examples

neuroepithelial bodies NEB innervated structures found in the intrapulmonary airways that produce neuropeptides

neuroepithelium (nu'ro-ep'i-tho'le-um) epithelial cells receptive to external stimuli

neuroepithelioma (nu'ro-ep'i-tho'le-o'ma) retinoblastoma

neurofibril (nu'ro-fi-bril) filamentous structures in the nerve cell

neurofibrillary tangles microtubule-associated proteins and neurofilaments, seen in Alzheimer's disease

neurofibroma (nu'ro-fi-bro'ma) schwannoma, a benign, non-encapsulated soft tumor due to proliferation of schwann cells; neurilemmoma. It presents with single or multiple nodules of variable size which are freely mobile

neurofibromatosis (nu'ro-fi-bro-ma-to'sis) multiple subcutaneous slow growing soft fibrous swellings that grow from nerves **generalised n** von Recklinghausen's disease, presence of multiple nodules all over the body with pale brown pigmentation of the skin **plexiform n** multiple fibromyxomatous masses hanging down loosely on folds of skin and subcutaneous tissue, usually on the face affecting the branches of trigeminal nerve

neurogenesis (nu'ro-jen'e-sis) formation of nervous tissue

neurogenic (nu'ro-jen'ik) originating in or caused by nervous system **flaccid n bladder** interference with voluntary and reflex control of urinary bladder from segmental lesions at S_2 to S_4 level. There is loss of the sensation of bladder fullness causing 'overflow' incontinence **n fracture** a fracture associated with the destruction of nerve supply to a specific bone **n abdominal pain** burning pain limited to the distribution of peripheral nerve **n arthropathy** painless disorganisation of joint **n claudication** symptoms of dysfunction of cauda equina appear on walking or prolonged standing and subside by rest **n shock** a form of shock resulting from peripheral vasodilation **spastic n bladder** loss of bladder control due to spinal lesion. It is accompanied by urgency, increased frequency decreased functional capacity, and spastic contractions and poor voluntary control

neuroglia (nu-rog′le-a) non-neuronal cellular elements of nervous system

neuroglycopaenia hypoglycaemia with blood glucose level below 50 mg/dL. It manifests as clouding of consciousness, convulsions and coma

neurography (nu′ro-g′rafe) the study of the action potentials of the nerves

neurohypophysis (nu′ro-hi-pof′i-sis) posterior lobe of pituitary, that is the source of antidiuretic hormone (ADH) and oxytocin

neurohormone (nu′ro-hor-mo′ne) a chemical messenger formed by neurosecretory cell such as acetylcholine, dopamine, epinephrine, norepinephrine and serotonin

neuroleptic (nu′ro-lep′tik) an agent causing analgesia, sedation and tranquilization; antipsychotic **n anaesthesia** a form of anaesthesia induced by injection of a butyrophenone derivative with a narcotic analgesic **n malignant syndrome** an acute or subacute reaction to therapy with neuroleptic medications characterized by extrapyramidal muscular rigidity, high core termperature, altered level of consciousness and elevated creatine kinase levels

neurologic (nu′r-o-loj′ik) pertaining to nervous system ı **assessment** an evaluation of the patient's neurologic status and symptoms **n examination** a systematic examination of nervous system which includes an assessment of higher functions, cranial nerves, motor and sensory systems, cerebellar functions and skull and spine, and carotid arteries

neurologist (nu-rol′o-jist) a specialist in neurology

neurology (nu-rol′o-je) the branch of medical science concerned with the nervous system and its disorders

neurolysis (nu-rol′i-sis) destruction of nerve tissue

neuron (nu′ron) a nerve cell arising from cells of nervous system

neuroma (nu-ro′ma) a combing word for a benign tumour of nerve tissue

neuromuscular (nu′ro-mus′ku-lar) referring to nerve and muscle **n blockade** the inhibition of a muscular contraction activated by nervous system **n blocking agent** a chemical substance that interferes locally with the transmission or reception of impulses from motor nerves to skeletal muscles **n junction** the point at which the impulse carried in a motor nerve fibre is transmitted to a muscle fibre, making it contract; motor end plate **n junction disease** *see* myasthenia gravis **n spindle** any one of a number of small bundles of delicate muscle fibres, enclosed by a capsule in which sensory nerve fibres terminate

neuromyasthenia (nu′ro-mias-the′ne-a) muscular weakness often of emotional origin

neuromyelitis (nu′ro-mie-li′tis) inflammation of nerve and spinal cord **n optica** acute demyelination of both optic nerves and large areas of spinal cord; Devic's disease, named after French Physician, Eugene Devic

neuromyopathy (nu′ro-mie′-o-pa-the) a disorder of muscle due to a disease of the nerve that supplies the muscle

neuromyxofibroma semisolid, slowly growing, painless lump that moves horizontally but not vertically which can arise in the vagus, hypoglossal, the sympathetic chain or a cord of brachial plexus

neurone (nu'ron) nerve cell, the basic unit of the nervous system consisting of nerve cell body, the axon and the dendrites **bipolar n** a neurone having one axon and one dendrite **motor n** neurone that transmits nerve impulses from the brain and the spinal cord to the muscles and the glandular tissue **multipolar n** neurone possessing one axon and several dendrites, most neurones in the brain and the spinal cord are examples **sensory n** neurone that transmits nerve impulses toward the spinal cord and the brain **unipolar n** embryonic structure whose dendrites and axons are fused into a single fibre, which after a short distance get separated into the two processes

neuronal (nu'ro-nul) pertaining to a neuron

neuronitis (nu'ro-ni'-tis) inflammation of nerve or a nerve cell especially the cells and roots of the spinal nerves

neuropathic arthropathy grossly distorted joints, *see* Charcot's joints

neuroptic (nu'ro-op'tik) pertaining to the CNS and eye

neuropharmacology (nu'ro-far'-ma-kol'o-je) the branch of pharmacology dealing with the effects of drugs on the nervous system

neuropathology (nu'ro-pa-thol'o-je) pathology of the nervous system

neuropathy (nu-rop'a-the) any disorder affecting any of the peripheral nerves **congenital n** hereditary sensory radicular neuropathy or hypertrophic interstitial neuropathy **entrapment n** compression of a peripheral nerve against bone or tendon. In early stages there is numbness and parasthesia and later a fixed sensory loss and muscle atrophy **peripheral n** non-acute traumatic degeneration of the nerves of the limbs. It includes rapid onset post-infective polyneuritis, slow onset hereditary sensorimotor neuropathy, subacute or chronic distal neuropathy and mononeuropathies **toxic n** tobacco, or alcohol-related amblyopia

neuropeptide biologically active polypeptide that functions as a neurotransmitter released from nerve endings or nerve fibres that innervate the CNS, airways and gastro-intestinal tract

neurophysiology (nu'ro-fiz'e-ol'o-je) physiology of the nervous system

neuroplegia (nu'rop-le'jea) nerve paralysis caused by disease, injury or the effect of neuroleptic drugs

neuropore (nu'p-o-por) the opening at each end of the neural tube during early embryonic development

neuropraxis (nu'ro-prak'sis) interruption of nerve conduction without break of axons

neuropsychiatry (nu'ro-si-ki'a-tre) the branch of medical science dealing with organic and functional diseases of the nervous system

neuroradiology (nu'ro-ra'de-ol'o-je) radiology concerned with the nervous system

neurorrhaphy (nu-ror'a-fe) joining together of a divided nerve by suture

neurosarcoma (nu'ro-sar-coma) a malignant tumour comprising nerve, connective and vascular tissues

neuroscience (nu'r-o-si'ens) the study of neurology and related subjects such as neuroanatomy, neurophysiology, neuropharmacology and neurosurgery

neurosecretion (nu'ro-se-kre'shun) the release of a chemical substance at the axon terminal

neurosecretory granule dense core granule; a round, membrane-bound vesicle surrounded by a clear space, in turn surrounded by a dark thin rim. They contain various hormones such as calcitonin, gastrin, glucagon and VIP

neurosis (nu-ro'sis) an emotional nervous disorder

neurosurgeon (nu-ro-sur'jun) a specialist in neurosurgery

neurosurgery (nu'ro-sur'jer-e) surgery of the nervous system

neurosyphilis (nu'ro-sif'i-lis) syphilitic involvement of the nervous system characterised by tabes dorsalis, and general paralysis of insane

neurotensin a neuropeptide that evokes vasodilation and inhibits gastric secretion and intestinal motility

neurothekoma nerve sheath myoxoma, occurring as a benign neural tumour of childhood affecting dermal-epidermal interface

neurotic (nu-rot'ik) relating to a neurosis

neurotomy (nu-rot'o-me) surgical division of a nerve

neurotonic (nu'ro-ton'ik) stimulating the impaired nervous system

neurotoxic (nu'ro-tok'sik) poisonous to the nervous system

neurotoxin (nu'ro-tok'sin) endotoxin which blocks conduction of the nerve impulse or block synaptic transmission

neurotransmitter (nu'ro-tran's-mi-ter) any chemical mediator released by a presynaptic cell, that is capable of transmitting an electrical impulse

neurotripsy (nu'ro-trip'se) surgical crushing of a nerve

neurotrophy (nu-rot'ro-fe) nutrition of tissue under the influence of nervous system

neurotropic (nu'tro-trop'ik) having affinity for nervous system **n factors** proteins that stimulate growth of nerve cells during normal development of foetus and after injury

neurovascular (nu'ro-vas'ku-lar) relating to the nerves supplying the blood vessels **n syndrome** the neurological syndrome produced by the occlusion of any vessel

neuter neither masculine or feminine

neutral (nu'tral) taking no part on either side; neither acid nor alkaline **n red test** virulent strains of tubercle bacillus are able to absorb phenothiazine dye from a neutral or slightly alkaline aqueous medium. The test helps to measure the virulence of *M. tuberculosis*

neutralisation (nu'tra'liz-ashun) rendering ineffective; change in reaction

neutralise (nu'tral-iz) to make neutral

neutralising antibody an immunoglobulin produced by the host as a defence against bacteria, that is capable of attenuating the infectivity of the microorganism.

neutron (nu-tro-n) particle of mass equal to proton without any charge

neutropaenia (nu-tro-pe'ne-a) an abnormal decrease in the number of neutrophils in the circulating blood **cyclical n** rare disorder showing periodic reduction in neutrophils at 3-4 week intervals **idiopathic benign n** fall in neutrophil count due to migration of neutrophils from circulating pool to the marginating pool. It is not associated with an increased tendency for infections **severe n** marked neutropaenia as a toxic reaction to several drugs or as a part of pancytopaenia

neutrophil (nu'tro-fil) a mature granulocytic white blood cell whose granules exhibit no special affinity to acid or basic dyes. It is responsbile for the body's protection against infection **n leucocytosis** increase in neutrophil count, occurs in many bacterial infections, inflammations, tissue necrosis, myeloproliferative disorders, acute haemorrhage and acute haemolysis

neutrophilia (nu'tro-fil'e-a) an increase in neutrophils in the circulating blood or cells

neutrotaxis (nu'tro-tak'sis) stimulation of the neutrophils by a substance under whose influence they may move towards it or away from it

newborn (nu'born) neonatal

newgrowth a neoplasm or tumour

New York Heart Association Classification a functional classification of dyspnoea as grade I (breathlessness on more than average work), grade II (breathlessness on accustomed work), grade III (breathlessness on less than average work) and grade IV (breathlessness at rest)

nexin a protein that is integral to axonemic structures in cilia and flagella **n links** links which interconnect the peripheral microtubular doublets of the core of axoneme of the cilia and sperm tail

nexus (nek'sus) junction; connection between two cells

Nezelof's syndrome progressively severe recurrent infections noted in infants and children due to absent T cell function, deficient B cell function, fairly normal level of immunoglobulins and failure to produce antibodies, named after C. Nezelof, French physician

ng nanogram

NG tube abbreviation for nasogastric tube

NHL non-Hodgkin's lymphoma

Ni chemical symbol for nickle

niacin (ni'a-sin) nicotinic acid and nicotinamide possessing equal biological potency, a part of Vitamin B complex. **n test** niacin is produced by *M. tuberculosis* hence niacin positive but *M. bovis* is negative

niacinamide (ni-a-sin-am'id) nicotinamide, biologically active form of nicotinic acid

niacytin an unabsorbable form of niacin, found in maize

niche (nich) a recess in a wall; an ulcerated or eroded region

Nicholas procedure a surgical procedure for repairing severe ligamentous injuries to the knee

Nicholson's method to overcome abdominal rigidity, the base of the palm of the left hand is placed upon the lower part of the sternum and increasing pressure is exerted. Eventually the examiner is leaning quite heavily on the chest with the result the patient breaths abdominally. While the patient draws his breath the abdominal muscles show a decrease in their tonicity whereupon the right hand palpates the abdomen, named after Neville Nicholson, English surgeon

nick (nik) break

nickle (nik'el) metal, Ni, atomic weight 58.7 **n dermatitis** an allergic contact dermatitis caused by the metal, nickle

niclosamide anthelminthic effective against tapeworms. It kills the scolex and segments on contact

nicotine (nik'o-ten) a poisonous volatile alkaloid from tobacco **n gum** nicotine polacrilex showing gum **n replacement therapy** use of nicotine gum to attenuate the symptoms of nicotine withdrawal

nicotinic (nik'o-ten'ik) nicotine-like **n acid** an integral part of nicotinamide adenine dinucleotide and its phosphate acts as coenzymes in the metabolic pathways of glucose and proteins. Dietary sources include liver, pulses, whole cereals, fish, meat, groundnuts, milk, and eggs. Daily requirement is 15 mg. Deficiency causes pellagra **n receptors** cholinergic receptors stimulated by nicotine

nictitate (nik-ti-tat) to wink

NICU abbreviation for neonatal intensive care unit

nidana (s) diagnosis and investigation into the causes of disease

nidation (ni-da'shun) embedding

NIDDM non-insulin-dependent diabetes mellitus, *see* diabetes mellitus

nidra (s) sleep

nidus (ni'dus) central point; point of lodgement; focus of infection

Niemann-Pick (ne'man pik) **disease** familial lipoidosis with accumulation of sphingomyelin in different tissues, named after Albert Niemann, German paediatrician and Ludwig Pick, German physician

nifedipine a calcium channel blocker

nigamana (s) conclusion

night the dark hours between sunset and sunrise **n blindness** decreased ability to see in dim light due to defective rod function with delayed dark adaptation and perceptual threshold. It is noted in deficiency of vitamin A, retinitis pigmentosa, late stages of glaucoma, cataract, optic atrophy and in retinal degeneration **n cry** involvement of articular cartilage in tuberculous arthritis causing pain which awakens the child from sleep **n guard** a dental prosthesis worn at night to prevent grinding of the teeth **n mare** a terrifying dream **n palsy** numbness of lower limb **n shade** a wild plant with berries having narcotic property **n soil** faecal material removed during the night **n stick fracture** an undisplaced fracture of the ulnar shaft caused by a direct blow **n sweat** profuse sweating during sleep **n walker** sleep walking; somnambulism

nightfall uncontrolled ejaculation during sleep

nigra black

nigraha (s) control, restraint

nigral (ni'gral) cell nerve cell of substantia nigra

NIH National Institutes of Health, located in Bethesda, Maryland, USA

nihilism (ni'hil-izm) delusion of non-existence; engagement in acts which are destructive

nihilistic delusion false feeling that self, others, or the world is non-existent or ending

nikethamide (ni-keth'a-mid) respiratory stimulant acting on respiratory centre

Nikolsky's (ni-kol'skez) **sign** in pemphigus, the external layer of the skin can be detached from the basal layer by slight friction or injury, named after Petr Nickolsky, Russian dermatologist

NIMHANS National Institute of Mental Health and Neuro-sciences, located in Bangalore

nimodipine (ni-mo-di-pine) calcium antagonist

NIN National Institute of Nutrition, located in Hyderabad

9+2 pattern Nine plus two arrangement. A configuration of nine peripheral microtubular doublets arranged in a circular fashion around a pair of central microtubules enclosed in a sheath, found in the core of the axoneme of cilia and the sperm tail by electron microscopy

nip to cut the edges

nipple (nip'l) papilla; the protuberance at the top of breast through which lactiferous ducts discharge. It contains erectile tissue and surrounded by pigmented areola **n discharge** serous and/or serosanguinous discharge from the breasts in peri- and post-menopausal women **n shield** a device to protect the nipples of a lactating woman **retracted n** a nipple whose tip lies below the level of surrounding skin

niridazole (ni-rid'ah-zol) anthelmintic used against schistosomes

Nirodh male condom

nirodha (s) full restraint

nirvikalpa (s) indeterminate

Nissl (nis'l) **granules** coarse RNA aggregations in cytoplasm of nerve cells which are the site of protein synthesis, named after Franz Nissl, German neurologist

nit an empty egg shell of louse attached to hair or clothing

nitrate (ni'trat) a vasodilator agent

nitric acid HNO_3, a colourless, corrosive liquid

nitric oxide NO, a gas normally produced in the body. It is a vasodilator produced by vascular endothelium

nitrite a salt of nitrous acid, used as a vasodilator and antispasmodic

nitrosamine (ni'tros-a-men) a toxic substance formed in the stomach and intestine from some food preservatives that may be a contributory factor for the development of cancer

nitrofurantoin (ni'tro-fu-ran'to-in) an urinary antiseptic

nitrogen (ni'tro-jen) a gaseous element which forms about 77 parts by weight of atmosphere **n gas** alkylating cytotoxic agent, mustine, war gas **n mustard** alkylating agent used in the treatment of malignant lymphoma

nitrogen balance a crude indicator of the adequacy of nutrition **negative n** loss of nitrogen excess intake as in aging, burns and protein-losing enteropathy **n cycle** the circulation of nitrogen through natural process

nitrogen dilution method a technique for measurement of static lung volumes

nitrogenous (ni-troj'e-nus) relating to or containing nitrogen

nitroglycerin (ni-tro'glis'erin) glycerol trinitrate. An organic nitrate used as a short acting vasodilator agent for the treatment of anginal pain

nitrosamine a carcinogen found in tobacco smoke

nitrosurea (nitro'so'oo-re'a) an alkylating agent used as an antineoplastic drug

nitrous (ni'trus) **oxide** N_2O, laughing gas, first general anaesthetic

niyama (s) rule, discipline

NK cell natural killer cell

NMR abbreviation for nuclear magnetic resonance

NNN Novy, MacNeal and Nicolle culture media for *Leishmania donovani* and *Trypanosoma cruzi*

NNRTI abbreviation for non-nucleoside reverse transcriptase inhibitor

Noble's plication operative procedure to free the peritoneal adhesions and stitching in a zigzag way so that there will not be any obstruction when adhesions recur

Nocardia (no'kar-de-a) a genus of aerobic nonmotile actinomycetes, of which *N. asteroids* and *N. brasiliensis* are pathogenic, named after Edmund-

Nocord, French veterinary pathologist. *Nocardia madurae* organism causes Madura foot

nocardiosis (no-kar-de-o'sis) a disease due to Nocardia involving the lungs and nervous system

noci - relating to injury or pain

nociceptive (no'se-sep'tiv) capable of appreciation or transmission of pain **n reflex** a reflex caused by a painful stimulus **n stimulus** a painful stimulus

nociceptor (no'se-sep'tor) a receptor to appreciate and transmit painful or injurious stimuli, located in periarticular and mucocutaneous regions

nocifensor (no'se-fen'sor) mechanism to protect the body from injury

noct a prefix referring 'to night'

nocte night

noctiphobia (nok'ti-fo'be-a) abnormal fear of night and darkness

nocturia (nok-tu're-a) increased urination at night disturbing a person's sleep. It can be an early symptom in diabetes mellitus, chronic renal insufficiency or early congestive heart failure

nocturnal (nok-tur'nal) pertaining to night or darkness **n emission** ejaculation during sleep often associated with an erotic dream **n enuresis** involuntary urination while asleep at night **n paroxysmal dyspnoea** sudden attacks of breathlessness, sweating, tachycardia and wheezing that awaken the person from sleep, seen in left ventricular failure and pulmonary oedema **n penile tumescence** NPT penile erection that occurs during sleep

nocuous (nok'u-us) harmful, injurious, poisonous

nodal (no'dal) relating to a node **n ectopics** premature beats arising in any part of the atrio-ventricular junctional tissue. The QRS complex is normal, but the P waves are inverted and occur just before, during or just after QRS complex **n osteoarthritis** a distinct form of osteoarthritis occurring predominantly in middle-aged women. It affects the terminal phalangeal joints of the fingers with the development of gelatinous cysts or bony outgrowths on the dorsal aspect of such joints **n rhythm** atrial excitation is retrograde and ECG usually shows an inverted P wave and a heart rate of 40 to 60 per minute. It is associated with sharp cannon waves in the neck **n tachycardia** a rapid discharge of impulses from an ectopic focus in the area of AV node

nodding (nod'ing) involuntary movement of the head downwards

node (nod) a small circumscribed mass of tissue **sinoatrial n** SA node, the intrinsic pacemaker of the heart composed of neural tissue; located at the junction of the superior vena cava with the right atrium and conducts impulses by way of three Purkinje fibre tracts to the atrioventricular nodes **atrioventricular n** AV node, located in the right posterior portion of the interventricular septum which in turn is continuous with the bundle of His

nodular (nod'u-lar) containing or resembling nodules **n adenosis** a benign, well circumscribed lesion of the breast **n fasciitis** an inflammation of the fascia that results in development of nodules **n goitre** end result of repeated cycles of hyperplasia and incomplete involution of thyroid **n melanoma** a melanoma that is uniformly pigmented and nodular

nodule (nod'ul) a small, rounded mass of tissue of variable size and shape

Noguchia (no-goo'che-a) gram-negative flagellated rods found in conjunctiva, named after Hideyo Noguchia, Japanese bacteriologist

noise sound of any sort **n induced hearing loss** reduction in auditory perception induced by loud sounds **n pollution** the presence of noise and sounds in the workplace and environment that is annoying

noma (no'ma) a gangrenous stomatitis; cancrum oris. An acute necrotising polymicrobial and ulcerating infection of the orofacial tissues seen in malnourished children, which rapidly erodes deep tissues exposing bone and teeth

nomenclature (no'men-kla'tur) a set system of names used in any science

Nomina Anatomia the book of official nomenclature, for anatomy formulated by the International Congress of Anatomists

nominal (no'mi-nal) **aphasia** inability to name objects

nomogram (nom'o-gram) a series of scales which are arranged in such a way so as to calculate the value of unknown parameter graphically

non A non B (NANB) **hepatitis** *see* hepatitis C

non-cirrhotic portal fibrosis an important cause of intrahepatic non-cirrhotic portal hypertension, which presents with gastrointestinal haemorrhage, splenomegaly runs a benign course and variceal bleeding has to be controlled

non-compliance failure of a patient to co-operate with treatment procedure or dietary advice

non-conductor (non'kon-duk'tor) a substance having no conductivity

non-disclosure the act of withholding relevant information

non-disease a form of iatrogenic illness created by misdiagnosis

non-disjunction (non'dis-junk'shun) failure of chromosome to separate during cell division resulting in passage of both chromosomes to the same daughter cell and result in serious genetic disorder.

non-essential amino acid any amino acid that can be synthesised in the body from available substrates

non-esterified fatty acids fatty acids not esterified to a glycerol and absorbed in the ileum as stearic and palmitic acids

non-gonococcal urethritis inflammation of the urethra caused by organisms other than bacteria that cause gonorrhoea, most commonly caused by *Chlamydia trachomatis* with features of dysuria, pyuria and symptoms similar to, but less intense than gonorrhoea

non-Hodgkin's lymphoma NHL any malignant condition of lymphoid tissue other than Hodgkin's disease. Most of them are B cell neoplasms. Unlike Hodgkin's lymphoma, the clinical picture is more variable and disease starts multicentrally. Extranodal involvement, and involvement of the blood and bone marrow are more common. The condition responds to radio-therapy in early stages and to chemotherapy in late stages

nonigravida (no'ni-gra'vi-da) a woman pregnant for the ninth time

non-insulin dependent diabetes mellitus (NIDDM) adult onset or type II diabetes mellitus

non-ionising radiation electromagnetic radiation, the photons of which have insufficient energy to ionise atoms

non-invasive any medical procedure that does not involve penetration of the skin or entry into the body; do not spread

nonipara (no-nip'ar-a) a woman who has given birth nine times

non-myelinated containing no myelin and nonmedullated, pertains to nerve fibres

non-nucleoside reverse transcriptase inhibitors, NNRTIs anti-HIV drugs such as efavirenz, delavirdine, nivirapine

non-parametric statistical methods that do not require restrictive assumptions about population distribution

non-photochromogen one group of atypical mycobacteria that has no capacity to produce pale yellow pigment. Exposure to light does not intensify the colour, a feature of *Mycobacterium avium-intracellulare*

non-proprietary name the chemical or generic name of a drug or device, as distinguished from a brand name or trade mark.

non-protein nitrogen NPN the nitrogen in the blood that is not a constituent of a protein such as nitrogen associated with urea, uric acid, creatinine and polypeptides

non-rapid eye movement NREM, *see* sleep

non-Q-wave infarction a subendocardial myocardial infarction in which ECG shows a persistent abnormal ST-segment depression in all but the aVR lead often accompanied by T-wave changes

non-self denotes antigenic constituents foreign to the organism which are eliminated through humoral or cell-mediated immunity

nonsense mutation a single DNA base change resulting in a premature stop codon

nonsense syndrome *Psy* a condition in which a person gives incorrect answers to simple questions

non-steroidal anti-inflammatory drugs NSAIDs; a pain killing drug that reduces inflammation in joints and muscles, by inhibiting prostagladin biosynthesis and by interfering with membrane bound reaction. It consists of aspirin, sodium salicylate, acetic acid analogues (indomethacin), propionic acid analogues (ibuprofen, naproxen), fenamic acid analogues (mefanamic acid) and enolic acid analogues (oxyphenbutazone, phenylbutazone)

non-stress test a non-invasive monitoring of the well-being of a foetus. It consists of monitoring of frequency of foetal movement, degree of heart rate acceleration and beat-to-beat variation of heart rate. It helps in determining the health of the placental vasculature

non-striated muscle smooth (involuntary) muscle controlling actions of the internal organs

non-tuberculous mycobacteria, NTM, atypical or anonymous mycobacteria that are weak pathogens and histologically distinct from *Myco-*

bacterium tuberculosis. They are ubiquitously distributed and may infect the skin, soft tissue, lymph nodes, lungs, implant devices, bones and joints. The organisms have been classified into four groups based on colony morphology pigmentation and growth characteristics as photochromogens (*M. kansasii*), scotochromogens (*M. scrofulaceum*), non-chromogens (*M. avium-intracellulare*) and rapid growers (*M. fortuitum, M. chelonei*).

non-tuberculous mycobacterial disease clinical infection by non-tuberculous mycobacteria and they may be in the form of chronic pulmonary infections, cervical lymphadenopathy, skin and soft tissue infections or disseminated infections

non-ulcer dyspepsia a condition characterised by peptic ulcer symptoms in the absence of gross ulceration. Endoscopy may show oedema, and erosions of the duodenal mucosa

non-union a fracture that is not united after nine 9 months.

non-verbal (non-vur'bal) **communication** the transmission of message without the use of words; body language

non-viable (non-viah-b'l) incapable of independent existence

Noone's (non'ez) **syndrome** pseudocerebral tumour exhibiting raised intracranial tension and papilloedema

Nonne-Milroy's (non'e-mil'roy'ez) **disease** familial lymphangiectatic swelling of legs, named after Max Nonne and William Milroy, US physicians.

Noonan's (noo'nenz) **syndrome** non-chromosomal Turner's syndrome, described by Jacqueline Noonan, American paediatrician. It is a male equivalent of Turner's syndrome exhibiting low set ears, webbing of the neck, cubitus valgus, congenital heart disease and sometimes severe mental retardation

noradrenaline (nor'ah-dren'a-lin) nor-epinephrine, adrenaline less N methyl group, a sympathetic neurotransmitter

norethandrolone (nor'eth-an'dro-lon) anabolic steroid

norethisterone (nor'eth'i-st-ron) progesterone with some androgenic activity

norfloxacin (nor-flok'sesin) a quinolone antibacterial agent used in the treatment of infections of urinary tract

norgestrel (nor'ges-trel) a progesterone used in oral contraceptive

norm normal; a standard for a specific group

norma basalis (nor'ma-basa'lis) the inferior surface of the base of the skull with the mandible removed

normal (nor'mal) healthy, usual, typical, as it ought to be **n saline** a 0.9% w/v sterile solution of sodium chloride in water that is isotonic with blood

normoblast (nor'mo-blast) a nucleated red blood cell and its presence suggests haemolysis; erythroblast

normocapnic (nor'mo-kap'nik) a normal level of arterial carbon dioxide in the blood

normochromia (nor'mo-kro'me-a) normal colour, pertains to red blood cell having normal colour by presence of an adequate amount of haemoglobin

normocyte (nor'mo-sit) normal mature red cell having a diameter of 7 microns

normoglycaemia (nor'mo-gli-se'me-a) normal blood sugar

normokalaemia (nor'mo-ka-le'me-a) a normal level of potassium in the blood

normotension (nor'mo-ten'shun) normal blood pressure

norplant levonorgestrel; an implantable contraceptive that prevents pregnancy by inhibiting ovulation and causing thickening of cervical mucosa

Norrie's (nor'iz) **disease** a rare form of sex-linked hereditary blindness due to malformation of retina, named after Gordon Norrie, Danish ophthalmologist

northern blotting procedure to transfer RNA from an agarose gel to a nylon membrane

nortryptiline (nor-trip'ti-len) a tricyclic antidepressant useful in mental depression

Norwalk virus a parvovirus causing epidemic gastroenteritis, first recognised in Norwalk town in Ohio, USA

nose (noz) nasus, a central projection of the face which acts as an organ of smell and the opening to the nasal cavities that warms, moistens and filters inhaled air as it moves into respiratory tract **n bleed** bleeding from nose from injury, hypertension, foreign body or fracture **saddle n** depressed bridge of nose due to erosion of nasal bones seen in congenital syphilis and leprosy

noso- a combining word for relating to disease

nosocomial (nos'o-ko'me-al) hospital acquired **n infection** an infection acquired in a hospital by pathogens that were not in incubation period when the person concerned was admitted for treatment

nosogenic (nos'o-jen'ik) pathogenic

nosology (no-sol'o-je) scientific classification of diseases

nostras locally derived, endemic

nostril (nos'tril) one of the external orifices of the nose

nostrum (nos'trum) a quack or secret medicine

notal relating to the back

notch an indentation or a depression in a bone or organ

notching small grooves on the anterior aspect of ribs on chest roentgenograms, seen in post-ductal coarctation of aorta

notch sign a short straight radiolucency that penetrates a relatively well circumscribed lung mass, seen in malignancy and granulomatous conditions

note-taking accurate record of history and physical signs suggesting the diagnosis

nothing by mouth; *non per os* an instruction which prohibits the patient to take food, beverage or medicine by mouth and is essential in a patient about to undergo surgery or diagnostic procedure requiring the alimentary tract to be empty or in acute abdomen

Nothnagel's (not'na-gelz) **syndrome** brain stem syndrome with lesion at the tectum of mid-brain often neoplasm, exhibiting ipsilateral ocular palsy and cerebellar ataxia, named after Wilhelm Nothnagel, German physician

notifiable diseases a group of communicable diseases which are considered to be serious menaces to public health

notification once a communicable disease is detected it should be notified immediately to the local health authorities to permit immediate action to control the spread of the disease

notalgia (no-tal'je-a) pain in the back

notch (noch) incisure

notochord (no'toko-rd) the axial fibrocellular structure around which the vertebral primardia develop

nourish (nur'ish) to provide essential nutrients for maintaining life

nourishment (nur'ish-ment) 1. the act of nourishing 2. any substance that nourishes and supports the life and growth of living organisms.

noxious (nok'shus) injurious

noy unit of loudness perceived by listener

NREM abbreviation for non rapid eye movements, a phase of sleep

NRTI abbreviation for nuceloside reverse transcriptase inhibitor

NSAID abbreviation for non-steroidal anti-inflammatory drug

NTM non-tuberculous mycobacteria

NTP National tuberculosis programme.

nucha (nu'ka) the back of the neck

nuchal (nu'kal) relating to the nucha

nuclear (nu'kle-ar) relating to or resembling a nucleus **n transplantation** taking the nucleus of one embryo cell and transplanting it into another embryo cell

nuclear magnetic resonance NMR non-invasive, imaging technique without use of ionising radiation.

nuclear: cytoplasmic ratio nuclei are proportionately larger than their accompanying cytoplasm as in malignant cells

nuclear family the core family unit consisting of parents and their direct genetic progeny

nuclear medicine an area of medicine that uses radioisotopes for the diagnosis and treatment of disease

nuclear roundness factor the degree to which a nucleus shows a perfect circle in cross section. Malignant conditions are associated with increased nuclear irregularity

nuclease (nu'kle-as) any enzyme catalysing the hydrolysis of nucleic acids, consists of DNAse (DNase) and RNAase (RNase) enzymes

nucleic (nu'kle'ik) **acid** polymer of nucleotide, DNA or RNA which possess a complex chemical structure consisting of pentoses (sugars), phosphoric acid and purines and pyramidines (nitrogenous bases)

nucleolar (nu-kle'o-lar) relating to a nucleolus

nucleolus (nu'kle'o-lus) a small round mass within the cell nucleus concerned with the production of nucleoprotein pl. **nucleoli**

nucleoprotein (nu'kle-o-pro'te-in) a complex of protein and nucleic acid

nucleorrhexis (nu'kle-o-rek'sis) fragmentation of a cell nucleus

nucleosidase (nu'kle-o-si'das) an enzyme catalysing hydrolysis of nucleotides into purine or pyrimidine bases

nucleoside (nu'kle-o-sid) a compound of sugar (ribose or deoxyribose) with a purine or pyrimidine base **n analogue** chemical that interferes with the replication of viruses **n base** chemical that forms the building blocks of DNA or RNA and their sequence gives the picture of genetic code

Nucleoside reverse transcriptase inhibitors, NRTIs anti-HIV drugs such as abacavir. didanosine, lamivudine,

stavudine, zalcitabine, and zidovudine

nucleosome an aggregate of highly basic proteins that is associated with chromosomes

nucleotidase (nu'kleot'i-das) an enzyme catalysing hydrolysis of nucleotides into phosphoric acid and nucleosides

nucleotide (nu'kle-o-tid) the basic unit of nucleic acids DNA/RNA, which is made up of a purine or pyrimidine base (A adenine, T thymine, U uracil, G guanine or C cytosine), a pentose sugar (ribose or deoxyribose) and a phosphate group **n analogue** a chemical substance that resembles a nucleotide

nucleus (nu'kle-us) oval mass containing chromatin and nucleoli which acts as the central unit of a living cell. pl. **nuclei n pulposus** central liquid area of intervertebral disc

nuclide (nu'klid) a species of atom characterised by the constitution of its nucleus in particular by the number of protons and neutrons

null cell a lymphocyte that develops in the bone marrow and lacks the characteristic surface markers of the T and B lymphocytes are known as natural killer or NK cells

null hypothesis *stat* the hypothesis that observe differences or variations in scores can be attributed to random sources. When null hypothesis is rejected, observed differences between groups are deemed to be improbable by chance alone

nulligravida a woman who has never conceived a child

nullipara (nu-lli'pa-ra) a woman who has never borne a child

nulliparity (nul'i-par'i-te) the condition of having borne no children

null phenotype the non-expression of a protein because of its corresponding gene is defective or absent on both inherited haplotypes. They involve the red blood cell as in blood group O

numb (num) insensible; inability to move

numbness (num'ness) partial or total loss of sensation due to impaired cutaneous perception and interference with passage of impulses along sensory nerves

nummular (num'u-lar) coin-shaped **n dermatitis** a skin disease exhibiting coin-shaped scaly eczema like lesions **n sputum** sputum in rounded disks, simulating coins

Nuremburg code a set of 10 ethical principles for medical research devised in 1947 by three US judges, and it is the first set of ethical guidelines protecting human research subjects

nurse (ners) a person involved in the care of the sick persons; a woman taking care of an infant or young child; to suckle a child **n midwife** a nurse involved in the care and education of women during pregnancy and labour, supervision of delivery and provision of postnatal care **registered n** a person who has passed general nursing and midwifery examination after training in a recognised school of nursing and has been granted a licence to practice nursing profession **wet n** a woman who breast-feeds a baby that is not her own

nursemaid's elbow subluxation of the head of the radius

nurses' aide trained women employed in hospitals to perform non-medical services such as making beds, serving meals etc.

nursing (nurs'ing) caring for the sick; breast feeding of an infant **n station** a centrally located health care facility in the ward or clinic that serves as the administrative centre for nursing care

nurture (nur'cher) to feed, foster or care for such as in the nourishment, and care of growing children

nutation (nu-ta'shun) nodding

nutmeg liver a liver with chronic passive congestion secondary to cardiac failure There is intense congestion with deep red, centrilobular zone, sharply demarcated from the pale peripheral zones

nutrient (nu'tre-ent) food material that is used by the body to sustain life and health and the examples are carbohydrates, fats, proteins, vitamins and minerals **n enema** introduction of saline or glucose into the body *via* the rectum **n medium** culture medium that provides the essential nutrients required for growth of microorganism, usually carbohydrates and proteins

nutrition (nu-tri'shun) food material that is metabolised by the body facilitating the building of tissue and liberation of energy **enteral n** introduction of nutrients, through a nasogastric tube

nutritional (nu'tre-sh'enal) pertaining to the quality of food **n anaemia** a disorder characterised by inadequate production of haemoglobin or erythrocytes from a nutritional deficiency of iron, folic acid or vitamin B_{12}

nux vomica (nuks vom'i-ka) vomiting nut, tree producing strychnine

nyctalgia (nik-tal'je-a) pain occurring at night

nyctalopia (nik'ta-lo'pe-ah) night blindness encountered in Vitamin A deficiency, retinitis pigmentosa and chorioretinitis

nycterohemeral (nik'ter-o-hem'er-al) relating to day and night

nyctophobia (nik'to-fo'be-a) abnormal fear of darkness

nycturia (nik-tu're-a) nocturnal frequency urine

NYHA New York Heart Association, adopted grading of cardiac status as grade 1. asymptomatic 2. symptoms on moderate or severe exertion 3. symptoms on slight exertion and 4. symptoms at rest.

nymph (nimf) a stage between larva and adult in the life cycle of certain arthropods

nympha (nim'fah) small folds of the labia minora

nymphectomy (nim-fek'to-me) excision of the hypertrophied labia minora

nymphomania (nim'fo-ma'ne-a) abnormally excessive sexual desire in women

nystagmoid (nis-tag'moyd) resembling nystagmus. A few irregular jerks of the eyes of brief duration may be seen in full lateral deviation in normal individuals

nystagmus (nis-tag'mus) involuntary, often rhythmic oscillation of the eye balls. The movements may be up-and-down, side-to-side or rotary. The speed of the movements may be the same in both directions, or quicker in one direction than another; in the latter case the quicker movements indicates the direction of the nystagmus. Nystagmus may be due to disorders of the vestibular system, lesions affecting the central pathways concerned in ocular movements or to weakness of ocular muscles **ataxic n** nystagmus in abducting eye than in adducting eye during lateral gaze noted in multiple sclerosis involving medial longitudinal fasciculus **cerebellar n** nystagmus in lateral lobe lesions with the fast component towards the side of lesion **downbeat n** nystagmus with fast phase downwards in a lesion at lower medulla **gaze-evoked n** nystagmus in the direction of gaze **horizontal n** nystagmus at extremes of gaze, often it has no pathologic significance **jerking n** nystagmus of constant direction irrespective of direction of gaze and suggests labyrinthine or cerebellar lesion **miner's n** nystagmus of retinal origin noted in miners who work in dimlight **optokinetic n** a normal reflex phenomenon involving occipital cortex and frontal eye fields. Nystagmus has a slow phase in the direction of movement of the rotating object and a quick corrective phase in opposite direction **pendular n** nystagmus of visual origin and often rotary on central fixation of the eyes. It has a smooth equal oscillation in either direction **positional n** nystagmus associated with benign epidemic vertigo and with posterior fossa tumours, may be induced only by certain movements of the head **rebound n** nystagmus that reverses direction as the eccentric gaze position is held, noted in cerebellar atrophy **rotary n** oscillatory movements of the eyeballs affecting more than one place **see-saw n** a rare variety in which one eye moves upwards while the other moves downwards, occurs in lesion of suprasellar region **vestibular n** occurs following damage to inner ear, eighth cranial nerve or its central connections. It is greater on looking away from the side of destructive lesion and the fast component is always directed away from the side of lesion **vertical n** nystagmus that locates the lesion to brain stem **upbeat n** nystagmus with fast components upwards due to lesions at level of superior colliculus

nystatin (nis'ta-tin) polyene antifungal agent for candida

Nysten's (ne-stanz) **law** as per law formulated by Pierre Nysten, French paediatrician, rigor mortis sets in the muscles of mastigation first and makes a progress from head downwards and last to involve are feet

Nyxis (nik'sis) piercing; puncturing

O

O$_2$ Chemical symbol for oxygen molecule

O$_3$ Chemical symbol for ozone

O **antigen** a bacterial lipopolysaccharide protein antigen used for serologic classification of enteric bacteria; a oligosaccharide precursor for the A and B antigens of the ABO blood group

oat a cereal **o cell carcinoma** a histologic subtype of small cell carcinoma of the lung **o meal** a porridge made by cooking oats

oath a solemn attestation or affirmation

OB obstetrics

obdormition (ob-dor-mish'un) numbness followed by tingling in an extremity from pressure on the sensory nerve

obduction (ob-duk'shun) a medicolegal autopsy

obelion (o-be'le-on) a craniometric point on the sagittal suture between the two parietal foramina

Ober's (ob'erz) **test** a diagnostic test for contracture of iliotibial tract and tensor fascia lata which occurs in residual poliomyelitis, named after Frank Ober, US orthopaedic surgeon

obese excessive fat.

obesitas obesity

obesity (o-be'si-te) an excessive accumulation of fat in the body resulting in an increase in body weight more than 20 per cent or more over the maximum desirable weight for his or her weight **endogenous o** obesity caused by a metabolic abnormality **exogenous o** obesity due to excessive intake of food **hypothalamic o** obesity due to a dysfunction of hypothalamus especially the appetite-regulating centre **o hypoventilation syndrome** alveolar hypoventilation during wakefulness and most of them have severe obstructive sleep apnoea

obex (o'beks) posterior limit of the fourth ventricle marking the beginning of the central canal

OB-Gyn abbreviation for obstetrics and gynaecology

obidoxime reactivator of acetylcholinesterase, used in the treatment of organophosphorous insecticide poisoning

object (ob'jekt) a thing visible; *Psy* something through which an instinct can achieve its goal.

objective (ob-jec-tiv) 1. lens in a microscope near the object that is being examined 2. appreciate the events or phenomenon by external senses 3. precise statements of numerically measurable outputs and inputs to be achieved by a specific deadline **oil immersion o** a microscope objective with the space between the objective lens and specimen is filled with oil **o sign** a clinical observation that can be seen, heard, measured or recorded. **o symptom** a symptom that is accompanied by signs

obligate (ob'li-gat) compulsory, ability to survive in a particular environment **o aerobe** an organism that cannot grow in the absence of oxygen **o anaerobe** an organism that cannot grow in the presence of oxygen such as Clostridia organisms **o parasite** an organism that depends entirely on its host for survival

oblique (ob-lik) slant or incline **o bandage** a circular bandage applied spirally in slanting turns, usually to a limb **o fissure** major fissure of the lungs separating the lower lobe from the upper lobe on left side and upper and middle lobes on the right side **o fracture** a slanting fracture of the shaft on the long axis of a bone **o presentation** a presentation in which the long axis of the foetus is oblique to the long axis of the mother

obliquity (ob-lik-wit-e) the state of being inclined or slanting

obliteration (ob-lit'er-a'shun) complete removal; filling

oblongata (ob'long-ga'ta) oblong; rather long **medulla o** cylindrical extension of the spinal cord as it enters the brain

obmutescence (ob'mu-tes'ens) aphonia

obsession (ob-sesh'un) *Psy* a recurrent, persistent thought, impulse or image which fills the mind despite one's efforts to ignore it

obscessive (ob-ses'siv) characterised by obsession

obscure (ob-skur') indistinct; hidden

observations the essential structural units which go to build the edifice of scientific knowledge

observer variation *stat* all observations are subject to variations (errors) **inter observer v** variation between different observers on the same subject or material **intra observer v** variation between repeated observations by the same observer on the same subject or material at the same time

obsessive-compulsive (ob-ses'iv-kom-pul'siv) *Psy* a disorder with persistent ideas making a person to undertake certain acts repeatedly and ritualistically to relieve anxiety. It may respond to certain tricyclic antidepressants

obsession (ob-sesh'un) *Psy* a mental state with an irresistable thought or feeling that cannnot be eliminated from consciousness by logical effort which is associated with anxiety

obsolete (ob'so-let) gone out of use

obstetric (obste'rik) pertaining to obstetrics and midwifery **o anaesthesia** any of various procedures used to provide anaesthesia for child birth **o forceps** forceps used to assist delivery of the foetal head. It consists of a pair of instruments comprising a handle, a long shank and a curved blade **o**

position lateral recumbent position wherein patient lies on the left side with the right thigh and knee drawn up

obstetrician (ob'ste-trish-an) a specialist in obstetrics **o's hand** contractions of the hand as in tetany

obstetrics (ob'ste'riks) branch of medical science concerned with the care of the pregnant women during pregnancy, labour and the puerperium. **obstetric, obstetrical,** adj.

obstinate (ob'sti'nate) intractable, refractory

obstipation (osti-pa'shun) severe constipation

obstructed labour condition in which spontaneous delivery through the natural passages is impossible

obstructed hernia irreducible hernia causing intestinal obstruction without affecting the blood supply

obstruction (ob-struk'shun) blockage **intestinal o** blockage of the lumen of the intestine **laryngeal o** obstruction to the larynx causing a prolonged inspiration **lymphatic o** obstruction to lymph flow giving rise to unilateral non-pitting oedema **pyloric o** complication of chronic duodenal ulcer, due to narrowing of the pyloric canal by fibrosis. There is failure of gastric emptying and patients complain of vomiting food eaten hours before

obstructive causing obstruction **o anuria** absence of urination caused by an obstruction of the urinary tract **o hydrocephalus** hydrocephalus due to interference with the flow of cerebrospinal fluid, resulting in enlargement of ventricles **o jaundice** obstruction to the flow of bile through any part of the biliary system, from liver to duodenum, resulting in cholestasis. The obstruction may be within the liver (intrahepatic) or outside (extrahepatic) chronic **o pulmonary disease** COPD a disorder characterised by abnormal tests of expiratory flow which do not change markedly over period of several months of observation. It includes chronic bronchitis, emphysema and small airway disease **o sleep apnoea** disturbed sleep and respiration due to obstruction to the extra-thoracic upper airway at the level of oropharynx. It is sucked in and closed when the patient breathes in during sleep. The cyclical respiratory contractions of the diaphragm and other respiratory muscles are present throughout the episodes of apnoea. They fail to elicit any airflow due to upper airway obstruction **o uropathy** any pathologic state that results in obstruction of the flow of urine

obstruent (ob'stroo-ent) any agent causing obstruction

obtund (ob-tund') to dull or blunt

obtundation (ob-tun-da'shun) clouding of consciousness

obtundent (ob-tun'dent) having the capacity to dull sensibility; a soothing agent

obturation (ob-tur-a'shun) occlusion or closure of a passage

obturator (ob'tu-rat'or) a disk or plate used in closing an opening or a cavity **o block** obturator nerve is blocked by an anaesthetic as it lies in the obturator canal for operations involving the knee joint and medial aspects of the thigh **o foramen** a membrane between the rami of hip bone **o externus** the flat triangular muscle covering the outer surface of the anterior wall of the pelvis **o internus** a muscle that covers a large part of the inferior aspect of the lesser pelvis, where it surrounds the obturator foramen **o membrane** a tough fibrous membrane covering the obturator foramen on either side of the pelvis **o muscles** two muscles on either side of the pelvis that rotate the thighs outward **o nerve** nerve to adductors of the lower limb and it arises from 3rd and 4th lumbar plexus **o neuralgia** paroxysmal stabbing pain in the dis-

tribution of the great auricular or occipital nerves. The affected nerve may be tender on palpation **o sign** a unilateral increase in the bulk of obturator muscle seen as a soft tissue bulge on inner pelvis with medial displacement of the normal fat line, radiologically it is a feature of infective arthritis **o test** on flexing the right thigh, and internally rotating the hip joint the obturator internus is flexed. An inflammed appendix in its contact causes pain in the hypogastrium

obtuse (ob-t-us') blunt; dull

obtusion (ob-tu'zhun) blunting of sensibility

occipital (ok-sip'i-tal) relating to the back of the head **o artery** a branch from the external carotid artery supplying parts of the head and scalp **o bone** bone in the back of the skull between the parietal and temporal bones **o horn** occipital exostoses that extend caudally from the base of the skull, a feature of X-linked type IX Ehlers-Danlos syndrome **o lobe** one of the sections or lobes of cerebrum located towards the back in the shape of three-sided pyramid **o pain** nerve root pain from the neck **o sinus** smallest of cranial sinuses located in the attached margin of the falx cerebelli

occipitalis (ok-sip'i-ta'lis) the posterior portion of the occipitofrontalis muscle at the back of the head

occipitalisation (ok-sipi-tal-i-za'shun) synostosis between the atlas and occipital bones

occipitobregmatic (ok-sip'it-o-bregmat'ik) pertaining to the occiput and the frontal bone

occipitocervical (ok-sip'it-o-ser'vi-kal) pertaining to the occiput and neck

occipitofrontal (ok-sip'it-o-fron'tal) pertaining to the occiput and the face

occipitofrontalis (ok-sip'it-o-fron'tal'is) one of a pair of thin, broad muscles covering the top of the skull consisting of an occipital belly and a frontal belly connected by an aponeurosis occipitomastoid (ok-sip'it-o-mas'toyd) pertaining to the occiput bone and mastoid process

occipitomental (ok-sip'it-o-ment'l) pertaining to the occiput and chin

occipitoparietal (ok-sip'i-to-pa'rie-tal) pertaining to the occiput and parietal bones or lobes of the brain

occiptotemporal (ok-sip'ito-tem'po-ral) pertaining to the occipital and temporal bones

occipitothalamic (ok-sip'ito-tha-lam'ik) pertaining to the occipital lobe and thalamus

occiput (ok'si-put) the back portion of the skull, adj. occipital

occlude (o-klood) to close; bring together; obstruct

occlusal (o-kloo'z'l) pertaining to a closure of an opening such as contact between the teeth of upper and lower jaws o adjustment the grinding of the occluding surfaces of teeth to improve the relation between opposing surface of teeth o contouring the modification by grinding of irregularities of occlusal tooth forms o form the shape of the occluding surfaces of a tooth or teeth o plane a plane passing through the occlusal surfaces of the teeth o rest a support which is part of a removable partial denture o surface the surfaces of teeth in one arch that makes contact with the corresponding surfaces of the teeth in the opposite arch o trauma injury to a tooth and surrounding structures caused by malocclusive stresses

occlusion (o-kloo'zhun) the act of closure; blockage of any channel or opening in the body o rim an artificial dental structure with occluding surfaces attached to temporary or permanent denture bases

occlusive (o-kloo'siv) helping to close o dressing dressing to occlude the area of skin bearing the lesion from external atmosphere. It helps in accumulation of sweat and water and raise humidity and cause maceration and damage to the epithelial barier

occult (ok-kult') concealed, obscure, hidden o blood the presence of blood in body fluids or in faeces that cannot be seen by the naked eye but can be detected by chemical tests o cancer a malignancy of unknown origin that first manifests itself as metastasis and it reflectes poor prognosis o fracture fracture that cannot be found by examination initially but may be evident in radiograph taken subsequently. o hydrocephalus normal pressure hydrocephalus wherein the ventricles are dilated without an increase in the intracranial pressure. It is associated with progressive dementia, ataxia and urinary incontinence in elderly persons o infection a bacterial infection in an obscure site presenting with polymorphonuclear leucocytosis and fever of unknown origin o pneumothorax pneumothorax seen only on the CT scan

occupancy (ok'yu-panse) the ratio of average daily hospital census to the number of beds maintained; an act of occupying

occupation (ok'u-pah-zhun) work; state of being employed

occupational pertaining to work o acne contact with heavy oils, waxes and tar producing acne form eruptions at the site of contact of skin o asthma a disease characterised by variable airflow limitation and/or airway hyper-responsiveness due to causes and conditions attributable to a particular occupational environment and not to stimuli, encountered outside the work place o disability a condition in which a worker is unable to perform the functions required to complete a job satisfactorily due to an occupational disease or an occupational accident o disease a disease caused by particular job unsually resuting from prolonged exposure to harmful substances in the work place o dystonias highly specific action dystonias of the upper limbs, closely related to skilled activities, writer's cramp is the example o **environment** the sum of the external conditions and influences which prevail at the place of work and which have a bearing on the health of working population o **hazards** industrial worker exposed to 5 types of hazards such as physical, chemical, biological, mechanical and psychosocial conditions o **health** application of preventive medicine in all places of employment o **lung disease** exposure to potentially harmful substances in the form of gas, fumes, smoke or dust in an environment where a person works, result in lung diseases due to its wide surface area, high blood flow and thin alveolar epithelium o **malignancy** asbestos exposure increases the risk of development of bronchogenic carcinoma and pleural mesothelioma o **neurosis** a functional disorder that may develop in persons in certain occupations o **therapist** a person who helps in self care, work, play and task performance skills of normal and disabled individuals and restore, develop and maintain their ability to accomplish the tasks o **therapy** utilisation of work, self care and play as therapeutic measures to increase the function, to enhance competence and to prevent disability

ochlesis (ok-le'sis) any disease due to overcrowding

ochlophobia (ok'lo-fo'be-a) abnormal fear of crowds

ochrometer (o-krom'it-er) an instrument to measure the capillary blood pressure

ochronosis (o'kro-n-o'sis) an inborn error of protein metabolism causing pigmentation of the body tissues by the deposition of alkapton bodies. There is dusky discolouration of the sclerae and ears, arthritis and darkening of urine on standing due to the presence of homogentisic acid. There is lack of homogentisic acid oxidase in the liver and kidney resulting in accumulation of homogentisic acid

Ochsner clasping test when hands are clasped index finger fails to flex and stands pointing in median nerve paralysis, described by Albert Ochsner, US surgeon

octa - combining word for the number eight or series of eight

octan (ok'tan) recurring every eighth day

octapeptide (ok'ta-pep'tid) a peptide containing eight aminoacids

octigravida (ok'ti-grav'i-da) a woman pregnant for the eighth time

octipara (ok-tip'a-ra) a woman who had eight pregnancies with viable offspring

octogenarian (ok'to-jen-er'ean) a person who is in eighties

octopamine (ok'to-pam'en) a sympathomimetic amine, a false neurotransmitter

octreotide (ok-tre'o-tid) a synthetic analogue of somatostatin having high affinity for growth hormone (GH). It causes decrease in serum GH and gives relief of symptoms in patients with acromegaly

ocular (ok'u-lar) 1. relating to the eye and its structure pl. **oculi**. 2. eye piece of a microscope o **bobbing** sudden, brisk, downward diving eye movements seen in pontine or cerebellar haemorrhage o **cysticercosis** cysticercosis of the eye may present as retinitis, uveitis, conjunctivitis or choroidal atrophy o **dysmetria** a visual disorder wherein the eyes are unable to fix the gaze on an object or follow a moving object properly o **fundi** examination with ophthalmoscope the optic disc, arteries, veins, haemorrhages and exudates o **herpes** a herpes virus infection of the eye o **hyperteleorism** markedly widened bridge of the nose and increased distance in between the eyes o **hypoteleorism** marked narrowing of the bridge of the nose and decreased distance between the eyes o **larva migrans** the larva of toxocara may affect eye producing a posterior chorioretinitis or an intraretinal granuloma **o movements** horizontal, vertical, diagonal or rotatory movements of the eye **o myopathy** slowly progressive weakness of ocular muscles exhibiting decreased movements of the eye and ptosis. It may be unilateral or bilateral **o tension** pressure in the eyeball roughly assessed by palpating the eyeball or accurately by tonometer

oculentum (ok'ulen-tum) an eye ointment

oculist (ok'u-list) ophthalmologist

oculistics (ok'u-lis'tiks) the treatment of disorders of the eye

oculo (ok'ulo) referable to the eye

oculocardiac (ok'u-lo-car'diak) **reflex** a variety of stimuli arising in or near the eye may cause abnormalities of the rate or rhythm of the heart

oculocephalic (ok'ulo-sefal'ik) **reflex** a test to determine the integrity of brainstem function. The eyes normally lag behind the head movement when the patient's head is quickly moved to one side and then to the other. The eyes slowly reach the midline position. In a lesion on the ipsilateral side of the brain stem, there is failure of the eyes which either lag properly or revert back to the midline

oculocerebrorenal syndrome X-linked recessive disorder characterised by cataract, mental deficiency, tubular dysfunction, areflexia, hypotonia, glaucoma and joint swelling; Lowe's syndrome

oculocutaneous (ok'u-lo-ku-ta'ne-us) pertaining to the eye and the skin

oculodental dysplasia (ok'u-lo-den'tal-dis'pla-zhea) an autosomal dominant disorder characterised by hypertension, microphthalmia, myopia, hypoplastic teeth, syndactyly, visceral malformation and no mental deficiency

oculofacial (ok'u-lo-fa'she-al) pertaining to the eye and face

oculogyration (ok'u-lo-ji-ra'shun) circular movement of the eyeball around its

anteroposteriar axis and fixation of the eyes up and sideways, adj. **oculogyric**

oculogyric (ok'u-lo-ji'rik) **crisis** a rare manifestation of post-encephalitic parkinsonism in which the eyes are held fixed usually up and sideways for a variable length of time

oculomotor (ok'u-lo-mot'or) relating to the movements of the eye **o nerve** third cranial nerve arising in the midbrain. It supplies the medial, superior and inferior recti, inferior oblique, levator palpebrum superioris, ciliary muscle and sphincter muscles of the iris. The nerve takes its origin form a series of nuclei in the midbrain. The nuclei in the front give parasympathetic innervation to the ciliary muscles and iris (Edinger-Westphal nucleus) and the nuclei behind are concerned with innervation to the extraocular muscles **o nucleus** a nucleus of a third cranial nerve in the midbrain **o palsy** the eye is deviated downwards and outwards. There will be paresis, pupils are dilated and fixed. There is an inability to move the eye ball inwards and upwards

oculomycosis (ok'u-lo-mi-ko'sis) a fungal disease of the eye

oculonasal (ok'u-lo-na'zal) pertaining to the eye and the nose

oculopharyngeal muscular dystrophy a rare late onset hereditary myopathy characterised by progressive ptosis and dysphagia

oculoplastics (ok'u-lo-plas-tiks) plastic surgery of the eyes to correct drooping lids, burns and other cosmetic errors

oculozygomatic (ok'u-lo-zi'go-mat'ik) pertaining to the eye and zygoma

oculus (ok'u-lus) eye, pl. **oculi o dexter** the right eye; **o sinister** the left eye

odaxesmus (o'dak-sez'mus) the biting of the tongue, lip or cheek during an epileptic attack

Oddi's (od'ez) **sphincter** muscular sphincter at the opening of the common bile duct and pancreatic duct into the duodenum, described by Italian physician, Ruggero Oddi

odds ratio *stat* a measure of the strength of the association between risk factor and outcome. It is closely related to relative risk

O'Donoghue's knee triad rupture of medial collateral ligament, damage to medial meniscus and rupture of anterior cruciate ligament, described by O'Donoghue, US orthopaedic surgeon

odont (odon-t) a tooth

odontagra (o-don-ta'gra) tooth ache especially when associated with gout

odontalgia (o'don-tal'je-a) toothache

odontatrophy (o'don'tat'ro-fe) imperfect development of the teeth

odontectomy (o'don-tek'to-me) excision of a tooth

odontexesis (o'don-tex-is) the removal of dental calculus and polishing of the teeth

odontic (o-don'tik) referring to tooth

odontitis (o'donti'tis) an inflammation of the odontoblasts resulting in an abnormal enlargement of a tooth

odontoblast (o-don'to-blast) cell concerned with deposition of dentin and with formation of the outer surface of the dental pulp

odontoblastoma (o-don'to-blas-to'ma) a tumour consisting of odontoblasts

odontoclast (o-don'to-klast) a cell responsible for absorption of the roots of the deciduous tooth

odontodynia (o-don'to-din'e-a) tooth ache

odontodysplasia (o-don'to-displa'zhea) an abnormality in the development of the teeth exhibiting deficient formation of enamel and dentin

odontogen (o-don'to-jen) the substance concerned with the formation of dentine of the teeth

odontogenesis (o-don'to-jen'i-sis) origin and development of the teeth

odontogenic (o-do'nto-jen'ik) forming teeth **o fibroma** a benign neoplasm of the jaw **o fibrosarcoma** a malignant neoplasm of the jaw

odontography (o-don-tog'ra-fe) a description of the teeth; tracing of the surface of the tooth

odontoid (o-don'toyd) tooth-like **o process** tooth-like projection from the upper surface of the body of second cervical vertebra (axis) which serves as a pivot for the rotation of the first cervical vertebra (atlas) allowing the head to turn

odontolith (o-don'to-lith) dental calculus

odontologist (o-don'tol-o-jist) a dentist; a dental surgeon

odontology (o'don-tol'o-je) dentistry

odontolysis (o-don-tol'i-sis) the resorption of tooth

odontoma (o'don-to'ma) benign tumour of tooth

odontonecrosis (o-don'to-ne-kro'sis) extensive decay of a tooth

odontopathy (o'don-top'a-the) any disease of the teeth

odontoplasty (o'don-top'la-ste) orthodontics

odontoprisis (o'don'to-pri'sis) grinding of the teeth

odontorrhagia (o-don'to-ra'je-a) haemorrhage from a tooth socket following extraction

odontoradiograph a roentgenograph of a tooth or of the teeth

odontoscopy (o'don-tos'ko-pe) obtaining impressions of the teeth; examination of teeth and oral cavity by an odontoscope

odontoseisis (o'don-to-se-sis) looseness of the teeth

odontosis (o'don-to'sis) formation of the teeth

odontotomy (o'don-tot'ah-me) cutting into the crown of a tooth

odour (o'der) smell. It may be spicy, flowery, fruity, resinous, foul and scorched. The sense of smell is activated when airborne molecules stimulate receptors of the olfactory nerve

odynia pain

odynophagia (o-din'o-fa'jah) painful swallowing of food characteristic of monilial and herpes oesophagitis

Oedipus (ed'i-pus) **complex** sexual feelings of a son towards his mother. Oedipus of Greek mythology killed his father unknowingly and married his mother

oedema (e-de'mah) accumulation of fluid in subcutaneous tissue due to extracellular volume expansion. There is swelling of tissues which can be demonstrated by pressing lightly with the thumb over a bony prominence **dependent o** oedema over the dorsum of the feet, around the ankles **non-pitting o** occurs in lymphatic obstruction, myxoedema and systemic sclerosis **pitting o** on pressure a pit appears for a while, noted in heart failure, nephrotic syndrome, cirrhosis of the liver, and hypoproteinaemia **sacral o** oedema over the sacrum in those confined to bed from gravitational effect **unilateral o** oedema in venous or lymphatic obstruction in one limb

Oerekermann's syndrome mucopolysaccharoidosis due to acid-alpha mannosidase deficiency

oesophageal (e-sof'ah-jial) pertaining to oesophagus **o atresia** malformation in which upper oesophagus ends in a blind pouch **o cancer** squamous cell cancer is most common type characterised by dysphagia, odynophagia, pain, aspiration, bleeding and anaemia. Alcohol, smoking, tobacco chewing, fungal contamination of food grains are implicated in its development **o diverticula** outpouching of the oesophageal wall from an area of muscular weakness **o reflux** normally prevented by the gastro-oesophageal sphincter. Patients with reflux exhibit repeated episodes of significant quantities of acid, bile and food regurgitating into the lower oesophagus **o ring** located in the squamo-columnar mucosal junction of the lower oesophagus and they possess squamous epithelium on the oesophageal side and columnar epithelium on the gastric side

o varices large anastomotic veins in and around lower half of oesophagus and cardia **o voice** produced by belching following laryngectomy **o web** occur in the upper oesophagus which are lined entirely by squamous epithelium. Usually they are acquired and may present with intermittent dysphagia

oesophagus (e-sof'ah-gus) muscular tube connecting the pharynx to the stomach. It is 25 cm long extending from cricopharyngeal sphincter at the level of the sixth cervical vertebra to the gastro-oesophageal junction **Barrett's o** metaplasia of the normal squamous epithelium of the oesophagus to form columnar epithelium as a consequence of chronic gastro-oesophageal reflux **corkscrew o** diffuse oesophageal spasm giving the appearance corkscrew of barium filled oesophagus

oesophagitis inflammation of the oesophagus secondary to reflux. Typical symptoms are heart burn, retrosternal pain and vomiting.

oesophagoscopy endoscopic examination of upper gastrointestinal tract

oestriasis (es-tri'ah-sis) infestation with larvae of flies belonging to genus *Oestrus*.

oestrodial secretion of ovarian theca cells which is converted in part to oestrone and oestriol by the liver

oestrogen replacement therapy hormone replacement therapy effective for menopausal symptoms and prevents osteoporosis. It may have benefit for coronary artery disease, with a small increase in risk of breast and endometrial cancer

oestrogens steroid hormones found during proliferative phase of menstrual cycle and synthetic equivalents **designer o** substances capable of mimicking oestrogen effects at some receptors but not at others

oestrous (es'trus) 'heat' during which the female will receive the male

offline not connected to a network or the Internet

ofloxacin (o-flok'sah-sin) an antibiotic effective against a wide variety of gram-negative organisms

ogawa a serotype of *Vibrio cholera*

Ogden plate a long metal plate with slots, used in fixing long bone fractures associated with preexisting intramedullary devices

Ogilvie's syndrome an acute intestinal pseudo obstruction from intestinal (mostly colon) dilatation, named after William Ogilvie, British physician.

Ogston's line a line from the tubercle of the femur to the intercondylar notch, named after Sir Alexandar Ogston, Scottish surgeon

Oguchi's nyctalopia familial night blindness seen in Japanese. The retina is pale and the condition is unresponsive to vitamin A, described by Japanese ophthalmologist, Chuta Oguchi

Ohio bed an open-sided bed for a baby in intensive care, that provides enough space around the baby for life support equipment and facilitates maintenance of baby's body temperature

Ohm (om) the SI unit of electrical resistance, named after a German physicist, Georg Ohm.

Ohmmeter (om'met-er) an instrument that measures electrical resistance in ohms

OI opportunistic infection

oid-oid disease a combination of exudative discoid dermatitis and lichenoid dermatitis

oil (oyl) 1. a liquid of animal, vegetable or mineral origin that is cumbustible and soluble in other but not in water 2. a fat that is liquid at room temperature

ointment (oint'ment) a semisolid medicinal preparation for external application to the body

ojas (s) vitality

ok-azaki fragments *Mol* DNA segments that are produced in discontinuous replication

okra sign radiologically the upper duo-denal bulb may appear mildly twisted and filled with air, whose cross-sectional view may appear like a transected okra *Hibiscus esculentus*

old tuberculin OT. A denatured mixture containing a large number of mycobacterial antigens obtained from culture filtrates of *Mycobacterium tuberculosis*. The active principle participating in the tuberculin test is present in the protein fraction

oleaginous (o'le-aj-i-nus) oily; greasy

oleander (o'le-an'der) a poisonous shrub containing cardiac glycoside

oleandomycin (o'le-an'do-mi'sin) an antimicrobial macrolide

oleate (o'le-at) a salt, ester or anion of oleic acid

olecranon (olek'rah-non) the proximal bony projection of the ulna in the region of the elbow and it fits into the olecranon fossa of the humerus when the forearm is extended **o bursa** the bursa of the elbow **o fossa** the depression in the posterior surface of the humerus that receives the olecranon of the ulna when the forearm is extended

oleic (o-le'ik) **acid** an organic acid prepared from animal fats and vegetable oils and it is used as an emulsifying agent

oleinitis (o-len-i'tis) inflammation of the elbow joint

oleo- referable to oil

oleotherapy (o-le-o-ther'ah-pe) treatment with oil

oleothorax (o-le-o-tho'raks) the therapeutic injection of oil into the pleural cavity

olestra a polymer of sucrose and triglycerides. It is not absorbed and acts like a 'fake fat ' to result in a decreased intake of fat and therefore, a reduction in total calories

oleum oil pl. **olea**

oleovitamin (o'le-ovi'ta-min) fish-liver oil or edible vegetable oil that contains one or more fat soluble vitamins

olfaction (ol-fak'shun) the sense of smell

olfactory (ol'fak-ter-e) relating to the sense

of smell **o bulb** the area of forebrain where the olfactory nerves terminate and olfactory tracts arise **o centre** neurones located near the junction of the temporal and parietal lobes responsible for appreciation of smell **o cortex** part of cerebral cortex, including the pyriform lobe and hippocampus formation concerned with the sense of smell **o foramen** one of several openings in the cribriform plate of the ethmoid bone **o hallucination** false perception of smelling a foul odour **o nerve** first cranial nerve that carries smell sensations from the nose to the brain. It arises from the sensory cells that ramify in the mucous membrane of the olfactory area in the upper part of the nasal fossa and reach the olfactory bulb after passing through the cribriform plate of ethmoid **o receptors** bipolar cells located in the nasal epithelium. Their axons become fibres of the olfactory nerve **o spectogram** test to determine the quality and quantity of sense of smell with seven primary odours - camphoraceous, ethereal, floral, musky, minty, pungent and putrid **o tract** the fibres forming the olfactory tract emerge from the olfactory bulb and reach the uncus of the hippocampal gyrus (olfactory area) in the cerebral cortex

oligaemia (ol'i-gem'e-ah) deficiency in the volume of the blood; an increased radiographic lucency

oligo a combining word for, scanty, little

oligochromaemia (ol'i-go-kro-mem'e-ah) deficiency of haemoglobin in the blood

oligodactyly (-dak'ti-le) congenital absence of one or more fingers or toes

oligodendrocyte (-den'dro-sit) a cell of the oligodendroglia. Its dendritic projections coil around axons of neural cells

oligodendroglia (-den'drog'le-ah) the nonneural cells of ectodermal origin becoming part of the neurolgia of the central nervous system

oligodendroglioma (-den'dro-glio-o'mah) a slow-growing neoplasm found on cerebral hemispheres, particularly the frontal lobes consisting of oligodendrocytes

oligodontia (-don'she-ah) presence of less than normal number of teeth

oligogene *Mol* a gene capable of producing major phenotypic alterations when mutated

oligohydramnios (-hi-dram'ne-os) the presence of abnormally small amount of amniotic fluid in the uterus during pregnancy. It can result in miscarriage, foetal deformities or foetal death; oligoamnios

oligomenorrhoea (-men'o-re'ah) markedly decreased menstrual flow

oligonucleotide (ol'i-go-nu' kle-o-tid) *Mol* small single stranded segments of DNA, required for DNA amplification and DNA sequencing, and contain 20-30 nucleotide bases

oligopnoea (ol-i-gop'ne-a) infrequent or shallow respiration

oligopontocerebellar (-pon'tosur'ibel'ar) of or pertaining to olivae, middle peduncles and the cerebellum

oligoptyalism (ol-i-go-ti'a-lizm) insufficient secretion of saliva.

oligosaccharide (ol'i-go-sak'a-rid) a compound made up of a small number of monosaccharide units

oligospermia (-sperm'e-ah) decrease in the number of spermatozoa in the semen. It forms a major cause of sterility

oligotrophia (-tro'fe-ah) poor nutritional state

oliguria (ol'i-gu're-ah) scanty urine. Amount of urine voided is less than 500 ml in every 24 hours, and is noted in peripheral circulatory failure, acute nephritis, dehydration and cardiac failure

olisthy (olis'the) the slippage of a bone from its normal anatomic position such as slipped disc

olivary (ol'i-var'e) olive-shaped **o body**

olivary nucleus as a collection of small densely packed nerve cells on the medulla oblongata

olive oil a vegetable oil that contains increased amount of monounsaturated fatty acids

olivopontocerebellar (ol'ivo-pon'to-sur'ibel'ar) of or pertaining to the olivae, the middle peduncles and the cerebellum o atrophy a multisystem atrophy characterised by cerebellar ataxia, dementia, spasticity, choreoathetosis, retinal degeneration and myelopathy

Ollier's (ol'e-az) disease a rare disorder of bone development wherein the epiphysis spreads through the bones causing abnormal, irregular growth and deformity, named after Louis Ollier, French surgeon

olophonia (ol'o-fo'ne-ah) defective speech due to malformed vocal cords

o m L. every morning

oma a suffix meaning tumour, neoplasm

omalgia (omal'jea) pain in the shoulder

omarthritis (o'marthri'tis) inflammation of the shoulder joint

omega-3 fatty acids polyunsaturated fatty acids with a double bond between carbons 3 and 4. Fish oils are examples which tend to raise HDL and decrease LDL

Omega sign facial expression with a furrowed brow caused by sustained contraction of the corrugator muscle, seen in melancholic patients

omental bursa a cavity in the peritoneum behind the stomach, the lesser omentum and the lower border of the liver and in front of the pancreas and duodenum

omental cake infiltration of the omental fat by material with soft-tissue density, noted in abdominal ultrasound or MR image, seen in secondary deposits in the omentum from tumours of the ovary, stomach and colon, and tuberculous peritonitis

omentectomy (o'men'tek'tah-me) excision

of all or part of the omentum

omentitis (o'men-tit'is) inflammation of the omentum

omentopexy (o-men'to-pek'se) fixing the omentum to some other tissue, and is performed to establish collateral circulation

omentorrhaphy (o'men-tor'ah-fe) repairs of the omentum

omentum (o'men'tum) a fold of peritoneum extending from the stomach to adjacent abdominal organs greater o an extension of the peritoneum covering the transverse colon and the coils of the small intestine. It is attached along the greater curvature of the stomach and the first part of the duodenum. There are blood vessels and fat pads between the layers of omentum lesser o a peritoneal extension from the peritoneal layers covering the stomach and the first part of the duodenum which extends from the portal fissure of the liver to the diaphragm where the layers separate to enclose the end of the oesophagus

omeprazole a drug that inhibits gastric secretion by altering the activity of the transmembrane proton pump, H^+/K^+ ATPase which is the final step in acid secretion in the parietal cells of the stomach

omission (omish'en) neglect to fulfil a duty required by law

omnifocal (om'nefo'kal) an eye glass useful for both near and far vision with the reading portion in a variable curve

omnipotence very powerful; identification with an idealised and powerful good object and denial of other aspects of internal and external reality, as a maniac defence

omnivorus (omni'vo-rus) eating both plants and animal flesh

omo - relation to shoulder

omoclavicular (o'mo-klah-vik'ul-er) pertaining to the shoulder and clavicle

omohyoid (-hi'oid) pertaining to the shoulder and the hyoid bone

omphal umbilicus

omphalic (omfal'ik) pertaining to the umbilicus

omphalectomy (om-fah-lek'tah-me) excision of the umbilicus

omphalelcosis (om'fal-el-ko'sis) ulceration of the umbilicus

omphalitis (om'fah-lit'is) inflammation of the umbilicus due to infection of the umbilical stump following its septic cutting and improper hygiene

omphalocoele (om'fah-lo-sel) protrusion of a part of the intestine at birth through a defect in the abdominal wall at the umbilicus

omphaloma (om'fah-lo-ma) a tumour at the site of the umbilicus

omphalophlebitis (-fle'bi'tis) inflammation of the umbilical veins

omphalorrhagia (-ra'je-ah) haemorrhage from the umbilicus

omphalorrhoea (-re'ah) discharge of lymph at the umbilicus

omphalorrhexis (-rek'sis) rupture of the umbilicus

omphalotomy (om'fah-lot'ah-me) the cutting of the umbilical cord at birth

omphalus (om'fah-lus) the umbilicus

ompholith (om'fah-lith) a mixture of accumulated sebaceous secretions with hair, dirt and desquamated epithelium and may present as a greyish brown or black stone in the umbilicus; umbolith

Omsk haemorrhagic fever a viral infection occurring in the summer in Western Siberia causing haemorrhage, fever and encephalitis. The disease spreads by tick

o n L. every night

o'nanism (o'nah-nizm) coitus interruptus

Onchocerca (ong'ko-ser'kah) a nematode whose adult, Onchocerca volvulus lives in subcutaneous tissues o dermopathy skin changes in onchocerca may be in the form of lizard skin (shiny), leopard skin (spotted) and elephant skin (thickened)

onchocerciasis (-ser-ki'ah-sis) infection by nematodes of genus Onchocerca. It presents with an itchy and erythematous rash, cutaneous lymphoedema with leathery thickening of the skin and impaired visual acuity. It is treated with diethyl carbamazine or ivermectin; river blindness

onco - relating to a tumour

oncocyte (ong'ko-sit') a large epithelial cell containing extremely acidophilic and granular cytoplasm with a large number of mitochondria. It exhibits a high ATPase and oxidative enzyme activity. These cells may increase with age and starvation

oncofetal antigens antigens that are expressed in the foetus during embryogenesis. They are produced in greater amounts in adults. However they may reappear during malignant dedifferentiation, in the form of -fetoprotein in hepatocellular carcinoma and as carcinoembryonic antigen in a variety of tumours and colonic adenocarcinoma

oncogene (ong-ko-jen) dominantly acting altered genes that are capable of inducing malignant transformation, such 'cancer genes' are derived from oncogenic RNA viruses and from normal genes

oncogenesis (-jeni-sis) the production of tumours, adj. oncogenetic

onchogenic (-jen'ik) causing tumour formation o virus any DNA virus (human papilloma virus) or RNA virus (retrovirus) that has the ability to cause malignant transformation of cells

oncology (ong-kol'ah-je) the study of neoplasms

oncologist (ong-kol'egist) a specialist in oncology

oncolysate (on-kol'i-sat) any agent that destroys tumour cells

oncolysis (ong-kol'i-sis) destruction of tumour cells

oncosphere (ong'-ko-sfer) larva of tapeworm which exists in the tissues of vertebrates and invertebrates

oncotherapy (ong'ko-the'rah-pe) the treatment of tumours

oncotic pressure the osmotic pressure of a colloid in solution

oncotomy (ong-kot'ah-me) the incision of a tumour

oncotropic (ang'ko-trop'ik) having affinity to tumour cells

oncovirus human T-cell leukaemia virus

Ondine's (ondenz') **curse** loss of automatic functions of the body leading to sleep apnoea syndrome, named after a watersprite in Greek mythology

one-and-a-half spica cast an orthopaedic plaster cast used for immobilising the trunk of the body cranially to the nipple line, one leg caudally as far as the toes, and the other leg caudally as far as the knee

one-and-one-half syndrome a unilateral pontine lesion producing ipsilateral gaze palsy and infranuclear ophthalmoplegia on the contralateral gaze with preservation of abduction

one-eyed vertebra unilateral destruction of a lumbar vertebral pedicle seen in AP film in metastatic carcinoma to vertebral body

oneiric (o-ni-rik) pertaining to dreaming.

oneirism (o-ni'rizm) a waking dream state

oneir – combining word for dream

onion bulbs segmental demyelination seen in peripheral nerves in chronic inflammatory demyelinating polyneuropathy, where schwann cells are arranged in lamellae resembling an onion skin

onion skinning a pattern of concentric laminations of differing radiologic (periosteal new bone formation) or histologic (concentric fibrosis of splenic arteries in lupus erythematosus, lamellar fibrosis surrounding medium sized bile ducts in the liver with sclerosing cholangitis, concentric arterial thickening in malignant hypertension) densities

onlay (on'la) a graft applied on the surface of an organ or structure; an occlu-sal rest portion of a removable partial denture, extended to cover the entire occlusal surface **o graft** a bone graft in which the transplanted tissue is laid directly onto the surface of the recipient bone

on-line a computer actively connected via a modem to the internet

on-off phenomenon periodic fluctuation in response to treatment with L-Dopa in Parkinson's disease; waxing and waning features of parkinsonism

onomatomania (on'ah-mat'ah-ma'ne-ah) a mental derangement regarding words or names

onset of action the time required after administration of a drug for a response to be observed

ontogeny (on-toj'i-ne) development of the individual organism **ontogenic**, adj

onychalgia (on'i-kal-jea) pain in the nails

onychatrophia (o-nik'ah-tro'fe-ah) atrophy of a nail

onychauxia (oni-kawk'sia) thickening of the nails

onychia (o-nik'e-ah) inflammation of the matrix of the nails, resulting in loss of the nail

onychocryptosis (oni-ko-krip-to'sis) ingrown nail

onychodystrophy malformed or discoloured finger nails or toe nails

onychogryphosis (oni-ko-gri-fo'sis) marked thickening and curvature of the nails

onycholysis (oni-kol'i-sis) separation of a nail from nail bed

onychomycosis (-mi-ko'sis) fungal infection of the nail; *Tinea unguium*

onychophagia (oni-kof'h-jah) biting of the nails

onychorrhexis (oni-ko-rek'sis) spontaneous breaking of nails

onychosis (oni-ko'sis) disease of the nail

onychotillomania (oni-ko-til'o-ma'neah) neurotic picking or tearing at the nails

onychotomy (onikot'ah-me) incision into the finger nail or toe nail

O'nyong-Nyong (o'ni-ang ni-ang) **disease**

a mosquito-borne dengue-like alpha virus infection seen in Uganda, characterised by weakening of the joints and generalized lymphadenopathy

oo- a prefix meaning 'of or pertaining to an egg or ovum'

oocyesis (o'si-e'sis) an ectopic ovarian pregnancy

oocyst (o'osist) the encysted zygote in the wall of a mosquito's stomach

oocyte (-sit) a developing egg cell

oogamy (o'og'ame) sexual reproduction by fertilisation of a large non-motile female gamete by a smaller, actively motile gamete

oogenesis (o'o-jen'e-sis) the process of formation of the female gametes or ova

ookinesis (-ki-ne'sis) the chromosomal movements of the egg during its maturation and fertilisation

ookinete (-ki-net') the fertilised form of the malarial parasite in the body of the mosquito

oophorectomy (o-of'ah-rek'tah-me) the surgical removal of the one or both ovaries; ovariectomy

oophoritis (-rit'is) inflammation of the ovary

oophorocystectomy (o-of'ah-ro-sis-tek'-tah-me) exision of an ovarian cyst

oophorocystosis (-sis-to'sis) the formation of ovarian cysts

oophoron (o-of'ah-ron) ovary

oophorosalpingectomy (o-of'ahrosal' pinjek'-tah-me) the surgical removal of one or both ovaries and the corresponding fallopian tubes

oophorosalpingitis (o-of'ah-rosal'pinje'itis) an inflammation of both the ovary and fallopian tube

oophorostomy (o-of'ah-ros'tah-me) incision of an ovarian cyst for drainage

ooplasm (o'o-plazm) cytoplasm of an ovum

oosperm (-sperm) a fertilised ovum

ootid (-tid) the mature ovum after penetration by spermatozoa and completion of second meiotic division

OP abbreviation for outpatient

opacification (o-pa'si-fi-ka'shun) the development of an opacity

opacity (o-pas'it-e) opaque

opalescent (o'pah-les'int) milky appearance

opaque (o-pak') impervious to light rays or to x-rays

OPD abbreviation for outpatient department

open amputation an amputation in which a straight guillotine cut is made without skin flaps

open bite an abnormal dental condition in which the anterior teeth do not occlude in any mandibular position

open dislocation a dislocation in which the skin is broken

open drop administration administration of chloroform and diethyl ether using a folded kerchief or mask

open heart surgery any surgical procedure performed on the heart in which the heart is temporarily stopped and its function is taken over by a mechanical pump

opening (o'pin-ing) orifice, aperture **o snap** a sharp, snapping sound audible in mitral stenosis when the stenotic mitral valve which is flung open is brought to abrupt halt. It is heard about midway between the second and third heart sounds in expiration at the lower left sternal edge

open-label a clinical trial where both the investigator and participants know who is taking the experimental therapy

open pneumothorax the presence of air in the pleural cavity as a result of an open wound in the chest wall

open wound a wound that disrupts the integrity of the skin

operable (op'er-ah-b'l) a condition wherein a surgical procedure can be undertaken with reasonable expectation of cure or relief

operant (op'er-ant) any response that recurs at a given rate without any specific external stimulus

operating (op'er-a-ting) **microscope** A binocular microscope used in delicate surgery especially surgery of the eye or ear

operation (op'er-a'shun) any surgical procedure **o theatre,** OT, area where minor and major surgical procedures are carried out

operculum (o-per'ku-lum) a lid or covering

operon (op'er-on) *Mol* a segment of chromosome consisting of an operator gene and closely linked structural gene possessing related function

ophiasis (o-fi'ah-sis) an extension of patches of hair loss into the actual hair margin especially in the temporal and occipital regions

ophidism (ofi-dizm) poisoning by snake venom

ophryon (of're-on) the point on midline of the forehead just above the glabella

ophryosis (of're-o'sis) spasm of the eyebrow

ophiotoxaemia poisoning by snake venom

ophthalmagra (of'thal-mag'rah) sudden pain in the eye

ophthalmalgia (of'thal-mal'jah) pain in the eye

ophthalmatrophia atrophy of the eye

ophthalmectomy (of'thal-mek'tah-me) enucleation of the eyeball

ophthalmencephalon (of'thal-men-sef'-ah-lon) the retina, optic nerve and visual apparatus of the brain

ophthalmia (of-thal'me-a) severe inflammation of the eye **o neonatorum** purulent infection of the eyes of the infant from gonococcus or chlamydia

ophthalmiatrics (of-thal-me-at'riks) the treatment of eye diseases

ophthalmic (of-thal'mik) relating to the eye **o nerve** the first division of the trigeminal nerve supplying the eyeball, forehead, scalp, lacrimal gland and duramater

ophthalmitis (of'thal-mi'tis) inflammation of the eye

ophthalmoblennorrhoea (of'thal'mo-blen'o-re'a) purulent infection of the eye

ophthalmodonesis (of'thal'mo-do-ne'sis) a trembling motion of the eyes

ophthalmodynamometer (of'thal'mo-di'nah-mom'e-ter) an instrument for measuring the retinal artery pressure

ophthalmodynamometry (of'thal'mo-di'nah-mom'e-tre) determination of the retinal artery pressure

ophthalmologist (of'thal'mol'o-jist) specialist trained in the diagnosis and management of diseases of the eye

ophthalmology (of'thal'mol'o-je) science dealing with the eye and its disorders

ophthalmomalacia (of'thal'mo-mah-la'she-a) abnormal softness of the eye

ophthalmometer (of'thal-mom'e-ter) instrument to measure refractive powers

ophthalmometry (of'thal-mom'e-tre) determination of the refractive powers and defects of the eye

ophthalmomyositis (of'thal'mo-mi'o-si'tis) inflammation of the eye muscles

ophthalmoplegia (of'thal'mo-ple'je-a) partial or total paralysis of the muscles that move the eyes

ophthalmoscope (of'thal'mo-skop) an illuminated viewing instrument to examine the retina

ophthalmoscopy (of'thal'mos'ko-pe) examination of the retina using an ophthalmoscope

opiate (o'pe-at) any natural or synthetic (fentanyl) semisynthetic (morphine) alkaloid narcotic possessing opium-like activity **o poisoning** toxic effects of the potent narcotic causing depression of brain centres and coma **o receptor any** of a group of cells in the brain that bind to opiate drugs

opioid (o'pe-yod) **peptides** endogenous opiates. They are natural polypeptide neurotransmitters that are involved in the perception of pain, response to stress, regulation of appetite and sleep, memory and learning

opisthenar (o-pis'the-nar) dorsum of the hand

Opisthorchis (o'pis-thor'kis) a genus of trematodes

opisthotonus (o'pis-thot'o-nos) a spasm wherein the head and the heels are bent back making the body like a bow noted in extreme cases of tetanus

Opitz-Frias syndrome the hypospadias, dysphagia syndrome, a rare congenital condition named after, J.M. Opitz, and Jaime Frias, Chilean Paediatricians

opium (o'pe-um) exudate from capsules of *Papaver somniferum.* Morphine, heroin and codeine are extracted from opium

Oppenheim's (op'en-himz) **reflex** an extension of big toe with slight dorsiflexion of the foot can be elicited by pressing with the thumb and the index finger along the medial border of the tibia, named after Herman Oppenheim, Berlin neurologist

opponens (o-po'nenz) opposing **o pollicis** muscle in the thumb tested by touching the top of the little finger with the point of the thumb

opportunistic (op'or-tu-nis'tik) **infections** infections caused by organisms which rarely produce disease in a healthy person but frequently cause disease in persons whose immune system is weakened by a disease such as AIDS or as a result of immunosuppressive therapy

opportunists (op'or-tu-nis'ts) taking advantage of the opportunity of impaired host defence mechanisms

opsin (op'sin) a transmembrane protein of retinal rods and cones

opsoclonus (op'so-clo'nus) conjugate, irregular and non-rhythmic jerky movements of the eyes

opsomania (op'so-ma'nea) a craving for some special food

opsonin (op-so'nin) a substance that binds to red cells, bacteria or other exogenous agents enhancing their susceptibility to phagocytosis

opsonization (op'so-ni-za'shun) rendering bacteria and other cells subject to phagocytosis

optic (op'tik) pertaining to the eyes or to sight **o atrophy** optic disc is paler than normal and may even be white **o chiasma** optic nerves of both sides meet at this point lying in close contact with pituitary gland and there is decussation of fibres from the inner half of each retina **o density** a number describing the blackening of an x-ray film in any specified location **o disc** pink, oval or circular prominent structure of retina whose margins are sharp with a small central depression **o disc drusen** condensations of hyaline-like material within the substance of the optic nerve head **o foramen** an aperture in the root of the lesser wing of the sphenoidal bone transmitting the optic nerve **o fundus** fundus of the eye **o glioma** a slow growing tumour on the optic nerve or in the chiasma. It consists of glial cells and presents with loss of vision, stabismus, exophthalmos and ocular paralysis **o nerve** second cranial nerve that transmits information about visual images received from the retina to the lateral geniculate body. It also acts as an afferent pathway for the pupillary reflexes. The fibres originating in the retina pass behind as optic nerve and enter cranial cavity through the optic foramen **o neuritis** inflammatory demyelinating or vascular disease affecting optic nerve leading to loss of vision **o radiation** axons of nerve cells of lateral geniculate body carrying visual information **o righting** a basic neuromuscular reaction enabling a person to change body position that involves a reflex that automatically orients the head to a new optical or visual fixation point, depending on the body position change **o stalk** one of a pair of slender embryonic structures that become the optic nerve **o tract** nerve fibres running backward and laterally around each cerebral peduncle from the optic chiasma to the lateral geniculate body

optical (op'ti-kal) pertaining to vision **o illusion** a false visual image obtained from a misinterpretation of sensory stimuli

optician (op-tish'an) person who fits and supplies spectacles or contact lenses

opticokinetic (op'ti-ko-ki-net'ik) concerning the movement of the eye

optics (op'tiks) science dealing with light and its relation to vision

optimism looking at the bright side of a condition or event

optimum (op'ti-mum) the most desirable state of affairs

opto - combining word for eye, vision

optometer (op-tom'e-ter) instrument measuring the power and range of vision

optometrist (op-tom'e-trist) a person trained to test the eyes and prescribe spectacles and other visual aids

optometry (op-tom-e-tre) measurement of the powers of vision and its adaptation to lenses **behavioural o** a special branch of optometry which recognizes that posture, general health and the environment can affect eyesight

OPV abbreviation for oral poliovirus vaccine

ora a margin or border

oral (or'al) pertaining to the mouth **o allergy syndrome** contact with certain fresh fruit juices results in urticaria and angiooedema of the lips and oropharynx **o cavity** the cavity of the mouth including the tongue and teeth **o cancer** a malignant neoplasm on the lip or in the mouth **o contraceptives** used as effective spacing method of contraception and they prevent release of the ovum from the ovary. Combined pill consisting of 30-35 mcg of a synthetic oestrogen with 0.5 to 1.0 mg progesterogen taken orally for 21 consecutive days beginning on the fifth day of the menstrual cycle, followed by a break of 7 days during which period menstruation occurs. Mini pill consists of progesterogen only and it is given throughout the cycle. Morning after pill or postcoital pill contains very high doses of oestrogen and is used in an unprotected intercourse **o glucose tolerance test** test to determine the ability to metabolise sugar. Performed in the morning after 3 days of unrestricted diet and physical activity, but the patient should be fasting at least 10 hours before and a loading dose of glucose of 75 g (adults) or 1.75 g/kg (children) given **o hygiene** maintenance of the tissues and structures of the mouth clean by brushing the teeth, massaging the gums **o hypoglycaemic agents** They are sulphonyl ureas (tolbutamide, chlorpropamide, glypizide, glibenclamide, glyclazide and glimepiride), biguanides (phenformin, metformin) guargum and acarbose **o poliovirus vaccine** an attenuated live poliovirus vaccine that confers immunity to poliomyelitis prepared by Albert Sabin, US virologist **o rehydration therapy** administration of 3.5, gm sodium chloride 2.5, gm sodium bicarbonate, 1.5, gm potassium chloride and 20, gm of glucose dissolved in one litre of water orally at frequent intervals to correct dehydration caused by diarrhoea **o surgery** surgery concerned with operations in and around the mouth **o temperature** recording of body temperature with the centrigrade clinical thermometer. Before its use, the thermometer should be washed with water and the mercury column brought down by shaking it. The thermometer should be kept beneath the tongue and the mouth closed. It must be allowed to stay for 1 to 2 minutes. The normal temperature is 37°C (98.6°F) with average from 36.6°C to 37.2°C (98-99°F) **o ulceration** ulceration in oral mucosa, which may occur as aphthous ulcers or in association with systemic disorders **o white patches** white lesions in the oral mucosa either due to candida infection or are rarely seen in SLE

orange peel skin appearance peau d'orange appearance as in skin overlying breast cancer

orange person syndrome a rare side effect of an overdose of rifampicin colouring the skin and body fluids a deep orange. The liver functions are abnormal and there is pruritus

orb a spherical body such as eye

orbicular (or-bik'u-lar) circular

orbicularis muscles in the face supplied by facial nerve o oculi muscle of the eye which helps in closing the eye tightly o oris muscle of lips that helps to purse the lips

orbit (or'bit) socket in the skull containing the eyeball, protective pads of fat, blood vessels, muscles and nerves

orbital (orbi-tal) concerning the orbit o aperture an opening in the cranium to the orbit of the eye o cholecystography opacification of the bile ducts following ingestion of iodinated contrast. The contrast is excreted by hepatocytes in the bile ducts o fissure the space between the floor and lateral wall of the orbit through which the nerves and blood vessels pass

orbitale (or'bita'le) lowest point along the inferior margin of the orbit

orchialgia (or-ke-al'je-a) pain in a testis

orchi - orchio - combining word for testicle

orchiectomy (or'ke-ek'to-ome) surgical removal of one or both testes

orchiepididymitis (or'ke-ep'i-did'i-mi'tis) inflammation of a testis and epididymis

orchiopexy (or'ke-o-pek'se) surgical fixation of an undescended testis into the scrotum

orchioschirrhus (or'ke-o-skir'rus) hardened testis from tumour formation

orchis (or'kis) testis

orchitis (or-kit'is) inflammation of one or both testes characterised by swelling and pain. Treatment includes support and elevation of the scrotum, cold packs and analgesics

order (or'der) arrangement or sequence of events, rules, regulations or procedures

ordinate (or'di-nat) line used as a base of reference o scale assessment of size of an organ as mild, moderate and massive, severity of pain, tenderness, muscle power, sugar and albumin in urine as 0, 1+, 2+, 3+ and 4+.

orf sheep pox

organ (or'gan) any part of the body performing a specific function o bank a repository for a long-term storage of certain tissues destined for transplantation o donation permission given by a person or from relatives after the death of a person for surgical removal of one or more organs for use in transplant surgery o recital giving a list of complaints from multiple organs and organ systems by a hypochondriac o transplantation transfer of an organ (kidney, heart, liver) between members of the same species

organelle (or'gan'el) a specific particle bound to membrane in a cell

organic (or-gan'ik) pertaining to an organ o amnestic syndrome a marked impairment of memory occurring in clear consciousness. It is associated with impairment of short-term memory. It may be noted in severe thiamine deficiency secondary to chronic alcohol abuse o brain syndrome cerebral degeneration in the form of cortical atrophy o delusional disorder a mental state dominated by delusions which are very often persecutory o·disease disorder accompanied by demonstrable changes in the body structure o dust dried particles of plants, animals, fungi or bacteria carried by wind. o mental disorders disorders characterised by progressive deterioration of the mental processes. They develop from brain dysfunction or brain damage

organism (or'gan-izm) any living individual either animal or plant. It is an organised system of parts that ordinarily work together in a unified manner

organ of Corti the true organ of hearing

named after Alfansi Corti, Italian anatomist. It is a spiral structure within the cochlea containing hair cells that are stimulated by sound vibrations. They are converted into nerve impulses and transmitted by cochlear portion of the auditory nerve to the brain

organogenesis (-jen'esis) the formation and differentiation of organs and organ systems during embryonic development

organoid (or'ga-noid) a synthetic organ exhibiting angiogenic and secretory capacities of an organ

organomegaly (or'ga-no-meg'a-le) the enlargement of visceral organs

organopexy (or'gan-o-pek'se) the surgical fixation of an organ that is detached from its place

organophosphates (-fos'fats) a class of anticholinesterase chemicals used as insecticides. They are heterogeneous group of compounds that are composed of a phosphoric acid derivative with two organic side chains and an additional side chain containing a cyanide, thiocyanate, halide, phosphate, phenoxy, thiophenoxy or carboxylate group. They are rapidly absorbed by all routes - dermal, respiratory, alimentary and conjunctival. They cause acetylcholinesterase inhibition in the nervous system resulting in accumulation of acetylcholine at synapses and the myoneural junction. They produce muscarine (sweating, miosis, lacrimation, excessive salivation, wheezing, vomiting, diarrhoea, bradycardia, blurred vision), nicotinic (fasciculations, cramps, tachycardia) and CNS (restlessness, ataxia, convulsions, coma) effects. The antidotal therapy consists of atropine and pralidoxime

organotherapy (or'gan-o-ther'a-pe) the treatment of disease by preparations of the endocrine glands of animals or by their extracts

orgasm (or'gazm) peak of sexual excitement, experienced as an intensely pleasurable sensation

orthodiagrphy an accurate tracing of the heart shadow

orthopnoea (or'thop-ne'ah) dyspnoea in the recumbent, but not in the upright position. It is usually relieved by two or three pillows under the head and back. It is a hallmark of pulmonary congestion that stiffens the lungs

orthotopic (or'tho-top'ik) in the correct place **o graft** transfer of grafts to anatomically similar positions in the recipient, as in skin to a bed prepared in the skin

oriental sore cutaneous leishmaniasis caused by *Leishmania tropica*

orientation (or'en-ta-shun) determination of one's position with respect to space and time

orifice (or'i-fis) the mouth, entrace or outlet of any anatomic structure

origin (or'i-jin) the point of beginning

ornithinaemia (or'ni-then-e'mea) **type I** an autosomal recessive condition with hyperornithinaemia, postprandial hyperammonaemia and homocitrullinaemia, HHH syndrome

ornithinaemia type II a condition exhibiting hyperornithinaemia with gyrate atrophy (HOGA syndrome) of the choroid and retina leading to slowly progressive loss of vision, myopia and nyctalopia and renal tubular dysfunction

ornithine (or'ni-thin) an amino acid formed on hydrolysis of arginine by arginase

ornithosis (oe'no-tho'sis) an acute generalised, infectious disease of birds transmitted to man and is caused by *Chlamydia psittaci*, psittacosis, parrot fever. Illness is like influenza and effective treatment is tetracycline or erythromycin.

oro- a combining word for related to mouth.

orofacial (or'o-fa-she-al) concerning the mouth and face

orolingual (or'o-ling'gwal) concerning the mouth and tongue

oromandibular-dystonia involuntary movement of the mouth and tongue

oronasal (or'o-na'zal) pertaining to the mouth and nose

oropharynx (or'o-far'inks) the region of pharynx lying between the soft palate and epiglottis

orphan destitute, a child whose parents have died or are not known **o disease** an illness due to its rarity has received less attention **o drugs** drugs used to treat rare diseases but are not profitable to the manfacturer **o virus** a virus that has been isolated and identified although it has not been associated with any particular disease

orrhodiagnosis (or'o-diag-no'sis) serum diagnosis

orrhorrhoea (or'o-roh'rea) a watery or serous discharge

orrhotherapy (or'oh-thera'py) serum therapy

ORS abbreviation for oral rehydration solution

ORT see oral rehydration therapy

ortho combining word for - straight.

orthochromatic (or'tho-kro-mat'ik) having normal colour or staining normally

orthodeoxia (or'tho-de-ok-sea) decreased arterial oxygen concentration while in an erect position

orthodontic (or'tho-don'tik) **appliance** any device used to modify tooth position

orthodontic band a thin metal ring of stainless steel, fitted over a tooth for securing orthodontic attachments to a tooth

orthodontics (or'tho-don'tiks) branch of dentistry referring to corrective dental work for irregularities of teeth; orthodontia

orthodontist (or'tho-don'tist) a dentist who has specialised in orthodontics

orthokeratosis (or'tho-ker'o-to-sis) hyperkeratosis in which nuclei are not retained in cornified cells

orthokinetic tactile stimulatory techniques employed to stimulate the proprioceptors of muscles and tendons

orthomyxoviruses (or'tho-mik'so-vi'rusus) a family of large, spherical viruses that includes influenza viruses

orthopaedics (or'tho-pe-diks) the branch of surgery concerned with the disease of the skeletal system

orthopaedic traction a procedure in which a patient is maintained in a device attached by ropes and pulleys to weights that exert a pulling force on a limb or body part while counter-traction is maintained.

orthopaedist (or'tho-pe-dist) a specialist in orthopaedics

orthopercussion (or'tho-per-kush'un) percussion wherein the terminal phalanx of the pleximeter finger is held perpendicular to the chest wall

orthopnoea (or'thop' ne-a) difficult breathing in recumbent position

orthopnoeic (or'thop'ne-ik) **position** a posture that enables to breath comfortably The patient sits and bends forwards with the arms supported on a table

orthopsia (or'thop'sea) the ability to see objects during twilight

orthoptic (or-thop'tik) producing normal binocular vision

orthoptics the science of correcting defects in binocular vision that have resulted from defects in optic musculature

orthoptist (or'thop'tist) a person who tests the strength of eye muscles and helps in strengthening the eye muscles by teaching exercises with supervision of an ophthalmologist

orthoreovirus a rare cause of enteritis and upper respiratory infection

orthosis (or-tho'sis) an orthopaedic appliance to correct deformities

orthostatic (or'tho-stat'ik) caused by standing erect **o hypotension** blood pressure falling when the individual assumes the standing posture; postural hypotension **o proteinuria** a benign condition where apparently healthy persons excrete small amounts of protein in relation to assuming erect posture

orthotic a device to control, correct or compensate for deformities of bones, muscles or joints

orthotics (or'thot'iks) the science dealing with orthopaedic appliances

orthotist (or'tho-tist) a person who designs, fabricates and fits orthopaedic devices prescribed by an orthopaedic surgeon

orthotolidine test test to determine both free and combined chlorine in water

orthotonus (or'tho-to'nus) a straight, rigid posture of the body caused by tetanic spasm, noted in the tetanus and strychnine poisoning

orthropsia (or'throp'sea) vision that is better at dawn or dusk than in bright sunlight

Ortner's syndrome huskiness of voice due to paralysis of the left recurrent laryngeal nerve in mitral stenosis. The nerve may be compressed by dilated left atrium. It can also occur by enlarged tracheobronchial lymph nodes and dilatation of the pulmonary artery, named after Norbert Ortner, Austrian physician

Ortolani click sound produced by head of the femur returning to the acetabulum, test used to determine for evidence of congenital dislocation of the hip, named after Marius Ortolani, Italian orthopaedic surgeon

os any orifice of the body, bone; mouth, opening

oscheal (os'ke-al) pertaining to the scrotum

oscheitis (os-ke-i'tis) inflammation of the scrotum

oschelephantiasis (osk'el-e-fan-ti'a-sis) elephantiasis of the scrotum

oscillation (os'sil-a'shun) a backward and forward movement like a pendulum

oscillograph (os'il-o-graf) an instrument useful to record electric oscillations

oscillometer (os-il-om'e-ter) an instrument to measure oscillations produced by changes in the volume

oscillopsia (o'-sil-o-p'sea) oscillating vision

oscitate (os'sit-at) to yawn

oscitation (os'sit-a-shun) yawning

osculum (os'ku-lum) minute opening

Osgood (oz'good) **osteotomy** a surgical procedure to correct malrotation of a femur

Osgood-Schlatter's disease apophysitis of the tibial tuberosity exhibiting tender, puffy swelling of the bony prominence just below the knee, described by Robert Osgood, US orthopaedic surgeon and Carl Schlatter, Zurich surgeon

Osler's nodes painful red transitory nodular swellings in the pulp of the fingers, thenar and hypothenar eminences and toes due to infected cutaneous emboli seen in infective endocarditis, described by Sir William Osler, American-British physician

Osler-Weber-Rendu syndrome haemorrhagic telangiectasis, named after Osler, Fredrick Weber, London physician and Henri Rendu, French physician. The condition is inherited as an autosomal dominant trait characterised by small red-to-violet lesions in the skin and mucous membrane. The thin dilated vessels may bleed spontaneously or as a result of minor trauma

osmatic (oz-mat'ik) refers to the sense of smell

osmesia (oz-me-sea) smelling.

osmesthesia (oz'mes-the'ze-a) ability to appreciate different odours

osmalagnia (oz-mo-lag'ne-a) sexual excitation produced by odour

osmolal gap (os'mo-lal-gap) an osmometer measurement indicating a serum osmolality that is more than 10 Osm/L greater than the calculated osmolality. It suggests the presence of an osmotically active substance that is not accounted for by the calculated osmolality. Ethanol produces an increase in measured osmolality over the calculated osmolality

osmolality (os'mo-lal'ite) a measurement of the amount of osmotically effective solute per 1000 grams of solvent (Osm). It is the molar equivalent of the number of molecular particles in a litre of water. It is measured either directly by determining the freezing point (osmometry) or by calculation. The formula for calculating osmolality is

Serum osmolality = 2×Na+(meq/L)

$$+\frac{BUN\,(mg\,/\,dl)}{2.8}+\frac{glucose\,(mg\,/\,dl)}{18}$$

where BUN is the blood urea nitrogen level. The normal serum osmolality is 280 to 295 mOsm/L

osmolar (oz-mo'lar) concerning the osmotic concentration of a solution

osmolarity (os'mo-lar'i-te) the number of osmotically active particles in a litre of solution expressed is osmol/kg of solvent. Osmolality is preferred to the term osmolarity.

osmolar gap the difference between the measured osmolality and the calculated osmolality

osmole the molecular weight of a solute in grams divided by the number of particles into which it dissociates in solution. When an osmol of a substance dissolved in one litre of water, it exerts an osmotic pressure of 22.4 atmosphere

osmology (ozmol'eje) the science of the sense of smell

osmometer (oz-mom'et-er) instrument useful to measure osmotic force or to measure the acuteness of the sense of smell

osmophilic affinity for solutions having a high osmotic pressure

osmoreceptor (oz mo-re-sep'tor) a sensory receptor stimulated by changes in the osmotic pressure or by sensation of odours

osmoregulation (oz'mo-reg'u-la'shun) maintenance of osmolarity

osmosis (oz-mo'sis) the passage of a solvent from a less concentrated solution to a concentrated one through a semipermeable membrane

osmotherapy (oz-mo-ther'a-pe) administration of hypertonic solutions to draw

water from brain due to osmotic gradient and reduce brain oedema

osmotic agent a substance that is used to induce drainage of fluid from one side of a cell membrane to another

osmotic diuresis diuresis occurring from presence of non-absorbable substances in the renal tubules such as mannitol

osmotic fragility normal red blood cells lyse in saline of strength 0.45% and 0.3%. It is increased in hereditary spherocytosis and decreased in thalassemia, jaundice, sickle cell anaemia and iron therapy

osmotic pressure pressure aquired to prevent migration of solvent into a compartment where the concentration of solute is higher across a membrane that is permeable to the solvent but not the the solute. It is measured as osmolarity

osphresis (os-fre'sis) the sense of smell

osphyarthrosis (os-fe-ar'tho-sis) inflammation of the hip joint.

ossein (os'e-in) the collagen of bone **o deformans** Paget's disease **o fibrosa cystica** hyperparathyroidism

osseous (os'e-us) bony **o labyrinth** the bony portion of the internal ear. It consists of three cavities: the vestibule, the semicircular canals, and the cochlea. They contain perilymph in which a membranous labyrinth is suspended

ossicle (os'i-kl) a small bone

ossiculectomy (os'ik-u -lek'to-me) surgical removal of an ossicle

ossiculum (o-sik'u-lum) a small bone

ossification (os'i-fi-ka'shun) the process of formation of bone; conversion of cartilage into bone **intramembranous o** preceded by membrane as in the formation of the roof and sides of the skull. **intracertilaginous o** preceded by cartilage as in the bones of the limb

ossifying developing into bone

ostalgia (os-tal'je-a) pain in a bone

osteal (os'te-al) bony

ostectomy (os-tek'to-me) the excision of a bone

osteitis (os-te-i-tis) inflammation of a bone **o deformans** see Paget's disease **o fibrosa cystica** see hyperparathyroidism. There is replacement of normal bone by cysts and fibrous tissue

**osteo - ** a prefix meaning of or relating to a bone

osteoarthritis (os'te-o-ar-thri'tis) degenerative joint disease characterised by both degeneration of articular cartilage and simultaneous proliferation of new bone, cartilage and connective tissue. The joints most frequently involved are those of the spine, hip, knees and hands. Radiographs show loss of joint space and formation of marginal osteophytes. Treatment is directed towards relieving symptoms and maintaining and improving joint function

osteoarthropathy (os'te-o-ar-throp'a-the) any disease of the joints and bones **hypertropic o** swelling around the wrists and ankles from periosteal thickening

osteoarthrosis (os'te-o-ar-thro'sis) non-inflammatory joint involvement

osteoarticular pertaining to the joints and bones

osteoblast (os'te-o-blast) cell arising from a fibroblast concerned with building new bone

osteoblastic tumours tumours producing substances with parathyroid hormone-like activity

osteoblastoma (os'te-o-blas-to-ma) a small, benign vascular tumour of the bone

osteocalcin a noncollagenous bone protein

osteochondrial pertaining to bone and cartilage

osteochondritis (os'te-o-kon-dri'tis) inflammation of bone and cartilage **o dissecans** a disorder following an injury, releasing small fragments of cartilage or bone into the joint space especially of the knee and elbow **o juvenilis** inflammation of a growing area of bone in a child or adolescent. It causes local pain and distortion of a joint

osteochondrodystrophy (os'te-o-kon-dro-dis'tro-fe) Morquio's syndrome

osteochondroma (os'te-o-kon-dro'ma) a benign tumour of bone originating from the growing epiphyseal cartilage. It grows outwards from the bone like a mushroom and is capped by cartilage

osteochondromatosis (-to'sis) rare disease of synovial membrane. Their villous folds become pedunculated and undergo change to cartilage. They get separated as free mobile bodies

osteochondropathy (os'te-o-kon-dro-pa'the) disorder affecting bone and cartilage

osteochondrosis (os'te-o-kon-dro'sis) a disease of ossification centre in children which exhibits degeneration followed by regeneration

osteoclasia (os'te-o-kla'ze-a) the absorption and destruction of bony tissue

osteoclasis (os'te-o-kla'sis) forcible bending or incomplete breaking of a bone to correct deformities of the long bones

osteoclast (os'te-o-klast) cell concerned with the absorption and removal of bone; an instrument useful in the surgical fractures of bone

osteoclast-like giant cell a multinucleated giant cell with abundant eosinophilic, finely granular or homogeneous cytoplasm containing nearly a hundred uniform oval nuclei

osteoclastoma (os'-te-o-klas-to'ma) giant cell tumour of bone. Though benign, it tends to recur after removal, noted in young adults. It presents with pain at the site of the tumour and a gradually increasing local swelling. There is destruction of the bone with expansion of the cortex

osteocranium (os'-te-o-kra'ne-um) the foetal cranium during the stages of ossification

osteocyte (os'-te-o-sit) an osteoblast within the bony matrix

osteodesmosis (os'-te-o-des-mo'sis) ossification of tendon

osteodynia (os'-te-o-din'e-a) pain in a bone

osteodystrophy (os'-te-o-dis'tro-fe) defective bone formation

osteoenchondroma (os'te-o-en-kandro'ma) a benign bone and cartilage tumour within a bone

osteofibrochondrosarcoma (-fi'brokon'dro-sarko-ma) a malignant tumour composed of bone, cartilage and fibrous tissues

osteofibroma (os'-te-o-fi-bro-ma) a tumour consisting of bone and fibrous tissue

osteoflurosis (os'-te-o-flu-ro'sis) bony changes exhibiting osteosclerosis due to excessive intake of fluorides over a long period of time

osteogenesis (os'-te-o-jen'e-sis) formation of bone **o imperfecta** a genetic disorder in which bones are abnormally soft and easily broken. It is associated with blue sclerae, deafness, scoliosis, thin hyperextensible skin, visceral herniation, ligamentous laxity and easy bruising; fragilitas ossium; brittle bone disease.

osteogenic sarcoma; osteosarcoma a malignant bone tumour of childhood or early adult life, may occur in later life as a complication of osteitis deformans. It arises from primitive bone forming cells commonly at the lower end of the femur and the upper end of the humerus. It begins in the metaphysis and destroys the bone substance. It presents with local pain and a diffuse firm thickening of bone. Radiograph shows irregular destruction of the metaphysis and later the cortex appears to have been 'burst open'. Occasionally well marked radiating spicules of new bone seen within the tumour gives a sun-ray appearance. It spreads rapidly to other parts of the body, especially the lungs

osteohalisteresis (os'-te-o-hal'is'ter-e-sis) deficient mineral content of bone, leading to softening of bones

osteohyoma (os'-te-o-hi-oma) an overgrowth of a bone

osteoid (os'-te-oyd) organic matrix of bone **o osteoma** a benign, circumscribed lesion of bone with a severe deep 'boring pain' which is ill-localised and worst at night. It has to be excised

osteologist (os'-te-ol-'o-jist) specialist in osteology

osteology (os'-te-ol'a-je) the scientific study of the bones

osteolysis (os'-te-ol'i-sis) degeneration and dissolution of bone, resulting from disease, infection or lack of a blood supply

osteolytic (os'te-o-lit'ik) causing osteolysis

osteoma (os'-te-o'ma) a bony tumour, that may occur on any bone. It may be composed of hard compact bone (**ivory o**) or of spongy bone (**cancellous o**)

osteomalacia (os'-te-o-mal-a-she-a) softening, weakening and demineralisation of adult bones due to vitamin D deficiency, phosphate depletion or chronic metabolic acidosis. It presents with bone pain and tenderness. There can be proximal myopathy. Radiologically the bones appear less dense than normal and the long bones may show areas of decalcification treated by Vitamin D2

osteomyelitis (os'-te-o-mi-el-i'tis) inflammation of bone and bone marrow due to a pyogenic infection **acute o** infection of the bone with pyogenic organisms - usually the *Staphylococcus aureus*. A minor injury to bone renders it vulnerable to infection by organisms circulating in the blood. Occurs in children, has rapid onset with pain over the affected bone and fever. There is exquisite tenderness over affected bone and later a fluctuant abscess may be present. Radiological changes occur two to three weeks later with diffuse rarefaction of metaphysis with new bone outlining the raised periosteum. The condition is treated by bed rest and systemic antibiotic therapy. The pus may have to be evacuated and limb splinted **chronic o** occurs as a sequel to acute osteomyelitis. It is common in long bones. The bone is thickened and denser than normal with presence of sequestra. Often a sinus track leads to skin surface. In addition to rest and antibiotics, the fragments of infected dead bone have to be removed

osteon (os'-te-on) the basic unit of structure of compact bone

osteonecrosis (os'te-o-ne-kro'sis) the death of a segment of bone

osteopath (os'-te-o-path) a practitioner of osteopathy

osteopathy (os'-te-op-a-the) any disease of a bone; a system of medicine relying on manipulation of various body parts to regain a state of wellness

osteopaenia (os'-te-o-pe'ne-a) decrease in the bony mass due to a decreased rate of osteoid synthesis

osteoperiostitis (os'-te-o-per'e-os-ti'tis) inflammation of a bone and its periosteum

osteopetrosis (os-te-o-pe-tro'sis) a rare genetic disorder showing abnormally hard, dense bone due to a faulty bone resorption. There is increased liability to fracture and anaemia

osteophone (os'-te-o-fun) a bone-crushing forceps

osteophyte (os'-te-o-fit) an overgrowth of a bone at the edge of a joint, seen in osteoarthritis.

osteopoikilosis (or'tho-poi-kil-o-sis) an uncommon, familial disorder characterised by uniform, punctate, round, oval or linear streaks of bone in the epiphysis and metaphysis of long bones and in the pelvic bones

osteoporosis (os-te-o-por-o'sis) a systemic skeletal disease characterised by low bone mass and microarchitectural deterioration with a consequent increase in bone fragility and susceptibility to fracture **senile o** diffuse osteoporosis of unknown cause affecting elderly, especially women. There is reduction of total bone mass and compression fracture of vertebrae may be noted

osteosarcoma (os'-te-o-sar-ko'ma) *see* osteogenic sarcoma.

osteosclerosis (os-te-o-skle-ro'sis) hardening or an abnormal density of bone

osteosis (os-te-o'sis) the formation of bony tissue

osteospondylomegaepiphysealdysplasia an autosomal recessive form of chandrodystrophy, characterised by dwarfism, deafness, deformed ears, saddle nose, leathery skin, soft tissue calcification and cleft palate

osteosynovitis (os-te-o-sin'o-vi'tis) occurrence of inflammation of synovium and bony tissue of the neighbouring bones

osteotabes (os-te-o-ta'bes) destruction of the cells of bone marrow in infants

osteotome (os-te-o-tom) a chisel-like knife useful to cut the bone

osteotomy (os-te-ot'o-me) the surgical cutting of a bone to correct a deformity or to change its length or to improve the joint stability

ostium (os-te-um) opening between cavities or an opening into a tube

ostomy (os'tome) a suffix meaning to 'form a new opening'; a surgical procedure in which an opening is made to facilitate the passage of urine from the bladder or of intestinal contents from the bowel to a stoma surgically created in the wall of abdomen

Ostwald coefficient the amount of gas which dissolves in a unit volume of solvent, measured under the conditions of temperature and pressure at which solution takes place, described by Wilhelm Ostwald, Russian-German physical chemist

OT old tuberculin; operation theatre

otalgia (os-tal'je-a) ear ache

otectomy (o-tek'to-me) excision of tissues of the internal and middle ear

Othello syndrome a delusional disorder with delusion that a spouse has been unfaithful and it usually afflicts males and usually with no prior psychiatric illness

otic (o'tik) pertaining to the ear

otitis (o-ti'tis) inflammation of the ear **o externa** inflammation of the outer part of the ear including the ear canal. **o media** inflammation of the middle ear. It may be acute, noted in children, characterised by severe pain, fever and varying degree of deafness. The tympanic membrane is bulging, reddish and sometimes pulsatile. It may resolve or lead to perforation. Chronic otitis media presents with continuous discharge of pus and deafness. There is a hole in the tympanic membrane

oto related to the ear

otoblennorrhoea (oto'blen'no-rhea) mucus discharge from the ear

otoencephalitis (o'to-en-sef'a-li-tis) inflammation of the brain occurring as an extension from an inflamed middle ear

otogenous (o-toj'en-us) originating within the ear

otolaryngology (o'to-lar'in-gol-o-je) branch of medical science dealing with the diseases of the ear, nose and throat

otolith (o'to-lith) a calcareous mass in the inner ear

otologic (o'to-loj-ik) referring to the ear

otologist a specialist in the diseases of the ear

otology (o-tol' o-je) branch of medical science dealing with the ear

otomyces (o'to-mi-sez) fungi infesting the ear

otomycosis (o'to-mi-ko'sis) fungal infection of the external ear and ear canal

otopalatodigital syndrome OPD syndrome X-linked disorder characterised by craniofacial deformity, short trunk, dwarfism and brachydactyly

otoplasty (o'to-plas-te) a reconstructive surgery of the cartilage in the ears

otorhinolaryngology (o'to-ri-no-lar-in-gel-o-je) branch of medicine dealing with the disease of ear, nose, pharynx and larynx

otorrhoea (oto-rea) a discharge from the ear. It may be serous, purulent or sanguinous

otoscope (o'to-sk-op) an instrument consisting of a light, magnifying lens and a device for insufflation, used to examine the external ear and tympanic membrane

otoscopy (oto'sko'pe) examination of deeper part of the external auditory canal and tympanic membrane under good illumination with a head mirror and an ear speculum

otosclerosis (o'to-skle-ro'sis) an inherited disorder exhibiting irregular ossification in the bony labyrinth of inner ear especially of the stapes, causing tinnitus and later deafness. Stapedectomy is necessary to restore hearing

ototoxic (o'to-tok'sik) having a toxic effect on the eighth cranial nerve or the organs of hearing and balance. Aminoglycoside antibiotics, aspirin, furosemide and quinine are some examples

ototoxicity (o'to-tok'sity) impaired hearing and balance from toxic effects of certain drugs

ouabaine (wa-ba'in) a rapid and short-acting digitalis preparation

Ouch-Ouch disease a form of renal osteodystrophy with marked bony pain, described in Japanese women due to accumulation of cadmium in bone from eating fish contaminated by industrial pollutants.

Ouchterlony double diffusion a gel diffusion technique in which antigen and antibody are allowed to diffuse towards each other, named after Orjan Ouchterlony, a Swedish bacteriologist

ounce (ouns) Oz a unit of weight equal to 28.349 grams.

-ous a combining word for an 'element or compound' with a valence lower than the corresponding one ending in-ic, such as ferrous

outbreak the sudden increase in the incidence of a disease or conditon in a specific area

outcome the result of an action; condition at the end of therapy or of a disease process

outcomes research a comprehensive approach to determine the effects of medical care

outercourse sexual behaviour that does not involve intercourse

outflow the passage of an impulse outwardly

outlet an opening through which something can escape

outline form the shape of the cavosurface of a tooth cavity

outpatient a patient who gets the diagnosis and treatment in a clinic or hospital without getting admitted

output (owt'poot) the yield; the total of any and all measurable liquids lost from the body

ova egg pl. **ovum**

oval (o'val) egg shaped

ovalbumin (o'val-bu'min) egg white

ovalocytes (o'val'o-sits) oval-shaped red blood cells with pale centres found occasionally in patients with haemolytic anaemia, thalassemias and hereditary elliptosis

oval window an oval-shaped aperture in the wall of the middle ear leading to the inner ear

ovarian (o-va're-an) concerned with ovary **o cycle** a sex cycle having a follicular phase and a luteal phase with ovulation intervening **o cyst** a globular sac filled with fluid or semisolid material that develops in or on the ovary **o hyperstimulation syndrome** ovarian enlargement, ascites, pleural effusion, hypovolaemia, haemoconcentration and oliguria. It is a serious complication of ovulation induction with human chorionic gonadotropin and occasionally clomiphene **o pregnancy** ectopic gestation on ovary **o vein** one of a pair of veins emerging from the plexus in the broad ligament near the ovaries and uterine tubes. The right ovarian vein opens into the inferior vena cava and the left into the renal vein **o tumour** a malignant tumour of the ovary that is diagnosed only in advanced

stage as a palpable abdominal or pelvic mass accompanied by irregular or excessive menses or postmenopausal bleeding. It spreads over the surface of peritoneum. It requires total abdominal hysterectomy and bilateral salpingo-oophorectomy with omentectomy **o vein syndrome** a disorder due to an enlarged and tortuous right ovarian vein with incompetent valves noted in pregnancy accompanied by hydronephrosis and pyelonephritis

ovariocyesis (o-va're-o-si-e'sis) ovarian pregnancy

ovariosalpingectomy (o-va're-o-sal'pin-jek-to-me) surgical removal of an ovary and fallopian tube

ovariectomy (o'va-re-ek'to-me) surgical removal of an ovary

ovarium (o-va're-um) female sexual gland

ovary (o'va-re) female gonad found on each side of the lower abdomen besides the uterus in a fold of the broad ligament. It is firm and smooth resembling an almond in size. An egg is extruded from a follicle on the surface of the ovary at the time of ovulation. The mature ovarian follicle secretes oestrogen and progesterogen which regulate the menstrual cycle

overactivity hyperactivity

overbite (o'verbit) vertical overlapping of lower teeth by upper teeth

overdenture (o'ver-den'cher) a complete or partial removable denture supported by retained roots to provide improved support and stability

overdose (-dos) consumption of much larger than recommended quantity of a drug or narcotic

overflow continuous escape of a fluid **o diarrhoea** secretory diarrhoea in which the fluid produced in the upper intestine exceeds the resorptive capacity of the lower intestine as seen in cholera **o incontinence** an overflow of urine from a distended paralysed bladder **o proteinuria** persistent proteinuria without glomerular disease. There is an increased production of filterable low molecular weight proteins, exceeding the resorptive capacities of the renal tubules as in Bence-Jones proteinuria

overgrowth an excessive growth

overhang an excess of dental filling material that projects beyond the margin of the associated tooth cavity

overhydration (o'ver-hidra'shun) an excess of water in the body

overinflation expansion

overjet a horizontal projection of upper teeth beyond lower teeth

overlap syndrome a combination of diseases, such as combinations of connective tissue diseases, Crohn's disease and ulcerative colitis, Parkinsonism plus syndromes and necrotising vasculitis and polyarteritis nodosa and Churg-Strauss disease

overlearning repetitions over and above those required for complete mastery

overload (o'ver-lod) a burden greater than the capacity of the system to move or process it

overpressure a stretch force applied to soft tissues at the end of the range of motion

overriding the overlapping or telescoping of body parts

overshoot alkalosis may be seen in lactic acidosis and in ketoacidosis when the lactic acid and ketoacids are oxidised to bicarbonate in response to a rapid-bolus administration of bicarbonate

overstretch a stretch beyond the normal range of motion of a joint and the surrounding soft tissues

overtone tone coming from the vibration of halves of a wire, a string, a reed or a bar of wood

overuse syndrome chronic trauma caused by repetitive forces on the musculotendinous region and chondro-osseous tissues resulting in inflammation, pain or dysfunction of the affected joint, bones and ligaments

overweight (o'ver-wat) more than normal in body weight after adjustment for age, height and build. It is 10 to 20 percent above the desirable weight

oviduct (o'vi-dukt) fallopian tube

oviparous (ovip'ares) giving birth to young by laying eggs

ovoid egg-shaped

ovulation (ov'u-la'shun) the discharge of a ovum from the graafian follicle of the ovary in a cyclic fashion. It usually occurs on the fourteenth day after the first day of the last menstrual period

ovule (o'vul) the ovum within the graafian follicle

ovum (o'vum) the female reproductive cell; an egg cell. pl. **ova**

owl eye appearance inclusion seen in cytomegalovirus (CMV) infection, wherein the CMV-infected epithelial cells, appear markedly enlarged and contain massive eosinophilic intranuclear inclusions and surrrounded by a clear halo

oxacillin (ok'sasil'in) a penicillinase-resistant penicillin antibiotic. Used in the treatment of severe infections caused by penicillinase-producing staphylococci

oxalate (ok'sa-lat) a salt of oxalic acid. The foodstuffs such an spinach, rhubarb and tea are high in oxalate

ox eye a progressively enlarged eye encountered in children with congenital glaucoma; buphthalmos

Oxford tube an inverted L-shaped intubation tube which conforms to the passage from mouth to trachea to prevent kinks even when the head is fully flexed

oxidant (ok'sident) an oxidising agent: a substance that contains oxygen and gives it up readily

oxidase (ok'si-das) an enzyme that catalyses the reduction of molecular oxygen.

oxidation (ok'si-da'shun) the chemical process of uniting with oxygen or burning **o pond** an open shallow pool with an inlet and outlet containing algae and bacteria which feed on decaying organic matter and sunlight. The organic matter in the sewage gets oxidised by bacteria to simple chemical compounds and algae utilise CO_2. It is a method of purifying sewage for small communities

oxycephaly (ok'se-sef'a-le) a malformed skull developing from premature closure of the coronal and sagittal sutures. There is an accelerated upward growth of the head giving it a long, narrow pointed appearance

oxygen (ok'si-jen) a colourless, odourless, tasteless gas that is essential for life. It is used in the cell mitochondria and energy is produced through citric acid cycle in the form of adenosine triphosphate **o capacity** the maximum amount of oxygen that can be made to combine chemically with haemoglobin. 1 gram of haemoglobin can bind a maximum of 1.34 ml of oxygen **o concentrator** a device that separates oxygen from the air **o consumption** utilisation of oxygen per minute by the metabolising tissues **o content** amount of total oxygen present in the blood **o cost of breathing** the rate at which the respiratory muscles consume oxygen as they ventilate the lungs **o debt** the differences, with time between the oxygen demand and the actual oxygen consumption per minute **o delivery** amount of oxygen delivered to the tissues and it depends on the total oxygen content of the blood and cardiac output **o delivery devices** devices to deliver oxygen such a cannulae, prongs and masks **o dissociation curve** a sigmoid curve that describes the relationship between haemoglobin oxygen saturation and tension. The curve shifts to the right indicating decreased haemoglobin affinity for oxygen as in decreased pH and it shifts to the left indicating increased oxygen affinity with increased pH; oxygen saturation curve **o elec-**trode a platinum cathode and a silver anode in a potassium hydroxide solution. Platinum gives up electrons to oxygen and the resulting voltage change can be measured and expressed in terms of oxygen tension **o free radicals** active sources of oxygen produced in the body by normal activity and by external agents that damage cells highly reactive, toxic molecules that appear when electrons are added to oxygen in the presence of hydrogen ions **o hood** a device placed over the head of neonatal patients to deliver high concentrations of oxygen **o mask** mask to deliver oxygen at high concentration. It may be simple without any valve or reservoir, partial rebreathing with a unidirectional valve on either side and air-entrainment type to provide a constant fraction of inspired oxygen regulated by venturi design **o ratio** estimated by dividing PaO_2 in mms Hg by inspired oxygen concentration (FiO_2) in per cent (PaO_2/FiO_2). Normally it is 4 **o saturation** the proportion of haemoglobin (Hb) combining with oxygen. It reflects the degree of oxygenation of the blood **o tension** partial pressure of oxygen in the arterial blood and it is 80 to 100 mmHg at sea level **o tent** a canopy that encloses the head and neck of a patient under high oxygen tension **o toxicity** occurrence of toxic features when the concentration of inhaled oxygen is high, and it causes damage to the pulmonary capillaries and alveolar epithelium

oxygenator (ok'si-je-na'tor) a mechanical device that oxygenates venous blood outside the body

oxyhaemoglobin (ok'se-hamo-glo'bin) oxygenated haemoglobin; oxygen combined with haemoglobin. HbO_2. Each gram of haemoglobin can bind 1.39 ml of oxygen

oxyhood a plastic hood that fits over the infant's head to deliver a constant con-

centration of oxygen to a spontaneously breathing infant

oxymetry (ok-sim′e-tre) sampling of blood for its oxygen content, using a device attached to the earlobe or finger tip

oximeter (ok-sim′e-tor) a photoelectric device useful in determination of oxygen saturation of blood. Light at certain wavelengths is shone on the the blood and the amount of light reflected or transmitted is measured

oxtriphylline (oks′trefil′en) a xanthine derivative, useful as a bronchodilator

oxyspec an oxygen device wherein the oxygen tubing is concealed in a thick rimmed frames of spectacles

oxytocia (ok′se-to′sia) rapid labour

oxytetracycline bacteriostatic antibiotic that inhibits growth of a wide range of gram-positive and gram-negative bacteria

oxytocin (ok′se-to-sin) a hypothalamic polypeptide hormone released into the pituitary gland that induces and stimulates the contraction of the uterus during labour and stimulates the flow of milk for breast feeding **o stress test** a clinical test to evaluate the ability of the foetus to withstand labour that uses oxytocin

oxyuriasis (ok′se-u-ri′as-is) infection with *Enterobius vermicularis.*

oxyuricide (ok′se-u′ri-sid) an agent causing destruction of threadworm

Oxyuris (ok′se-ur′is) an intestinal nematode

ozone (o′zon) O_3, a form of oxygen present in upper atmosphere that protects Earth from the harmful effects of ultraviolet radiation of the sun

ozostomia (o′zo-sto′me-a) foul breath

P

P symbol for phosphate, phosphorus, probability, pressure, para, posterior

P_2 pulmonic second sound

P symbol for Pico, proton, the short arm of chromosome

P24 antigen the core antigen of the human immunodeficiency virus type 1, (HIV-1), which is held responsible for AIDS

P_{53} a protein produced by tumour suppressor gene which has a role in the birth and death of the cells

PA abbreviation for pulmonary artery; posteroanterior

P (A-a) O_2 oxygen pressure gradient between the alveoli and the arterial blood

pabulum (pab'u-lum) food; nourishment

Pacchionian (pak-e-o'ni-an) corpuscles prominent arachnoid valli, named after Antonio Pacchioni, Italian anatomist

pacemaker 1. any rhythmic centre that establishes a pace of activity 2. an electronic device used to stimulate or regulate the heart beat p syndrome a complication of implanted pacemakers, characterised by vertigo, syncope, dyspnoea, weakness, postural hypotension, decreased effort tolerance and palpable hepatic and jugular pulsations, and it is due to alternating atrioventricular asynchrony wandering p a disturbance of the normal cardiac rhythm in which the site that controls the pacemaker shifts from beat to beat usually between the sinus and AV nodes

pachaka (s) digestive

pachakagni (s) digestive fire or juice

pachana (s) digestion

pachy combining word for 'thick'

pachyblepharon (pak'e-blef'a-ron) thickening of the tarsal border of the eyelids

pachycephaly (-sef'a-le) abnormal thickness of the bones of the skull

pachychelia (-ki'le-a) thickening of the lips

pachychromatic (-kro-mat'ik) having a coarse chromatin reticulum

pachydactyly (-dak'ti-le) enlargement of the fingers or toes

pachyderma (-der'-ma) abnormal thickening of the skin

pachydermatocoele (-der-mat'ah-sel) 1. increased amount of skin hanging in folds 2. huge neurofibroma

pachydermoperiostosis (-durm'o-pe're-os-to'sis) abnormal thickening of the skin in natural folds, accentuation of the creases of the face and scalp, thickening of the bones of the distal extremities and clubbed digits

pachydermy (-der'mi) leathery subcutaneous thickening due to accumulation of inelastic connective tissue as in acromegaly or due to protein-rich mucin as in myxoedema

pachyglossia (-glos'se-a) abnormally thick tongue

pachyleptomeningitis (-lep'to-men'in-jit'is) inflammation of the dura mater and pia mater of the brain and spinal cord

pachymeningitis (-men'in-jit'is) inflammation of the dura mater

pachymeninx (-me'ninks) pl. pachymeninges the dura mater

pachynsis (pa-kin'sis) an abnormal thickening

pachyonychia (pak'e-o-nik'e-a) abnormal thickening of the finger nails or toe nails

pachyperiostitis (pak'i-pe're-os-ti'tis) periostitis of the long bones resulting in the thickness of affected bones

pachyperitonitis (-pe'ri-to-ni'tis) inflammation and thickening of the peritoneum

pachypleuritis (-ploor-it'is) inflammation and thickening of pleura

pachysalpingitis (-sal'pin-jit'is) chronic inflammation of fallopian tube with thickening

pachysalpingoovaritis (-sal-ping'go-o'varitis) chronic inflammation of the ovary and fallopian tube with thickening

pachytene (pak'i-ten) the stage of prophase in meiosis in which the pairing of homologous chromosomes is complete. They may twine about each other and undergo longitudinal cleavage to become a set of four intertwined chromatids

pachyvaginalitis (pak'i-vaj'in-ilit'is) inflammation and thickening of the tunica vaginalis testis

pachyvaginitis (-vaj'i-ni'tis) chronic inflammation of the vagina with thickening of the vaginal walls

pacing (pas'ing) use of electric pacemaker to maintain normal cardiac rhythm

Pacinian (pa-sin'e-an) **corpuscles** large encapsulated touch receptors especially of skin, named after Filippo Pacini, Italian anatomist

pack (pak) 1. to wrap the body in a sheet, or blanket 2. to fill up a cavity with cotton or gauze

package insert a paper giving details of the full product information that accompanies a prescription drug

packed cell volume PCV the percentage of volume of red blood cells in the blood determined by using Wintrobe's haematocrit tube. Normal PCV is 45%

packed red cells a concentrated unit of red blood cells obtained from a unit of whole blood by removing most of the volume

packer (pak'er) an instrument for packing a cavity or a wound

packing (-ing) 1. filling a cavity or a wound with gauze piece 2. material used to fill a cavity or a wound

pack years a crude indicator of a person's cigarette consumption; the number of packs of cigarettes smoked per day multiplied by the length of consumption in years

PaCO₂ partial pressure of carbon dioxide in the arterial blood

pad 1. a cushion of soft material used to apply or relieve pressure on a part or organ 2. a fatty mass **p sign** padded-out appearance of duodenal loop in carcinoma of head of pancreas on barium meal

pada (s) feet

padmasana (s) the lotus posture in hatha yoga

paediatric (pe-di-at'rik) relating to paediatrics **p advanced life support** PALS, the treatment measures including the basic and advanced life support required to stabilise critically ill child

paediatrician (pe'di-a-trish'an) a specialist in paediatrics

paediatrics (pe'de-at'riks) the medical specialty concerned with the development and care of children and the diagnosis and management of their diseases

paedophilia sexual attraction to prepubertal children usually of opposite sex

paenia combining word for deficiency

PAF abbreviation for 1. platelet activating factor 2. paroxysmal atrial fibrillation

PAF acether platelet activating factor, structurally acetyl and an ether linked to glyceryl and phosphocholine

pain (pan) the sensation of marked discomfort that is either sharp and well localised or dull and diffuse **abdominal p** pain in the abdomen due to a variety of conditions **acute p** sudden pain of variable intensity **after p's** painful contractions of the uterus occurring after childbirth **agonizing p** intense severe pain **bearing down p's** a uterine contraction with pain and straining in the second stage of labour **chest p** severe pain in the chest **chronic p** slow onset of mild to severe pain **expulsive p** effective labour pain associated with uterine contraction **false p** ineffective uterine contraction without any cervical dilatation **girdle p** painful sensation like a constricting cord around the trunk **growing p's** aching pain felt at night in the limbs of growing children **hunger p**

pain in the epigastrium associated with hunger **intermenstrual p** pelvic pain occurring at midpoint of menstruation **intractable p** severe pain seen in neoplastic conditions, which is not easily relieved **labour p** rhythmic uterine contractions that normally increase in quality, frequency and duration due to contraction of the uterus at child birth **phantom limb p** pain felt as though arising in an amputated limb **precordial p** pain over the heart **psychologic p** pain having a mental origin **referred p** pain felt as coming from an area remote from its actual site of origin **rest p** pain due to ischaemia occurring when sitting or lying **shooting p** lightning pain

painful crisis one of the crises seen in sickle cell anaemia where sludging of sickled red cell causes capillary stasis and infarction. It causes severe musculoskeletal pain, referral type organ pain, haemoptysis, haematuria, melena and CNS symptoms

painful fat syndrome chronic, symmetric swelling and tenderness of the legs due to lipoedema, noted in adolescent females

painful heel tenderness of heel with focal oedema often with calcaneal spur in elderly men

painful red leg syndrome increased sensitivity to skin temperature above 32°C, characterised by focal vasodilatation and a burning sensation; erythromelia

Pagets' disease of bone a condition characterised by increased and disorganised bone resorption and bone formation throughout the skeleton. It affects pelvis, femur, tibia, lumbar spine, skull and scapula and the condition does not spread to new bones after diagnosis. There is bone deformity, warmth of the skin over affected bones and pathological fractures. Alkaline phosphatase is raised in presence of normal levels of serum calcium and phosphates, described by Sir James Paget, UK surgeon

Paget's disease of the breast a weeping

eczematoid erosive lesion of the nipple that is associated with underlying intraductal breast carcinoma

pain a sensation of marked discomfort that is either sharp and well-localised, or dull and diffuse **p receptors** basic nerve endings in the skin and other organs, however they are not present everywhere in the body

paint (pant) a solution of medicaments for application to the skin

painter's colic lead colic from lead paints

pair (per) a combination of two or anything similar in shape, size and conformation

paired organs organs of which the body has a pair such as eyes, kidneys, sex glands and lungs

palatal (pal'a-tal) pertaining to the palate **p myoclonus** rhythmic contraction of one side of soft palate due to damage of dentate and olivary nuclei

palate (pal'it) roof of the mouth, the partition separating the nasal and oral cavities **bony p** the concave bony plate formed by maxilla and palatine bones and it forms the anterior portion of the palate **cleft p** congenital fissure in the midline of the palate which often is associated with cleft lips **gothic p** an excessively high arched palate **hard p** bony palate **pendulous p** uvula **soft p** posterior muscular portion of the palate that separates the mouth and pharynx

palatine (pal'a-tin) 1. palatal 2. palate bones **p tonsil** tonsil

palatitis (pal'ah-tit'is) inflammation of the palate

palatoglossal (pal'k-to-glos'al) pertaining to the palate and tongue

palatoglossus (pal'a-toglos'us) *see* table of muscles

palatognathous (pal'a-tog'na-thus) having a congenitally cleft palate

palatopharyngoplasty a surgical procedure for the soft palate and pharynx to eliminate redundant mucosa

palatoplasty (pal'a-to-plas'te) surgical reconstruction of the palate

palatoplegia (pal'a-to-ple'jah) paralysis of the palate

palatorrhaphy (pal-a-tor'a-fe) surgical repair of a cleft palate

palatoschisis (pal-a-tos'ki-sis) cleft palate

paleocerebellum (pa'le-o-ser'a-bel'um) medial part of the cerebellum comprising vermis and adjacent medial zone of cerebellar hemisphere having spino-cerebellar fibres and is concerned with equilibrium and movements of locomotion

paleocortex (-kor'teks) cerebral hemisphere represented by the olfactory cortex

paleopathology (pa'le-o-pa-thol-a-je) study of disease process in the corpse preserved from ancient times

paleostriatum (-stri-at'um) the globus pallidus

paleothalamus (-thal'a-mus) the medial portion of the thalamus

palindromia (pal'in-dro'me-a) intermittent recurring episodes

palinopsia (-op'se-a) persistence of a visual sensation after the stimulus has gone

palinopsis (pal'i-no-p-sis) persistent or recurrent visual images, following removal of the exciting stimulus

palisading arrangement of elongated and compressed epithelial cells that are perpendicular to a surface **p granuloma** presence of histiocytic nuclei lying at right angles to the surface of necrotic material as in rheumatoid nodules and necrobiosis lipoidica

pallanaesthesia (pal'an-es-the'zhah) loss of sense of vibration

pallesthesia (pal'es-the'zhah) ability to appreciate mechanical vibrations on or near the body such as placing a vibrating tuning fork over a bony prominence

palliation treatment which improves the patient's feelings without curing underlying disease

palliative (pal'e-a'tiv) 1. giving relief 2. a drug giving relief **p care** improvement of the quality of life when treatment to cure disease and prolong life is no longer a realistic objective **p surgery** a therapeutic procedure undertaken to reduce the severity of symptoms and improve the quality of life in presence of advanced stage of malignancy **p therapy** any treatment of a terminally-ill patient to alleviate pain and suffering without undertaking any aggressive procedures

pallid (pal'id) pale, lacking colour

pallidectomy (pal'i-dek'ta-me) surgical removal of the globus pallidus

pallidotomy (pal'i-dot-a-me) a stereotaxic surgical procedure for production of lesions in the globus pallidus to relieve involuntary movements or muscular rigidity

pallidum (pal'i-dum) the globus pallidus **pallidal** adj.

pallium (pal'e-um) the cerebral cortex

pallor (pal'er) paleness as of skin and mucus membrane

palm (pam) the flexor surface of the hand **palmar** adj.

palma (pah'mah) palm

palmaris (pah-mar'is) palmar

palmar keratosis squamous keratosis

palmitic (pa-mit'ik) **acid** a 16 carbon saturated fatty acid found in most oils and fats

palmoplantar pustulosis PPP a phenomenon of recurrent sterile pustules, erythema and scaling affecting the palms and soles

palmus (pa'mus) 1. palpitation 2. clonic spasm of leg muscles

palpation (pal-pa'shun) the act of feeling with the hand, one of the cardinal methods of physical examination

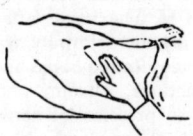

Palpation of the liver

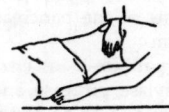

Palpation of the spleen

palpebra (pal'pe-bra) pl. palpebrae eyelid palpebral adj.

palpebralis (pal'pa-bral'is) palpebral

palpebritis (pal'pa-brit'is) inflammation of the eyelids; blepharitis

palpitation (pal'pi-ta'shun) a subjective feeling of an unusually rapid or irregular heart beat

palsy (pawl'ze) paralysis Bells' facial paralysis see Bell's palsy birth p obstetric paralysis, from an injury received at birth or due to anoxic injury of the foetal brain in utero bulbar p progressive muscular paralysis occurring due to degeneration of the nuclei of lower cranial nerves cerebral p see cerebral palsy Erb's p see Erb's paralysis facial p Bell's palsy pressure p temporary paralysis due to pressure on nerve trunk Saturday night p see Saturday night paralysis shaking p paralysis agitans

PAM abbreviation for 1. penicillin aluminium monostearate 2. pyridine aldoxime methochloride 3. pregnancy associated macroglobulinaemia 4. pulmonary alveolar macrophage

pampiniform (pam-pini-form) shaped like a tendril p flexus abundant veins of spermatic cord

PAN abbreviation for polyarteritis nodosa

pan combining form for all

pan betel-leaf with arecanut and lime

panacea (pan-a-se'a) cure all, remedy, single solution for multiple problems a remedy claimed to be curative to all ills.

panacinar emphysema, see emphysema

panagglutinin (pan'a-gloo'ti-nin) an agglutinin capable of agglutinating the red blood cells of all human blood groups

panagraphy (pan-a'gra-fe) view of all teeth in one jaw with x-ray source in mouth and film in cassette wrapped round jaw

panarteritis (pan'ar-te-ri'tis) polyarteritis

panarthritis (pan'ar-thri'tis) 1. inflammation of all joints of the body 2. Inflammation of all parts of a joint

panatrophy (pan-a'trah-fe) diffuse atrophy

pancake omentum an omentum that has undergone marked thickening and induration secondary to diffuse infiltration from any malignancy

pancarditis (pan'kar-dit'is) diffuse inflammation of all tissues of the heart as in rheumatic fever

panchakarma (s) five cleansing actions of vomiting, enemas, purgation, blood letting and nasal medications used as therapy

panchakarma (s) five-fold threrapy

panchendriya (s) five senses

Pancoast's tumour bronchogenic carcinoma of the apex of the lung which grows upwards to invade brachial plexus and cervical sympathetic chain on the same side, named after Henry Pancoast, US radiologist

pancolectomy (-ko-lek'ta-me) surgical removal of the entire colon with creation of an ileostomy

pancreas (pan'kre-as) a lobulated gland functioning as an exocrine and endocrine organ, devoid of capsule, extending from the concavity of the duodenum to the spleen in a horizontal position in front of first and second lumbar vertebrae. It is divided into head attached to the duodenum, body and tail reaching the spleen. The exocrine portion consists of acini which secrete pancreatic juice which drain into main pancreatic duct. It joins the common bile duct and empties into the duodenum. The islets of Langerhans distributed throughout the gland have alpha, beta and delta cells secreting glucagon, insulin and somatostatin respectively and function as an endocrine gland

pancreatectomy (pan'kre-a-tek-ta-me) excision of the pancreas

pancreat, pancreatic (o) combining word for pancreas; pancreatic duct

pancreatic (pan'kre-at'ik) relating to pancreas **p alpha cells** cells secrete glucagon **p beta cells** cells secrete insulin **p cholera syndrome** condition characterised by diarrhoea from endocrine tumours of the pancreas, such as vasoactive intestinal peptide-producing pancreatic tumour **p delta cells** cells secrete somatostatin **p elastase** (pan'kre-at'ik-e-las'tas) a peptidase catalysing the breakdown of specific peptide bonds in the protein digestion **p endocrine tumours** a group of tumours of pancreas such as APUDoma, islet cell tumour and nesidioblastoma found in its body and tail, where there is a greater concentration of islets of Langerhans **p pseudocyst** a localised collection of pancreatic juice enclosed by a wall of fibrosis or granulation cyst arising as a consequence of pancreatitis, pancreatic trauma or neoplastic obstruction of the pancreatic duct. The cyst persists as long as there is communication with the pancreatic duct **p pseudopseudocyst** occurrence of acute fluid collection early in the course of severe form of acute pancreatitis and it does not possess a wall of fibrous or granulation tissue. It represents a serous or exudative reaction to pancreatic or peripancreatic trauma **p rest** a focus of ectopic pancreatic tissue in the stomach, small intestine or Meckel's diverticulum.

pancreaticoduodenal (pan'kre-at'i-ko-doo'a-de'nil) pertaining to the pancreas and duodenum

pancreaticoduodenostomy (-doo'o-de-nos'ta-me) anastomosis of the pancreatic duct to a different location on the duodenum

pancreaticoenterostomy (-en'ter-os'ta-me) anastomosis of the pancreatic duct to the intestine

pancreaticogastrostomy (-gas-tros-ta-me) anastomosis of the pancreatic duct to the stomach

pancreaticojejunostomy (-je'joo-nos'ta-me) anastomosis of the pancreatic duct to the jejunum

pancreatin (pan'kre-it-in) enzymes containing amylase, protease, and lipase obtained from hog or ox and used to facilitate digestion

pancreatitis (pan'kre-a-ti'tis) inflammation of the pancreas **acute p** pancreatitis due to interstitial inflammation, oedema, necrosis and haemorrhage. There is premature release of proteases which digest the pancreas and surrounding tissue and the condition is characterised by severe constant upper abdominal pain, nausea, vomiting and marked epigastric tenderness **chronic p** a chronic inflammatory disease characterised by fibrosis and destruction of exocrine pancreatic tissue, resulting from alcohol abuse in majority of cases

pancreatoduodenectomy (pan'kre-a-to-doo'o-de-nek'ta-me) surgical removal of the head of the pancreas along with the encircling loop of the duodenum

pancreatogenous (-toj'i-nus) arising in the pancreas

pancreatography (-tog-ra-fe) imaging of the pancreas and its network of ducts

pancreatolithectomy (-to-li-thek'ta-me) excision of a stone from the pancreas

pancreatolithiasis (-li-thi'a-sis) presence of stone in the parenchyma or ducts of the pancreas

pancreatolithotomy (-li-thot'o-me) removal of stone by incising the pancreas

pancreatolysis (pan'kre-a-tol'i-sis) destruction of pancreatic tissue

pancreatotomy (-tot'a-me) incision of the pancreas

pancreatotropic (pan'kre-it-o-trop'ik) possessing an affinity for pancreas

pancreoprivic (pan'kre-o-priv'ik) not having a pancreas

pancreozymin (-zi'min) a duodenal hormone that stimulates the pancreas for production of amylase

pancurorium (pan'ku-ro'ne-um) a skeletal muscle relaxant used as an adjunct to anaesthesia

pancystitis (pan'sis-ti-tis) inflammation involving the entire thickness of the wall of the urinary bladder

pancytopaenia (-sit-o-pe'ne-a) hypoplasia or aplasia of bone marrow resulting in deficiency of all types of blood cells

pandemic (pan-dem'ik) a widespread epidemic disease affecting a large number of people at the same time and in many geographic regions

pakshaghata (s) hemiplegia

pandu (s) anaemia

Pandy's (pan'dez) **test** presence of globulin in CSF tested by addition of 7% phenol which produces turbidity, named after Kalman Pandy, Hungarian psychiatrist

panencephalitis (pan'en-sef'a-lit'is) encephalitis producing lesions of both the gray and white matter of the brain

panendoscopy (pan-en'do-sko-pe) fibreoptic endoscopic study of oesophagus, stomach and duodenum at one sitting

Paneth's (pah'natz) **cells** large cells with eosinophilic granules in the epithelium of small intestine crypts, described by Josef Paneth, German physician

pang 1. a sudden sharp pain 2. A sudden attack of any emotion

panhypopituitarism (-hi'po-pi-tu'-it-er-izm) a condition in which there is an inadequate or absent secretion of all anterior pituitary hormones as a result of destruction of anterior pituitary gland

panhysterectomy (-his-ter-ek'to-me) surgical removal of the entire uterus including the cervix uteri

panhysterosalpingectomy (-his-ter-o-sal'pin-jek'ta-me) surgical removal of the uterus, cervix and fallopian tubes

panhysterosalpingoophorectomy (-salping'go-o'of-a-rek'to-me) surgical removal of the uterus, cervix, fallopian tubes and ovaries

panic (pan'ik) fear, widespread terror, frightening **attack** acute, episodic, intense attack of anxiety with overwhelming feelings of dread and autonomic discharge

panniculectomy (pa-nik'u-lek'ta-me) surgical removal of the abdominal fat in obese individuals

panniculitis (pan-nik'u-li'tis) inflammation of subcutaenous fat in the anterior wall of the abdomen

panniculus (pa-nik'u-lus) a layer of membrane, such as subcutaneous fat layer

pannus (pan'us) 1. fibrovascular proliferative response occurring in the cornea and conjunctiva due to *Chlamydia trachomatis* 2. a nonspecific immune response in the form of a reticulated membrane of granulation tissue in chronic prolifero-destructive phase of rheumatoid arthritis

panography (pan-og'ra-fe) a radiologic technique providing full view of an entire dental arch on one film

panophthalmitis (pan'of-thal-mit'is) inflammation of all parts of the eye

panotitis (-o-tit'is) inflammation of all parts or structures of the ear

panplegia (pan-ple'je-a) total paralysis

pansinusitis (pan'si-nus-i'tis) inflammation of all paranasal sinuses

pansystolic murmur holosystolic murmur extending from first to second heart sound

pant 1. to gasp for breath 2. to breath rapidly and shallowly

pantaloon hernia *see* hernia

pantothenate (pan'to-then'at) any salt of pantothenic acid

pantothenic acid a member of vitamin B complex, widespread in food that helps in the release of energy in the cells

PaO₂ partial pressure of oxygen in arterial blood

papain (pa-pa'in) a proteolytic enzyme from *Carica papaya* which catalyses the hydrolysis of proteins and polypeptides to amino acids

Papanicolaou test pap smear-a cytologic sampling from the uterine cervix that serves to detect dysplasia and squamous cell carcinoma of the cervix, described by George Papanicolaou, Greek-US physician

papaverine (pa-pav'er-in) isoquinoline alkaloid found in opium, a smooth muscle relaxant

paper (pa'per) a material produced in thin sheets from fibrous substances reduced to pulp **filter p** a porous unglazed paper used for filtration **litmus p** paper impregnated with litmus solution which becomes blue in alkaline solution and red in acidic solution **test p** paper impregnated with a compound which changes its colour when exposed to a certain pH or to chemicals

papilla (pa-pil'ah) pl. **papillae** a small nipple-shaped projection **papillary** adj. **circumvallate p** large papillae found near the base on the dorsal surface of the tongue arranged in a V-shape **conical p** numerous projections on the dorsum of the tongue **dental p** a mesenchymal tissue giving rise to dentine and dental tissue **duodenal p** the point of opening of the common bile duct into the duodenum **filiform p** elongated conical projection on the dorsum of the tongue **foliate p** numerous projections arranged in several folds in the lateral margins of the tongue **fungiform p** numerous minute flat papillae on the dorsum of the tongue resembling a fungus **gingival p** gingival tissue between the adjacent teeth **hair p** a conical projection containing capillaries at the bottom of hair follicles **incisive p** a slight projection of mucosa on the anterior portion of raphe of the palate **interdental p** the gingiva that fills the space between adjacent teeth **lacrimal p** a slight projection from the margin of each eyelid near the medial commissure, in the centre of which there is opening of the lacrimal duct **lingual p** any of the tiny projections such as conical, filiform, fungiform and vallate papillae covering the anterior two-thirds of the

tongue **optic p** optic disc **p basilaris** organ of corti **p mamma** nipple, teat **parotid p** the projection at the opening of the parotid duct into the mouth opposite second upper molar tooth **p pili** hair papilla **renal p** the apex of a renal pyramid which projects into a minor calyx **tactile p** a dermal papilla containing a tactile cell or corpuscle **urethral p** a slight projection in the vestibule of the vagina marking the urethral orifice **vallate p** circumvallate papilla

papillary (pap'i-lar-e) relating to or resembling papillae **p carcinoma** slow growing tumour of thyroid **p necrosis** a coagulation necrosis of the renal pyramids with preservation of the outlines of the tubules that occurs as a complication of acute pyelonephritis

papillitis (pap'i-lits) 1. inflammation of a papilla 2. a type of optic neuritis affecting the optic disc

papilloedema oedematous swelling of optic disc due to raised intracranial tension

papilloma (pap'il-o'ma) 1. a benign epithelial tumour 2. epithelial tumour of skin or mucous membrane consisting of villous outgrowths such as warts, polyps or condylomas

papillomatosis (pap'il-o'ma-to'sis) development of multiple papilloma

papillomavirinae (pap'i-lo-ma-vir-i'ne) papillomaviruses belonging to the family of Papovaviridae

papillomavirus (pap'i-lo'ma-vir'rus) any virus of the subfamily of Papillomavirinae **human p** HPV virus inducing development of warts, particularly plantar and genital warts on the skin and mucous membranes

papilloretinitis (pap'il-o-ret'i-ni'tis) inflammation of the optic disc and retina

papillotomy (pap'il-ot'a-me) incision of a papilla.

papovaviridae (pa-po'vah-vir'i-de) papovaviruses which are potentially oncogenic. It includes two subfamilies – Papillomavirinae and Polyomavirinae

papovavirus (pa-po'vah-vi'rus) any virus of the family Papovaviridae

Pappenheimer bodies small basophilic iron-containing granules in red blood cells, often noted after splenectomy, named after A. Pappenheimer, US biochemist

papulation (pap'ul-a'shun) the occurrence of papules

papule (pap'ul) a small, circumscribed, solid, elevated lesion of the skin. **papular** adj

papulosis (pap'ul-o'sis) the presence of multiple papules

papyraceous (pap'i-ra'shus) like paper

para (par'ah) a woman who has produced viable young regardless of whether the child was alive at birth used with Roman numerals to designate such pregnancies as para 0 (none-nullipara), para 1 (one–primipara), para 2 (two-secondipara), para 3 (three-tripara), para 4 (four-quadripara) etc. A multiple birth is considered as a single parous experience

para- combining word for beside; near; resembling, accessory to

para-aminobenzoic (par'a-a-mi'no-benzo'ik) **acid**, PABA, a folic acid precursor

para-aminohippuric acid PAH, substance cleared entirely from plasma while passing through the kidney

para-aminosalicylic acid PAS a bacteriostatic antituberculosis drug. It acts by affecting the intermediate metabolism of the folic acid system of mycobacteria and inhibits growth of virulent mycobacteria

paraanaesthesia (par'a-an'es-the'zhah) anaesthesia of the lower part of the body

paraaortic body one of the small masses of chromatin tissue lying along the abdominal aorta

parabiosis (-bi-o'sis) 1. the union of two individuals, as conjoined twins 2. temporary suppression of conductivity and excitability

paracentesis (-sen-te'sis) a procedure in which a body cavity is punctured from outside with a needle or trocar to remove fluid for therapeutic and diagnostic purpose

paracentral (par'a-sen'tral) situated near the centre

paracetamol (par'a-sit'a-mol) analgesic similar in effects to that of aspirin

paracholera (-kol'er-a) a disease resembling cholera

parachute mitral valve Chordae tendinae of both of the leaflets of the mitral valve inserted into the left ventricular papillary muscle causing obstruction of the blood flow

paraclinical (-klin'i-k'l) 1. subjects of study during training in the mid-career of a medical student, such as pharmacology, pathology, microbiology and forensic medicine 2. pertaining to the morphologic and/or biochemical abnormalities underlying clinical manifestations

paracolic (-ko-li'k) vertical peritoneal gutters lateral to ascending and descending colons

paracolitis (-kol-it's) inflammation of the outercoat of the colon

paracrine (par'a-krin) action of hormones on cells close to secreting cells

paracusis (par-a-ku'sis) any perversion of hearing

paradidymis (-did'i-mis) a small vestigeal structure in the spermatic cord

paradigm a widely accepted explanation for a set of biomedical phenomenon, which becomes accepted when data accumulates to corroborate aspects of the paradigm's theory

paradox (par'a-doks) contradiction

paradoxical different from normal expectation **p embolism** emboli that occur when thrombotic material passes through right-to-left cardiac shunts **p hypertension** a hypertensive episode that develops two or three days following surgery in elderly patients for coarctation of the aorta due to increased pressure in visceral arteries **p hypoxia** administration of oxygen may lead to temporary deterioration of conscious-ness **p incontinence** dribbling of urine due to chronic overdistension of the bladder **p movement** 1. chest wall movement in flail chest 2. in neonate with inspiration the anterior thorax draws inward and the abdomen pro-trudes and it is normal as breathing is entirely diaphragmatic **p pulse** a de-crease of greater than 10 mm in the systolic blood pressure upon inspiration

paraffin (par'a-fin) 1. a hydrocarbon wax used for embedding histological speci-mens 2. a light mineral oil as liquid paraffin **p section** a stained section of tissue mounted on a glass slide and ex-amined by light microscopy

paraffinoma (par-a-fi-no'ma) a granuloma produced by prolonged exposure to par-affin

parafollicular cells calcitonin-secreting C-cells of thyroid

paraganglioma (-gang'gle-o'ma) a neural crest tumour that occurs in the head and neck

paraganglion (-gang'gle-on) pl. **paraganglia** a collection of chromaffin cells derived from neural ectoderm. They are found outside the adrenal medulla near the sympathetic ganglia

parageusia (-goo'ze-a) perversion of the taste sensation

paragonimiasis (-gon'i-mi-a-sis) infestation with flukes belonging to the genus *Paragonimus. P. westermani* cysts in the lung presents with haemoptysis and clubbing. Liver and brain may be af-fected. Praziquantel is used in the treat-ment

Paragonimus (-gon-i-mis) a genus of trematode parasite *P. westermani*, most common fluke that live in the lungs, whose ova are expectorated or elimi-nated in faeces. Miracidia emerge in water from these eggs and are taken by fresh-water snail. The larvae emerging from snail encyst in freshwater crabs as Metacercariae, which when eaten raw or undercooked, can infect man

paragranuloma (-gran'u-lo'ma) a benign form of Hodgkin's disease affecting lymph nodes

parahaemophilia (-hem'o-fil'e-a) a heredi-tary haemorrhagic tendency due to de-ficiency of coagulation factor V

parahormone (-hor'mon) a substance ex-hibiting hormone-like action

para influenza viruses a group of viruses responsible for acute respiratory infec-tions in children

parakeratosis (-ker'a-to'sis) retention of nuclei in keratinised cells of epidermis

parakinesia (-ki-ne'se-a) any motor abnor-mality

paralalia (-lal'e-a) any speech defect wherein one letter is habitually substi-tuted for another

paraldehyde (par-al'de-hid) hypnotic and anticonvulsant possessing a peculiar smell

paralagma (par'a-lag'ma) displacement of a bone or its broken fragments

parallergy (par-al'er-je) an allergic condi-tion in which body becomes predis-posed to non-specific stimuli after hav-ing been sensitised with a specific aller-gen

paralysis (pa-ral'i-sis) loss of power of mo-tor system concerned with voluntary movement in a muscle due to a lesion of neural or muscular mechanism **acute ascending p** rapidly progressive paraly-sis beginning in the legs and involving progressively the trunk, arms and neck **bulbar p** progressive bulbar palsy **compressive p** paralysis caused by pres-sure on a nerve **conjugate p** paralysis of the conjugate movement of the eyes due to paralysis of one or more extraocular muscles **crossed p, cruciate p** paralysis affecting one side of the face and limbs on the opposite side of the body **crutch p** paralysis due to pressure on nerves in the axilla due to improper use of a crutch **decubitus p** paralysis due to pressure on a nerve due to lying in one position for a long period **diphtheritic p** paralysis of the muscles of palate, accommodation and limbs as a late manifestation of diphtheria **Duchenne's p** pseudohypertrophic muscular paralysis **Duchenne-Erb p, Erb p** paralysis of the muscles of the arm due to involvement of fifth and sixth roots of the brachial plexus **facial p** facial palsy **flaccid p** loss of muscle tone, loss of deep tendon reflexes from lesions of lower motor neurones of spinal cord **hyperkalaemic periodic p** periodic paralysis of brief duration and attack is precipitated by administration of potassium **hypokalaemic periodic p** periodic paralysis coming after strenuous exercise and low level of serum potassium **hysterical p** loss of movement without any organic cause **infantile p** poliomyelitis **Klumpke's p** paralysis and wasting of the small muscles of the hand and of forearm due to paralysis of cervical eighth and first thoracic nerves **Landry's p** acute ascending paralysis **p agitans** classic Parkinsonism **progressive bulbar p** paralysis of muscles of tongue, lips, palate, pharynx and larynx due to atrophic degeneration of neurones innervating these muscles **pseudobulbar p** spastic weakness of the muscles of the face, pharynx and tongue due to cerebral lesions involving the upper motor neurones bilaterally. There is difficulty in speech, and swallowing with emotional instability **sensory p** loss of sensation **spinal p** loss of motor power due to lesion of spinal cord **supranuclear p** paralysis from disorders in pathways or centres above the nuclei of origin **Todd's p** transient paralysis after an epileptic seizure **vasomotor p** paralysis of vasmotor centres

paralytic ileus a situation in which the peristalsis of the intestine slow down or stop, noted following abdominal surgery, electrolyte abnormalities (hypokalaemia) or peritonitis

paralysant (par'a-liz'ant) 1. causing paralysis 2. a drug that causes paralysis.

paramastitis (-mas-tit'is) inflammation of tissues around the mammary gland

Paramecium (par-a-me'se-um) a genus of ciliate protozoa

paramedian incision a vertical incision 1 to 2.5 cm away from midline of abdomen with lateral retraction of rectus muscle

paramedic a person trained to provide emergency medical care, such as resuscitation following an accident

paramedical 1. professions allied to medicine 2. services related to medicine and performed by technically trained persons

paramenia (-me'ne-a) disordered or difficult menstruation

paramesonephric duct *see* Mullerian duct

parameter (pa-ram'it-er) one of many ways of measuring an object or evaluating a person

parametric (-met'rik) 1. situated near the uterus 2. pertaining to a parameter

parametritis (-me-tri'tis) inflammation of the parametrium

parametrium (-me'tre-um) loose connective tissue in broad ligament beside cervix and fornices

paramimia (-mim'e-a) the use of wrong or improper gestures in speaking

paramnesia (par'am-ne'zhah) recall of events that have not taken place

paramucin (-mu'sin) a glycoprotein found in ovarian and some other cysts. It is not soluble in water but gets precipitated by tannin

paramyloidosis (par-am'i–loi-do'sis) accumulation of an atypical form of amyloid in tissues

paramyoclonus (par-a-mi-ok'lo-nus) myoclonus in a widely different group of muscles

paramyotonia (-mi'o-to'ne-a) muscle spasm induced by cold.

Paramyxoviridae (-mik'so-vir'i-de) the paramyxomaviruses; a family of RNA viruses including the genera Paramyxovirus, Morbilivirus and Pneumovirus

paramyxovirus (mik'so-vi'rus) paramyxoviruses a genus of viruses belonging to the family Paramyxoviridae, responsible for respiratory infections, measles and mumps.

paraneoplastic (-ne'o-plas'tik) pertaining to changes produced in tissues remote from a tumour or its metastases **p syndrome (s)** comorbid conditions due to remote or biologic effects of malignancy, which may be the first sign of a neoplasm or its recurrence.

paranephric (-nef'rik) 1. near the kidney 2. adrenal gland

paranephritis (-ne-frit'is) 1. inflammation of the connective tissue around the kidney 2. inflammation of the adrenal gland

paranephros (-nef'ros) an adrenal gland

paranoia (par'a-noi-a) a disorder characterised by the false belief that people or events are in some way related to oneself

paranoid delusions *see* delusions

paranoid ideation suspiciousness of less than delusional proportion

paranoid personality a person of suspicious opinionated and is either over-sensitive or aggressive

paranoid schizophrenia schizophrenia in which delusions of persecution are predominant

paraoesophageal by the side of oesophagus **p hernia** rolling hiatus hernia

paranomia (par'a-no'me-a) aphasia in which there is an inability to remember correct names of the objects seen

paranucleus (-noo'kle-is) a small chromatin lying near a nucleus

paraparesis (-pa-re'sis) symmetrical partial paralysis of the lower limbs

parapertusis (-per-tus'is) an acute respiratory illness caused by *Bordetella parapertusis*. The clinical features simulate mild form of pertusis

paraphasia (-fa'ze-a) production of incoherent speech

paraphemia (-fe'me-a) paraphasia

paraphia (par-a'fe-a) perversion of sense of touch

paraphilia (par'a-fil'e-a) abnormal desires, usually limited to sexual perversion

paraphimosis constriction of the glans penis by a tight foreskin that has been pulled back; causing swelling and pain

paraplasm (par'a-plazm) 1. any abnormal growth 2. protoplasmic fluid of a cell

paraplectic (par'a-plek'tik) paraplegic

paraplegia (-ple-jah) paralysis of the lower limbs **paraplegia** adj

para-polio a pseudodisease which mimics the symptoms of polio

parapraxia (-prak'se-a) inaccurate performance of purposive acts such as slips of the tongue, tendency to misplace things

paraproxis (-prak'sis) substitution of different action for intended one

paraprotein (-pro'ten) various proteins found in large amounts in blood or urine in disease and not normal constituent

paraproteinaemia (-pro'ten-e'me-a) presence of abnormal proteins in the blood due to plasma cell dyscrasias

parapsis (par-ap'sis) paraphia, any disorder of the touch sensation

parapsoriasis (par'a-sor-i'a-sas) a chronic maculopapular scaly erythroderma appearing in persistent and often enlarging plaques

paraquat (par'a-qwaht) a powerful herbicide and fatal poisoning can occur by its accidental ingestion. It acts like a corrosive poison and causes hepatic and renal damage. Lung involvement leads to inexorable pulmonary fibrosis

pararrhythmia (-rith'me-a) parasystole

parasexual (-sek'shoo-l) other than sexual means

parasitaemia (par'a-si-te'me-a) the presence of parasites, especially malarial parasites, in the blood

parasite (par'a-sit) organisms that live in or on other organisms; some of which cause disease in people **external p** a parasite that lives on the skin such as lice, fleas, ticks or mites **facultative p** an organism capable of living independently of its host at times **incidental p** a parasite that normally lives on another than its present host **internal p** a parasite such as a protozoon or worm that lives within the body of the host **malarial p** any one of the species of plasmodium that can cause malaria **obligate p** a parasite that is entirely dependent on the host **specific p** a parasite needing a specific host to complete its life cycle

parasitic foetus one of the twin foetus lacking heart but surviving on circulation maintained by normal twin

parasitism (par'a-si'tizm) 1. infestation by a parasite 2. a symbiotic relationship wherein the parasite gets benefit from the host

parasitogenic (par-a-sit-a-jen'ik) due to parasites

parasitology (-si-tol'a-je) the scientific study of parasites and parasitism

paraspadias (-spa'de-as) a congenital condition in which urethra opens through one side of the penis

parasuicide (-soo'i-sid) an apparent attempt at suicide by self-poisoning or self-mutilation

parasympathetic (-sim-pa-thet'ik) pertaining to a division of autonomic nervous system

parasympathomimetic (-tho-mi-met'ik) 1. producing effects resembling those resulting from stimulation of parasympathetic nervous system 2. relating to an agent producing features resembling that caused by stimulation of the parasympathetic nervous system

parasynapsis (-si-nap'sis) side-to-side union of chromosomes during meiosis

parasystole (-sis'tah-le) additional source of regular rhythmic contraction, independent of sinus

paratenon (-ten'on) connective tissue immediately surrounding tendon

parathion (-thi'on) an acetyl-cholinesterase- inhibiting organophosphate insecticide

parathormone (-thor'mon) parathyroid hormone

parathymia (-thi'me-a) perverted or inappropriate mood

parathyroid (-th'roid) 1. situated beside thyroid gland 2. one of the four small endocrine glands on the back of or at lower edge of thyroid gland or embedded within its substance. They secrete parathyroid hormone that regulates calcium and phosphorus metabolism

parathyrotropic (-thi'ro-trop'ik) having an affinity for the parathyroid glands

paratope (par'a-top) the site on the antibody that attaches to an antigen

paratrophy (par-a'tra-fe) dystrophy

paratuberculosis (par'a-too-burk'ul-o'sis) a tuberculosis-like disease not due to *Mycobacterium tuberculosis*

paratyphoid (-ti'foid) milder form of typhoid due to *Salmonella paratyphii* A and B

paravaccinia (-vak-sin'e-a) a disease due to paravaccinia virus affecting the udders of cows. It may be transmitted to the hands of humans milking infected cows. It produces painless warty lesions in the hands as milker's nodules

paravaginitis (-vaj'i-ni'tis) inflammation of the tissues by the side of vagina

parboiled rice paddy steamed before husking

paravertebral (per-a-ver'te-bral) by the side of the vertebral column

paregoric (par'i-gor'ik) 1. camphorated tincture of opium used as an anti-peristaltic agent in diarrhoea 2. soothing

parenchyma (pa-reng'ki-ma) the essential part of an organ consisting of functional elements as distinguished from its framework

parenteral (pa-ren'ter-il) administration of drugs, nutrients or other substances by any other route other than the digestive tract

paraepididymis (par'ep-i-did'i-mis) paradidymis

paresis (pa-re'sis) partial paralysis

paresthesia (par'es-the'zhah) a tingling in the skin; a 'pins and needles' sensation.

paribhasha (s) terminology

paries (par'e-ez) a wall

parietal (par-ri'e-t'l) 1. of or pertaining to the walls of a cavity 2. pertaining to or located near the parietal bone **p cell** large eosinophilic cell of gastric glands concerned with production of hydrochloric acid **p layer** serosal lining of the external surface of the cavity **p lobe** part of each cerebral hemisphere that is involved in pain and touch sensations, speech and control of spatial orientation

parietofrontal (pa-ri'e-to-front'l) pertaining to the parietal and frontal bones, gyri or fissures

pariksha (s) examination

parinama (s) result; effect

Parinaud's syndrome inability to elevate or depress gaze at will due to midbrain lesion, named after Henri Parinaud, French ophthalmologist

parite an intraarterial fibrous plaque in atherosclerosis

parity (par'it-e) 1. the condition of having given birth to an offspring alive or dead. Multiple births are considered as a single para 2. equality or similarity

Parkin (par'kin) gene on chromosome 6, involved in degradation of protein, whose mutation cause early onset form of inherited Parkinson's disease

Parkinsonism (par'kin-sin-izm) a degenerative disease affecting the basal ganglia presenting with slowness of movement (bradykinesia), increased tone (rigidity), tremor and loss of postural reflexes **secondary p** Parkinsonism developing from definable causes, such as drugs (phenothiazines, reserpine, lithium), toxins (manganese, 1-methyl 4-phenyl tetrahydropyridine), carbon monoxide, encephalitis lethargica, atherosclerosis, Wilson's disease or head injury (punch-drunk syndrome).

Parkinson's disease paralysis agitans idiopathic, starts insidiously, tremor, rigidity, akinesia and postural distur-

bances are the major clinical manifestations. The face is expressionless, tremors are resting and suppressed by voluntary movement. Rigidity affects entire range of movements. There is postural instability and gait difficulty. There is degeneration of nigrostrial tract. The degenerating neurones contain Lewy bodies and neurofibrillar tangles, named after James Parkinson, British physician

paroccipital (par'ok-sip'it'l) beside the occipital bone

paromomycin (par'a-mo-mi'sin) an aminoglycoside antibiotic useful in treating amoebiasis

paronychia (par'o-nik'e-a) an infection of the nail fold especially of the lateral, and it becomes red, swollen, tender and very painful. It involves a single nail at a time **chronic p** asymptomatic erythematous swelling of the posterior nail fold of one or more fingers

paronychial (-a-nik'e-al) pertaining to paronychia or to the nail folds.

parophthalmia (-of-thal'me-a) inflammation of the connective tissue around the eye

parorchidium (-or-kid'e-im) displacement of a testis or testes

parotid (pa-rot'id) near the ear **p glands** the largest pair of salivary glands which are present on either side of the face, just below and in front of the ear

parotitis (par'o-tit'is) inflammation of the parotid gland

parovarian (par'o-var'e-in) beside the ovary

paroxysm (par'ok-sizm) a sudden attack or worsening or recurrence of symptoms or of a disease or a spasm or seizure

parrot fever psittacosis

pars a part or portion of a structure

parthenium grass weed *Parthenium hysterophorus* growing wild in India. The pollens are potential sources of allergic airway disease

partial mastectomy surgical removal of a breast cancer along with the overlying

skin, a portion of surrounding tissues and some of the underlying muscles

partial seizure a localised abnormal electrical discharge in the brain that affects isolated body or mental functions

partial thromboplastin time activated partial thromboplastin time (aPPT) a one-stage coagulation test that is sensitive to deficiencies of antihaemophilic factors

particle (part'ik'l) a very small part or piece of anything

partitioning (par-tish'un-ing) dividing into parts

parturient (par-tur'e-int) relating to childbirth

parturiometer (par-tir'e-om'it-er) a device to determine the force of uterine contractions in childbirth.

parturition (par'tu-ri'shun) childbirth

parulis (pa-roo'lis) a subperiosteal abscess of the gum

parvicellular (par'vi-sel'u-lar) pertaining to or composed of cells of small size

Parvoviridae (par'vo-vir'i-de) family of viruses with single-stranded DNA that replicate in the nucleus of infected cells. It includes the genera *Parvovirus* and *Densovirus*

Parvovirus (par'vo-vi'rus) a genus of viruses similar to adeno-associated viruses, pathogenic to animals and humans, and produce erythema infectiosum, aplastic anaemia, hydrops foetalis and foetal death

PAS abbreviation for para aminosalicylic acid; periodic acid-Schiff (stain)

PASA – abbreviation for para aminosalicylic acid

Pascal (pas-kal) pressure expressed in newtons per square metre, named after Blaise Pascal French scientist

passive (pas'iv) not active; submissive

passive exercise exercise using external force or other muscles with body to restore muscle strength

passive smoking inhalation of tobacco smoke from other people's cigarettes or *beedies* and it increases the risk of respiratory disorders including malignancy

paste a soft semisolid that flows slowly .

Pasteurella (pas'ter-el'a) a genus of gram-negative bacteria belonging to the family Pasteurellaceae, and it includes *P. multocida,* named after Louis Pasteur French chemist and bacteriologist

pasteurellosis (pas'ter-e-lo'sis) infection with bacteria belonging to the genus *Pasteurella*

pasteurisation (pas'cher-i-za'shun) the process of heating of milk or other liquids for about 30 minutes at 60°C which kills the bacteria and prevents the spread of milk-borne pathogens

past pointing misjudging the distances in cerebellar lesions, resulting in missing the target

Patau's syndrome trisomy 13 presenting with cleft lip and palate, polydactyly, small head and congenital heart disease named after Klaus Patau, German born US geneticist.

patch (pach) a small circumscribed area differing from the surrounding surface

p test application of allergens to the skin of the back to detect type IV hypersensitivity used in the diagnosis and as a test for safety of drugs

patella (pa-tel'a) the knee cap, *see* table of bones **patellar** adj Table of

patellectomy (pat'il-ek'ta-me) excision of the patella

patency (pa'ten-si) the state of being freely open

patent (pat'nt) 1. open or unobstructed **p ductus arteriosus** (PDA) during foetal life, the blood from the pulmonary artery passes through the ductus arteriosus into the aorta, that closes after birth. It may remain persistent producing a continuous murmur and enlarged pulmonary artery. Later there can be reversed shunt **p foramen ovale** persistent ostium secondum 2. an arrangement to protect a discovery for the benefit of the discoverer

paternity testing the use of DNA fingerprints to help whether or not a particular individual is the father of a particular child.

pathergy (path'er-je) reactions of all kinds resulting from a state of altered activity

pathfinder (path'find'er) a filiform bougie for introduction through a narrow stricture. It acts as a guide for introduction of a larger sound or catheter

pathobiology (-bi-ol'a-je) pathology with emphasis on biological aspects

pathogen (path'a-jen) any diseaseproducing agent or microorganism **pathogenic** adj

pathogenesis (path'a-jen'e-sis) the process by which a disease originates and develops

pathognomonic (path'ug-no-man'ih) characteristic of a disease

pathologic (path'a-loj'ik) relating to disease

pathology (pa-thol'a-je) branch of medical science dealing with the structural and functional changes that result from disease process **cellular p** interpretation of diseases on the basis of cellular alterations **clinical p** use of laboratory methods as pertains to diagnosis of the disease **comparative p** the disease of animals especially in relation to human pathology **oral p** morbid anatomic or functional changes due to diseases of oral and paraoral structures **speech p** functional and organic speech defects and disorders **surgical p** examination of tissues removed from living patients for the purpose of diagnosis

pathomimesis (path'o-mi-me'sis) mimicry of disease

pathomorphism (-mor'fizm) abnormal morphology

pathophysiology (-fiz'e-ol'a-je) the physiology of disordered function

pathopsychology (-si-kol'a-je) the psychology of mental disease

pathosis (pa-tho'sis) a diseased condition

pathway (pay'wa) 1. a path or a course, a collection of axons of nerve cells over which impulses pass from their point of origin to their destination 2. any sequence of chemical reactions leading from one compound to another **afferent p** the nerve pathway through which a sensory impulse is transmitted from receptor to cerebral cortex **arachidonic acid metabolic p** stimulation of release of arachidonic acid from phospholipid component of cell membrane resulting in activation of 5 lipoxygenase and cyclo-oxygenase pathways **central p** pathway within the brain and spinal cord **complement alternative p** a pathway of complement activation initiated by a variety of factors other than those initiating the classic pathway **complement classic p** a first complement cascade initiated by an antigen-antibody reaction that activates complement factor 1 (C_1) **efferent p** the nerve structures through which an impulse passes away from the brain for innervation of muscles, glands or other effector organs **Embden-Myerhof p** the enzymatic reactions in anaerobic conversion of glucose to lactic acid and in production of ATP **extrinsic p of coagulation** production of fibrin rapidly following tissue injury by formation of an activated complex between tissue factor and factor VII **intrinsic p of coagulation** occurrence of a sequence of reactions that lead to formation of fibrin. It begins with contact of activating factor XII and later ending with activation of factor X **metabolic p** occurrence of a sequential chemical reactions during the metabolism **sensory p** an afferent pathway over which sensory impulses are conveyed from sense organs or receptors to sensory or reflex centres in the spinal cord or brain

pathya (s) diet

patient (pa'shent) a person who is suffering from a disease or disorder and undergoing treatment for it **p satisfaction** patients' subjective evaluation of their health care

patrilineal (pat'ri-lin'e-il) descended through the male line

patulous (pach'il-is) patent

pauci – combining word for few

Paul-Bunnell test test to detect heterophile antibody in sera in infectious mononucleosis, named after John Paul and Walls Bunnell, US physicians

pause (pawz) temporary stop or cessation.

pavor (pa'vor) terror

PAWP abbreviation for pulmonary artery wedge pressure

Pb chemical symbol for lead (plumbum)

PBI abbreviation for protein-bound iodine

P.C. post cibal, L after food

PaCO₂ abbreviation for arterial carbon-dioxide tension

PCO₂ abbreviation for carbon dioxide partial pressure

PCP Pneumocystis carinii pneumonia

PCR abbreviation for polymerase chain reaction

PCV abbreviation for packed cell volume

PCWP abbreviation for pulmonary capillary wedge pressure

p.d. prism diopter

Peaked T Wave ECG abnormality in hyperkalaemia.

pearl (perl) 1. a small, thin glass globule containing volatile medicine, which is crushed in a handkerchief and inhaled, such as amyl nitrite 2. a rounded thick mass of sputum as seen in bronchial asthma **epithelial p** central area of keratinisation within concentric layers of abnormal squamous cells, found in squamous cell carcinoma

Peau d'orange (po'do-ranj) multiple dimples seen in the skin resembling an orange, due to lymphatic oedema

pecten (pek'ten) a structure possessing comb-like processes or projections

pectenosis (pek'te-no'sis) stenosis of the anal canal

pectin (pek'tin) a polymer of sugar acids of fruit, especially the extract from peel of citrus fruits or from the pulp of apple. It forms a gel when cooked with sugar at proper pH

pectinate (pek'ti-nat) comb-shaped

pectineal (pek-tin'e-il) pertaining to the os pubis

pectiniform (pek-tin'i-form) comb-shaped

pectoral (pek'ter-il) relating to the chest

pectoralis (pek'ta-ra'lis) *see* Table of muscles.

pectoriloquy (pek-to-ril'o-kwi) an increased vocal resonance with transmission of voice sounds through the pulmonary structures **spoken p** spoken words are clearly audible as if speaking right into the listener's ears **whispering p** distinctly audible syllables of the whispering sounds, heard over an area of consolidation, or over a big cavity communicating with a patent bronchus

pectus (pek'tus) chest, thorax or the breast **p carinatum** pigeon chest **p excavatum** funnel chest

pedal (ped'l) pertaining to the foot or feet

pederasty (ped'er-as'te) anal intercourse, especially when practised on boys

pedicel (ped'i-sil) 1. foot process; foot plate 2. the secondary process of a podocyte

pedicellation (ped'i-sil-a'shun) formation of a pedicle, or peduncle

pedicle (ped'ik'l) a foot-like structure 1. a stalk by which a tumour attaches to the normal tissue 2. a stalk through which a skin flap in plastic surgery receives its blood supply

pedicular (pe-dik'ul-er) 1. pertaining to a stalk 2. concerning to lice

pediculation (pe-dik'ul-a'shun) 1. process of developing a stalk 2. infestation with lice

pediculicide (pe-dik'ul-i-sid) 1. destroying the lice 2. an agent that destroys lice

pediculosis (pe-dik'u-lo'sis) an infestation caused by lice **p capitis** infestation by head louse, *Pediculus humanis capitis* affecting scalp hair, transmitted by close contact. The lice are brown in colour and live on the scalp and lay eggs (nits), which stick to hairs. It causes severe itching **p corporis** caused by body louse *P. humanis corporis*. It is white in colour and lives in seams of the clothes, causes itching and severe excoriations, transmitted by close contact in individuals with poor hygiene **p pubis** caused by *Pthirus pubis* which infests hairs in the pubic region, moustache, beard, axillae and eye lashes and causes intense itching often transmitted by sexual contact

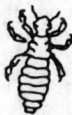

Pediculus humanis capitis

pediculous (pe-dik'ul-is) infested with lice

pediculus (pe-dik'u-lus) 1. a genus of lice belonging to the family Pediculidae that live on hair and feed periodically on blood 2. a stalk

pedigree (ped'i-gre) a table or chart giving the details of ancestors, that is helpful in analysis of Mendelian inheritance

pedodontics (pe-do-don'tiks) the branch of dentistry dealing with dental care and treatment of children

pedodontist a dentist practising pedodontics

pedophilia (-fil'e-a) 1. abnormal fondness for children by an adult for sexual purpose 2. *psy* a sexual perversion to have sexual relations with children

pedorthics (pe-dor'thiks) the process of production of shoes and other foot appliances to give relief to painful conditions of the foot and leg

peduncle (pe-dung'k'l) 1. pedicle 2. band of connecting nerve fibres **cerebellar p** three sets of band of nerve fibres connecting cerebellum with spinal cord and medulla (inferior), pons (middle) and midbrain (superior) **cerebral p** a pair of white bundles connecting midbrain to the cerebrum and consists of anterior (crus cerebri) and posterior (tegmentum) parts **mamillary p** a band of fibres connecting the tegmentum of the midbrain to the mamillary body **olfactory p** the long stalk of the olfactory bulb **pineal p** a band from either side of pineal gland extending to the fornix **thalamic p** one of the four radiations extending from the thalamus to the cerebral cortex

pedunculus (pe-dung'ku-lus) pl. **pendunculi** peduncle

PEEP positive end- expiratory pressure.

peg a projecting structure **p teeth** incisons with a barrel-shaped deformity

Pel-Ebstein fever febrile state for several days alternating with variable periods of pyrexia and apyrexia as in Hogdkin's disease, named after Pieter Pel, Dutch physician and Wilhelm Ebstein, German physician

pelage (pel'aj) collective term for hair of the body including scalp

peliosis (pel'e-o'sis) purpura

pellagra (pe-lag'-ra) a syndrome due to niacin deficiency in individuals with high intake of maize (deficient in tryptophan) or *jowar* (high leucine content) characterised by dermatitis on exposed parts of the body, diarrhoea and mental changes

pellagroid (pe-lag'roid) resembling pellegra

pellicle (pel'ik'l) 1. a thin piece of skin 2. a thin film on the surface of liquids

pellet (pel'et) a small pill of medicine

pellucid (pel-oo'sid) translucent

pelvic pertaining to the pelvis **p examination** examination of a woman's external and internal genitalia **p floor** a region bordered anteriorly by the pubis and posteriorly by the sacrum, laterally by the ischial and iliac bones superiorly by the peritoneum and inferiorly by the levator ani and coccygeus muscles. It contains uterus and adnexae, the bladder, and rectum **p floor exercise** voluntary contraction of muscles at the floor of the pelvis to strengthen and tone them **p inflammatory disease** infection of the internal female reproductive organs such as fallopian tube, ovary, uterus and it forms the most common cause of infertility in women

pelvicalyceal (pel'vi-kal'i-se-il) pertaining to the renal pelves and calices

pelvicephalometry (-sef'a-lom'i-tre) measurement of the foetal head in relation the maternal pelvis

pelvifixation (-fik-sa'shun) surgical fixation of a floating pelvic organ

pelvimetry (pel-vim'i-tre) measurement of the diameters of the pelvis

pelviotomy (pel've-ot'a-me) 1. enlargement of the pelvic outlet by incision into symphysis pubis 2. an incision into the pelvis of the kidney

pelvis (pel'vis) pl. **pelves** the basin-shaped bony structure at the base of the spine consisting of the ilium (hip bone), the sacrum and coccyx. 2. a cup shaped cavity as the pelvis of the kidney. **android p** a masculine pelvis **anthropometric p** a female pelvis with a long anteroposterior diameter and a narrow transverse diameter **assimilation p** a deformity in which transverse processes, of the last lumbar vertebra are fused with the sacrum or the last sacral with the first coccygeal body. Pelvis with pelvic bone laterally compressed **beaked p** osteomalacic pelvis **branchypellic p** pelvis with transverse diameter exceeding the anteroposterior diameter **champagne glass p** pelvic radiograph exhibiting flattening of the iliac wings with pelvic inlet resembling a champagne bottle, noted in achondroplasia **contracted p** pelvis with less than normal measurements in all dimensions **cordate p** sacrum projecting forward between the ilia, making the brim of pelvis heart shaped **dolichopellic p** an elongated pelvis with the anteroposterior diameter being greater than the transverse diameter **false p** pelvis major **flat p** a pelvis in which the anteroposterior diameter is uniformly contracted **funnel-shaped p** pelvis with normal inlet but a greatly narrowed outlet **gynaecoid p** normal female pelvis, a rounded oval pelvis with rounded anterior and posterior segments **infantile p** generally contracted pelvis with oval shape with slender bones **p justo major** an unusally large gynaecoid pelvis with all dimensions increased **p justo minor** a small gynaecoid pelvis with all its diameters smaller than normal **kyphotic p** backward curvature of lumbar spine making pelvis contracted **p female** pelvis resembling that of a male pelvis and it is narrower, funnel-shaped, large with heavy bones **mesatipellic p** a pelvis with equal anteroposterior and transverse diameters **osteomalacic p** beaked pelvis, pelvic aperture with the shape of a heart of clover leaf and pubic bones beak-shaped, a deformity due to osteomalacia **p girdle** the ring of bones which form the hips and lower abdominal area **p major** false pelvis, the expanded portion of pelvis above brim **masculine p** minor true pelvis, the cavity of pelvis below the brim **platypellic p** a flat oval pelvis in which the transverse diameter is longer than the anteroposterior diameter **rachitic p** a contracted and deformed pelvis **renal p** flat, funnel-shaped expansion of the upper end of the ureter receiving the calices of the kidney **split p** absence of symphysis pubis with separated pelvic bones **spondylolisthetic p** pelvic brim being occluded by a dislocation forward of body of the lower lumbar vertebra **true p** pelvis minor

pelvispondylitis (pel'vi-spon'di-li'tis) a rheumatoid spondylitis affecting pelvic portion of the spine

pemphigoid (pem'fi-goid) occurrence of tense large blisters associated with an erythematous discolouration of skin **bullous p** large tense and unilocular blisters in and around axilla and limbs **p gestationis** blistering condition affecting periumbilical region and limbs, in young pregnant females

pemphigus (-gus) an autoimmune disease caused by reaction of IgG with a protein (glycocalyx) found on the surface of the epidermal cells. It leads to activation of some proteases, which cause separation of epidermal cells from one another (acantholysis) and formation of intraepidermal bullae **p erythematosus**

lesions surrounded by erythema and found on the butterfly area of the face **p vegetans** lesions are vegetating growths in the skin folds such as axillae and groins. Bullae are less in numbers **p vulgaris** an auto-immune disorder with appearance of crops of intraepidermal bullae in the mouth, face, neck and trunk. Pressure on bullae enlarge them due to splitting of the skin. Bullae contain clear or purulent fluid which on healing leave behind pigmentation and scarring

pendelluft (pen'del-looft) movement of air in the conducting system (nose, mouth, pharynx, larynx, bronchi and bronchioles) not participating in the gas exchange

Pendred's syndrome a congenital disorder characterised by goitrous hypothyroidism due to a block in the synthesis of thyroid hormone, with deafness or deaf-mutism, named after Vaughan Pendred, British physician.

pendulous (pen'dul-us) swinging freely from the attached part

penem a member of β-lactam antibiotic acting on the bacterial cell wall. It causes lysis of bacteria that are in the resting phase

penetrance (pen'i-trans) 1. the frequency with which a mutant gene produces its characteristic effect in those possessing it 2. the extent to which something enters an object or part

penetrometer (pen'i-trom'it-er) a device for measuring penetrating power of x-rays

penicillamine (pen'i-sil'a-men) a hydrolytic degradation product of penicillin used to facilitate urinary excretion of heavy metals such as copper, mercury, zinc or lead

penicillic (pen-i-sil'ik) **acid** an antibiotic substance isolated from cultures of different species of penicillium and aspergillus

penicillin (pen'i-sil'in) antibiotic with a basic structure of a four-membered β-lactam ring produced by the molds,

Pencillium notatum and *P. chrysogenum*. It is bactericidal killing bacteria by interfering with their cell wall synthesis. It acts on both gram-positive and certain gram-negative organisms. Penicillinase is capable of inactivating the penicillin. Hypersensitivity forms the most important adverse reaction.

penicillinase (pan'i-sil'i-nas) a β-lactamase which can cleave the β-lactam ring and inactivate penicillin. The plasmids which code for the enzyme are transmissible between bacteria

penicillium (-sil'e-um) a genus of fungi belonging to class Ascomycetes or the order Aspergillales yielding many antibiotic substances

penicillus (pen'i-sil'us) a group of branches of arteries in the spleen that are arranged like the bristles of a brush

penile (pe'nil) of or pertaining to the penis **p implant** a silicone splint or an inflatable device inserted into the pelvis to enable a man who is impotent to have intercourse

penis (pe'nis) the male organ of copulation and urination. It is suspended from the front and sides of pubic arch and is composed of erectile tissue arranged in three columns. There are two lateral columns, called corpora cavernosa and a median column corpus spongiosum containing urethra. Glans penis is a cone-shaped head of the penis containing urethral orifice, and is covered by the foreskin (prepuce). Sexual excitement causes hyperaemia facilitating filling of corpora cavernosa and erection. It becomes flaccid on subsidence of hyperaemia

penitis (pe-nit'is) inflammation of the penis

penniform (pen'i-form) shaped like a feather

penta – combining word for 'five'

pentadactyl (pen'ta-ak'til) having five digits on each hand and foot

pentaerythritol (pen'ta-e-rith'ri-tol) **tetranitrate** an organic nitrate used in the treatment of angina pectoris

pentagastrin (-gas'trin) a synthetic gastrin used to test the ability of the stomach to secrete hydrochloric acid

pentamidine (-am'i-dine) an antiparasitic agent used in the treatment of *Pneumocystis carinii* pneumonia, visceral leishmaniasis and sleeping sickness

pentazocine (pen-taz'o-sen) a synthetic narcotic analgesic agent

pentetic (pen-tet'ik) **acid** a chelating agent

pentobarbital (pen'to-bar'bi-tal) a hypnotic barbiturate

pentose (pen'tos) a monosaccharide containing five carbon atoms in a molecule.

pentosuria (pen'to-su're-a) the excretion of one or more pentoses in the urine

peotillomania (pe'o-til'o-ma-ne-a) a nervous habit of constant pulling of thepenis

peplos (pep'los) lipoprotein envelope surrounding certain virions

peotomy (pe'ot'o-me) surgical removal of penis

pepsin (pep'sin) the principal enzyme secreted in the stomach that helps in digestion of protein. It is formed from pepsinogen by the chief cells of gastric glands and reduces proteins to smaller molecules such as proteoses and pentoses

pepsinogen (pep-sin'a-jin) a proenzyme secreted by the chief cells of the gastric mucosa

peptic (pep'tik) 1. relating to gastric digestion 2. pertaining to pepsin **p ulcer** an ulcer in the lower oesophagus, stomach or duodenum, in the jejunum following surgical anastomosis to the stomach or rarely in the ileum adjacent to a Meckel's diverticulum. Chronic peptic ulcer presents with pain in the epigastrium, clock like regularity of pain in relation to intake of food - on eating (gastric) and on empty stomach (duodenal)

peptidase (pep'ti-das) an enzyme capable of hydrolysing one of the peptide links of a peptide to produce an amino acid

peptide (pep'tid) a compound of two or more amino acids wherein −carboxyl group of one is united with the −amino group of the other

peptidergic (pep'ti-der'jik) referring to nerve cells of fibres using small peptide molecules as neurotransmitters

peptidoglycan (pep'ti-do-gli'kan) a compound containing amino acids or peptides joined with sugars. It is the essential constituent of the cell wall of most bacteria

peptococcus (pep'to-kok'us) an anaerobic gram-positive coccus that can produce infections synergistically with other organisms

peptogenic (pep'to-jen'ik) 1. producing peptones 2. promoting digestion

peptolysis (pep-tol'i-sis) the splitting up of peptones **peptolytic** adj

peptone (pep'ton) intermediate polypeptide products formed in partial hydrolysis of proteins

peptostreptococcus (pep'to-strep'to-kok'us) a genus of gram-positive anaerobic cocci, which act as opportunistic pathogens

peracute (per'a-kut) very acute

per anum (pera'num) through the anus

per rectum (per-rek'tum) through the rectum

per vagina (pervaj'i-na) through the vagina

percept (per'sept) the mental image of an object seen

perception (per-sep'shun) process of transferring physical stimulation into psychological information; mental process by which sensory stimuli are brought to awareness

perceptivity (per'sep-tiv'it-e) the ability to receive sensory impressions

percolate (per'kah-lat)1. to allow a fluid to seep through a powdered substance; to strain 2. any fluid that has been percolated or filtered

percolation (per'kah-la'shun) 1. filtration 2. the process of extraction of soluble portions of a powdered drug by passing a solvent liquid through it

per contiguum (per kon-tig'u-um) in contiguity; touching, as in spread of an inflammatory process or malignancy from one part to an adjacent structure

per continuum (per kon-tin'u-um) in continuity; continuous, as in spread of an inflammatory or malignant process from one part to an adjacent part.

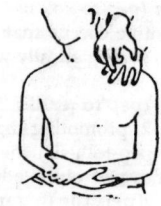

Percussion of the apex

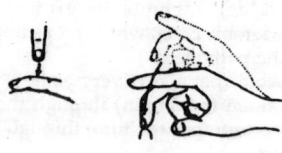

Percussion-position of pleximeter and plexor

percussion (per-kush'in) a technique to produce sound waves by tapping the surface with the finger and it varies in its quality depending on the density of the underlying tissues **auscultatory p** auscultation of the sounds produced by percussion **direct p** percussion wherein the finger strikes directly over the bony region without the intervention of any other finger as on clavicle **immediate p** direct percussion **radiate p** digitodigital percussion where percussion is done by using the middle finger of one hand as a plexor and of the middle finger of other hand applied firmly on the surface as pleximeter

percussor (per-kus'or) 1. a device consisting of a hammer with rubber head used for diagnostic percussion

percutaneous (per'ku-ta'ne-us) performed through the skin **p transluminal coronary angioplasty** (PTCA) an interventional procedure consisting of balloon expansion of one or more stenosed coronary arteries

per diem L. per day

perforans (per'fo-ranz) penetrating

perfusate (per-fu'zat) fluid used to perfuse a tissue or organ

perfusion (-zhun) 1. the passage of blood or other fluid through a vascular bed of an organ or tissue 2. pouring of a fluid 3. supply of nutrients to an organ by injecting into an artery

peri - combining word for around, near

periacinal (per'e-as'i-nal) around an acinus

periadenitis (-ad'e-ni'tis) inflammation of tissues around a gland

periampullary (-am'pul-e-re) around an ampulla

periapical (-a'pi-ki) surrounding the apex of the root of a tooth

periappendicitis (-a-pen'di-sit'is) inflammation of the tissues around the appendix

periarteritis (-ar'-te-ri'tis) inflammation of the outer coat of an artery

periarthritis (-ar-thrit'is) inflammation of tissues around a joint

periarticular (-ar-tik'u-ler) around a joint

peribronchiolitis (pep'i-bronk'-e-o-lit'is) inflammation of tissues around the bronchioles

peribronchitis (-bronk-it'is) inflammation of tissues around the bronchi

pericaliceal (-kal'i-se'al) located near a renal calyx

pericallosal (-ka-lo'sl) located around the corpus callosum

pericardiectomy (-kar-de-ek'ta-me) surgical removal of a portion of the pericardium

pericardiocentesis (-kar-de-o-sen-te'sis) paracentesis of the pericardium

pericardiolysis (-kar'de-ol'i-sis) the operative separation of adhesions between the visceral and the parietal pericardium

pericardiophrenic (-kar'de-o-fren'ik) pertaining to the pericardium and diaphragm

pericardiorrhaphy (-kar'de-ox'a-fe) suture of the pericardium

pericardiostomy (-kar'de-os'ta-me) creation of an opening into the pericardium

pericardiotomy (-kar'de-ot'a-me) incision of the pericardium

pericarditis (-kar-di'tis) inflammation of the pericardium due to infection, immunological reaction, trauma or malignancy and sometimes unexplained cause characterised by retrosternal pain, fever and pericardial rub **acute fibrinous p** pericarditis with a fibrinous exudate **adhesive p** fibrinous pericarditis leading to varying degrees of adhesion formation between the two layers of the pericardium or between the pericardium and the heart or the neighbouring structures **constrictive p** progressive thickening, fibrosis and calcification of the pericardium **fibrinous p** acute pericarditis with fibrinous exudate **haemorrhagic p** haemorrhagic effusion in the pericardium often due to malignant disease **purulent p** purulent collection of fluid in pericardium as a complication of septicemia or by direct spread of an intrathoracic infection **serous p** a large effusion of turbid, straw-coloured fluid in the pericardium

pericardium (-kar'de-um) the fibroserous membrane covering the heart and the beginning of the aorta and pulmonary artery. It consists of a serous visceral layer surrounding the heart and the parietal layer composed of fibrous tissue whose inner surface is lined by a serous membrane, and forms a potential space with serous fluid

pericaecitis (-se-sit'is) inflammation of the tissues around caecum.

pericementitis (-se'men-tit'is) periodontitis

pericholangitis (-ko'lan-jit'is) inflammation of the tissues around the bile ducts

pericholecystitis (-ko'le-sis-tis'is) inflammation of the tissues around the gall bladder

perichondrium (-kon'dre-um) a membrane of fibrous connective tissue around cartilage

perichordal (-kor'd'l) surrounding the notochord

perichoroidal (-ko-roid'l) around the choroid coat

pericolitis (-ko-li'tis) inflammation around the colon

pericolpitis (-kol-pit'is) inflammation of tissues around the vagina

pericoronal (-ko-no'n-l) around the crown of a tooth

pericranium (-kra'ne-um) the periosteum of the skull **pericranial** adj

pericyte (per'i-sit) an elongated contractile cell found in close association to the outside of capillary wall

pericytial (per'i-si-shal) around a cell

periderm (per'i-durm) a thin layer of flat cells covering the epidermis in the foetus, that disappears before birth

peridesmium (per'i-dez'me-um) the connective tissue membrane covering a ligament

perididymis (-did'i-mis) tunica vaginalis.

perididymitis (-did'i-mit'is) inflammation of the tunica vaginalis

peridiverticulits (-di'ver-tik'u-li'tis) inflammation of tissues around an intestinal diverticulum

periduodenitis (-doo'o-den-it'is) inflammation around the duodenum

periencephalitis (per'e-en-sef'a-li'tis) meningoencephalitis

perienteritis (-en'ter-it'is) inflammation of the peritoneum of the intestine

perifolliculitis (per'i-fa-lik'ul-it is) inflammation surrounding the hair follicles

perigangliitis (-gang'gle-it'is) inflammation of tissues surrounding a ganglia

perigastritis (-gas-trit'is) inflammation of the peritoneal coat of the stomach

perihepatitis (-hep'a-titis) inflammation of the peritoneal covering of the liver

periislet (pere'i'lit) tissue located around the islets of Langerhans

perijejunitis (per'i-je'joo-nit'is) inflammation around jejunum

perikaryon (-kar'e-on) 1. the cytoplasm around a nucleus, 2. the cell body of a nerve cell as distinguished from its axon and dendrites 3. an odontoblast excluding the dentinal fibre

perikymata (-ki'ma-ta) numerous transverse grooves found on the enamel of newly erupted teeth

perilabyrinthitis (-lab'i-rin-thit'is) inflammation of the tissues surrounding the labyrinth

perilaryngitis (-lar'in-jit'is) inflammation of the tissues surrounding the larynx

perilymph (pe'ri-limf) fluid found within the space between membranous and bony labyrinths of the ear

perilymphangitis (-lim-fan-jit'is) inflammation of the tissues surrounding a lymphatic vessel

perimeningitis (-men'in-jit'is) pachy meningitis

perimenopause the period immediately prior to the menopause and the first year after the last menstrual period

perimeter 1. boundary of an area 2. instrument for perimetry

perimetrium (-me'tre-im) the serous membrane covering the uterus

perimetry measurement of field of vision

perimyelitis (-mi'il-it'is) 1. inflammation of pia mater and arachnoid of the spinal cord 2. inflammation of the membrane surrounding medullary cavity of a bone

perimyositis (-mi-a-sit'is) inflammation of the connective tissue surrounding a muscle

perimysitis (-mis'e-it'is) inflammation of the perimysium; myofibrositis

perimysium (-mis'e-um) the fibrous sheath surrounding each of the primary bundles of skeletal muscle fibres

perinatal (-nat'l) relating to the period just before, during or just after birth. It pertains to the period beginning after 28th week of pregnancy to one to four weeks after birth

perinatology (-na-tol'a-je) a subspeciality of paediatrics concerned with the care of the foetus and infant during perinatal period

perineal (-ne'il) pertaining to the perineum **p body** midline tendon of pelvic floor **p prostatectomy** surgical removal of prostate by an approach between rectum and urethra

perineocoele (-ne'a-sel) a hernia in the perineal region that can occur either between rectum and the vagina or the rectum and the bladder

perineoplasty (-ne'a-plas'te) surgical repair of the perineum

perineorrhaphy (-ne-or'a-fe) suture of the perineum

perineotomy (-ne-ot'a-me) incision of the perineum

perineovaginal (-ne'a-vaj'i-nal) pertaining to the perineum and vagina

perinephritis (-ne-frit'is) the inflammation of perinephric tissue

perinephrium (-nef're-um) the connective tissue and fat surrounding the kidney

perineum (-ne'um) 1. the tissue between the external genitalia and the anus that extends internally upto the muscles at the base of the pelvis and the surrounding bony structures 2. superficial area corresponding to the inferior outlet of pelvis

perineuritis (-noor-it'is) inflammation of perineurium

perineurium (-noor'e-um) fibrous sheath of separate fascicles in a peripheral nerve

period (per'e-id) 1. the interval of time between a regularly occurring event or phenomenon 2. the menses 3. time taken by a disease or by a stage of a disease **child bearing p** puberty to menopause **critical p** the time during gestation when important organs are being developed and the foetus is vulnerable to the effects of environmental factors **ejection p** the period in the cardiac cycle when the blood is discharged into the aorta and pulmonary artery. It consists of a rapid ejection phase followed by reduced ejection **fertile p** the time during the menstrual cycle when the ovum can be fertilised **gestation p** the period of pregnancy, measured from the onset of the last menstruation **incubation p** the time from the entry of infection to the appearance of clinical manifestations **induction p** the interval between an injection of antigen and the appearance of antibodies in the blood **isoelectric p** the time when no electric energy being produced in muscle contraction. In ECG, the interval between the end of S wave and beginning of T wave, where the tracing is at zero, as there is no difference in potential under the two electrodes **isometric p** a short period in the diastole in which the muscle fibres do not shorten although the cardiac muscle is excited and the period extends from the closure of AV valves to the opening of semilunar valves **latent p** 1. the time interval between the stimulation and the beginning of response 2. incubation period 3. the time interval between exposure to ionising radiation and appearance of visible signs of effects **missed p** menstruation not occurring at an expected time **monthly p** the time of menstruation **puerperal p** the time interval from the delivery of a child to complete involution of the uterus **refractory p** the period that follows an effective stimulation during which an excitable tissue fails to respond to a stimulus **safe p** the period during the menstrual cycle when the conception is least likely to occur

periodicity (per'e-a-dis'it-e) the tendency to recur at regular intervals

periodontal (per'e-o-don'tal) around a tooth concerning the periodontium

periodontics (per'e-o-don'tiks) the branch of dentistry concerned with the study of the tissues situated immediately about the teeth

periodontitis (-don-ti'tis) a disease of the tissues that surround and support the teeth characterised by inflammation of gingivae, degeneration and resorption of dental periosteum, alveolar bone and cementum. There is loosening of teeth and recession of gingivae

periodontium (-don'she-um) the tissues that surround and support the teeth. They are gingivae, cementum, periodontal membrane and alveolar bone

periodontosis (-don-to'sis) a degenerative disorder of periodontal structures that leads to looseness and migration of teeth

perionychia (-nik'i-a) inflammation around a nail

perionychium (-o-nik'e-um) epidermis surrounding a nail

perioophoritis (-o-of'or-it'is) inflammation of the tissues around the ovary

perioophorosalpingitis (-o-of'ar-o-sal-pin-jit'is) inflammation of tissues around an ovary and fallopian tube

perioperative (-op'er-it-iv) pertaining to any event that occurs during the period of operation

periophthalmic (-of-thal'mik) around the eye

perioptometry (per'e-op-tom'i-tre) measurement of the limits of the visual field

periorbita (-or'bit-a) 1. the periosteum of the bones of the orbit 2. orbital fascia **periorbital** adj

periorbititis (-or'bi-ti'tis) inflammation of the orbital fascia

periorchitis (-or-kit'is) inflammation of the tunica vaginalis testis

periosteitis (-os'te-it'is) periostitis

periosteoma (-os-te-o'ma) a tumour from the periosteum

periosteomyelitis (-os'te-o-mi'e-li'tis) inflammation of the bone, including the periosteum and marrow

periosteophyte (-os'te-o-fit) a bony growth on the periosteum

periosteotomy (-os'te-ot'a-me) cutting through the periosteum

periosteum (-os'te-im) the thick, fibrous membrane that covers the bones except the articular cartilage. It consists of two layers – an inner osteogenic layer forming new bone tissue and an outer connective tissue layer containing blood vessels and nerves

periostitis (-os-tit'is) painful inflammation of the periosteum, resulting from injury or infection

periostosis (-os-to'sis) an abnormal deposition of periosteal bone

periotic (-ot'ik) 1. situated around a ear, especially inner ear 2. the mastoid and petrous portions of the temporal bone

peripapillary (per'i-pap'i-le're) around a papilla

peripartum (-part'um) the period pertaining to the last month of pregnancy or the first few months after delivery

periphacitis (-fa-sit'is) inflammation of the capsule of the lens of the eye

peripherad (per-uf'er-ad) towards the periphery

peripheral 1. situated at the periphery 2. part away from the centre **p nerve** consists of two principal cellular structures-the axon, with the anterior horn cell, and the myelin sheath **p nervous system** all the nerves that fan out from the central nervous system to the rest of the body **p neuropathy** a pathological process affecting a peripheral nerve **p vascular disease** disease of the blood vessels of the extremities, especially those conditions which interfere with adequate blood supply, such as atherosclerosis with narrowing of the arterial lumen

periphery (per-if'er-e) 1. the outer part of surface of a body 2. the pathway from the centre

periphlebitis (per'i-fle-bit'is) inflammation of tissues around a vein or of the outer coat of vein

periplasmic (-plas'mik) around a plasma membrane

periproctitis (-prok-tit'is) inflammation of the tissues around the rectum and anus

periprostatitis (-pros'ta-ti'tis) inflammation of tissues around the prostate

peripylephlebitis (-pi'le-fle-bit'is) inflammation of tissues around the portal vein

perirectitis (-rek-tit'is) periproctitis

perisalpingitis (-sal'pin-jit'is) inflammation of tissues around the fallopian tube

perisigmoiditis (-sig'moid-it'is) inflammation of the peritoneum of the sigmoid flexure

perisinusitis (-si'nis-it'is) inflammation of tissues about a sinus, especially a venous sinus of a dura mater

perispermatitis (-spurm'a-tit'is) inflammation of the tissues surrounding the spermatic cord

perisplanchnitis (-splank-nit'is) inflammation of tissues around viscera

perisplenitis (-splin-it'is) inflammation of the peritoneal covering of the spleen

perispondylitis (-spon'di-lit'is) inflammation of the tissues around a vertebra

peristalsis (-stal'sis) involuntary, wave like alternate contraction and relaxation occurring in tubular structures, especially alimentary canal by which the contents are propelled onward **mass p** forced peristaltic movements of short duration seen in large intestine which allows the movement of its contents from one part to another **reversed p** peristalsis in a direction, the reverse of the normal, which forces the contents backward

peristaphyline (-staf'i-lin) around the uvula

peritectomy (-tek'ta-me) surgical removal of a ring of conjunctiva around the cornea to correct pannus

peritendineum (-ten-din'e-um) one of the fibrous sheaths covering tendons and extending between the fibres composing the tendon

peritendinitis (-ten'di-ni'tis) inflammation of the sheath of a tendon

peritenonitis (-ten'o-ni'tis) peritendinitis

perithelioma (-thel'e-o'ma) a tumour arising from the perithelium of smaller blood vessels

perithelium (-thel'e-im) the fibrous connective tissue layer surrounding small blood vessels and capillaries

perithyroiditis (-thi'roid-it'is) inflammation of the capsule or tissues surrounding the thyroid gland

peritomy (per-it'a-me) 1. excision of a ring of conjunctiva around the cornea 2. circumcision

peritoneal (per'it-o-ne'il) pertaining to the peritoneum **p dialysis** a treatment modality to clear toxic substances from the body in patients who are in terminal renal failure. The procedure may be intermittent or continuous ambulatory

peritonealgia (per'it-o-ne-al'jah) pain in the peritoneum

peritoneocentesis (per'it-o-ne'o-sen-te-sis) paracentesis of the abdominal cavity

peritoneoclysis (per'it-o-ne-ok'li-sis) introduction of fluid into the peritoneal cavity

peritoneoscope (per'i-to'ne-o-skop) a long, slender telescope with a light at one end and an eye piece at the other. It facilitates inspection of the peritoneal cavity through a small incision in the abdominal wall

peritoneoscopy (per'it-o-ne-os'ko-pe) examination of the contents of the peritoneal cavity with a peritoneoscope introduced through the abdominal wall

peritoneotomy (peri'it-o-ne-ot'a-me) incision into the peritoneum

peritoneovenous (perit-o-ne'o-ve'nus) communication between the peritoneal cavity and the venous system

peritoneum (per'it-o-ne'um) the serous membrane lining the wall of the abdominal cavity (**parietal p**) and pelvic cavities and reflecting over the viscera contained therein (**visceral p**) and it forms two sacs, the peritoneal (greater) sac and the omental bursa (lesser sac) connected by the foramen epiploicum

peritonitis (per'i-to-ni'tis) inflammation of the peritoneum

peritonisillar (per'i-ton'si-lar) around a tonsil

peritonsillitis (per'i-ton'si-li'tis) inflammation of peritonsillar tissue

peritracheal (per'i-tra'ke-al) around the trachea

peritrichous (pe-ri'tri-kus) microorganism having cilia or flagella around the entire surface

peritrochanteric (per'i-tro'kan-ter'ik) around a trochanter

perityphlic (per'i-tif'lik) around the caecum

perityphlitis (per'i-tif-li'tis) appendicitis

periumbilical (per'e-um-bil'ik'l) around the umbilicus

periungual (per'e-ung'gwal) around a nail

periureteral (per'e-u-re'ter-al) around a ureter

periureteritis (per'e-u-re'ter-i'tis) inflammation of tissues around the ureter

periurethral (per'e-u-re'thral) around the urethra

periurethritis (per'e-u're-thri'tis) inflammation of the tissues around the urethera

periuterine (per'e-u-teri-in) around the uterus

perivaginal (per'i-vaji'-nal) around the vagina

perivaginitis (per'i-vaj'i-ni'tis) inflammation of the region around the vagina

perivascular (per'i-vas'ku-lar) around a vessel especially a blood vessel

perivasculitis (per'i-vas'ku-li'tis) inflammation of the tissues surrounding a blood vessel

perivenous (per'i-ve'nus) around a vein

perivertebral (per'i-ver'te-bral) around a vertebra

perivesicle (per'i-ves'i-kal) around a bladder especially urinary bladder

perivesiculitis (per'i-ve-sik'u-li'tis) inflammation of tissues around a seminal vesicle

perivisceral (per'i-vis'er-al) around the viscera or a seminal vesicle

perixenitis (per'i-ze-ni'tis) inflammation around a foreign body in a tissue or organ

perle (perl) a soft capsule containing medicine

perleche (per-lesh) *Fr* inflammation with

exudation, epithelial desquamation and fissuring at the corners of the mouth, especially in children.

perlingual (per-ling'gwal) by way of the tongue to administer medicine

permanent (per'ma-nent) unchanged; enduring

permanganate (per-man'ga-nat) a salt of permanganic acid

permeability (per'me-a-bil'i-te) a quality of being permeable **capillary p** capillary wall allowing substances to diffuse into tissue spaces or into cells or *vice versa*

permeable (per'me-a-b'l) permitting the movement of fluids or substances in solution

permeation (per'me-a'shun) penetration and spread throughout an organ, tissue or space

permutation (per'mu-ta'shun) transformation

pernicious (per-nish'us) fatal; harmful **p anaemia** anaemia due to intrinsic factor deficiency **p trend** *psy* departure from usual ideas and social interests

pernio (per'ne-o) chilblain; congestion and swelling of the skin from cold

pero - combining word for deformity; deformed

perobrachius (pe'ro-bra'ke-us) a person with congenitally deformed forearms and hands

perocephalus (pe'ro-sef'a-lus) a person with a congenitally deformed head

perochirus (pe'ro-ki'rus) a person with a congenitally deformed fingers or toes

perocormus (pe'ro-kor'mus) a person with a congenitally deformed trunk

perodactylus (pe'ro-dak'ti-lus) a person with congenitally deformed fingers or toes

peromelia (pe'ro-me'le-a) a congenital deformity of the limbs

peromelus (pe'rom'e-lus) a person with congenitally malformed limbs

perone (per-o'ne) the fibula

peroneal (per'o-ne'al) pertaining to the fibula **p atrophy** progressive peroneal muscle atrophy **p nerve palsy** entrapment neuropathy causing foot drop, dorsiflexion and eversion of foot

peroneotibial (per'o-ne'o-tib'e-al) pertaining to the fibula and tibia

peroral (per-or'al) administered through the mouth

per os L. by mouth

perosomus (pe'ro-so'mus) a person with congenitally defective body

perosseous (per-os'e-us) through bone

peroxidase (per-ok'si-das) iron-porphyrin enzyme facilitating the transfer of oxygen from peroxide to a tissue requiring oxygen

peroxide (per-ok'sid) oxide of any element containing more oxygen

peroxisome (pe-roks'i-som) membrane-bound vesicles containing enzymes such as perioxidase, catalase and d-amino oxidase, concentrated in liver and kidney cells

perphenazine (per-fen'a-zen) a tranquilizer used as an antipsychotic and as an anti emetic

per primam intentionem (per pri'mam inten'she-o'nem) L. by first intention as in healing

per rectum (per rek'tum) through the rectum

per se L by , in or of itself, intrinsically, essentially

per secundum (per se-kun'dam) **intentionem** L. by second intention as in healing

perseveration persisting response to a prior stimulus after a new stimulus has been presented, often associated with organic brain disease.

persistent vegetative state a persistent loss of upper cortical function where the patient is bed ridden who does not require respiratory support or circulatory assistance for survival. Their nutritional support is totally passive. They are in a state of chronic wakefulness without awareness; cognitive death

person a human being

persona the personality presented by a person to others

personality (pers'in-al'it-e) the characteristics, attitude, intellectual qualities, emotional dispositions and behaviour of an individual which sets him/her apart from others. It refers chiefly to the mental aspects than the physique **alternating p** a disorder in which a person exhibits two or more personalities, each with unique behaviour and social relationship **borderline p** a personality disorder exhibiting difficulty in maintaining a stable mood, self-image and interpersonal relationships **compulsive p** a personality exhibiting compulsions to repetitively perform certain acts **dual p** multiple personality **extroverted p** a type of personality in which activities are directed to other individuals or the environment **inadequate p** a personality in which the person is ineffective and physically and emotionally unstable exhibiting difficulty to cope with normal stress of living **introvert p** type of personality in which the activities are directed to the person himself or herself **multiple p** alternating personality **obsessive-compulsive p** compulsive personality **psycopathic p** a personality exhibiting marked egocentricity, lack of feelings and lack of guilt and show little or no regard for the rights or convenience of others **type A p** action-oriented personality, aggressive, impatient, struggling to achieve their goals **type B p** relaxed, less aggressive and less concerned to achieve their goals

personality disorder a pathological disturbance of a person's thinking, and feeling **antisocial p d** a personality disorder in which there is an inability to conform to the social norms. The person exhibits an antisocial behaviour **avoidant p d** a personality disorder leading a socially withdrawn life **borderline p d** a personality disorder exhibiting difficulty in maintaining stable interpersonal relationship and self image **dependent p d** a personality disorder showing feelings of helplessness

histrionic p d a personality disorder showing excessive emotionalism and attention-seeking **narcissistic p d** a personality disorder exhibiting a heightened sense of self-importance and grandiose feelings of uniqueness **obsessive-compulsive p d** a personality disorder characterised by emotional constriction, orderliness, perseverance and stubbornness. **paranoid pd** a personality disorder characterised by suspiciousness and mistrust of others. They refuse responsibility for their own feelings and assign responsibility to others. **passive aggressive p d** a personality disorder characterised by obstructionism, stubbornness and inefficiency **schizoid p d** a personality disorder exhibiting marked deficits in interpersonal relationships and social withdrawal

perspiration (per'spi-ra'shun) 1.sweating; the secretion of the sweat glands of the skin. 2.sweat, a weak solution of sodium chloride **insensible p** evaporation of water vapour from the body without producing any moisture on the skin **sensible p** perspiration producing moisture on the skin.

perspire (per'spir) sweat

persuation (per-swa'zhun) *psy* influencing the behaviour by reason or argument

per tertiam (per ter'she-am) **intentioneum** L. healing by third intention

pertain to relate, to concern, to have reference

Perthes' (per'tez) **disease** osteochondritis deformans juvenilis, named after Georg Perthes, German surgeon

per tubam (pertu'bam) through a tube

perturbation (per'ter-ba'shun) being disturbed or agitated

pertusis (per-tus'is) *see* whooping cough

pertussoid (per-tus'oyd) 1.resembling whooping cough 2. a cough similar to that of whooping cough

pervasive spreading throughout, permeating

per vaginum (per-va-ji'num) through the vagina

perversion (per-ver'zhun) deviation from the normal course **sexual p** seeking sexual satisfaction in ways deviating from the accepted norm

pervert to turn from the acceptable norm or course

per vias naturrales (per ve'as nat'u-ra'lez) L. through the natural ways

pervious (per've-us) permeable

pes pl **pedes** 1. the foot 2. any foot like process **p anserinus** 1. the three main branches of the facial nerve 2. the tendinous expansions of the sartorius, gracilis and semitendinosus muscles **p cavus** marked concavity of the sole of the foot **p contortus** talipes equinovarus **p equinovalgus** a deformity in which heel is elevated and turned outward **p equinovarus** a deformity in which heel is turned inward and foot is plantar flexed **p equinus** a deformity in which heel does not touch the ground while walking **p hippocampi** the lower part of hippocampus major **p planus** flat foot **p valgus** talipes valgus **p varus** talipes varus

pesi (s) muscle.

pessary (pes'a-re) 1. a device placed in the vagina to support the uterus or rectum or as a contraceptive device 2. a medicated vaginal suppository

pessimism a gloomly or negativistic approach toward life and thoughts

pest 1.a fatal epidemic disease 2.a destructive insect

pesticide (pes'ti-sid) any chemical agent used to kill pests. They are in the form of fumigants, fungicides, herbicides or insecticides.

pestilence (pes'til-ens) a contagious epidemic disease

pestis (pes'tis) plague

pestle (pes'l) a device for pounding drugs in a mortar

PET abbreviation for positron emission tomography a non-invasive imaging modality that utilises radionuclides to detect biochemical and pathological abnormalities in living tissues, especially cerebral cortex

petechiae small capillary haemorrhages due to an endothelial damage

Peter's anomaly central corneal opacity due to a congenital gap in Descemet's membrane, named after Peter, US ophthalmologist

pethidine a morphine substitute

petiole (pet'e-ol) a stalk or pedicle

petiolus (pa-ti-ah-ol-us) petiole

petit mal (pe-te-mahl) 1. epilepsy without major fits 2. epileptic fit without loss of consciousness

Petit's triangle a triangular area bounded by iliac crest, latissimus dorsi and external oblique, a site where spinal abscesses occasionally point, named after Jean Petit, French surgeon

petri dish a container with two flattened clear glass or plastic plates allowing examination of bacterial culture devised by R J Petri, asistant to Robert Koch in Berlin

petrissage (pa'tre-sahzh) kneading of tissues in massage

petrolatum (pe'tro-la'tum) soft paraffin

petroleum jelly a semisolid mixture of hydrocarbons obtained from petroleum used as a base for ointment

petromastoid (-mas'toid) relating to the petrous portion of the temporal bone and its mastoid process

petrooccipital (-ok-sip'it'l) relating to the petrous portion of the temporal bone and to the occipital bone

petrosal (pe-tro'sil) relating to petrous portion of the temporal bone

petrositis (pe'tro-sit'is) inflammation of the petrous portion of the temporal bone

petrosphenoid (-sfe'noid) relating to the petrous portion of the temporal bone and to the sphenoid bone

petrosquamous (-skwa'mis) relating to the petrous and squamous portions of the temporal bone

petrous 1. stony 2. solid basal mass of temporal bone

Peutz-Jeghers syndrome familial jejunal polypi with pigmented spots in and around mouth, named after Johannes

Peutz, Dutch physician and Herold Jeghers, US physician

pexis (pek'sis) fixation, usually surgical, of substances in a tissue.

-pexy combining word for surgical fixation

Peyer's patches submucosal lymphoid aggregates of ileal mucosa, named after Johann Peyer, Swiss physician

Peyronie's disease fibromatous contracture of penis due to hardening of the corpora cavernosa of the penis, named after Francois Peyronie, French surgeon

Pfeiffer's bacillus *Haemophilus influenzae*, named after R. Pfeiffer, German bacteriologist

pH potential of hydrogen. It is the symbol for the logarithm of the reciprocal of the H ion concentration. It is expressed in molarity. A solution with a pH 7.4 is neutral, above it is alkaline and below it is acidic.

PHA abbreviation for phytohaemagglutinin

phac (o) combining word for lens or lens-shaped

phacoanaphylaxis (fak'o-aṇ-a-fi-lak'sis) hypersensitivity to the protein of the lens of eye that has been escaped from the lens capsule

phacocoele (fak'o-sel) hernia of the eye lens

phacocystectomy (fak'o-sis-tek'to-me) surgical removal of a part of the lens capsule for cataract

phacocystitis (-sis-tit'is) inflammation of the capsule of the lens of the eye

phacoemulsification (-i-mul'si-fi-ka'shun) a method of fragmentation, emulsification and aspiration of a cataract by using a low-frequency ultrasonic vibrations

phacoerysis (-e-re'sis) removal of the lens by means of suction

phacoid (fak'oid) shaped like a lens

phacoiditis (fak'oid-it'is) inflammation of the lens of the eye

phacoidoscope (fa-koid'a-skop) phacoscope

phacolysis (fa-kol'i-sis) operative break down and removal of the eye lens

phacomalacia (fak'o-ma-la'she-a) softening of the eye lens; a soft cataract

phacometachoresis (-met'a-kor-e'sis) displacement of the lens of the eye

phacomatosis (-ma-to'sis) a group of hereditary diseases characterised by hamartomas in the tissues of ectodermal origin

phacosclerosis (-skle-ro'sis) hardening of the eye lens; a hard cataract

phacoscope (fak'o-skop) an instrument to note the changes in the eye lens during accommodation

phacotoxic (fak'o-tok'sik) having a deleterious effect upon the eye lens

phag (o) combining word for eating, ingestion

phage (faj) bacteriophage **p typing** a technique that characterises certain strains of bacteria using bacteriorhages

phage-combining word for one that eats or destroys

phagia combining word for eating; swallowing

phagocyte (fag'o-sit) a cell of the immune system that can surround, engulf and digest microorganisms, foreign particles and cellular debris

phagocytin (fag'o-sit'in) a bactericidal substance from polymorphonuclear leucocytes

phagocytolysis (si-tol'i-sis) destruction of phagocytes

phagocytosis (-si-to'sis) the process of engulfing of microorganisms, necrotic tissue or other foreign bodies by phagocytes and their digestion

phagosome (fag'o-som) a membrane-bound vesicle around a particle within the phagocyte - its digestion is aided by the fusion of the vacuole with the lysosome and is then called a phagolysosome

phagotype (-tip) phage type

-phagy *see* phagia

phak (o) *see* phac (o)

phakitis (fa-kit'is) inflammation of the eye lens

phakoma (fa-ko-ma) a hamartoma found in phacomatosis.

phakomatosis (fak'o-ma-to'sis) phacomatosis

phala (s) result

phalang (o) combining word for phalanx or phalanges

phalangeal (fa-lan'jé-il) pertaining to a phalanx

phalangectomy (fal'an-jek-ta-me) excision of a phalanx

phalangitis (-jit'is) inflammation of one or more phalanges

phalanx (fa'lang-ks) 1. one of the bones of the fingers or toes, two for the thumb or big toe, and three each for other digits, are referred as proximal, middle and distal, beginning from the metacarpus 2. one of a set of plates made up of inner and outer phalangeal cells forming the reticular membrane of organ of Corti

phallectomy (fal-ek'ta-me) amputation of the penis

phallitis (fal-it'is) inflammation of the penis

phallus (fal'us) penis **phallic** adj

phanerosis (fan'er-o'sis) the process of becoming apparent

phantasm (fan'tazm) a mental image not evoked by actual stimuli

phantom (fant'um) 1. model of organs or of the body **p bone disease** disappearing bone disease characterised by extensive bone resorption **p limb** the perception that a limb is present after it has been amputated **p tumour** a well circumscribed accumulation of fluid in the interlobar spaces seen on chest radiographs which may occur in congestive heart failure

phantosmia (fan-toz'me-a) a parosmia where a smell is felt in the absence of any external stimulus

pharm pharmacy; pharmaceutical; pharmacopoeia

pharmaceutical (far'ma-soot'itkil) relating to pharmacy or drugs.

pharmacist (far'ma-sist) a person qualified in pharmacy who is licensed to prepare and dispense drugs

pharmaco - combining word for drug; medicine

pharmacoangiography (far'ma-ko-anje-og'ra-fe) an angiography in which the visualisation is enhanced by administering vasodilator or vasoconstrictor agents

pharmacodynamics (-di-nam'iks) the study of the effects of a given concentration of drug at its site of action

pharmacoepidemiology the study of the usage, acceptability, efficacy, safety, complementarity and cost-effectiveness of drugs in a large number of people

pharmacogenetics (-ji-net'iks) the study of the relation between the genetic factors and the response to drugs

pharmacognosy (far'ma-kog'na-se) a branch of pharmacology concerned with the natural drugs and their characteristics and source

pharmacokinetics (for'ma-ko-ki-net'iks) movement and concentrations of drugs in relevant tissues as function of time

pharmacologist a person qualified in pharmacology who can undertake research and evaluate drugs and therapeutic agents

pharmacology (far'ma-kol'a-je) the science concerned with the study of drugs, their structure, absorption, distribution, biotransformation, effects and side effects **molecular p** pharmacology that considers molecules as the fundamental functional units. It explains the pharmacological effects of biologically active compounds at the molecular level

pharmacopoeia (far'ma-ko-pe-a) a standard text giving a detailed description of drugs, their actions, indications, dosage, methods of preparation and side effects

pharmacopsychosis (-si-ko'sis) a mental disorder produced by a drug, alcohol or a poison

pharmacotherapy (-ther'a-pe) treatment of diseases by drugs

pharmacy (far'ma-se) 1. the branch of health sciences concerned with the preparation, dispensing and utilisation of drugs 2. a place where drugs are prepared and dispensed 3. a drug store

pharyng (o) combining word for pharynx.

pharyngalgia (far'ing-gal'je-a) pain in the pharynx

pharyngeal (fa-rin'je-al) pertaining to the pharynx **p arches** series of primitive structures appearing in the fourth and fifth week of the embryo and give rise to major structures of the head and neck **p bursa** 1. a midline recess over nasopharyngeal tonsil 2. a groove in embryonic pharyngeal wall representing pharyngeal cleft **p clefts** primitive structures seen in the five-week embryo, one of which (first) gives rise to external auditory canal **p pouches** embryonic structures occurring as outpouchings along the lateral wall of the pharyngeal cleft

pharyngectomy (far'in-jek'ta-me) excision of part of the pharynx

pharyngemphraxis (far'in-jem-frak'sis) a pharyngeal obstruction

pharyngismus (far'in-jiz'mis) spasm of the pharyngeal muscles

pharyngitis (far'in-jit'is) inflammation of the pharynx

pharyngocoele (fa-ring'go-sel) a herniation or a diverticulum of the pharynx

pharyngoconjunctival fever infection from adenovirus, sometimes, coxsackie virus in children characterised by fever, pharyngitis and conjunctivitis

pharyngomycosis (fa-ring'go-mi-ko'sis) any fungal infection of the pharynx

pharyngooesophageal (fa-ring'go-e-sof'a-je'al) pertaining to the pharynx and oesophagus

pharyngoperistole (-pe-ris'ta-le) narrowing or stricture of the pharynx

pharyngoplegia (-ple'jah) paralysis of the muscles of the pharynx

pharyngorrhoea (-re'a) discharge of mucus from the pharynx

pharyngoscope (fa'ring'go-skop) an instrument for direct visual examination of the pharynx

pharyngoscopy (far'ing-gos'ka-pe) direct examination of the pharynx using a pharyngoscope

pharyngostenosis (fa-ring'go-sten-o'sis) stricture of the pharynx

pharyngotomy (far-ing-got'a-me) incision of the pharynx

pharynx (far'inks) the throat; the passage that connects the back of the mouth and nose to oesophagus and trachea

phase (faz) 1. one of the stages during the course of development or change 2. a homogeneous material separable from a heterogeneous system 3. a time relationship between two or more events

phase 1, 2 and 3 studies a series of clinical trials referring to the efficacy and safety of a new drug under investigation which involves many subjects/patients at different phases

phase contrast microscope a microscope that converts the differences in refractive index into variations of light intensity enabling visualisation of structural details

phenacetin (fe-nas'e-tin) an analgesic and antipyretic

phenindione (fen'in-di'on) a rapid onset and short active anticoagulant

pheniramine (fen'ir'a-men) an antihistamine

phenobarbital (fe'no-bar'bi-tal) a long acting barbiturate used as a sedative and hypnotic

phenocopy the appearance of a trait strongly resembling one attributed to a specific genetic aetiology, but it is actually the result of environmental or random effects

phenol (fe'nol) phenyl alcohol; phenic or carbolic acid, used as an antiseptic and disinfectant. It can be ingested in 3 to 4% solution to cause neurolysis

phenolphthalein (fe'nol-thal'en) bright red crystalline powder used as an indicator in tissue culture media, and by parenteral injection as a test for renal function. It is also a laxative

phenomenon (fe-nom'e-non) pl. **phenomena** 1. an observable change noticed in an organ or vital function 2. a sign or a symptom **breakaway p** persons flying in outer space experiencing a sense of losing contact with other persons **dawn p** an early morning increase in the plasma glucose concentration necessitating an increased requirement of insulin in patients with NIDDM **Donath Landsteiner p** haemolysis of blood of a patient of paroxysmal haemoglobinuria when the sample is cooled to around 5°C and then warmed again *dejavu p see* dejavu **Goldblatt p** hypertension occurring from partial occlusion of a renal artery **Koebner's p** *see* Koebner's phenomenon **Marcuss Gun p** jaw winking syndrome **on-off p** rapid fluctuation of akinetic (off) and choreoathetotic (on) movements during treatment of Parkinson's disease by l-dopa **Raynaud's p** blanching and numbness of fingers due to spasm of digital arteries **Somogyi p** excessive glucose counter-regulation may result in hyperglycaemia in type I diabetes mellitus by inducing insulin resistance after hypoglycaemia

phenothiazine (fe'no-thi'a-zin) the parent compound for synthesis of a variety of antipsychotic agents such as chlorpromazine, mepazine and prochloroperazine

phenotype (fe'nah-tip) all the observable characteristics of an organism as determined by the genetic and environmental factors

phenoxybenzamine (fe-nok'se-ben'zamen) an alpha–adrenergic receptor blocking agent and is used to treat hypertension

phensuximide (fen-suk'si-mid) an anticonvulsant used in petit mal epilepsy

phentolamine (fen-tol'a-men) a potent alpha-adrenergic blocking agent useful in treatment of hypertension due to pheochromocytoma

phenyl (fen'il) the universal radical of phenol, C_6H_5

phenylacetic (fen'il-a-se'tik) **acid** a catabolite of phenylalanine, that appears in the urine in phenylketonuria.

phenylalanine (-al'a-nen) an essential amino acid in proteins

phenylbutazone (-bu'ta-zon) an analgesic, anti-inflammatory and anti-pyretic agent used in treatment of rheumatoid arthritis

phenylephrine (-ef'rin) an adrenergic compound used to produce nasal decongestion

phenylketonuria (-ke-to-nu'rea) a genetic disorder in which the body is not capable of oxidising the amino acid phenylalanine to tyrosine and it leads to severe mental retardation. Dietary restriction of phenylalanine is vital in the treatment

phenylpropanolamine (-pro'pa-nol'a-men) a sympathomimetic nasal decongestant

phenytoin (fen'i-to-in) an anticonvulsant and anti-arrhythmic agent

pheochromoblast (fe'o-kro'ma-blast) an embryonic cell developing into pheochromocyte

pheochromocyte (-kro'mo-sit) a chromaffin cell, found in adrenal medulla

pheochromocytoma (-kro'ma-si-to-ma) a benign tumour of adrenal medulla that secretes the hormones adrenaline and nor adrenaline, leading to intermittent, life threatening increase in blood pressure **p triad** headaches, sweating and tachycardia in a patient with hypertension

pheromone (far'a-mon) a hormone released by an organism that is capable of evoking a response in a member of the same species

pheromones (fer'o-mons) individual smell of a person

PhD Doctor of Philosophy

Philadelphia chromosome a defective chromosome (distal long arm of chromosome 22 that is transferred to the long arm of chromosome 9) found in patients with chronic myeloid leukaemia

philtrum (fil'trum) the median groove on the outer surface of the lip

phimosis (fi-mo'sis) tightness of foreskin preventing it from being drawn back over the head of the penis

phiranga roga (s) syphilis

phleb (o) – combining word for vein.

phlebangioma (fleb'an-je-o'ma) an aneurysmal dilatation of a vein

phlebarteriectasia (-ar-ter'e-ek-ta'ze-a) vasodilatation

phlebectasia (-ek-ta'zhah) dilatation of a vein

phlebectomy (fle-bek'ta-me) excision of a segment of a vein

phebemphraxis (fleb'em-frak'sis) venous thrombosis

phlebitis (fle'-bit'is) inflammation of a vein, which often leads to development of a blood clot

phleboclysis (fle-bok'li-sis) intravenous injection of a fluid in quantity such as glucose, saline

phlebography (fle-bog'ra-fe) 1. the recording of the venous pulse 2. the radiography of a vein filled with contrast media

phlebolithiasis (fleb'o-li-thi'a-sis) development of calcareous deposit in the venous wall

phlebomanometer (-me-nom'e-ter) a manometer for measuring the venous blood pressure

phleborrhaphy (fle-bor'a-fe) suture of a vein

phlebosclerosis (fleb'o-skle-ro'sis) fibrous thickening of the walls of a vein

phlebostasis (fle-bos'ta-sis) 1. markedly slow movement of blood in veins. 2. a temporary stoppage of venous return to the heart by compression of veins of extremities with tourniquets

phlebothrombosis (fleb'o-throm-bo'sis) a condition in which a blood clot forms in a vein without any inflammation

Phlebotomus (fle-bot'a-mus) a genus of blood sucking sand flies which transmit diseases such as kala azar, cutaneous leishmaniasis and phlebotomus fever

phlebotomy (fle-bot'a-me) venesection; incision of a vein to withdraw blood

phlegm (flem) sputum 1. viscid mucus, especially from respiratory tract 2. one of the four humours of the body

phlegmasia (fleg-ma'ze-a) inflammation **p alba dolens** milk leg, markedly swollen leg following child birth due to thrombosis of veins draining the part **p cerulea dolens** a deep vein thrombosis of the limb with sudden severe pain, oedematous swelling and cyanosis

phlegmatic (fleg-mat'ik) person of apathetic, calm and sluggish temperament

plegmon (fleg'mon) acute suppurative inflammation of the subcutaneous connective tissue

phlog (o) combining word for inflammation

phlogogenic (flog'a-jen'ik) causing inflammation

phlyctena (flik-te'na) a small vesicle following first degree burns

phlyctenular (flik-ten'u-lar) relating to or marked by presense of phlyctenule **p conjunctivitis** tiny vesicles containing lymph in conjunctiva

phlyctenule (flik'tin-ul) a small vesicle as on cornea or conjunctiva

phobia (fo'be-a) a persistent, irrational fear of a particular object, person, place or situation

phocomelia (fo'ka-me'le-a) a congenital skeletal limb deformity due to the idiopathic absence of the radial elements of a limb bud

phocomelus (fo-kom'il-is) a person exhibiting phocomelia

phonasthenia (fo'nas-the'ne-a) weakness of voice

phonation (fo-na'shun) the production of sounds by means of vocal cords

phonendoscope (fo-nen'da-skop) a stethoscope that intensifies auscultatory sounds

phoniatrics (fo'ne-a-triks) the science concerned with speech and speech habits

phon (o) combining word for sound, speech, voice

phonocardiography (fo'no-kar'de-og'ra-fe) recording of heart sounds with a phonocardiograph

phonomyoclonus (-mi-ok'la-nis) fibrillary muscular contractions audible on auscultation

phonomyography (-mi-og'ra-fe) recording of the sounds produced by muscle contraction

phonostethograph (-steth'o-graf) an instrument that amplifies the respiratory sounds

phonosurgery a surgical procedure done on the vocal cords and adjacent tissue to improve the timbre, tone and quality of the voice

Phoparan disease a state of failure of acclimatisation to high altitudes, immigrants to Himalayas manifesting with hypoxia, polycythaemia, pulmonary arterial hypertension, right ventricular hypertrophy and gross proteinuria, named after a military picket, Phoparan, Laddakh, India.

-phore combining word for a carrier

-phoresis combining word for transmission

phosgene (fos'gen) carbon chloride $COCl_2$ a highly poisonous gas, used in chemical warfare

phosphatase (fos-fa-tas) any of a group of enzymes that catalyse the hydrolysis of phosphonic acid esters **acid p** a phosphatase acting at an optimum pH of 5.4 and is present in prostate gland **alkaline p** a phosphatase acting at an optimum pH of 8.6. It is present in teeth, developing bone, plasma, kidney and intestine. The level is very high in infancy which gradually decreases later

phosphate (fos'fat) a salt or ester of phosphoric acid

phosphataemia (fos'fa-tem'e-a) an increased amount of inorganic phosphates in the blood

phosphaturia (fos'fa-tur'e-a) elimination of an increased amount of phosphates in the urine

phosphodiesterase (-di-es'ter-as) an enzyme that catalyses the breakdown of cyclic adenosine monophosphate

phosphoglycerides (-glis'er-id's) phospholipids containing glycerol phosphate

phospholipase (-lip'as) an enzyme that catalyses the hydrolysis of a phospholipid

phospholipid (-lip'id) a lipid containing phosphorus. It includes lecithin and sphingomyelin. The lipid portion of cell membranes are essentially made up of phospholipids

phosphoric (fos'for'ik) **acid** a solvent. A dilute solution used to remove necrotic debris

phosphorus (fos'fer-us) a non-metallic chemical, symbol P, at no. 15. It occurs as phosphate in all living cells and forms major component of mineral phase of bone. It is actively involved in metabolic process

phosphorylase (fos-for'i-las) 1. a transferase, as involved in transfer of an inorganic phosphate group to some organic acceptor 2. any of the group of enzymes that catalyse phosphorylysis

phosphorylation (fos'for-i-la'shun) the metabolic process of addition of phosphate to an organic compound **oxidative p** the formation of high energy phosphate bonds by phosphorylation of ADP to ATP

phot (o) combining word for light

photalgia (fo-tal'jah) pain caused by light as in eye

photoactivators ingested substances that increase the deleterious effect of light

photoactive (-ak'tiv) reacting chemically to sunlight or ultraviolet radiation

photoallergen (-al'er-jen) an agent eliciting an allergic response to light

photoallergy (-al'er-je) a delayed immunologic type of photosensitivity produced by the interaction of light and certain chemicals to which the individual has been previously become sensitised

photocatalysis (-ka'tal'i-sis) promotion of a chemical reaction by light

photocatalyst (-kat'a-list) a substance that causes a chemical reaction to light, chlorophyll

photochemotherapy (-ke'mo-the'ra-pe) the use of light and chemicals in the treatment

photochromogen (-kro-ma-jen) microorganism in which pigment develops when grown in presence of light, such as *Mycobacterium kansasii*

photocoagulation (-ko-ag'ul-a'shun) destruction of tissue by heating effect of intensely focussed light

photodermatitis (-der'ma-tit'is) dermatitis caused by exposure to ultraviolet light

photodynamic therapy a treatment modality in which tumour cells that concentrate a photocsensitiser, are destroyed following exposure to light at an appropriate wavelength

photogenic (-jen'ik) 1. light producing 2. produced by light

photoinactivation (fo'to-in-ak-ti-va'shun) inactivation by light

photolysis (fo-tol'i-sis) decomposition of a chemical compound by the action of light

photometry (fo-tom'i-tre) measurement of the intensity of light

photomicrograph (fo'to-mi'kro-graf) an enlarged photograph of an object viewed with a microscope

photon (fo'ton) a particle of radiant energy

photoparoxysmal (fo'to-par'oks-iz'mil) an abnormal EEG response to brief flashes of light. There is diffuse paroxysmal discharge in the form of spike complexes

photoperiod (fo'to-per'e-id) the daily duration of exposure of an organism to light

photopheresis (-fe-re'sis) a method of treatment of cutaneous T lymphoma where a photoactive chemical is administered and then blood is removed and circulated through a source of ultraviolet radiation, and then returned to the patient

photophilic (-fil'ik) seeking light

photophobic abnormal sensitivity of the eyes to the light

photophthalmia (fot'of-thal'me-a) an inflammatory reaction of the eye due to exposure to intense light as in snow blindness

photopia (fo-to'pe-a) adjustment of the eye for vision in bright light

photopigment (fo'to-pig'ment) a pigment that is unstable in the presence of light

photoprotection protection of cells from ultra-violet light-induced damage

photopsia (fo-top'se-a) a subjective sensation of lights, sparks or colour in retinal irritation

photopsin (fo-top'sin) the protein moiety of the pigment (iodopsin) in the cones of the retina.

photoptarmosis (fo'to-tar-mo'sis) reflex sneezing in presence of bright light

photoptometer (fo'top-tom'iter) an instrument for determination of the smallest amount of light that will make the object visible

photoreaction (fo'to-re-ak'shun) a reaction caused by light

photoreactivation (fo'to-re-ak'ti-va'shun) activation by light of a process previously inactivated

photoreceptor (-re-sep'ter) a receptor that is sensitive to light, such as retinal rods and cones

photoretinitis (-ret'in-it'is) decreased visual acuity from a macular burn due to excessive exposure to sunlight or other intense light

photoscan (-skan) scintiscan, a representation of a radioisotope outlining of an organ in the body

photosensitive (-sen'sit-iv) exhibiting abnormal sensitivity to light

photosensitivity abnormal reaction to exposure to sunlight, usually in the form of rash. It can result from some disorders or from ingestion of particular drugs

photosensitization (-sen'sit'iz-a'shun) an abnormally heightened reactivity of skin to sunlight

photostable (fot'o-sta'b'l) unchanged by exposure to light

photosynthesis (fo'to-sin'thi-sis) the process by which plants are able to produce carbohydrates by combining carbon dioxide and water in the chlorophyll tissue under the influence of light

phototaxis (-tak'sis) reaction of living protoplasm to the stimulus of light

phototherapy (-ther'a-pe) 1. treatment of diseases by exposure to light 2. use of light to treat hyperbilirubinaemia

phototoxic (-tok'sik) pertaining to the harmful reaction produced by exposure to light

phototropism (fo-ta'tra-pizm) the movement of an organism toward or away from light

phren (o) combining word for diaphragm; phrenic nerve; mind

phrenetic (fre-net'ik) maniacal

phrenic (fen'ik) pertaining to the diaphragm or mind

phrenicectomy (fen'i-sek'ta-me) resection of a part of phrenic nerve

phreniclasia (fren'i-kla'zah) phrenic nerve crush with a clamp causing paralysis of the diaphragm

phrenico-exeresis (fren'i-ko-ek-ser'e-sis) avulsion of the phrenic nerve

phrenicotomy (-kot'a-me) sectioning of the phrenic nerve

phrenocolic (fren'o-kol'ik) pertaining to the diaphragm and colon

phrenogastric (-gas'trik) pertaining to the diaphragm and stomach

phrenohepatic (-he-pat'ik) pertaining to the diaphragm and liver

phrenology (fre'nol-o-gi)art of determining a persons' mental characteristics and personality by studying the shape and contours of the skull

phrenoplegia (-ple'ja) paralysis of the diaphragm

phrenotropic (fren'o-trop'ik) exerting its effect on the mind

phrynoderma (frin'o-de'r-ma) a follicular hyperkeratosis due to a deficiency of vitamin A or of essential fatty acids

phthiriasis (thi-ri'a-sis) infestation with *Phthirus pubis*

phthirus (thir'is) a genus of lice including *Phthirus pubis* which infect pubic hairs, eyebrows and eyelashes

phthisis (thi'sis) 1. a wasting disease of the body 2. tuberculosis **p bulbi** degen-

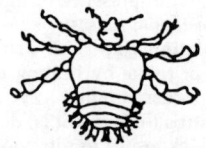

Phthirus pubis

eration of the ocular globe accompanied by retinal necrosis, atrophy, thickening of sclera, and loss of function

phyco – combining word for algae

phycomycetes (fi'ko-mi-set'ez) a class of saprophobic pathogenic fungi

phycomycosis (-mi-ko'sis) an acute fungal disease caused by phycomycetes

phylogeny (fi-loj'i-ne) the evolutionary development of any organism

phylum (fi'lum) a taxonomic division below kingdom and above class

physiatrics (fiz'e-a'triks) physical therapy.

physiatrist (-trist) a physician specialised in physical medicine

physiatry (-tre) physical medicine

physical (fiz'ik-l) relating to the body **p dependence** need to continue using a drug to maintain normal body function and to avoid withdrawal illness ; addiction **p examination** examination of the body by inspection, palpation, percussion and auscultation **p fitness** the ability to undertake daily tasks without undue fatigue **p therapy** treatment using physical methods such as exercise or agents such as heat, light or water

physician (fi-zish'in) 1. a person who has successfully completed the prescribed medical curriculum in a medical institution recognised by the medical council and who has obtained the licence from the medical council to practice medicine 2. a person who practices medicine as distinct from surgery

physicochemical (fiz'i-ko-kem'ik'il) pertaining to the application of the laws of physics to chemical reaction

physics (fiz'iks) the branch of science concerned with the laws and phenomena of nature

physi (o) combining word for nature; physical; physiology

physiochemical (fiz'o-p-kem'ik-il) pertaining to physiology and chemistry

physiognomy (fiz'e-og'na-me) 1. the countenance or face. 2. the facial expression and appearance

physiologic (fiz'e-o-loj'ik) physiological

physiological (-loj'i–kal) pertaining to normal physiology

physiologist (fiz'e-ol'a-jist) a specialist in physiology

physiology (-je) the science concerned with the normal functions of the living organism and its components including the physical and chemical processes involved

physiopathologic (fiz'e-o-path-a'-loj'ik) 1. pertaining to physiology and pathology 2. pertaining to a pathologic alteration in a normal function

physiotherapist (-the'ra-pist) physical therapist

physiotherapy (-the'ra-pe) physical therapy

physique (fi-zek) the build; the physical or bodily structure

physohaematometra (fi'so-hem'a-to-me'tra) distension of uterine cavity with gas and blood

physohydrometra (-hi'dro-me'tra) distension of uterine cavity with gas and serous fluid

physometra (-me'tra) distension of uterine cavity with air or gas

physopyosalpinx (-pi'o-sal'pinks) pyosalpinx accompanied by formation of gas in the tube

physostigmine (-stig'men) a cholinergic alkaloid inactivating cholinesterase, thus prolonging the action of acetylcholine

phytic (fi'tik) **acid** a hexaphosphoric acid ester of inositol

phyt (o) combining word for plant

phytobezoar (fi'to-be'zor) food ball, a gastric concretion composed of vegetable fibres with seeds and skin of fruits.

phytohaemagglutinin (-hem'a-gloot'in-in) a phytomitogen from plants that agglutinates red blood cells

phytohormone (-hor'mon) plant hormone

phytol (fi-tol) an unsaturated aliphatic alcohol from chlorophyll used for synthesis of vitamin E and K

phytotherapy (fy'to-ther-api) herbal medicine

phytotoxin (fi'to-tok'sin) any toxin of plant origin

pia (pi'a) pia mater

pia-arachnitis (pi'a-a-rak-ni'tis) leptomeningitis

pia-arachnoid (pi'a-a-rak-noyd) leptomeninges

pia mater (pi'a-ma'ter) the innermost of the three meninges covering the brain and spinal cord. It is a delicate vascular fibrous membrane

piarachnoid (pia-rak'noyd) pia-arachnoid

pica (pi'ka) a perverted appetite with craving for unnatural articles as food

pick 1. a sharp pointed curved instrument used to explore teeth surfaces 2. to remove bits of food from teeth

Pick (pik) **bodies** presence of intracytoplasmic globular blue inclusions, named after Arnold Pick, Czeck physician

Pick cells ballooned neurons with abundant cytoplasm and eccentric nuclei, named after Ludwig Pick, German physician.

Pick's disease a form of presenile dementia affecting frontal and temporal lobes, and characterised by personality change, named after Ludwig Pick, German physician

Pick's disease chronic pericarditis of unknown aetiology, named after Arnold Pick, Czeck physician

Pickwickian syndrome a disorder characterised by obesity, excessive day time sleepiness, sleep apnoea, named after a obese character in Pickwick papers by Charles Dickens

pico – combining word meaning small.

picogram (pi'ko-gram) pg one trillionth of (10^{-12}) a gram

picometre (pi'ko-me-ter) Pm one trillionth of (10^{-12}) a metre

picornovirus (pi-kor′na-vi′rus) an extremely small non-enveloped virus having a core of single-stained RNA. It includes polioviruses, coxsackie viruses and echoviruses

picrate (pik′rat) a salt of picric acid

picric acid trinitrophenol used in application in burns, eczema and pruritus

picrotoxin (pik′ro-tok′sn) a bitter principle obtained from seed of *Anamirta cocculus*, was earlier used as central and respiratory stimulant in babiturate poisoning

PID abbreviation for pelvic inflammatory disease.

PIE abbreviation for pulmonary infiltrates with eosinophilia

piedra (pe-a′dra) a fungal disease of the beard and moustache in which the fungi form sheath-like nodular masses

piesthesia (pi-e-zes-the′ze-a) the sense by which pressure stimuli are appreciated

piesimeter (pi′e-sim′e-ter) an instrument to measure sensitiveness of the skin to pressure

piezoelectric crystals crystals that produce a partial separation of electrical charge when they are deformed

pigeon chest *see* chest

pigeon fancier′s lung people exposed to pigeon droppings are sensitised to avian serum proteins resulting in extrinsic allergic alveolitis

pigment (pig′mint) 1. any colouring matter of the body 2. a stain used in histologic work 3. a medicinal preparation for external use, applied to the skin like a paint **pigmentary** adj. **bile p′s** a complex, highly coloured substances such as bilirubin, biliverdin and their derivatives such as urobilinogen, urobilin, and impart brown colour to intestinal contents and faeces **blood p** a pigment in red blood cell (haemoglobin) and a derivative of it (haematin, methaemoglobin, haemosiderin) **respiratory p′s** the oxygen carrying pigments such as haemoglobin, myoglobin or cytochromes participating in the oxidative processes of the body **retinal p** visual pigment **skin p** melanin and carotene **urinary p** urochrome and sometimes urobilin **uveal p** melanin in the choroid layer of the eye, ciliary processes and the posterior surface of the iris **visual p′s** the photopigment of retinal cones (photopsins) and rods (scotopsins) that absorb light and initiate the phenomenon of vision **wear and tear p** accumulation of lipofuscine in aging cells

pigmentary (pig′men-ter′e) relating to a pigment.

pigmentation (pig′men-ta′shun) colouration of skin or tissues due to deposition of pigment

pigmented (pigment′ed) coloured by a deposit of pigment

pigmentolysin (pig-men-tol′i-sin) a substance causing destruction of a pigment

pigtail catheter a drainage catheter with side holes

pilar, piliary (pil′er; pil′a-re) relating to the hair

pill (pil) 1. a little ball of medicine 2. oral contraceptive agent **p box** a box for holding pills **pep p** stimulating drugs used to keep the person from falling asleep

pill-rolling a circular movement of the tips of the thumb and index finger in Parkinson′s disease

pil (o) combining word for hair

pilobezoar (pi-lo-be′zor) trichobezoar

pilocarpine (pi′lo-kar′pen) a cholinergic alkaloid from leaves of pilocarpus, used as an ophthalmic miotic agent in glaucoma

pilocystic (-sis′tik) a cyst-like structure containing hair.

piloerection (-e-rek′shun) erection of the hair

piloid hair-like

pilomotor (-mo′ter) referring to the arrector muscles, whose contraction results in goose flesh and piloerection

pilonidal (-nid′l) referring to a growth of hair in deeper layer of skin or in a dermoid cyst pilose (pi'los) hairy

pilosebaceous (pi'lo-si-ba'shus) pertaining to the hair follicles and the sebaceous glands

pilus (pi'lus) 1. a hair 2. one of the minute filamentous appendages of certain bacteria

pimelitis (pim'il-it'is) 1. inflammation of the adipose tissue 2. inflammation of conjunctival tissue

pimelopterygium (pim'il-o-ter-ij'e-um) a pterygium containing fat

pimelosis (-o'sis) 1. fatty degeneration 2. adiposis

pimple (pim'pl) a papule or a small pustule

pin (pin) a slender elongated metal piece used for fixation of parts **endodontic p** a straight or threaded pin passed through the root canal to the alveolar bone **Steinmann p** a metal rod for internal fixation of fractures

pin and plate devices for internal fixation of extra capsular fracture of the neck of femur with pin in neck and plate screwed to shaft

pincer nail an increased transverse curvature of the nail bed with severe pain and loss of soft tissue at the finger tips

pinch 1. a method of holding things between the thumb and index finger, teeth, the jaws of an instrument 2. to compress, constrict or squeeze painfully **p cock** a clamp for compressing a flexible tube in order to regulate or stop the flow of fluid.

pindaka (s) poultice

pindolol a beta-adrenergic blocking agent

pineal (pin-e-al) 1. shaped like a pine cone 2. pertaining to the pineal gland **p calcification** marker of brain shifts in adults, on skull radiograph

pinealectomy (pin'e-al-ek-to-me) excision of the pineal gland

pineal gland a cone-shaped gland located in the roof of the third ventricle

pinealoblastoma (pin'e-a-lo-blas-to'ma) a malignant tumour of pineal gland often occur in childhood or young adults

pinealocyte (pin'e-o-lo'sit) the principal cell of pineal gland, which contains a pale-staining cytoplasm, and produces hormones

pinealoma (pin'e-a-lo'ma) an encapsulated tumour of pineal gland, that may present with precocious puberty

pineoblastoma (pin'e-o-blas-to'ma) pinealocytoma

pineocytoma a malignant tumour of the pineal gland

ping-ponging the spread of an infectious disease, especially sexually transmitted *Trichomonas vaginalis* infection disease between two persons. The first person who had a cure, can get reinfection from his sexual partner, in a fashion likened to a pingpong ball

pinguicula yellowish raised area of degenerated collagen under conjunctiva near limbus

pinhole (pin'hol) a small perforation of the size of a pin **p meatus** pinhole opening of urethra **p os** a very small opening to the uterus from the vagina

piniform (pin'i-form) conical

pink disease acrodynia

pink eye acute contagious conjunctivitis by *Haemophilus aegypticus* or *H. ducreyi*

pink puffer a patient with COPD, severe emphysema exhibiting hyperventilation and shortness of breath

pinna (pin'a) pl. **pinnae** 1. the auricle or projected part of the external ear composed of elastic cartilage and covered by skin, that collects and directs sound waves into the external auditory meatus 2. a feather or wing **p nasi** a protruding cartilaginous extension on each nostril

pinpoint 1. the point of a pin 2. marked constriction of pupil to that size

pinprick any minute puncture made by a pin

pinocytosis (pi'no-si-to'sis) the process by which cells ingest liquid to form small vesicles

pinosome (pi'no-som) fluid-filled vacuole formed during pinocytosis

pins and needles a subjective sensation in

the peripheral parts of the limb experienced in peripheral neuropathy

pinta (pen'ta) a non-venereal disease caused by the spirochaete, *Treponema carateum*, transmitted by direct mucocutaneous inoculation

pintid (pin'tid) a flat red skin lesion in second stage of pinta

pinus (pi'nus) pertaining to the pineal gland

pinworm *Enterobius vermicularis*, causing Enterobiasis

pioepithelium (pi'o-ep'i-the'le-um) epithelium containing fat globules

pipe a hollow cylinder of metal, wood or other material used for conveying water, gas or steam **p stem** the stem of a tobacco pipe, colon in ulcerative colitis may resemble it

piperazine (pi'per-a-zen) anthelmintic used in the treatment of round worm and thread worm infestation

pipette (pi-pet) a narrow graduated glass tube with both ends open, used for measuring and transferring liquids from one vessel to another

pirbuterol b_2-adrenergic receptor agonist used in bronchial asthma

piriform (pir-i-form) pear-shaped

piri formis syndrome an entrapment neuropathy of sciatic nerve characterised by pain in the hip and buttock that radiate up into the lower back and down the leg

Pirogoff's (pir'o-gofs) **amputation** amputation of foot at the ankle with removal of a part of calcaneal bone, devised by Nikolai Pirogoff, Russian surgeon

piroxicam an analgesic and anti-inflammatory agent

Pirquet's (per-kaz) **test** a tuberculin skin test, named after Chemens Pirquet, Austrian paediatrician

Pisiform (pi'si-form) pea-shaped

pistol shot sound *see* sound

pit 1. a tiny hollow 2. a shallow depression on pressure in oedema 3. a small depression in the enamel surface of a tooth

pitapat with a quick succession of beats or taps

pitch (pich) 1. to fix or set in array 2. the quality of sound that is dependent on the frequency of vibration of the waves producing it 3. residue from coal distillation

pithing (pith'ing) destruction of CNS by piercing brain or spinal cord

pitta (s) biological fire humour; bile *pachaka p* pitta governing digestion

pitting 1. the formation of a small depression, usually by scarring 2. a splenic function removing intracytoplasmic inclusions such as siderotic granules or Howell-Jolly bodies 3. remaining indented for some time after removal of firm finger pressure, as in oedema

Pittsburg brain stem score a scale to determine the clinical status of a victim of cerebral trauma

pituicyte (pi-tu'i-sit) supporting cell of posterior pituitary gland

pituitary (pi-tu'i-tar'e) the pituitary gland; hypophysis **p apoplexy** haemorrhage into pituitary may have catastrophic effects with neurologic signs of an expanding sellar mass and rapid evolution of hypopitutarism **p gland** master of endocrine orchestra, a pea-sized structure lying in the sella turcica of the sphenoid bone and attached to the hypothalamus by the infundibulum. The pituitary gland has two anatomically and functionally separate portions. The anterior pituitary is derived from an outgrowth of ectoderm (Rathke's pouch) in the roof of the mouth and contains many glandular epithelial cells. The secretions regulate a wide range of bodily activities. The hormones are human growth hormone (hGH) prolactin, adrenocorticotropic hormone (ACTH), thyroid-stimulating hormone (TSH), follicle-stimulating hormone (FSH), luteinizing hormone (LH) and melanocyte-stimulating hormone (MSH). The posterior pituitary arises as an outgrowth of neurohypophyseal bud. Though it does not synthesise hormones, it is concerned with storage and release of oxytocin and antidiuretic hormone (ADH). In addition there is an atrophied intermediate lobe (pars intermedia) **p dwarfism** a condition caused by hyposecretion of human growth hormone during growth years **p tumour** mostly benign adenomas, may be hormonally silent or hormonally active

pityriasis (pit'i-ri'a-sis) a non-inflammatory skin disorder with scale formation **p alba** a condition characterised by ill-defined, hypopigmented macules, located on the cheeks, noted before puberty, probably because of lack of sebaceous secretion; pityriasis simplex **p capitis** dandruff **P rosea** a condition characterised by sudden eruption of asymptomatic, oval or circular erythematous, scaly lesions where margins are more prominent and pink and are found on the upper trunk and arms. A herald patch appears two to three days before appearance of eruptions **p rubra pilaris** a follicular keratotic condition characterised by skin coloured follicular papules on the extremities and trunk **p versicolor** tinea versicolor, a fungal infection caused by *Pityrosporum orbiculare (Malassezia furfur)* which affects the stratum corneum in the form of discrete hypo- or hyperpigmented macules with overlying scales over the trunk, arms and face

pivot (piv'ut) pin or a short shaft on the end of which something rests and turns **p joint** a synovial joint in which a rounded or conical surface of one bone articulates with a ring formed partly by another bone and partly by a ligament, as in the joint between the atlas and axis, and between the proximal ends of radius and ulna

pix (piks) pitch; tar

pK dissociation constant (K) expressed a minus log to base 10

pKa measure of dissociation of acids

PKU phenylketonuria

PLAB Professional and Linguistics Assessment Board

placebo (pla-se'bo) 1. a substance having no pharmacological effect but given merely to satisfy a patient who considers it to be a medicine 2. a substance having no pharmacological effect but administered as a control in testing experimentally or clinically the efficacy of a biologically active preparation **p effect** a positive or negative response to a drug resulting from a person's expectations rather than from any real chemical effects

placenta (pla-sen'ta) a special structure through which the exchange of materials between foetal and maternal circulation occurs **p accreta** firm attachment of placenta to the uterine wall preventing its separation at labour **p praevia** implantation of placenta in lower uterine segments

placental (pla-sen'tal) pertaining to the placenta **p grading** maturity of placenta determined by ultrasound. It depends on degree and pattern of calcification **p insufficiency** inability of the placenta to supply the needs of foetus

placentation (pla'sen-ta'shun) the process of formation and attachment of the placenta

placentitis (pla'sen-ti'tis) inflammation of the placenta

placentography (pla'sen-tag'ra-fe) radiographic examination of the placenta

Placido's (pla-se'doz) **disc** defects in curvature of the cornea giving large black and white circles, named after Antonio. Placido, Portugese oculist

placode (plak'od) a plate-like thickening of the epithelium, usually the ectoderm

placoid (plad'oyd) platelike

pladaroma (plad-a-ro'ma) a wart-like soft growth on the eyelid

plagio combining word for slanting; oblique

plagiocephaly (pla-je-o-sef'a-le) oblique skull showing bulge anteriorly on one side and posteriorly on other side

plague (plag) a communicable disease caused by *Yersinia pestis* acquired by humans from rats or by droplet infection **bubonic p** condition acquired by bite of infected fleas (xenopsiella) carrying disease from dying rats. It has a sudden onset with high fever, dry skin, headache and swelling at the site of the affected lymph node (bubo). The condition may lead to toxaemia and death **domestic p** plaque spread by rodents living with man **pneumonic p** spread of plague between humans by droplets containing *Y. pestis*. It is characterised by cough and dyspnoea, expectoration of highly frothy blood-stained sputum **septicaemic p** patients with plague exhibiting severe toxaemia, hypotension and mental confusion **wild sylvitic p** plague afflicting mainly rodents and independent of human population

plan a design of future states

planchet (plan'chet) a small flat container used to place radioactive material

plane (plan) 1. a flat, relatively smooth surface 2. a specified level, as the plane of anaesthesia 3. between the tissue layers **p wart** a variety of viral papilloma of the skin exhibiting several small round flat plaques on the face and back of hands

planigraphy (pla-nig'ra-fe) body section by radiography

planimeter (pla-nim'e-tor) a mechanical device to measure the area of a plane figure by passing a tracer round its periphery

planing (pla'ning) 1. abrasion of disfigured skin to promote reepithelisation with minimal scarring 2. deep scaling procedure in dentistry

planned parenthood the methods of practice by which the parents regulate the number and frequency of their children

planocellular (pla'no-sel'u-lar) composed of flat cells

planoconcave (pla'no-kon'kav) pertaining to a lens that is plane on one side and concave on the other

planoconvex (pla'no-kon'veks) pertaining to a lens that is plane on one side and convex on the other

Planorbis (plan-or'bis) a genus of fresh water snails that act as intermediate hosts for certain species of schistosoma (blood flukes)

planotopokinesia (pla'no-top'o-ki-ne'ze-a) loss of orientation in space

plant a living thing containing chlorophyll that synthesises carbohydrates and oxygen from carbon dioxide and water

planta pedis (plan'ta-pe'dus) pl. **plantae** the sole of the foot

plantalgia (plan-tal'je-a) pain in the sole of the foot

plantar (plan'tar) pertaining to the sole of the foot **equivocal p response** stroking of the outer side of the sole of the foot may elicit only dorsiflexion of big toe without any fanning of the toes or fanning of the toes without dorsiflexion of the big toe; it is noted in early pyramidal disease or in its minimal involvement **extensor p response** extension of big toe at the metatarsophalangeal joint due to the contraction of the extensor hallucis longus, and extension and spread of the other toes like a fan when

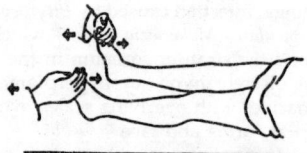

Plantar flexion

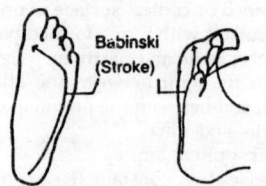

Plantar response

the outer side of the sole of the foot is stroked. It indicates disease involving the corticospinal tract **p fasciitis** tenderness under the heel from plantar fibromatosis or tear of plantar fascia **p flexion** bending of the foot in the direction of the sole **p response** there is flexion of the great toe at the metatarsophalangeal joint and flexion and abduction of other toes when the outer side of the sole of the foot is stroked lightly **p wart** a hard, horny, rough surfaced area on the sole of the foot caused by papovavirus.

plantaris (plan-tar'is) *see* Table of Muscles.

plantation (plan-ta'shun) insertion or transplantationof a tooth into the bony socket

plantigrade foot posture in which the entire sole of the foot is placed on the ground

planula (plan'u-la) the larval stage of coelenterate

planum (pla'num) pl. **plana** a flat surface; a plane

planuria (pla-nu're-a) passage of urine from an abnormal passage

plaque (plak) 1. a cholesterol-containing mass in the tunica media of arteries 2. a mass of bacterial cells, polysaccharide and other debris that adheres to the teeth 3. areas of demyelination in disseminated sclerosis

plasia combining word for formation; growth; proliferation

plasm (plazm) plasma

plasm combining word for living substance; tissue.

plasma (palz'ma) the extracellular fluid found in blood vessels and lymphatics **p cell** plasmacyte with abundant RNA in cytoplasm **p exchange therapy** removal of plasma from the body and replacement with normal plasma **p thromboplastin** antecedent clotting factor XI that activates Christmas factor **p thromboplastin component** Christmas factor IX

plasmablast (plaz'ma-blast) an undifferentiated cell that matures into a plasma cell

plasmacyte (-sit) a plasma cell, found in the bone marrow and connective tissue capable of producing antibodies

plasmacytoma (-si-to'ma) a tumour composed of plasma cells

plasmacytosis (-si-to'sis) presence of increased number of plasma cells in the blood

plasmagel (plaze'ma-jel) the peripheral portion of endoplasm that has the consistency of gel, such as in amoeba

plasmagene (plaz'ma-jen) a cytoplasmic hereditary determiner

plasmapheresis (plaz'ma-fer-e'sis) a procedure in which blood is removed from the body, its components are separated, disease causing components such as toxins, metabolic products and antibodies are removed, and the remainder is returned to the body

plasmasome (plaz-ma-som) a leucocyte granule

plasmatherapy (plaz'ma-ther'a-pe) use of blood plasma as a therapy, in conditions such as shock

plasmatic (plaz-mat'ik) relating to plasma.

plasmatogamy (-ma-tog'a-me) union of cytoplasm of two or more cells without an union of nuclei

plasmatorrhexis (plaz'ma-to-rek'sis) rupture of a cell with loss of its contents

plasma volume extender high molecular weight solutions such as dextran used intravenously in the treatment of shock

plasmid cytoplasmic, autonomously replicating extrachromosomal circular DNA molecule. It is used as vectors for cloning. They are found in bacteria where they can code for antibiotic resistance factors

plasmin (plaz'min) fibrinolytic enzyme derived from plasma plasminogen

plasminogen (plaz'min'o-jen) the blood substance that when activated forms plasmin

plasmocyte (plaz'mo-sit) an abnormal leucocyte found in bone marrow, connective tissue and sometimes in plasma; and is a major constituent of plasma cell myeloma

plasmodial (plaz-mo-de'al) concerning plasmodia

plasmodicidal (plaz'mo-di-si-dal) killing plasmodia

plasmodium (plaz-mo'de-um) pl. **plasmodia** a genus of protozoa belonging to subphylum sporozoa. It includes the malarial parasite *P. falciparum* the causative agent of malignant tertian malaria *P. malariae* the causative agent of quartan malaria *P. ovale* the causative agent of benign tertian malaria *P vivax* the causative agent of benign tertian malaria

plasmogamy (plas-mog'a-me) the fusion of cells

plasmolysis (plaz'mol'i-sis) shrinkage of cytoplasm of the cell due to loss of water

plasmoma (plaz-mo'ma) 1. a collection of plasma cells 2. plasmacytoma

plasmoptysis (plaz-mop'ti-sis) the bursting of protoplasm from a cell due to rupture of the cell wall from a high osmotic pressure within the cell

plasmorrhexis (plaz-mo-rek'sis) the rupture of a cell with loss of its contents

plastein (plas'tein) polypeptides formed by proteolytic enzymes following the peptic digestion of proteins

plaster 1. a solid material which can be spread when heated and which becomes adhesive at the body temperature 2. a topical preparation used to apply drugs to the surface to obtain their systemic effects **adhesive p** a plaster made of a strong cloth that has a coating of an adhesive substance on one side. It is used to keep the edges of a wound in apposition, and to protect raw surfaces **dental p** a semi-solid paste that hardens to a model material **p cast** a rigid dressing made of gauze impregnated with plaster of Paris used in immobili-

sation of bone fractures **P lung** extensive pulmonary consolidation seen in *Klebsiella pneumonia* infection **P of Paris** exsiccated calcium sulphate (gypsum cement) which when mixed with water forms a paste that sets rapidly. It is used for casts.

plastic (plas'tik) 1. capable of being moulded; pliable 2. a synthetic substance that can be shaped to form a cavity or mould **p surgery** surgery aimed at restoring the lost functions and in some instances improving personal appearance.

plasticity (plas-tis'i-te) the ability to be moulded

plastid (plas'tid) a cytoplasmic organoid found in plant cells

plastron the sternum and attached cartilages

-plast combining word for moulding; surgical forming

plate (plat) 1. a thin flattened part especially of a bone 2. a shallow covered dish for culturing bacteria 3. To inoculate micro-organisms in a culture plate 4. a denture

plateau 1. an elevated flat area **p pulse** a sustained peak with a slow upstroke and a downstroke as in aortic stenosis **p stage** second stage of sexual response pattern; a levelling off of arousal immediately before orgasm **ventricular p** the flat portion of the interventricular pressure record during the end of the ejection by the ventricle

platelet (plat'let) a round or oval disc of 2 to 4 mm in diameter, found in the blood and their number varies from 1,50,000 to 4,00,000/mm³. They are fragments of megakaryocytes. They play an important role in blood coagulation, haemostasis and formation of thrombus **p activating factor** (PAF) a phospholipid synthesised by leucocytes, macrophages and endothelial cells that produces platelet aggregation, neutrophal release of enzymes and amines, and increased vascular permeability **p plug** aggregation platelets at a damaged blood vessel to prevent loss of blood

plateletpheresis a procedure in which the platelets are removed from the donor blood and the remaining blood is transfused back

plating inoculation of culture media with micro-organisms

platinic (pla-tin'ik) a compound containing quadrivalent platinum

platinosis allergic reaction in the skin and respiratory tract from exposure to platinum salts.

platinous (plat-i-nus) a compound containing divalent platinum

platinum (palt'i-num) a heavy silver white metal at no. 78, symbol Pt, highly resistant to corrosion

platonic close association between two people that does not include a sexual relationship

platy a combining word for broad

platybasia (plat'e-ba'se-a) a malformation where the base of the skull is flattened on the cervical spine

platycoelous (plat-e-se'lus) ventral concavity and dorsal convexity, such as vertebrates.

platycephalous (plat'e-sef'a-lus) having a broad skull with a vertical index less than 70

platycephaly (plat'e-sef'a-le) flattening of the skull

platycnemia (plt'ik-ne'me-a) 1. unusually broad tibia 2. condition with broad legs

platycoria (pat'e-kor-e'a) dilated pupils

platycrania (plat'e-kra'ne-a) a broad skull

platyglossal (plat'e-glos'al) a broad tongue

platyhelminth (plat'e-hel-minth) flat worm.

platyhelminthes (plat'e-hel-min'thez) a phyllum of flat worms that includes flukes (Trematoda) and tapeworms (Cestoidea)

platyhieric (plat'e-hi-er'ik) a broad sacrum with a sacral index greater than 100

platymeric (plat'e-me'rik) broad femur

platymorphia (plat'e-mor'fe-a) an eye with short anteroposterior diameter

platyopia (plat'e-o'pe-a) a broad, flat face

platyopic (plat'e-op'ik) having a broad flat face

platypellic (plat'e-pel'ik) flattened with reduced anteroposterior diameters as in pelvis

platypnoea (pla'tip'ne-a) dyspnoea on standing erect

platyrrhine (plat'ir-in) wide nose

platysma myoides (pla-tiz'ma-mi-oy-dez) a broad thin plate-like muscle, *see* table of muscles

platyspondylia (plat'e-spon-dil'e-a) flat vertebral bodies

platystencephaly (plat-i-sten-sef'a-le) a skull with wide occiput

play sport or recreational activity

pleasure the feeling of delight or pleasure.

pledget (plej'et) 1. a small compress of gauze or absorbent cotton that is used to absorb fluid or as a protective 2. a small spherical mass of cotton used with forceps for topical application of medicinal substances

plegophonia (pleg'a-fo'ne-a) an auscultatory sound heard on percussion of the larynx

-plegia combining word for paralysis; stroke

pleio, pleo, plio combing word for more

pleiotropy (pli'o-tro'pe) different effects of a gene on apparently unrelated characteristics such as the phenotype, organ systems or functions

pleiotropism (pli-ot'ro-pizm) pleiotropy

Pleistophora a genus of microsporidia

pleochroic (ple'o-kro'ik) refers to property of crystals that give different colours when viewed from different axes

pleocytosis (ple'o-si-to'sis) increase in the number of cells, especially in CSF

pleomorphic (ple-o-mor'fik) existing in many forms

pleomorphism (ple-o-mor'fizm) 1. the occurrence of more than one form in a life cycle 2. the property of crystallising into two or more different forms.

pleomorphous (ple-o-mor'fus) polymorphic

pleonasm (ple'o-nazm) 1. the state of having more than the normal number of organs or parts 2. the use of more number of words to express an idea

pleonexia (ple'o-nek'se-a) a morbid desire for possession of material things

pleonosteosis (ple'on-os'te-o'sis) markedly increased ossification

pleoptics (ple-op'tiks) ocular exercises to stimulate and train an amblyopic eye

plerocercoid larval tapeworm of *Diphyllobothrium latum* found in fish, which develops into adult when eaten by men

plesiomorphism (ple'se-o-mor'fizm) similarity of form

plesiopia (ple'se-o'pe-a) an increased convexity of the lens of the eye

plessesthesia (ples'es-the'ze-a) percussion of the left middle finger pressed against the body surface by the right middle finger

plessimeter (ple-sim'e-ter) pleximeter

plessor (ples'or) plexor

plethora (pleth'o-ra) 1. excess amount of fluid 2. appearance of having more blood

plethoric (ple-thor'ik) characterised by plethora

plethysmograph (ple'thiz'mo-graf) instrument for measuring changes in the size of part or whole body

plethysmography (pleth'iz-mogira-fe) a technique that measures the changes in the volume of an organ, limb or the body **impendance p** measurement of changes in limb volume with each arterial pulse and during occlusion of the cuff of the venous return from a limb to determine the acute venous obstruction or vascular insufficiency in an extremity **whole body p** measurement of thoracic gas volume and airway resistance

pleur (o) combining word for pleura; rib; side

pleura (ploo'ra) pl. **pleurae** the serous membrane that covers the lungs and lines the chest wall and the diaphragm **parietal p** the membrane lining the inner surface of chest wall, cervical tissues, mediastinum and diaphragm **visceral p** the membrane encasing the lung including the interlobar fissures

pleuracotomy (ploor'a-kot'o-me) incision of the pleura through the chest wall

pleural (ploo'ral) concerning the pleura **p cavity** small potential space between the visceral and parietal pleurae **p effusion** a collection of fluid in the pleural space and the fluid may be exudate, transudate, haemorrhagic or chylous **p fibrosis** thickened pleura often with obliteration of the pleural cavity **p plaque** areas of localised pleural thickening that occur as discrete elevated whitish gray lesions distributed in an irregular fashion, extra pleurally, and asbestos is a potent stimulus for its formation **p thickening** focal or diffuse thickening of visceral pleura

pleuralgia (ploo-ral'je-a) pain in the pleura or the side.

pleurapophysis (ploo-ra'-pof'i-sis) a rib or a vertebral lateral process

pleurectomy (ploo-rek'to-me) surgical removal of part of the pleura

pleurisy (ploo'ris-e) inflammation of the pleura

pleuritic (ploo-rit'ik) pertaining to the pleura

pleuritis (ploo-ri'tis) pleurisy

pleuritogenous (ploor'i-toj'e-nus) causing pleurisy

pleurocoele (ploo'ro-sel) 1. hernia of the lungs and pleura 2. collection of serous fluid in the pleural cavity

pleurocentesis (ploo'ro-sen-te'sis) thoracentesis

pleurodesis (ploo'ro-de'sis) production of adhesions between the parietal and visceral pleura **chemical p** instillation of chemical irritants such as quinacrine, tetra-cycline, cyclophosphamide or iodised talc into the pleural space to produce pleural irritation, fibrosis and adhesion.

pleurodynia (ploo'ro-din'e-a) sharp pain in the intercostal muscles **epidemic p** Bornholm's disease

pleurogenic (ploo-roj'en-ic) arising in the pleura

pleurohepatitis (ploo'ro-hep'a-ti'tis) inflammation of the pleura and the liver

pleurolysis (ploo-rol'i-sis) loosening of parietal pleura from intrathoracic fascia.

pleuroparietopexy (ploo'ro-par-i'et-o-pek'se) fixation of the lung to the chest wall by adhesion of visceral and parietal pleura

pleuropericardial (ploor'o-per-i-kar'de-al) concerning the pleura and pericardium

pleuropericarditis (ploo'ro-per'i-kar-di'tis) pleuritis and pericarditis

pleuroperitoneal (ploo'ro-per'i-to-ne'al) concerning the pleura and peritoneum

pleurisy (ploo'ris-i) inflammation of the pleura

pleuropneumonia (ploo'ro-ne-mo'ne-a) pleurisy in association with pneumonia

pleuropneumolysis (ploo're-nu'mo-li'sis) resection of one or more ribs from one side to cause collapse of the lung

pleuropulmonary (ploor'o-pul'mo-ner'e) concerning the pleura and the lung

pleurorrhoea (plor'o-re'a) effusion of fluid into the pleural cavity

pleuroscopy (ploo-ros'ko-pe) visualisation of the pleural surface by a pleuroscope or a flexible fiberoptic bronchoscope

pleurothotonus (ploo'ro-thoto-nus) a tetanic spasm in which body is arched to a side

pleurotomy (ploo-rot'o-me) incision of the pleura

pleurovisceral (ploo'ro-vis'er-al) concerning the pleura and viscera

plexal (plek'sal) pl. **plexus** pertaining to or of the nature of a plexus

plexectomy (plek-sek'to-me) operative removal of a plexus

plexiform (plek-si-form) resembling a plexus of a network

pleximeter (pleks-im'e-ter) a finger or a device held over the surface of the body for receiving the blow of a finger or the percussion hammer, in mediate percussion

plexitis (plek-si'tis) inflammation of a nerve plexus

plexometer (plek-som'e-ter) pleximeter

plexopathy a disorder affecting either the brachial or lumbosacral plexus from injury, infiltration by malignancy or radiation therapy

plexor (pleks'or) a hammer or a finger for striking on the pleximeter in percussion

plexus (pleks'us) a network of nerves or of blood vessels or lymphatics

pliability (pli'a-bil'i-te) capacity of being bent

pliant flexible

plica (pli'ka) pl. **plicae** a fold

plicate (pli'kat) folded or plaited

plication (pli-ka-shun) the stitching of folds or tucks in the wall of organ to decrease its size

plicotomy (pli-kot'a-me) surgical division of the posterior fold of tympanic membrane

pliha (s) spleen

plinth a table or seat on which a patient lies or sits while performing exercises

ploidy (ploy'de) the number of chromosome sets in a cell. Haploidy, diploidy and triploidy refer to one, two and three sets of chromosomes respectively

plombage (plom-bazh) a method of causing collapse of the diseased lung by stripping parietal pleura from the chest wall and packing the space by small plastic balls

plug a mass obstructing a hole

plugger a device for condensing amalgam or gold foil in the cavity of a tooth

plumbic (plum'bik) pertaining to or containing lead

plumbism (plum'bizm) poisoning from lead

plumbum (plum'bum) lead

Plummer-Vinson (plum'er-vin'sun) **syndrome** an iron deficiency anaemia associated with dysphagia and koilonychia, named after Henry Plummer, US physician and Porter Vinson, US surgeon

plumose (plu'mus) a delicate feathery growth

plumper (plum'per) a pad to fill sunken cheek

pluri - combining word for several; more

pluriceptor (ploo'ri-sep'tor) a receptor that has more than two groups uniting with the complement

pluriglandular (ploo'ri-gland'u-lar) polyglandular

plurigravida (ploo'ri-grav'i-da) a pregnant woman who has had three or more pregnancies

plurilocular (ploor'i-lok'u-lar) multilocular

plurinuclear (ploor'i-nu'kle-ar) having many nuclei

pluripara (ploo-rip'a-pa) a woman who has given birth three or more times

pluriparity (ploo'ri-par'i-te) the condition of having three or more pregnancies that have reached a point of viability regardless of the outcome

pluripotent (ploo-rip'o-tent) 1. an embryonic cell capable of developing into defferent kinds of cells 2. capable of different actions **p haematopoietic stem cell** an immature stem cell in the bone marrow that gives rise to the precursors of all different mature cells

pluriresistant (ploor'i-re'-zis'tant) resistant to the action of several agents, especially antibiotics

plutonium (ploo-to'ne-um) chemical element from uranium at weight 244 at. no. 94, symbol Pu

PMF progressive massive fibrosis

PMNs polymorphonuclear leucocytes

pneo - (ne'o) combining word for breath; breathing

pneum-, pneuma-, pneumato- combing word for air, gas, respiration

pneumarthrogram (nu-mɔr'thro-gram) radiograph of a synovial joint following injection of air

pneumarthrography (nu'mar-throg'ra-fe) radiograph of a synovial joint following injection of air

pneumarthrosis (nu-mar-thro'sis) gas or air in a joint

pneumatic (nu-mat'ik) pertaining to gas or air or respiration

pneumatisation (nu'mo-ti-za'shun) the formation of air-filled cells or cavities, usually in bone such as paranasal sinuses and mastoid process of temporal bone

pneumatocardia (nu-mat'o-kar'de-a) air or gas in the cardiac chambers

pneumotocoele (nu-mot'o-sel) 1. hernia of the lung 2. a thin-walled air containing cyst in the parenchyma of the lung most often in staphylococcal pneumonia 3. a gaseous swelling in the scrotum

pneumatodyspnoea (nu'mat-o-disp'ne-a) dyspnoea due to a respiratory condition

pneumatology (nu'ma-tol'o-je) the science dealing with the study of air and gases

pneumatosis (nu'ma-to'sis) the presence of air or gas in unusual location in the body **p cystoides intestinalis** presence of thin-walled gas containing cysts in the wall of intestines

pneumatograph (nu-mat'o-graf) a device to record the movements of the chest wall in respiration

pneumatotherapy (nu'mat-o-ther'a-pe) 1. treatment of the diseases of the lung 2. treatment of diseases by rarefied condensed gases

pneumaturia (nu'mat-u're-a) excretion of urine containing gas

pneumatype (nu'ma-tip) the deposition of moisture on a glass from the breath exhaled through the nostrils with mouth closed

pneumectomy (nu-mek'to-me) excision of all or part of lung

pneumo-, pneumono- combining word for air, lung

pneumoangiography (nu'mo-an'je-o'g'ra-fe) a radiographic study of vessels of the lung using a contrast medium

pneumoarthrography (nu'mo-ar-throg'ra-fe) pneumarthrography

pneumobulbar (nu'mo-bul'bar) pertaining to the lungs and the respiratory centre in the medulla oblongata

pneumocentesis (nu'mo-sen-te'sis) puncture of a lung cavity to remove its contents

pneumocephalus (nu'mo-sef'a-lus) gas or air in the intracranial cavity

pneumocholecystitis (nu'mo-ko'le-sis-ti'tis) cholecystitis with presence of gas in the gall bladder

pneumococcal (nu'mo-kok'al) pertaining to or caused by pneumococci

pneumococcaemia (nu'mo-kok-se'ome-a) the presence of pneumococci in the blood

pneumococci (nu'mo-kok'si) plural of pneumococcus.

pneumococcidal (nu'mo-kok-si'dal) destroying pneumococci

Pneumococcus (nu'mo-kok'us) an oval-shaped, encapsulated, gram-positive organism occuppying in pairs (diplococcus) and having a lancet-shaped ends. There are more than 80 serologic types of pneumococci and cause pneumonia, otitis media, bronchitis, and meningitis

pneumocolon (nu'mo-ko'lon) distension of the colon with air

pneumoconiosis (nu'mo-ko'ne-o'sis) occupational pulmonary diseases caused by prolonged inhalation of dusts which accumulate in lungs causing tissue reactions, in the form of fibrosis, pneumonia, bronchiolitis, extrinsic allergic alveolitis and asthma

pneumocranium (nu'mo-kra'ne-um) pneumocephalus

Pneumocystis carinii (nu'mo-sis'tis-ka-ri'ne-i) a round or elongated organism of 2 to 4 microns length that causes an opportunistic infection in an immunocompromised host. AIDS patients develop pneumonia from its infection. The infection is limited to the lungs

pneumocystography (nu'mo-sis-tog'ra-fe) a cystogram performed after introduction of air into the urinary bladder

pneumocystosis (nu'mo-sis-to'sis) *Pneumocystis carinii* pneumonia

pneumocyte alveolar lining cell; type I membranous, simple thin lining cell; type II granular surfactant secreting and type III pyramidal, scanty

pneumoderma (nu'mo-der'ma) subcutaneous emphysema

pneumodynamics (nu'mo-di-nam'iks) the branch of science concerned with the study of force used in respiration

pneumoempyema (nu'mo-em-pi-e'ma) pyopneumothorax

pneumoencephalogram (nu'mo-en-sef'a-lo-gram) a radiograph of the subarachnoid space and the ventricles of the brain during pneumoencephalography

pneumoencephalography (-log'ra-fe) radiography of the subarachnoid space and the ventricles following removal of CSF and injection of air or oxygen via lumbar puncture

pneumogalactocoele (nu'mo-gal-ak'to-sel) a swelling in the breast containing milk and air

pneumogastric (nu'mo-gas'trik) pertaining to the lungs and stomach **p nerve** vagus nerve

pneumogastrography (nu'mo-gas-trog'ra-fe) a radiographic study of the stomach following introduction of air into it

pneumogram (nu'mo-gram) 1. a graphic record of respiratory movements 2. a radiograph after injection of gas or air

pneumography (nu'mo-grafe) 1. an anatomical description of the lungs 2. graphic recording of respiratory movements 3. radiography of a part or organ after injection of air

pneumohaemopericardium (pnu'mo-hem'o-per-i-kar'de-um) presence of air and blood in the pericardial cavity

pneumohaemorrhagica (nu'mo-hem-o-ra'ji-ka) haemorrhage into the alveoli

pneumohaemothorax (nu'mo-hem'o-tho'raks) presence of gas or air and blood in the pleural cavity

pneumohydrometra (nu'mo-hi'dro-me'tra) accumulation of gas and fluid in the uterus

pneumohydropericardium (nu'mo-hi'dro-per-i-kar'de-um) presence of air and fluid in the pericardial cavity

pneumohydrothorax (-tho'raks) hydropneumothorax; presence of air or gas and fluid in the pleural cavity

pneumohypoderma (nu'mo-hi'po-der'ma) subcutaneous emphysema

pneumokidney (nu'mo-kid'ne) air in the pelvis of the kidney

pneumolith (nu'mo-lith) a concretion in the lung

pneumolithiasis (nu'mo-lith-i'as-is) formation of concretions in the lung

pneumomassage (nu'mo-ma-saz) massage of tympanum with air to facilitate movement of the ossicles of the inner ear

pneumomediastinum (nu'mo-me'de-as-ti'num) the presence of air or gas in the mediastinum

pneumomelanosis (nu'mo-mel-an-o'sis) pigmentation of the lung

pneumometer (nu-mom'et-ér) spirometer

pneumomycosis (nu'mo-mi-ko'sis) any fungal disease of the lungs

pneumomyelography (nu'mo-mi-el-og'rafe) radiography of the spinal canal following injection of air *via* lumbar puncture

pneumonectasia (nu'mon-ek-ta-ze-a) distension of the lungs

pneumonectomy (nu'mon-ek'to-me) excision of all or part of the lung

pneumonia (nu-mo'ne-a) consolidation of a part or the whole of the lung from an acute inflammatory exudate into the alveolar spaces **acute eosinophilic p** acute respiratory failure with marked eosinophilia **aspiration p** pneumonia resulting from aspiration of foreign material, usually food particles or vomit into the bronchi **atypical p** pneumonia caused by virus or mycoplasma **bacterial p** bacterial infection of the alveoli **bronchial p** bronchopneumonia **chlamydial p** pneumonia produced by *Chlamydia pneumoniae* **chronic eosinophilic p** insidious condition with dyspnoea, non-productive cough, eosinophilia and radiologic peripheral homogeneous density **community acquired p** pneumonia developing from infection acquired from patients or convalescent carriers through droplets **desquamative interstitial p** diffuse proliferation of alveolar lining cells which desquamate into the air sacs that produce a gradual onset of dyspnoea and dry cough **double p** lobar pneumonia affecting both lungs **gram negative p** infection from aerobic gram-negative organisms in situations of poor resistance and altered defense mechanisms **hypostatic p** pneumonia occuring in elderly or bed-ridden patients **influenzal p** 1. P neumonia due to *Haemophilus influenzae* 2. pneumonia complicating influenza **Klebsiella p** infection from *Klebsiella pneumoniae* with a necrotising pneumonia **Legionella p** infection by *Legionella pneumophila* **lipoid p** diffuse pneumonia or fibrotic granuloma from inhalation of oil into the lungs **lobar p** pneumonia involving one or more lobes of the lung, usually caused by *Streptococcus pneumoniae* **mycoplasmal p** pneumonia caused by *Mycoplasma pneumoniae* **non-bacterial p** pneumonia involving interstitium of the lungs **nosocomial p** pneumonia developing after hospitalisation provided the infection was not incubating at the time of admission **pneumococcal p** the commonest bacterial pneumonia caused by *Streptococcus pneumoniae* characterised by chills, fever, chest pain, cough and rusty sputum **Pneumocystic carinii p** pulmonary infection from *Pneumocystis carinii* in immunocompromised patients especially those with AIDS **radiation p** an inflammatory condition of the lung caused by thoracic irradiation **rickettsial p** infection from *Coxiella burnetti* developing in persons with history of contact with cattle or sheep **staphylococcal p** pneumonia in infants and children by *Staphylococcus aureus* **streptococcal p** pneumonia occurring as a complication of viral infections (*Streptococcus pyogenes*) or following secondary invasion during lowered resistance (*Streptococcus viridans*) **tuberculous p** pneumonia caused by *M. tuberculosis* with rapid and widespread inflammatory exudate **varicella p** involvement of lungs during the course of chickenpox that may leave behind multiple calcification **viral p** occurrence of pneumonia as a primary viral infection in infants (respiratory syncytial virus and para influenza virus) and in elderly, debilitated individuals (adenovirus and influenza virus)

pneumonic (nu-mon'ik) pertaining to the lungs or pneumonia

pneumonitis (nu'mo-ni'tis) inflammation of the lung usually as a hypersensitivity reactions to the organic dusts or chemicals

pneumono – pneumo

pneumonocoele (nu-mon'o-sel) pneumatocele

pneumonocentesis (nu-mo'no-sen-te'sis) pneumocentesis

pneumonoconiosis (nu-mo'no-ko'ne-o'sis) pneumoconiosis

pneumonocyte pneumocyte

pneumonolysis (nu'mo-nol'i-sis) division of tissues attaching the lung to the walls of thoracic cavity to allow its collapse **extrapleural p** separation of parietal pleura from the chest wall **intrapleural p** separation of adhering visceral and parietal pleura

pneumonopathy (nu'mo-nop'ath-e) any disease of the lungs

pneumonoperitonitis (nu'mo-no-per'i-to-ni'tis) peritonitis with gas in the peritoneal cavity

pneumonopexy (nu-mo'no-pek'se) surgical fixation of the lung to the chest wall

pneumonopleuritis (nu-mo'no-ploo-ri'tis) inflammation of the lung and pleura

pneumonorrhaphy (nu'mo-nor'a-fe) suture of a lung

pneumonotomy (nu-mo-not'o-me) incision of a lung

pneumopericardium (nu'mo-per-i-kar'de-um) presence of air or gas in the pericardial cavity

pneumoperitoneography radiographic examination of the peritoneum and abdominal organs after introduction of air into the peritoneal cavity

pneumoperitoneum (nu'mo-per-i-to-ne'um) air or gas in the peritoneal cavity, as in laparoscopic procedure

pneumoperitonitis (nu'mo-per-i-to-ni'tis) peritonitis with accumulation of gas or air in the peritoneal cavity

pneumopexy (nu'no-peks'e) pneumonopexy

pneumopleuritis (nu'mo-ploo-ri'tis) inflammation of the lung and pleura

pneumopleuroparietopexy (nu'mo-ploor'ro-pa-ri'et-o-pek'se) the operative attachment of the lung with its pleura to the margin of the thoracic wound

pneumopyelography (nu'mo-pi-e-log'ra-fe) radiography of the renal pelvis and ureters after injection of air or oxygen into the renal pelvis

pneumopyopericardium (nu'mo-pi'o-per-i-kar'de-um) accumulation of gas or air and pus in the peritoneal cavity

pneumopyothorax (nu'mo-pi'o-tho'raks) accumulation of gas or air and pus in the pleural cavity

pneumoradiography (nu'mo-ra-de-og'ra-fe) radiography of a part following injection of air or oxygen

pneumorrhachis (nu'mo-ra'kis) accumulation of gas in the spinal canal

pneumorrhagia (nu'mo-ra'je-a) bleeding from the lungs

pneumotachograph (-tak'a-graf) an instrument to record the velocity of respired air

pneumotachometer (-ta-kom'it-er) a transducer to measure expired airflow

pneumosilicosis (nu'mo-sil'i-ko'sis) silicosis

pneumotaxic (nu'mo-tak'sik) pertaining to the regulation of breathing

pneumotherapy (nu-mo-ther'a-pe) 1. treatment of the diseases of the lung 2. treatment of disease by rarefied or condensed gases

pneumothorax (nu-mo-tho'raks) presence of air in the pleural space where air (gas) can enter either from the lung parenchyma and airways (internal) or from outside (external) **artificial p** deliberate introduction of air into the pleural space **catamanial p** pneumothorax during menstruation **closed p** pneumothorax with the opening sealed by deposition of fibrin and the pleural pressure is negative **noisy p** a shallow left sided pneumothorax producing a crunching or clicking sounds near the apex of the cardia **shallow p** pneumothorax with at least 300 to 500 ml of air in the pleural cavity **open p** pneumothorax with communication between the lung and the pleural space that remains patent, allowing free movement of air in and out of pleural cavity during respiration **simple p** closed pneumothorax **spontaneous p** spontaneous occurrence of pneumothorax developing secondary to an underlying pulmonary lesion or from congenital weakness of the pleura **tension p** a flap of opening acting as a check valve allowing entry of air into pleural cavity during inspiration. There is progressive increase in size of pneumothorax with positive intrapleural pressure and shift of mediastinum to the opposite side **traumatic p** pneumothorax that develops following injuries over the chest or rib fractures **valvular p** tension pneumothorax

pneumotomy (nu'mot'o-me) pneumonotomy

pneumoventricle (nu'mo-ven'tri-k'l) accumulation of air in the ventricles of the brain

pneumoventriculography (nu'mo-ventrik'u-log'ra-fe) radiography of the ventricles of the brain following introduction of air

pneumovirus respiratory syncytial virus

PO₂ partial pressure of oxygen

po *per os*, by mouth

pock (pok) a pustule of eruptive fever, or small p(x

pocket (pok'et) a sac-like cavity **p dosimeter** *radiol* a small ionising chamber worn by persons exposed to ionising radiation

pockmarked a depressed scar left by pustule as in small pox.

Poculum Diogenes (pok'u-lum'di-oj'e-nis) the concavity formed by the contracting muscles of the hand making the palm cupped, name derived from Diogenes, Greek philosopher

podagra (po-dag'ra) joint pain in the big toe especially in gout

podalgia (po-dal'je-a) pain in the foot

podalic (po-dal'ik) 1. pertaining to the feet 2. of or in the direction of feet especially the use of feet in version during labour

podencephalus (pod'en-sef'a-lus) a malformed foetus with most of the brain outside the skull

podiatrist (po-di'a-trist) health professional specialised in the treatment of ailments of the feet

podiatry (po-di'a-tre) chiropody; the study and care of the foot

podium (po'de-um) a foot-like projection

podo- combining word for foot

podocyte (pod'o-sit) epithelial cell with many foot plates, that form the inner layer of Bowman's capsule of renal glomerulus which have spaces for the passage of glomerular filtrate

pododynamometer (pod'o-di-na'mom'e-ter) a device to test the strength of the muscles of the leg and foot

podophyllum (pod-o-fil'um) the dried rhizome and roots of *Podophyllum peltatum* used to treat certain papillomas by direct application

POEMS an acronym for polyneuropathy, organomegaly, endocrinopathy, monoclonal gammopathy and skin changes

pogoniasis (po'go-ni'a-sis) growth of beard on a woman

pogonion (po-go'ne-on) the most anterior point on the mandible in the midline.

-poiesis combining word as a suffix for formation, production

poikilo- combining word for irregular, varied

poikilocyte an irregularly shaped red blood cell

poikilocytosis (poy'kil-o-si-to'sis) a pear-shaped erythrocyte, seen in myelofibrosis

poikilodentosis (poy'ki-lo-den-to'sis) mottling of the teeth by presence of excess amount of fluoride in the drinking water

poikiloderma (poy'ki-lo-derma) a mottled appearance of the skin due to hyper-pigmentation followed by atrophy

poikilotherm (poy-kil'o-therm) a cold blooded animal whose body temperature varies according to the temperature of the environment

poikilothrombocyte (pong-kil'o-throm'bosit) an abnormal-shaped platelet

point (poynt) 1. a spot or small area 2. the sharp end of any object 3. to approach the surface as in an abscess about to rupture 4. a position of space, time or degree **p mutation** a change in one of the nucleotides on the double stranded DNA molecule **p prevalence** prevalence at point in time

pointer contusion at a bony eminence

pointillage (pwan'ti-yazh) massage with finger tips

pointing 1. reaching a point 2. an abscess in contact with the skin that is about to burst **p sign** ability of patient to localise pain by pointing with one finger in peptic ulcer or appendicitis

poise (poyz) unit of viscosity of a liquid, being number of grams per centimetre per second, named after Jean Poiseuille, French physiologist

Poiseuille's (pwa-zu'yez) **law** a formula stating rate of flow of liquid through small vessels is directly proportional to pressure and fourth power of radius of the tube and inversely proportional to the viscosity of the fluid and length of the tube, described by Jean Poiseuille, French physiologist

Poiseuille's space the capillary current showing slow movement of leucocytes near the wall; and of rapid movement

of the erythrocytes in the middle current

poison (poy'zn) a chemical substance that usually kills, injures or impairs an organism

poisoning clinical symptomatology from poison. It may be accidental, unintentional or unaware of toxic exposure

poisonous (poy'zon-us) possessing the properties of a poison

poker back stiffness of the spine

pol **gene** gene that encodes reverse transcriptase enzyme of a retrovirus

Poland's syndrome syndactyly with absence of sternal head of pectoralis major muscle on the same side, named after Alfred Poland, UK physician

polar concerning a pole **p body** one of the two small bodies containing chromosomes discarded from ovum during meiotic division

polarimeter (po-lar-im'e-ter) an instrument for measuring the amout of polarisation of light or rotation of plane of polarisation of the light

polarimetry (po'lar-im'e-tre) measurement of the rotation of plane of polarised light

polariscope (po-lar'i-skop) an apparatus used for the measurement of polarised light

polariscopy (po-lar-is'ko-pe) the study of polarised light by the use of a polariscope

polarity (po-lar'i-te) 1. the condition of having poles 2. the exhibition of opposite effects at the two extremities 3. the orientation of intracellular structures to the tissues

polarisation (po-lar-i-za'shun) 1. the presence of polarity 2. a condition in light in which vibrations occur in one plane only 3. the process of separation of positive and negative charges in the body 4. the electrical state existing at the cell membrane of an excitable cell at rest

polarised a condition in which opposite effects or states exist at the same time, such as positive and negative electric charges

polariser (po'lar-riz'er) the part of a polariscope that polarises light

polio poliomyelitis

polio- combining word for gray

polioclastic (pol'e-o-klas'tik) destructive to the gray matter of nervous system

polioencephalitis (pol'e-o-en-sef'a-li'tis) inflammation of the gray matter of the brain

polioencephalomeningomyelitis (pol'e-o-en-sef'al-o-men-in'go-mi'el-i'tis) inflammation of the gray matter of the brain and spinal cord and their meninges

polioencephalomyelitis (pol'e-o-en-sef'al-o-mi'el-i'tis) inflammation of the gray matter of the brain and spinal cord

polioencephalopathy (pol'e-o-en-sef'a-of'a-the) disease of the gray matter of the brain

poliomyelencephalitis (pol'e-o-ni-elen-sef'al-i'tis) poliomyelitis and polioencephalitis

poliomyelitis (pol'e-o-mi'el-i-tis) an acute disease caused by one of three polioviruses. The virus infects the gray matter of the spinal cord, brain stem and cortex and has a particular propensity to damage anterior horn cells. After an incubation period of 1–2 weeks it presents as a febrile illness or as an aseptic meningitis or encephalitis from which many patients recover. In some weakness may develop in one muscle group and can lead to widespread paresis, and cause residual disability. In early stages bed rest is necessary as exercise may worsen the paralysis or precipitate it. Residual disability needs physiotherapy and orthopaedic measures. The condition is prevented by immunisation with oral polio vaccine

poliosis (pol'e-o'sis) grey or whiteness of hair

poliovirus (po'le-o-vi'rus) the causative agent of poliomyelitis. It consists of three serotypes named type I, II and III and belong to the enteroviruses group. In fection occurs through the nasopharynx. Widesread use of oral vaccines through pulse polio programme is expected to eliminate the infection

polishing (pol'ish-ing) producing a smooth glassy finish on a denture.

Politzer (pol'it-zer) **bag** a soft rubber bag with a rubber tap for inflation of the Eustachian tube, named after Adam Politzer, Hugarian otologist

polkissen (pol-kis'en) *Ger* juxtaglomerular cells

pollen (pol'en) microspores of seed plants that are carried by wind or insects. Many air-borne pollens act as allergens

pollenogenic (pol'en-o-jen'ik) caused by the pollen of plants

pollex (pol'eks) the thumb **p valgus** deviation of the thumb toward the ulnar side **p varus** deviation of the thumb toward the radial side

pollinosis (pol'in-o'sis) a hypersensitivity reaction to pollen; hay fever

pollution (pol-loo'shun) the state of making impure or unclean with dirty or toxic substances

polocyte (po'la-sit) polar body

polus (po'lus) pl. **poll** pole

poly (pol'e) polymorphonuclear leucocyte

poly- combining word for many, much

polyacrylic acid acrylic acid polymers, used in ion exchange

polyadenitis (pol'e-ad'e-ni'tis) inflammation of several lymph nodes, especially cervical lymph nodes

polyadenomatosis (pol'e-ad'e-no-ma-to'sis) adenoma of several glands particularly endocrine glands

polyadenopathy (pol'e-ad'e-nop'a-the) any disease affecting many glands

polyadenous (pol'e-ad'e-nus) involving or pertaining to many glands

polyagglutination agglutination of red blood cells by a large proportion of human sera

polyalgesia (pol'e-al-je'se-a) a single stimulus to a part producing sensation of many parts

polyamine (-amen) any compound containing two or more amino groups

polyandry (pol'i-an'dri) the practice of having more than one husband at the same time

polyangiitis (pol'e-an'je-i'tis) inflammation of multiple blood vessels

polyarteritis (pol'e-ar'ter-i-tis) **nodosa** a systemic necrotising arteritis that affects muscular arteries throughout the body especially in the kidneys, heart, gastrointestinal tract and peripheral nervous system. The clinical features include fever, myalgia, weight loss, rashes, gangrene, manoneuritis multiplex, haematuria, loin pain, acute and chronic renal failure, abdominal pain and hypertension

polyarthritis (pol-e-ar-thri'tis) inflammation of several joints

polyarticular (-ar-tik'lar) pertaining to or affecting several joints

polyavitaminosis (pol'e-a-vita-min-o'sis) a deficiency of several vitamins

polybasic (pol'e-ba'sik) an acid having two or more hydrogen ions that will combine with a base

polyblast (pol'e-blast) mononucleated phagocytic cell found in inflammatory exudates

polyblennia (pol'e-ble'ne-a) secretion of an abnormal amount of mucus

polycarbophil (pol'e-kar'bo-fil) a hydrophilic substance used in the production of bulk forming laxative

polycentric (pol'e-sen'trik) the condition of having many centres

polycheiria (pol'e-ki're-a) having more than two hands

polychemotherapy (pol'e-ke'mo-ther'a-pe) use of many chemotherapeutic agents at a time in the treatment

polychondritis (pol'e-kon-dri'tis) a widespread inflammation of cartilage

polychromasia (pol'e-kro-ma'se-a) staining readily with acid, basic and neutral dyes

polychromatic (pol'e-kro-mat'ik) multicoloured especially of histological dyes, staining with more than one colour

polychromatocyte (pol'e-kro-mat'o-sit) a cell having an affinity for different stains.

polychromatophil (pol'e-kro-mat'o-fil) a cell, especially a red blood cell, that is stained by different stains

polychromatophilia (-fil'ea) 1. a property of certain cells to stain with acidic and basic dyes 2. an affinity exhibited by red cell for acid, basic or neutral stains

polychylia (pol'e-ki'le-a) excessive secretion of chyle

polyclinic (pol'e-klin'ik) a dispensary for the treatment of all kinds of diseases

polyclonal (pol'e-klon'al) arising from more than one cell lines **p antibodies** immunoglobulins produced by multiple, usually non-malignant clones of cells. They elicit multiple clonal expansions, each responding to a different epitope on the antigen

polycoria (pol'e-ko're-a) presence of two or more pupils in one iris

polycrotic (pol'e'krat'ik) relating to or marked by polycrotism

polycrotism (pol-ik'ro'tizm) the tendency of having many secondary waves in the descending limb of the pulse tracing.

polycystic (pol'e-sis'tik) having many cysts **p kidney** cystic disease of the kidney that may be juvenile with a recessive inheritance or adult with dominant inheritance. It may present with abdominal lump, haematuria, hypertension, and chronic renal failure. **p liver** multiple cysts of variable size lined by cuboidal epithelium

polycystic ovary syndrome endocrinopathy characterised by oligomenorrhoea, androgen excess and a high prevalence of glucose intolerance and type 2 diabetes mellitus

polycythaemia (pol'e-si-the'me-a) an increase in the number of red blood cells **p rubra vera** a malignant myeloproliferative disorder with predominant expansion of mature erythroid cell population. It presents with splenomegaly, pruritus, hyperviscosity and gastrointestinal bleeding **secondary p** increased red cell mass due to a raised level of erythropoietin

polydactylism (pol′e-dak′ti-lizm) polydactyly

polydactyly (pol′e-dak′ti-le) presence of more than five digits on either hand or foot

polydipsia (pol′e-dip′se-a) frequent drinking from excessive thirst

polydysplasia (pol′e-dis-pla′ze-a) faulty development of tissues or organs

polydystrophy (pol′e-dis′tro-fe) a condition exhibiting multiple congenital abnormalities of the connective tissue

polyene (pol-e′in) an organic compound having multiple double bonds, especially antifungal agents such as amphotericin B and nystatin

polyesters polymers of dicarboxylic acids and polyalcohols

polyesthesia (pol′i-es-the′ze-a) a disorder of sensation in which a stimulus at one point elicits a sensation as if several points are touched

polyethylene (pol′e-eth′i-len) polymerised ethylene

polygalactia (pal′e-ga-tak′she-a) excessive secretion of milk especially at the weaning period

polygamy (po-lig′a-me) having several wives or husbands at the same time

polyganglionic (pol′e-gang′gli-on′ik) concerning many ganglia

polygastria (pol′e-ga′tre-a) increased secretion of gastric juice

polygene (pol′e-jen) one of a group of genes acting together to bring about quantitative changes of a particular character

polygenic (pol′e-jen′ik) control of a normal character by interaction of genes at more than one locus which results from an interaction of multiple genes at different loci **p inheritance** a phenomenon of a trait being governed by many genes each contributing a minor effect in expression of that trait

polyglandular (pol′e-glan′du-lar) pertaining to or affecting several glands

polyglycolic acid a polymer of glycolic acid anhydride used in the production of surgical suture material

polygnathus (po-lig′na-thus) conjoined twins of unequal size in which the smaller is attached to the jaw of the bigger

polygram (pol′e-gram) a record made by a polygraph

polygraph (po′e-graf) 1. an instrument to obtain simultaneous recording of blood pressure, pulse and respiration 2. lie detector, an instrument for recording of physiologic changes as indicators of emotional reactions

polygyny having more than one female mate at a time

polgyria (pol′e-ji′re-a) an excessive number of convolutions in the brain

polyhedral (pol′e-he′dral) having many sides or surfaces

polyhydramnios (pol′e-hi-dram′ne-os) an excess in the amount of amniotic fluid

polyhydric (pol′e-hi′drik) having more than two hydroxyl groups

polyhydruria (pol′e-hi-dro-re-a) passage of excess amount of water in the urine

polyhypermenorrhoea (pol′e-hi′per-men′o-re-a) frequent menstruation with an increased flow

polyhypomenorrhoea (pol′e-hi′pa-men′o-re′a) frequent menstruation with a scanty flow

polyidrosis (pol′e-id-ro′sis) hyperhidrosis

polyinfection (pol′e-in-fek′shun) infection with more than one micro-organism

polykaryocyte (pol′e-kar′e-o-sit) a cell containing many nuclei

polykaryon (-kar′e-on) multinucleate cell

polykarysome (-kar′e-som) a cell with multiple nuclei due to cell fusion induced by infection with *Herpes simplex*

polylysine (pol′e-li′sin) a polypeptide having two lysine molecules that are linked by a peptide

polymastia (pol′e-mas′te-a) presence of supernumerary breasts

polymastigote (pol′e-mas′ti-got) having several flagella

polymazia polymastia

polymelus (pol′e-me′lus) presence of supernumerary limbs

polymenorrhoea (pol′e-men-o-re′a) abnormally frequent menstruation

polymer (pol′i-mer) a substance formed by a combination of simple molecules (monomeres)

polymerase (pol-im′er-as) an enzyme that catalyses polymerisation **DNA p** enzymes which can synthesise DNA from four nucleotide precursors provided a template or primer is available to initiate the process. These polymerases participate in DNA repair and DNA replication. Reverse transcriptase is a DNA polymerase **p chain reaction** a DNA method which allows amplification of a targeted DNA sequence **RNA p** enzymes which catalyse the formation of RNA using DNA as a template

polymeria (pol-i-me′re-a) an excess number of parts, limbs or organs of the body

polymeric (pol′i-mer′ik) exhibiting the characteristics of a polymer

polymerism (pol′i-mer′izm) polymeria

polymerisation (pol′i-mer′i-za′shun) the combining of several simpler compounds to form a substance of higher molecular weight

polymerise (pol′i-mer-iz) to bring about polymerisation

polymicrobial (pol′e-mi-kro′be-al) presence of several species of micro-organisms

polymicrogyria (pol′e-mi′kro-ji′re-a) presence of numerous of convolutions of the brain

polymorph (pol′i-morf) a polymorphonuclear leucocyte

polymorphic (pol′i-morfik) 1. occurring in several forms 2. appearing in different forms in different stages of development **p genell** gene having multiple allels at one locus

polymorphism 1. a part of the DNA sequence that can occur in two forms 2. occurrence in more than one form

polymorphocellular (pol′e-mor′fo-sel′ular) cells of different kinds

polymorphonuclear (-nu′kle-ar) having a deeply lobed nucleus **p leucocyte** neutrophil

polymorphous (pol′e-mor′fus) polymorphic

polymyalgia rheumatica a condition of undetermined aetiology, seen in elderly characterised by sudden pain and severe stiffness of proximal muscles and periarticular tissues.

polymyoclonus (pol′e-mi-ok-lo-nus) myoclonus occurring in several muscles simultaneously or in rapid succession

polymyositis (pol′e-mi-si′tis) an inflammatory muscle disease presenting with progressive painful , proximal upper and lower limb weakness, dysphagia and respiratory muscle weakness. There is arthralgia, malaise and fever

polymyxin (pol′i-miks′in) polypeptide antibiotic from *Bacillus aerosporus*, active against many gram-negative bacteria

polynesic occurring in several septic foci

polyneural (pol′i-nu′ral) relating to, supplied by, or affecting several nerves

polyneuralgia (pol′i-nu′ral′je-a) neuralgia of several nerves

polyneuritis (pol′i-nu′ri′tis) inflammation of several peripheral nerves simultaneously

polyneuromyositis (pol′i-nu′ro-mi′o-si′tis) a condition of polyneuritis and polymyositis occurring together

polyneuropathy (pol′i-nu-rop′a-the) neuropathy of several peripheral nerves simultaneously **acute inflammatory p** Guillain-Barre syndrome, an acute demyelinating predominantly motor polyradiculoneuropathy

polyneuroradiculitis (pol′i-nu′ro-ra-dik′u-li′tis) inflammation of the nerve roots, the peripheral nerves and spinal ganglia.

polynuclear (pol′e-nu′kle-ar) multinuclear

polynucleotidase (pol′e-nu′k′e-o′ti-das) an enzyme catalysing hydrolysis of polynucleotides to oligonucleotides or to mononucleotides

polyodontia (pol'e-o-don'she-a) presence of supernumerary teeth

polyomavirus (pol'e-o-ma-vi'rus) any member of the subfamily Polyomavirinae

polyonychia (pol'e-a-nik'e-a) presence of supernumerary nails on fingers or toes

polypharmacy treatment with multiple drugs

polyopsia (pol'e-op'se-a) the perception of several images of the same object

polyorchidism (pol'e-or'ki-dism) presence of one or more supernumerary testes

polyorchis (pol'e-or'kis) a person exhibiting polyorchidism

polyostatic (pol'e-os-tet'ik) involving more than one bone

polyotia (pol'e-o'she-a) a person having supernumerary auricle on one or both sides of the head

polyovulatory (pol'e-ov'u-la-to're) discharging several ova in one ovarian cycle.

polyp (pol'ip) a growth with a pedicle protruding from a mucous membrane commonly found in structures which are vascular such as nose, uterus, colon and rectum. They bleed easily and may become malignant

polypectomy (pol'i-pek'to-me) excision of a polyp

polypeptidaemia (pol'e-pep'ti-dem'e-a) presence of polypeptides in the blood

polypeptidase (pol'e-pep'ts-das) an enzyme that catalyses the hydrolysis of peptides

polypeptide (pol'e-pep'tid) a peptide formed by the union of a large number of aminoacids

polyphagia (-fa-jah) excessive eating

polyphalangia (-fa-lan'jah) increase in the number of phalanges such as side-by side duplication

polyphalangism (-fal-lan'jizm) polyphalangia

polypharmacy (-far-ma'se) treatment with multiple drugs

polyphobia (-fo'be-a) an abnormal fear of a number of things

polyphrasia (-fra'zi-a) excessive talkativeness

polyplastic (-plas'tik) containing many constituent elements

polyploidy (-ploi'de) a cell nucleus having multiple of the euploid (correct number) number of chromosomes

polypnoea (pol'ip-ne'a) tachypnoea

polypoid (pol'i-poid) resembling a polyp

polyporous (pol-ip'or-us) having many small pores

polyposis (pol'i-po'sis) multiple polyps **familial adenomatous p** an autosomal dominant disorder from germ line cell mutation of the APC gene on chromosome S, and develop in the colon, stomach and duodenum **juvenile p** mucusfilled hamartomatous polyps found in the colon and rectum

polypous (pol'i-pus) pertaining to or characterised by the presence of a polyp or polyps

polypropylene (pol'i-pro'pi-len) a synthetic, thermoplastic, polymer used in surgical casts and in membrane oxygenators

polyptychial (-ti'ke-al) arranged in several layers

polypus (pol'i-pus) pl. **polypi** a polyp

polyradiculoneuritis (-ra-dik'u-lo-noori'tis) inflammation of peripheral nerves and spinal nerve roots

polyradiculoneuropathy (-noo-rop'a-the) any disease of peripheral nerves and spinal roots

polyribosome (pol'e-ri'bo-sum) two or more ribosomes connected by a messenger RNA that takes part in peptide synthesis

polysaccharide (-sak'a-rid) a carbohydrate which on hydrolysis yields many molecules of monosaccharides

polyserositis (-ser'o-sit'is) fibrotic thickening of serosa of multiple sacs with effusion

polysinusitis inflammation of two or more sinuses simultaneously

polysome (pol'e-sum) aggregate of ribosome around a messenger RNA molecule

polysomnography (pol'e-som-nog'ra-fe) method to study sleep and its distribution among different stages, degree of sleep fragmentation and occurrence of apnoea by continuous monitoring by ECG, EEG, electrooculogram (EOG) and electromyogram (EMG)

polysomy (-so'me) presence of chromosome more than one normal pair

polyspermia (-sper'mi-a) 1. an abnormally profuse secretion of seminal fluid 2. polyspermy

polyspermy (-sper'me) fertilisation of an ovum by many spermatozoa

polystichia (pol-i-stik'i-a) presence of two or more rows of eyelashes

polystyrene (-sti'ren) a synthetic resin produced by polymerisation of styrene, used in the construction of dental bases

polysynaptic (-si'nap'tik) pertaining to nerve pathways formed by a chain of many synaptically connected nerve cells

polysyndactyly (-sin-dak'ti-le) polydactyly associated with syndactyly

polytenosynovitis (pol'e-ten'o-sin'o-vit'is) inflammation of several tendon sheaths simultaneously

polytetrafluoroethylene a highly stable plastic material

polythelia (-thel'e-a) presence of supernumerary nipples on the breast or elsewhere

polythetic classification using multiple criteria

polythiazide (-thi'a-zid) a long acting thiazid diuretic

polytomogram (-tom'a-gram) record produced by polytomography

polytomography (-to-mog'ra-fi) body section radiography

polytrauma (traw'ma) multiple injuries affecting many systems

polytrichia (-trik'e-a) excessive hairyness

polyunsaturated (-unsach'er-at-ed) **fatty acid** a fatty acid with two or more double-bonded carbons, abundant in corn oil, safflower oil and cottonseed oil

polyuria (-ur'e-a) passage of excess amount of urine noted in excess fluid intake, hyperglycaemia and diabetes insipidus

polyvalent (-va'lent) 1. multivalent 2. pertaining to a polyvalent serum

polyvinyl (-vi'nil) a compound containing a number of vinyl groups in polymerised form **p chloride** (PVC) a thermoplastic polymer formed from vinyl chloride

Pomeroy sterilisation laparotomy and excision of middle of fallopian tubes with ligation, named after R. Pomeroy, US gynaecologist

Pompe's disease a glycogen storage disease type 2, characterised by muscle weakness and mental defect that is rapidly fatal in infants, named after Johann Pompe, Dutch physician

pompholyx (pom'fo-liks) intense pruritus of the palmoplantar surfaces, with crops of vesicles and bullae, and it can be provoked by heat, stress and nickel ingestion

pomum (po'mum) an apple **p adami** prominent thyroid cartilage

ponderal (pon'der-al) relating to weight

pons (ponz) 1. the portion of the brain stem that forms a 'bridge' between the medulla and the midbrain, anterior to the cerebellum. It contains fibre tracts connecting the medulla and cerebellum with the upper portions of the brain. The abducens, facial and cochlear division of the eight nerve take their origin in pons 2. any bridge-like structure connecting parts of the same structure or organ

pontic (pon'tik) an artificial tooth on a fixed partial denture

ponticulus (pon-tik'u-lus) a bridge-like structure

pontine (pon'tin) pertaining to the pons

pont (o) combining word for the pons

pontobulbar (pon'to-bul'bar) pertaining to the pons and medulla

pontocerebellar (-ser'i-bel'er) pertaining to the pons and cerebellum

pool 1. a collection of blood in any region of the body 2. to mix blood from many donors

POP 1. plaster of Paris 2. persistent occipito-posterior

popcorn a radiologic abnormality with features simulating the solitary kernels of 'popped corn' **p calcification** 1. clusters of small scalloped radiolucencies with sclerotic margins, seen in epiphysis and metaphysis of children with osteogenesis imperfecta 2. puffed and lobulated appearance of calcified hemartoma of the lung

popliteal (pop'lit'e-al) relating to the area behind the knee **p cyst** cyst communicating with knee, but fluid is prevented from returning to the joint by valve-like mechanism; Baker's cyst

population (pop-u-la'shun) 1. the number of inhabitants of any place 2. *stat* the entire collection of a set of objects having same definition **p genetics** a disease gene is very much less common in the population than the normal gene, hence heterozygotes are more common than homozygotes **p medicine** scientific discipline concerned with promotion of health and prevention of disease **p survey** survey for evaluating the health status of a population, that involves community diagnosis of problems of health and disease

poradentis (por'ad-e-ni'tis) inflammation of the iliac glands with multiple small abscesses

porcelain doll face the puffy, pale facies in adults with myxoedema due to accumulation of glycosaminoglycans

porcine (por'sin) relating to pig

pore (por) 1. a small opening of the secretory duct of the sweat gland 2. a minute opening on an epithelial surface **alveolar p's** openings between adjacent pulmonary alveoli **gustatory p's** external opening of taste buds **nuclear p** a small octagonal opening where the inner and outer membranes of the nuclear envelopes are continuous **p's of Kohn** alveolar pores, named after Hans Kohn, German pathologist **slit p's** small slit-like spaces between the interdigitating

pedicles of podocytes of the renal glomerulus.

porencephalitis (por'en-sef'a-li'tis) inflammation of the brain resulting in cavities in the brain substance

porencephaly (-en-sef'a-le) presence of abnormal cavity(ies) in the brain filled with CSF

porin a voltage-gated membrane channel in the outer membrane of gram-negative bacterial walls that acts as a diffusional pathway

por (o) combining word for duct; passage; opening; pore

pork tapeworm *Taenia solium*

porokeratosis (por'o-ker'a-to'sis) a dermatosis characterised by thickening of the stratum corneum followed by its progressive centrifugal atrophy

poroma (por-o'ma) 1. callosity 2. exostosis 3. a tumour of cells lining the skin openings of sweat glands

porosis (por-o'sis) 1. callus formation in the repair of a fractured bone 2. cavity formation

porosity (por-os'it-e) a porous condition

porotomy (por-ot'a-me) meatotomy

porous (por'is) having pores that pass through a substance

porphin (por'fin) a tetrapyrole nucleus forming the basis of porphyrins.

porphobilin (por'fo-bi'lin) a porphin derivative

porphobilinogen (por'fo-bi'lin-o-jin) an intermediate product in haeme synthesis. It is found in the urine in large quantities in cases of acute porphyria

porphyrias (por-fir'e-as) a heterogeneous group of disorders due to inherited or acquired abnormalities of enzymes involved in the biosynthesis of haem resulting in excess production, accumulation and excretion of intermediate compounds, the porphyrins, and/or its precursors - delta aminolevulinic acid and porphobilinogen **acute intermittent p** hereditary hepatic porphyria with an increased production of 8-aminolevulinic acid. It is associated with abdominal colic, intermittent hypertension, psychosis and neuropathy. There is increased urinary excretion of 8-aminolevulinic acid and porphobilinogen **congenital erythropoietic p** increased formation of porphyrin by erythroid cells in the bone marrow leading to severe porphyrinuria. There is an increased cutaneous photosensitivity **p cutanea tarda** a condition noted in middle aged, often in males with bullous skin eruptions on exposure to sunlight, which heal by scarring. It develops in those with liver dysfunction in whom alcohol acts as a precipitating agent **hepatic p** acute intermittent porphyria **symptomatic p** cutaneous hepatic porphyria **variegate p** increased production of protoporphyrin exhibiting clinical features of acute porphyria with those of cutaneous porphyria

porphyrins (por'fi-rins) pigments consisting of four pyrroles joined in a ring of porphyrin structure and are categorised as uro-, copro- or protoporphyrins depending on their structure. Both uro- and coproporphyrins can be eliminated in the urine. An increased production of protoporphyrins is associated with its excretion in the urine

porphyrinuria (por'fi-ri-nu're-a) an increased elimination of uro- and coproporphyrins; and an increased elimination of protoporphyrins in the urine turn reddish-brown on standing

Porro's (por'oz) **operation** Caesarean section followed by removal of uterus, fallopian tubes and ovaries, named after Edoardo Porro, Italian obstetrician.

porta (por'ta) pl. **portae** hilum; the point of entry of the blood vessels and nerves to an organ **p hepatis** a transverse fissure on the visceral surface of the liver where portal vein and hepatic artery enter as the hepatic duct leaves **p lienis** the hilus of the spleen **p pulmonis** pulmonary hilus for entry and exit of bronchi, vessels and nerves. **p renis** the hilus of the kidney

portocaval (port'a-ka'val) pertaining to the portal vein and inferior vena cava **p shunt** a surgical procedure that diverts blood away from the portal venous system into the inferior vena cava, reducing portal hypertension

portal (port'l) 1. relating to any porta 2. the point of entry into the body of a pathogenic microorganism 3. the point of exit of the infectious agent from a carrier **p cirrhosis** diffuse process of fibrosis that converts the liver into structurally abnormal nodules **p hypertension** obstruction to the portal vein or its radicals leading to development of back pressure and rise in the pressure and its radicals. There is splenomegaly and development of collaterals between the radicals of the portal vein and systemic veins as varices **p pyaemia** suppurative infection of portal veins especially within the liver **p venous thrombosis** a complication of portal hypertension presenting with abdominal pain and diarrhoea. It may lead to bowel infarction **p vein** *see* table of veins

portio (por'she-o) 1. a part 2. referring to a portion of a structure or organ **p supravaginalis** the part of the cervix uteri lying above the vagina **p vaginalis** the part of the cervix uteri that projects into the vagina

portoenterostomy (port'o-en'ter-os'to-me) a surgical procedure to establish a passage for bile flow in an infant with biliary atresia. A loop of jejunum is anastomosed to the structures of porta hepatis

portogram (por'to-gram) the radiograph obtained after portography

portography (por-tog'ra-fe) radiography of the portal circulation following injection of a radioopaque contrast medium into the spleen or into the portal vein

portosystemic (por'to-sis-tem'ik) relating to connections between the portal and systemic venous systems **p encephalopathy** a neuropsychiatric syndrome caused by liver disease

port-wine naevus naevus flammeus; a congenital neurovascular malformation that appears as deep red-purple macular lesions

port wine urine transparent red urine found in myoglobinuria

porus (por'us) a pore, meatus or foramen **p acousticus externus** the orifice of the external acoustic meatus in the tympanic portion of the temporal bone **p acousticus internus** the opening of the internal acoustic meatus on the posterior surface of the petrous part of the temporal bone **p opticus** the opening in the sclera for the passage of retinal vessels

-posis combining word for intake of fluids

poshaka (s) promote

position (po-zish'un) 1. an attitude, posture or place occupied 2. the relation of a given point of the presenting part of the foetus to right or left side of the maternal pelvis (*see* table of positions of foetus in the uterus) 3. the manner in which the body is arranged for examination **anatomical p** the position of the body standing erect with the face directed forward, the arms at the side and the palms of the hands facing forward **anteroposterior p** a position adapted during radiological examination in which the central ray enters the front of the body and exits from the back **axial p** a position adapted during radiological examination in which the central ray enters the body at an angle **Bozeman's p** knee-elbow position, the patient being strapped to supports **Brickner's p** obtaining traction in abduction and external rotation by tying the wrist to the elevated head of the bed **decubitus p** position of the body lying on a flat surface, designated according to the aspect of the body touching the surface as left lateral decubitus (on the left side), right lateral decubitus (on the right side), dorsal decubitus (on the back) and ventral decubitus (on the abdomen) **enface p** a position in which the mother and infant are face to face **Fowler's p** an in-

clined position obtained by raising the head of the bed with lower extremities moderately flexed. It facilitates application of obstetric forceps, repair of vaginal lesions, and vaginal examination **genucubital p** knee-elbow position **genupectoral p** knee-chest position **knee chest p** the patient resting on his knees and upper part of the chest for gynaecologic or rectal examination **knee elbow p** the patient resting on his knees and elbows with the chest elevated **lateral p** a side-lying position in radiological examination which allows the central ray to enter the upright side **lithotomy p** supine position with hips and knees fully flexed and thigh abducted and externally rotated **Mayo-Robson's p** a supine position with a thick pad beneath the loin causing marked lordosis in that region, adapted in operations on gall bladder **occlusal p** the relation of the upper and lower jaw when jaws are closed and the teeth are in contact **p sense** a deep sensation to demonstrate the integrity of the posterior column. One limb of the patient is kept in a particular position while the eyes are closed and the patient is then asked to keep other limb in a similar position. In the absence of paralysis of the limb, the individual must be able to bring the limb in the same position as the other limb **Rose's p** full extension **Sim's p** the patient on his left side and chest, the right knee and thigh drawn up, the left arm along the back, to facilitate vaginal examination **Trendelenburg p** the patient supine on a surface inclined at an angle of 45° so that the pelvis is higher than the head, used during and after operations in the pelvis or for shock **Valentine's p** a supine position on a table with double inclined place causing flexion at the hips, used during urethral irrigation **Water's p** a radiographic position giving a posteroanterior view of the maxillary sinus, maxilla, orbits and zygomatic arches

Table 9: Positions of foetus in the uterus

Presentation and point of designation	Position	abbreviation
Cephalic		
a) Vertex (occiput)	left occipitoanterior	LOA
	right occipitoanterior	ROA
	left occipitoposterior	LOP
	right occipitoposterior	ROP
	occipitoanterior	OA
	occipitoposterior	OP
	left occipitotransverse	LOT
	right occipitotransverse	ROT
b) face (chin)	left mentoanterior	LMA
	right mentoanterior	RMA
	left mentoposterior	LMP
	right mentoposterior	RMP
	mentoanterior	MA
	mentoposterior	MP
	left mentotransverse	LMT
	right mentotransverse	RMT
Pelvic (breech)		
sacrum	left sacroanterior	LSA
	right sacroanterior	RSA
	left sacroposterior	LSP
	right sacroposterior	RSP
	sacroanterior	SA
	sacroposterior	SP
	left sacrotransverse	LST
	right sacrotransverse	RST
Transverse		
shoulder (scapula)	left scapuloanterior	L Sc A
	right scapuloanterior	R Sc A
	left scapuloposterior	L Sc P
	right scapuloposterior	R Sc P

positive (pos′it-iv) 1. affirmative; definite 2. having a value greater than zero **p end expiratory pressure** (PEEP) a special wave form with application of positive pressure during the entire expiratory phase to secure adequate oxygenation when the patients are not able to obtain satisfactory oxygenation on volume-cycled ventilators **p predictive value** *stat* the number of true positives divided by the sum of true positives and false positives

positron (pos′i-tron) a subatomic particle of the same mass as the electron but of the opposite charge **p emission transaxial tomography** PET scanning, a non-invasive imaging modality that uses radionuclides to detect biochemical and pathological abnormalities in living tissues, such as cerebral cortex

posology (pa-sol′a-je) the science of dosage of remedies

post - combining word for, after

postabortal (post′a-bor′tal) following abortion

postacetabular (post'ac-e-tab'u-lar) behind the acetabulum

postadolescent (post'ad-o-les'ent) a person who has passed adolescence

postanaesthetic (post'an-es-thet'ik) pertaining to the period following anaesthesia

postanal (post-a'nal) behind the anus

postapoplectic (post'ap-o-plek'tik) pertaining to the period immediately after a stroke

postaxial (post-ak'se-al) situated behind an axis

postbrachial (post-bre'ke-al) pertaining to the posterior part of the arm

postcapillary (post-kap'il-la-re) venous capillary

postcardial (post-kar'de-al) behind the heart

postcardiotomy (post-kar'de-ot'o-me) pertaining to the period after open heart surgery p syndrome occurrence of pericarditis, pleurisy and fever following cardiac surgery

postcaval pertaining to the postcava, the inferior vena cava

postcentral (post-sen'tral) 1. behind a centre 2. behind the fissure of Rolando

postcibal (post-si'bal) after food

postclavicular (post'kla-vik'u-lar) behind the clavicle

postclimacteric (post'kli-mak-ter'ik) after menopause

postcoital (post-ko'it-al) following sexual intercourse p syndrome use of drugs such as high dose of norethisterone to prevent implantation p test examination of cervical mucus for motile sperms

postconnubial (post'kon-u'be-al) after marriage

postconvulsive (post'kon-vul'siv) after a convulsion

postcricoid web a fold of oesophageal mucosa causing dysphagia in iron deficiency anaemia

postdiastolic (post'di-as-tol'ik) after diastole

postdicrotic (post'di-krot'ik) after the dicrotic pulse wave

postdiphtheritic (post'dif-ther-it'ik) following diphtheria

postductal coarctation constriction of aorta beyond ductus arteriosus

postencephalitis (post'en-sef-a-li'tis) after encephalitis

postepileptic (post'ep-i-lep'tik) following an epileptic attack

posterior (pos-te're-ur) 1. toward the back or dorsal 2. situated behind 3. toward the caudal end

postero (pos'ter-o) combining word for posterior; situated behind; toward the back

posteroanterior (pos'ter-o-an'ter-e-or) from behind to the front, pertaining to flow or movement

posteroexternal (-ex-ter'nal) toward the back and lateral side

posteroinferior (-in-fer'e-or) posterior and inferior

posterointernal toward the back and medial side

posterolateral posteroexternal

posteromedial (pos'ter-o'me'de-al) postero- internal

posteromedian located posteriorly and in the median plane

posteroparietal behind the parietal bone

posterosuperior posterior and superior

posterotemporal behind the temporal bone

posteruption a stage of eruption of tooth in which the tooth has reached the occlusal plane

postethmoid (post'eth'moyd) behind the ethmoid bone

postfebrile (post-fe'bril) occurring after a fever

postganglionic (post'gan-gle-on'ik) distal to the ganglia

posthaemorrhagic (post-haem'o-rig'ik) after haemorrhage

posthemiplegic (post'hem-i-ple'jik) after hemiplegia

posthepatitis (post'hep-a-tit'is) occurring after hepatitis

posthitis (pos-thi'tis) inflammation of the foreskin

posthumous (pos-tu-mus) 1. occurring after death 2. born after the death of the father 3. Caesarean delivery after death of the mother

posthypnotic (post'hip-not'ik) subsequent to hypnotic state

postictal (post'ik-tal) following seizure or a stroke **p confusion** confusion that follows a seizure

posticteric (post'ik-ter'ik) after jaundice

postload increased cardiac work due to changes on output side

postmalarial (post'ma-la're-al) after malaria

postmature (post'ma-tur) 1. referring to an infant born after 42 weeks of gestation 2. referring to an infant born after the calculated due date

postmaturity after 42 weeks of gestation

postmediastinal (post'me-di-as-ti-nal) behind the mediastinum

postmenopausal (post'men-o-paw'zal) after menopause

postmortem 1. autopsy 2. occurring or performed after death

postmyocardial infarction syndrome presence of persistent fever, pericarditis and pleurisy occurring a few weeks or months after a myocardial infarction, probably due to autoimmunity; Dressler's syndrome

postnasal (post-na'sal) behind the nose

postnatal occurring after birth

postnecrotic (post'ne-krot'ik) after the death of a tissue or part

postocular (post-ok'u-lar) behind the eye **p neuritis** inflammation of the optic nerve behind the eyeball

postoesophageal (post'e-sof'a-je-al) behind the oesophagus

postolivary (post-ol'i-va-re) behind the olivary body

postoperative following operation **p care** care undertaken after a surgical operation

postoral (post'or-al) behind or posterior part of the oral cavity

postorbital (post-or'bi-tal) behind the orbit of the eye

postpalatine (post-pal'a-tin) behind the palate

postpallium (post-pal'e-um) referring the cerebral cortex present behind the fissure of Rolando

postpaludal (post-pal'u-dal) following an attack of malaria

postparalytic (post-par-a-lit'ic) following an attack of paralysis.

postpartal (post-par-tal) following child birth **p period** the time following the childbirth

postpartum (post-par'tum) after childbirth

postprandial (post-pran'de-al) postcibal; after taking food **p syndrome** symptoms suggestive of, but not actually due to hypoglycaemia occurring 1-2 hours after the food

postprimary tuberculosis tuberculosis that occur after the first few weeks of primary infection when immunity to the mycobacteria has developed

postpubertal (-pu'ber-al) postpubescent

postpubescent (post'pu-bes'ent) subsequent to the pubertal period

postrenal (post-re'nal) beyond the kidney **p failure** uraemia developing from obstruction of both ureters or urethra

postsinusoidal (post'si-nu-soi-dal) located behind a sinusoid

postsphygmic (post-sfig'mik) after a pulse wave

poststenotic (post'ste-not'ik) distal to a stenosed or a constricted area, especially of an artery

postsynaptic (-si-nap'tik) distal to a synapse

postterm (post-term) pregnancy continuing beyond the beginning of 42nd week of gestation

posttraumatic following or related to trauma **p stress disorder** a delayed and protracted response to a stressful event of a catastrophic nature, such as natural calamities, terrorist activity, serious accidents and witnessing violent deaths. There is flashback of traumatic episode, sleep disturbance, nightmares, emotional blunting numbing of responsiveness to such reminders, and persistent hyperarousal, and avoidance of any situation that evokes memories of the trauma

postulate (pos'choo-lat) a statement or formula offered as the basis of theory **Koch's p's** experimental proof to establish the aetiologic relationship of a given microbe to a specific disease. It is by demonstrating the microorganism in the blood, sputum, urine or cerebrospinal fluid, growing in the artificial laboratory medium and reproducing the disease in the experimental animal, described by Robert Koch, German bacteriologist

postural (pos'tu-ral) relating to the posture **p drainage** drainage of secretions from the bronchi or abscess cavity in the lung by positioning the patient in such a way so that gravity will allow drainage from the involved segment or lobe

posture (pos'tur) position of the limbs **round-back p**. a posture characterised by an increased thoracic curve, protracted scapula and a forward head

postvaccinal (post-vak'si-nil) following vaccination **p encephalitis** severe form of demyelinating encephalitis developing 10 days after vaccination

postvalvular relating to a position distal to the pulmonary or aortic valves

potable (po'ta-bl) drinkable; fit to drink **p water** safe, odourless, drinking water

potash (pot'ash) potassium carbonate **caustic p** potassium hydroxide

potassaemia (pot'a-se-me-ah) an excess amount of potassium in the blood

potassium (pot'tas'e-um) an alkaline metallic element at. no. 19; symbol K (kalium)

potato tumour chemodactoma of carotid body

potency (po'ten-se) 1. power, force or strength 2. strength of a medicine 3. a condition being potent **sexual p** the ability of a man to carry out sexual act

potential (po-ten'shul) 1. capable of doing; latent existing in possibility 2. a state of tension in an electric source, capable of doing work

potentiation (po-ten'she-e'shun) a degree of synergism that is greater than additive

potion (po'shun) a drink; a dose of liquid medicine or poison

Pott's disease caries spine, named after Sir Percivall Pott, British surgeon

Pott's fracture fracture of the lower end of the fibula and medial malleolus of the tibia with dislocation of the foot outward and backward

pouch (powch) a pocket; cul-de-sac

pouchitis (pouch-i'tis) an acute inflammation of the surgically created pouch

poudrage (poo-drash') powdering; application of an irritant; non-toxic powder to the pleural space of the lung to produce pleural adhesions

poultice (pol'tis) a soft, moist, hot mass of mustard, linseed or soap and oil between layers of gauze or linen applied to the skin to create moist local heat or counter irritation

Poupart's (pu-parz') **ligament** inguinal ligament, named after Francis Poupart, French anatomist

poverty absence or scarcity of, requisite substance or ingredient **emotional p** diminution in normal emotional qualities such as love, sympathy **p of movement** hypokinesia as in Parkinsonism

powder 1. an aggregation of minute separate particles 2. finely-divided, relatively dry, particulate matter 3. a dose of such a powder

power 1. potency 2. capacity for action 3. the rate at which work is carried out 4. degree to which a lens magnifies 5. the number of times the diameter of an object is magnified in microscopy

pox (poks) any infectious disease with pustular skin eruption

poxvirus large, brick-shaped viruses with double-stranded DNA, causing small pox, vaccinia and molluscum contagiosum

PP punctum proximum, the near point of visual accommodation

PPD purified protein derivative, substance used in the skin test for tuberculosis

PPH 1. postpartum haemorrhage 2. primary pulmonary hypertension

PPM parts per million

PP oma a pancreatic polypeptide producing islet cell tumour exhibiting hyperglycaemia, hypercalcaemia, hypomagnesaemia and muscular weakness

P protein a regulatory protein that is capable of reactivating glutamine synthetase after inactivation through adenylation

ppt precipitate

P pulmonale *ECG* a sharply peaked P wave in COPD

PR 1. *ECG* interval or segment 2. per rectum

pr punctum remotum, the far point of visual accommodation

practice (prak'tis) exercise of the medical profession to provide a comprehensive health care

practitioner (prak'tish'un-er) a person who practises medicine or an allied health care profession

practolol Beta-adrenergic blocking agent used in resistant ventricular arrhythmias

praecox (pre'koks) early; premature

Prader-Willi syndrome a genetic mutation disorder characterised by obesity, hypogonadism and mental retardation due to lack of paternal contribution to the chromosome 15 region, named after Andrea Prader, and Heinrich Willi, Swiss Paediatricians

praevia (pre've-a) preceding

pragbhakta (s) before meals

pragmatanosia (prag'mat-ag-no'ze-a) inability to recognise a familiar object

pragmatamnesia (prag'mat-am-ne'ze-a) loss of ability to recognise the appearance of objects

pragmatic an approach judged by practical results

pragmatism (prag'ma-tizm) an approach

that emphasises practical applications and consequences

pralidoxime a cholinesterase reactivator used in the treatment of organophosphorous insecticide poisoning

prakasha (s) light

prakriti (s) constitution; natural state nature, temperament *p pariksha* constitutional examination

pralapa (s) delirium

prameha (s) urinary disorder

prana (s) life force *p vayu* oxygen

pranayama (s) breath control

pranijanya (s) animal product

prasara (s) spread

prash (s) ayurvedic herbal jelly

prasna (s) enquiry

prandial (pran'de-al) relating to a meal

prashtha (s) back

Prausnitz-Kustner (prows'nits-kist'ner) **reaction** a skin reaction to detect IgE, or reaginic antibody, named after Carl Prausnitz, German bacteriologist and Heinz Kustner, German gynaecologist

pravistatin a cholesterol lowering agent inhibiting HMG-CoA(3-hydroxy 3 methyl glutaryl coenzyme A) reductase, the rate limiting enzyme of cholesterol synthesis

praxinoscope (prak-sin'o-skop) an instrument to study the larynx

praxiology (prak'se-ol'o-je) the study of conduct of an individual

praxis (prak'sis) ability to perform coordinated movement

-praxis combining word for act; activity; use; practice

praziquantel an anti-parasitic agent used in the treatment of Schistosomiasis (*S. haematobium, S. japonicum*). flukes (*Clonorchis sinensis, Paragonimus buski*) and tapeworms (*Hymenolepsis nana* and *Taenia solium*)

prazosin alpha-blocking vasodilator used as an antihypertensive agent

pre - prefix indicating before, in front of

preagonal (pre-ag'o-nal) immediately preceding death

preanal (pre-a'nal) in front of the anus

preanaesthesia (pre'an-es-the'ze-a) before anaesthesia

preanaesthetic (pre-an-es-thet'ik) an agent administered to facilitate induction of general anaesthesia

preaortic (pre'a-or'tik) in front of the aorta

preataxic (pre-a-tak'sik) before occurrence of ataxia

preauricular (pre'aw-rik'u-lar) in front of the ear

preaxial (pre-ak'se-al) anterior to the axis of the body or a limb

prebeta lipoprotein very low density lipoprotein

precancer (pre-kan-ser) premalignant

precancerous (pre-kan'ser-us) pertaining to any lesion that is considered as a precancer

precapillary preceding a capillary referring to the branches of an arteriole or venule

precautions a preventive measure; caution

precartilage an aggregation of mesenchymal cells before differentiation into embryonic cartilage

precava (pre-ka'va) superior vena cava

precentral (pre-sen'tral) in front of a centre, as in central fissure of the brain p convolution the ascending frontal convolution of the brain

prechordal (pre-kor'dal) in front of the notochord

precipitable (pre-sip'i-ta-b'l) capable of being precipitated

precipitant (pre-sip'i-tant) a substance causing a precipitation from a solution.

precipitate (pre-sip'i-tat) 1. to cause a substance in solution to settle down in solid particles 2. a deposit made by precipitation 3. occurring very rapidly as precipitate labour

precipitation (pre-sip'i-ta'shun) the process of forming a precipitate

precipitin (pre-sip'i-tin) an antibody that interacts with an antigen forming a precipitate that sediments out of solution

precipitinogen (pre-sip'i-tin'o-jen) an antigen that stimulates the production of specific precipitin following injection into the animal body

precipitum (pre-sip'i-tum) the precipitate produced by the action of a precipitin

precision a measurement of the reproducibility of a test or assay

preclinical (pre-klin'i-kal) 1. before the onset of disease 2. a period of medical education prior to clinical studies, during which the student studies anatomy, physiology, biochemistry and preventive medicine 3. of in vitro research or research involving animals undertaken prior to research in humans

preclival (pre-kli'val) in front of cerebellar clivus

precocious (pre-ko'shus) developing very early p puberty appearance of secondary sexual characteristics before age of 8 years in the girls and age 9 in boys

precocity (pre-kos'i-te) unusually early or rapid development of physical or mental traits

precognition (pre-kog-nish'un) an extrasensory perception of a future event

precoital (pre-ko'i-tal) before sexual intercourse

precoma (pre-ko'ma) before coma

preconscious (pre-kon'shus) a psyche wherein the past experiences and memory impressions can be consciously recalled

preconvulsive (pre'kon-vul'siv) before an epileptic seizure

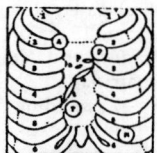

Precordia: Position of valves and auscultatory areas

Valves: tricuspid (t) mitral (m) aortic (a) pulmonary (p)

areas: tricuspid (T) mitral (M) aortic (A) pulmonary (P)

precordia (pre-kor'de-a) the anterior surface of the lower part of the chest and the epigastrium

precordial (pre-kor'de-al) relating to the precordia

precornu (pre-kor'nu) the anterior horn of the lateral ventricle of the brain

precose an alpha-glycosidase inhibitor that reduces postprandial glucose levels

precostal (pre-kos'tal) in front of the ribs

precuneus (pre-ku'ne-us) a divison of the medial surface of a cerebral hemisphere between the cuneus and paracentral lobule

precursor (pre-ker'ser) 1. anything that precedes another 2. a substance synthesised from another

predentin the organic fibrillar matrix of the dentin prior to calcification

prediabetes (pre-di'a-be'tez) condition prior to the development of diabetes

prediastole (pre'di-as'to-le) the interval in the cardiac rhythm immediately before diastole

prediastolic (pre'di-a-stol'ik) relating to the interval before diastole

predicrotic (pre'di-krot'ik) preceding the dicrotic wave of the sphygmographic tracing

predigestion (pre-di-jes'chun) artificial digestion of proteins and starches before ingestion

predisposition (pre'dis-pozish'un) a tendency or susceptibility to a disease

prednisolone (pred-nis'o-lon) synthetic glucocorticoid with minimum mineral activity

prednisone (pred'ni-son) synthetic glucocorticoid that is converted to prednisolone in the body

preductal coarctation constriction of the aorta above the ductus arteriosus resulting in cyanosis of the lower half of the body.

preeclampsia (pre'e-klamp'se-a) a triad of oedema, proteinuria and hypertension during pregnancy and it may be progressive, presenting increased risk to the foetus and mother

preembryo egg in early embryogenesis, used in *in vitro* fertilisation

preeruption (pre'e-rup'shun) 1. before an eruption 2. stage of tooth eruption when the tooth bud is in the bony socket

preexcitation (pre-ek'si-ta'shun) premature activation of a portion of the ventricle by the impulses transmitted along an accessory pathway

prefrontal (pre-fron'tal) situated in the anterior part of the frontal lobe or region **p leucotomy** extensive division of white matter of frontal lobes to reduce tension in schizophrenia

preganglionic (pre'gang-le-on'ik) situated proximal to or preceding a ganglion

pregenital (pre-jen'i-tal) before the emergence of normal adult sexual impulses

pregnancy (preg'nan-se) gestation; the state of a woman after conception until the birth of the baby **abdominal p** implantation and development of the ovum in the peritoneal cavity **ampullary p** tubal pregnancy in the ampulla of the fallopian tube **bigeminal p** pregnancy with twins in utero **cervical p** implantation of the ovum in cervical canal **cornual p** development of impregnated ovum in one of the cornua of the uterus **ectopic p** development of an impregnated ovum outside the cavity of the uterus **false p** pseudocyesis **heterotropic p** combined intrauterine and extrauterine pregnancies **high risk p** pregnancy with coexisting diseases causing a greater risk to the health of the mother, embryo or both **hydatid p** pregnancy leading to the development of hydatidiform mole **intraligamentary p** ectopic pregnancy within the broad ligament **intramural p** development of the fertilised ovum in the uterine portion of the fallopian tube **membranous p** embryo lying in direct contact with the uterine wall **molar p** ovum developing into a mole instead of an embryo **multiple p** presence of two or more foetuses simultaneously in the uterus **ovarian p** development of a fertilised ovum in an ovarian follicle **postdate p** pregnancy that extends beyond 42 weeks of gestation **tubal p** development of embryo in the fallopian tube **tuboabdominal p** development of an ectopic pregnancy partly in the tube and partly in the abdominal cavity **tuboovarian p** development of the fertilised ovum at the fimbriated end of the fallopian tube and involving ovary **uteroabdominal p** twin pregnancy with one embryo developing in the uterus and other in the abdominal cavity

pregnandiol (preg'nan-di'ol) product of progesterone excreted in urine, the amount is markedly increased in late pregnancy

pregnanetriol (preg'nan-tri'ol) a urinary metabolite of 17-hydroxy progesterone that is biologically inactive

pregnenolone (preg-nen'o-lon) an intermediate in the synthesis of steroid hormone

pregnant (preg'nant) gravid; referring a female carrying within her the product of conception

pregnane (preg'nen) parent hydrocarbon of steroids

pregravidic (pre-gra-vid'ik) before pregnancy

prehallux (pre-hal'uks) a supernumerary bone growing from medial border of scaphoid

prehemiplegic (pre'hem-i-ple'jik) before an attack of hemiplegia

prehensile (pre-hen'sil) adapted for grasping or holding

prehormone a secretion of an endocrine gland having no inherent biological potency

prehyoid (pre-hi'oyd) in front of the hyoid bone

prehypophysis (pre'hi-pof'i-sis) the anterior lobe of the pituitary gland

preictal (pre-ik'tal) before a convulsion or stroke

preicteric (pre-ik-ter'ik) before appearance of jaundice

preinvasive (pre'in-va'siv) a state of malignancy in which metastasis has not taken place **p carcinoma** carcinoma *in-situ*

Preiser's disease aseptic necrosis of scaphoid bone, named after Georg Preiser, German radiologist

preleukaemia presence of increased numbers of immature cells in the blood or bone marrow

preload extent of stretch of heart muscle immediately before systole

prelymphoma condition with monotonous aggregates of lymphocytes with a tendency to evolve to lymphoma

premalignancy any lesion with a tendency to undergo malignant degeneration

premaniacal (pre'ma-ni'a-kal) before the attack of mania

premature (pre-ma-chur) 1. born before 37th week, but mature enough to survive 2. occurring before the usual or expected time **p rupture of membranes** the occurrence of rupture of amniotic membranes in pregnancy, before the time of labour expected **p ventricular contraction** contraction of ventricle prior to the normal time due to premature discharge of a ventricular ectopic focus. It may be isolated or frequent and the abnormal pattern may be similar in morphology in ECG if it is unifocal or show varying morphology if multifocal

prematurity an infant delivered before 37 weeks of gestation, who is often also immature

premaxilla (pre'mak-sil'a) an element from medial nasal process, earlier called incisive bone, fusing with the maxilla

premaxillary (pre-mak'si-ler'e) before the maxilla

premedication (pre'med-i-ka'shun) drugs administered in preparation for anaesthesia

premelanosome an oval structure with a dense grainy matrix and cross striations of melanocytes.

premenarchal (pre'me-nar'kal) before establishment of menstruation

premenstrual (pre-men'stroo-al) relating to the period before menstruation **p**

dysphoric disorder occurrence of depressed mood, anxiety, marked affective lability and decreased interest in activities before menstruation **p tension syndrome** premenstrual dysphoric disorder

premenstruum (pre-men'stroo-um) the period preceding menstruation

premolar (pre-mo'ler) 1. anterior to a molar tooth 2. a bicuspid tooth

premonition (pre-me-nish'um) a feeling of what is going to happen; presentiment

premonitory (pre-mon'i-to-re) giving warning or notice before hand

premonocyte an immature monocyte

premorbid (pre-mor'bid) before development of disease

premunition immunity against major infectious disease due to persistent subclinical infection

premyeloblast (pre-mi'e-lo-blast) the earliest precursor of the myelocyte

premyelocyte (pre-mi'el-o-sit) promyelocyte, precursor of myelocyte

prenarcosis (pre-nar-ko'sis) premedication

prenatal (pre-na'tl) antenatal; preceding birth **p care** care of the woman during pregnancy **p diagnosis** diagnosis of a disease or malformation while the foetus in utero **p surgery** interauterine surgical procedures

preoperative before undertaking surgery **p care** care of the patient before operative procedure

preoptic (pre-op'tik) in front of the optic chiasma

preoral (pre-o'ral) in front of the mouth

prep preparation for surgery

prepalatal (pre-pal'a-tal) in front of the teeth

preparalytic (pre-par-a-lit'ik) before the manifestation of paralysis

preparation (prep-a-ra'shun) making ready before hand such as medicine for use, patient for operation, or specimen set up for demonstration

prepatellar (pre'pa-tel'ar) in front of the patella **p bursitis** inflammation of prepatellar bursa; house maid's knee

prepatent before becoming evident or manifest **p period** an interval between infection and demonstration of organisms

preperception (pre'per-sep'shun) before being perceived by means of the senses

preperitoneal (pre'per-i-to-ne'al) in front of the peritoneum

preplacental (pre'pla-sen'tal) occurring before formation of the placenta

prepotent (pre-po'tent) an ability possessed by one parent in greater degree than the other, of transmitting heritable characteristics to the progeny

preprandial (pre-pran'de-al) before a meal

preprotein an inactive precursor of a secretory protein

prepubertal (pre-pu'ber-tal) before puberty

prepubescent (pre'pu-bes'ent) immediately before the beginning of puberty

prepuce (pre'pus) foreskin; the free fold of skin that covers the glans penis

preputial (pre-pu'shal) relating to prepuce **p gland** modified sebaceous gland on the inner surface of prepuce secreting smegma **p sinus** space between foreskin and glans

preputium (pre-pu'she-um) prepuce **p clitoridis** the external fold of the labia minora forming a cap over the clitoris

prepyloric (pre'pi-lor'ik) just proximal to the pylorus

prerectal (pre-rek'tal) in front of the rectum

prerenal (pre-re'nal) in front of the kidney **p failure** uraemia due to loss of excretory function of healthy kidney, due to inadequate perfusion from decreased volume of blood or fall in blood pressure

preretinal (pre ret'i-nal) between retina and vitreous **p haemorrhage** large haemorrhage near optic disc with meniscus

presacral (pre-sa'kral) in front of the sacrum **p plexus** superior hypogastric sympathetic plexus in front of first lumbar vertebra

presby - combining word for old

presbyacusia (prez'be-a-ku'se-a) loss of ability to perceive or discriminate sounds with ageing

presbyatrics (prez-be-at'riks) geriatrics

presbycardia (prez-bi-kar'de-a) impaired cardiac function due to ageing

presbycusis (prez-bi-ku'sis) presbyacusia

presbyopia (prez-be-o'pe-a) age-related loss of range of visual accommodation

presbyopic (pres'be-op'ik) relating to or having presbyopia

presbyatrics (prez'bi-at'riks) geriatrics

prescribe (pre-skrib) to give directions for the preparation and administration of a medication

prescription (pre-skrip'shun) 1. a written direction for the preparation and administration of any medication 2. a medicinal preparation compounded according to directions. It consists of subscription (to take, with symbol R_x), inscription (ingredients), subscription (direction regarding preparation) and signature (direction on the manner of taking and signature of the prescribing physician)

presenile (pre-se'nil) exhibiting presenility

presenility (pre'se-nil'i-ti) premature old age

presenium (pre-se'ne-um) just before the onset of senility

present appear; to introduce into the presence of; to lay before for examination

presentation (pre-zen-ta'shun) 1. lie 2. the position of the foetus presenting itself to the examining finger of obstetrician 3. the relationship of the long axis of the foetus to that of the mother antigen p presentation of antigen at the surface of macrophages to lymphocytes for induction of an immune response breech p presentation of the foetal buttocks in labour. It may be complete (thighs of the foetus flexed on the abdomen and legs flexed upon the thighs), frank (legs extended against the trunk and feet lying against the face) or incomplete (prolapse of the feet or knees into maternal vagina) brow p presentation of foetal brow or face in labour cephalic p pres-

entation of any part of the foetal head during labour compound p prolapse of an extremity of the foetus along side the head in cephalic presentation or arm alongside the breech at the commencement of the labour face p presentation of face footling p presentation of the feet funic p presentation of umbilical cord in labour longitudinal p presentation in which the long axis of the foetus is parallel to the long axis of the mother oblique p presentation in which the long axis of the foetus is oblique to that of the mother pelvic p breech presentation placental p placenta praevia shoulder p presentation of the foetal shoulder during labour vertex p presentation of the upper and back portion of foetal head in labour

preservative (pre-zer'va-tiv) a substance that is added to the medicines or foods to prevent them from spoiling

presomite (pro-so'mit) an embryonic stage before the appearance of somites

presphenoid (pre-sfe'noyd) the anterior portion of the body of the sphenoid bone

presphygmic (pre-sfig'mik) preceding the pulse beat

prespinal (pre-spi'nal) in front of the spine

prespondylolisthesis (pre-spon'dil-o-lis-the'sis) a congenital abnormality of the pedicles of the fifth lumbar vertebra leading to spondylolisthesis

pressor (pres'or) 1. exciting to vasomotor activity 2. producing increased blood pressure

pressoreceptive (pres'o-re-sep'tiv) sensitive to pressure stimuli

pressoreceptor (pres'o-re-sep'tor) baroreceptor responding to changes in blood pressure, found in the aorta and carotid sinus

pressure (presh'ur) 1. a stress or force acting against resistance 2. the force per unit area exerted by a gas or liquid against the walls of its container atmospheric p pressure of the weight of the atmosphere which at the sea level is 760 mmHg **back p** pressure exerted upstream in the circulation due to obstruction for forward flow **blood p** the tension of the blood within the arteries maintained by the left ventricular contraction, resistance of the arterioles and capillaries, elasticity of the arterial walls, viscosity and volume of the blood **capillary p** blood pressure in the capillaries **central venous p** (CVP) the pressure of blood within the vena cavae, and the right atrium. Normally it is between 4 and 10 cm of water **cerebrospinal p** pressure of cerebrospinal fluid, it is normally 100 to 150 mm of water **diastolic p** the lowest blood pressure reached during ventricular cycle **effective osmotic p** that part of the total osmotic pressure of a solution that determines the tendency of its solvent to pass across a boundary **end diastolic p** blood pressure in a ventricle of the heart at the end of diastole **hydrostatic p** the pressure exerted by a fluid within a closed container **intraabdominal p** pressure within the abdominal cavity **intracranial p** the pressure of CSF in the subarachnoid space between the skull and the brain **intraocular p** the pressure of the intraocular fluid within the eye, approximately 12 to 20 mm Hg **intrapleural p** pressure between two pleural membranes which is normally negative, lower than atmosphere **occlusal p** biting pressure **oncotic p** osmotic pressure exerted by the colloids in solution **osmotic p** pressure that must be applied to a solution to prevent the passage into it of a solvent when in solution **partial p** the pressure exerted by a single component of gases. It is expressed in mm of Hg or torr **Positive end-expiratory pressure** (PEEP) maintenance of positive pressure constantly in the airways on ventilator **pulmonary capillary wedge p** (PCWP) left atrial pressure obtained by wedging a catheter into a small pulmonary artery **pulse p** the difference between systolic and diastolic pressure **systolic p** the highest blood pressure reached during ventricular cycle

pressure point a location used for exertion of pressure to control bleeding

pressure ring site of constriction in strangulation

pressure sore a bed sore; a decubital ulcer appearing on dependent sites usually on lumbosacral region, most common in bed-ridden elderly persons

presternum (pre-ster'num) manubrium sterni

presuppurative (pre-sup'u-ra'tiv) an early stage in an inflammation before the formation of pus

presylvian (pre'sil've-an) **fissure** the anterior division of the sylvian fissure

presymptomatic (pre'sim-to-mat'ik) the state of health before the manifestations of a disease

presynaptic (pre'si-nap'tik) situated or occurring proximal to a synapse **p knob** swelling of axon end in contact with synaptic cleft

presyncope fainting

presystole (pre-sis'to-le) late diastole; relating to the period immediately before systole

presystolic (pre-sis-tol'ik) late diastolic; relating to the period immediately before systole

pretarsal (pre-tar'sal) anterior or inferior portion of tarsus

preterm premature; occurring prior to the 37th week of gestation **p birth** delivery occurring between 20 and 38 weeks of gestation **p labour** labour that begins between 20 and 38 weeks of gestation

pretibial (pre-tib'e-al) in front of the tibia **p fever** leptospirosis **p myxoedema** a red-brown infiltration on the shins which can become lumpy and tender, in hyperthyroidism

pretympanic (pre'tim-pan'ik) situated in front of the tympanic membrane

preurethritis (pre'u-re-thri'tis) inflammation around the urethral orifice of the vaginal vestibule

prevalence (prev'a-lens) the number of existing cases of a disease in a given population at a specific time. It is obtained by the number of cases of a disease divided by the total number of subjects in a population **point p** the number of all current cases of a disease at a point of time in relation to a defined population **period p** the frequency of all current cases existing during a defined period of time

prevention act of preventing **primary p** interventions prior to the onset of the disease preventing the possibility of occurrence of the disease **secondary p** interventions halting the progression of the disease at its incipient stage and preventing complications **tertiary p** interventions reducing impairments and disabilities from the disease

preventive (pre-ven'tiv) 1. prophylactic 2. anything that causes arrest of threatened onset of a disease **p medicine** organised activities of the community to prevent occurrence as well as progression of disease and disability and timely application of all means to promote health of individuals and of the community as a whole

prevertebral (pre-ver'te-bral) in front of a vertebrta

prevertiginous (pre-ver-tij'i-nus) a tendency to fall forward

prevesical (pre-vesi'kl) anterior to the bladder

previa (pre've-a) praevia

previable not sufficiently mature to survive

previus (pre'vi-us) refers to anything obstructing the passages in child birth

prezonular pertaining to the space between the iris and suspensory ligament in the posterior chamber

prezygote occurring before completion of fertilisation

priapism (pri'a-pizm) prolonged and unusually painful penile erection occurring in the absence of sexual excitement or desire

priapitis (pri-a-pi'tis) inflammation of the penis

priapus (pri'a-pus) the penis

prickle cell keratinocyte

prickly heat miliaria; papular itching eruption of the skin due to blockage of sweat ducts

prick test a test for immediate hypersensitivity in which a diluted allergen is placed on the skin and a sterile needle is used to prick the epidermal surface

priest's knee infrapatellar bursitis

primal 1. primary or first 2. primordia

primaquine (prim'a-kwin) 8 aminoquinoline, antimalarial agent, active against exoerythrocytic parasites, used in eradication of parasites

primary (pri-ma-re) first 1. original seat of disease 2. not secondary to anything known **p aldosteronism** Conn's syndrome **p amenorrhoea** never having menstruated **p apnoea** absence of breath in first minutes of birth **p autonomic dysfunction** a disorder of autonomic nervous system characterised by postural hypotension, decreased sweating, heat intolerance, gastrointestinal symptoms, impotence, urinary and faecal incontinence **p bile acids** cholic and chenodeoxycholic acids formed by the liver **p biliary cirrhosis** a progressive destruction of bile ducts eventually leading to cirrhosis. It may be asymptomatic or present with pruritus, jaundice and hepatomegaly **p bubo** an inflammed lymph node occurring as initial lesion in syphilis **p care** least specialised level of medical care rendered by a primary physician **p chancre** initial sore of syphilis **p complex** tuberculous lesion at a subpleural location, often in the middle to lower zones of the lung, draining lymphatics of the area and regional lymph nodes **p dysmenorrhoea** spasmodic painful menstruation noted soon after menarche **p haemorrhage** bleeding from wound **p health care** the first level contact between the individual and health system where essential health care is provided **p hydrocephalus** obstructive hydrocephalus **p hypertension** essential hypertension **p infertility** having never achieved pregnancy **p optic atrophy** a condition without any preceding ophthalmic changes, where disc margins are clear and disc is pale **p polycythaemia** erythraemia **p response** the response exhibited by the immune system when it is exposed to an antigen **p sore** original site of infection as in chancre of syphilis **p tuberculosis** lesions due to an infection with *M. tuberculosis* in individuals who have never had previous experience with tubercle bacilli **p tumour** malignant growth at site of origin

primate (pri'mat) an individual of the order primates including man, apes, monkeys and lemures

prime (prim) 1. first in order of time, rank of importance 2. full health and strength 3. an initial treatment that is carried out before administering a large dose of the same or different medicine

prime-boost an immunization strategy to boost the immune response, which uses two different vaccines, each of which includes the same protein from a pathogen that the immune system will target and remember

primed having undergone initial exposure, there is likelihood of production of immune reaction on re-exposure in the cells of immune system

primer a short oligonucleotide segment which pairs with a complementary single-stranded DNA sequence

primidone (prim'i-don) an antiepileptic agent

primigravida (pri-mi-grav'i-da) a woman who is pregnant for the first time **elderly p** a woman who is 35 years of age or above becoming pregnant for the first time

primipara (pri-mip'ara) a woman who has given birth for the first time to an infant or infants

primiparous (pri-mip'a-rus) denoting a primipara

primitive (pri'mi-tiv) structures in the earliest stage of development

primordial (pri-mor'de-al) 1. relating to primordium 2. primitive

primordium (pri-mor'de-um) earliest recognisable embryological stage

primum non nocere (pri'mum non no'sere) as foremost consideration, do not make matters worse

princeps (prin'seps) 1. principal; chief 2. name of certain arteries

principal (prin'si-pal) 1. chief 2. principal of a school or college

principle (prin'si-pl) 1. force 2. essential ingredient in a drug or chemical compound 3. a law of conduct

Prinzmetal's angina anginal attacks at rest with ST elevation, due probably to coronary spasm, named after Myron Prinzmetal, US cardiologist

prion (pre'on) non-nucleic acid protein, apparently capable of reproduction without DNA or RNA infective agent of slow viruses **p diseases** neurological diseases developing many months or years after infection with prions. They bring about neuronal loss, spongiform change and gliosis with deposition of a characteristic prion protein. The examples of the diseases are Kuru, and Creutzfeldt-Jokob disease

prism (prizm) a transparent solid whose ends are similar, equal and parallel planes and whose sides are parallelograms

prismatic (priz-mat'ik) resembling or pertaining to a prism

prismoid (priz'moyd) resembling a prism

privacy 1. secrecy 2. respect for the confidential nature of the physician-patient relationship

private practice the practice by a physician or dentist practising independently under state licencing laws

previleged sites sites where no immune reaction to graft occurs, such as cartilage and cornea

p.r.n. pro re nata as needed; as circumstances may require

pro - prefix denoting before, forward; in front of; for; from

proaccelerin clotting factor V, on activation it accelerates conversion of prothrombin to thrombin

proactivator (pre-ak'ti-va-tor) a fragment obtained on chemically splitting a substance capable of rendering another substance chemically active

proagglutinoid (pro'a-gloo'ti-noyd) an agglutinoid with a greater affinity for the agglutinogen

proal (pro'al) concerning to forward movement

proantithrombin (pro'an-ti-throm'bin) a substance found in the blood which gets converted into antithrombin by heparin

proarrhythmia a situation likely to lead for development of an arrhythmia

probability *stat* proportion of positive results to be expected if trial were repeated any number of times

proband the affected individual from which a pedigree is constructed

probang (pro'bang) a flexible thin rod with a sponge attached to the end useful for application of medicine and to determine the site of stricture

probationer (pro-ba'shun-er) one who is on probation, before confirmation of his service

probe (prob) 1., a single stranded segment of DNA/RNA which is labelled with a radioactive substance or chemical and it will bind to its complementary single-stranded target sequence 2. a slender rod with a blunt bulbous tip; used for exploring an open body part

probenecid 1. uricosuric agent used in gout 2. concomitant use with benzyl penicillin, raises the blood levels of penicillin by delaying its excretion by the kidney

problem-based learning (PBL) the learning that results from the process of working towards the understanding or resolution of a problem

problem-based medical curriculum integration of basic medical sciences across disciplines and early patient contract in a longitudinal course

problem-oriented medical record a formally organised medical record containing the details of the patient's conditions, often organised in the form of subjective criteria, and objective criteria

probucol anticholesteraemic agent, increasing excretion of bile

procainamide a cardiac depressant used in arrhythmias especially originating in the ventricle

procaine (pro'kan) **hydrochloride** short-acting local anaesthetic

procaine penicillin long acting procaine benzyl penicillin.

procarbazine (pro-kar'ba-zen) cytotoxic agent inhibiting DNA synthesis

procarcinogen substance converted to carcinogen in body

procaryote (pro-kar'e-ot) prokaryote

procaspid (pro-kap'sid) a protein shell lacking a virus genome

procedure (pro-se'dur) act or conduct of a treatment or an operation **universal p** a strategy for controlling infection in which medical professionals use gloves and other protective equipments while in contact with every patient

procentriole (pro-sen'tre-ol) the early stage in the development of centrioles from the centrosphere

procephalic (pro'se-fal'ik) relating to the anterior part of the head

procercoid (pro-ser'koyd) the first larval stage of cestodes following ingestion of the newly hatched larva (coracidium) by a water flea

procerus muscle a muscle arising from the skin over the nose. It is connected to the forehead. It draws the eyebrows down

process (pros'es) 1. a prominence or projection as from a bone 2. a method of action 3. progress, as of a disease

processing changing a latent film image into a visible image, as in radiology by using a developer, fixer, washer and dryer

processor 1. an automatic machine used in radiology that helps in the conversion of latent image into a visible image 2. the central processing unit (CPU) of a computer

processus (pro-ses'us) process **p vaginalis** peritoneal outpouching that precedes descent of testis and it becomes tunica vaginalis with rest being obliterated

procheilon (pro-ki'lon) a prominence in the central portion of the upper lip

prochlorperazine a phenothiazine drug used in the treatment of nausea and vomiting

prochondral (pro-kon'dral) a developmental stage before the formation of cartilage

prochordal (pro-kor'dal) in front of the notochord

procidentia (pro'si-den'she-a) a prolapse of any organ or part as in uterus

proclination outward inclination, as of teeth

proclivity natural tendency, bent, inclination, learning

procollagen (pro-kol'a-jen) precursor of collagen

proconversion (pro'kon-ver'tin) clotting factor VII

procreate (pro'kre-at) to beget; to produce by sexual act

procreation (pro'kre-a'shun) reproduction

proctagra (prok'tag'ra) sudden pain in the rectum

proctalgia (prok-tal'je-a) pain in the anus or in the rectum **p fugax** brief attacks of severe pain in rectal region

proctectasia (prok'tek-ta'se-a) dilatation of anus or rectum

proctectomy (prok-tek'to-mi) surgical resection of the rectum

proctenclisis (prok'ten-kli'sis) stricture of anus or rectum

procteurynter (prok'tu-rin'ter) an inflatable bag for dilating the rectum

proctitis (prok-ti'tis) inflammation of the mucous membrane of the rectum

proct (o) combining word for anus, rectum

proctocoele (prok'to-sel) prolapse or herniation of the rectum

proctocylisis (prok-tok'li-sis) infusion of fluid such as saline into rectum

proctococcypexia (prok'to-kok-si-pek'se-a) suture of a prolapsing rectum to the structures in front of coccyx

proctocolectomy (prok'to-ko-lek'to-mi) surgical resection of the rectum and part or all of the colon

proctocolitis (prok'to-ko-li'tis) inflammation of the rectum and colon

proctocolonoscopy (prok'to-ko'lon-os'kope) inspection of interior of rectum and colon

proctocolpoplasty (-kol'po-plas'ti) surgical closure of a rectovaginal fistula

proctocystoplasty (prok'to-sis-to-plas'te) surgical closure of rectovesical fistula

proctocystotomy (prok'to-sis-tot'o-me) incision into the bladder through the rectum

proctodeum (prok-to-de'um) anal pit; an ectodermally lined depression at the terminal portion of embryonic hindgut from which anal and urogenital external orifices are developed

proctodynia (prok'to-din'e-a) pain in the rectum or anus

proctologic (prok'to-loj'ik) relating to proctology

proctologist (prok'tol'o-jist) a person specialised in the diseases of colon, rectum and anus

proctology (prok-tol'o-je) a surgical speciality concerned with the diseases of colon, rectum and anus

proctoparalysis (prok'to-par-al'i-sis) paralysis of the anal sphincter leading to incontinence of faeces

proctoperineoplasty (prok'to-per'i-ne'o-plas'te) plastic surgery of anus and rectum

proctoperineorrhaphy (-per'i-ne-or'a-fe) proctoperineoplasty

proctopexy (-pek'se) surgical fixation of a prolapsing rectum

proctoplasty (-plas'te) plastic surgery of the anus or of the rectum proctoptosis (prok'top-to'sis) prolapse of the rectum and anus

proctorrhagia (prok'to-ra'je-a) bleeding from the rectum

proctorrhaphy (prok-tor'a-fe) suturing of a rectum or anus

proctorrhoea (prok-tor-e'a) a mucus discharge from the rectum

proctoscope (prok'to-skop) a speculum for inspection of the rectum

proctoscopy (prok'tos'ko-pe) inspection of the rectum with proctoscope

procotosigmoidectomy (prok'to-sig'moy-dek'to-me) excision of the rectum and sigmoid colon

proctosigmoiditis (-sig'moyd-i-tis) inflammation of rectum and sigmoid colon

proctosigmoidoscopy (-os'ko-pe) inspection of rectum and sigmoid colon through sigmoidoscope

proctospasm (prok'to-spazm) spasmodic contraction of the rectum

proctostasis (prok'to-sta'sis) constipation due to failure of rectum to defecation stimulus

proctostenosis (prok'to-sten-o'sis) stricture of the rectum or anus

proctostomy (prok-tos'to-me) surgical creation of an artificial opening into the rectum

proctotome (prok'to-tom) a knife for incision into the rectum

proctotresia (prok-to-tro'se-a) surgical correction of an imperforate anus

proctovalvotomy (prok'to-val-vot'o-me) incision of rectal valves

procurement the process of obtaining organs for transplantation

procumbent (pro-kum'bent) in a prone position; lying face down

procursive (pro-kur'sive) an involuntary tendency to run forward

procurvation (pro'kur-va'shun) bending forward

procyclidine anticholinergic agent used in the treatment of Parkinsonism

prodromal (pro-dro'mal) pertaining to the early stage of a disease

prodrome (pro'drom) an early or premonitory symptom of a disease

prodrug a substance which requires metabolic transformation into active form in the body

product (prod'ukt) anything made or produced

production (pro-duk'shun) development of a substance either naturally or artificially

productive (pro-duk'tiv) producing or capable of producing

proencephalus (pro'en-sef'a-lus) a deformed foetus with brain protruding through a fissure in the frontal region

proenzyme (pro-en'zim) inactive precursor of an enzyme, requiring some change to make it active; zymogen

proerythroblast (pro'e-rith'ro-blast) earliest recognisable cell of red cell series

proerythrocyte an immature red cell with a nucleus, precursor of an erythrocyte

proestrus (pro-es'trus) development of ovarian follicles and endometrium preceding estrus

professional (pro-fesh'un-al) 1. pertaining to a profession 2. a person who is a specialist in a particular field

profibrinolysin (pro'fi-bri-no-li'sin) plasminogen

profile (pro'fil) 1. a group of screening tests selected to establish a baseline and to get maximum diagnostic information 2. a cross-sectional aggregation of health care data applied to any segment

profilin a protein found in platelets and neutrophils that regulates the length of actin filaments involved in bringing about changes in cell shape in carcinogenesis and thrombogenesis

profluvium (pro-floo've-um) an increased flow or discharge

profunda deeply located

profundus (pro-fun'dus) deep

progastrin (pro-gas'trin) inactive precursor of gastrin

progenitor (pro-jen'itor) an ancestor; a precursor

progeny (proj'e-ne) offspring; descendents

progeria (pro-je're-a) a condition characterised by markedly premature ageing of childhood onset, in which the morbid conditions encountered in elderly are noted during puberty and death from old age occurs by 20

progestational (pro'jes-ta'shun-al) a phase of menstrual cycle prior to menstruation when endometrium is fully prepared for implantation of a fertilised ovum

progesterone (pro-jes'ter-on) steroid hormone of secretory phase of menstrual cycle

progestin (pro-jes'tin) any natural or synthetic compound with progesterone-like activity

progestogen (pro-jes'to-jen) a hormonal substance that produces effects similar to those due to progesterone

proglossis (pro-glos'is) tip of the tongue

proglottid (pro-glot'id) one of the segments of a tapeworm containing the reproductive organs

proglottis (pro-glot'tis) pl. **proglottides** proglottid

prognathic (prog-na'thick) 1. having a projecting jaw 2. referring to a forward projection of either or both of the jaws

prognathism (prog'na-thizm) the condition of being prognathic

prognathous (prog'na-thus) prognathic

prognose (prog-nos) to predict the course of the disease

prognosis (prog-no'sis) to forecast the outcome of the disease

prognosticate (prog-nos'ti-at) to give a prognosis

prognostic scoring system; an analytic system attempting to predict outcome of the condition

program a plan giving the outline of the procedure

programmed killing selective destruction of the neurones that are overproduced in early brain development

progranulocyte (pro-gran'u-lo-sit) promyelocyte

progravid (pro-grav'id) preceding pregnancy

progress the sequence of events of an ongoing disease process

progression (pro-gresh'un) moving forward

progressive (pro-gres'iv) advancing, referring to a disease from bad to worse **p bulbar palsy** lower motor neuron palsy affecting ninth, tenth, eleventh and twelfth cranial nerves producing dysphagia and dysarthria. The tongue is wasted and fasciculating **p massive fibrosis** the nodular densities in silicosis becoming larger leading to contraction of the upper lobes, presenting with progressive dyspnoea, cough and respiratory failure **p muscular atrophy** motor neuron disease affecting predominantly spinal motor neurones, with weakness and wasting of distal muscles, fasciculations and absence of tendon jerks

proguanil antimalarial used chiefly in prophylaxis

prohormone (pro-hor'mon) immediate precursor of active hormone **p systemic sclerosis** systemic sclerosis

proinsulin precursor of insulin consisting of A and B chains linked by C-peptide

projection 1. the act of throwing forward 2. a prominence 3. the referring of sensation to the object producing it 4. localisation of visual impressions 5. the act of extending 6. an unconscious defence mechanism

projectile vomiting violent vomiting without antecedent nausea, occurring in conditions with raised intracranial tension

prokaryon (pro-kar'e-on) nuclear material scattered throughout the cytoplasm of the cell and is not bounded by a cell membrane

prokaryote (pro-kar'e-ot) bacteria and certain algae with cells that are not nucleated

prolabium (pro-la'be-um) the prominent central part of the upper lip

prolactin (pro-lak'tin) anterior pituitary hormone concerned with maintenance of lactation

prolactinoma a pituitary adenoma that produces prolactin

prolapse (pro-laps) abnormal descent of a structure, usually within or into cavity due to laxity of its attachments **p of cord** appearance of umbilical cord in vagina before birth of child

prolapsus prolapse

prolepsis (pro-lep'sis) recurrence of the paroxysm at successively shorter intervals

proleptic relating to prolepsis

proleucocyte an undeveloped leucocyte

prolidase enzyme splitting proline and hydroxy proline dipeptides

proliferate (pro-lif'er-at) to increase by reproduction of similar forms

proliferation (pro-lif'er-a'shun) growth and reproduction of similar forms

proliferative phase preovulation phase of the menstrual cycle where the endometrium undergoes regeneration in preparation for implantation of an egg **p endometrium** active growth of endometrium from end of menstruation to the time of ovulation and it pertains to oestrogen phase of active growth **p retinopathy** a complication of diabetes with growth of new vessels increasing the chance of risk of haemorrhage or retinal detachment

proliferous reproductive, increasing the number of similar tissue cells

prolific reproductive

proline (pro-len) amino acid derived from glutamic acid

prolymphocyte (pro'limf'o-sit) an intermediate cell between a lymphoblast and a lymphocyte

PROM premature rupture of membranes leading to leakage of amniotic fluid prior to the onset of labour

promazine (pro'ma-zen) antipsychotic and antiemetic agent

promegakaryocyte (pro-meg'a-kar'e-o-sit) a precursor of a megakaryocyte

promegaloblast (pro-meg'a-lo-blast) a cell of erythrocyte series preceding the megaloblast

prometaphase (pro-met'a-faz) the stage of mitosis in which the nuclear membrane undergoes disintegration, and chromosomes move toward the equatorial plate.

promethazine (pro-meth'a-zen) antihistamine agent

prominence (prom'i-nens) a projection or protrusion

prominentia (prom'i-nen'she-a) a projection

promonocyte (pro-mon'o-sit) an intermediate cell between a monoblast and a monocyte

promontory (prom'on-tor'e) 1. bulge above the oval window in the middle ear, marking the basal turn of cochlea 2. upper anterior edge of first sacral segment

promoter (pro-mo'ter) 1. the site on the DNA double helix where RNA polymerases bind and initiate gene transcription 2. a substance that helps a catalyst to act

prompt acting with alacrity

promyelocyte (pro-mi'e-lo-sit) early precursor of granulocytes

pronasion (pro-na'zi-on) the point of the angle between the septum of the nose and the surface of upper lip

pronate (pro'nat) to assume or to place in a prone position

pronation (pro-na'shun) the act of assuming or of being placed in a prone position

pronator a muscle which turns a part into prone position **p syndrome** entrapment of median nerve at the elbow with pain in the wrist, paresthesia of the hand and tenderness of proximal thenar muscles

pronaus (pro-na'us) the vagina

prone (pron) 1. lying face downward 2. denoting a hand with the palm or a foot with sole turned downward

pronephric (pro-nef'rik) pertaining to the pronephros

pronephros (pro-nef'ros) the primordial kidney consisting of a series of tortuous tubules emptying into the cloaca by a primary nephric duct

prong 1. the spike of a fork or similar instrument 2. a cone-shaped body such as the root of a tooth

pronometer (pro-nom'e-ter) a device to determine the extent of pronation and supination of the forearm

pronormoblast (pro-nor'mo-blast) proerythroblast, the earliest stage in the development of normoblast

pronucleus (pro-nu'kle-us) the nuclear material of the sperm or of the ovum after fertilisation of the ovum; each carriesa haploid number of chromosomes

prootic (pro-ot'ik) in front of the ear

prop a metal frame used to give support; anything on which body rests for supports, as of pillows

propalinal (pro-pal'i-nal) a backward and forward movement, as of the jaws.

propane (pro'opan) $CH_3CH_2CH_3$; an alkane hydrocarbon found in natural gas

propantheline (pro-pan'the-len) an anticholinergic agent

propepsin (pro-pep'sin) pepsinogen

propeptone (pro-pep'ton) an intermediate product in the digestion of protein, which gets converted into peptone

properdin (pro-perd'in) a globulin fraction of serum that participates in the alternate pathway to activate the terminal components of complement

prophase (pro'faz) the first phase of mitosis or meiosis that consists of increase in thickness of chromosomes, division of centriole and migration of the two daughter centrioles toward either pole of the cell

prophylactic (pro-fi-lak'tik) 1. preventing disease 2. an agent that helps in the prevention of infection or disease

prophylaxis (pro-fi-lak'sis) the prevention of the disease

propionibacterium (pro-pi-on-i-bak-ter'i-um) a saprophytic gram-positive bacteria found in dairy products, on the skin and the intestinal tract and may be pathogenic

proplasmacyte (pro-plaz'ma-sit) precursor of the plasma cell

propositus (pro-poz'i-tus) 1. proband 2. a premise

propoxycaine (pro-pok'se-ken) a local anaesthetic

propoxyphane (-fen) an analgesic agent

propranolol a beta-adrenergic blocking agent used in the treatment of angina pectoris, cardiac arrhythmia and hypertension

proprietary name the patented name of the drug under which a manufacturer markets the product

proprioception (pro'pre-o-sep'shun) sensation pertaining to stimuli arising from within the body giving an awareness of posture, movements, and changes in the equilibrium

proprioceptor (pro'pre-o-sep'tor) one of a variety of sensory receptor that responds to stimuli originating within the body, as to pressure, position or stretch

proptometer (prop-tom'e-ter) an instrument for the measurement of proptosis

proptosis (prop-to'sis) a forward displacement of any organ, as in exophthalmus

propulsion (pro-pul'shun) a tendency to fall forward in walking , encountered in Parkinson's disease

propyl (pro'pil) the radical of propyl alcohol or propane, $CH_3CH_2CH_2$

propylene (prop'i-len) glycol; a colourless viscous liquid

propylhexedrine (pro'pil-hek'se-dren) a sympathomimetic agent decreasing nasal congestion

propylthiouracil (pro'pil-thi'o-u'ra-sil) an inhibitor of thyroid biosynthesis

pro re nata (pro-re-na'ta) (prn) L. as required

prorrhaphy (pro'ra-fe) insertion of a muscle or tendon to a point further away by surgery

prorsad (pror'sad) in a forward direction

prorubricyte (pro-roo'bri-sit) a basophilic normoblast

prosecretin (pro'se-kre-'tin) precursor of secretin found in the duodenal mucosa

prosection (pro-sek'shun) dissection of a cadaver or any part for an anatomical demonstration

prosector (pro-sek'tor) a person who dissects or prepares material for an anatomical demonstration

prosencephalon (pros'en-sef'a-lon) the embryonic forebrain which undergoes division into diencephalon and telencephalon

proso- combining word for forward, anterior

prosodemic (pros'o-dem'ik) refers to disease that is trasmitted directly from person to person

prosody (pros'a-de) the normal rhythm, melody and accent of speech

prosopagnosia (pros'o-pag-no'se-a) an inability to recognise familiar faces

prosopalgia (pros'o-pal'je-a) trigeminal neuralgia

prosopectasia (pro'o-pek-ta'ze-a) abnormal enlargement of the face

prosopic (pro'sop'ik) referring to the face that is convex anteriorly

prosoplasia (pros'o-pla'se-a) progressive transformation of cells

prosopodiplegia (pros'o-po-di-ple'je-a) bilateral facial paralysis

prosopodynia (pros'o-po-din'e-a) trigeminal neuralgia

prosoponeuralgia (pros'o-po-nu-ral'je-a) trigeminal neuralgia

prosopopagus (pros'o-pop'a-gus) an unequal conjoined twins in which the parasite is attached to some part of the upper face

prosopoplegia (pros'o-po-ple'je-a) facial paralysis

prosoposchisis (pros-o-pos'ki-sis) a congenital facial cleft

prosopospasm (pros'o-po-spazm) facial tic.

prosopotocia (pro'o-po-to'she-a) presentation of face in parturition

prospective study a study designed to determine the relationship between a condition and a characteristic shared by some members of a group

prospermia (pro-sper'mi-a) premature ejaculation

prostacyclin (pros-ta-si'klin) a derivator of prostaglandin that inhibits platelet aggregation and acts as a vasodilator

prostaglandin (-glan'din) (PG) oxidative metabolic product of arachidonic acid

by cyclooxygenase enzymes. The important examples are PGE_2, PGF_{2a}, PGD_2, PGI_2 (prostacyclin). Prostaglandins have a variety of biological effects and act as local intracellular or intercellular modulators of biochemical activity of the tissues in which they are formed

prostanoid (pros'ta-noid) any of a group of complex fatty acids derived from arachidonic acid that includes prostaglandins, prostanoic acid and the thromboxanes

prostalgia (pros-ta-ta'je-a) pain in the prostate gland

prostate (pros-tat) a gland having a median lobe and two lateral lobes surrounding the neck of the bladder and urethra in the male. It is partly muscular and partly glandular. The secretion from the gland drains into the prostatic portion of the urethra. The secretion is thin opalescent fluid forming part of the semen

prostatectomy (pros'ta-tek'to-me) surgical removal of part or all of the prostate

prostatic (pros-tat'ik) concerning the prostate gland

prostatism (pros'ta-tizm) a disorder characterised by obstruction to urinary flow due to enlargement of the prostate gland

prostatitis (pros'ta-ti'tis) inflammation of the prostate

prostatocystitis (pros'ta-to-sis-ti'tis) inflammation of the prostate and the bladder.

prostatocystotomy (pros'ta-to-sis-tot'o-me) incision through the prostate and bladder wall

prostatodynia (pros'ta-to-din'e-a) pain in the prostate gland without features of inflammation

prostatolith (pros-tat'o-lith) a concretion formed in the prostate gland

prostatolithotomy (pros-tat'o-lithot'o-me) incision of prostate for removal of a calculus

prostatomegaly (pros'ta-to-meg'a-le) enlargement of the prostate gland

prostatomy (pros-tat'o-me) an incision into the prostate

prostatomyomectomy (pros'ta-to-mi'o-mek'to-me) excision of a prostatic myoma

prostatorrhoea (pros'ta-to-re'a) an abnormal discharge from prostate gland

prostatovesiculectomy (pro'ta-to-ve-sik'u-lek'to-me) excision of the prostate gland and seminal vesicles

prostheon (pros'the-on) the midpoint of the lower border of the upper alveolar arch of the jaw

prosthesis (pros'the-sis) pl. **prostheses** device that replaces organ or part of the body such as a limb, tooth, eye or heart valve and performs some of its function

prosthetic (pros-thet'ik) relating to a prosthesis **p anaemia** mild form of haemolytic anaemia in patients with artificial heart valves

prosthetics (pros-that'iks) a branch of surgery concerned with the design, construction and attachment of artificial limbs or other parts to replace function of a missing part of the body

prosthetist (pros'the-tist) a person who fabricates and fits artificial limbs and similar devices under the direction of an orthopaedic surgeon

prosthetosclerokeratoplasty (pros'the-to-skle'ro-ker'o-to-plas'te) a surgical procedure for removal of damaged sclera and cornea with implantation of a transparent prosthesis

prosthion (pros'the-on) the lowest point on the maxillary alveolar process in the midline

prosthodontics (pros'tho-don'tiks) a branch of dentistry concerned with the construction of artificial appliances that replace missing teeth or restore facial parts

prosthodontist (pros'tho-don'tist) a dentist specialised in prosthodontics

prosthokeratoplasty (pros'tho-ker'a-to-plas'te) surgical replacement of a damaged cornea with a transparent prosthesis

prostitute (pros'ti-tut) a person who solicits sexual relations with monetary gains

prostitution (pros'ti-tu'shun) the act or practice of prostituting

prostrate (pros'trat) 1. lying at length 2. to exhaust

prostrated exhausted

prostration (pros-tra'shun) a condition of extreme exhaustion; marked loss of strength

protal (pro'tal) congenital

protamine (pro'ta-min) a heparin antagonist **p zinc insulin** a long-acting insulin

protanope (pro'ta-nop) a colour blindness with a defect in perception of red colour

protanopia (pro-tan-o'pe-a) a form of colour blindness where a person is not capable of distinguishing shades of red colour

protean (pro'te-an) having the ability to change the body form like the amoeba

protease (pro'te-as) an enzyme acting as a catalyst in the breakdown of protein **p inhibitor** anti-HIV drugs such as amprenavir, atazanavir, indinavir, lopinavir, nelfinavir, ritonavir, and sequinavir

protective (pro-tek'tiv) guarding from danger or injury by providing a safe environment **p efficiency rate** percentage of susceptibles rendered non-susceptible by procedure under test

proteidogenous (pro'te-id-oj'en-us) producing proteins

protein (pro'ten) any of a group of complex nitrogenous compounds containing carbon, hydrogen, oxygen, nitrogen and sulphur. They are the essential constituents of protoplasm of all cells and consist of amino acids joined by peptide linkages. They serve as enzymes, hormones, immunoglobulins and are involved in oxygen transport, electron transport and muscle contraction **p energy malnutrition** (PEM) a variety of interrelated clinical syndromes that occur as a result of lack of protein and calories in proper proportions. Occurs most frequently in infants and young children and presents with loss of subcutaneous fat and muscle wasting (marasmus) or with oedema, hepatomegaly, skin and hair changes (kwashiorkor) **p losing enteropathy** a condition exhibiting an increased transmucosal efflux of plasma proteins from the intestinal lumen due to increased permeability **p sparing** addition of carbohydrates and fats to a low-protein diet to minimise protein catabolism

proteinaceous (pro'te-in-a'shus) resembling a protein

proteinase (pro'te-in-as) a proteolytic enzyme that catalyses hydrolysis of native protein or polypeptides

protein C a potent anticoagulant which inactivates coagulation factors V and VIII

proteinogenous (pro'te-in-oj'en-us) developing from a protein

proteinosis (pro'te-in-o'sis) an accumulation of excess amount of protein in the tissues **lipid p** yellow deposits of hyaline lipid-carbohydrate mixture on inner surface of the lips, under the tongue, on the oropharynx and larynx and skin **pulmonary alveolar p** *see* pulmonary alveolar proteinosis

proteinuria (pro'te-in-u're-a) excretion of protein in the urine **proteoglycan** a high molecular weight glycoprotein located on the plasma membranes of cells and in the extracellular matrix

proteoglycan (pro'te-og'li-kan) a high molecular weight glycoprotein found on the plasma membranes and in the extracellular matrix

proteolipid (pro'te-o-lip'id) a lipid-soluble protein

proteolysin (pro'te-ol'i-sin) a substance causing decomposition of proteins

proteolysis (pro'te-ol'i-sis) hydrolysis of protein

proteolytic (pro'te-o'lit'ik) relating to or causing proteolysis

proteometabolism (pro'te-o-me-tab'o-lizm) protein metabolism

proteomics (pro'te-o-mix) analysis of complete components of protein

proteopepsis (pro'te-o-pep'sis) digestion of proteins

proteopeptic (pro'te-o-pep'tik) pertaining to the digestion of protein

proteopexy (pro'o-peks'e) the fixation of proteins within the body

proteose (pro'te-us) a mixture of intermediate products of proteolysis between protein and peptone

proteosuria (pro'te-os-u're-a) presence of protein in urine

Proteus (pro'te-us) a genus of gram-negative motile bacilli found in faecal matter and decaying material. It includes *P. mirabilis* and *P. vulgaris*

prothrombin a plasma protein precursor of thrombin. It is synthesised in the liver if there is adequate amount of vitamin K **p time** the time taken for clotting following addition of thromboplastin and calcium to decalcified plasma

prothrombinase (pro-throm'bin-as) thromboplastin

prothrombinaemia presence of prothrombin in the blood

prothrombinopaenia a deficiency of prothrombin in the blood

prothymocyte a precursor cell that develops into a T-lymphocyte

protide (pro'tid) protein

proto- 1. combining word for first 2. prefix for the lowest of a series of compounds having the same elements

protobiology (pro'to-bi-ol'o-je) a branch of science concerned with the study of minute life forms.

protocol (pro'to-kol) detailed description of methods used in an investigation

protodiastole (pro'to-di-as'to-le) earliest phase of ventricular diastole immediately following second heart sound

protoduodenum (pro'to-du-o-de'num) the first part of the duodenum derived from embryonic foregut extending from the pylorus to papilla duodeni

protoleucocyte (pro'to-lu'ko-sit) a minute lymphoid cell in the red bone marrow and spleen

protomastigida (pro'to-mas-ij'i-da) a flagellate protozoa that includes leishmania and trypanosoma

proton (pro'ton) a positively charged particle found in the nucleus of all atoms. The number of protons in the nucleus of an atom equals the atomic number of the element **p pump** an ATP dependent H+ ion transporter

proto-oncogenes normal genes involved in cellular proliferation

protopathic (pro'topath'ik) pertaining to the somatic sensations of pain and temperature

protoplasia (pro-to-plas'ze-a) the primary formation of tissue

protoplasm (pro'to-plasm) the living substance of a cell consisting of water, mineral and organic compounds

protoplast (pro'to-plast) 1. the protoplasm of a cell without its containing membrane 2. the original

protoporphyria (pro'to-por-fir'e-a) increased levels of protoporphyrin in the blood and faeces

protoporphyrin (pro'to-por'fi-rin) a porphyrin that combines with iron and protein to produce haemoglobin, myoglobin and catalase.

protoporphyrinuria (pro'to-por'fi-rin-u're-a) presence of protoporphyrins in the urine

protospasm (pro'to-spazm) a spasm beginning in one region and extending to other regions

prototype (pro'to-tip) the primitive form: the original type from which subsequent types arise.

protozoa pl. **protozoon** simplest organisms of animal kingdom consisting of unicellular organisms. They possess a flexible membrane and ability to move. Common examples are plasmodium, entamoeba, giardia, and leishmania

protozoal (pro'to-zo'al) pertaining to protozoa

protozoan (pro'ta-zo'an) 1. a member of protozoa 2. relating to protozoa

protract (pro-trak't) to prolong, to lengthen

protraction (pro-trak'shun) extension forward into a position anterior to normal, such as teeth or structures of jaw

protractor (pro-trak'tor) 1. a muscle drawing a part forward as against a retractor 2. an instrument for removal of foreign bodies from wounds

protrude to project; to extend beyond limit

protrusion (pro-troo'zhun) 1. the state of being thrust forward or projected 2. a forward position of the mandible

protuberance (pro-tu'ber-ans) a prominence, eminence or projection

protuberant (pro-tu'ber-ant) bulging, prominent, sticking out

proud flesh an exuberant granulation tissue found in a poorly healed wound

proviral DNA the chemical form in which the genetic information of a virus is stored within the infected cells

provirus a virus that is integrated into a host cell's genome and can be transmitted vertically to the host's progeny during cell division.

provisional (pro-vizh'un-al) 1. temporary 2. conclusion on available clinical findings 3. tentative

provitamin (pro-vi'ta-min) an inactive substance that can be converted in the body to a corresponding active vitamin

provocative tests tests designed to establish diagnosis by temporarily increasing signs and symptoms of the disease

proxemics study of a particular area of body language

proximad (prok'sim-ad) toward the central point

proximal (prok'sim-al) nearest to a centre or median line **proximate** (prok'sim-at) nearer to a point of reference usually the trunk of the body

proximoataxia (prok'si-mo-a-tak'se-a) inco- ordination of the muscles of the proximal portions of the extremities

proximobuccal (prok'si-mo-buk'al) pertaining to the proximal and buccal surfaces of a tooth

proximolabial (-la'be-al) pertaining to the proximal and labial surface of a tooth

proximolingual (-ling'gwal) pertaining to the proximal and lingual surface of a tooth

prozone (pro'zon) failure of an immunological reaction from an excessive amount of antigen or antibody, especially of antibody excess in precipitin reactions.

prozymogen (pro-zi'mo-jen) a precursor of zymogen found in the nucleus

prune belly absence of muscles of the abdominal wall, giving a rugose, prune-like appearance to the flaccid abdominal wall.

pruned tree appearance pulmonary angiographic appearance of central pulmonary thromboembolism

prune juice discharge dark brown vaginal discharge of hydatiform mole.

pruriginous (proo-rij'i-nus) pertaining to or of the nature of prurigo

prurigo (pro-ri'go) any of the several constantly recurring, discrete pale, deep seated, intensely itchy papules on the extensor surface of the limbs, followed by crusting and lichenification. **pruriginous** adj

pruritogenic (pro'ri-to-jen'ik) causing pruritus

pruritus (proo-ritus) severe itching, **pruritic** adj. **p ani** intense itching around the anus **p vulvae** intense itching of female external genitalia

Prussian blue a chemical stain, used to demonstrate copper by developing bright blue colour, named after Prussia, Germany.

PSA prostate specific antigen a glycoprotein serine protease secreted exclusively by the prostate epithelium. It is responsible for lysis of the seminal coagulum

psalterium (sal-te're-um) commissure of the fornix of the brain

psammoma (sam-o'ma) a neoplasm containing psammoma bodies, that occurs in meninges, choroid plexus, pineal body and ovaries **p bodies** round laminated calcified masses due to degenerated papillary clusters of cellular debris in benign prostatic hypertrophy

psammosarcoma (sam'o-sar-ko'ma) a sarcoma

psammous (sam'us) sandy

psellism (sel'izm) defective pronunciation, stuttering or stammering

pseudacousma (soo'da-kooz'ma) false hearing of sounds

pseudoankylosis (soo'dang-ki-lo'sis) fibrous ankylosis

pseudoarthritis (soo'dar-thri'tis) a condition simulating arthritis

pseudarthrosis (soo'dar-thro'sis) a new false joint arising at the site of ununited fracture

pseudo- (soo'do) combining word for false

pseudoacanthosis nigricans hyperpigmented patches in obese, dark skinned persons

pseudoachondroplasia decreased limb growth, flattened vertebrae, lumbar lordosis, scoliosis, kyphosis, short hands and feet

pseudoallergy a nonimmunologic, anaphylaxis like reaction of sudden onset, often associated with food

pseudoanaemia (soo'do-a-ne'me-a) pallor of skin and mucous membrane without other features of anaemia

pseudoaneurysm (soo'do-an'u-rizm) a dilatation or tortuosity in a vessel

pseudoangina (soo'do-an'ji-na) heart-burn

pseudoankylosis (soo'do-ang'ki-lo'sis) a false joint

pseudoapoplexy (soo'do-ap'o-plek'se) a condition resembling apoplexy but not accompanied by haemorrhage

pseudoarthrosis non-union of two fractured ends of long bones

pseudoblepsis (soo'do-blep'se-a) false vision

pseudobubo massive inguinal lymphadenopathy caused by *Calymmatobacterium granulomatis*, the causative agent of granuloma inguinale

pseudobulbar palsy multifocal infarction in the brain resulting in dysarthria, dysphonia, dysphagia, bilateral facial weakness and lack of emotional expression or exhibit inappropriate responses to environmental cues

pseudocapsule a partial fibrous fissure covering of neoplasms

pseudocast (soo'do-kast) a urinary sediment composed of epithelial cells

pseudocholera infantum white stool diarrhoea

pseudocholesteatoma (soo'do-ko 'les-te-a-to'ma) a hard epithelial mass resembling cholesteatoma in the tympanic cavity in chronic inflammation of the middle ear

pseudocholinesterase (soo'do-ko'lines'ter'as) an enzyme found in the liver and plasma that hydrolyses succinylcholine and acetylcholine

pseudochorea (soo'do-ko-re'a) a hysterial picture resembling chorea

pseudochylous effusion a milky-white pleural effusion resembling chylothorax, associated with high lipid levels

pseudocirrhosis (soo'do-sir-o'-sis) a condition caused by any process that causes obstruction to the venous flow from the liver

pseudoclaudication (soo'do-klaw'di-ka'shun) patients with lumbar spondylosis exhibiting unilateral or bilateral pain, paresthesia and weakness in the lower limbs exaggerated by walking and relieved by rest

pseudocoma a condition mimicking unconsciousness with intact self-awareness

pseudocrisis (soo'do-kri'sis) a temporary fall in the body temperature to be followed by a rise

pseudocroup (soo'do-kroop) laryngismus stridulus

pseudocryptorchidism a testicle drawn into the inguinal canal by cold temperature, fear or genital manipulation

pseudo-Cushing's syndrome presence of truncal obesity and purple striae, and raised levels of urinary cortisol in young obese individuals

pseudocyesis (soo'do-si-e'sis) women having a strong and unfulfilled desire for children exhibiting amenorrhoea, morning sickness and increased abdominal girth

pseudocyst (soo'do-sist) a dilated space that is not lined by epithelium or mesothelium, seen in acute pancreatitis

pseudodementia (soo'do-de-men'she-a) dementia-like symptoms due to psychological impairment. There is cognitive impairment with preservation of attention and ability to concentrate

pseudodiabetes defective carbohydrate metabolism with reduced glucose tolerance as in chronic renal failure

pseudodiphtheria (soo'do-dif*-the're-a) a condition resembling diphtheria

pseudoemphysema (soo'do-em-fi-ze'ma) a condition simulating emphysema caused by temporary obstruction of the bronchi

pseudofracture (soo'do-frak'chur) a thin radiolucent line that mimics a true fracture

pseudogene a DNA sequence having a sequence similar to that of a known gene, but does not encode a protein, often called 'junk' gene

pseudoglandular (sud'o-glan-du-lar) a structure that resembles an authentic gland

pseudoglioma (soo'do-gli-o-ma) choreoretinal lesions

pseudogoitre excessive cervical lordosis of the cervical spine

pseudogout (soo'do-gowt) an arthropathy in elderly females characterised by deposition of calcium pyrophosphate dihydrate crystals in large joints

pseudogynaecomastia (soo'do-jin'e-ko-mas'te-a) increased adipose tissue in male breast without an increase in glandular tissue

pseudohaematuria (soo'do-he'ma-tu're-a) urine looking like blood due to red pigment, as in intake of rifampicin

pseudohaemoptysis (soo'do-he'mop' tisis) sputum having a red colour as in Serratia infection

pseudohermaphrodite (soo'do-her-maf'ro-dit) a person having sex glands of only one sex but exhibiting some of the physical features of an individual of opposite sex **female p** a condition caused by a relative excess of androgen in utero resulting in a phenotypic male with genital ambiguity and/or virilisation **male p** a condition caused by a relative deficiency of androgens in utero resulting in a phenotypic female with ambiguous genitalia in a genotypic male

pseudo-Hirschsprung's disease colonic inertia in children possibly of psychogenic origin

pseudohyperaldosteronism an autosomal dominant condition with an excess resorption of sodium by the distal renal tubules, loss of potassium and hypertension mimicking primaryaldosteronism

pseudohyperparathyroidism hypercalcaemia of malignancy

pseudohypertension elderly persons exhibiting increased blood pressure due to extensive atherosclerosis

pseudohypertrophy (soo'do-hi-per' tro-fe) increase in the size of an organ or structure due to hypertrophy or hyperplasia of the supporting structure and not of parenchyma

pseudohypoparathyroidism (soo'do-hi'po-par'a-thi roi-dizm) a situation of a congenital endorgan resistance to parathormone with features of round face, short neck and short metacarpals and short metatarsals. There is hypocalcaemia and hyperphosphataemia

pseudoincontinence an inability to retain urine due to difficulty in reaching the toilet

pseudoinfarct an ECG Q wave inversion in Wolff-Parkinson-White syndrome, cardiac amyloidosis and hypertrophic cardiomyopathy

pseudoinsomnia subjective difficulty in falling asleep

pseudojaundice (soo'do-jown'dis) skin pigmentation as in carotenaemia that resembles jaundice

pseudolymphoma a lymphoid hyperplasia with a relatively monotonous population of lymphocytes

pseudomania (soo'do-ma'ne-a) 1. a false or pretended psychosis 2. pathologic lying

pseudomembrane (soo'do-mem'bran) a thin, adherent, gray-white exudate in the oropharynx, whose removal causes bleeding. It is composed of necrotic debris and neutrophils

pseudomembranous colitis an acute often severe diarrhoea following antibiotic therapy due to elimination of patient's native bacterial flora and super infection by *Clostridium difficile*

pseudomeningitis (soo'do-men-in-ji'tis) a condition resembling meningitis without meningeal inflammation

pseudomenstruation (soo-do-men'stroa'shun) uterine bleeding without the usual changes in the endometrium

pseudomonas (soo-do-mo'nas) a genus of small, motile gram-negative bacilli with polar flagella. They exist as saprophytes, but can be sometimes pathogenic such as *P. aeruginosa, P. pseudomallei*

pseudomyxoma peritonei a condition with poorly-circumscribed gelatinous masses containing mucin-secreting cells that may arise from the ovary

pseudoneuritis (soo'do-nu-ri'tis) pseudopapilloedema

pseudopapilloedema (soo'do-pap'i-le-de ma) a swelling of the optic nerve head with blurring of disc margins and is not caused by optic neuritis

pseudoparalysis (soo'do-pa-r al'i-sis) loss of motor power of hysterical origin

pseudopodium (soo'do-po'de-um) a temporary protruding process of an amoeba or of a leucocyte

pseudopolyp (soo'do-pol'ip) an hypertrophy of mucosa resembling polyp

pseudoprecocity sexual maturation in female children by functional ovarian tumours

pseudopseudohȳpoparthyroidism persons exhibiting skeletal features of pseudohypoparathyroidism without metabolic abnormalities

pseudopuberty growth of pubic hair and enlargement of penis in male infants from Leydig cell tumour

pseudotumour cerebri benign intracranial hypertension

pseudoxanthoma elasticum a rare condition affecting the connective tissue of the skin, cardiovascular system, joints and eyes with features of lax, yellow plaques on the skin, angioid streaks of the optic fundus, hypertension, cerebral and gastrointestinal haemorrhage

psi phenomenon, events or actions that have no logical explanation

psittacosis (sit-a-ko'sis) an acute systemic infection due to *Chalamydia psittaci* transmitted by infected parrots, parakeets and fowls. *C psittaci* is gram-negative intracellular bacteria and produces clinical manifestations varying from a flu- like illness to severe fatal pneumonia

psoas (so'as) one of the two muscles of the loins *see* table of muscles **p sign** loss of the sharp delineation of the psoas muscle border on a plain erect abdominal film, indicative of the presence of intra abdominal or retroperitoreal condition

psoitis (so-i'tis) inflammation of psoas muscles

psomophagia (so'mo-fa'je-a) ·swallowing food without properly chewing it

psoralen a photosensitive substance extracted from plants especially Psoralea, used in the treatment of psoriasis

psorelcosis (so'rel-ko'sis) ulceration resulting from scabies

psoriasis (so-ri'a-sis) a chronic disorder characterised by well defined, scaly, erthematous plaques on the extensor surfaces of the extremities like elbows and knees, trunk, back and scalp. It may be localised or generalised and is considered as an autoimmune disease **exfoliative p** sudden widespread involvement of psoriasis after abrupt dis-

continuation of treatment associated with itching and burning **guttate p** sudden crops of erythematous shiny papules on the trunk and proximal part of extremities in children and young adults **pustular p** tiny, superficial, sterile pustules appearing either on the surface of psoriatic lesions or on previously unaffected skin **p. vulgaris** erythematous, scaly, well defined plaques on extremities, trunk and scalp and nail involvement is common

psoriatic (sori-at'ik) relating to psoriasis **p arthritis** seronegative polyarthritis affecting distal interphalangeal joints of the fingers and toes in association with psoriatic lesions of the skin and nails

psorophthalmia (so'rof-thal'me-a) inflammation of the margin of the eyelids with ulceration

psorous (so'rus) relating to, or affected with, itch

psych (o) combining word for mind; mental process

psychalgia (si-kal'je-a) a functional pain in the absence of any organic cause, usually associated with acute anxiety

psychataxia (si'ka-tak'se-a) inability to fix the attention

psyche (si'ke) mind

psychiatric (si-ke-a'trik) pertaining to psychiatry

psychiatrist (si-ki'a-trist) a specialist in psychiatry

psychiatry (si-ki'a-tre) medical specialty concerned with mental disorders or diseases, and problems of emotional character

psychic (si'-kik) 1. pertaining to the mind 2. a person sensitive to non-physical forces

psychoactive (si'ko-ak'tiv) pertaining to a pharmaceutical agent that affects normal mental functions such as mood, behaviour or thinking process, examples are stimulants, sedatives and hallucinogens

psychoanaleptic (si'ko-an'alep'tik) exhibiting a stimulatory effect on the mind

psychoanalysis (si'ko-a-nal'i-sis) a division of psychiatry concerned with exploration of patient's personality

psychoanalyst (si'ko-an'a-list) a psychiatrist trained in psychoanalysis and applies techniques of psychoanalytic theory

psychobiology (si'-ko-bi-ol'o-je) the study of the biology of the mind

psychocatharsis (si'ko-ka-thar'sis) a process of bringing of traumatic experiences into consciousness

psychochrome (si'ko-krom) colour impression produced by the stimulus of a sense organ other than that of vision

psychocoma (si'ko-ko'ma) mental stupor

psychocortical (si'ko-kor'ti-kal) pertaining to the cerebral cortex concerned with the sensory motor and psychic functions

psychodiagnosis (psi'ko-di-ag-no'sis) use of psychological testing methods to diagnose mental disorders

psychodynamics (si'ko-di-nam'iks) the study of the forces that motivate behaviour

psychogalvanometer (si'ko-gal'va-nom'e-ter) a device to determine the alterations in the electrical resistance of the skin in response to emotional stimuli

psychogenesis (si'ko-jen'e-sis) 1. The development of the mind or mental process 2. the occurrence of physical symptoms from a psychic origin

psychogenetic (si'ko-jen-et'ik) 1. of mental origin 2. relating to psychogenesis

psychogenic (si-ko-jen'ik) psychogenetic

psychogeriatric concerning to an elderly person having a psychiatric disorder

psychogeusic (si'ko-gu'sik) pertaining to taste perception

psychograph (si'ko-graf) a profile or graph indicating personality traits of an individual

psychokinesis (si-ko-ki-ne'sis) 1. impulsive behaviour 2. influence of mind upon a physical matter

psycholagny (si'ko-lag'ne) sexual excitement caused by mental imagery

psychological (si-ko-loj'i-kal) relating to psychology or to the mental processes

p autopsy an autopsy analysing the cause of death by examining both the body and the circumstances that led to death p testing a group of tests to determine a person's perceptual-motor integrity, intelligence quotient, potential achievement and sense of reality

psychologist (si-kol'o-jist) a person, not a physician, who has been trained in the study of human behaviour and psychology

psychology (si-kol'o-je) 1. the study of behaviour and of functions and processes of the mind, and its relation to the social and physical environment of an individual or a group of individuals 2. a profession dealing with understanding of, prevention of and finding a solution to individual or social problems

psychometry (si-kom'e-tre) psychological and mental testing and analysis of individual's attitudes or mental processes

psychomotor (si'ko-mo'tor) pertaining to or causing voluntary movements associated with mental processes

psychoneurosis (si'ko-nu-ro'sis) an emotional or behavioural disorder arising from unresolved unconscious conflicts

psychoneurotic (si'ko-nu-rot'ik) 1. pertaining to a functional disorder of psychic origin 2. a person suffering from psychoneurosis

psychopath (si-ko-path) a person exhibiting an antisocial behaviour

psychopathic (si'ko-path'ik) relating to psychopathy

psychopathology (si'ko-path-ol'o-je) 1. the study of the aetiology, processes, and features of mental disorders 2. the behavioural manifestation of any mental disorder

psychopathy (si-kop'a-the) any disease of the mind, not necessarily associated with subnormal intelligence

psychopharmacology (si-ko-far'ma-kol'o-je) the scientific study of the effect of drugs on behaviour and normal and abnormal mental functions

psychophysical (si'ko-fiz'i-kal) concerning the relationships between physical stimuli and sensory responses

psychophysics (si'ko-fiz'iks) the branch of psychology dealing with the relationships between physical stimuli and sensory responses

psychophysiological (si'ko-fiz'e-o-loj'-kal) pertaining to psychophysiology **p disorder** one of a large group of mental disorders exhibiting dysfunction of an organ or organ systems innervated by autonomic nervous system, which may be caused or aggravated by emotional factors

psychophysiology (si-ko-fiz'e-ol'o-je) physiology of the mind

psychoplegic (si'ko-ple'jik) an agent causing reduction of excitability of the mental process

psychoprophylaxis (si'ko-pro'fi-lak'sis) a system of prenatal education preparing for natural childbirth

psychosensory (si'ko-sen'so-re) concerning the perceptions not arising in sensory organs, as hallucinations

psychosexual (si'ko-seks'u-al) pertaining to the psychologic and emotional components of sex

psychosis (si-ko'sis) any mental disorder of organic or emotional origin exhibiting a gross impairment in reality testing. The person fails to evaluate the correctness of his or her perceptions and thoughts and makes incorrect references about the reality even when it is contrary

psychosocial (si'ko-so'shal) relating to both psychological and social factors

psychosomatic (si'ko-so-mat'ik) 1. bodily diseases stimulated, or caused by mental factors 2. the expression of emotional conflict through physical symptoms 3. of or pertaining to psychosomatic medicine

psychosurgery (si-ko-sur'jer-e) operative treatment designed to correct psychological diseases

psychotherapy (si-ko-ther'a-pe) treatment

aimed at helping the patient to solve his psychiatric and emotional problems

psychotic (si-kat 'ik) 1. relating to or affected by psychosis 2. a person exhibiting the characteristics of a psychosis

psychotogenic (si-kot'o-jen'ik) inducing psychosis

psychotomimetic (si-kot'o-mi-me'tik) a drug or other agent whose effects simulate the symptoms of psychosis

psychotropic drug drug altering emotional and behavioural response

psychr (o) combining word for cold

psychroalgia (si'kro-al'je-a) a painful sensation of cold

psychroesthesia (si'kro-es-the'ze-a) a subjective sensation of cold in a part of the body

psychrometer (si-krom'e-ter) a device to measure relative humidity of the atmosphere

psychrophilic (si-kro-fil'ik) preferring cold, refers to the bacteria thriving at low temperatures

psychrophobia (si-kro-fo'be-a) abnormal sensitiveness to cold

psychrophore (si'kro-for) a double-lumen catheter through which cold water is circulated to apply cold to a canal like urethra

psychrotherapy (si'kro-ther'a-pe) the treatment of disease by use of cold.

Pt symbol for platinum

PTAH stain phosphotungstic acid haematoxylin stain used in histology to delineate different structures

ptarmic (tar'mik) 1. causing sneezing 2. an agent that causes sneezing

ptarmus (tar'mus) spasmodic sneezing

PTC percutaneous transhepatic cholangiography; plasma thromboplastin component

PTCA percutaneous transluminal coronary angioplasty

pterion (te're-on) point of suture of frontal, parietal, temporal and sphenoid bones

pternalgia (ter-nal'je-a) pain in the heel

pterygium (ter-ji'e-um) a thick triangular

tissue that extends medially from the nasal border of the cornea to the inner canthus of the eye

pterygoid (ter'i-goyd) wing-shaped **p hamulus** a small bony projection on pterygoid process to which tensor veli palantini muscle is attached

pterygomandibular (ter'i-go-man-dib'u-lar) pertaining to the pterygoid process of the sphenoid bone and the mandible

pterygomaxillary (-mak'si-ler'e) pertaining to the pterygoid process and the maxilla

pterygopalatine (-pal'a-tin) pertaining to the pterygoid process and the palate

PTH parathyroid hormone

ptilosis (ti-lo'sis) loss of eyelashes

ptomaine (to'man) a nitrogenous substance produced by putrefactive bacteria acting on proteins and aminoacids

ptosis (to'sis) drooping of an organ or part such as upper eyelid or visceral organs

PTT partial thromboplastin time

ptyalectasis (tia'lek'ta-sis) dilatation of a salivary duct

ptyalin (ti'a-lin) an enzyme found in the saliva that hydrolyses starch and glycogen

ptyalism (ti'a-lizm) excessive salivary secretion

ptyalith (ti'a-lith) a salivary calculus

ptyalocoele (ti-al'o-sel) a cystic dilatation of a salivary duct

ptyalogenic   (ti-al'o-jen'ik)   of salivary origin

ptyalogogue (ti-al'o-gog) an agent that stimulates flow of saliva

ptyalography (ti-al-og'ra-fe) sialography

ptyalolithiasis (ti'al-o-li-thi'a-sis) concretion in a salivary gland or duct

ptyalorrhoea (ti'a-lo-re-a) an increased flow of saliva

ptyocrinous (ti-ok'ri-nus) discharge of contents of the cell in the secretion of the gland

ptysis (ti'sis) spitting

Pn symbol for plutoneum

pubarche (pu-bar'ke) 1. the beginning of puberty 2. appearance of pubic hair

puber (pu'ber) one at the onset of puberty

puberal (pu'ber-al) pubertal

pubertal pertaining to puberty

pubertas (pu'ber-tas) puberty **p praecox** precocious puberty

puberty (pu'ber-te) transformation of a child into an young adult at which the individual becomes capable of reproduction **precocious p** development of pubertal changes at an unusually early age.

pubes (pu'bez) 1. the anterior part of the innominate bone 2. the pubic region 3. the pubic hair

pubescence (pu-bes'ens) 1. puberty 2. the covering of fine, soft hairs on the body

pubetrotomy (pu'be-trot'o-me) section through the pelvic bone and lower abdominal wall

pubic (pu'bik) pertaining to the pubes **p bone** the lower anterior part of innominate bone **p hair** hair over the pubes that appears at onset of sexual maturity

pubio - pubo combining word for pubic bone, pubic region

pubiotomy (pu-be-ot'o-me) incision across pubis undertaken to enlarge the pelvic passage to facilitate the delivery of foetus in malformed pelvis

pubis (pu'bis) pl. **pubes** pubic bone

public health the science and art of preventing disease, prolonging life and promoting health through organised community efforts

pubococcygeal (pu'bo-kok-sij'e-al) pertaining to the pubis and coccyx

pubofemoral (-fem'or-al) pertaining to the pubis and femur

pubomadesis loss or absence of pubic hair

puboprostatic (-pros-tat'ik) pertaining to the pubis and prostate gland

puborectal (-rek'tal) pertaining to the pubis and rectum

pubovesical (-ves'i'kl) pertaining to the pubis and bladder

Puddle's sign percussion of the umbilical area in knee chest position when there is suspicion of a small amount of fluid in the abdomen, and it gives a dull note

pudenda (pu-den'da) vulva

pudendagra (pu'den-dag'ra) pain in the external genitalia

pudendal (pu-den'dal) pertaining to the female external genitals **p femininum** vulva **p muliebre** female external genitals

purile (pu'e-ril) concerning a child; childlike

puerilism (pu-er-il-izm) childishness

puerperal (pu-er'per-al) concerning the puerperium **p eclampsia** eclampsia during puerperium **p fever** septicemia following child birth

puerperalism (pu-er'per-al-izm) a pathologic condition noted at child birth

puerperant (pu-er'per-ant) 1. a woman in labour 2. woman who has recently given birth

puerperium (pu'er-pe're-um) the period from the termination of labour to complete involution of the uterus, lasting approximately 6 weeks

PUFA polyunsaturated fatty acids

puff sudden forceful breath inhaling medication mist by actuating metered dose inhalers or dry powder inhalers

puffy tumour a fluctuant swelling overlying frontal bones affected by osteomyelitis

PUGH sydrome a condition of pseudouveitis, glaucoma and hyphaema with neovascularisation of iris and occlusion of the central retinal vein

pulicatio (pu'li-ka'te-o) infested with fleas

pulicidae (pu-lis'i-de) a family of fleas belonging to the order of Siphonaptera, that includes Xenopsylla

pulicide (pu'li-sid) an agent that destroys fleas

pullulate (pul'i-lat) to bud or germinate

pullulation (pul'i-la'shun) the act of budding or germinating

pulmo a combining word for lung

pulmoaortic (pul'mo-a-or'tik) 1. pertaining to the lungs and aorta 2. pertaining to the pulmonary artery and aorta

pulmometry (pul-mom'e-tre) determination of the lung capacity

pulmonary (pul'mo-ne-re) pertaining to the lungs or respiratory system. **noncardiogenic p oedema** *see* ARDS **p agenesis** a congenital anomaly exhibiting failure of development of the primitive lung bud **p alveolar microlithiasis** a condition characterised by the intra-alveolar deposition of a large number of minute calcific concretions uniformly throughout both the lungs **p alveolar proteinosis** a non-inflammatory progressive pulmonary disease presenting with dyspnoea due to intra-alveolar extracellular deposition of granular lipoproteinaceous material **p amyloidosis** extracellular deposition of fibrils derived from light chain of a mononuclear immunoglobulin that is converted into amyloid, and it gives rise to parenchymal nodules **p angiitis** tissue reactions characterised by focal destructive and infiltrative vascular disease in the lung **p artery** *see* table of arteries **p atresia** atretic pulmonary valve with hypoplastic pulmonary artery **p congestion** an excessive accumulation of fluid in the lungs, usually associated with either an inflammation or congestive heart failure **p dirofilariasis** a granulomatous reaction in the lung for a filarial nematode, *Dirofilaria immitis* **p echinococcosis** hydatid disease of the lung **p embolism** pulmonary thromboembolism **p eosinophil syndrome** pulmonary disorders affecting major airways or parenchyma of the lung or both associated with excess of blood or tissue eosinophilia or both **p haemosiderosis** recurrent haemoptysis and iron deficiency due to intrapulmonary haemorrhage **p hyper sensitivity** immunologically mediated reactions in the respiratory system due to inhaled organic dusts **p hypertension** marked narrowing of pulmonary vascular bed from anatomic or vasomotor mechanisms, either singly or together result in an increased vascular resistance to the blood flow through the lung and pulmonary hypertension

infarction complete necrosis of lung parenchyma in submassive pulmonary embolism when embolus obstructs completely distal branches of the pulmonary circulation **p lymphangioleiomyomatosis** disorder occurring only in women in child bearing age characterised by perivascular, perilymphatic and peribronchial smooth muscle proliferation, presenting with progressive dyspnoea, chylous effusion and pneumothorax **p meliodosis** a chronic pulmonary infection from *Pseudomonas pseudomallei* an aerobic gram-negative bacillus **p metastases** metastatic spread of malignancy to the lung from carcinomatous conditions in different parts of the body **p oedema** increased pulmonary capillary pressure leading to accumulation of extra vascular fluid in the lung tissue and alveoli commonly from congestive heart failure **p oxygen toxicity** oxygen poisoning by breathing high concentrations of oxygen **p regurgitation** pulmonary incompetence from pulmonary artery dilatation due to pulmonary hypertension **p stenosis** narrowing of pulmonary valve orifice **p thromboembolism** a condition associated with the obstruction of pulmonary artery by a thrombus arising from an extrapulmonary source **solitary p nodule** single small round or oval shadow in the lung parenchyma

pulmonectomy (pul'mo-nek'to-me) pneumonectomy

pulmonic (pul-mon'ik) pertaining to the lungs or pulmonary valve or pulmonary artery

pulmonitis (pul-mo-no'tis) pneumonia

pulmonologist a physician specialised in pulmonary diseases

pulmotor (pul'mo-tor) an apparatus for induction of artificial respiration by forcing air or oxygen into the lungs

pulp 1. soft part of an organ. 2. soft part of a fruit 3. a mass of partially digested food 4. the soft vascular part of the centre of tooth

pulpa (pul'pa) pulp

pulpal (pul'pal) relating to pulp

pulpalgia (pul-pal'je-a) pain in the pulp of a tooth

pulpectomy (pul-pek'to-me) surgical removal of pulp from a tooth

pulpitis (pul-pi'tis) inflammation of the pulp of a tooth

pulpy (pul'pe) flabby

pulsate (pul'sat) rhythmic beating

pulsatile (pul'sa-til) pulsating

pulsation (pul-sa'shun) the rhythmic beat, as of the heart and blood vessels

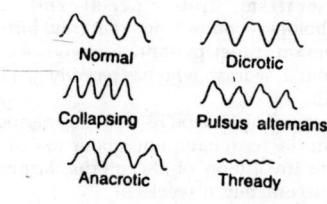

Pulse

pulse a wave of expansion felt due to systolic ejection of the left ventricle in already filled arteries **anacrotic p** a prominent initial tidal wave than the main wave **capillary p** pulsations noted in the regions adjoining the poorly vascular and richly vascular areas of the capillary systems, commonly in the nailbed **carotid p** pulsations noted in the carotid artery **collapsing p** pulse showing a rapid upstroke due to markedly increased stroke volume and a fall due to regurgitation of blood back into the left ventricle during diastole and to decreased systemic vascular resistance, seen in aortic incompetence and hyperdynamic circulatory states **dicrotic p** a double arterial pulse due to an exaggerated dicrotic wave in the early diastole **plateau p** a sustained peak with a slow upstroke and a downstroke as in aortic stenosis **p deficit** radial pulse being less than ventricular rate as in atrial fibrillation **p pressure** the difference between the systolic and diastolic pressures, normally a value of about 40 mmHg **radial p** normal pulse felt in the radial artery at the wrist **venous p** pulsations in the jugular vein exhibiting a wavy pattern with three distinct positive waves during each cardiac cycle and are better seen than felt **thready p** rapid pulse with low volume and low force as in shock **unequal p** a pulse in which beats vary in force **waterhammer p** collapsing pulse appreciated when the arm of the patient is raised above the level of the head

pulseless disease Takayasu's arteritis

pulsion (pul'shun) driving in any direction

pulsus (pul'sus) pulse **p alternans** the successive beats of the ventricle being strong and weak in an alternating manner due to alternate strong and weak ventricular contraction, a manifestation of left ventricular failure **p bigeminus** an arrhythmia in which two beats come in couples, noted in partial heart block and digoxin toxicity **p bisferiens** a double systolic impulse with features of a slow upstroke and a collapsing pulse as in aortic stenosis and aortic incompetence and in idiopathic subaortic stenosis **p paradoxus** an exaggerated inspiratory fall in blood pressure during quiet breathing and there is a decrease in the pulse amplitude or disappearance of pulse during quiet breathing **p parvus** small volume of pulse with a slow upstroke due to slow ejection of blood from the left ventricle and a downstroke, as in aortic stenosis **p tardus** pulsus parvus

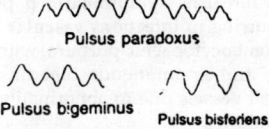

Pulsus paradoxus

Pulsus bigeminus   Pulsus bisferiens

Pulsus

pulv powder

pulverisation (pul'ver-i-za'shun) the crushing of a substance to powder or smaller particles

pulverulent (pul-ver'u-lent) resembling powder

pulvinar (pul-vi-nar) a part of thalamus comprising a portion of the posterior nucleus

pulvinate (pul'vi-nat) convex; shaped like a cushion

pulvis powder

pumis (pum'is) complex silicate used as an abrasive

pump 1. an apparatus that transfers fluids or gases by pressure or suction 2. to force air or fluid along a pathway, such as heart pumping blood into the blood vessels

pump-oxygenator a device that pumps and oxygenates blood

punch an instrument to make a small circular hole in a material or tissue **p biopsy** removal of a living tissue for microscopic examination by a punch, as in bone marrow aspirates

punch-drunk a concussion syndrome from multiple trauma to the head as in boxers

punched out appearing as if holes have been made, a radiologic appearance of bones in multiple myeloma

puncta (punk'ta) points

punctate (punk'tat) having pinpoint depressions or punctures on the surface

punctiform (-ti-form) 1. formed like a point 2. pinpoint colonies

punctio (punk'she-o) the act of puncturing or pricking

punctum (punk'tum) pl. **puncta** point

puncture (punk'chur) 1. a hole made by a sharp pointed instrument 2. to make a hole by a pointed instrument

pungency (pun'jen-se) its quality of being sharp, strong or bitter as an odour or taste

pungent (pun'jent) acrid or sharp, as applied to an odour or taste

PUO pyrexia of unknown origin

pupa (pu'pa) a stage in metamorphosis of an insect between a larva and adult

pupil the contractile circular opening in the centre of the iris of the eye. It lies behind the anterior chamber of the eye and the cornea and in front of the lens. It contracts when exposed to strong light and when focussed on a near object and dilates in the dark and when focussed on a distant object

pupilla (pu-pil'a) the pupil of the eye

pupillary (pu-pi-ler-e) pertaining to the pupil

pupillography recording the movements of the pupil

pupillometer (pu-pil-om'e-ter) a device for measuring the diameter of the pupil

pupillometry (pu-pil-om'e-tre) measurement of the diameter of the pupil

pupilloplegia (pu'pi-lo-ple'je-a) slow reaction of the pupil of the eye

pupilloscopy (pu'pil-s-ko-pe) examination of the pupil

pupphusa (s) lungs

pure (pur) free from pollution; uncontaminated

purgation (pur-ga'shun) 1. cleaning 2. evacuation of the bowel by a purgative

purgative (pur'ga-tiv) 1. cleansing 2. an agent stimulating the bowel movements **cholagogue p** a purgative stimulating the flow of bile **drastic p** a purgative causing violent bowel movements **saline p** a purgative producing large amount of watery discharges **p enema** a strong, high bowel purgative as an enema

purge (purj) 1. to evacuate the bowels by a cathartic 2. a drug that causes evacuation of the bowels

puriform (pu'ri-form) resembling pus

purinase (pu-ri-nas) an enzyme that catalyses purine metabolism

purine (pu'ren) any one of a large group of nitrogenous compounds. They are end products in the digestion of certain proteins in the diet, and some are synthesised in the body **p base** any of the purine derivates such as zanthine and uric acid

purisha (s) faeces

purishavaha srotas (s) excretory system

purity the state of being clean and free form contamination

Purkinje (pur-kin'je) **cell** large neuron of the cerebellar cortex, named after Johannes Purkinje, Polish physiologist

Purkinje fibres myocardial fibres that are a continuation of the bundle branches and extend into the ventricular walls

purohepatitis (pu'ro-hep'a-ti-tis) purulent inflammation of the liver

puromucous (pu'ro-mu'kus) mucopurulent

purple a colour from a mixture of red and blue **visual p** rhodopsin

purpura (pur'pu-ra) a disorder characterised by bleeding into the skin often associated with bleeding from mucous membranes. It is caused by thrombocytopaenia or thrombocytopathy or primary disorders affecting the blood vessels. The bleeding is circumscribed showing a clearcut margin with the surface and not blanching on application of pressure **anaphylactoid p** an immune complex-mediated disease associated with vasculitis involving small blood vessels **drug-induced p** vascular purpura following exposure to drugs such as penicillin, sulphonamides, aspirin and sedatives **Henoch-Schonlein p** anaphylactoid purpura **immune thrombocytopaenic p** condition exhibiting antibodies directed against platelet components. There are purpuric spots and ecchymoses over limbs, chest and back. There is marked reduction in the number of platelets **senile p** chronic disorder in elderly with purpura and ecchymoses on the extensor surfaces of the forearms **symptomatic p** purpura occurring in infections **vascular p** nonthrombocytopaenic purpura, with bruising and spontaneous bleeding from small vessels due to abnormality in the capillaries

purpuric (pur-pu'rik) pertaining to resembling or suffering from pupura

pursed-lip breathing deep inspirations followed by prolonged expiration through pursed lips

purulence (pur'u-lens) the state of containing pus

purulency (pur'u-len'se) purulence

purulent (pur'u-lent) suppurative; forming or containing pus

puruloid (pur'u-loyd) like pus

purusha (s) 1. man 2. inner self

purvarupa (s) premonitory manifestations

pus a pale yellow or green creamy liquid consisting of dead leucocytes that occurs at the site of bacterial infection

pustula (pus'tu-la) pustule

pustulant (pus'tu-lant) causing pustules

pustular (pus'tu-lar) pertaining to, or characterised by pustules

pustulation (pus'tu-la'shun) the development of pustules

pustule (pus'tul) a small circumscribed elevation of the skin containing purulent fluid

pustulocrustaceous (pus'tu-lo-krus-ta'shus) characterised by formation of pustules and crusts

pustulosis (pus'tu-lo'sis) a generalised eruption of pustules

putamen (pu-ta'men) a part of the lentiform nucleus situated lateral to the globus pallidus

putrefaction (pu'tre-fak'shun) decomposition of animal matter

putrefactive (pu'tre-fak'tiv) causing or pertaining to putrefaction

putrefy (pu'tre-fi) to undergo putrefaction

putrescence (pu-tres'ens) decay

putrid (pu'trid) decayed; foul

PUVA therapy treatment of psoriasis by psoralen and ultraviolet - A light

p value *stat* the statistical probability of occurrence of a given finding by chance alone in comparison with the known distribution of possible findings

PVC 1. premature ventricular contraction 2. polyvinyl chloride

p wave the deflection wave of an ECG that records atrial depolarisation

pyaemia (pi-e'me-a) septicaemia due to pyogenic organisms in the blood causing multiple abscesses.

pyaemic (pi-e'mik) relating to pyaemia

pyarthrosis (pi-ar-thro'sis) pus in a joint cavity

pycn (o) combining word for dense, thick, frequent, compact

pyecchysis (pi-ek'i-sis) a purulent effusion

pyelectasia (pi'e-lek-ta'ze-a) dilatation of the renal pelvis

pyelitic (pi'e-lit'ik) realting to pyelitis

pyelitis (pi'e-li'tis) inflammation of the pelvis of the kidney and its calices

pyel (o) combining word for pelvis

pyelocaliectasis (pi'ea-lo-kal'e-ek'ta-sis) dilatation of the pelvis and calices of the kidney

pyelocystitis (-sis-ti'tis) inflammation of the renal pelvis and the bladder

pyelocystostomosis (-sis-to-sto-mo'sis) the surgical creation of a communication between the kidney and bladder

pyelogram (pi'e-lo-gram) radiography of the renal pelves and ureters following intravenous injection of a radioopaque substance

pyelography (pi'e-log'ra-fe) radiography of the renal pelves and ureters following injection of a radioopaque contrast substance

pyelolithotomy (pi'elo-lith-ot'o-me) the surgical removal of calculus from the pelvis of a kidney

pyelonephritis (pi-e-lo-ne-fri'tis) inflammation of the kidney and renal pelvis

pyelonephrosis (pi'e-lo-ne-fro'sis) any disease affecting the pelvis of the kidney

pyeloplasty (pi'e-lo-plas'te) surgical repair of the pelvis of the kidney

pyelostomy (pi'e-los'to-me) creation of an opening into the renal pelvis

pyelotomy (pi'e-lot'o-me) incision of the renal pelvis

pyeloureterectasis dilatation of the pelvis of the kidney and ureter

pyencephalus (pi'en-sef'a-lus) an abscess of the brain with suppuration within the skull

pygal (pi'jal) concerning the buttocks

pygalgia (pi-gal'je-a) pain in the buttocks

Pygmalionism (pig-ma'le-on-izm) a psychopathic condition of falling in love with one's own creation, named after Greek sculptor, Pygmalion, who fell in love a figure he carved

pygmy (pig'me) dwarf

pyknic (pik'nik) a body structure characterised by short, round limbs, a full face, short neck, stockiness and tendency toward obesity

pykn (o) combining word for thick, compact, dense, frequent *see* pycno

pyknocyte (pik'no-sit) a spiculed red blood cell

pyknodysostosis (pik'no-dis'os-to'sis) an autosomal recessive disorder characterised by short stature, delayed closure of fontanelles, hypoplasia of facial bones and phalanges and blue sclerae

pyknophrasia (pik'no-fra'ze-a) thickness of words uttered in speech

pyknosis (pik-no'sis) reduction in the size of the cell or its nucleus, usually associated with hyperchromatosis

pylemphroxis (pi'lem-frak'sis) occlusion of the portal vein

pylephlebectasia (pi'le-fle-bek-ta'ze-a) distension of the portal vein

pylephlebitis (pi'le-fle-bi'tis) inflammation of the portal vein

pylethrombophlebitis (pi'le-throm'bo-fle-bi'tis) thrombosis and inflammation of the portal vein

pylorectomy (pi'lo-rek'to-me) operative removal of the pylorus

pyloric (pi-lor'ik) pertaining to the distal portion of the stomach **p sphincter** a thick, circular muscle in the distal end of the stomach that controls the passage of food into the small intestine

pyloristenosis (pi-lor'i-sten-o'sis) constriction of the pylorus

pyloritis (pi'lo-ri'tis) inflammation of the pylorus

pylorodiosis (pi-lo'ro-di-o'sis) dilatation of the pylorus of the stomach

pyloroduodenitis (pi-lor'o-du'o-de-ni'tis) inflammation of the mucosa of the pylorus and duodenum

pylorogastrectomy (pi-lor'o-gas-trek'to-me) excision of the pyloric portion of the stomach

pyloromyotomy (-mi-ot'o-me) incision and suture of the pyloric sphincter

pyloroplasty (-plas'te) a surgical procedure to widen the muscular outlet from the stomach

pylorospasm (-spazm) spasmodic contraction of the pyloric orifice

pylorostenosis (-sten-o'sis) stricture of the pyloric orifice

pylorostomy (pi-lor-os'to-me) creation of an opening through the abdominal wall into the pylorus

pylorus (pi-lor'us) the inferior region of the stomach that connects to the duodenum. It has two parts, the pyloric antrum which connects to the body of the stomach and the pyloric canal which leads into the duodenum. Pylorus has a sphincter at the site of its communication with the duodenum

pyo combining word for pus

pyocephalus (-sef-a-lus) purulent material within the cranium

pyococcus (-kok-us) a micrococcus causing pus formation such as *Streptococcus pyogenes*

pyocoele (pi'o-sel) a hydrocoele where the fluid has become purulent due to secondary infection. It is an acutely tender swelling with positive fluctuation but negative transillumination test

pyocolpocoele (-kol'po-sel) a vaginal swelling containing pus

pyocyanic (-si-an'ik) pertaining to pyocyanin or blue pus

pyocyst (pi'o-sist) a cyst containing pus

pyoderma (pi'o-derma) any purulent skin disease, such as impetigo

pyodermatitis (pi'o-der-ma-ti'tis) pyogenic infection of the skin resulting in dermatitis

pyodermia (pi'o-der'me-a) any suppurative skin disorder

pyogenesis (pi'o-jen'e-sis) the formation of pus

pyogenic (pi-o-jen'ik) producing pus **p** **microorganism** a microorganism producing pus

pyohaemothorax (pi'o-he'mo-tho'raks) presence of pus and blood in the pleural cavity

pyoid (pi'oyd) resembling pus

pyolabyrinthitis (pi'o-lab'i-rin-thi'tis) an inflammation with suppuration of the labyrinth of the ear

pyometra (pi'o-me'tra) accumulation of pus in the uterine cavity

pyometritis (pio'-me-tri'tis) purulent inflammation of the uterus

pyonephritis (pi'o-nef-ri'tis) purulent inflammation of the kidney

pyonephrosis (pi'o-ref-ro'sis) accumulation of pus in the renal pelvis

pyoovarium (pi'o-o-va're-um) formation of abscess in an ovary

pyopericarditis (pi'o-per'i-kar-di'tis) suppurative inflammation of the pericardium

pyopericardium (-de-um) pus collection in the pericardial cavity

pyoperitonitis (pi'o-per'into-ni'tis) suppurative inflammation of the peritoneum

pyophthalmia (pi'of-thal-me-a) pyophthalmitis

pyophthalmitis (-mi'tis) suppurative inflammation of the eye

pyophysometra (pi'o-fi'so-me'tra) collection of pus and gas in the uterus

pyopneumocholecystitis (pi'o-nu'mo-ko-le-sis-ti'tis) distension of the gall bladder with pus and gas

pyopneumocyst (pi'o-nu'mo-sist) a cyst containing pus and gas

pyopneumohepatitis (-hep'a-ti'tis) an abscess in the liver containing gas

pyopneumopericardium (-per'i-kar'de-um) collection of pus and gas or air in the pericardial cavity

pyopneumoperitoneum (-per'i-to-ne'um) collection of pus and gas or air in the peritoneal cavity

pyopneumoperitonitis (-ni'tis) peritonitis with collection of pus and gas or air in the peritoneal cavity

pyopneumothorax (pi'o-nu'mo-tho'raks) the collection of pus and gas in the pleural cavity

pyoptysis (pi-op'ti-sis) coughing of pus

pyopylectosis (pi'o-pi'e-lek'ta-sis) pus in the dilated renal pelvis

pyorrhoea (pi'o-re-a) discharge of pus

pyosalphingitis (pi-'o-sal'pin-ji'tis) inflammation of the fallopian tube with collection of pus

pyosalphingo-oophoritis (pi'o-sal-pin'go-o'of-o-ri'tis) inflammation of the ovary and fallopian tube with collection of pus

pyosalpinx (pi'o-sal'pinks) collection of pus in the fallopian tube

pyosemia (pi'o-seme-a) discharge of pus in the semen

pyostatic (pi'o-stat'ik) 1. preventing the formation of pus 2. an agent having such an effect

pyothorax (pi'o-tho'raks) empyema thoracis

pyotorrhoea (pi'o-to-re-a) purulent discharge from the ear

pyourachus (pi'o-u-ra-kus) collection of pus in the urachus

pyoureter (pi'o-u-re'ter) collection of pus in the ureter

pyramid (pir'a-mid) a mass of tissue rising to an apex as in cerebellum and kidneys.

pyramidal (pi-ram'i-dal) in the shape of a pyramid

pyramidalis (-dal'is) *see* table of muscles

pyramidotomy (-dot'o-me) excision of the pyramidal tract

pyrantel pamoate (pi-ran'tel-pam'o-a-te) an anthelmintic used in the treatment of infestation by round worms or thread worms

pyrazinamide (pi'ra-zin'a-mid) a bactericidal antituberculosis drug that has action more marked on intracellular bacilli and in an acid medium. It has a potent sterilising action on slowly multiplying bacilli inside the macrophages

pyrectic (pi-rek'tik) referring to fever

pyrenaemia (pi-rene'me-a) presence of nucleated red blood cells in the blood

pyretherapy (pi-re-thre'a-pe) treatment by raising the body temperature

pyrethrins (pi-re'thrinz) substances obtained by pyrethrum flowers such as Chrysanthemums

pyreto (pi-ret'o) a prefix for fever

pyretogenesis (pi-re-to-jen'e-sis) production of fever

pyretolysis (pi're-to-ti-fo'sis) delirious state induced by high fever

pyrexia (pi-ek-se'a) fever

pyridine (pir'i-din) a colourless volatile liquid obtained by distillation of nitrogen-containing organic matter

pyridostigmine (per'a-do-stig'men) an anticholinesterase used in the treatment of myasthenia

pyridoxine (pi-ri-doks'en) a water soluble vitamin, part of the B complex group derived from pyridine. It functions as coenzyme for the synthesis and breakdown of aminoacids, the conversion of tryptophan to niacin, the breakdown of glycogen to glucose-1 phosphate and the formation of haeme in haemoglobin

pyriform (pir'i-form) pear-shaped

pyrimethamine (pir'i-meth'a-men) a prophylactic antimalarial agent

pyrimidine (pi-rim'id-in) an organic compound of heterocyclic nitrogen found in nucleic acids and in antiviral drugs

pyro (pi'ro) prefix for heat, fire

pyrogen (pi'ro-jen) an agent inducing fever

pyrogenic (pi'ro-jen'ik) inducing fever

pyroglobulinaemia (pi'ro-glob'u-li'ne-me-a) presence of an abnormal globulin in the blood that precipitates irreversibly on heating to 56°C

pyrolysis (pi-rol'i-sis) decomposition of organic matter when there is rise in temperature

pyromania (pi-'ro-ma'ne-a) an impulse-control disorder with an uncontrollable urge to set fires

pyrometer (pi-rom'e-ter) a device for measurement of temperature

pyronine (pi-ro-nin) a stain to demonstrate RNA and DNA

pyronyxis (-nek-sis) cauterisation by hot needles

pyrophobia (-fo'be-a) abnormal fear of fire

pyrophosphate (-fos'fat) any salt of phosphoric acid

pyropuncture (pi'ro-punk'chur) treatment by puncturing with hot needles

pyrosis (pi-ro'sis) heart burn

pyrotic (pi-rot'ik) 1. caustic 2. burning 3. pertaining to pyrosis

pyrotoxin (pi'ro-tok'sin) a toxin produced during fever

pyrrole (per'ol) a heterocyclic substance found in the body, and it provides building blocks for haeme and porphyrin

pyruvate (pi'roo-vat) a salt of pyruvic acid **p kinase** an enzyme essential for anaerobic glycolysis in red blood cells

pyruvic (pi-roo'vik) **acid** an end product of glycolysis in the anaerobic metabolism of glucose

pyrvinium (pir-vin'e-um) **pamoate** a cyanine dye derived drug used in the treatment of threadworm infestation

pythogenesis (pi'tho-jen'e-sis) originating in decaying material

pyuria (pi-u're-a) discharge of pus in the urine and is a sign of urinary tract infection

PZI protamine zinc insulin

Q

Q symbol for blood volume, rate of blood flow, perfusion, electric quantity

q symbol for long arm of a chromosome, electric charge

q.4h *Pres* abbreviation for L. *quaque quarta hora* every four hours

Q angle obtuse angle formed by patellar tendon and patellar ligament

QA abbreviation for quality assurance

QAP abbreviation for quality assurance programme

Q band fluorescent bands that appear at constant sites when chromosomes are stained with quinacrine, a fluorescent dye, which inserts into the DNA helix

QCO_2 microlitres of CO_2 given off per milligram of dry weight of tissue per hour.

q.d. *Pres* abbreviation for L. *quaque die*, every day

Q fever query or Queensland fever. An acute zoonotic rickettsial infection caused by *Coxiella burnetti*. It follows an occupational contact work with livestock and presents with influenza-like picture which may progress to pneumonia. It responds to tetracycline or doxycycline

q. h. *Pres* abbreviation for L. *quaque hora*, every hour

q.i.d. *Pres* abbreviation for L. *quater in die*, four times a day

q.l. *Pres* abbreviation for L. *quantum libet*, as much as one desires

q.n.s. *Pres* abbreviation for quantity not sufficient

QO_2 critical threshold for oxygen delivery: oxygen consumption; the number of microlitres of oxygen taken up per milligram of dry weight of tissue per hour

q.q.h. *Pres* abbreviation for L. *quaque quarta hora*, every four hours

q.q.hor *Pres* abbreviation for L. *quaque hora* every hour

QRS axis *ECG* the mean frontal plane vector of QRS complex which normally lies between 0° and 90°. It can be estimated roughly by seeing which limb lead has the biggest R wave in electrocardiogram

QRS complex *ECG* a complex consisting of a positive deflection R, preceded and followed by negative deflections Q and S respectively in the electrocardiogram. It is produced by ventricular activation

QRS interval *ECG* time taken for ventricular depolarisation and it is measured from the beginning of the Q wave to the end of S wave in the electrocardiogram having its upper limit 0.1 second

QRST complex *ECG* the Q, R, S and T waves of an electrocardiogram. The T wave following the QRS complex, reflects ventricular repolarisation.

QRST interval *ECG* the electrocardiographic period of ventricular electrical activity

q.s. *Pres* abbreviation for L. *quantum sufficit*, as much as it suffices

q-sort (ku'sort) a technique of assessment of personality

Qs flow of blood *via* shunts

Qs/Qt shunt fraction, venous admixure, wasted perfusion, perfusion of poorly ventilated alveoli

Q wave *ECG* a small negative deflection preceding R wave in electrocardiogram which is caused by activation from left to right of the interventricular system

QS wave *ECG* QRS complex in the electrocardiogram without any positive R wave and the whole complex is a negative wave

Qt total blood flow from the right ventricle

QT interval *ECG* duration of ventricular systole is measured in the electrocardiogram from the beginning of the Q wave to the end of T wave and it varies with the heart beat. It represents repolarisation of the heart

QT syndrome *ECG* a combination of prolonged QT interval and *torsades de pointes*

quack (kwak) charlatan; a person who pretends to possess medical knowledge and experience which he does not possess

quackery (kwak'er-i) charlatanism; false representation of a substance, device or therapeutic system, as being beneficial in treating a medical condition

quacksalver (kwak'sal'var) a quack doctor

quadpack quadruple pack; a plastic blood collection bag that has three peripheral bags facilitating the sterile collection and separation of a unit of whole blood (500 ml) into four 125 ml aliquots, useful in transfusion for neonates

quadragenarian (kowd'rajanar'e-an) 40 years of age

quadrangular (kwod-rang'u-ler) having four angles **q lobe** a region forming the superior portion of each cerebellar hemisphere **q membrane** the upper portion of the elastic membrane of the larynx

quadrant (kwod'rant) 1. one quarter of a circle 2. one of the corresponding parts, as of the surface of the abdomen or of the visual field **dental q** one quarter of the mouth, where each arch is divided in half

quadrantanopsia (kwod'rantan-op'sia) blindness in one-fourth of the visual field

quadrantectomy (kwod'ran-tak'ta-me) partial surgical removal of a quadrant of breast

quadrate (kwod'rat) square, four equal sided, rectangular **q lobe** a small lobe of liver located on the visceral surface, lying in contact with pylorus and duodenum

quadratus (kwod'ratus) four-sided

quadri combing word for four

quadriceps (kwod'ri-seps) having four heads **q femoris** powerful anterior thigh muscle with four heads (rectus femoris, vastus lateralis, vastus medialis and vastus intermedius) that extends the knee joint **q reflex** extension of the leg following contraction of quadriceps muscle from patellar tap

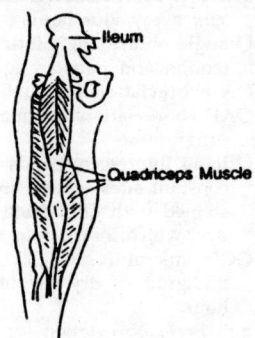

quadricuspid (kwod'ri-kus'pid) having four cusps as in a tooth

quadridigitate (kwod'ri-dij'i-tat) having only four fingers or four toes

quadrigemina (kwod'ri-jem'in-a) four eminences of mid-brain containing accumulations of nerve cells

quadrigeminal (kwod- jem'inal) four-fold, occurring in a group of four **q pulse a** pulse in which a pause occurs after every fourth beat

quadrigeminy (kwod'ri-jemi-ne) occurrence of four beats of the pulse followed by a pause

quadrigeminum (kwod'-ri-jem'-inum) one of the corpora quadrigemina.

quadrigeminus (kwod'ri-jem'i-nus) composed of four parts

quadrilateral (kwod'ri-lat-er-al') having four sides **Celsus q** four signs of inflammation, redness, swelling, heat and pain described by Celsus, Roman medical encyclopaedist in the first century

q socket a four-sided prosthetic socket design for people with above knee amputations

quadrilemmal (kwod'ri-lem'mal) **body** a crystalloid structure seen within mitochondria that is composed of four sets of parallel lines, seen by electron microscopy

quadripara (kwod-ripa-ra) a woman who has had four pregnancies that resulted in giving birth to four viable offsprings, para IV

quadripartite (kwod'ri-par-tit) divided into four parts

quadriparesis (kwod'ri-par-e-sis) weakness of all four limbs

quadriplegia (kwod'ri-ple'je-a) 1. paralysis of all four limbs 2. tetraplegia **flaccid q** can occur in brain stem lesions with neuronal shock, polyneuropathy, due to Guillain-Barre syndrome, diphtheria, or porphyria, myasthenic crisis, periodic dyskalaemic paralysis and polymyositis. **spastic q** can occur in high cervical cord lesions such as cervical spondylosis, craniovertebral anomalies, fracture dislocation of cervical spine, haematomyelia and cervical cord tumours, brain stem lesions such as vertebrobasilar insufficiency, motorneuron disease, disseminated sclerosis, bulbar poliomyelitis and brain stem tumours, or in cortical lesions such as cerebral palsy or decerebrate rigidity

quadriplegic (kwod'ri-ple'jik) referring to quadriplegia

quadrisect (kowd'ri-sekt') to divide into four equal parts

quadrisection (kwod'ri-sek'shun) dividing into four parts

quadritubercular (kwod'ri-tuber'ku-ler) having four tubercles

quadrivalent (kwod'-ri-va'lent) having a combining power or chemical valence of four

quadruped (kwod'-roo-ped) an animal having four feet; assuming a position with hands and feet on floor

quadruple (kwod'roo-ple) four-fold **q syndrome** an autosomal dominant condition characterised by cleft palate, popliteal webbing, lip pitting and genital malformations

quadruplet (kwod'-roo-plet) one of four offsprings from a single gestation

Quain's degeneration degeneration of muscle of the heart, described by Richard Quain, British physician

quale (kwa'le) the quality of a thing especially of the sensation

qualitative (kwol'i-ta'tive) referring to the quality of anything **q data** recording of presence or absence of a characteristic without stating its magnitude

quality (kwol'-te) character, property or attribute **q adjusted life year** QALY a way of assigning a numerical value to the quality of any extra years of life which a particular person's treatment, if successful, is likely to yield **q assurance** QA a formal and systematic set of activities that provides a continuous audit against an established standard quality and which provides a means for correcting deviations from the standard so that a product maintains its quality **q assurance programme** QAP programme to ensure the quality of care, with quality having the characteristics of excellence. It involves five stages - criteria development, description of actual practice, evaluation, corrective action and reassessment **q control** a system to verify and maintain a desired level of quality in a product or process; the assessment of actual performance in relation to performance goals. **q factor** evaluation of the biologic damage that radiation can produce **q of life** a measure of optimal energy or force that endows a person with the power to cope successfully with the full range of challenges encountered in life

qualm (kwam) an uneasy feeling

quantify ('kwon'-ti-fie) to determine quantity

quantimeter (kwon-tim'et-er) device to measure quantity of roentgen rays to which a subject is exposed

quantitative (kwon'ti-ta-tiv) that which is estimated by quantity **q test** result of a measurement on a continuous scale

quantity (kwon'ti-te) amount

quantum (kwon'tum) pl. **quanta** 1. a unit of measure of the amount or quantity 2. a definite amount. *q libet* as much as desired *q sufficit* as much as it suffices

quarantine (kwor'an-ten) 1. isolation or detention of a person who has been exposed to a communicable disease, which is imposed for the maximal incubation period with the purpose of preventing its further dissemination 2. period of detention for vessels, or travellers coming from infected or suspected ports or places

quarry (kwor'e) an excavation usually open to air from which stone is obtained by cutting and blasting; anything eagerly persued

quart (kwort) a unit of measure; two pints, one fourth of a gallon

quartan (kwor'tan) recurring at 72 hour intervals **q fever** the fever caused by *Plasmodium malariae* in which fever spikes appear every third day

quarter (kwor-ter) 1. one fourth 2. the part of a horse's hoof between the toe and the heel; a place to stay in **q moon sign** collection of barium with a smooth inner margin with the concavity towards the lumen as in benign gastric ulcers

quarterly once in three months

quartile (kwar'til) one-fourth of the distribution scores

quartipara (kwor-tip-a-ra) a woman who has had four pregnancies that have resulted in giving birth to four viable offsprigs.

quartisect (kwor'ti-sekt) to cut into four parts

quartz (kworts) silica, a crystalline form of silicon dioxide, principal ingredient of sandstone

quasi- (kwa-si) a prefix which means almost, seemingly but not actually resembling **q species** a mixed population of viruses that have multiple variant nucleic acid sequences as in HIV-1

Quasimodo (kwa-si'mo-do) **syndrome** a disorder characterised by severe kyphoscoliosis, dyspnoea with associated hypoxaemia and altered sleep pattern. It is likened to the symptoms suffered by Victor Hugo's Quasimodo, the hunch back

quassation (kwo-sa'-shun) crushing of drugs

quassia (kwosh'e-a) wood of a tree *Quassia amara* used in the treatment of fever

quasu (kwo'su) bitter wood whose extract acts as an insecticide

quater in die (kwah'ter in de'a) *Pres* qid four times a day

quaternary (kwo'ter-na-re) 1. fourth in order 2. pertaining to a chemical compound in which four atoms or groups of elements are bonded to one atom.

queasy a feeling of sickness in the stomach

Queckenstedt's (kwek'en-stets) **test** absence of variation in pressure of the cerebrospinal fluid when the jugular veins are compressed. It indicates a block in the vertebral canal and was described by German physician, Hans Queckenstedt

queer; abnormal; homosexual

quell (kwel) to suppress

quellung (kwel'ung) swelling of encapsulated bacteria **q reaction** a swelling of the capsule of the bacteria on exposure to specific antisera

quench (kwench) allay, satisfy

quenching (kwench'ing) any interference with the transfer of energy; cooling something that is hot

quengle (kwen'gel) **cast** a two-section, hinged orthopaedic cast for immobilising the lower extremities and used for correction of knee contractures

Quenu-Mayo operation excision of the rectum, together with neighbouring lymph nodes for cancer, described by Andre Quenu, French surgeon and William Mayo, American surgeon

querulent (kever'u-lent) complaining

Quervain's (ker'vanz) **disease** painful tenosynovitis affecting narrow tendon of abductor pollicis longus and extensor pollicis brevis, described by Fritz de Quervain, Swiss surgeon

query (kwer'e) a question, an enquiry

quest search or pursuit

questionnaire (kwes'chenar') a list of questions

Quetelet index body mass index, described by Lumbert Quetelet, Belgian mathematician. The weight in kg is divided by height in metres squared

quick (kwik) fast, sensitive, flesh deep to nails

quickening (kwik'en-ing) a subjective feeling caused by the foetal movement within the uterus, usually noted early in the fifth month of pregnancy as 'fluttering of a bird' by the mother

quicklime calcium oxide, CaO

quicksilver mercury

Quick's (kwiks) **test** one stage prothombin test, time to clot after addition of thromboplastin and calcium. It was described by US physician, Armand Quick

Quick tourniquet test test to determine capillary fragility when the circulation is obstructed in forearm by applying a blood pressure cuff to upper arm and noting the number of petechiae that have appeared

quidding (kwid'ing) a condition wherein the horses take food into the mouth, repeatedly chew and then expel

quid-pro quo-d L one thing in return for another, something for something

quiescence quiet state

quiescent (kwees'ant) quiet, being at rest, still inactive

quiet (kwi'it) making no disturbance **q zone** silent zone, the terminal airways of less than 2 mm in diameter contributing little to the total airflow resistance

quietus put an end to life; release from life

quin one of five children at birth

quinacrine (kwin'ah-krin) an alkaloid used in the suppressive treatment of malaria, and in the treatment of tape worm infestation and giardiasis; mepacrine

quinagolide (kwi'na-go-lide) a non-ergot, dopamine agonist used in the treatment of prolactinoma

quinapril (kwin'ah-pril) an angiotensin-converting enzyme inhibitor used in the treatment of hypertension

quinaquina cinchona

Quincke's (kwink'ez) **disease** angioneurotic oedema, named after German physician, Heinrich Quincke who described it

Quincke's pulse alternate pallor and reddening of capillary areas in the nail bed noted in aortic incompetence; capillary pulse

Quincke's puncture lumbar puncture

quinestrol (kwin-es'trol) a long-acting oestrogen

quinghaosu a Chinese compound extracted from *Artimisia*, useful against multidrug resistant infection with *P. falciparum*

quinidine (kwin'i-din) an alkaloid isomeric with quinine, used to regulate heart rhythm in cardiac arrhythmias. It suppresses excitability and slows conduction in atrial or ventricular muscle

quinine (kwi'nin) an alkaloid obtained from cinchona bark. Its hydrochloride and sulphate preparations are used in treatment of chloroquin-resistant malaria

quininism (kwin'-i-nizm) cinchonism, poisoning by cinchona or its alkaloids

quinoline (kwin'o-len) alkaloid derived from quinine or coal tar possessing antiseptic and antipyretic properties

quinolone (kwin'o-lon) broad spectrum antibiotic related structurally to nalidixic acid with high activity against aerobic gram-negative bacilli and also active against chlamydia and mycoplasmas. Ciprofloxacin, ofloxacin, norfloxacin, pefloxacin, and aerosoxacin are some of examples of quinolone antibiotics. The quinolones target bacterial gyrase

quinone (kwi-non) any of a group of highly aromatic compounds derived from benzene or multiple ring hydrocarbons

quinqu - combining word for, five

Quinquaud's (kan-koz') **sign** feeling trembling of fingers in alcoholism, described by Charles Quinquaud, French physician

quinquecuspid (kwin'kwe-kus'pid) having five cusps

quinquina (kwin-kwi'na) cinchona

quinsy (kwin'ze) 1. painful abscess of tonsils 2. suppurative tonsillitis with peritonsillar abscess

quint – combining word for, five, fifth.

quintan (kwin'tan) recurring at about 96 hours intervals

quintana fever trench fever

quintessence (kwin-tes'ens) a highly concentrated extract of any substance

quinti – combining word for, fifth.

quintipara (kwin-tip'a-ra) a woman who has had five pregnancies which resulted in live births; para V

quintuplet (kwin'tu-plet) one of five offsprings from a single gestation

quirk a peculiarity in action, behaviour, personality or manner

quittor (kwit'er) a fistulous ulcer on the quarters

quiver tremble, vibrate

quoadvitum (kwo'advi'tam) referring to the length of life

quotid daily

quotidian (kwo-tid'e-an) occur daily **q fever** a malarial fever with daily occurrence

quotient (kwo'shent) a number obtained as a result of division **achievement q** the achievement age in learning divided by the mental age **caloric q** the heat generated (in calories) divided by the oxygen consumed (in milligrams) in metabolism **intelligence q** (IQ), a measure of intelligence obtained by dividing mental age by the chronological age and multiplying the result by 100 **respiratory q** (RQ), the ratio of the volume of carbon dioxide liberated by the body tissues to the volume of oxygen absorbed by them **spinal q** a quotient obtained by dividing cerebrospinal fluid pressure after removal of 10 ml of cerebrospinal fluid by that noted before such removal and multiplied by 10. Normally it is 5.5 to 6.5. The quotient is low in subarachnoid block and high in hydrocephalus or meningitis, named after Ayala, Italian neurologist as Ayala quotient

q v *Pres* abbreviation for L. *quantus vis.* as much as you please

Q wave infarct *ECG* a myocardial infarct involving the entire thickness of the myocardium (transmural) which occur from thrombotic occlusion of the proximal coronary arteries. The ECG shows prominent and prolonged Q waves, decreased amplitude of R wave, hyper acute ST elevation and prominent peaked T waves

q w every week

R

Rx recipe, prescription

R symbol for Roentgen

RA abbreviation for rheumatoid arthritis; right atrium

r symbol for ribose, recombinant

Ra radium

RAA renin-angiotensin–aldosterone

rabbit fever *see* tularemia

rabbit nose nose twitching and wrinkling by children with allergic rhinitis. There is upward rubbing of the nose and it may result in a groove formation at the tip of the nose

rabbit syndrome a rare drug induced extra-pyramidal syndrome where the patient makes rapid chewing movements similar to those made by rabbits

rabbetting (rab'et-ing) interlocking of the jagged edges of a fractured bone.

rabid (rab'id) pertaining to or affected with rabies

rabies (ra-bez) hydrophobia, a highly fatal infection caused by a bullet-shaped neurotropic rhabdovirus transmitted by the bite of carnivorous animals. The incubation period, during which the virus is spreading centripetally along axons to the brain varies from 4 to 8 weeks or longer. Though a proportion of people bitten by a rabid animal develop the disease, but once manifest it is almost invariably fatal. The patient becomes increasingly anxious and develops characteristic fear of water, hydrophobia. Any attempt at drinking provokes violent contractions of the diaphragm and other inspiratory muscles. Even the sight or sound of water may precipitate distressing spasms and attacks of panic. There is cranial nerve lesions and hyperpyrexia. Death occurs within a week of the onset of symptoms. The wounds should be thoroughly cleaned; damaged tissue excised and the wound left unsutured. Post exposure prophylaxis is by administration of human diploid cell strain vaccine; 1.0 ml given intramuscularly on days 0, 3, 7, 14, and 28.

race (ras) a class of individuals having common somatic inherited features.

raccoon sign periorbital ecchymosis and it may be a feature of basilar skull fracture; black eyes

racemic (ra-se-mik) compound made up of levorotatory isomers, which is optically inactive under polarised light

racemose (ras'e-mos) branching with nodular ends, resembling a bunch of grapes r aneurysm marked dilatation of lengthened and tortuous blood vessels

rachi pertaining to spine

rachial (ra'ke-al) pertaining to spinal column

rachialgia (ra-ke-al'je-a) pain in the spine

rachianalgesia (ra'ke-an-al-je'ze-a) spinal analgesia

rachicentesis (ra-ki-sen-te'sis) lumbar puncture

rachiometer (ra-ke-om'e-ter) instrument to measure the curvature of the spine

rachigraph (ra'ki-graf) a graph recording the curves of the vertebrae

rachiotomy (ra-ki-ot'mi) laminectomy

rachis (ra'kis) the spinal column

rachitic (ra-kit'ik) rickety; pertaining to rickets r dwarf a person whose retarded growth is caused by rickets r rosary bulbous widening of the costochondral junction due to softened epiphysis, seen in vitamin D-deficient rickets, childhood hypophosphataemia and in adenosine deaminase deficiency

rachitis (ra-kit'is) 1. rickets 2. an inflammatory condition of vertebral column

racial (ra'sheal) **immunity** a form of natural immunity to certain diseases shared by a genetically related population

racquet cells cells in rhabdomyosarcoma which demonstrate a globose swelling at one end, tapering into elongated wispy cytoplasm

racquet finger nail distal phalanx of the thumb being shorter and wider than normal resulting in a shorter and wider than normal nail with a loss of its curvature, may be seen in tertiary hypoparathyroidism

rad a unit to measure the dose absorbed from ionising radiation

radial (ra'di-al) lateral aspect of the upper limb; relating to the radius **r artery** an artery in the forearm, beginning at the bifurcation of the brachial artery giving branches to the forearm, wrist and hand **r bursa** tendon sheath of flexor pollicis in palm and thumb **r immunodiffusion** a method for quantifying serum proteins, complement proteins and immunoglobulins **r keratotomy** tiny shallow incisions made on the cornea to make it bulge slightly to correct for near- sightedness **r nerve** the largest branch of the brachial plexus. The nerve supplies the skin of the arm and forearm and, in the arm triceps, brachialis, brachioradialis, extensor carpi longus *et* brevis and anconeus and in the forearm the extensor group of muscles including supinator **r nerve palsy** weakness of extension of wrist and fingers due to paralysis of wrist and finger extensors and supinator. The condition is often precipitated by sleeping in abnormal posture **r pulse** the pulse of the radial artery felt at the wrist over the radius **r reflex** reflex elicited by tapping over the distal radius with the response being flexion of the forearm

radiant (ra'di-ant) pertaining to any object giving out rays

radiate (ra'de-at) 1. to spread in all directions from a centre 2. to emit radiation

r ligament a ligament that connects the head of a rib with a vertebra and an associated intervertebral disc

radiation (ra-de-a'shun) 1. sending forth of energy in the form of x-rays, radiowaves, visible light, ultraviolet light· and gamma rays 2. the act of diverging in all directions from a centre **r burn** a burn resulting from exposure to radiant energy (sunlight, x-ray or nuclear emissions) **r cataract** a cataract developing after an excessive exposure of the eye to x-rays or other type of radiation **r dermatitis** inflammation of the skin caused by exposure to ionising radiation **r exposure** a measure of the ionisation produced in air by x-rays or gamma rays **r fibrosis** development of fibrosis in all patients with radiation pneumonitis 6-12 month after radiotherapy **r pneumonitis** radiation injury of the lung developing 2 to 6 months following radiation therapy **r oncologist** a physician trained in the use of ionising radiation to treat cancer **r oncology** the study of the treatment of cancer using ionising radiation **r sickness** acute radiation injury presenting with anorexia, nausea, vomiting, fatigue, leucopaenia and thrombocytopaenia **r symbol** a symbol consisting of a purple popeller pattern of three fan- shaped images as if radiating from a solid dark circle on a yellow background

radical (rad'I-kal) 1. a group of atoms acting as a single unit, which do not change while passing from one compound to another 2. oriented towards the root **r dissection** the surgical excision of tissue in an extensive area surrounding the operative site. It is undertaken in malignancy to decrease the chance of recurrence **r mastectomy** excision of entire breast, axillary lymph nodes, pectoral muscles and all fat, fascia and adjacent tissues in cancer of the breast

radicula (ra-dik'u-la) a spinal nerve root

radicular (ra-dik'u-lar) referring to the root of a tooth, or of a spinal nerve **r cyst** a cyst attached to the apex of the root of a tooth with dead pulp

radiculitis (ra-dik-ụ-li-tis) inflammation of a spinal nerve root present within the dura, accompanied by pain and hyperaesthesia

radiculomyelopathy (ra-dik'u-lo-mi'e-lop-a-the) disease affecting spinal cord and spinal nerve root

radiculography introduction of contrast liquid into subarachnoid space to visualise lumbosacral roots

radiculopathy (ra-dik'u-lop'a-the) a disease of the spinal nerve roots

radioactive (ra'de-o-ak-tiv) possessing radioactivity **r decay** changes occurring in the nucleus of a radioactive isotope which result in the liberation of neutrons, protons and electrons **r element** an element subject to spontaneous degeneration of its nucleus accompanied by the emission of alpha particles, beta particles or gamma rays **r iodine** a radioactive isotope of iodine used as a tracer. It is used in management of hyperthyroidism where it acts by destroying functioning thyroid cells or by inhibiting their ability to replicate

radioactivity (ra'de-o-ak-tiv'i-te) the property of emission of rays (alpha, beta, gamma) as a consequence of its nuclear degeneration

radioallergosorbent (ra'de-o'alur'gosor'bent) **test** a test to detect presence of IgE antibodies in blood to various allergens by a technique of radioimmunoassay; RAST

radiobiology (ra'de-o'bi-ol'eje) the biologic study of the effects of ionising radiation upon living organisms

radiocarpal relating to the radius and the bones of the carpus **r articulation** the wrist joint that connects the radius and distal surface of an articular disc with scaphoid, lunate and triquetral bones

radiocinematography (ra'de-o-cin'e-ma-tog-ra-fi) taking a moving picture of the movements of the organs in a radiologic examination

radiodermatitis dermatitis due to exposure to ionising radiation

radio-diagnosis diagnosis by x-rays

radio-femoral delay delay of the femoral pulse compared to the radial pulse in coarctation of the aorta

radiogram (ra'de-o-gram) radiograph

radiograph (ra'de-o-graf) roentgenogram wherein a shadow image is produced on a sensitised film by radiography

radiographer (ra'de-og'rafer) a paramedical professional using radiographic imaging modalities as directed by a physician

radiography (rade-og'ra-fi) roentgenography; production of images upon a photographic plate of film of any region of the body by passing x-rays

radioimmunoassay (ra'de-o-im'no-as'sa) RIA, an immunologic procedure utilising a radioisotope substance to measure the amount of specific antibodies or antigens present in the test fluid

radioimmunoelectrophoresis (ra'de-o-im'u-no-e-lek'tro-fo-re'sis) electrophoresis procedure of an antigen or antibody labelled with a radioisotope

radioimmunosorbent (ra'de-o-im'uno-sor'bent) **assay test** a test that uses serum immunoglobulin E to detect allergies to different substances

radioimmunoprecipitation assay RIPA, a technique to identify antibodies to specific viral components and it requires an electrophoretic separation step

radioisotope (ra-de-o-i'so-top) an unstable isotope that decays to a stable state by emitting radiation

radioligand (ra-de-o–lig'and) a molecule with a radionuclide tracer attached

radiologist (ra'de-o-lo jist) roentgenologist, a specialist in radiography

radiology (ra'de-olo'ji) roentgenology, a branch of science concerned with radiant energy

radiolucency (ra'de'-o-loo'sensi) material allowing x-rays to pass through them to produce relatively dark images

radiolucent (ra'de-olu'-sent) pertaining to

materials that allow radiation to penetrate with a minimum of absorption

radiometer (ra'di-o-me-ter) a device to determine the penetrative pow.er of x-rays

radiomimetic drug an immunosuppressive agent which has effects on nucleic acid, and used in the treatment of malignancy

radionecrosis necrosis occurring after excessive exposure to radiation

radionuclide (rade-o-noo'klid) an isotope exhibiting radioactivity **r imaging** examination of different parts of the body especially the heart using thallium 201

radiopaque (ra-de-o-pak) relatively impenetrable to radiation and such substances are used to make organs to stand out more clearly on x-ray images **r dye** a chemical substance that does not permit the passage of x-rays

radioresistant (ra'de-o-resis'tent) unaffected by radiation

radiosensitive (ra'de-o-sen'sitis) affected by radiation

radiosensitivity the relative susceptibility of cells and tissues to irreversible damage by radiation

radiotherapist a specialist in therapeutic use of radiant energy

radiotherapy (ra'de-o-ther'epe) the medical speciality concerned with use of radiant energy from a cobolt source in the treatment of disease; exposure of a defined area of the body to a source of ionising radiation under carefully controlled conditions

radish bacillus a non-photochromogen, *Mycobacterium terrae* isolated from soil and vegetables. It is non-pathogenic

radium (ra'de-um) a radioactive metallic element, symbol Ra, atomic no. 88 **r insertion** an introduction of metallic radium into body cavity, such as uterus or cervix to treat cancer **r therapy** the use of radium and its radioactive emissions to treat malignant condition

radius (radi-us) 1. the lateral short bone of the forearm lying parallel to the ulna. Its small proximal end forms part of the elbow joint and the large distal end forms a part of the wrist joint. 2. a straight line drawn from the centre to the periphery of a circle pl. **radii**

radix root

radon a radioactive gas resulting from the decay of uranium. Symbol Rn, atomic no. 86 **r daughters** electrically charged ions that are decay products of radon gas that are potential health hazard **r seed** a small sealed tube containing radon for insertion into body tissues in the treatment of malignancies

RADS reactive airway dysfunction syndrome

ragged red fibre disease a mitochondrial myopathy exhibiting extensive cell destruction at the skeletal muscle cell periphery with vacuolated fibres which are 'ragged'

rajas (s) menstrual blood

ragocyte an atypical neutrophil containing IgM rheumatoid factor, IgG complement and fibrin, seen in rheumatoid arthritis

Rai staging system five-stage to determine survival of untreated patients with chronic lymphocytic leukaemia

railroad track appearance parallel, relatively straight line radio-opacities or radiolucencies of varying length

Raji cell a B lymphoblastic cell with minimal or no surface immunoglobulin, low avidity Fc receptors and a high density of C3 receptors, used to detect circulating immunoglobulins in serum

rakta (s) blood *pitta* haematemesis *r mokshana* blood letting

rale (rahl) crepitation; crackles heard as a moist adventitious sounds on auscultation of the chest

raloxifene selective oestrogen receptor modulator

ramification (ram-I-fi-ka'shun) branching

ramify (ram-i-fi) to branch

ramipril an ACE inhibitor

Ramsay Hunt's syndrome herpes zoster infection of the geniculate ganglion, characterised by rash over the palate and over external ear, severe ear pain, vertigo, hearing loss and lower motor neuron facial palsy, named after James Ramsay Hunt, US neurologist

RAMTES abbreviation for regulated activated normal T cells expressed secreted

ramus (ra'mus) a branch pl. **rami**

rancid (ran'sid) 1. stinking 2. a disagreeable odour and taste

random controlled trial a study plan for a new treatment modality where the subjects are assigned on a random basis where the experimental group receives new treatment and the control group a placebo

random variable *stat* a variable for which the variation is determined by chance

Randomisation allocation of the patients taking part in the trial at random to treatment group or the control group

range (ranj) a statistical measure of dispersion of values determined by the end point values **r of accommodation** the distance between the far point that an object can be seen clearly with accommodation fully relaxed and the nearest distance that an object can be seen with full accommodation **r of motion** the range of movement of a joint from a maximum extension to maximum flexion

ranine (ra'nin) relating to the under-surface of the tongue

ranitidine (ranit'iden) a histamine H_2 receptor antagonist indicated in the treatment of peptic ulcers and gastric hyper-secretory states

Ranke (ran'ke) **complex** parenchymal calcification plus scattered calcification of a hilar or mediastinal draining lymph nodes, named after Karl Ranke, German physician

Ranson (ran'sun) **criteria** scoring system to predict morbidity and mortality of alcohol-induced acute pancreatitis attack

ranula (ran'u-la) sublingual cyst. A mucocele in the floor of the mouth caused by obstruction of the ducts of sublingual salivary glands

Ranvier's (ranve'az) **nodes** constrictions in the myelin substance of a nerve fibre at regular intervals, described by Louis Ranvier, French pathologist

rape (rap) a physical and emotional outrage that assaults psychological well-being in a particular way. It is a sexual assault and there is sexual intercourse with a woman by force or without her legal consent **aquaintance r** forced sexual intercourse between individuals who know each other.

raphe (ra'fe) a line of union of two contiguous bilaterally symmetrical structures **r of tongue** a fibrous wall forming a line of union between the right and left sides of the tongue

rapid card test test to detect circulating *W bancrofti*-specific antigen

rapinirole a non-ergoline dopamine agonist

rapport (rap-or') a sense of mutuality and understanding underlying a relationship between two persons

raptus (rap'tus) a state of intense emotional or mental excitement

rarefaction (rar'e-fak'shun) a condition of becoming light or less dense

rasa (s) taste, juice, chyle, essence.

rasa sala (s) alchemist's laboratory.

rasavaidya (s) system of therapeutic alchemy

ras genes a family of oncogenes and proto-oncogenes first identified in a rat sarcoma, which encode oncoproteins or proto-oncoproteins

rash a cutaneous eruption

raspberry tongue bright red tongue with oedematous white papillae seen in scarlet fever

raspberry tumour umbilical adenoma occurs due to prolapse of the mucosa of unobliterated distal part of the vitellointestinal duct, seen in infants as a pedunculated raspberry-coloured mass with a tendency to bleed

ras proteins proteins carrying guanosine-diphosphate (GDP). It is converted to GTP by activated upstream signalling molecules

RAST radio allergosorbent test

rat-bite fever febrile illness following rat bite carrying *Spirillum minus* or *Streptobacillus moniliformis*. It is characterised by fever, headache, malaise, nausea, vomiting and rash. There is a swelling at the site of the wound and regional lymphadenopathy. It responds to penicillin

rate (rat) measurement of an event in relation to some fixed standard

Rathke's (rat'kez) **pouch** a depression that forms the roof of the mouth of an embryo. The walls of the diverticulum develop into the anterior lobe of the pituitary gland, described by Martin Rathke, German anatomist

ratio (ra'shi-o) an expression used to relate one quantity to another

rational (rash'en-el) 1. of or pertaining to a method, or procedure based on reason 2. normal reasoning or behaviour

rationale (rash'-en-al) a system of reasoning used in explaining data or phenomenon

rationalisation (rash'enal'iza-shun) a defence mechanism wherein an individual justifies ideas, actions or feelings with seemingly acceptable reasons or explanation

rattle a coarse vibratory sound heard by auscultation

rattle snake a poisonous pit viper with a series of loosely connected horny segments at the end of the tail

rauwolfia (rowol'fe-a) dried roots of *Rauwolfia serpentina* that provide extracts for antihypertensive agents and tranquillising alkaloids like reserpine, named after Leonhard Rauwolf, German botanist

raw milk unpasteurised milk

ray a line of light, heat or other forms of radiation

Raynaud's (ra-noz') **disease** a disorder wherein exposure to cold causes sudden contraction of small arteries supplying the fingers and toes, named after Maurice Raynaud, French physician

Raynaud's phenomenon abnormal sensitivity in response to exposure to cold causing intense vasospasm of peripheral arteries. It affects hands and passes through three stages with sudden onset precipitated by cold, stage of blanching due to local syncope, stage of dusky cyanosis from local asphyxia and stage of red engorgement and recovery. They are usually accompanied by numbness, tingling, burning and often pain. Warmth restores normal colour and sensation. It is noted in systemic sclerosis, SLE, thoracic outlet syndrome, drug intoxication and trauma, named after Maurice Raynaud, French physician

RBBB abbreviation for right bundle branch block

RBC abbreviation for red blood cell or red blood corpuscle

RCA right coronary artery

reabsorption (re'absorp-sh-en) the process of something being absorbed again

reaction (re-ak-shun) a response in opposition to a stimulus, substance or treatment

reactivate (re-ak'ti-vat) to make active again adj. **reactivity**

reactivation restoration of a cell or molecule's functional activity

reading disorder a language disorder in which one's reading ability is markedly below intellectual capacity

Read method a method of psychophysical preparation for natural childbirth, designed by Grantly Dick-Read

reagent (re-a'-jent) a chemical substance known to react in a specific way

reagin (re'ajin) an initiator of the immediate hypersensitivity reaction; IgE

reality testing *Psy* the objective evaluation and judgement of the world outside the self

real time imaging visualisation of a dynamic process within microseconds after its occurrence. It is a modality requiring very rapid information processing as in 'B' mode ultrasound

reapproximate (re'aprok'simat) to rejoin the tissues separated by surgery or trauma

reattachment (re'atach'ment) the rejoining of accidentally severed body parts

rebase (rebas) a process of refitting a denture by replacing or adding to its base material without changing the occlusal relationship of teeth

rebound tenderness deep pressure is exerted over the site of pain on the abdomen. The hand is removed suddenly and the patient experiences sharp pain indicating inflammation of the parietal peritoneum

rebreathing (re-bre'thing) inhalation of gas previously exhaled as in breathing into a closed system **r bag** a flexible bag attached to a mask. It serves as a reservoir for anaesthetic gases or for oxygen

recalcification (re-kal'si-fika'shen) the replacement of lost calcium salts in the body

recall the process of remembering thoughts, words and actions of a past event

recanalization (re-kan'ah-li-za'shun) restoration of the continuity of the lumen

recannulate (rekan'yulat) to make a new opening through an organ or tissue

receptor (re-sep'tor) a nerve cell responding to a specific stimulus by producing nerve impulses or an area on the surface of a cell to which a chemical substance binds to have its effect **r defect** a defect in a receptor that prevents the chemical that normally binds to it from having its effect **r site** a location on a cell surface where certain molecules attach to interact with cellular components

recess (re'ses) a small hollow cavity

recession (re-sesh'un) retraction or withdrawal

recessive (re-ses'iv) 1. receeding 2. suppressed 3. pertaining to gene whose effect is masked or hidden in presence of a dominant gene at the same locus **r gene** the member of a pair of genes that lacks the ability to express itself in presence of its more dominant allele. It is a trait expressed in individuals who are homozygous for a particular gene but not seen in heterozygote **r inheritance** a pattern of inheritance wherein a person inherits two copies of a particular recessive gene (one from each parent) to be affected by it. The parents are unaffected **r trait** a genetically determined characteristic that is expressed only when present in the homozygotic state

receipe (res'i-pi) 1. a prescription or formula 2. take; superscription of a prescription

recipient (ris'i-pe-ant) the person who receives a blood transfusion, or tissue graft or organ

reclination (rek'li-na-shun) to bend back.

recombinant (re-kombi-nent) *mol* obtaining genetic material from a different strain or inserting a new sequence into a chain **r DNA** a DNA molecule in which rearrangement of the genes has been artificially induced by enzymes **r DNA technology** technique that consist of 'gene engineering' in which a gene producing a protein of interest from one organism is spliced into the genome of another organism **r pharmacology** use of recombinant DNA techniques to produce DNA-derived biological products for use in disease states or to increase a desired biologic function

recombination (re'kom-bin-a-shun) a normal meiotic process wherein the genes from two genetically distinct individuals are mixed, to result in progeny that differs from parents

recon (re'kon) *mol* the smallest unit of recombination between two homologous chromosomes

reconstitution (re'kons-tit-oo'shen) the continuous repair of damaged tissue

reconstructive surgery surgical procedure attempting to restore a tissue close to its original structure

record (ri-cord) a written document of information relevant to the care of a patient

recoup to recover, to regain, to make up for

recovery room an area adjacent to the operation theatre in which surgical patients are taken care while still under effects of anaesthesia before being returned to the ward

recreational drug any substance with pharmacologic effects that is taken voluntarily for personal pleasure

recrement (rek're-ment) a secretion

recrudescence (re-kru-des'ens) a recurrence of a morbid process or its symptoms following a period of improvement

rectal (rek'tal) relating to the rectum **r abscess** an abscess in the perianal region **r alimentation** administration of nourishment in a concentrated form by instillation through rectum **r bleeding** bleeding from rectum from injury, polyp, carcinoma, ulcerative colitis and prolapse **r carcinoma** a primary adenocarcinoma which gives a rapidly growing bulky mass and present with bleeding rectum, sense of incomplete defection and altered bowel habit **r prolapse** a descent of the bowel through the anal opening. It is incomplete if only mucosa is prolapsing and complete if entire wall of the rectum protrudes **r reflex** defecation response to the presence of an accumulation of faeces in the rectum; defecation reflex **r temperature** temperature measured in the rectum, which is generally 0.3 to 0.4°C or 0.5 to 0.75°F higher than mouth temperature **r thermometer** a

clinical thermometer suitable for measuring body temperature rectally **r tube** a flexible tube inserted into the rectum to assist in the relief of gas

rectify (rek'ti-fi) to correct

rectilinear (rek'tilin'e-ar) **scanner** a device generating an image of an anatomical structure by detecting radioactivity within the structure

rectocoele (rek't-o-sel) a protrusion of the rectum and the posterior wall of the vagina into the vagina.

rectoscope (rek'to-skop) proctoscope

rectosigmoid (rek-to-sig'moyd) pertaining to rectum and sigmoid colon

rectosigmoidoscopy (-o-s'kape) the examination of the rectum and sigmoid colon with a sigmoidoscope

rectovaginal (-vaj'i-nal) pertaining to rectum and vagina **r fistula** an abnormal passage between the rectum and vagina

rectum (rek'tum) the terminal part of the alimentary tract extending from the sigmoid colon to the anal canal where faeces collect before being eliminated. It is about 12 cm long and contains three transverse semilunar folds which overlap when the intestine is empty

recumbent (re-kum'bent) to lie back

recuperate (re-ku'per-at) to recover one's health and strength

recuperation (re-u'per-a-shun) the process of recovering health and strength

recurrence (re-kur'ens) 1. relapse 2. return of symptoms of a disease after a period of remission

recurrent (re-kur'ent) 1. reappearance of symptoms or lesion after an interval 2. turning back on oneself **r bandage** a bandage that is wrapped several times around itself as in head or an amputated stump

red blood cell one of the doughnut-shaped cells in the blood concerned with the transportation of oxygen from lungs to body tissues

red cell fragmentation syndrome a haemolytic condition caused by mechanical intravascular destruction of red cells as seen in valvular heart disease, prosthetic valves, malignant hypertension or thrombotic thrombocytopaenic anaemia

red cell preservative maintenance of a unit of packed red cells in fluid state until the time of transfusion by addition of preservative such as citrate, phosphate, and dextrose with adenine

Red Cross International an international Geneva-based organisation which endeavours to prevent and alleviate human sufferings wherever it may be found, to protect life and health and to ensure respect for human being

red degeneration necrosis seen in uterine leiomyomas or fibromas in pregnancy

red diaper syndrome a rare type of gastroenteritis seen in early infancy due to *Serratia marcescens* which produces a red pigment

red eye an inflammed eye caused by conjunctivitis

red hepatization second stage in the development of lobar pneumonia wherein the lung is red due to extravasation of erythrocytes and becomes liver-like due to accumulation of fibrin

red hot throat erythematous, acutely inflammed oropharynx seen in various infections

red infarct a pathologic change that occurs in brain that has been rendered ischaemic by lack of blood

red marrow the red vascular substance found in the cavities of many bones. It is concerned with the production and release of erythrocytes and leucocytes into the blood stream

redirection activity *Psy* the venting of one's drive from two or more incompatible, but simultaneously activated, drives on some third object

redman syndrome an abrupt onset of maculopapular erythema with hypotension may develop following rapid intravenous infusion of vancomycin for gram-negative septicemia in neutro-

paenic patients which is associated with release of histamine

red nucleus a prominent mass in the tegmentum of the midbrain

redon (re'don) *mol* the smallest unit of the DNA molecule capable of recombination

redox an abbreviation for reduction-oxidation reaction

red pulp a histologically distinct zone of the spleen which conditions the reticulocytes and removes defective erythrocytes and helps in reutilisation of iron

red,white and blue sign spider bite causing central blistering with ecchymosis surrounded by blanched skin, which in turn is surrounded by erythema

reduce (rid'oos) 1. the restoration of a part to its original position after displacement 2. to decrease the amount, size, extent or number of something

reducibility a lump when compressed gently moves into the adjoining cavity from which it has come out, and is a cardinal sign of uncomplicated hernia

reduction (re-duk'shun) 1. repositioning 2. restoration 3. gain one or more electrons by a compound 4. addition of a hydrogen to a substance 5. removal of oxygen from a substance 6. the correction of a fracture, hernia or luxation **r diet** a diet that is low in calories, used for reduction of body weight **r of fracture** the technique of manipulating or surgically realigning displaced broken bony ends

reduplication (re-du-pli-ka'shun) doubling

Reed-Sternberg cell a large, multinucleated reticuloendothelial cell found in Hodgkin's disease, named afer Dorothy Reed, US pathologist and Karl Sternberg, Austrian pathologist

reentry (re'en'tri) return of the same impulse into an area of heart and cause its reactivation **r tear** the most distal intimal tear in a dissecting aortic aneurysm, allowing the blood to return to the circulation

reference range a set of values established as reasonable maximums or minimums for a given analyte

referral referring a patient for second opinion or treatment to a specialist

referred pain pain felt at a distance from its real site as in pain from inflamed diaphragm being felt at the tip of the shoulder, or pain from myocardial infarct referred to the jaw and upper arm

reflection (re'flek'shun) 1. bending back 2. sending back of light or other form of radiant energy from a surface

reflectors substances which when present on the skin surface reflect the rays of light in other directions and prevent their entry into the skin. The examples are titanium dioxide, tannic oxide and calamina

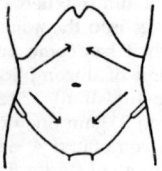

Abdominal reflex

reflex (re'fleks) an involuntary motor response in response to a stimulus. It is dependent on the integrity of a sensory receptor, an afferent pathway in the peripheral or cranial nerve, centre in the spinal cord, brain stem or midbrain, path in the peripheral or cranial nerve and an effector in the muscle **abdominal r** reflex elicited by scratching the abdominal wall with a blunt point when the patient is recumbent and relaxed. There is contraction of abdominal muscles with drawing of the *linea alba* and the umbilicus towards the stimulus. The reflex is lost in upper motor neuron lesions, acute abdominal conditions and in abdominal distension **anal r** scratching the skin around the anus results in immediate contraction of the voluntary anal sphincter **biceps r** *see* biceps jerk **brachioradialis r** *see* brachioradialis jerk **ciliospinal r** normally pupil dilates when the skin of the neck is pinched, due to reflex excitation of the pupil-dilating fibres in cervical sympathetic. It is lost in the lesions of the sympathetic tract and pathway in the spinal cord. The loss of reflex is useful to assess the depth of coma and to diagnose brain death **cremasteric r** it is elicited by stroking the inner parts of the upper thigh in male patients. There is drawing of the testicle upwards due to contraction of *dortos* muscle. It is not elicited in pyramidal tract lesion and in conditions associated with hydrocoele, or orchitis and in elderly men **deep r** muscle or monosynaptic stretch reflex, a single sharp tap with a soft rubber hammer on the tendon of a slightly stretched muscle results in a brief contraction of the muscle **glabellar r** there is blinking when the middle of the forehead above the level of the nose is tapped with the finger. Normally it stops quickly on continuing tapping, but it continues to occur rhythmically in senile dementia and Parkinsonism **Gonda's r** extension of big toe with slight dorsiflexion of the foot occur on squeezing the calf in gross lesions of corticospinal tract **grading of r** tendon reflexes are graded on their briskness as 0 (absent), 1 (normal), 2 (brisk), 3 (very brisk) and 4 (clonus) **grasp r** grasping of the examiner's finger when it is drawn across the patient's palm between the thumb and index fingers in lesions of contralateral frontal lobe; reflex is normally present in infancy **myotonic r** delayed return of contracted muscle to the resting phase as in myxoedema **organic r** act of swallowing, micturition and defecation are a reflex phenomenon and depend on complex movement of striated and unstriated muscles **palatal r** reflex contraction and elevation of soft palate and uvula on touching posterior wall of the pharynx **reinforcement of r** *see* Jendrassik's manoeuvre, **released r** certain reflexes released from the control of higher centres are elicitable in patients with dementia and organic confusional states **superficial r** reflexes elicited by stimulating an area of skin (scratching), or mucous membrane (touching), the examples are corneal, conjunctival, palatal, ciliospinal, abdominal, cremasteric reflexes and plantar response **visceral r** organic reflex

reflex arc a neurologic unit of a sensory neuron that carries a sensory impulse to the spinal cord where it connects to a motor neuron that carries the reflex impulse back to an appropriate muscle or gland

reflex emesis vomiting induced by touching the mucous membrane of the throat

reflex hammer a percussion mallet with a rubber head that is used to tap tendons or muscles to elicit reflex reaction

reflexogenic (re'flok-so-jenik) causing a reflex

reflexology an ancient form of healing which uses pressure particularly on the feet

reflux (re-fluks) a backward flow **bile r** duodenogastric bile reflux leading to chronic gastritis. It may be asymptomatic or present with dyspepsia **hepatojugular r** firm pressure over the right upper abdomen or elsewhere in the abdomen of a recumbent patient with neck at 45° angle while breathing normally will cause distension of the neck veins and moving up of the level of venous pulsation indicating early right heart failure **gastrooesophageal r** a backflow of acid from the stomach into the lower part of the oesophagus.

It occurs due to inefficiency of gastro-oesophageal sphincter **r oesophagitis** oesophageal irritation and inflammation that occurs from reflux of stomach contents into the oesophagus

refract (re'frakt) a bend of a ray of light

refraction (re-frak'shun) 1. deflection of a ray of light when it passes from one medium to another of different optical density 2. determination of the nature and extent of the refractive errors in the eyes and its connection by lenses

refractionist (re-frak'shun-ist) a person trained in the measurement of the refraction of the eye and to determine the proper corrective lenses

refractive (re-frak'tiv) **error** a defect in the ability of the lens of the eye to focus an image accurately **r index** a numerical expression of the refractive power of a medium **r surgery** a surgical technique performed on the cornea to correct myopia by changing the configuration of the cornea

refractometer (re-frak-tom'e-ter) an instrument to measure the degree of refraction in translucent substances especially the media of the eye

refractory (re-frak'to-ri) pertaining to a disorder that is resistant to the treatment; intractable

refracture (re-frak'chur) breaking a bone that had been united after a fracture

refrigeration (re-fri'jer-a'shun) the act of cooling

Refsum's (ref'soomz) **disease** a rare hereditary disorder of lipid metabolism with accumulation of phytic acid resulting in ataxia, retinitis pigmentosa, polyneuropathy and a raised CSF protein. Treatment is avoiding substances rich in diet such as butter, animal fat and vegetables, named after Sigvald Refsum, Norwegian physician

regeneration (rejen-er-a'shun) reproduction or reconstitution of a lost or injured part. There is a high rate of regrowth of cells in bone marrow, gastrointestinal tract, liver and skin

regimen (rej'i-men) a regulation of the mode of living, diet, exercise etc. for health or therapy

region (re'jun) a portion of the body

regional (re'je-nal) of or pertaining to a geographic area or to a part of the body **r anaesthesia** anaesthesia of an area of the body by injecting a local anaesthetic agent to block a group of sensory nerve fibres **r enteritis** *see* Crohn's disease

registered medical practitioner a medical professional who has completed a course of study at a recognised medical institution and registered in the medical council of the state or country

regression (re-gresh'un) 1. subsidence 2. relapse 3. return **r line** *stat* a line that defines the amount of change in one variable per unit change in the other

regulation (regu-la'shun) control

regurgitant (re-garji-tant) backward flow **r murmur** a cardiac murmur caused by a defective valve allowing blood flow backwards as in pansystolic murmur of mitral incompetence and early diastolic murmur of aortic incompetence

regurgitate (re-ger'ji-tat) to flow backward

regurgitation (re-ger'ji-ta'shun) a backward flow as in return of swallowed food or drink from the stomach back into the mouth or the backflow of blood through an incompetent valve

rehabilitation (re-ha-bil'i-ta'shun) restoration of ability to function

rehydration (re-hi-dra'shun) the return of water to a system following its loss **r solution** any fluid that is used to treat severe diarrhoea. Two types of solutions commonly used are glucose-based which increases intestinal resorption of fluids and electrolytes, and rice-syrup based solution which in addition decreases the stool output

Reid index hypertrophy of mucus glands in chronic bronchitis can be quantified. It is based on ratio of the thickness of the submucous glands to that of the bronchial wall (from the basement membrane of epithelium to cartilage). Normally it is less than 0.4. It reaches 0.7 to 0.8 in chronic bronchitis as the gland thickness exceeds two-thirds of the lumen of proximal airways, described by Lynn Reid, a pathologist

reinfection (re-infe'shun) a second infection by the same micro-organism after recovery from a primary infection

reinforcement an increase of force or strength

reinnervation (re'in-ner-va'shun) restoration of nerve supply

reintegration (re'in-te-gra'shun) return of well adjusted functions after disturbances due to a mental disorder

Reiter's (ri'terz) **syndrome** occurrence of urethritis, conjunctivitis and arthritis. It usually follows a case of nongonococcal urethritis, named after Hans Reiter, German hygienist

rejection (re-jek'shun) 1. refuse to accept 2. incompatibility in a transplanted organ 3. an immune reaction evoked by allografted organs

rejuvenation (re-ju've-na'shun) restoration of health and vitality

relapse (re'laps) recurrence or recrudescence

relapsing fevers a group of diseases due to infection by spirochaetes of the genus Borrelia transmitted by body lice or soft ticks; vagabond fever

relapsing polychondritis recurrent inflammation and destruction of cartilaginous and other connective tissue structures

relation (re-la'shun) a connection between people or objects

relative bradycardia normally for each half degree centigrade rise of temperature the pulse rate quickens by 10 beats. The pulse-temperature relationship is not maintained in typhoid, meningitis, cerebral abscess, dengue fever, hepatitis and burns where the pulse rate is relatively slow when compared to the temperature

relative risk the ratio of the frequency of a certain disorder in groups exposed and groups not exposed to a particular hereditary or environment factor

relative tachycardia the pulse rate quickens out of proportion to the temperature in cases of rheumatic fever, diphtheria, clostridial infections, tuberculosis and thyrotoxicosis

relaxant relaxing

relaxation (re'lak-sa'shun) loosening, lengthening or dilatation; any conversion of a system to a state requiring less energy

relaxin an insulin-like polypeptide produced by the corpus luteum that relaxes ligaments at symphysis pubis and sacroiliac joints

releasing hormone RH one of several peptides produced by the hypothalamus and secreted directly into the interior of pituitary through a connecting vein

reliability 1. *stat* the extent to which a measuring procedure yields consistent results on repeated trials 2. repeatability, stability **r of a measurement** the ratio of variance due to differences among subjects divided by the total variance

relieve (re-lev') to free from

REM 1. rapid eye movement **REM sleep** rapid eye movement sleep. A segment of normal sleep cycle where eye muscles contract rapidly and dreaming occurs in which the usual high amplitude slow brain waves seen by EEG are replaced by rapid eye movement, rapid, low voltage irregular EEG activity, a pattern similar to that seen in an awake person

remedy (rem'e-di) an agent that cures the disease or relieves its symptoms

remineralisation (re'min'er-al-I-za'shun) replenishment of the minerals lost through disease or dietary deficiencies

remission (re-mish'un) partial or complete disappearance of symptoms or lesions

remittent temporary relief of the symptoms **r fever** *see* fever

renal relating to kidney **r anuria** cessation of urine production due to diseases of the kidney **r arteriography** injection of contrast material into the aorta to investigate suspected renal artery stenosis or haemorrhage **r artery** *see* arteries **r artery stenosis** atheromatous narrowing of the renal artery leading to secondary hypertension **r biopsy** study of renal tissue to establish the nature and extent of renal disease **r calculus** renal stone, may be of calcium oxalate, phosphate, uric acid and urates, cystine or rarely xanthine indigo matrix stone, may be asymptomatic or present with dull aching pain **r calyx** the first part in the system of ducts in the kidney carrying urine from the renal pyramid of the cortex to the renal pelvis for excretion through the ureters **r capsule** a connective tissue capsule surrounding the kidney **r colic** a gripping pain which comes in waves with freedom from pain between the attacks. It starts in loin and then radiaties downwards obliquely across abdomen towards groin and the patient is found rolling in bed **r dialysis** treatment method used in the management of acute or chronic renal failure where the excretory function of the kidney are partially replaced by dialysis wherein the blood is diffused across a semipermeable membrane **r failure** failure of excretory function of the kidneys, leading to retention of nitrogen waste products of metabolism. Acute renal failure (ARC) is a sudden and usually reversible loss of renal function, which develops over a period of days or weeks. Biochemically there is increase in plasma creatinine concentration to greater then 200 m mol/l. The cause of it can't be rapidly corrected, it has to be managed by dialysis. Chronic renal failure (CRF) is an irreversible deterioration in renal function which develops over a period of years. The condition is caused by any condition which destroys the normal architecture and function of the kidney **r function** kidney regulates the volume and composition of body fluids. It is the main source of erythropoietin. Kidney is essential for the metabolism of vitamin D and it secretes renin **r hypertension** hypertension resulting from kidney disease **r glycosuria** an autosomal recessive condition in which there is glycosuria without hyperglycaemia. The patients are asymptomatic and have a normal glucose tolerance test **r osteodystrophy** a metabolic bone disease accompanying CRF. It consists of a mixture of osteomalacia, osteitis fibrosa, osteoporosis and osteosclerosis **r papillary necrosis** an analgesic nephropathy developing from long continued ingestion of analgesic drugs **r papilloma** a premalignant growth arising in the renal pelvis that presents as painless, profuse and paroxysmal haematuria **r pelvis** a funnel-shaped dilatation that drains urine from the kidney to ureter **r pyramid** one of the conical masses of tissue that form the kidney medulla that consist of the loops of the Henle and the collecting tubules of nephrons **r rickets** a condition characterised by rachitic changes in the skeleton due to chronic nephritis **r sclerosis** atherosclerosis of the arterioles of the kidney **r tuberculosis** occurs secondarily to the presence of primary lesion elsewhere, presents with increased frequency of micturation both during day and night and urine is sterile on ordinary culture **r tubular acidosis** a condition caused by functional defects in the distal renal tubules with loss of ability to form ammonia and to exchange hydrogen ions. The glomerular filtration rate is normal, but there is persistent metabolic acidosis and hyperchloraemia and markedly decreased urinary excretion of acid **r tubule** the part of nephron that leads from the glomerulus to the collecting tubules **r ultrasound** a quick, non-invasive method of renal imaging. It shows renal size and position, dilatation of the collecting system, tumours and cysts **r vein** *see* veins **r transplantation** kidney graft to restore normal kidney function and to correct the metabolic abnormalities of CRF

reniform kidney-shaped

renin (re'nin) proteolytic enzyme produced in the juxtaglomerular apparatus that converts angiotensinogen to angiotensin. It occurs in response to a reduction in renal perfusion pressure

renin-angiotensin-aldosterone system RAA system plays a major role in the humoral control of blood pressure and volume

Rendu-Osler-Weber disease familial telangiectasia affecting the skin, mucous membranes and other organs. The telangiectasia appear in childhood and later in life. The lesions may bleed, named after Henri Rendu, French physician, Sir William Osler, Candian-born US-British physician and Frederick Weber, British physician

rennin (ren'in) a milk-curdling enzyme found in the gastric juices of infants

renogram the assessment of kidney function by external radiation detectors

renography (re'nog'ra-fi) radiography of the kidney

renomegaly (re'no-meg'a-li) enlargement of the kidney

renovascular hypertension RVH systemic hypertension due to renal artery obstruction by atherosclerosis, fibroplastic disease or embolism

reovirus (re-o-vi'rus) a double stranded RNA virus family which is not enveloped (naked) which includes orthoreovirus, orbivirus and rotovirus, which may produce gastroenteritis, or rhinopharyngitis

repaglinide a beta-cell stimulator hypoglycaemic agent

repair (re-par) restoration of damaged tissues

repellent repulsive

repetitive strain injury injury to a part of the body caused by persistent repetition of the same movement. It can affect the muscles, tendons, tendon sheaths, bones or nerves

replacement (re-plas'-ment) the substitution of a missing substance or part with a similar substance or structure **r therapy** use of a medicinal product to replace a natural hormone or enzyme that the body is not able to produce in sufficient amount **r transfusion** the removal of all or most of a patient's diseased blood and its simultaneous replacement with an equal volume of normal blood

replenish to provide a new supply for

replicate (rep'li-kat) to produce an exact copy

replication (rep'li-ka'shun) the process of copying, reproducing or duplicating; the process of synthesising a daughter DNA molecule from a parent DNA 'template'

repolarization (re'po-lar-i-za'shun) the process by which the membrane cell or fibre gets repolarized

repositioning the restoration of an organ or body part to its natural position

repression (re-presh'un) removal of ideas, impulses or affects from consciousness

reproducibility the extent to which the test consistently gives similar results when administered on several occasions to stable subjects; stability; precision

reproduction (re-pro-duk'shun) procreation

reproductive history a woman's obstetric history giving parity and gravidity

reproductive system the male and female organs and connecting tubes and glands necessary for sexual intercourse and production of offspring **female r** consists of the ovaries, fallopian tubes, uterus, vagina, clitoris and vulva **male r** consists of the testes, epididymis, vas

deferens, seminal vesicles, ejaculatory duct, prostate and penis

repulsion (re-pul'shun) 1. aversion 2. to drive away

RES abbreviation for reticuloendothelial system

res ipsa loquitur L the fact speaks for itself

resection (re-sek'shun) 1. surgical removal 2. excision

resectoscope (re-sek'to-skop) an endoscope for transurethral removal of lesions in the urethra, prostate or bladder

reserpine (re-ser'pin) an alkaloid isolated from *Rauwolfia serpentina* used as an anti- hypertensive

reserve (re-zerv) availability of something for later use

reservoir (rez'er-vor) a receptacle or chamber **r bag** a component of an anaesthesia machine in which gas accumulates, forming a reserve supply of gas for use when the quantity of flow is insufficient **r host** a non-human host that serves as a means of sustaining an infective agent and act as a potential source of human infection

residency a period of formal graduate medical education programme that consists of on-the-job training in a teaching hospital following a one-year internship. The period is of three years duration

resident (rezi-dent) a house officer working in a hospital

residual volume RV the volume of gas present in the lungs (and airways) following a maximal voluntary expiration. It is calculated as the difference between the functional residual capacity and the expiratory reserve volume

residue (rez'idu) that which remains after removal

resistance (re-zis'tans) ability to remain unaffected **r ratio** (RR) a ratio of the minimal inhibitory concentration of a test strain to that of the control strain

resolution regression; the minimum distance or degree of separation between two points that can be identified as distinct

resonance (rez'o-nans) sound obtained on percussing a part which vibrates freely

resorb (ri-sorb') to reabsorb

resorption (ri-sorp'shun) act of removal by absorption

respiration (res-pi-ra'shun) a process involving ventilation concerned with the movement of gases along the airways to-and-out of the alveoli, intrapulmonary distribution of air and adequate perfusion of capillaries, matching ventilation and perfusion thus diffusion of gases (oxygen and carbon dioxide) over the wide area of the alveolar-capillary membrane **r rate** the number of inspirations per minute

respirator ventilator **r brain** global necrotic softening of the cerebral cortex. It is noted in 'brain dead' persons who are kept alive by ventilatory support

respiratory pertaining to respiratory system **r acidosis** an acid base disturbance developing from an increase in $PaCO_2$. It is caused in situations of reduced alveolar ventilation and ventilation-perfusion imbalance. It can be acute or chronic. In acute condition there is an abrupt elevation of $PaCO_2$, accumulation of H^+ ions and fall in pH. In a sustained elevation in $PaCO_2$ there is a rise in the level of plasma bicarbonate **r alkalosis** an acid base disturbance where CO_2 in the arterial blood is below normal range. There is hyperventilation causing an increased elimination of CO_2. There is reduction in H^+ ions and pH is raised **r alternans** alternately occurring abdominal and thoracic cage movements during inspiration **r arrest** the cessation of breathing **r burst** an abrupt increase in the consumption of oxygen which is followed by a sequence of metabolic events in neutrophils and monocytes prior to bacteriolysis **r centre** a group of nerve cells in the pons and medulla of the brain that control the rhythm of

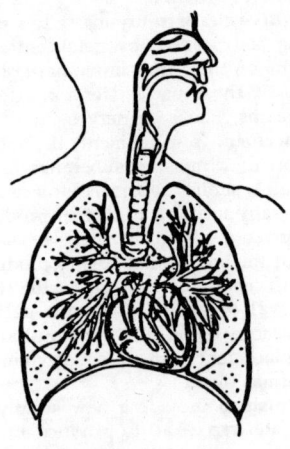

Respiratory tract

respiration in response to the changes in the level of oxygen and carbon dioxide in the blood and cerebrospinal fluid **r cycle** an inspiration followed by an expiration **r distress syndrome, acute** ARDS a severe, life-threatening catastrophe occuring suddenly in patients without any evidence of previous lung diseases. The condition is characterised by marked dyspnoea, progressive hypoxaemia, reduced pulmonary compliance, marked impairment in oxygen transportation despite ventilatory assistance and roentgenographic evidence of bilateral pulmonary infiltrates. It needs ventilatory support and PEEP **r distress syndrome of new born** hyaline membrane disease; a complex disorder characterised by loss of alveolar stability leading to progressive atelectasis of the affected lung presenting as respiratory distress at or shortly after birth. It is seen most frequently in premature infants of less than 37 weeks gestation **r endurance** ability of the respiratory muscles to withstand the respiratory loads **r failure** an inability of the respiratory system to keep the arterial blood gases at normal level while breathing ambient air at rest at sea level and the individual exhibits the partial pressure of oxygen below 60 mmHg with or without an elevation of carbon dioxide tension above 49 mmHg in the arterial blood. It may be acute with threat to life within minutes to hours or days or chronic developing over a prolonged period due to smouldering disease in the lung. Acute respiratory failure may develop from inadequate gas exchange and/or inadequate ventilation **r muscles** the muscles that produce volume changes of thorax during breathing **r quotient** RQ ratio of the volume of CO_2 produced to the volume of O_2 consumed per unit of time at steady state conditions **r rhythm** a regular oscillating cycle of inspiration and expiration **r syncytial virus** most frequent cause of lower respiratory tract disease of infants and children **r syndrome** an immune response to high-dose rifampicin therapy characterised by a flu-like complex, dyspnoea, wheezing, leucopaenia and thrombocytopaenia **r system** organs responsible for exchange of gases between inspired air and blood in the alveolar capillaries. They provide a surface for transfer of gases through which blood gets rid of carbon dioxide and absorbs oxygen. It maintains the arterial oxygen and carbon dioxide tensions at constant levels of 100 mm and 40 mm respectively with variations in a very narrow range and maintenance of normal acid-base balance of the body **r therapy** any treatment that maintains or improves the ventilatory function of the respiratory tract **r tract** a continuous tract responsible for carrying oxygen from air and expelled CO_2. It is divided as upper and lower respiratory tracts using cricoid cartilage as

the separating landmark. The nose, nasal sinuses, nasopharynx and larynx form the upper respiratory tract. The lower respiratory tract includes the trachea and bronchi

response (re-spons') reaction to any stimulus

responsiveness stat the ability of a test to detect clinically meaningful changes

restenosis recurrence of stenosis following corrective surgery

resting pulse the pulse rate of a person who is at rest both physically and emotionally

restless leg syndrome a disorder characterised by nocturnal cramping of the calf muscles, restlessness, a feeling of heaviness, painful parasthesia, tingling and twitching of the legs interfering with sleep

restoration (res-to-ra'shun) replacement of the lost structure

rest pain severe relentless, continuous pain occurring even at rest in severely ischaemic limb which keeps the patient awake at night. It is probably due to ischaemic changes in the somatic nerves

restraint any device used to restrict the free movement of patients with behavioural problems

restricted affect a reduction in intensity of feeling tone

restrictive cardiomyopathy *see* cardiomyopathy

restrictive disease a respiratory disorder characterised by restriction of expansion of the lungs or chest wall resulting in diminished lung volumes or capacities

resume summary, abridgement, recapitulation

resuscitate (re-sus-i-tat) to revive

resuscitation (re-sus-i-ta'shun) sustenance of vital function of a person in respiratory or cardiac failure while reviving by use of techniques of artificial respiration and cardiac massage, correction of acid base imbalance and treatment of cause of failure

retardation (re-tar-da'shun) a slowness of development

rete (re'te) net, network

retch an involuntary effort to vomit

retching dry vomiting –

retention (re-ten'shun) a holding back; retaining

reticular formation a small, thick cluster of neurones within the brain stem controlling breathing, heart beat, blood pressure and consciousness

reticular pattern mesh-like with curvilinear densities surrounding air-filled alveoli. The radiologic densities may be graded as fine, medium or coarse

reticulation (re-tik-u-la'shun) formation of a network

reticulin (re-tik'u-lin) a scleroprotein present in the connective tissue framework.

reticulocyte (re-tik'u-lo-sit) a young red blood cell containing residual ribosomal RNA **r count** enumeration of reticulocytes to evaluate red cell production in the bone marrow

reticulocytopaenia (re-tik'u-lo-si-to-pen-ia) a decrease in the number of circulating reticulocytes

reticulocytosis (retik'u-lo-si-to'sis) an increase in the number of circulating reticulocytes

reticuloendothelial (re-tik'u-lo-endo-thelial) referring to a reticuloendothelium **r system** a system involved in defence against infection and disposal of the products of breakdown of cells

reticuloendotheliosis (re-tik'u-lo-en'do-theli-o-sis) proliferation of reticuoendothelial system

reticuloendothelium (re-tik'u-lo-en-do-the'li-um) referring to the cells of reticuloendothelial system

reticulosis (re-tik'u-lo-sis) proliferation of reticuloendothelial cells such as histiocytes, or monocytes

reticulum (re-tik-u-lum) a fine network of connective tissue fibres between cells

retina (ret-i-na) the light-sensitive membrane which lines the inside of the back of the eye, on which light rays are focussed. It is 10-layered and continuous with the optic nerve, and transmits the visual impulses through the optic nerve to the brain

retinaculum (ret-i-nak'u-lum) a strong fibrous band

retinal detachment a separation of the retina from the choroid in the back of the eye

retinitis (ret-i-nitis) inflammation of the retina **r pigmentosa** retinal degeneration characterised by night blindness, and progressive centripetal loss of visual fields progressing to blindness **r proliferans** serous products leaking from new vessels formed in diabetic retinopathy stimulate a connective tissue reaction

retinoblastoma (ret-i-no-blas-to'ma) a malignant tumour of the retina that affects infants and children

retinoic acid a molecule involved in vertebrate development **r embryopathy** a teratogenic complex induced by a vitamin A derived product.

retinoid a synthetic compound similar to vitamin A, that is used to treat skin conditions such as acne and psoriasis

retinol (reti-nol) vitamin A

retinopathy (ret-i-nop'a-thi) a degenerative disorder of the retina **diabetic r** a common cause of blindness. Initial abnormality is microaneurysms appearing as minute, discrete, circular dark red spots near to retinal vessels, later occurrence of haemorrhages in the deeper layers of the retina. There are hard exudates from leakage of plasma from abnormal retinal capillaries and soft exudates as cotton wool spots. Ischaemic retina leads to proliferative diabetic retinopathy. The veins undergo beading and tortuosity. There is widespread capillary non-perfusion. Retinal photocoagulation is indicated at an early stage of development **hypertensive r** a condition developing in individuals having prolonged hypertension. It consists of arteriolar narrowing due to vasoconstriction and intimal hyalinisation (Grade 1),extensive vascular thickening imparting a copper (column of blood still visible) or silver (no longer visible) 'wire' appearance with 'nicking' of the veins where they are crossed by arteries (Grade II), haemorrhages within the nerve fibre layer, exudates and marked nicking (Grade III) and oedema of optic disc (Grade IV)

retinoschisis (ret'i-nes'ki-sis) splitting of sensory layers of the retina resulting in a fixed, smooth, convex, transparent elevation

retinoscope (reti-no-skop) an optical device used in retinoscopy

retinoscopy (reti-no-skop-pi) detection of errors of refraction by illuminating the retina and noting the reflections of the light back through the pupil when the mirror or retinoscope is rotated

retirement syndrome *Psy* acute or chronic maladjustment to retirement characterised by apathy, asthenia andnon-specific autonomic nervous system complaints

retraction (re-trak'shun) 1. drawing back 2. posterior movement

retractor (re-trak'tor) an instrument to draw aside the structures

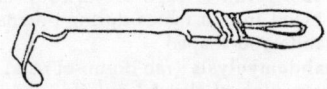

Retractor

retrieval (re-tre'val) memory process to bring back into consciousness of the stored information

retro - combining word for backward; behind

retro echoing the past

retrobulbar pertaining to area behind the eyeball **r neuritis** neuropathy affecting the optic nerve

retrocaecal (re-tro-se'kal) pertaining to the region behind the caecum

retroflexion (re-tro-flek'shun) backward bending

retrognathia (ret'ro-na'the-a) a condition in which either or both jaws recede with respect to the frontal plane of forehead

retrograde (re-tro-grad) moving backward; degenerative **r amnesia** loss of memory regarding the events preceding the accident **r ejaculation** an ejaculation of semen in a reverse direction into the urinary bladder **r flow** regurgitation **r infection** an infection that spreads along a tube or duct against the flow of secretions or excretions **r pyelography** a radiologic technique to examine the structures of the collecting system of the kidneys, wherein a radiopaque contrast medium is injected through a urinary catheter into the ureters and calyces of the pelves of the kidney. It is useful in locating a urinary tract obstruction

retrogression (re-tro-gresh'un) degeneration or deterioration

retrolental fibroplasia variable degree of blindness noted after administration of high concentrations of oxygen in the neonatal period

retromammary behind the breast **r abscess** a cold abscess secondary to collection of pus in the cellular tissue behind the breast due to tuberculosis of the rib or spine

retroperitoneal (retro-per'i-to-ne-al) behind the peritoneum **r fibrosis** a chronic inflammatory process of unknown aetiology in which fibrous tissue surrounds the large blood vessels in the lower lumbar region

retroperitonitis (retro-per'i-to-ni'tis) inflammation of the tissue behind the peritoneum

retropharyngeal behind the pharynx **r abscess** abscess developing from suppuration of retropharyngeal lymph nodes that are situated one side of the central septum (acute) or from caries of upper cervical vertebrae in the midline behind prevertebral fascia and in front of the body of the vertebra (chronic)

retroposition (retro-po-zish'un) backward displacement of a structure or organ

retropulsion (retro-pul'shun) an involuntary backward walking

retrospective falsification recollection of a true memory to which the patient adds false details

retrosternal behind the sternum **r goitre** goitre arising from the lower pole of the nodular goitre that can be partly palpable just above the sternum (substernal) or intrathoracic which can (plunging) or can't be forced back into the neck by coughing

retroversion (re-tro-ver'zhun) turning backward

retrovirus (re-tro-vi-rus) an RNA virus possessing reverse transcriptase. It is capable of inserting and efficiently expressing its own genetic-information in a host cell's genome by transcribing its own RNA to DNA that is integrated with a host cells genome

revascularization (re-vas'ki-lar-za'shun) reestablishment of blood supply to a part

reversal (re-ver'sal) a turning in opposite direction

reverse transcriptase *mol* an RNA dependent DNA polymerase that is capable of copying genomic RNA into DNA, catalysing the synthesis of DNA using retroviral RNA as a template **r t inhibitors** agents preventing the spread of infectious virus to uninfected cells but do not affect replication of the HIV genome once integrated into the host cell

reverse transcription the copying of single stranded retroviral RNA into double-stranded DNA catalysed by reverse transcriptase. Normal transcription is from DNA to RNA

reversible ischaemic neurological disability RIND an ischaemia-induced focal loss of neurologic function of abrupt onset with disability lasting more than 24 hours but less than 3 weeks. It is considered a variant of a transient ischaemic attack

reversion (re-ver'zhun) return of the earlier features which were not apparent

Reye's syndrome occurrence of brain and liver damage following a viral infection and it may be related to taking aspirin for treatment of infection. There is vomiting, hepatic dysfunction, and minimal neurologic impairment often preceded by viral upper respiratory tract infection. It affects children under 15, is named after Ralph Reye, Australian pathologist

RFLP restriction fragment length polymorphism, used identification of a portion of an individual's DNA

r factor an episome in bacteria that is responsible for drug resistance

Rh Rhesus **Rh blood group** a blood group classified by the presence or absence of a Rh factor on the surface of red blood cells: people with the substance are Rh positive and those without it are Rh negative **Rh sensitised** description of a woman with Rh-negative blood who has developed permanent antibodies against Rh-positive blood as a result of exposure to Rh-positive blood from a foetus during pregnancy

rhabdo rod-shaped

rhabdomyolysis (rab'do-mi-ol'i-sis) destruction of skeletal muscle exhibiting myoglobinaemia and myoglobinuria

rhabdomyoma (rab'do-mi-o'ma) a benign tumour of skeletal muscle

rhabdomyosarcoma (rab'do-mi-o-sar-ka'ma) a malignant tumour of the skeletal muscle

rhabdovirus a family of single-stranded RNA viruses that includes the rabies virus

rhagades (rag'a-des) cracks or fissures at mucocutaneous junctions

rhegma (reg'ma) a fissure.

rheo blood flow

rheology (re-ol'o-ji) the study of the deformation and flow of materials

rhesus system blood group system dependent on three genes designated by the letters C, D and E and their alleles by the small letters c, d and e

rheumatalgia (ru-ma-tal'ji-a) rheumatic pain

rheumatic (ru-mati'k) relating to rheumatism **r fever** a condition affecting children or young adults that is triggered by infection with group A streptococci which possess antigens that cross-react with human connective tissue particularly heart valve glycoprotein. It is a systemic illness presenting with fever, anorexia, lethargy and joint pains. The diagnosis is based on Jones Criteria (*see* Jones Criteria) **r heart disease** damage to heart valves and heart muscle resulting from rheumatic fever

rheumatism (ru'ma-tizm) a painful condition arising from articular or other elements of musculoskeletal system

rheumatoid (ru'ma-toyd) resembling rheumatism **r arthritis** an autoimmune inflammatory arthropathy presenting with morning stiffness in and around joints lasting at least one hour before maximum improvement, soft tissue swelling of three or more joints, swelling of the proximal interphalangeal, metacarpophalangeal or wrist joints, symmetric arthritis, rheumatoid nodules, presence of rheumatoid factor and roentgenographic erosions and/or periarticular osteopaenia **r factors** RF polyclonal IgM antibodies produced by synovial neutrophils in a majority of patients with rheumatoid arthritis, which may be demonstrated by erythrocyte agglutination (Rose-Waaler test) or latex agglutination test **r nodule** a mass consisting of central necrosis surrounded by successive rims of fibrinoid degeneration, fibrosis and palisaded serous membranes and lung parenchyma in some patients with rheuma-

toid arthritis **r pneumonitis** diffuse interstitial fibrosis encountered infrequently in rheumatoid arthritis

rheumatologist (ru-ma-tol'o-jist) a specialist in the diagnosis and management of rheumatic conditions

rhexis (rek'sis) rupture of a vessel or organ

Rh factor an antigenic substance present in the erythrocytes. The person having the factor is Rh⁺ (Rh positive), a person lacking the factor is Rh⁻ (Rh negative)

Rh immune globulin an Rh immune globulin concentrate used to prevent the maternal immunisation against the infant's Rh group D antigen

Rh incompatibility a lack of compatibility between two groups of blood cells that are antigenically different due to the presence of the Rh factor in one group and absence of the Rh factor in another

rhinal (ri-'nal) nasal

rhinalgia (ri-nal'ji-a) pain in the nose

rhinencephalon (ri-nen-sef'a-lon) that part of the cerebral hemisphere containing structures of the sense of the smell

rhinitis (ri-ni'tis) inflammation of nasal mucosa, which causes sneezing, nasal discharge and facial discomfort **allergic r** occurs as an immediate hypersensitivity reaction to allergens in the nasal mucosa. Grass pollens are common allergens. It is associated with nasal congestion, watery nasal discharge and sneezing. It may be seasonal or perennial **vasomotor r** rhinitis caused by physical or chemical irritants

rhino- referring to nose

rhinoedema (rin-e-de'ma) swelling of the nasal mucosa

rhinolalia (ri'no-la'li-a) nasal speech

rhinolaryngitis (rino-lar-in-ji'tis) inflammation of the nasal and laryngeal mucosa

rhinolaryngology (rino-lar-ing-gol'o-ji) study of nasal and laryngeal structures and functions

rhinolith (rino-lith) nasal calculus

rhinology (rino'lo-ji) medical science concerned with the nose and its diseases

rhinomycosis (ri'no-mi-kosis) fungal infection of the nasal mucous membrane

rhinophyma (ri'no-fi-ma) bulbous deformity and redness of the nose. It occurs as a severe complication of rosacea, occurring primarily in elderly men

rhinoplasty (rino-plas-ti) a surgical procedure to change the structure of the nose either for cosmetic purpose or to correct an injury or deformity

rhinorrhagia (ri-no-ra'ji-a) nose bleed

rhinorrhoea (ri-no-re'ah) a discharge from the nasal mucosa

rhinosalpingitis (rino-sal-pin-ji'tis) inflammation of the mucous membrane of the nose and eustachian tube

rhinoscleroma (ri-no-skle-ro'ma) a chronic granulomatous condition affecting the nose, upper lip, oral cavity and upper air ways

rhinoscope (ri'no-skop) a small mirror having an angled handle to visualise the posterior part of the nasal cavity

rhinoscopy (ri'no-skopi) visualisation of the nasal cavity **anterior r** examination of anterior part of the nasal cavity by nasal speculum under good illumination **posterior r** visualisation of posterior nares by placing a mirror behind the uvula and soft palate

rhinosporidiosis (rino-spo-rid-i-o'sis) chronic granulomatous condition of nasal mucosa due to *Rhinosporidium seeberi*, an yeast-like organism

rhinostenosis (ri-no-ste-no'sis) nasal obstruction

rhinovirus (ri'no-virus) virus associated with common cold

rhizo a combining word for root

rhizoid (ri'zoyd) root-like

rhizotomy (ri-zot'o-mi) section of the nerve roots

rhodo a combining word for red colour

Rhodococcus equi a plemorphic gram-positive, weakly acid-fast cocco-bacillus and a facultative intracellular pathogen that develops as an opportunistic pathogenin patients receiving immunosuppressive therapy or in those infected by HIV

Rhodococcus pneumonia, *R. equi* infection with an insidious onset exhibiting fever, cough and expectoration involves upper lobes of the lung, treated with erythromycin and/or rifampicin

rhodopsin (ro-dop'sin) visual purple

rhomboid (rom'boyd) oblique with unequal sides

rhonchus (rong'kus) wheezy continuous, dry adventitious respiratory sound having a musical pitch pl. **ronchi**. It is produced by an acoustic mechanism similar to that of a simple uncoupled oscillating reed. The airways narrowed to the point of closure, make their opposing walls to come in close contact and oscillate like reed of a musical instrument. The walls are set in oscillation by the turbulent air flow within their lumen **sibilant r** obstruction of smaller bronchi result in high-pitched rhonchi as whistling or squeaking sounds **sonorous r** obstruction of larger bronchi producing low pitched, snoring quality sounds

rhythm (rithm) the regular alteration of motion of two different or opposite states **r method** a contraceptive method where unprotected intercourse is allowed shortly after a menstrual period or before the onset of the next period

RIA radioimmunoassay

rib costa, one of the 12 pairs of elastic bony structure forming thoracic cage **r cage** the bony framework of bones attached to the spine and the sternum that supports the chest wall and protects the heart, lungs and other organs in the chest

ribavirin a synthetic nucleoside having a broad spectrum of antiviral activity against both DNA and RNA viruses

riboflavin *see* vitamin B$_2$

ribonuclease (ri-bo-nu'kle-as) Rnase, an enzyme that catalyses the hydrolysis of ribonucleic acid

ribonucleic (ribo-nu-kle'ik) **acid**, RNA, a ribonucleoside present in all cells in the nuclei and cytoplasm that helps to decode the genetic instructions carried in the DNA of cells

ribonucleoprotein (ri'bo-nu'kle-o-pro'ten) a combination of protein and RNA

ribonucleotide (ri'bo-nu'kle-o-tid) a nucleotide containing ribose **r reductase** an enzyme needed by all proliferating cells to catalyse the synthesis of deoxyribonucleotide precursors for DNA

ribose (ri'bos) pentose present in RNA

ribosome (ri-bo-som) a particle of ribonucleoprotein found inside cells which plays an important role in the protein synthesis

rib-tip syndrome sharp episodic pain at the costal margin caused by hypermotility of the anterior end of tenth rib, often due to trauma

rice bodies elongated and indurated oval-to-round rice-like masses composed of collagen, which may occur in the joints of patients with rheumatoid arthritis, LE, septic arthritis and synovial chondromatosis

rice water stools clear and watery diarrhoea with flecks of mucus giving an appearance of water boiled rice, an appearance seen in cholera

Richter's (rik'terz) **syndrome** a large cell lymphamatous transformation as a terminal event in chronic lymphoctic leukaemia described by August Richter, US pathologist

rickets (rik'ets) a vitamin D deficiency seen primarily in infancy and childhood associated with excess production and deficient calcification of osteoid tissue resulting in bony deformities, like bow legs and knock knee, nodular enlargements on the ends and sides of the bones, muscle pain, enlarged skull, chest deformities, spinal curvature, hepatosplenomegaly and profuse sweating. It responds to vitamin D and calcium supplementation

Rickettsia (riket'sia) pl. **rickettsiae** a gram-negative micro-organism which spreads to men from lice, fleas, ticks and mites where it is intracytoplasmic, named after Howard Ricketts, US pathologist

rickettsial (ri-ket-si-al) caused by rickettsiae **r infections** infections in humans by rickettsiae are conveyed through the skin from excreta of arthropods. Epidemic and endemic typhus and Rocky Mountain spotted fever, scrub typhus and trench fever are examples

rickettsialpox a mite-borne infectious disease caused by Rickettsis akari

rickettsiosis (ri-ket-si-o'sis) infection with rickettsia

Richter's hernia a hernia wherein a portion of the circumference of the bowel is strangulated. It is common in femoral hernia. The diagnosis is delayed as the patient is able to pass flatus and faeces, named after August Richter, German surgeon

Riedel's disease iigneous thyroiditis. Stony hard goitre which is not very large but causes tracheal compression early in the course of the disease. It occurs in young adults of either sex, described by Bernhard Riedel, surgeon at Breslau.

Riedel's (re'delz) lobe a tongue-shaped projection of the right lobe of the liver which may be mistaken for gall bladder

rifampicin highly potent antibiotic against *Mycobacterium tuberculosis* where it interferes with the synthesis of RNA, quickly absorbed on oral administration on an empty stomach. It penetrates well into the tissues and cells. Being scarlet coloured imparts red colour to the urine. It is active against staphylococci, *M. Leprae*, *Legionella* and *Melliodosis pseudomallei*

right bundle branch block RBBB interruption of the right branch of bundle of His delays activation of right ventricle. ECG shows broadened QRS complexes with 'M' shaped configuration in leads V1 and V2, and a wide

S wave in lead 1 noted in right ventricular hypertrophy or strain as in pulmonary embolism, or coronary artery disease or ASD

right heart failure a condition with decreased right ventricular output. There is congestion and elevation in pressure in systemic veins. Isolated right heart failure is noted in chronic lung diseases (cor pulmonale), multiple pulmonary emboli and pulmonary valve stenosis. It commonly occurs secondary to left heart failure

right-to-left shunt blood flow from right to left side due to intracardiac or intrapulmonary shunts

right ventricle thin-walled chamber of the heart that pumps blood received from right atrium into the pulmonary arteries to the lungs for oxygenation

rigidity (ri-jid-i-ti) 1. stiffness 2. assumption of a rigid posture, against all efforts to be moved 3. an increase in tone and resistance in all groups of muscles (agonists and antagonists) to an equal degree and is a sign of disease of basal ganglia (**extrapyramidal r**) **cogwheel r** resistance less uniform and diminishing in jerky steps when the rigidity and tremors co-exist **hysterical r** resistance to passive movements is proportional to the amount of force applied **leadpipe r** resistance felt to the same degree throughout passive movement **paratonic r** an uniform resistance during all phases of passive movements as in catatonic states and dementia

rigid-spine syndrome severe muscular contracture affecting the spine and other joints

rigor (rig'er) 1. stiff 2. violent attack of shivering.

rigor mortis stiffening of muscles that occurs after death. There is rigid contraction of skeletal muscles that is first seen in the jaw 2-4 hours after death, later appearing on the trunk and extremities, reaching its peak at 48 hours,

disappearing in the same order of its development

rima a narrow elongated opening between two symmetric margins

rimantidine an antiviral agent that is a structural analogue of amantadine

rimose fissured

ring a circular band or structure **r abscess** histological appearance of an abscess seen in infective endocarditis which consists of a central focus of neutrophils, necrosis and bacteria surrounded by fibroblasts and fibrosis **r enhancement** CT finding in the brain consisting of a radiolucent zone surrounded by a faint radiodense rim, which in turn is surrounded by a second radiolucent zone outside of the rim. These rings correspond to regional oedema, hyper vascularity, and hypercellularity **r shadows** annular thickening of the bronchial walls seen by a plain roentgenogram in bronchiectasis

Ringer's lactate solution a physiologic solution containing calcium chloride, potassium chloride, sodium chloride and sodium lactate, which contains 1.35 mmol/L calcium, 4 mmol/L potassium and 130 mmol/L sodium, used to restore the fluid volume named after Sydney Ringer, English physiologist

ringworm dermatophyte, tinea capable of invading the keratinised tissue of skin, nail or hair. The lesions begin as a scaly plaque spreading centrifugally with central clearing

Rinne's test normally the sound is conducted better through the air than bone. A vibrating tuning fork is placed on the mastoid process on one side while the other ear is closed. When the patient stops hearing the sound, the tines of the fork are brought near the ear and noted whether the patient still hears the sound. In diseases of middle ear the bone conduction is better than air conduction. In nerve deafness both are lost, named after Heinrich Rinne, German otologist

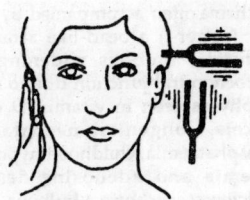

Rinne's test

risk the probability of suffering from a particular disease **r assessment** the process by which new chemical substances are evaluated for their potential impact on human health **r management** activities involved in reducing the risks of injury to the patients

risperidone a benzisoxazole preparation for psychosis

Risser cast a plaster of Paris cast to immobilise the trunk of the body in the treatment of scoliosis, named after Joseph Risser, American surgeon

risus sardonicus grinning facial expression seen in tetanus

ritonavir a protease inhibitor antiretroviral agent

Ritters' (rit'terz) syndrome Staphylococcal scalded skin syndrome, a neonatal disease, described by Gottfried Ritter, German physician

ritual *Psy* automatic activity compulsive in nature

ritualisation *Psy* process of a behaviour pattern being incorporated through evolution into a primary signalling function

rivalry (ri'val-ri) competition between two or more persons for the same object

river blindness infection with filarial worm, Onchocerca, causing blindness due to punctate keratitia, corneal fibrosis, iridocyclitis, glaucoma and optic atrophy

Robin Hood syndrome reduction of blood flow to relatively well oxygenated tissue by vasoconstriction, and diverting that blood to ischaemic tissues. The term has come from the English folk hero Robin Hood who allegedly stole from the rich to give to the poor

Rocky Mountain spotted fever an infectious disease caused by *R. rickettsii* transmitted by ticks and characterised by small pink spots on the wrists and ankle, enlargement of regional lymph nodes. It responds to tetracycline or chloramphenicol

rod 1. a straight slender cylinder. 2. photosensitive cell of the retina, that contains rhodopsin which adapts the eye to detect low intensity light

rodenticide (ro-den'ti-sid) an agent lethal to rodents

rodent ulcer a deeply invasive basal cell carcinoma

RMP registered medical practitioner

RN abbreviation for registered nurse

RNA ribonucleic acid **RNA polymerase** enzyme that copy strands of RNA from DNA template

Rnase abbreviation for ribonuclease

road to health a growth chart is a visible display of the child's physical growth and development. It is designed primarily for longitudinal follow-up of a child, so that changes over time can be interpreted

roentgen (ront'gen) the international unit of dose exposure to x- or gamma-radiation, named after the discoverer of x-rays, Wilhelm Conrad Roentgen, German physicist

roentgenogram (rent'gen-o-gram) radiograph

roentgenography (rent'gen-og'ra-fi) radiography

roentgenologist (rent'gen-ol'o-jist) radiologist

roentgenology (rent'gen-olo-ji) radiology concerned with study of the diagnostic and therapeutic uses of x-rays

roga (s) disease ailment *r. marga* route of entry of disease

rogi pariksha (s) examination of the patient

Rolando's fissure the central sulcus of the cerebrum, named after Luigi Rolando, Italian anatomist

roller bandage a long tightly wound strip of material applied as a circular bandage

ROM range of motion. The amount of angular motion allowed at the joint between any two bony levers

roma (s) hair

Romana's sign unilateral firm reddish swelling of the lids in Chaga's disease, described by Cecilio Romana, Argentine physician

Romberg sign a special test to demonstrate incoordination in the lower limbs, especially sensory ataxia. The patient loses balance when standing erect, feet together and eyes closed, named after Moritz' Romberg, German physician

rongeur (ron-zhur) forceps useful to nip the bone

R-on-T phenomenon *ECG* a premature venticular depolarisation which occurs very early in the cardiac cycle, that it falls on the apex of the preceding T wave

room temperature the air temperature as measured in a specific region of a room

root canal a tooth exhibiting well advanced decay which requires opening, cleaning and sterilising the root canal and closing and filling it with an impervious material **r file** a small metal hand instrument used for cleaning and shaping a root canal **r filling** a material placed in the root canal of a tooth to seal the space previously occupied by the dental pulp

rooting reflex a normal response in new borns when the cheek is touched or stroked along the side of the mouth to turn the head towards the stimulated side and to begin to suck. It disappears by 3 to 4 months of age

Rorschach (ror'shak) **test** *Psy* a psychological projective assessment test in which a person is asked to respond to a series of ink blots by saying what image or emotion each one evokes; ink blot test named after Hermann Rorschach, Swiss psychiatrist

rosacea (ro-za'she-a) a chronic inflammatory facial eruption consisting of erythema often accompanied by papules

rosary (ro'zer-i) a bead-like arrangement **rachitic r** bulbous widening of the costochondral junction due to softened epiphyses seen in vitamin D deficient rickets, congenital neonatal hypophosphataemia, childhood hypophosphataemia and adenosine deaminase deficiency **scorbutic r** bulbous enlargement of costochondral junction seen in scurvy. The angulation of the scorbutic 'beads' is sharper than in rickets **r bead appearance** an exaggerated haustral contractions seen in barium studies of irritable bowel syndrome **r bead oesophagus** corkscrew oesophagus

roseola (ro-ze'o-la) rose-red coloured small eruptions **r infantum** an infectious disease that primarily affects young children and is characterised by irritability, fever and rash

rose spots an erythematous maculopapular rash that blanches on pressure. They are located on the lower chest and upper abdomen and are due to bacterial emboli in cutaneous vessels seen in typhoid fever during the first week of disease

rosette (ro-zet) a group of cells wherein a number of nuclei form a ring; a segmented phase in the development of *Plasmodium malariae*

Rose-Waaler test an anti-immunoglobulin test with sheep erythrocytes sensitised with rabbit anti-sheep erythrocyte IgE. If the test serum contains rheumatoid factor it combines with the membrane-bound IgE and causes agglutination

Ross river virus a mosquito-borne virus causing headache, myalgia, arthritis, and pruritic rash, in Australia, Fizi and New Guinea

rostellum (ros-tel'um) the anterior part of the scolex of a tapeworm with a row of hooks

rostrum (ros'trum) beak-like structure

Rossolimo's (ros'o-le'moz) **reflex** on tapping the plantar surface of the toes, there is plantar flexion in pyramidal lesions, named after Gregori Rossolimo, Russian neurologist

rotahaler a breath-actuated device used as a dry power inhaler

rotameter (rotam'et-er) a device operated by a needle valve in an anaesthetic machine that measures gases by speed of flow.

rotating tourniquet one of the four constricting devices used in a rotating order to pool blood in the extremities to relieve congestion in the lungs

rotation (rota'shun) 1. a turning around an axis 2. one of the four basic kinds of movement allowed by various joints

rotator a muscle that helps a part to turn circularly **r cuff** the musculotendinous covering of the shoulder joint, bounded inferiorly by the subscapularis muscle, superiorly by the supraspinatus muscle and posteriorly by the infraspinatus and teres muscles

rotavirus an encapsulated double-stranded RNA virus belonging to reovirus family that causes gastroenteritis in infants

Roth's spots round or oval white spots seen in the retina in subacute bacterial endocarditis, named after Moritz Roth, Swiss physician.

rotor syndrome an autosomal dominant condition with defective bilirubin uptake and reduced intrahepatic binding exhibiting conjugated hyperbilirubinaemia. The condition is mild and does not affect life span

roughage (ruf'ij) indigestible food material

rouleaux (roolo') stacking of red blood cells occurring in presence of increased plasma fibrinogen and globulins

round cells small leucocytes of 10 to 20 microns with a single round-to-oval nucleus. It includes lymphocytes, monocytes, plasma cells and occasionally epitheloid cells and histiocytes

round ligament 1. fibromuscular band extending from the anterior surface of the uterus through the inguinal canal to labium majus 2. a curved fibrous band between the head of the femur and the transverse ligament of the acetabulum

rounds bedside visits by a physician to evaluate treatment, assess the current course and document the patient's progress. It forms a teaching activity

round window a round opening in the medial wall of the middle ear leading into the cochlea

roundworm a nematode belonging to the phylum Nemathelminthes

route of administration any one of the ways in which a drug may be administered such as intramuscular, intranasal, intravenous, oral, rectal, subcutaneous, sublingual, topical or vaginal

Roux-enY (roo'enwi') an anastomosis of the small intestine in the shape of the letter Y. The proximal end of the divided intestine is anastomosed end into side to the distal loop and a portion of distal loop is anastomosed to another part of digestive tract, named after Cesar Roux, Swiss surgeon.

Rovsing's (rov'sing∠) **sign** application of pressure on the left iliac fossa causes pain in the right iliac fossa in acute appendicitis, named after Nils Rovsing, Danish surgeon.

RQ respiratory quotient

R-R interval *ECG* the interval from the peak of one QRS complex to the peak of the next useful in assessing ventricular rate

RSP abbreviation for respirable suspended particles

RSV respiratory syncytial virus.

rubber dam a thin sheet of latex rubber for isolating one or more teeth during a dental procedure

rub friction noted in moving one part of the body over another

rubefacient (ru-be-fa'shent) 1. agent causing a reddening of the skin 2. a counter irritant producing redness on application to the skin surface rubella (Ru-bel'ah) see German measles r embryopathy any congenital abnormality in infant caused by maternal rubella in early stages of pregnancy

rubeola (ru-be'o-la) see measles

rubeosis (ru-be-o'sis) reddish discoloration of the skin

Rubin's test a test to assess patency of the fallopian tubes by introducing carbon dioxide gas under high pressure through a canula inserted into the cervix. If the tubes are patent gas enters the abdominal cavity which is reflected by fall in monometric pressure, high pitched bubbling sound audible over abdomen and pain in the shoulder and gas under diaphragm visible on x-ray, named after Isador Rubin, American gynaecologist

rubor (ru'ber) redness

rubricyte (roo'bri-sit) a nucleated red blood cell in the bone marrow

rudiment (ru'di-men-t) an organ or structure that is incompletely developed

rudimentary something vestigial or embryonic

rudhi (s) convention, habit

Ruffini's (roo-fe'nez) corpuscles certain nerve endings concerned in the perception of pressure and warmth, named after Angelo Ruffini, Italian anatomist

ruga a fold; a wrinkle, pl. rugae

rugose (ru'gos) wrinkle or fold

RUL right upper lobe of a lung

rule (rul) criterion or standard palm of the hand rule rule of nine used to assess extent of burns in adults can't be applied to children as their head is proportionately large, the size of the palm is equivalent to 1% of body surface r of bigeminy tendency of a lengthened ventricular cycle to precipitate ventricular premature complex of confidentiality a principle that personal information about patients should not be revealed to persons not authorised to receive such information rule of forceps a rule giving a hint about the handle of the forceps to be used on

which side of the mother to be: left blade, left handle and left side of mother; right blade, right handle and right side of mother of nine a quick method to assess the extent of burns on the skin surface. The head, upper extremities on either side, anterior or posterior surface of lower extremities on either side, represent 9% of skin surface, the anterior and posterior trunk represent 18% each and the inguinal area 1% of thirds body water accounts for two-thirds of the total body weight; one third is extracellular and two-thirds is intracellular: of the extracellular fluid one third is intracellular and two-thirds is plasma of twos Meckel's diverticulum is two feet from the ileocaecal valve, two inches long, two cm in diameter, found in two per cent of the population and twice common in males

rum fits generalised alcohol withdrawal-released convulsions seen in chronic alcoholics

ruminant (roo'mi-nant) an animal that chews the cud

rumination syndrome regurgitation of food 10-15 minutes following deglutition, which may be brought out or chewed and swallowed may be noted in those with emotional and intellectual defects or in children with marasmus

rumy the buttock or gluteal region

runner's knee pain on the outside of the knee caused by a strain in the fibrous tissue supporting the knee joint and it may occur in long distance runners

running long distance running. The energy expended during running is a function of the time the foot applies force to the ground during each stride

Runyon group a classification of atypical mycobacteria as photochromogens (Group I) e.g. M. kansasii, scotochromogens (Group II) e.g. M. scrofulaceum, non-pigmented organisms (Group III)

M. avium-intracellulare and rapid growers (Group IV) *M. fortuitum, M. cheloni, M. smegmatis, M. phlei,* named after Ernest Runyon, US microbiologist

rupia (ru'pia) ulcers covered with yellowish brown crusts, noted in syphilis and yaws

rupture (rup'chur) a break or a tear in continuity of an organ or body tissue

rusty lungs brown induration of the lungs due to accumulation of haemosiderin-laden macrophages

rusty sputum sputum composed of bacteria, haemorrhage, mucus and sloughed tissue seen in pneumonia produced by *Streptococcus pneumoniae*

RV residual volume

r-value *stat* correlation coefficient that determines the relatedness to a maximum of +1 to unrelatedness to a minimum of −1 of two series of data

R wave *ECG* the first positive deflection in the QRS complex, representing ventricular activation. In most leads there is upright R wave from the left ventricle

R'wave *ECG* the second positive deflection in the QRS complex after an S wave.

Rye classification division of Hodgkin's disease into four distinct clinicopathological categories as lymphocytic predominant (10% of cases more common in young adult males, low stage of disease), nodular sclerosing (40% of cases more common in young adult females, low stage of disease), mixed cellularity (40% of cases more common in young adult males, stage II-III disease) and lymphocyte depleted (10% of cases, more common in older adult males, stage III-IV disease), named after Rye, New York where a conference in 1965 adopted the classification

Ryle's tube a thin, flexible rubber tube of 75 cm length, having markings at 30.5 cms, 40 cm and 57 cm indicating the position of the tip of the tube in the cardiac end of the stomach, in the stomach and duodenum respectively when each mark is opposite the teeth. The tube has a blind bulbous end containing a lead shot and is perforated by a number of small holes at the sides 2 cm from the tip, named after John Ryle, professor of Social Medicine at Oxford

S

S symbol for sulphur, sacral vertebrae (S₁-S₅), spherical lens, smooth, sacral nerve (S₁-S₅), Svedberg unit

S₁ first heart sound

S₂ second heart sound

S₃ third heart sound; ventricular gallop

S₄ fourth heart sound; atrial gallop

SA abbreviation for sinoatrial; sino-auricular

Sa abbreviation for arterial saturation

sabda (s) sound

SAARD abbreviation for slow-acting antirheumatic drug

saber shin thickened, anteriorly-bowed tibial cortex caused by chronic periostitis seen in congenital or advanced acquired syphilis

Sabin vaccine a live oral vaccine to prevent poliomyelitis prepared by Albert Sabin, Russian-born US virologist.

sabot heart a heart with boot-like, radiologic silhouette, noted in Fallot's tetrology

Sabouraud's medium culture medium containing peptose, maltose and agar for culture of fungi, named after Raymond Sabouraud, French dermatologist

Sabraze's test ability to hold breath for 25 seconds as a respiratory function, named after J. Sabraze, French physician

sabulous (sab'u-lus) gritty or sandy

sac (sak) a pouch; a bag-like organ or structure air s alveolar sac allantoic s expanded portion of the allontois that becomes part of the placenta in many mammals alveolar s's air sacs from which alveoli arise. Alveoli are the terminal, blind-ending structures. They are connected with the respiratory bronchiole through alveolar ducts. Alveoli have a continuous layer of epithelial cells. The elastic reticular framework, small arterioles and a meshwork of capillaries surround the alveoli. Gas exchange occurs mostly in blind-ended alveolar ductal system and alveoli amniotic s amnion chorionic s chorion that encloses developing embryo conjunctival s the potential space lined by conjunctiva between the eyelids and the anterior surface of the eye ball dental s the mesenchymal tissue surrounding a developing tooth endolymphatic s the blind expanded distal end of the endolymphatic duct heart s pericardium hernial s a sac-like protrusion of peritoneum containing a herniated structure lacrimal s dilated upper end of the nasolacrimal duct situated in the groove of the lacrimal bone lesser peritoneal s omental bursa yolk s the extra embryonic membrane that connects with the midgut

saccade (sa-kad') rapid, involuntary movements of the eyes as they change from one point of gaze to another, noted in cerebellar hemisphere lesions

saccate (sak'at) 1. shaped like a sac 2. encysted

saccharase (sak'a-ras) an enzyme that catalyses the breakdown of disaccharides to monosaccharides such as sucrose to dextrose

saccharide (sak'a-rid) one of a series of carbohydrates such as monosaccharides, disaccharides, oligosaccharides and polysaccharides

saccharin (sak'a-rin) a white synthetic crystalline compound that is sweeter than sugar, and used as a non-nutritive sweetener s clearance time test to measure rate of ciliary movement of mucus by putting a saccharin tablet on inferior turbinate and appreciating sweet taste in the pharynx

saccharo combining word for sugar

saccharogalactorrhoea (sak'a-ro-ga-lak-to-re'a) excess secretion of lactose in milk.

saccharolytic (sak'a-ro-lit'ik) capable of splitting sugar

Saccharomyces (-mi'sez) a genus of yeasts

saccharomycosis (-mi-ko'sis) any disease produced by yeast

saccharopine (-pen) an intermediate in the metabolism of lysine

saccharum (sak'a-rum) sugar

sacciform (sak'si-form) shaped like a bag or sac

saccular (sak'u-lar) sac-like

sacculated (sak'u-lat'ed) containing small sacs

sacculation (sak'u-la-shun) 1. formation into a sac or sacs 2. a structure formed by a group of sacs

saccule (sak'ul) 1. a small sac 2. the smaller of the two divisions of the membranous labyrinth occupying the vestibule of the ear laryngeal s a small diverticulum extending from the laryngeal ventricle

sacculocochlear (sak'u-lo-kok'le-er) pertaining to the saccule and cochlea of the ear

sacculotomy (sak'u-lat'a-mi) puncture of the sacculus to relieve endolymphic hydrops

sacculus (sak'u-lus) pl. sacculi saccule

saccus (sak'us) pl. sacci a sac

SACE abbreviation for serum angiotensin converting enzyme.

sacrad (sa'krad) toward the sacrum

sacral (sa'kral) 1. pertaining to the sacrum 2. relating to or in the neighbourhood of sacrum s bone sacrum s flexure rectal curve in front of the sacrum s index sacral breadth multiplied by 100 and divided by sacral length s nerves see nerves s plexus a nerve plexus formed by the ventral branches of the fourth and fifth lumbar nerves and the first four sacral nerves from which the sciatic nerve takes its origin s vertebra one of the fused vertebrae forming the sacrum

sacralgia (sa-kra'l'je-a) pain in the sacrum

sacralisation (sa'kral-i-za'shun) fusion of the fifth lumbar vertebra with the sacrum

sacrectomy (sa-krek'to-me) excision of the sacrum, to facilitate an operation

sacrifice killing of laboratory animals on completion of experiment or as part of an experimental protocol that necessitates examination of internal organs

sacro - combining word for sacrum

sacroanterior (sa'kro-an-te're-or) direction of foetal sacrum anteriorly

sacrococcygeal (sa'kro-kok-sij-e-al) pertaining to the sacrum and coccyx

sacrococcygeus (sak'ro-kok-sij'e-us) one of the two small muscles extending from the sacrum to the coccyx

sacrocoxalgia (sak'ro-koks-al'je-a) pain in the sacroiliac joint

sacrocoxitis (sak'ro-koks-i'tis) inflammation of the sacroiliac joint

sacrodynia (sak'ro-din'e-a) pain in the region of the sacrum

sacroiliac (-il'e-ak) pertaining to the sacrum and ilium s joint a pair of rigid joints in the lower back that are located between each side of the sacrum and the innominate bone of the pelvis

sacroiliitis (-il'e-i'tis) inflammation of the sacroiliac joints, usually caused by ankylosing spondylitis, that causes aching pain in the lower back

sacrolisthesis (sak'ro-lis-the'sis) a deformity in which sacrum is present in front of the fifth lumbar vertebra

sacrolumbar (sak'ro-lum'ber) pertaining to the sacrum and lumbar region

sacroposterior (sak'ro-pos-te're-or) direction of foetal sacrum posteriorly

sacrosciatic (sak'ro-si-at'ik) pertaining to the sacrum and ischium

sacrospinal (sak'ro-spi'nal) pertaining to the sacrum and spinal column

sacrospinalis see table of muscles

sacrotomy (sa-krot'o-me) excision of the lower part of the sacrum

sacrouterine (sak'ro-u'ter-in) pertaining to the sacrum and uterus

sacrovertebral (sak'ro-ver'te-bral) pertaining to the sacrum and vertebral column **s angle** the angle formed by the base of the sacrum and the fifth lumbar vertebra

sacrum (sa'krum) the large, triangular bone in the lower part of the spine consisting of five united vertebrae that sits like a wedge between the two iliac bones and its articulations form the sacroiliac joints, name borrowed from Egyptians who considered the bone was sacred to Osiris, their God of resurrection **scimitar s** a deformed sacrum resembling a short curved sword accompanied by anorectal or neural anomalies

sactosalpinx (sak'to-sal'pin-ks) a dilated fallopian tube from retained secretions

SAD abbreviation for 1. small airway disease 2. seasonal affective disorder

saddle sella 1. a structure resembling the seat used to ride a horse 2. the base of artificial dentures **s area** the portion of the buttocks, perineum and thighs that comes in contact with the seat of the saddle **s back** lordosis **s back anaesthesia** the production of anaesthesia in the saddle area by introducing the anaesthetic agent low in the dural sac **s back fever** *see* fever **s bag hernia** inguinal hernia with two sacs on either side of inferior epigastric artery **s embolus** embolus lodged at the bifurcation and obstructing both branches as in aorta or pulmonary artery **s joint** a joint at the base of the thumb that has two inter-locking saddle-shaped surfaces **s nose deformity** destruction of nasal cartilage with collapse of bridge by Wegener's granulomatosis, and tertiary syphilis

sadhya (s) possible; favourable

sadism (sad'izm) sexual gratification by inflicting mental or physical pain on others, named after Marquis de Sade, French author

sadist (sad'ist) a person practising sadism

sadness a normal emotional feeling of sorrow or dejection

sadomasochism (sa'do-mas'e-kizm) a form of sexual perversion marked by love of cruelty in its active and/or passive form

Saemisch's (sa'mish-es) **ulcer** serpiginous infectious ulcer of the cornea, named after Edwin Saemisch, German ophthalmologist

safe blood packed red cells and blood products obtained from subjects with no known risks for exposure to transfusion-transmissible microorganisms

safe light a darkroom device emitting light that causes less fogging of underdeveloped film

safe sex the practice of protecting oneself and one's partner from sexually transmitted diseases by using condoms

safety pin bodies arrangement of Donovan bodies of granuloma inguinale within the macrophages

safflower oil the oil extracted from the seeds of safflower plant, *Cathamus tinctorius*. It is rich in linoleic acid and low in saturated fatty acids.

sagittal (saj'i-t'l) 1. arrow-like 2. situated in the direction of the sagittal suture 3. in an anteroposterior direction **s outlet diameter** of pelvic brim from lower end of sacrum to lower edge of symphysis **s plane** a vertical plane through the longitudinal axis of the trunk dividing the body into two parts **s sulcus** a groove in the inner surface of the parietal bones, forming a channel for the superior sagittal sinus **s suture** interparietal suture, line of union between two parietal bones

sagittalis (saj'i-ta'lis) sagittal

sago (sa'go) a starchy preparation from palm plant. It is a demulcent and a food with little residue **s spleen** splenic amyloid with discrete translucent bodies

sahaja (s) natural

sahajanya (s) inherited

Sahli's (sah'lez) **method** conversion of haemoglobin into acid haematin by adding HCl and comparing the colour with a standard colour scale to estimate haemoglobin, named after Herman Sahli, Bern physician

Saint's triad hiatus hernia, gall stones and diverticulosis, named after ℣. Saint, South African surgeon

Saint Vitus dance Sydenham's chorea

sakha (s) branch

sal salt

salaam (sa-lom) convulsion; nodding spasm of early infancy that disappears by age two or evolves into grand mal seizures with marked mental retardation. The lightning quick movement of the head, and flexion and extension of the trunk and arms simulate Arab way of greeting and prayer

salakya tantra (s) treatment of diseases of ear, nose and throat

salbutamol (sal-bu-to'mol) a beta-2 adrenergic agent that combines with beta-2 receptors on bronchial smooth muscle to increase production of cyclic AMP and reverse airway obstruction used as a bronchodilator

salicylamide (sali-sil-am'id) an amide salt of salicylic acid used as an analgesic and antipyretic

salicylate (sal'i-sil'at) a salt of salicylic acid **methyl** s oil of winter green used externally as a counter-irritant **sodium** s a white crystalline substance used as an analgesic and antipyretic

salicylic (sal'i-sil'ik) **acid** a white crystalline acid derived from phenol. Its salt as sodium salicylate acts as an analgesic. Topically it is a keratolytic agent

salicylism (sal'i-sil'ism) a toxic condition caused by an overdose of salicylic acid or its salts presenting with tinnitus, nausea and vomiting. There is a severe metabolic acidosis and a large anion gap

salicyluric (sal'i-si-lu'rik) **acid** a compound of glycol and salicylic acid found in the urine following intake of salicylic acid or its salts

salient prominent, conspicuous

saline (sa'lin) salty; containing salt or a salt solution **hypertonic** s an aqueous solution of sodium chloride of greater than 0.85% **hypotonic** s an aqueous solution of sodium chloride of less than 0.85% **isotonic** s a 0.9% solution of sodium chloride with an osmolality similar to that of blood serum **physiological** s an isotonic aqueous solution of sodium chloride s **cathartic** a salt capable of evacuation of the bowel s **enema** enema containing sodium chloride solution to induce peristalsis and evacuation

saliva (sa-li'va) a secretion of salivary glands and oral mucous glands. It consists of inorganic substances and enzymes and daily secretion is about 1.5 litre. It initiates digestion of starches, moistens the oral mucosa, and food for tasting, chewing and swallowing **salivary** adj. s **ejector** a device used during dental work to remove saliva

salivant (sa-li'vant) a substance provoking the flow of saliva

salivary (sal'i-ver-e) pertaining to the production of saliva s **digestion** digestion of starch initiated in the mouth by salivary amylase (ptyalin) s **glands** three pairs of glands - parotid, submandibular and sublingual glands - that secrete saliva to initiate digestion. The saliva travels from the glands through ducts into the mouth

salivation (sal'i-va'shun) 1. the act of secretion of saliva 2. excessive secretion of saliva

Salk (so'lk) **vaccine** an injectable, formalin-inactivated vaccine of poliomyelitis viruses, used to induce immunity against the disease, prepared by Jonas Salk, US microbiologist

sallow (sal'o) yellow complexion

Salmonella (sal'mo-nel'a) a genus of gram-negative, motile bacteria belonging to the family Enterobacteriaceae. The pathogenic species cause food poisoning and enteric fever. The organisms are, named after Daniel Salmon, US veterinarian *S. chol'erae suis* a species occurring in pigs which may cause gastroenteritis in humans *S. enteritidis* a species causing gastroenteritis and food poisoning *S. paratyphi* a group of organisms of salmonella types A, B, and C causing paratyphoid fever *S. typhi* a species causing typhoid fever *S. typhimurium* a species responsible for acute gastroenteritis

salmonellosis (sal-mo-ne-lo'sis) infection with organisms of the genus Salmonella *Salmonella* species other than *S. typhi* are very common causes of food poisoning

salpingectomy (sal'pin-jek'to-me) surgical removal of one or both fallopian tubes; tubectomy

salpingemphraxis (sol'pin-jem-frak'sis) an obstruction of eustachian tube

salpingian (sal'pin-je-an) pertaining to the eustachian tube or a fallopian tube

salpingion (sal'pin-je-on) a point at the inferior surface of the apex of the petrous portion of a temporal bone

salpingitis (sal'pin-ji'tis) inflammation or infection of fallopian tube or the eustachian tube

salpingo combining word for tube (usually fallopian or occasionally eustachian tube)

salpingocatheterism (sal'ping'go-kath'et-er-izm) catheterisation of the eustachian tube.

salpingocoele (sal'ping'go-sel) the hernial protrusion of a fallopian tube

salpingocyesis (sal'ping'o-si-e-sis) tubal pregnancy

salpingography (sal'ping-gog'ra-fe) radiographic examination of fallopian tubes after injection of a radiopaque contrast medium. It is performed to test the patency of the tubes

salpingolithiasis (sal'ping-go-li-thi'a-sis) the presense of calcareous substance in a fallopian tube

salpingolysis (sal'ping-gol'i-sis) surgical removal of scar tissue that has formed between a fallopian tube and surrounding tissues

salpingo-oophorectomy (sal-ping'go-o'of-o-rek'to-me) surgical removal of one or both of fallopian tubes and ovaries

salpingo-oophoritis (sal-ping'go-o'of-o-ri'tis) inflammation of a fallopian tube and an ovary

salpingo-oophorocoele (sal-ping'go-o'of'or-o-sel) a hernia containing a fallopian tube and ovary

salpingopexy (sal-ping'o-pek'se) operative fixation of a fallopian tube

salpingopharyngeal (sal-ping'go-fa-rin'je-al) pertaining to the eustachian tube and the pharynx

salpingopharyngeus (sal-ping'go-far-in'je-us) *see* Table of muscles

salpingoplasty (sal-ping'go-plas'te) plastic repair of a fallopian tube, undertaken to treat female infertility; tuboplasty

salpingorrhaphy (sal-ping'gor'a-fe) suture of a fallopian tube

salpingosalpingostomy (sal-ping'go-sal'ping-gos'to-me) a surgical procedure of attaching one fallopian tube to the other

salpingoscope (sal-ping'go-skop) an instrument for examining the nasopharynx and the eustachian tube

salpingostenochoria (sal-ping'go-sten'o-kor'e-a) a stricture or stenosis of the eustachian tube

salpingostomy (sal-pingo-os'to-me) a surgical procedure to make an opening in a blocked fallopian tube

salpinx (sal'pinks) a tube referring to a fallopian tube or eustachian tube

salt 1. common salt, sodium chloride (NaCl) 2. any compound formed by interaction of a base and an acid 3. in plural, any mineral salt or saline mixture used as a cathartic **bile** s a salt of glycocholic acid and taurocholic acid found in bile **buffer** s a salt that fixes excess amounts of acid or alkali without causing a change in pH **Epsom** s magnesium sulphate **Glauber's** s sodium sulphate **hypochlorite** s a salt of hypochlorous acid used as a bleaching agent **iodised** s a salt containing 1 part sodium or potassium iodide in 10000 parts of sodium chloride **rock** s natural sodium chloride **sea** s common salt obtained from sea water. It forms an important source of iodine and prevents goitre due to iodine deficiency **smelling** s aromatised ammonium carbonate used as a stimulant **substitute** s a substance that has a flavour similar to that of salt but low in sodium

salt and pepper pattern punctate and granular decalcification in x-ray of skull of advanced stage of primary hyperparathyroidism

saltation (sal-ta'shun) 1. leaping or jerky dancing as in chorea 2. a mutation 3. a sudden alteration in the course of a disease

saltatory conduction the transmission of a nerve impulse along a myelinated nerve fibre

salt free diet a low sodium diet that allows 500 mg or less salt per day ·

salt wasting disease a condition of excessive loss of sodium from the body seen in patients with renal cystic disease, obstructive uropathy, tubulointestinal disease, adrenocortical insufficiency or gastrointestinal disease. These patients require a high sodium and water intake to prevent fluid depletion and worsening of renal function; Salt losing syndrome

saltpeter (sawlt-pe'ter), potassium nitrate

salubrious (sa-loo'bre-us) conducive to health usually in reference to climate; wholesome

saluresis (sal'u-re'sis) urinary excretion of sodium and chloride ions **saluretic** adj

saluretic (sal-u-ret'ik) facilitating the renal excretion of sodium

salutary (sal'u-ta're) promoting health; curative

salvage (sal'va-j) to rescue or save from destruction s **therapy** any treatment regimen used after a number of particular regimens have failed to show the result

salvarsan (sal'var-san) an arsenic preparation, developed by Paul Ehrlich, for treatment of syphilis

salve (sav) a thick ointment made with a base of fat, oil petroleum or resin

salya tantra (s) surgery; operative procedure

sambandha (s) relation

sample 1. a subset of observations selected from a population 2. a portion of a whole that demonstrates the characteristics of the whole.

sampling (sam'pling) the process of selecting a portion to represent the whole s **error** impression of measurements made on sample when applied to whole population

samsaya (s) doubt

samyoga (s) conjugation; combination; union

sanative (san'a-tive) curative

sanatorium (san'a-to're-un) an institution for treatment of sick persons with chronic diseases such as tuberculosis or mental disorders, and for recuperation of health under medical supervision

sanatory (san'a-to're) conducive to health

sanchaya (s) accumulation

sanctuary (sangk'choo-ar'e) an area in body where a drug tends to accumulate without undergoing metabolic breakdown

sand fine gritty particles **auditory** s crystals of calcium carbonate in the utricle and saccule of the inner ear **brain** s heaped up concretion near the base of pineal gland **urinary** s multiple small calculous particles passed in the urine

sandfly any of various two-winged flies belonging to the genus Phlebotomus that transmit leishmaniasis, and sandfly **fever** s **fever** a mild viral illness resembling influenza without respiratory manifestations, transmitted by sandfly *Phlebotomus papatasi*

sandhi (s) joint

sandpaper skin coarse, bumpy, cool, pale hypotrichous skin in hypothyroidism

sandwich vertebrae increased density of

the vertebral end plates with normal bodies and preservation of intervertebral spaces, seen in osteopetrosis

sane (san) sound in mind

sangraha (s) compilation

sangui combining word for blood

sanguicolous (sang-gwik'o-lus) inhabiting the blood, as a parasite

sanguifacient (sang-gwi-fa'shent) agent promoting the formation of red blood cells

sanguiferous (sang-gwif'er-us) conducting or containing blood

sanguine (sang'gwin) 1. consisting of blood 2. plethoric or bloody 3. cheerful

sanguineous (sang-gwin'e-us) 1. pertaining to blood 2. abundance of blood

sanguinopurulent (sang'gwi-no-pu'roolent) containing blood and pus

sanguis (sang'gwis) blood

sanguisuga (sang'gwi-su'ga) a leech or blood sucker

sanies (sa'ne-ez) a foetid discharge containing serum, pus and blood

sanitarian (san-i-ta're-un) a person trained in sanitation and public health

sanitarium (san'i-tar'e-um) *see* sanatorium

sanitary (san-i-ta-re) 1. promoting or pertaining to health 2. clean, free of dirt, conducive to health s napkin perineal pad, used for absorbing menstrual fluid s latrine a latrine where excreta does not contaminate the ground or surface water s well well properly located, well constructed and protected against contamination with a view to yield a supply of safe water

sanitation (san'i-ta'shun) the establishment of conditions favourable to health, especially public health

sanitisation (san'i-ti-za'shun) the process of making sanitary

sanitiser an agent that reduces the number of bacterial contamination to safe level

sanity (san'i-te) soundness of mind, emotions and behaviour

SA node sinoatrial node of the heart

SaO$_2$ the arterial oxygen saturation expressed as a percentage. It is monitored non-invasively with a pulse oximeter

sap 1. any fluid essential and vital to life 2. to cause weakness or gradual exhaustion

saphena (sa-fe'na) a saphenous vein s varix single varix formed at origin of great saphenous vein

saphenectomy (saf'e-nek'to-me) the surgical removal of saphenous vein

saphenous (sa-fe'nus) pertaining to a saphenous vein or nerve in the leg s nerve *see* nerves s opening an oval aperture in the fascia in the inner and upper part of the thigh transmitting the saphenous vein s vein *see* table of veins

sapid 1.tasty 2. detectable by sense of taste

saponification (sa-pon'i-fi-ka'shun) conversion of an oil or fat into a soap by combining with an alkali

saponify (sa-pon'i-fi) to convert into a soap

saponin (sap'o-nin) glycoside found in roots of some plants which cause haemolysis in high dilutions

sapophore (sap'o-for) the molecular component that gives a substance its taste

saporific (sap'o-rifik) imparting a taste or flavour

saprobe (sa'prob) an organism that lives upon dead organic material such as fungi which do not possess photosynthetic material

saprogenic (sap'ro-jen'ik) causing putrefaction

saprophilous (sap'rof'il-us) living on decaying substances

saprophyte (sap'ro-fit) any organism living on decaying or dead organic matter such as higher fungi saprophytic adj

saprozoic (sap'ro-zo'ik) living in decaying organic matter

sarad (s) autumn

saralasin (sar-al'a-sin) an angiotensin II antagonist used as an antihypertensive agent

Sarcina (sar'si-na) a genus of spherical saprophytic bacteria of the family Micrococcaceae, found in soil and water

sarcitis (sar-si'tis) inflammation of muscle tissue; myositis

sarco - combining word for flesh

sarcoblast (sar'ko-blast) a primitive cell which develops into a muscle cell; myoblast

sarcoadenoma (sar'ko-ad'en-o'ma) a fleshy tumour of a gland

sarcocarcinoma (sar'ko-kar'sin'o-ma) a malignant tumour consisting of sarcomatous and carcinomatous tissue

sarcocoele (sar'ko-sel) fleshy tumour of the testis

sarcocyst (sar'ko-sist) 1. a protozoan parasite of the genus Sarcocystis 2. a cylindrical body with spores found in the muscles infected with Sarcocystis

Sarcocystis (sar'ko-sis'tis) a genus of parasitic protozoa found in the muscles

sarcocystosis (-sis-to'sis) infection with Sarcocystis that may remain asymptomatic or manifested with muscle cysts with myositis

sarcoid (sar'koid) 1. a small epithelioid tubercle-like lesion characteristic of sarcoidosis 2. muscle-like

sarcoidosis (sar'koi-do'sis) a chronic progressive multisystem granulomatous disorder of unknown aetiology characterised by enhanced cell-mediated immune processes at the site of involvement. There is widespread non-caseating granulomas and the histologic pattern is uniformly the same in all affected organs. It affects especially the lungs, lymph nodes, liver, skin and eyes. Intrathoracic involvement is noted in 90% of all patients of sarcoidosis. Cough and progressively increasing breathlessness are most common respiratory symptoms. Erythema nodosum, fever, polyarthralgia and hilar adenopathy are characteristics during the early stages of disease

sarcolemma (sar'ko-lem'a) the plasma membrane of a striated muscle fibre

sarcolysis (sar'ko-li-sis) decomposition of soft tissues

sarcoma (sar-ko'ma) a cancer arising from any tissue including muscle, fat, bone or blood vessels other than skin and mucous membranes

sarcomatoid (-toid) resembling a sarcoma

sarcomatosis (sar'ko-ma-to'sis) a condition characterised by the presence and spread of a sarcoma

sarcomatous (sar'ko-ma-tus) pertaining to or of the nature of a sarcoma

sarcomere (sar'ko-mer) the contractile unit of a myofibril. It consists of myosin and actin filaments arranged between two Z discs

sarcomphalocoele (sar'kom-fal-o-sel) a fleshy tumour of the umbilicus

sarcoplasm (sar'ko-plazm) the cytoplasm of striated muscle

sarcoplast (-plast) an interstitial cell of muscle, which can get transformed into muscle

Sarcoptes (sar-kop'tez) a genus of Acarina that includes the mites that infest humans and animals. *Sarcoptes scabiei* causes scabies in humans

Sarcoptes scabiei

sarcosis (sar-ko'sis) abnormal formation of flesh

sarcosporidiasis (sar'ko-spo-rid'e-o'sis) infection with protozoa (Sarcosporidia) in the muscle

sarcostosis (sar'kos-to-sis) ossification of muscular tissue

sarcotubule (sar'ko-tu-bul) a canalicular network around each myofibril

sarcous (sar'kus) pertaining to flesh or muscle tissue

sargramostin (sar-gram′o-stin) granu-locyte-macrophage colony stimulating factor developed by recombinant technology that can hasten recovery of haemopoietic system

sarira (s) body

SARS *abb.* Severe acute respiratory syndrome

sartorius (sar-to′re-us) the longest muscle in the body, *see* table of muscles

satellite (sat′l-it) 1. a small structure around a large one 2. lesions, masses, patterns or radiologic densities that surround a central point 3. a minute body attached to a chromosome

satellitism (sat′el-i-tizm) the phenomenon in which certain bacterial species grow better in the vicinity of colonies of other unrelated species as some species of Haemophilus in the vicinity of Staphylococci

satellitosis (sat′el-i-to′sis) accumulation of neuroglial cells about neurones especially seen during latter's damage

satiety (sa-ti′et-e) being full to satisfaction, especially with food s centre an area in hypothalamus that senses a feeling of satiety following a meal and inhibits the feeding centre located in the hypothalamus

satratoxin (sat′ra-tok-sin) mycotoxin from Stachbotrys atra

sattva bala (s) power of endurance

saturated (sat′u-ra′ted) 1. holding all that can be absorbed 2. a solution in which no more of a substance can be dissolved

saturation (sat′u-ra′shun) the state of being saturated s index the amount of haemoglobin present in a known volume of blood compared with the normal oxygen s the ratio of amount of oxygen found in a known volume of blood to amount of oxygen that could be carried by that volume of blood s time the time required for the arterial blood to get saturated on inhalation of oxygen

Saturday night palsy ischaemic neuropathy affecting radial nerve from drunken sleep with arm over back of chair

saturnine (sat′ur-nin) pertaining to or produced by lead

saturnism (sat′ur-nizm) lead poisoning; plumbism

Satyr ear a congenital abnormality of the auricle where helix lacks the usually rolled contour and tubercle is unusually prominent as in minor deities of Greek mythology

satyriasis (sat′i-ri′-a-sis) an excessive and often uncontrollable sexual desire in the male

saucerisation (saw-ser-i-za′shun) 1. the creation of a shallow depression to facilitate drainage 2. a disciform defect that parallels the shaft of long bones on a plain film in fibrosarcoma with bony involvement

sauna an enclosed area where a person is exposed to moderate to high termperatures and high humidity

SA/V ratio surface area/volume

saumya (s) mild

sausage link pattern marked dilatation and tortuosity of retinal veins that are totally segmented at arteriovenous crossings in the optic fundus in grade II hypertensive retinopathy, in non-proliferative diabetic retinopathy and in hyperviscosity syndrome or Waldenstrom's macroglobulinaemia

saw a cutting instrument with a serrated edge

sawfish pattern jagged systolic narrowing of the left anterior descending coronary artery in angiography, characteristic of hypertrophic cardiomyopathy

saw-tooth pattern 1. a histopathologic appearance as a jagged and thickened dermal-epidermal junction in lichen planus 2. a jagged radiocontrast column, seen by barium studies of the colon in ischaemic colitis, or necrotising enterocolitis

saxitoxin (sak′si-tok′sin) a powerful

neurotoxin synthesised by dino-flagellates which can accumulate in the shell fish feeding on dinoflagellates

Sayre's (sarz) jacket a jacket of plaster of Paris worn to support the spine, named after Lewis Sayre, US surgeon

Sb symbol for the element antimony (stibium)

SBE subacute bacterial endocarditis

SC subcutaneous or subcutaneously

scab (skab) crust of a wound, ulcer

scabicide (ska'bi-sid) an agent that kills mites such as causative agents of scabies

scabbard trachea flattened by external pressure especially retrosternal goitre

scabies (ska'bez) a condition caused by itch mite, *Sarcoptes scabiei hominis*. It is transmitted by direct contact and causes an intensely pruritic linear eruption corresponding to the tracks of the burrowing mite, commonly affects children and pruritus results in excoriation and secondary pyoderma

scabrities (ska-bri'te-ez) a scaly, roughened condition of the skin

scaffold any structural matrix providing physical support for a functional system

scala (ska'la) any one of the three spiral passages of the cochlea of the inner ear **s media** the cochlear duct lying between the scala tympani and scala vestibuli. Its floor contains the spiral organ of Corti **s tympani** the cochlear duct filled with perilymph lying below the spiral lamina **s vestibuli** the cochlear duct forming the upper portion of the bony canal. It extends from the oval window to the tip of the cochlea

scald (skold) a burn to the skin and underlying tissues caused by moist heat and steam

scalded skin syndrome necrosis of the epidermal layer of the skin. The underlying dermis is intact. There is fever, rash and extremely tender skin. The bullae are filled with clear fluid.

It is due to the exotoxin of staphylococci

scale (skal) 1. a small, dry, thin exfoliation occurring from the upper layers of the skin 2. a film of tartar encrusting the teeth 3. an instrument for weighing 4. a graduated measure

scalene (ska-len') 1. having unequal sides and angles 2. refers to scalenus muscle **s node** small lymph node over scalenus anterior muscle, often taken as a marker of lung cancer spread

scalenectomy (ska'le-nek'to-me) resection of any of the scalene muscles

scalenotomy (ska-le'not'o-me) one of the three deeply situated neck muscles extending from the tubercles of the transverse processes of first or second rib. The three muscles are scalenus anterior, medius and posterior. **s syndrome** a symptom complex exhibiting brachial neuritis, with or without vasomotor disturbances

scaler (ska'ler) an instrument used for removal of stains and adherent deposits on the teeth

scaling (skal'ing) removal of adherent deposits (plaque, tartar or calculus) from the crown of a tooth and root surfaces

scalp (ska'lp) the hairy integument of the head **s electrode** applied following rupture of membranes to the foetal head for continuous recording of foetal heart rate in high risk labour **s tourniquet** a tourniquet applied to the scalp during intravenous administration of antineoplastic agents to restrict the blood flow to the hair bearing portion of the scalp and to prevent alopaecia

scalpel (skal'pel) a small, straight surgical knife

scalprum (skal'prum) pl. **scalpra** 1. a large scalpel 2. a toothed instrument for removal of of carious bone

scaly (ska'le) characterised by scales

scan an image obtained from computed tomography, ultrasound or magnetic resonance imaging

scanning 1. the process of obtaining images of an anatomical part through computed tomography, ultrasound or magnetic resonance imaging 2. the lowest magnification power used in diagnostic pathology in surveying tissues s speech a slurring speech with tendency to separate syllables in cerebellar diseases

scanty (skana'te) small in amount

scapha (ska'fa) an elongated depression of the ear between the helix and antihelix

scapho - boat-shaped

scaphocephaly (skaf'o-sef'a-le) a deformed head projecting like the kneel of a boat. Sagittal fusion results in long narrow skull with sagittal ridge

scaphoid (skaf'oyd) depression s abdomen sunken abdomen where the anterior abdominal wall is hollowed in and presents a concavity to the horizontal plane when looked at from the sides s fracture commonest carpal fracture produced by fall on outstretched hand

scaphoiditis (skaf'oyd-i-tis) inflammation of the scaphoid bone

scaption (ska'p-shun) elevation of the humerus in the plane of the scapula that is 30 to 45 degrees anterior to the frontal plane

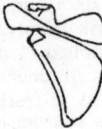

Scapula

scapula (skap'u-la) pl. scapulae the large triangular bone that forms the posterior part of the shoulder. It articulates with clavicle and the humerus winged s prominent medial border of the scapula, may be due to paralysis of serratus anterior or trapezius muscles

scapular (skap'u-lar) pertaining to the shoulder blade

scapulectomy (skap'u-lek'ta-me) resection of the scapula

scapuloclavicular (skap'u-lo-kla-vik'u-ler) pertaining to the scapula and clavicle

scapulohumeral (-hu'mer-al) pertaining to the scapula and humerus

scapulopexy (skap'u-lo-pek'se) surgical fixation of the scapula

scapus (ska'pus) shaft

scar (skar) cicatrix; fibrous trace of destructive lesion of tissue s cancer lung cancer developing in preexisting scars

scarification (skar'ifi-ka'shun) making multiple small skin incisions with a sharp point

scarifier (skar'i-fi'er) an instrument with many sharp points used in scarification

scarlatina (skar'la-te'na) scarlet fever due to haemolytic streptococcus

scarlet fever erythrogenic toxin produced by *Streptococcus pyogenes* causing pharyngitis, strawberry tongue, generalised blanching erythema of face with circumoral pallor and linear petechiae

Scarpa's triangle femoral triangle named after Antony Scarpa, Italian surgeon

SCAT sheep cell agglutination test

scataemia (ska-te'me-a) intestinal autointoxication

scatole (ska-tol) oxidation product of tryptophane responsible for much of faecal odour

scatology (ska-tol'-je) study and analysis faeces

scatoscopy (ska-tos'ko-pe) examination of faeces

scattergram a plot of data points in a coordinate system to determine existence of any correlation between two variables on the X and Y axes

SCC small cell carcinoma

s cell secretin producing endocrine cell in the mucosa of the upper small intestine

schema 1. synopsis 2. essential features of class 3. preliminary outline 4. a plan or outline

Schick's test intradermal injection of diphtheria toxin to determine immunity status. Lack of antibody is indicated by erythema, named after Bela Schick, Hungarian US paediatrician

Schilling test a test using radioactive vitamin B$_{12}$ to assess the gastrointestinal absorption of vitamin B$_{12}$ to diagnose primary pernicious anaemia, named after Robert Schilling, US haematologist.

Schimmelbusch mask wire frame to hold gauge, used to administer volatile anaesthetics, named after Curt Schimmelbusch, German surgeon

Schiotz tonometer instrument to measure intraocular pressure from indentation of cornea produced by standard weight, named after Hjalmar Schiotz, Norwegian ophthalmologist

Schirmer test test to determine lacrimal secretion and it measures length of wetting of strip of filter hooked over lower eyelid, named after Rudolf Schirmer, German ophthalmologist

schindylesis (skin'di-le'sis) an articulation in which one bone is received into a cleft of another

schist (o) combining word for cleft or split

schistocephalus (shis'to-sef'a-lus) a foetus with a cleft head

schistocoelia (-se'le-a) congenital fissure of the abdomen

schistocyte (shis'to-sit) fragmented red blood cell that arises from either an increase in cell fragility or from trauma caused by intravascular rugosities seen in haemolytic anaemia, trauma, prosthetic heart valves, disseminated intravascular coagulation and megaloblastic anaemia

schistocytosis (shis 'to-si-to'sis) presence of a large number of schistocytes in the blood

schistomelus (shis-tom'e-lus) a foetus with a cleft limb

Schistosoma (-so'ma) a genus of blood flukes that cause infection in man on entry through the skin. It includes *S. haematobium*, *S. japanicum* and *S. mansoni*. They belong to phylum **Platyhelminthes, class Trematoda**

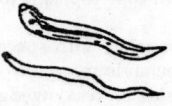

Schistosoma haematobium

schistosomiasis (shis'to-so-mi-a-sis) Three species of the genus Schistosoma (*S. haematobium*, *S. mansoni* and *S. japanicum*) are the causative agents of schistosomiasis. The ovum passed in the urine or faeces of infected persons gains entry into fresh water. A ciliated miracidium is liberated and it enters an intermediate host, a freshwater snail where it multiplies. A large number of cercariae are liberated which penetrate the skin or mucosa of definite host, human where they pass through the lung and reach liver and mature. The manifestations are painless terminal haematuria, frequency of micturition, pain, pyelonephritis, hydronephrosis, and uraemia (*S. haematobium*), abdominal pain, frequent stools with blood-stained mucus, hepatomegaly, portal hypertension, haematemesis and ascites (*S. mansoni*) features resembling infection with *S. mansoni* with added neurologic features (*S. japanicum*)

schistosomicide (-so-mi-sid) an agent lethal to schistosomes

schistothorax (-thor'ks) congenital fissure of the sternum

schizamnion (shiz-am'ne-on) an amnion developing by formation of a cavity within the inner cell mass

schiz (o) combining word for division, splitting

schizocyte schistocyte

schizogenesis (skiz'o-jen'e-sis) reproduction by fission. **schizogenous** adj

schizogony (ski'zog'a-ne) the asexual reproduction of a sporozoon parasite by multiple fission of the nucleus and later segmentation of cytoplasm to produce merozoites

schizoid personality introspective, solitary, shy behaviour

schizogyria (skiz'o-j're-a) wedge-shaped cracks in the cerebral convolutions

schizoid (skiz'oid) 1. schizophrenia-like trait 2. trait characterising the schizoid personality

schizont (skiz'ont) multinucleated stage during schizogony

schizonychia (skiz'o-nik'e-a) splitting of the nails

schizophasia (-fa'zhah) disordered speech

schizophrenia (skiz'o-fre'ne-a) a disorder of thinking and perception, and inappropriate or blunted mood **catatonic s** marked psychomotor disturbance which alternates between hyperkinesis and stupor **chronic s** schizophrenia exhibiting thought disorder and negative symptoms of underactivity, lack of drive, social withdrawal and emotional emptiness **hebephrenic s** schizophrenia characterised by a markedly shallow and in- appropriate mood **negative s** schizophrenia having a slow and insidious onset, apathy, social withdrawal, lack of motivation and underlying abnormalities of brain structure **paranoid s** schizophrenia with insidious onset, with delusions of persecutory nature with hallucinatory voices **positive s** schizophrenia with acute onset, with prominent delusions and hallucinations and normal structure of the brain **simple s** schizophrenia exhibiting insidious deterioration of the personality

Schonlein's purpura anaphylactoid purpura associated with joint lesions, named after Johann Schonlein , German physician

'School of fish' appearance microscopic appearance characterised by multiple, discrete oval to elongated structures arranged in long roughly parallel fascicles seen in malignant fibrous histiocytoma or *Haemophilus ducrey* bacillus

Schuffner's dots stippling of red cells in vivax malaria, named after Wilhelm Schuffner, German parasitologist

schizotrichia (skiz'o-trik'e-a) splitting of hairs at their ends

schizotypei (shiz'o-ti'pi) abnormal behaviour and style similar to those of schizophrenic. However the features are mild

Schwann cell one of the cells of the peripheral nervous system producing myelin sheath and neurilemma of peripheral nerve fibres, named after Theodor Schwann, German anatomist

schwannoma (skwan'o-ma) a tumour of Schwann cells; neurilemmomas are **benign s** and true or **malignant s** are Schwannomas, occurring as malignant peripheral nerve sheath tumours

Schwartze mastoidectomy surgical removal of all accessible mastoid cells and antrum without touching middle ear, named after Hermann Schwartze, German otologist

Schwartze sign bright pink colour seen through tympanic membrane in otosclerosis

sciatic (si-at'ik) pertaining to the ischium or hip *see* table of nerves

sciatica (si'al'i-ka) pain in the distribution of sciatic nerve due to lateral disc protrusion on L_4 and/or L_5 spinal nerve roots

science (si'ens) knowledge systematised; pursuit of knowledge

scieropia (si'er-o'pe-a) abnormal vision in which the things appear to be a shadow.

scimitar syndrome a rare vascular anomaly where the pulmonary veins drain into the inferior vena cava which appears as a curved (scimitar-shaped) radio-opacity adjacent to the right cardiac border

scintigram (sin'ti-gram) scintiscan

scintigraphy (sin-tig'ra-fe) production of two-dimensional images of the distribution of radioactivity in tissues after administration of a radiopharmaceutical imaging agent

scintillation (sin'ti-la'shun) 1. a subjective sensation of sparks or flashes of light 2. the light emitted when an X- or gamma- ray is absorbed by a crystal or liquid radiator detector

scintiscan (sin'ti-skan) the record obtained by scanning, that gives a photographic display of the distribution of internally administered radiopharmaceutical

scintiscanner (sin-ti-skan'er) the apparatus used to make a scintiscan

scirrhous (skir'us) hard; indurated

SCLC small cell lung cancer

sclera (skler'a) white of the eye; a fibrous tunic forming the outer envelope of the eye

scler (o) combining word for hard; sclera

scleradenitis (skler'ad-e-ni'tis) inflammation and hardening of a gland

sclerectasia (-ek-ta'zhah) a localised bulge of the sclera

sclerectoiridectomy (skle'rek'to-ir'i-dek'ta-me) excision of a portion of the sclera and of the iris

sclerectomy (skle-rek'ta-me) excision of a portion of the sclera

scleredema (skler'e-de-ma) a condition exhibiting oedema and induration following an acute infection

sclerema (skl-re'ma) induration of the subcutaneous fat

scleriritomy (skler'i-rit'a-me) incision of the iris and sclera

scleritis (skle-ritis) inflammation of the sclera **anterior s** inflammation affecting the sclera adjoining the limbus of the cornea **posterior s** inflammation of the sclera underlying retina and choroid

scleroblastema (skler'o-blas-te'ma) the embryonic tissue from which bone is formed

sclerochoroiditis (-kor'oi-di'tis) inflammation of the sclera and choroid

sclerocornea (-kor'ne-a) 1. hard outer coat of the eye formed by the sclera and cornea 2. a congenital anomaly in which cornea is opaque resembling the sclera

sclerodactyly (-dak'ti-le) acrosclerosis

scleroderma (-der'ma) widespread thickening and fibrosis of the skin due to accumulation of excess collagen and polyglycans, a manifestation of systemic sclerosis

sclerogenous (skle-roj'e-nus) producing sclerosis

scleroiritis (skler'o-i-ri'tis) inflammation of the sclera and iris

sclerokeratitis (-ker'a-ti'tis) inflammation of the sclera and cornea

scleroma (skle-ro'ma) a circumscribed indurated focus of granulation tissue in the skin of mucous membrane

scleromalacia (skler'o-ma-la'shah) degeneration and softening of the sclera

scleromere (skler'o-mer) any homologous segment of the skeleton, such as vertebral segment

scleromyxedema (skler'o-mik'se-de'ma) lichen myxedematosus exhibiting thickening of the skin under the papules

scleronyxis (-nik'sis) induration and thickening of the nails

sclero-oophoritis (-o'of-a-ri'tis) inflammatory induration of the ovary

sclerophthalmia (skler'of-thal'me-a) a congenital abnormality in which the opacity of the sclera has extended over the cornea leaving only a small central area of the latter transparent

scleroprotein protein capable of forming insoluble structural material

sclerogenous (skle-roj'e-nus) producing sclerosis

sclerosant (skle-ro'sant) a chemical injected into a vein to produce inflammation and ultimately fibrosis and obliteration of the lumen; used in the treatment of varicose veins

sclerose (skle-ros) to become hardened or sclerotic

sclerosing adenosis hyperplasia of the

glandular component of the breast, having indurated, often small multinodular lesions without any trabecular formations **s cholangitis** bile duct inflammation with cholestasis, presenting with jaundice, pruritis and portal hypertension **s epithelial hamartoma** a benign hair follicle tumour noted on the face of the young **s haemangioma** a well-circumscribed benign lesion in the lung arising from type II pneumocytes **s peritonitis** extensive peritoneal fibrosis occurring in response to asbestos **s retroperitonitis** idiopathic proliferation of fibrous tissue in the retroperitoneum that encases ureters causing renal failure.

sclerosis (skle-ro′sis) 1. an induration of tissue due to excess fibrosis 2. induration of nervous structures 3. thickening and hardening of the layers in the wall of an artery **amyotrophic lateral s** a variant of motor neuron disease causing degeneration of motor tracts of the lateral columns, distal and proximal muscle wasting and weakness, fasciculations, spasticity, exaggerated reflexes and extensor plantars **arterial s** arteriosclerosis **lateral s** sclerosis of the lateral column of the spinal cord **multiple s** occurrence of plaque of inflammatory demyelination in more than one anatomical site at more than one time such as periventricular regions of the brain, the optic nerves and subpial regions of the spinal cord. It presents a relapsing and remitting clinical course with optic neuritis, relapsing and remitting sensory symptoms, and acute brain non-compressive paraparesis **systemic s** a generalised disorder of connective tissue characterised by widespread thickening and fibrosis of the skin and obliterative lesions of the arterioles and capillaries. It presents with Raynaud's phenomenon, sclerodactyly, tightness, telangiectasias, arthralgia, dysphagia, interstitial pulmonary fibrosis **tuber-**

ous s an abnormal development of mesodermal tissue occurring as a genetic defect involving skin and the nervous system manifesting with features of epilepsy, mental retardation and adenoma sebaceum at an early age

sclerostenosis (skler′o-ste-no′sis) an autosomal recessive condition characterised by deafness, asymmetrically enlarged mandible, syndactyly and onychodysplasia

sclerostomy (skle-ros′ta-me) a surgical creation of an opening in the sclera, undertaken in the treatment of glaucoma

sclerotherapy (skler′o-ther′a-pe) injection of sclerosing agents in the treatment of piles or varicose veins

sclerotic (skle-rot′ik) 1. relating to or characterised by sclerosis 2. scleral

sclerotica (skl-rot′i-ka) sclera

sclerotitis (skler′o-ti′tis) scleritis

sclerotium (skl-ro′she-um) a hard mass formed by the growth of certain fungi

sclerotome (skler′o-tom) 1. knife used in sclerotomy 2. a group of mesenchymal cells migrating from mesodermal somite towards notochord

sclerotomy (skl-rot′a-me) incision of the sclera

sclerous (skler′us) hard; indurated

scolex (sko′leks) pl. **scoleces** head of tapeworm, attached by suckers and frequently, by rostellar hooks to the wall of intestine

scolio - combining word for twisted, crooked

scoliokyphosis (sko′le-o-ki-fo′sis) having lateral and posterior curvature of the vertebral column

scoliosiometry (-se-om′e-tre) measurement of spinal curvature

scoliosis (sko′le-o′sis) lateral curvature of the vertebral column. **scoliotic adj functional s** a non-structural reversible lateral curvature of the spine. **structural s.** an irreversible lateral curvature of the spine with fixed rotation of the vertebrae

scoliotic (sko'le-ot'ik) pertaining to or characterised by scoliosis

scolopsia (sko-lop'se-a) a suture between two bones that allows movement of one on the other

scoop (skoop) a spoon like instrument for evacuating cavities

scopalamine (sko-pol'a-men) an anticholinergic alkaloid obtained from different solanaceous plants; hyoscine

scopophilia (sko'po-fil'e-a) 1. voyeurism 2. exhibitionism

scopophobia (-fo'be-a) irrational fear of being seen

-scopy combining word for examination of

scorbutic (skor-bu'tik) pertaining to or affected by scurvy

scorbutigenic (skor-bu'ti-jen'ik) producing scurvy

scorbutus (skor-bu'tus) scurvy

scordinema (skor'di-ne'ma) heaviness of head accompanied by yawning and stretching

score (skor) a mark or notch for keeping count

scorpion (skor'pe-on) an arthropod having a venomous sting

scot (o) combining word for darkness

scotch tape test retrieval of eggs of *Enterobius vermicularis* from the perianal region in children by application of an adhesive tape

scotochromogen (sko'to-kro'mo-jen) an organism such as *M. scrofulaceum* growing slowly in culture, and producing colonies even in darkness. It turns orange on exposure to light

scotodinia (-din'e-a) dizziness, blurred vision and headache

scotoma (sko-to'ma) pl. **scotomata** localised loss of vision within otherwise normal lung fields

scotomagraph (-graf) an instrument for recording a scotoma

scotometry (sko-tom'e-tre) the measurement of scotomas

scotomisation (sko'ta-mi-za'shun) development of scotomata, especially mental scotomata wherein the patient attempts to deny existence of everything that conflicts with his ego.

scotopic vision vision with full dark adaptation

scotophilia (sko'to-fil'e-a) preference for the night or darkness

scotophobia (-fo'be-a) irrational fear of darkness

scotopia (sko-to'pe-a) scotopic vision

scotopsin (sko-top'sin) the protein moiety of the pigment in the rods of the retina

scourge cause of suffering or death, affliction

scout films any preliminary x-ray film taken of a body region prior to undertaking a definitive imaging study and it serves to establish a baseline

scrapie (skra'pe) a prion-induced infection which causes fatal neurologic degeneration in sheep and goats, who scrape themselves on rocks

screen (skren) 1. examination for presence of certain diseases or characteristics 2. a flat surface on which slides or movies are viewed 3. a structure used to protect from damaging influence such as x-ray or sun rays

screening (skren'ing) 1. a process in which a large population group is evaluated for the possible presence of a morbid condition by measuring clinical parameters 2. initial patient evaluation 3. a fluoroscopic examination

scrobiculate (skro-bik'u-lat) finely pitted

scrobiculus (-lus) pit s **cordis** epigastric fossa; pit of the stomach

scrofuloderma (-lo-der'ma) cutaneous tuberculosis

scrotectomy (skro-tek'ta-me) partial or total excision of the scrotum

scrotitis (-ti'tis) inflammation of the scrotum

scrub nurse a nurse who participates in a sterile surgical operation

scrub typhus rickettsial infection caused by *R. tsutsugamushi* transmitted by mites

scruff nape, back part of the neck

scrotocoele (skro'to-sel) scrotal hernia

scrotoplasty (-plaste) surgical reconstruction of the scrotum

scrotum (skro'tum) a musculocutaneous sac containing testes. It is formed of skin, a network of nonstriated muscle fibres (dartos), cremasteric muscle and fascia and serous coverings of the testes and epididymis **scrotal** adj. **lymph s** elephantiasis of the scrotum **s tongue** grooved or fissured tongue, which allows food particles to stick and later colonised by bacteria **watering-can s** presence of multiple sinuses on the under surface of the scrotum and the perineum discharging urine

scurvy (sker've) vitamin C deficiency manifesting in children with features of irritability, enlargement of ends of long bones, beading of costochondral junctions, subcutaneous echymosis, swollen gums and haemorrhage

scute (skut) a thin lamina or plate

scutiform (sku'ti-form) having a shape like a shield

scutum (sku'tum) 1. scale-like structure 2. a hard chitinous plate on the dorsal surface of hard-bodied ticks

scybalum (sib'a-lum) hard mass of faecal material in the intestine

scyphoid (si'foid) shaped like a cup

SD standard deviation; skin dose; surface density

SE standard error

Se chemical symbol, selenium

sealed envelope appearance high power light microscopic appearance of *Pneumocystis carinii* when stained with Gomori-methenamine silver stain. The envelope's flap corresponds to the organism's folded membrane

seam (sem) a line of union

searcher (serch'er) a form of sound used to determine the presence of a calculus in the bladder

seat worm (set'werm) *Enterobius vermicularis*

sebaceous (se-ba'shus) pertaining to or secreting sebum

sebiparous (se-bip'a-rus) producing oily secretion

sebolith (seb'o-lith) calculus in a sebaceous gland

seborrhoea (seb'o-re'a) excessive secretion of sebum **seborrhoeic** adj. **s sicca** 1. an accumulation on the skin, especially the scalp, of dry scales 2. dandruff

seborrhoeic dermatitis a chronic dermatitis affecting areas rich in sebaceous glands and presents with erythematous papulosquamous lesions with greasy scales

sebum (se'bum) oily secretion of the sebaceous glands, composed of fat and epithelial debris

seclude to isolate, to withdraw from others

secobarbital (sek'o-bar'bi-tal) a short acting barbiturate used as a hypnotic and sedative

second messenger chemical that sends genetic instructions after those received from messenger RNA, which enables turning genes on or off

secondary 1. arising from some earlier event or condition 2. later in time 3. metastasis of a tumour **s adrenal failure** pituitary deficiency causing adrenal insufficiency and is characterised by pallor **s amenorrhoea** cessation of menstruation after being once established **s bacterial infection** bacterial infection that develops as a consequence of a primary infection **s care** health care provided by a specialist in a community hospital to a patient who has been referred by a primary care physician **s deficiency** a nutritional deficiency resulting from either an increased requirement of a substance as in pregnancy or decreased availability or wastage of the nutrient as in proteinuria in a nephrotic syndrome **s gains** the benefits from being stricken by illness **s haemorrhage** bleeding from infection of wound with damage to vessels **s hydrocephalus** increase in volume of cerebrospinal fluid due to shrinkage of brain **s lesion** appearing as a result of the changes taking place in the primary lesion such as desquamation, scabs, crusts, ulceration or scar **s malignancy** a malignant neoplasm which arises in the background of another malignancy treated by radiotherapy or chemotherapy **s obesity** obesity as a symptom of other conditions **s optic atrophy** optic atrophy due to loss of retinal ganglion cells

second opinion an advice from a second health professional as to the correctness of the diagnosis and appropriateness of suggested line of treatment

secreta (se-kre'ta) products of secretion

secretagogue (se-kret'a-gog) 1. stimulating secretion 2. an agent that stimulates secretion

secrete (se-kret) to produce and release a secretion

secretin (se-kre'tin) a helical peptide produced by S cells in the upper small intestine, released by acid, bile or fat into the intestinal lumen, stimulating the release of water and bicarbonate from pancreas, neutralising gastric acid, stimulating intestinal motility and release of bile and gastric acid and inhibiting gastrin

secretion (-shun) 1. material produced by and separated from gland or cell 2. the process involved in it

secretogogue an agent that increases gastrointestinal secretion of electrolyte and fluid by increasing adenylate cyclase activity or by increasing calcium in the cytosol

secretoinhibitory (se-kro'to-hib'i-tor'e) inhibiting secretion

secretomotor (-mo'ter) stimulating secretion, refers to nerves

secretor (se-kre'ter) 1. a person who secretes ABH antigens of the ABO blood group in the saliva, gastric juice or semen 2. the process of producing specific products by the glands

secretory (se-kre'ta-re) pertaining to secretions **s endometrial carcinoma** a well-differentiated endometrial carcinoma in which cells have vacuolated or clear cytoplasm resembling normal secretory endometrium **s piece** a short polypetide carried by IgA.

sectio (sek'she-o) section

section (sek'shun) 1. an act of cutting 2. a cut surface 3. a segment or subdivision of an organ. **abdominal s** laparotomy **caesarian s** incision through the abdominal wall and uterus for extraction of the foetus **cross s** a section perpendicular to the long axis of an organ **frozen s** a thin section of tissue cut from a frozen specimen, used for rapid histologic diagnosis **perineal s** section through the perineum **serial s** one of a number of consecutive sections

secundigravida (se-kun'di-grav'i-da) gravida II; a woman becoming pregnant second time

secundines (se-kun'dinz) after birth

secular time related especially of long times

secundipara (se'kun-dip'a-ra) para II; a woman having had two pregnancies resulting in viable offspring

sedation (se-da'shun) making calm, allaying irritability or excitation by drugs

sedative (sed'a-tiv) 1. calming; quieting 2 an agent causing such an effect

sedentary (sed'en-tar'e) 1. sitting much 2. passed chiefly in sitting 3. mode of living with minimal exercise

sediment (sed'i-ment) 1. a precipitate that has formed spontaneously 2. an insoluble material that sinks to the bottom of a liquid

sedimentation (sed'i-men-ta'shun) the settling out of sediment

seed (sed) 1. male fecunding fluid, sperm 2. substance produced by the plants and animals from which new plants or animals are generated 3. capsule containing radon or radium **s calculi** a large number of small calculi that may form in a markedly hydronephrotic renal pelvis in ureteropelvic obstruction

seeding spread of tumour within the cavities

segment (seg'ment) **segmental** adj. 1. a part or section of an organ or body 2. one of the serial divisions of an animal **bronchopulmonary s** a wedge-shaped lung supplied by segmental bronchus **hepatic s** segment of the liver made up of smaller units (lobules) comprising of a central vein, radiating sinusoids separated from each other by hepatocytes and peripheral portal tracts **internodal s** the portion of a myelinated nerve between two successive nodes **mesode:mal s** a somite **uterine s** the lower end of the uterus joining with the cervical canal, which during pregnancy expands to become lower part of the uterine cavity and the upper part of the gravid uterus becomes thicker whose contractions provide the expulsory force in labour

segmentation (seg'men-ta'shun) 1. division into similiar parts 2. cleavage **s of colon** slow formation and relaxation of contraction rings in colon

segmentum (seg-men'tum) pl. **segmenta** segment

segregation (seg're-ga'shun) separation of two alleles of each gene at meiosis

seizure (se-shur) 1. the sudden attack or recurrence of a disease 2. an episode caused by an electrical discharge from the brain **absence s** petit mal. The attacks are brief and more frequent, and are caused by a general discharge which does not spread out of the hemisphere and there is no loss of posture **complex partial s** black-out; episodes of altered consciousness without collapsing to the ground **major s** loss of consciousness with patient falling to the ground **minor s** alteration of consciousness without the patient falling to the ground **partial motor s** rhythmical jerking or sustained spasm of contralateral face, arm, trunk and leg

as the electrical activity arises in precentral gyrus **partial sensory s** seizures arising in the sensory cortex exhibit unpleasant tingling or electric sensations in the contralateral face and limbs **partial visual s** electrical discharge from occipital lobe causing visual hallucinations **tonic clonic s** an aura followed by rigidity, unconsciousness, which a few moments later is periodically relaxed causing clonic jerks **versive s** electrical discharge from frontal lobe causing forced deviation of the eyes to the opposite side and may be followed by a tonic clonic seizure

Seldinger needle a needle used for arterial catheterisation. A guide wire is passed through the needle and catheter is introduced over guide wire, named after Sven Seldinger, Swedish physician

selectins a family of cell adhesion molecules or glycoproteins which are essential in the interactions between endothelium and cells in circulation

selection (se-lek'shun) to pick out from a number by preference

selegiline (se-lej'i-len) a selective monoamine oxidase type B inhibitor enhancing action of dopamine used in the symptomatic treatment of Parkinsonism

selenium (se-le'ne-um) an element of sulphur group, at. no. 34. a trace mineral, its, deficiency may cause dilated cardiomyopathy **s sulphide** used as a shampoo in seborrhoea

self actualisation Psy process of living upto one's full potential as a unique human being

self awareness aware of one's existence as an individual

self conscious 1 self awareness 2 sense of embarassment

self healing basic principle behind many traditional forms of medicine

self limited (self-lim'it-ed) referring to disease that tends to recede after a definite period

self mobilising techniques whereby the patient is taught to apply joint mobilisation techniques to restricted joints using proper gliding techniques

self mutilation *psy* an auto-destructive act related to self confinement, deprivation and depression

self one's own person

self realisation spiritual enlightenment or sense of inner understanding

self stretching technique whereby the patient is taught to stretch a joint or soft tissue passively using another part of the body for applying the stretch force

self tolerence (-tol'er-ans) immunological tolerance to auto-antigens

sella (sel'a) a saddle-shaped depression **sellar** adj. **s turcica** pituitary fossa

SEM 1. standard error of mean 2. scanning electron microscope

semantics the study of the significance and development of the meaning of words

semeiography (se'mi-og'ra-fe) a description of signs and symptoms or clinical feature of a disease

semeiotic (se'mi-ot'ik) 1. pertaining to signs and symptoms 2. pathognomonic

semeiotics (-iks) symptomatology

semelincident (sem'el-in'si-dent) attacking only once such as induction of immunity following an infectious disease

semen (se'men) material of male ejaculation containing secretions from seminal vesicle and prostate

semi- combining word for half

semicanal (semi-ka-nal) half canal; a deep groove on the edge of a bone, uniting with a similar groove of an adjoining bone

semicoma (-ko'ma) a stupor from which the patient may be aroused. **semicomatose** adj

semidominance (-dom'i-nans) incomplete dominance

semiflexion (-flek'shun) position of a limb midway between flexion and extension

semilente amorphous form of zinc-insulin complex that is more rapidily absorbed

semilunar (-loo'nar) half moon; crescent

semimembranous (-mem'bra-nus) composed partly of a membrane **s bursitis** bursa behind hamstring communicating with knee joint

seminiferous (-nif'er-us) carrying or conducting the semen, referring to the tubules of the testis

seminoma (-no'ma) testicular tumour presenting in the fourth decade of life as chronic painless enlargement of testicle. Testis is uniformly enlarged, and smooth. There is loss of testicular sensation

seminuria (se'mi-nu're-a) discharge of semen in the urine

semipermeable (sem'i-per'me-a-b'l) allowing passage only of certain molecules

semiquantitative (-kwon'ti-ta'tiv) amount of a substance falling short a quantitative result

semis (sem'is) half

semisulcus (sem'i-sul'kus) a slight groove on the edge of a bone or structure,

semisupination (-soo'pi-na'shun) half way between supination and pronation

semisynthetic (-sin-thet'ik) a chemical compound derived from a natural substance that is subjected to one or more synthetic steps to impart desired qualities

Semon's law loss of abduction before adduction in progressive recurrent laryngeal paralysis, named after Felix. Semon, British otologist

Semple vaccine anti-rabies vaccine containing infected rabbit brain inactivated with phenol, named after David. Semple, British microbiologist.

senescence (se'nes'ens) the process of growing old **replication s** human diploid fibroblasts at the end of their proliferative lifespan, remain alive in an arrested state and it occurs after about 60 cell divisions

Sengstaken-Blackmore tube a gastric tube with two oesophageal balloons to control bleeding from oesophageal varices, named after Robert Sengstaken, and Arthur Blackmore, American surgeons

senile (se'nil) pertaining to old age **s cataract** common type of granular cataract involving posterior central subcapasular area **s dementia** progressive neurodegenerative disease which may be primary (Alzheimer's disease) or secondary to vascular degeneration from atherosclerosis **s miosis** pupil becoming small and irregular in old age **s plaque** neuritic plaque composed of a core of extracellular amyloid surrounded by a spherical mass of axons and dendrites in the grey matter **s purpura** easy bruising and bleeding into the skin due to atrophy of the vascular supporting tissue

senilism (se'nil-izm) premature old age

senility (se-nil'i-te) old age; the sum of the physical and mental changes noted in advanced life

senna (sen'ah) extract of leaves or pods of *Cassia angustifolia* used as purgative

sennoside (sen'o-sid) arthraquinone glucosides found in senna that is used as a purgative

senopia (se-no'pe-a) an improvement in near vision in elderly due to myopia of increasing lenticular nuclear sclerosis. Ultimately it causes nuclear cataract.

sensation (sen-sa'shun) appreciation of sensation obtained from sources outside and inside the body **cortical s** stereognosis, tactile sensation and two-point discrimination **cutaneous s** the sense of light touch, pain and temperature **deep s** sense of position, passive movements, vibration and pressure **discriminatory s** stereognosis, tactile localisation and discrimination **exteroceptive s** sensations obtained from sources outside the body **kinesthetic s** deep sensation **proprioceptive s** sensations obtained from sources inside the body

sense (sens) feeling; a faculty by which

objects are perceived **colour s** the ability to distinguish differences in colour **joint s** sense of passive movement **kinesthetic s** muscular sense. **light s** ability to distinguish the degree of intensity of light **muscular s** a consciousness of the muscular movement needed in a given act **pain s** ability to appreciate prick of a pin **position s** ability to place a limb in a particular position **pressure s** ability to feel different degrees of pressure on the body surface **special s** one of the five senses related to the organs of sight, hearing, smell, taste and touch **static s** the sense that makes it possible to maintain equilibrium **temperature s** the ability to detect temperature **time s** ability to detect differences in time intervals **touch s** a primary sensation to recognise touch when different dermatomes are touched **vibration s** appreciation of vibrations **visceral s** the perception of existence of the internal organs

sensibility (sen'si-bil'i-te) the capability of perceiving sensory stimuli

sensible (sen'si-b'l) 1. perceptible to senses 2. capable of sensation

sensitive (sen'si-tiv) 1. capable of perceiving sensations 2. responding to a stimulus 3. a person rendered susceptible by previous exposure

sensitivity (sen'si-tiv'i-te) *stat* the degree to which a test or clinical assay is capable of confirming or supporting the diagnosis of a disease

sensitisation (sen'si-tiza'shun) 1. a condition of being made sensitive to a specific antigen such as a protein or pollen 2. the process of making an individual susceptible to a substance by repeated injections

sensitiser a substance that increases the susceptibility to a stimulus

sensomobile (sen'so-mo'bl) moving in response to a stimulus

sensomotor (-mo'tor) sensorimotor

sensorial (sen-sor'e-al) pertaining to the sensorium

sensorimotor (sen'sor-e-mo'ter) both sensory and motor

sensorineural (-noor'al) of or pertaining to a sensory nerve

sensorium (sen-sor'e-um) 1. an organ of sensation 2. *psy* consciousness

sensors (sen'surs) devices capable of detecting and measuring biological, chemical, electrical or other physical signals that are associated in health care

sensory (sen'sor-e) pertaining to sensation **s ataxia** ataxia due to posterior column lesions increased with eyes closed **s deafness** sensorineural deafness **s dysphasia** receptive dysphasia **s discrimination** ability to discriminate between the stimulus of two blunt points of a divider or two pins when applied simultaneously over the skin while the eyes are closed **s extinction** failure to perceive the stimulus such as touch or pinprick applied simultaneously, occurs in parietal lobe lesions

sensual (sen'shu-al) concerning or consisting in the gratification of the senses

sentient (sen'she-ent) able to feel; sensitive

sentinel clot an adherent blood clot or a prominent blood vessel in peptic ulcers which had bled earlier seen in upper gastrointestinal endoscopy

sentinel loop a dilated segment of jejunum in upper gastrointestinal radiocontrast series, seen in acute pancreatitis

sentinel node 1. an isolated enlarged left sided supraclavicular lymph node, associated with metastatic gastric carcinoma and its presence implies nonresectability of the growth 2. a node draining gall bladder lymph at cystic - common bile duct junction

sentinel pile skin tag at the lower end of a chronic anal fissure

separation process of disconnecting or severing

sepsis (sep'sis) presence of pathogens or their toxins in the blood or tissues **s syndrome** a systemic inflammatory response to infection exhibiting hypothermia or hyperthermia, tachycardia, tachypnoea, a focus of infection, positive blood cultures, one or more end organ dysfunction, hypoxaemia, and oliguria, initiating a systemic inflammatory response that adversely affects the blood flow to the vital organs

septa (sep'ta) pl. **septum**, partition dividing two cavities

septal (sep'tal) pertaining to a septum **s defect** an opening in the septum (interatrial or interventricular) between the left and right sides of the heart

septate (sep'tat) divided by a septum

septectomy (sep-tek'ta-me) excision of part of a nasal septum

septic (sep'tik) pertaining to sepsis **s arthritis** inflammation of joint by infection **s tank** a water-tight masonry tank into which household sewage is admitted for treatment **s shock** a septic shock syndrome with hypotension

septicemia (sep'ti-se'me-a) disease produced by multiplication of pathogenic organisms in the circulating blood

septicopyaemia (-ko-pi-e'me-a) septicemia and pyaemia together

septomarginal (sep'to-mar'ji-n'l) pertaining to the margin of a septum

septonasal (-na'z'l) pertaining to the nasal septum

septoplasty (sep'toplas'te) surgical reconstruction of the nasal septum

septostomy (sep'tos'ta-me) surgical creation of an opening in the septum

septotomy (sep-tot'a-me) incision of the nasal septum

septulum (sep'tu-lum) pl. **septula** partition

septum (sep'tum) pl. **septa** a thin wall dividing two cavities or masses of soft tissue. **s primum defect** a hole low in the interatrial septum, often involving AV valves **s secondum defect** a hole in the middle of the interatrial septum

septuplet (sep-tup'let) one of seven offsprings produced at one birth

sequel (se'k wel) sequela

sequela (se-kwe'la) pl. **sequelae** late complications or permanent ill-effects of a disease

sequence (se'kwens) order of succession; a series of things following in a certain order

sequential analysis *stat* continuous analysis of results to take action as soon as significance is reached

sequester (se-kwes'ter) 1. to isolate 2. sequestrum

sequestrant (se-kwes'trant) a sequestring agent such as cholestyramine which binds bile acids in the intestine preventing their absorption

sequestration (se'kwes-tra'shun) 1. a part separated from the surrounding healthy tissue 2. loss of blood or its fluid not participating in the circulation. **bronchopulmonary s** an area of nonfunctioning abnormal segment of lung parenchyma receiving its blood supply from a systemic artery and has no connection with tracheobronchial tree

sequestrectomy (-trek'ta-me) surgical removal of a sequestrum

sequestrum (se-kwes'trum) pl. **sequestra** a piece of necrosed tissue, usually bone separated from the surrounding healthy tissue

sequoiosis (se'kwoi-o'sis) extrinsic allergic alveolitis from redwood dust

sera (se'ra) pl. **serum**

serendipity (ser'en-dip'i-te) an unexpected reaction or result producing new insights

serial passage the repeated transfer of subpopulations of a pathogenic organism through a series of animals, tissue culture cells or growth media to attenuate the virulence of the organism while maintaining the immunogenicity.

series (se'rez) a succession of things connected by some likeness; sequence **erythrocytic s** the group of immature cells that develop into mature erythrocytes **granulocytic s** the immature cells in the bone marrow that develop into mature granular leucocytes

serine (ser'en) a non-essential amino acid found in many proteins **s proteases** a family of proteolytic enzymes that include coagulation cascade enzymes, trypsin and chymotrypsin

serocolitis (ser'o-ko-li'tis) inflammation of the serous coat of the colon

seroconversion (-con-ver'zhun) the change of an immune status from that of non-production of a particular antibody to a state of detectable production

serodiagnosis (-di'ag-no'sis) diagnosis of disease based on the serologic tests **serodiagnostic** adj

seroenteritis (-en'te-ri'tis) inflammation of the serous coat of the intestine

serofibrinous (-fi'bri-nus) composed of serum and fibrin, as in serofibrinous exudate

serogroup (ser'o-group) a group of bacteria containing a common antigen

serology (ser-ol'a-je) 1. study of serum in immunological aspects 2. results of immunological tests on the serum **serologic** adj

seroma (ser-o'ma) an area of graft filled with watery exudate

seromembranous (ser'o-mem'bra-nus) pertaining to or composed of serous membrane

seromucous (-mu'kus) both serous and mucous

seromuscular (-mis'ku-ler) pertaining to serous and muscular coats of the intestine

seronegative (-ne'ga-tiv) giving negative reaction to some serologic tests **s spondyloarthritis** diseases in which there is involvement of the spine and pauciarticular peripheral involvement with absence of rheumatoid factor, but positive for HLA B27. The examples are ankylosing spondylitis, psoriatic arthritis, Reiter's disease and Behcet's disease

seropositive (-poz'i-tiv) giving positive reaction to some serologic tests

seropurulent (-pu'roo-lent) both serous and purulent

seropus (ser'o-pus) serum mixed with pus

seroreaction (ser'o-re-ak'shun) any reaction occurring in or involving serum

serosa (se-ro'sa) 1. any flattened cell layer lining serous membranes 2. the chorion **serosal** adj

serosanguinous (ser'o-sang-gwin'o-us) composed of serum and blood

seroserous (-se'rus) pertaining to two or more serous membranes

serositis (-si'tis) pl. **serositides** inflammation of a serous membrane

serosurvey (-sur'va) a serologic screening test undertaken in persons at risks to determine susceptibility to a particular disease

serosynovitis (-sin'o-vi'tis) synovial inflammation with effusion of serum

serotherapy (-ther'a-pe) treatment of an infection by injection of immune serum or antitoxin

serotonin (ser'to'nin) 5 hydroxytryptamine, a molecule secreted by activated platelets. It is a potent vasoconstrictor and a neurotransmitter in CNS

serotoninergic (ser'o-to'nin-er'jik) 1. containing or activated by serotonin 2. pertaining to neurons that secrete serotonin

serotype (ser'o-tip) the type of a microorganism determined by its constituent antigens

serous (ser'us) 1. pertaining to or resembling serum 2. producing or containing serum 3. serosal 4. secreting watery fluid as parotid gland **s cystadenoma** ovarian cyst with watery contents and papillary in-growth into the cavity **s membrane** a membrane that lines a body cavity, such as pleural, pericardial and peritoneal cavities that does not open to the exterior

serovaccination (ser'o-vak'si-na'shun) a process to produce mixed immunity by injection of a serum to secure passive immunity and by vaccination with a modified or killed organism to acquire active immunity later

serovar serological variant of microbes

serpentine cords end-to-end arrangement of M. tuberculosis giving a beaded appearance

serpiginous (ser-pig'i-nus) creeping, having a wavy or serrated margin **s tract** a twisted vermiform radiolucency surrounded by a sclerotic rim in long bones in pyogenic osteomyelitis **s ulcer** ulcer of irregular shape which shows healing in one area while spreading in another

serpins a group of serine protease inhibitor proteins (antithrombins)

serrated (ser'at-ed) having a saw-like edge

serratia (se-ra'shea) a genus of Enterobacteria, a gram-negative organism, producing a red pigment **s marcescens** an important agent causing septicemia and lung infection in immunocompromised patients

serration (se-ra'shun) the state of being serrated or notched

serratus muscle any of the several muscles taking origin from ribs or vertebrae by separate slips

Sertoli cells supporting cells of testicular germinal layers, named after Enrice Sertoli, Italian physician

Sertoli tumour a benign testicular tumour secreting oestrogens

sertraline (ser'tra-len) a selective inhibitor of the reuptake of serotonin

serum (ser'um) pl. **sera** the fluid component of blood from which the coagulation factors have been removed **s hepatitis** type B viral hepatitis **s protein** any protein in the blood serum **s sickness** an immune response noted after reexposure to an antigen to which a person has been previously sensitised. The presence of soluble circulating immune complexes cause urticaria, fever, adenopathy and occasionally arthritis

serumal (se-roo'mal) pertaining to or formed from serum

serumfast (ser'um-fast) resistant to the effects of serum

server a computer that controls users' access to a network

sesamoid (ses'a-moid) sesame seed-like, bony nodule within the tendons

sesamoiditis (ses'a-moi-di'tis) inflammation of a sesamoid bone

sessile (ses'il) attached to a structure by a broad base

set 1. to fix firmly in place, as of reduction of fracture 2. to allow plaster to harden

setaceous (se-ta'shus) bristle-like

setaria (se-tar'e-a) a genus of filarial nematodes

setpoint (set'point) the target value of a controlled variable maintained by the control mechanisms of the body

setting sun sign inferior ocular deviation seen in severe infantile hydrocephalus

severe combined immunodeficiency SCID. A disease affecting the immune system and it is fatal if the affected person does not receive bone marrow transplantation

sewage the mixture of human excreta, urine and wash water, carried through underground sewers to the sewage treatment plant for final disposal

sex (seks) 1. the character that distinguishes between male and female based on sex chromosomes, the gonads and accessory genital organs 2. behaviour related to reproduction and/or sexual pleasure **s chromosomes** The 23rd pair of chromosomes, designated X and Y, which determine the genetic sex of an individual **s flush** reddish skin response that results from increasing sexual arousal **s ratio** the ratio of females to males, expressed as X women for every 1000 men

sexduction (-dwk'shun) the process of transfer of bacterial genes from one cell to another by sex factors

sex-conditioned (-kon-dish'und) sex-influenced

sex-influenced (-in'floo-ens'd) an autosomal trait that is expressed differently in either sex

sex-limited (-lim'i-ted) occurring in one sex only

sex-linked (seks'linkd) transmitted by a gene located on the X-chromosome, hence carried by the mother and expressed by the son

sexology (sek-sol'a-je) the scientific study of sex and sexuality

sextuplet (seks-tup'let) one of the six offsprings produced at one birth

sexual (sek'shoo-al) pertaining to sex **s abuse** sexual assault, rape or sexual molestation **s dysfunction** failure to enjoy sexual activity **s fantasies** fantasies with sexual themes **s harassment** unwanted attention of a sexual nature that creates embarrassment. **s intercourse** the insertion of erect penis of a male into the vagina of a female; coitus **s orientation** the sex to which one is attracted. **s precocity** development of secondary sexual characters before the age of 8 in boys and 6 in girls **s reassignment** the surgical conversion of an individual's secondary sexual characteristics to those of the opposite sex **s victimisation** sexual abuse of children, family members or subordinates by a person in a position of power

sexuality (sek'shoo-al'i-te) the human sexual response and the ability to produce and respond to gonadotropin-releasing hormone

sexually transmitted disease (STD) infections, and certain tumours that are transmitted by direct genital and orogenital contact

Sezary cell a T-lymphocyte containing large number of vacuoles filled with mucopolysaccharide, named after A. Sezary, French dermatologist

Sezary tumour T-cell lymphocytic tumour of the skin

sGaw specific airway conductance

SGOT serum glutamic oxaloacetic transaminase, named as aspartate transaminase

SGPT serum glutamic pyruvic transaminase, named as serum alanine transaminase

shaft an elongated rod-like structure as in long bone between the epiphyseal ends

shagreen patch indurated flesh-coloured clusters of papules on the back and lumbosacral region in tuberous sclerosis. It is likened to untanned leather prepared from the skin of horses

Shahade-Shah technique method to catheterise ruptured urethra by guiding metal bougie by little finger introduced suprapubically, devised by Indian surgeons

Sharma-Jhaver's technique minimum dissection in hydrocoele operation where testis is drawn out and placed in between fascia of scrotum devised by Indian surgeons

shakti (s) power; energy

shamana (s) palliation therapy

shank (shangk) a leg; leg-like part

shape (shap) 1. contour; outward form 2. to mould to a particular form

shaping (shap'ing) a technique of behaviour therapy to produce new behaviour

shavasana (s) corpse-pose in *hatha* yoga, posture taken by lying on the back on a hard surface with the feet apart and relaxed; the arms should lie easily at a natural distance from the body with palms up; the eyes are closed

shear (sher) a force applied parallel to the planes of an object, but opposite in direction

sheath (sheth) a tubular covering, shell or protective layer

shedding 1. casting off, such as surface layer of epidermis 2. loss of deciduous teeth

Sheehan's syndrome hypopituitarism due to an infarct of the pituitary following postpartum haemorrhage, manifesting in partial or total loss of thyroid, adrenocortical and gonadal functions, named after Harold Sheehan, British pathologist.

sheep cell agglutination test Rose-Waaler test

sheet (shet) 1. a linen or cotton bed covering 2. any structure resembling such a covering **draw s** a sheet folded under a patient's body that it may be withdrawn with minimal disturbance to the patient

Shefield splint splint for finger and metacarpal fractures

shelf life length of time that a therapeutic agent or blood product may be stored under appropriate conditions before it must be discarded

shelf operation bone graft to enlarge upper lip of acetabulum in congenital dislocation of hip

Shiastu (shi-a-stu') acupressure, a form of deep massage that focuses on special pressure points-meridians

shield (sheld) any protecting structure

shift a change or deviation **chloride s** the shift of chloride ions from the plasma into red blood cells on addition of CO_2 from the tissue and its reversal in the lungs on release of CO_2 **s to the left** a marked increase in the percentage of immature white cells in the circulating blood **s to the right** absence of young and immature white cells in the peripheral blood

shifting dullness free fluid in the peritoneal or pleural cavity shifts its position because of gravity when the patient turns his sides

Shiga bacillus *Shigella dysenteriae*, named after Kiyoshi Shiga, Japanese bacteriologist

Shiga dysentery infection with *S. dysenteriae*

Shigella (shi-gel'ah) genus of gram-negative non-motile bacilli, cause bacillary dysentery **S. boydii** agent causing dysentery; **S. dysenteriae** shiga bacillus responsible for most severe dysentery; **S. flexneri** Flexnor bacillus; **S. shiga, S. dysenteriae S. sonnei** agents causing mild dysentery.

Shigellosis (shi'gel-lo'sis) infection with shigella organisms; bacillary dysentery

shin the prominent anterior margin of the tibia or leg

shingles (shing'g'lz) herpes zoster; band-like involvement of neurocutaneous tissues

shin-splints pain in the region of tibia following strenuous exercise

Shirodkar operation purse-string suture to narrow internal os in habitual abortion. It is inserted early in pregnancy and removed near term, named after V.N. Shirodkar, Indian obstetrician

shita (s) cool;cold

shivering (shiv'er-ing) involuntary contraction of muscles that generate heat

shock (shok) 1. a profound haemodynamic disturbance characterised by failure of the circulatory system to maintain adequate perfusion of vital organs 2. a sudden disturbance of mental equilibrium **anaphylactic s** an immediate hypersensitivity reaction following exposure to a specific antigen by a sensitised individual **cardiogenic s** shock resulting from failure to maintain circulation or mechanical obstruction of the heart **electric s** shock resulting from passage of electric current through any part of the body **haemorrhagic s** condition due to insufficient amount of blood in the circulatory system **insulin s** condition resulting from overdose of insulin causing reduction of blood sugar below normal level **mental s** shock due to emotional stress **neurogenic s** shock due to decreased peripheral vascular resistance from damage to brain or the spinal cord **s lung** ARDS **septic s** shock associated with overwhelming infection **spinal s** flaccid paralysis and loss of all sensations and reflex activity below the level of injury to spinal cord **traumatic s** shock due to injury or surgery.

short bowel syndrome occurrence of multiple nutritional deficiencies following resection of large segments of small intestine

short sightedness myopia

Short's syndrome sick-sinus syndrome, named after British cardiologist

shotgun sequencing breaking of the genes into conveniently sized chunks

short stature stunted growth leading to dwarfism

shotty (shot'e) **lymphadenopathy** clusters of multiple small contiguous and indurated lymph nodes from viral infections, syphilis and carcinomatous metastases

shoulder (shol'der) the junction of clavicle and scapula where the arm joins the trunk **frozen s** adhesive capsulitis **s blade** scapula **s hand syndrome** swollen painful claw hand and shoulder pain, with limitation of movements **s pad sign** enlargement of glenohumeral joint due to periarticular accumulation of amyloid

show (sho) appearance of blood-stained cervical mucus fore running menstruation or labour

shredded appearance necrosis with irregular transverse bands of dense material separated by lighter areas in a skeletal muscle exposed to extreme heat or cold

'shrinking field' technique a method used in radiotherapy to treat large mediastinal lymph node malignancy in which treatment field and dose are reduced in size and amount respectively as the tumour responds

shrinking lungs raised diaphragm as in SLE, pleural adhesions, plate-like atelectasis and interstitial fibrosis resulting in small lungs

shukra (s) semen

shukraraha sratas (s) reproductive system

shunt diversion of blood from existing or normal channel to another. **arteriovenous s** the passage of blood directly from arteries to veins without passing through the capillary network **left-to- right s** acyanotic shunt wherein the right and left sides of heart communicate by an atrial or ventricular septal defect and patent ductus arteriosus. It leads to pulmonary congestion and later pulmonary hypertension **mesocaval s** anastomosis of the side of superior mesentric vein to the inferior vena cava to control portal hypertension **portacaval s** surgical anastomosis between the portal vein and inferior vena cava **right-to-left s** cyanotic shunt with a variable degree of pulmonary circulation bypass the lungs accompanied by obstruction to blood flow into the pulmonary circulation as in Fallot's tetrology, transposition of great vessels, tricuspid atresia, and truncus arteriosus, and in intrapulmonary shunting of blood as in ARDS **splenorenal s** end-to-end anastomosis of the splenic vein to left renal vein for control of portal hypertension

Shy-Dagger syndrome neuronal loss in central regions of autonomic nervous system, intermediolateral columns of thoracic spinal cord, peripheral autonomic ganglia and degeneration in caudate nucleus, substantia nigra and cerebellum, characterised by Parkinsonian symptoms, postural hypotension with syncope, dizziness, urinary incontinence, impotence and anhidrosis, named after George Shy, American neurologist and G. Dragger, American physician

SI 1. sacroiliac 2. systeme international d'unites which is a revised metric system for standardisation of units of measurement

SIADH syndrome of inappropriate antidiuretic hormone secretion. It is characterised by excess secretion of vasopressin, low plasma osmolarity, water retention and dilutional hyponatraemia noted as an ectopic hormone production in carcinoma, ACTH, deficiency, untreated Addison's disease, pneumonia, tuberculosis, use of PEEP and chromophobe adenoma

sialadenitis (si-al-ad'en-it'is) inflammation of a salivary gland

sialadenoma (-ad'e-no'ma) a benign tumour of the salivary gland

sialadenopathy (-ad'e-nop'a-the) enlargement of salivary glands

sialadenosis (-ad'en-o'sis) sialadenitis

sialagogue (si-al'a-gog) an agent which stimulates the salivary secretion **sialogogic** adj

sialectasia (si'al-ek-ta'zhah) dilatation of a salivary duct

sialic (si-al'ik) salivary

sialic (si-al'ik) **acid** ester of N-acetyl neuraminic acid, a component of various mucoproteins

sialine (si'a-lin) pertaining to the saliva

sialismus (si-al-iz'mus) excessive secretion of saliva

sialitis (si'a-li'tis) inflammation of a salivary gland or a salivary duct

sial (o) combining word for saliva; salivary glands

sialoadenectomy (si'a-lo-ad'en-ek'ta-me) excision of a salivary gland

sialoadenotomy (-ad'en-ot'a-me) incision and drainage of a salivary gland

sialoaerophagia (-ar'o-fa'jah) the swallowing of saliva and air

sialoangiectasis (-an'je-ek'ta-sis) dilatation of a salivary duct

sialoangiitis (-an'je-i'tis) inflammation of a salivary duct

sialoangiography (-an'je-og'ra-fe) radiography of the salivary ducts following injection of radiopaque material

sialocoele (si'a-lo-sel) a salivary cyst

sialodochitis (si'a-lo-do-ki'tis) inflammation of a salivary duct

sialodochoplasty (-do'ko-plas'te) surgical repair of a salivary duct

sialogram contrast radiograph of the salivary ducts

sialoductitis (-duk-ti'tis) sialodochitis

sialogenous (si'a-loj'e-nus) producing saliva

sialogram (si'a-log'ram) contrast radiograph of salivary ducts

sialography (si'a-log'ra-fe) sialoangiography

sialolith (si-al'o-lith) a calculus in the salivary ducts or glands sialolithiasis (si-al'o-li-thi'a-sis) the formation of salivary calculi

sialolithotomy (-li-thot'a-me) removal of a salivary calculus

sialometaplasia (-met'a-pla'zhah) metaplasia of the salivary glands

sialomucin (-mu'sin) a mucopolysaccharide containing sialic acid

sialorrhoea (-re'a) increased flow of saliva

sialoschesis (si'a-los'ke-sis) suppression of salivary secretion

sialosis (si'a-lo'sis) enlargement of salivary glands

sialosyrinx (-ser'inks) a salivary fistula

Siamese twins conjoined gestational products due to a failure in division of the yolk sac or due to a delay in monovular separation, mostly they are joined in the chest. Chang and Eng Bunker were most famous twins born in Siam (now Thailand)

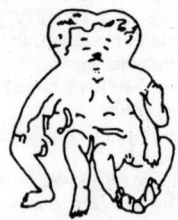

Siamese twins

sib person related especially by blood

sibilant (sib'i-lant) whistling; hissing s rhonchi high-pitched rhonchi as whistling or squeaking sounds and arise from obstruction of smaller bronchi

sibling (sib'i-ling) offspring of same two parents

sibship (-ship) brothers and sisters of a single family

sicca syndrome Sjogren's syndrome presenting with dry mouth and dry conjunctiva

siccus (sik'us) dry

sick building syndrome a group of symptoms noted in persons working in large, energy-efficient buildings. There is increased frequency of headaches, lethargy, dry skin , and allergic alveolitis

sick 1. unwell; ill; suffering from disease 2. nauseated

sick cell syndrome failure of sodium pump in chronic debilitating disease characterised by a rise in sodium and fall in potassium content of cells.

sicklaemia (sik-le'mi-a) presence of sickle-shaped erythrocytes in the peripheral blood, seen in sickle cell anaemia and sickle cell trait

sickle cell the distorted sickle-shaped red blood cells, that result when the haemoglobin (has an altered aminoacid structure of polypeptide) is deoxygenated, molecules of haemoglobin polymerise to form pseudocrystalline structures (tactoids) which distort red cell membrane and the process gets reversed when reoxygenated. The distortion of red cell membrane may become permanent to make the red cells to assume sickle shape constantly. Such cells increase blood viscosity, traverse capillaries poorly and obstruct the blood flow s anaemia a homozygous haemoglobin - S disease and most red cells contain haemoglobin S. The cells are prone to sickle in the region of microhyvasculature where the flow is sluggish and obstruct blood flow leading to thrombosis and infarction. There is severe pain, swelling and tenderness, and haemolysis s disease a congenital haemoglobinopathy caused by a point mutation on the gene that encodes haemoglobin resulting in a defective functioning of haemoglobin causing the red blood cells to ' sickle' when deoxygenated, that includes sickle cell anaemia s trait a heterozygous condition where the red blood cell has both normal haemoglobin A and abnormal haemoglobin S and the genotype is depicted as AS unlike a normal adult represented by genotype AA. The patient is relatively resistant to lethal effects of falciparum malaria in early childhood

sickness (sik'nes) a state of ill health

sick sinus syndrome sinoatrial disease characterised by a variety of arrhythmias and may present with palpitation, dizzy spells or syncope

sickle-form malarial crescent

sickling (sik'ling) production of sickle-shaped erythrocytes in the peripheral blood

sickness disease; ill-health

siddha professional medicine outside Vedic tradition with a strong tantric orientation, practised in Tamil Nadu, India, whose origin is obscure

side effect (side-fekt) an action or effect of a drug other than desired

siderate sudden; fulminating

siden (o) combining word for iron; stars

sideroblast (sid'er-o-blast) red cell precursor with haemosiderin granules in the cytoplasm

sideroblastic anaemia a refractory anaemia with hypochromic microcytic anaemia and ring sideroblasts due to inadequate utilisation of iron

siderocyte (-sit) red blood cell with iron containing granules

sideroderma (sid'er-o-der'ma) bronzed skin

siderofibrosis (-fi-bro'sis) fibrosis associated with iron deposits

sideromycin (-mi'sin) an antibiotic that inhibits the bacterial growth interfering with iron uptake

sideropaenia (-pe'ne-a) iron deficiency in the body or blood **sideropaenic** adj

siderophil (sid'er-o-fil) 1. a cell that contains iron 2. absorbing iron

siderophilous (sid'er-of'i-lus) siderophil

siderophore (sid'er-o-for) a mononuclear phagocyte containing haemosiderin

siderosis (sid'er-o'sis) 1. iron overload 2. pneumoconiosis from inhalation of dust or fumes containing iron particles

sidestream smoke the smoke that comes from the burning end of a cigarette, cigar or pipe

SIDS sudden infant death syndrome; due to deficiency of thiamine; cot death

Siegel's speculum a magnifying glass and a rubber bulb to apply air pressure to ear drum.

Siemens (se'menz) (s) a unit referring to the conductance of one ampere per volt in a body with an ohm resistance

Sievert (SV) a measure of absorbed dose of radiation energy

sight (sit) vision **far s** hyperopia **near s** myopia **night s** hemaralopia

SIg surface immunoglobulin of B lymphocytes

SIgA secretory immunoglobulin A found in lacrimal and salivary secretions

sigmatism (sig'ma-tizm) excessive or defective use of 'S' sounds in speech

sigmoid (sig'moid) 1. shaped like the letter C or S 2. the sigmoid colon **s colon** the S-shaped portion of large intestine that begins at the level of the left iliac crest, projects inward to the midline, and terminates at the rectum.

sigmoidectomy (sig'moi-dek'ta-me) surgical removal of a part or whole of the sigmoid colon

sigmoiditis (sig'moi-di'tis) inflammation of sigmoid colon

sigmoidopexy (sig-moid'o-pek'se) surgical fixation of sigmoid colon

sigmoidoproctostomy (sig-moid'o-proktos'ta-me) surgical anastomosis of the sigmoid colon to the rectum

sigmoidoscope rigid tubular speculum introduced through anus to visualise sigmoid colon

sigmoidoscopy (sig'moi-dos'ka-pe) examination of the interior of sigmoid colon by a sigmoidoscope

sigmoidostomy (sig'moi-dos'ta-me) creation of an artificial anus by opening into sigmoid colon

sigmoidotomy (sig'moi-dot'a-me) incision of sigmoid colon

sign (sin) finding elicited by making a general and systemic examination and it represents the objective evidence of disease 2. a conventional or arbitrary mark, figure or symbol used technically as an arbitrary or conventional symbol

signa (sig'na) a term used in prescriptions meaning to label to the subscription according to the dose, frequency and route of administration

signal averaging *ECG* the averaging of the root mean square voltages of 100 or more consecutive similar beats so that background activity is masked and repetitive activity amplified useful in recognition of ventricular late potentials.

Table 10: signs and symbols

+	death
O→	male
O₊	female
+	excess of acid reaction, positive reaction
−	deficiency of alkaline reaction, negative reaction
a c	before meals, ante cibum
Ag	silver, argentums
Al	aluminium
aq	water, aqua
aq dist	distilled water
As	arsenic
Au	gold, aurum
Ba	barium
Bi	bismuth
b I d	twice a day, bis in die
Br	bromine
C	carbon
c	with, cum
Ca	calcium
Cap	capsule
Cd	cadmium
cib	food or meals, cibum
Cl	chlorine
Cm	curium
Co	cobalt
c/o	complains of
coch	spoonful, cochleare
Cr	cromium
Cu	copper, caprum
d	day
D & C	dilatation and curettage

D/s	dextrose in saline
D/w	dextrose in water
Dx	diagnosis
et al	and others, et alit; elsewhere et alibi
ex aq	with water
F	fluorine
Fe	iron, ferrum
Ga	gallium,
gt	drops, guttae
H	hydrogen
He	helium
Hg	mercury, hydrargyrum
h s	at bed time, just before going to sleep, hora somni
Hx	history
I	iodine
K	potassium, kalium
Kr	krypton
Li	lithium
Mg	magnesium
mst	mixture, mistura
Mn	manganese
N	nitrogen
Na	sodium, natrium
Nd	neodymium
Ni	nickel
NR	do not repeat, non repetatur
O	oxygen
O D	right eye, ocular dexter
O d	once daily,
O h	every hour. amni hora
O n	every night , omni nocte
O S	left eye, oculus sinister
O u	in each eye, oculo ultra
P	phosphorus
Pb	lead, plumbum
pc	after food, post cibum
P o	by mouth, per os
PR	through the rectum, per rectum
P r n	as occasion arises, given when necessary, pro re nata
Pulv	powder, pulvis

PV	through the vagina, per vagina
Px	past history
Q2h	every second hour, quaque secunda hora
Q3h	every third hour, quaque tertia hora
Q4h	every fourth hour, quaque quarta hora
Q d	every day, quaque die
Q h	every hour, quaque hora
Q i d	four times a day , quarter in die
Q n	every night, quaque note
Q s	as much as will suffice, quantum sufficit
Rx	take though, sign of Jupiter, used to propitate the god in writing a prescription
Rh-	Rhesus(factor) negative
Rh+	Rhesus(factor) positive
R/O	rule out
S	signa, signetur label indicating directions to be written on a package or label for the use of the patient
S & s	signs and symptoms
S1	first heart sound
S2	second heart sound
S3	third heart sound
S4	fourth heart sound
Si op sit	if it is necessary, si opus sit
sol	solution, solutio
S O S	if needed, si opus sit
S s	one half, semis
SD	Standard deviation stat SD, an interval consisting of the 95 percent of observed values
Stat	immediately, statim
Syr	syrup, syrupus
t i d	three times a day, ter in die
Tin	tincture, tincutra
Ung	ointment, unguentum
Ut	dict, as directed, ut dictum
W/v	weight in volume
W/w	weight in weight
X	sex chromosome, female will have two X chromosomes
XX	chromosome pair resulting in offspring with female characteristics
XY	chromosome pair resulting in offspring with male characteristics
Y	sex chromosome, male will have one X and one Y chromosome

signature (-chur) 1. the part of prescription giving instructions to the patient 2. writing one's name to certify the validity of the document

signet ring cells malignant cells distended with mucus and the nucleus pressed to one side, seen in scirrhous carcinoma of stomach

significant 1. important 2. *stat* a difference is considered statistically significant if the results have little probability of having occurred owing to chance

silapada (s) elephantiasis

silent gap auscultatory gap evident in some patients with high blood pressure. During deflation of the cuff, the sounds may disappear suddenly and make their reappearance later at a much lower level of blood pressure. The error is overcome by noting the blood pressure by the palpatory method before auscultation is carried out

silastic (si-las'tik) silicone rubber of high stability

sildenafil (sil-den'a-fil) a selective phosphodiesterase-5 inhibitor that releases nitric oxide so as to improve erectile dysfunction.

silent infarction occurrence of myocardial infarction without pain, common among patients with diabetes and hypertension

silica (sil'i-ka) (SiO$_2$) silicon dioxide, SiO$_2$. It is formed in the earth's crust under increased heat and pressure. It exists in nature in three crystalline forms: quartz, tridymite, and cristobalite

silicoanthracosis (sil'i-ko-an'thra-ko'sis) silicosis combined with anthracosis, in coal miners

silicon (sil'i-kon) a non-metallic element, at. weight 28, abundant as silica and silicates

silicone (sil'i-kon) a plastic compound of silicon oxides

silicosiderosis (sil'i-ko-sid'er-o'sis) silicosis due to inhalation of iron and silica dust

silicosis (sil'i-ko'sis) a chronic fibrosis of the lungs caused by prolonged exposure to free silica. Radiologically it shows finely nodular, rounded opacities predominantly in the upper lung zones. The condition may progress to massive fibrosis **accelerated s** upper zone fibrosis progressing at an intermediate rate **acute s** silicoproteinosis developing in individuals in overwhelming exposure of pure silica particles **chronic s** progressive, nodular interstitial fibrosis from inhalation of low concentrations of silica **conglomerate s** presence of both small nodules of simple silicosis and confluent nodules

silicotuberculosis (sil'i-ko-tu'ber-ku-lo'-sis) silicosis associated with pulmonary tuberculosis

siliquose (sil'i-kwos) a form of cataract resulting in shrivelling of lens

silo (sail-au) store, pit or structure holding animal fodder or grain

silo-filler's disease damage to the lungs produced in silo workers, when exposed to nitrogen dioxide

silvastic infections spreading among wild animals

silver (sil'ver) a non-toxic metal, at. no. 47, symbol Au (argyr) **s impregnation** silver complexes applied to demonstrate reticulin **s nitrate** an antiseptic and astringent

simethicone (si-meth'i-kon) a mixture of dimethyl polysiloxanes and silica gel, an antiflatulent preparation

simian related to or affecting monkeys **crease** single crease, seen in mongolism

similia similibus curantur The homoeopathic principles expressing the doctrine that any drug which is capable of producing symptoms in a healthy person will remove similar symptoms occurring as a manifestation of disease; likes are cured by likes

simplex virus (sim'pleks-vi'rus) herpes simplex virus

Sims position a semiprone position with the patient on the left side, right knee and thigh drawn up, left along the patient's back and chest inclined forward position used while administering enema, rectal examination, and curettement of uterus, named after James Sims, US gynaecologist

Simmonds' disease a condition of atrophy of pituitary causing loss of function of thyroid, adrenals and gonads, cachexia and premature senility, named after Morris Simmonds, German physician

simul (sim'ul) at the same time or at once

simulation (sim'u-la'shun) imitation, refers to a disease or symptom that resembles another

simulator (sim'u-la-tor) any situation or device that creates a situation or condition similar to one that might be encountered

simvastatin (sim'va-stat'in) a lipid lowering agent, that inhibits HMG-CoA (3-hydroxy-3-methyl glutaryl Coenzyme A) reductase, the rate limiting enzyme of cholesterol synthesis, effective in hypercholestrolaemia

sinciput (sin'si-put) 1. forehead 2. bregma

sine qua non (sine-kwa'nun) L something indispensable, necessary condition

sinew (sin'u) a tendon of a muscle **weeping s** an encysted ganglion containing synovial fluid

sine wave ECG disappearance of P wave and merging of the ORS complex and T wave in an oscillating pattern, in severe hyperkalaemia

singer's nodes small nodules, such as keratosis papilloma or fibrous polyp on vocal cords, related to overuse of voice

singlehood the state of not being married

single nucleotide polymorphism Snip brings variation in individuals and it occurs about once every 1000 base pairs in the genome

singultus (sing-gul'tus) hiccup

sinister (sin'is-ter) left; on the left side

sinistrad (sin'is-trad) toward the left

sinistral (-tral) 1. pertaining to the left side 2. a left handed person

sinistrality (sin'is-tral'i-te) the preferential use, in voluntary motor activities, of the organ on the left side

sinistraural (sin'is-traw'ral) hearing better with the left ear

sinister (o) combining word for left; left side

sinisterocerebral (sin'is-tro-ser'e-bral) pertaining to or situated in left cerebral hemisphere

sinistrogyration (sin'is-tro-ji-ra'shun) a turning around to the left

sinistromanual (-man'u-al) left-handed

sinistropedal (sin'is-trop'e-dal) using left foot in preference to the right

sinistrotorsion (sin'is-tro-tor'shun) a twisting toward the left

sinogram contrast x-ray of sinus, especially cavernous sinus

sinography visualisation of sinus by x-ray after injection of contrast

sinoatrial (si'no-a'tre-al) pertaining to sinus venosus and right atrium of the heart **s2 node** modified muscle cells with spontaneous rhythm acting as cardiac pacemaker, located in the right atrium beneath the opening of superior vena cava

sinopulmonary (-pul'ma-nar-e) involving the paranasal sinuses and the lungs

sinuous (sin'u-us) winding

sinus (si'nus) 1. a hollow in a bone, as paranasal sinus 2. a channel for blood as vascular sinus 3. any cavity having a narrow opening **accessory nasal s** one of the paranasal sinuses: frontal, maxillary, ethmoidal and sphnoidal **anal s** the grooves between the anal columns **aortic s** the space between each semilunar valve and the wall of the aorta **carotid s** dilatation of the common carotid artery at its bifurcation, that contains baroreceptters **cav-**

ernous s a paired dural sinus on either side of sella turcica and communicating across the midline, containing internal carotid artery and abducent nerve **coronary s** a short venous trunk receiving the veins of the heart, that runs in the posterior part of coronary sulcus and empties into the right atrium **dural s's** endothelium lined venous channels in the dura mater **ethmoidal s's** paranasal sinuses in the ethmoidal bone **frontal s** one of the paired paranasal sinuses in the frontal bone each communicating with the middle meatus of the ipsilateral nasal cavity **intercavernous s's** the anterior and posterior anastomoses between the cavernous sinuses **lactiferous s** a circumscribed spindle-shaped dilatation of the lactiferous duct prior to its entry into the nipple **lymphatic s** irregular tortuous spaces within the lymph nodes through which lymph passes **mastoid s's** numerous small intercommunicating cavities in the mastoid process of temporal bone **maxillary s** the air cavity in the body of its maxilla communicating with the middle meatus of the nose **occipital s** a venous sinus in the attached margin of falx cerebelli extending to the foramen magnum **paranasal s's** accessory nasal sinuses **pilonidal s** a pit in the sacral region **pleural s** pleural cavity **prostatic s** groove on either side of the urethral crest in the prostatic part of the urethra **rectus s** a venous sinus at the junction of the falx cerebri and the cerebellar tentorium **renal s** the cavity of the kidney containing calyces and pelvis **sagittal s** an unpaired dural sinus in the lower margin of the falx cerebri (inferior) and in the sagittal groove (superior) **sigmoid s** S-shaped dural sinus lying on the mastoid process of the occipital bone **s of valsalva** aortic sinus **s of venaecavae** the portion of the cavity of right atrium of the heart receiving the blood from venae

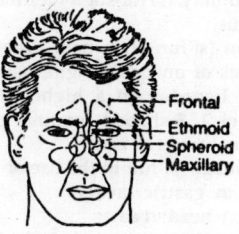

Paranasal sinuses

cavae **sphenoidal s** one of a pair of cavities in the sphenoid bone communicating with the nasal cavity **sphenoparietal s** either of two sinuses of dura mater draining into the cavernous sinus **splenic s** a dilated venous sinus in the substance of spleen **straight s** rectus sinus **s venosus** a cavity at the caudal end of embryonic cardiac tube **tarsal s** a canal formed by the groove of the talus and the groove of calcaneum **transverse s** 1. a sinus that unites the two inferior petrosal sinuses of the cranium 2. venous network in the dura over the basilar process of occipital bone 3. passage in the pericardium between the origins of great vessels and atria **tympanic s** a deep recess in the posterior part of the tympanic cavity **urogenital s** the ventral part of the cloaca that gives rise to lower part of the bladder in both sexes, the prostatic portion of male urethra, and to urethra and vestibule in the female **uterine s** a small vascular channel in the endometrium **venous s** a sinus carrying venous blood.

sinusitis (si'nu-si'tis) inflammation of the mucous membrane of a paranasal sinus

sinusoid (si'nu-soid) a microscopic space or passage for blood in organs like liver or spleen

sinusoidal (si'nu-soi'dal) relating to a sinusoid

sinusotomy (si'nu-sot'a-me) incision of a sinus

siphon (si'fun) 1. a bent tube with two arms of unequal length, used to transfer liquid from a higher to a lower level 2. $-shaped terminal part of internal carotid artery

siphonage (si-fun-ij) the use of the siphon as in gastric lavage

sira (s) head; vein

sirenomelus (si'ren-om'e-lus) a foetus with fused legs without feet; mermaid legs

-sis a combining word for state; condition

sisira (s) late winter

sister (sis'ter) 1. the nurse incharge of a hospital ward 2. any registered nurse **s chromatid(s)** a pair of metaphase chromosomes or nucleoproteins that are joined at the centre **s chromatid exchange** crossing-over between chromatids of same pair **s Mary Joseph nodule** a nonulcerating periumbilical nodule that is a metastatic mass originating from an adenocarcinoma of the stomach, colon, ovary or pancreas. Sister Mary Joseph was nursing superintendent, US

sita (s) cold; cool

sitala (s) chickenpox

site (sit) place; seat; location **s of election** most favourable position, usually for incision

sit (o) combining word for food

sitology (si-tol'a-je) dietetics

sitomania (sito-ma'ne-a) excessive hunger

sitophobia fear of eating due to unpleasant symptoms, a feature of chemotherapy induced anorexia

sitosterolaemia (si-tos'ter-ol-e'me-a) presence of excess amount of plant sterols especially sitosterol, in the blood

sitotherapy (si'to-ther'a-pe) dietery treatment

sitotropism (si-tot'ro-pizm) response of living cells to the presence of nutritive substances

Sjogren's syndrome an autoimmune disorder characterised by lymphocytic infiltration of salivary and lacrimal glands leading to xerostomia and keratoconjunctivitis sicca, named after Henrick Sjogren, Swedish ophthalmologist

situs (si'tus) site or position **s inversus** mirror-image transposition of viscera of the thorax and abdomen **s perversus** dislocation of any viscera

skatole (skat'ol) methylindole produced by decomposition of proteins, especially tryptophan, in the intestine.

skelalgia (skel-al'jah) pain in the leg

Skene's glands minute mucous glands in the female urethra, named after Alexander Skene, US gynaecologist; paraurethral glands

skeletisation (skel'e-ti-za'sun) 1. extreme emaciation 2. removal of soft parts from the skeleton

skeletogenous (skel'e-toj'e-nus) producing skeletal structures

skeleton (skel'e-ton) 1. the bony framework of the body in vertebrates (endoskeleton) or hard outer envelope of insects (exoskeleton) 2. all dry parts of the body after removal of soft parts 3. all bones of the body taken together **appendicular s** the bones of the limbs including the pectoral and pelvic girdles **axial s** the bones of the head and trunk excluding the pectoral and pelvic girdles

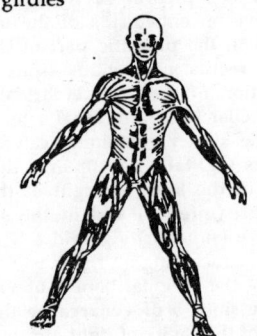

Skeleton

skenitis (sken-i'tis) inflammation of Skene's glands

skew (skyu) deviating from a straight line

skiagram (ski'a-gram) a roentgenogram

skiagraphy (ski'og'ra-fe) roentgenography

skiascopy (ski-as'ko-pe) 1. retinoscopy 2. examination of the body by x-ray

skimming (skim'ing) the removing of floating matter from a liquid

skin the largest organ in the body consisting of epidermis and dermis. The epidermis is continuously renewing, stratified squamous epithelium that keratinises. Innermost layer of epidermis is stratum germinativum in which keratinocytes are formed. Above it stratum spinosum is present in which progressive stages of keratinisation occurs. Stratum granulosum overlies this layer where the cells become flat and contain keratohyalin granules. Stratum lucidum and stratum corneum are the most superficial layers

skingraft skin used to cover the skin surfaces with third degree burns

skinfold measurement of thickness of pinched-up fold of skin of the upper arm or abdomen as an index of nutrition

skinny needle a 22-gauge needle used for percutaneous biopsies

skin traction extension of fracture by pulling on the adhesive plaster applied to the skin

skip lesion smaller lesions separated by normal mucosa from the main lesion as in Crohn's disease

skip metastases the metastatic spread in which contiguous regions are skipped although distant foci are present.

Skodiac resonance a hyperresonant note of a boxy quality above the level of pleural effusion and consolidation; it arises from the relaxed lung still containing air or from the lung showing compensatory emphysema, described by Josef Skoda, Austrian physician

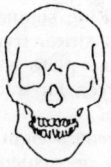

Skull-front view

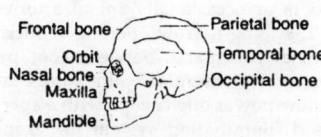

Skull-lateral view

skull (skul) the cranium; the bony framework of the head composed of cranial and facial bones

slant culture a bacterial culture grown on agar-based growth medium poured in a test tube and allowed to solidity at a slanting angle

sleshma (s) phlegm, expectoration

SLE systemic lupus erythematosus

sleep (slep) to take rest by relaxation of consciousness; to slumber. It is a non-homogeneous phenomenon having two distinct forms: rapid eye movement (REM) sleep and non-rapid eye movement (NREM) sleep, REM sleep shows bursts of rapid eye movements. The skeletal muscle tone is decreased. NREM sleep exhibits four stages demonstrating a progression in a cyclic fashion throughout the night in a normal adult and are governed by the 100 minute ultradian rhythm **s apnoea** absence of airflow at the nose and mouth for at least 10 seconds during sleep. The apnoeic episodes are repetitive and result in sleep arousal and they occur at a rate greater than 20 episodes per hour of sleep **s paralysis** shortlived paralysis immediately on waking **s walking** somnambulism

sleeping sickness African trypanosomiasis

slide (slīd) a glass plate on which substance are placed for microscopic examination

slim disease extreme weight loss in AIDS

sling a bandage or suspensor for supporting structures of the body.

slipped disc herniation of nucleus pulposus of the intervertebral disc through its capsule, and press on ligaments, nerve roots or occasionally spinal arteries

slit 1. A long narrow opening or incision 2. narrow spaces between foot processes of glomerular epithelium **s lamp** a low power microscope with a specialised illuminating system for examining the anterior segment of the eye

slough (sluf) necrotic tissue that is getting cast off from viable part of the body

sludge (sluj) a suspension of solid or semisolid particles in a fluid.

sludging (sluj'ing) setting out of solid particles from solution

slur smear or stain

small airway peripheral conducting airways, that are non-alveolated of less than 2 mm internal diameter and the respiratory bronchioles **s disease** disease affecting the silent zone of the lungs

small cell carcinoma tumour of the lung arising from the bronchial epithelium that grows rapidly and metastatise to hilar lymph nodes and mediastinum. The cells are loosely arranged and contain oval, round or fusiform nuclei with finely stippled chromatin. The cytoplasm is scanty. They contain neurosecretory granules and often produce the endocrine paraneoplastic manifestations; SSC

small cuff hypertension recording of raised blood pressure by use of very small sphygmomanometer cuff

small intestine a long tube of the alimentary tract that begins at the pyloric sphincter of the stomach, coils through the central and lower part of the abdominal cavity and ends at large intestine. It consists of three segments: duodenum, jejunum and ileum

smallpox (small'poks) **variola** a disease eradicated from the globe. An acute eruptive contagious disease caused by pox virus marked by fever, chills, headache followed by papules which become umbilicated vesicles and later pustules. They get dried and form scab and fall leaving a permanent mark on the skin

small stomach syndrome an inability to tolerate any but small meals after gastric surgery; small capacity syndrome

slow viruses a group of viruses responsible for fatal infectious encephalitis after prolonged latency periods. *see* Prions

slow vital capacity (SVC) test used when FVC is reduced and obstruction is suspected with slow exhalation, as there is less airway narrowing a patient can exhale a larger volume in airflow obstruction

smear (smer) a specimen for microscopic examination prepared by spreading the material across the glass slide

smudge cell degenerated lymphocytes and nucleated erythrocytes appearing as red-purple nuclear debris with clumped chromatin and rounded nucleolar remnants

smegma (smeg'ma) sebum and keratinous debris collected under foreskin

Smith Petersen nail three-finned nail for femoral neck fracture, named after Smith Petersen, American orthopaedic surgeon.

smooth muscle an organ specialised for contraction, composed of smooth muscle fibres, located in the walls of hollow internal structures **s antibodies** IgM or IgG autoantibodies found in chronic active hepatitis and biliary cirrhosis

Sn chemical symbol, tin; stannum

snake (snak) a class of reptiles, in shape limbless and much elongated, includes cobras, kraits, Russell's viper, saw-scaled vipers, and sea snakes. Bite from a poisonous snake results in neurotoxicity with paralysis (cobra), coagulopathy and bleeding (vipers), and paralysis, myoglobinuria and renal failure (sea snake)

smog atmospheric pollution from smoke and fog

snap a short, sharp sound **opening** s a high pitched, short snapping sound heard as an extra sound in the early part of the diastole, in mitral stenosis and rarely in tricuspid stenosis

snare (snar) a wire loop for removing polyps by encircling them at the base and closing the loop

snapping finger trigger finger

Sneddon's syndrome antiphospholipid antibodies associated with recurrent cerebral ischaemia, livedo reticularis and hypertension

snehana (s) OU massage; oleation therapy

Snellen's chart to test visual acuity by asking the patient to read letters on the chart at a distance of six metres. The construction of the letters is such that the test letter is visible to the normal eye at 60 metres and the seventh (penultimate) line can be read at a distance of six metres. The individual who can read all letters, has a visual acuity of 6/6 named after Herman Snellen, Dutch ophthalmologist

snayu (s) ligament

sneeze (s) an involuntary sudden, violent and audible expulsion of air through the mouth and nose

snore (snor) a harsh buzzing noise in a sleeping person from vibration of redundant soft palate

snow blindness ultraviolet keratitis and severe blepherospasm

soap (sop) any compound of one or more fatty acids with an alkali; used for cleansing purposes and as an excipient in making of pills and suppositories

SOB shortness of breath

socialisation (so'shal-i-zol'shun) adaptation of an individual toward getting along with others

social medicine branch of medicine concerned with identification and modification of features of social organisation that promote illness

sociology (so'se-ol'a-je) the science that treats man as a social being, in the origins organisation, and development of human society and human culture

sociometry (so'se-om'e-tre) the branch of sociology dealing with the measurement of human social behaviour

sociopathy (so'so-op'a-the) anti-social personality disorder

sociotherapy (so'se-o-ther'a-pe) a treatment advising modification of the environment and improvement in interpersonal relationships

socket (sok'it) a hollow or depression into which a corresponding part fits **tooth** s the cavities in upper and lower jaw in which teeth are embedded

soda sodium bicarbonate, sodium hydroxide and sodium carbonate

sodium alkaline metal, at. no. 11, symbol Na s **bicarbonate** $NaHCO_3$, baking soda used as a gastric and systemic antacid, to alkalise urine s **carbonate** washing soda, used in scaly skin diseases s **chloride** NaCl, common table salt, used in preparing isotonic and physiological salt solution s **cyclamate** salt of cyclamic acid, a non-caloric artificial sweetener s **flumide** a white crystalline powder used as a dental prophylactic of caries s **hydroxide** caustic soda NaOH, a caustic s **nitrate** antidote for cyanide poisoning s **nitroprusside** an antihypertensive and a powerful vasodilator s **pump** ATPase-based enzyme active transport system of cell membrane that actively moves sodium ions out of the cell and potassium ions into the cell at the expense of cellular ATP. It enables to keep the ionic concentrations at physiological levels **s salicylate** analgesic and antipyretic **s sulphate** a saline cathartic **s thiosulphate** antidote for cyanide poisoning

sodomy (so'a-me) anal intercourses, copulation of man and animal

sofa (s) oedema

soft cataract cortical cataract

soft chancre chancroid

soft palate the muscular posterior portion of the roof of the mouth, extending posteriorly from the palatine bones to the uvula

soft x-rays of long wave length and low penetration

softening (sof'en-ing) a process of becoming soft

SOL space occupying lesion

sɔl a liquid colloidal solution

solace (sol-as) consolation, comfort in grief or trouble

solar (so'ler) 1. pertaining to the sun 2. great sympathetic plexus and its ganglia with radiating nerves **s cataract** cortical cataract **s keratosis** actinic keratitis

solation (so-la'shun) the liquefaction of a gel

soiling the bedding and bedsheets becoming dirty and contaminated by urine, stools, vomitus or secretions

solitaire single cholesterol gallstone

sole (sol) the bottom of the foot

solubility (sol'u-bil'i-te) property of being soluble

soluble (sol'u-b'l) capable of being dissolved **fat s** soluble in fats and oils **water s** soluble in water

solum (so'lum) the bottom

solute (sol'ut) substances that are dissolved by a solvent

solution (sa-loo'shun) a homogeneous molecular or ionic dispersion of one or more solutes usually in a solvent

solvent (sol'vent) a liquid dissolving medium, such as water, alcohol or oils

soma (so'ma) 1. the body as distinguished from mind 2. the body tissue 3. the cell body

somasthenia (so'mas-the'ne-ah) long standing weakness and fatigability

somatalgia (so'ma-tal'jah) bodily pain

somatesthesia (so'mat-es-the'zhah) the consciousness of having a body

somatic (so-mat'ik) pertaining to body or body wall **s cell** any cell in an organism which is not a germ cell **s cell division** in which the parent cell duplicates itself to produce two daughter cells **s cell genetic disorder** defects in DNA in specific somatic cells (cancer) **s cell hybrid** a hybrid formed from fusion together of different cells from different species. Human and rodent hybrids are used for human gene mapping **s mutation** a mutation which occurs in any cell that will not become a germ cell **s nervous system** the portion of peripheral nervous system consisting of somatic efferent fibres that run between the CNS and the skeletal muscles and skin

somatisation (so'ma-tiza'shun) expression of mental disorder as apparent physical disease

somat (o) combining word for body; viscera

somatochrome (so-mat'o-krom) a nerve cell possessing a well-marked cell body surrounding the nucleus

somatoform (so-mat'o-for) mental disorder presenting as an organic disease **s autonomic dysfunction** a somatic form disorder in which symptoms are referred to organs which are largely under autonomic control such as psychogenic hyperventilation, psychogenic vomiting, irritable bowel syndrome or cardiac neurosis **s pain disorder** severe persistent pain which cannot be explained by a physical illness or physiological disturbance.

somatogenic (so-ma-to-jen'ik) originating in the body

somatognosis (so'ma-tog-no'sis) general feeling of the existence of one's body and of the functioning of the organs

somatology (so'ma-tol'a-je) the study of the anatomy and physiology of the body

somatomedin (so'ma-to-me'din) peptide acting as intermediary between growth hormone and tissues. It is produced by the liver in response to stimulation by human growth hormone

somatometry (so'ma-tom'e-tre) measurement of the body

somatopagus (so'-ma-top'a-gus) a double foetus with trunks fused

somatopathy (so'ma-top'a-the) a bodily disorder

somatoplasm (so-mat'o-plazm) the protoplasm of the body cells

somatopleure (-ploor) the embryonic body wall made of ectoderm and somatic mesoderm

somatopsychic (so'ma-to-si'kik) pertaining to both body and mind

somatoscopy (so'ma-tos'ka-pe) examination of the body

somatosensory (so'ma-to-sen'so-re) pertaining to the sensations received in the skin and deep tissues

somatosexual (-sek'shoo-al) pertaining to both physical and sex characteristics

somatostatin (-stat'in) a hormone that inhibits the release of somatotropin, and secretion of insulin and gastrin. It is produced by the hypothalamus and delta cells of pancreas

somatostinoma non-functioning delta cell tumour, found in the duodenal wall, may present with diabetes, cholelithiasis and steatorrhoea

somatotherapy (-ther'a-pe) biological treatment of bodily disorders

somatotopic (-top'ik) pertaining to the relationship between relative positions of cerebral neurones and relative positions of parts of the body they are connected to

somatotrope (so-mat'o-trop) somatotroph

somatotroph (-trof) a cell of the anterior pituitary producing somatotropin

somatotrophic (so'ma-to-trof'ik) having a stimulatory effect on the nutrition and growth of the body

somatotrophin (-tro'fin) pituitary growth hormone

somatotropic (-trop'ik) 1. having affinity for the body or body cells 2. having the properties of somatotropin

somatotropin (-tro'pin) growth hormone

somatotype (so-mat'o-tip) body configuration. It may be ectomorph, endomorph or mesomorph

somesthesia (so'mes-the'zhah) the consciousness of having a body

somite (so'mit) block of mesodermal cells in a developing embryo that forms skeletal muscles (myotome), a connective tissue (dermatome) and vertebrae (sclerotome)

somnambulism (som-nam'bu-lizm) sleep walking

Somogyi phenomenon transient hyperglycaemia and ketosis after a hypoglycaemic episode in insulin treated diabetic patients, named after Micheal Somogyi, US biochemist

somnifacient (som'ni-fa'shint) hypnotic

somniferous (som-nif'er-us) producing sleep

somniloquism (som-nil'o-kwism) talking in one's sleep

somnolence (som'no-lens) sleepiness

somnolentia (som'no-len'shah) drowsiness

sonication (son'i-ka'shun) dispersion of solid material in the fluid by ultrasound

sonita (s) ovum

Sonne dysentery mild form of dysentery due to *Shigella sonne*, named after C. Sonne, Danish bacteriologist

sonitus (son'i-tus) a sounding or tinkling in the ears

sonography (so-nog'ra-fe) ultrasonography **sonographic** adj

sonolucent (so'no-loo'sent) producing no echoes to ultrasound

sopha (s) inflammation

sopar (so'par) deep sleep

soporific (sop'o-rif'ik) 1. producing deep sleep 2. an agent that produces deep sleep

soporous (so'por-us) associated with deep sleep

sorb to attract and retain substances by absorption

sorbefacient (sor'be-fa'shint) 1. promoting absorption 2. an agent that promotes absorption

sorbent (sor'bent) causing or facilitating absorption

sorbic (sor'bik) **acid** a hexadienoic acid' used as a preservative

sorbitan (sor'bi-tan) an anhydride of sorbitol

sorbitol (soı'bi-tol) hexahydroxyhexane, a sugar substitute for diabetics s **cataract** due to excess sorbitol in the lens in hyperglycaemic state

sordes (sor'dez) a dark brown crust-like collection on the lips, teeth and gums of a person with dehydration in chronic debilitating disease

sore (sor) 1. a lesion of the skin or mucous membrane 2. a wound, ulcer 3. painful

sore throat inflammation of the pharynx, larynx and tonsils often caused by haemolytic streptococcus or adenovirus

sorption (sorp'shun) absorption; adsorption

SOS si o'pus sit; if necessary

sosha (s) phthisis, emaciation

soshana (s) absorption

sotha (s) drops

soufle (soofl) systolic bruit audible with the bell of a stethoscope over an artery **mammary** s systolic bruit over lactating breast **uterine** s systolic bruit audible over pregnant uterus

sotalol beta-blocker used in hypertension

sound 1. noise; vibrations produced by a sounding body transmitted by the air and perceived by the internal ear 2. an elongated cylindrical usually curved instrument is used for exploring the bladder or other cavities of the body, dilating strictures of the urethra or oesophagus, or detecting the presence of a foreign body in a body cavity 3. healthy **amphoric breath** s a variant of bronchial breathing where a number of high-pitched sounds overlap the fundamental low-pitched sounds **bowel s'**

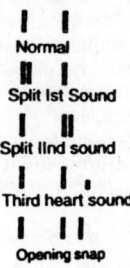

Heart sounds

s gurgling and bubbling sounds (borborygmi) due to the peristaltic action of the intestinal wall on the contents (fluid and air) within **breath s's** sounds due to the penetration of the air into the normal lung tissue and its expulsion, **bronchial s** an abnormal breath sound with a pause between inspiration and expiration and expiratory phase being longer and harsher than inspiratory phase **bronchovesicular breath s** an intermediate type of breathing having features of vesicular and bronchial breathing **cavernous breath s** a low-pitched bronchial breath sound **cracked pot s** a tympanitic percussion note in internal hydrocephalus in children with separation of sutures from raised intracranial tension **ejection s** a high-pitched clicking sound heard just after the first heart sound **first s** sound due to the closure of atrioventricular valves and it heralds the beginning of the ventricular systole **foetal heart s** sound produced by contraction of the foetal heart **fourth h s** sound occurs from the vibrations generated from vigourous contraction of the artria and is heard in late diastole **friction s** friction rub produced by inflammed opposing pleural surfaces **heart s ' s** one of the sounds heard on auscultation over the heart

Korotkoff's s sounds heard over an artery when blood pressure is measured by the auscultatory method **pistol shot s** sound coinciding first heart sound audible over brachial and femoral artery in hyperkinetic circulatory states and aortic incompetence **second h s** sound due to the closure of the aortic and pulmonary valves and it occurs at the end of the systole **succussion s** a splashing sound elicited in a patient with hydro-or pyo pneumothorax **tambours s** a heart sound from aortic or pulmonary valve closure giving a booming and ringing quality like that of a drum **third h s** sound produced by the ventricular wall during transition in from rapid early diastolic flow to the slow rate of passive distension of the ventricle and it occurs early in the diastole **tracheal breath s** loud, low-pitched breath sounds audible over trachea **tubular breath s** a high-pitched bronchial breath sound **urethral s** a device to explore urethra **vesicular breath s** normal breath sound **white s** a sound made up of all audible frequencies

Southern blot technique of transferring DNA fragments from gel after electrophoresis to cellulose nitrate filter paper named after Southern UK zoologist

Soutter's tube cylinder of spiral wire introduced into the oesophagus to preserve its lumen in inoperable carcinoma, named after H. Soutter, UK surgeon

space (spas) an actual or potential cavity of the body **alveolar dead s** ventilation of relatively underperfused or nonperfused alveoli **anatomical dead s** the air present in the conducting system (nose, mouth, pharynx, larynx, bronchi and bronchioles) does not participate in gas exchange and that part is considered as wasted **apical s** the space between the alveolar wall and the apex of the root of a tooth **axillary s** axilla **circumlental s** the space between the equator of the lens and the ciliary body **dead s.** 1. an anatomical and physiological dead space 2. an unobliterated space remaining after closure of a wound **epidural s** the space between the dura mater and the bones of the cranium and/or vertebral column **extracellular s** the space between the cells **intercostal s** the interval between the ribs **interpleural s** the mediastinum **interproximal s** the space between adjacent teeth in a dental arch **inter- radicular s** the space between the roots of multirooted teeth **intervillous s** the space between placental villi containing maternal blood **mediastinal s** mediastinum **medullary s** the marrow containing area of the cancellous bone **palmar s** one of the two fascial spaces in the palm (midpalmar and thenar spaces) **perilymphatic s** the space between the bony and membranous portions of the labyrinth **perineal s** spaces on either side of the inferior fascia of the urogenital diaphragm, the deep between it and the superficial fascia, the superficial between it and superficial perineal space **perivascular s** spaces within the adventitia of large blood vessels of the brain **physiological dead s** tidal volume which does not participate in gas exchange and it includes anatomic and alveolar dead spaces **plantar s** one of the four areas between fascial layers in the foot **popliteal s** the space in the back of the knee joint **retroperitoneal s** the potential space between the parietal peritoneum and the muscles and bones of posterior abdominal wall **retropharyngeal s** the space behind the pharynxseparating paravertebral from visceral fascia **subarachnoid s** space between the arachnoid and pia mater filled with cerebrospinal fluid **subdural s** the narrow space between the dura and arachnoid **subphrenic s** space between the diaphragm and the abdominal organs **suprasternal s** triangular space above the manubrium sterni between layers of deep cervical fascia **Tennon's s** lymph space between the sclera and tennon's capsule **thenar s** a deep palmar space in the hand lying anterior to adductor pollicis muscle **tissue s** any space within the tissues not lined by the epithelium and containing tissue fluid **zonular s'** s the spaces between the fibres of zonula ciliaris at the equator of lens of the eye

Spadling's sign foetal death demonstrated by overlapping of skull bones on x-ray, named after A. Spadling, US obstetrician

span length between the tips of the middle fingers of both outstretched and abducted upper limbs. Normally it is equal to the total height of the body

spanda (s) movement

sparaxis laceration

spargnosis an immature tapeworm developing in humans, usually subcutaneously

sparsha (s) touch

spasm (spazm) an involuntary contraction of the muscles occurring in an exaggerated form as in tetanus, hydrophobia, strychnine poisoning **clonic s** spasm interrupted by relaxations **tonic s** continuous contractions of the muscles

spasmodic (spaz-mod'ik) on the nature of spasm **s dysmenorrhoea** colicky menstruation especially noted near menarche **s dysphonia** a chronic phonatory disorder with jerky, effortful strained sounds with laryngeal discomfort **s torticollis** intermittent turning of head to one side with muscle contractions

spasmolysis (spaz-mol'i-sis) the arrest of a spasm **spasmolytic** adj

spasmus (spaz'mus) spasm

spastic (spas'tik) an increase in muscle tone (stiffness) **s colon** irritable bowel syndrome **s diplegia** cerebral palsy

spasticity (spas-tis'i-te) increase in the muscle tone due to lesions of pyramidal tract **clasp-knife s** resistance being felt at the beginning of passive flexion in spasticity and it gives way suddenly on continued pressure. The muscles feel firm

spatium (spa'she-um) a space

spatula (spach'u-la) a flat, blunt instrument for spreading plasters and for mixing ointments

spatulate (spach'u-lat) 1. having a flat blunt end 2. to mix or manipulate with spatula

spavin (spav'in) an exostosis of the tarsus of equines distal to the tibiotarsal articulation

spay (spa) to remove the ovaries

specialist (spesh'a-list) a person who is an expert in a recognised field of medicine

specialty (spesh'ul-te) the field of practice of a specialist

species (spe'shez) a taxonomic category subordinate to a genus and superior to subspecies **s specific** characteristic of a particular species

specific (spe-sif'ik) 1. pertaining to a species 2. produced by a single kind of microorganism 3. pertaining to the special affinity of antigen for the corresponding antibody **s gravity** a measure of solutes in a fluid

specificity (spas'i-fis'i-te) 1. the degree of an enzyme's selectivity for a substrate 2. the avidity of an antibody for an antigen. 3. the condition of being specific, of having a fixed relation to a single cause or to a definite result 4. the proportion of individuals with negative test results for the disease that the test is intended to reveal

specimen (spes'i-men) a small part or sample, of any substance or material obtained for testing

SPECT single photon emission computerized tomography, a method for reconstructing cross-sectional images of

radiotracer distribution in an organ, used to evaluate acute ischaemic episodes of the brain, vascular dementia, and myocardial perfusion

spectacles (spek'ta-k'lz) a pair of lenses mounted in a frame to assist vision

spectinomycin (spek'ti-no-mi'sin) an aminocyclitol antibiotic used in penicillin-resistant gonorrhoea

spectra (spek'tra) plural of spectrum

spectral (spek'tral) pertaining to a spectrum

spectrin (spek'trin) fibrous protein supporting red cell envelope

spectrometry (spek-trom'e-tre) the process of determining the wavelength of light rays by use of a spectrometer

spectrophotometer (spek'tro-fo-tom'e-ter) an instrument for measuring the intensity of light of definite wavelength transmitted by a substance or solution It gives a quantitative measure of amount of material in the solution absorbing the light

spectroscope (spek'tro-skop) an instrument for forming and examining spectra of luminous bodies

spectrum (spek'trum) 1. breakdown of white light into coloured bands 2. the range of effectiveness of drugs

speculum (spek'u-lum) pl **specula** an instrument for exposing the interior of a passage or cavity of the body

speech (spech) that which is spoken; the power of speaking **s audiometry** determination of percentage of words recognised at varying levels of loudness **s centre** formation of speech is a cortical function and the centres are situated in the left hemisphere in the right handed individuals as the dominant hemisphere. The centre is situated in the form of a quadrilateral consisting of visual area (calcarine sulcus of the occipital lobe), auditory area (superior temporal gyrus), Broca's area (3rd frontal convolution), writing centre (2nd frontal convolution) and their associated fibres in between

spell episode of sickness

sperm 1. spermatozoon 2. semen **s antibody** an antibody directed against the sperm heads or tails

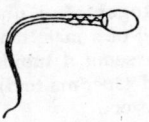

Sperm

spermatic (sper-mat'ik) pertaining to the semen; seminal **s cord** a supporting structure extending from a testis to the deep inguinal ring, that includes vas deferens, arteries, veins, lymphatics, nerves, cremaster muscle and connective tissue

spermatid (sper'ma-tid) spermatoblast; a cell derived from spermatocyte, and develops into spermatozoon

spermatitis (sper'ma-ti'tis) inflammation of a vas deferens

spermat (o) combining word for seed; male germ

spermatoblast (sper-mat'o-blast) spermatid

spermatocoele (-sel) a cystic tumour of epididymis containing spermatozoa

spermatocoelectomy (sper'ma-to-se-lek'to-me) surgical removal of a spermatocoele

spermaticidal (-si'd'l) an agent causing destruction of sperm

spermatocyst (sper-mat'o-sist) 1. a seminal vesicle 2. a spermatocoele

spermatocystectomy (sper'ma-to-sis-tek'ta-me) excision of the seminal vesicles

spermatocystotomy (-sis-tot'o-me) an incision into the seminal vesicles for drainage

spermatocyte (sper-mat'o-sit) a cell developing from a spermatogonium that gives rise to spermatozoa

spermatocytogenesis (sper'ma-to-si'to-jen'e-sis) spermatogenesis

spermatogenesis (-jen'e-sis) the formation and development of spermatozoa in the seminiferous tubules of the testes

spermatogenic (-jen'ik) producing semen or spermatozoa

spermatogonium (-go'ne-um) pl **spermatogonia** an undifferentiated germ cell of a male that takes its origin in a seminal tubule

spermatoid (sper'ma-toid) resembling a spermatozoon

spermatolysis (sper'ma-tol'i-sis) **spermatolytic** adj. destruction of spermatozoa

spermatopathia (sper'ma-to-path'e-a) abnormality of the semen

spermatorrhoea (-re'a) involuntary and excessive discharge of semen without orgasm

spermatoschesis (sper'ma-tos'ke-sis) suppression of production of semen

spermatozoicide (sper'ma-to-zo'i-sid) spermicide

spermatozoon (-zo'on) a mature sperm cell

spermaturia (sper'ma-to're-a) a discharge of semen with urine

spermectomy (sper-mek'to-me) excision of a portion of the spermatic cord

spermicide (sper'-mi-sid) an agent that kills spermatozoa

spermiduct (-dukt) the ejaculatory duct and vas deferens together

spermiogenesis (sper'me-o-jen'e-sis) the maturation of spermatids into spermatozoa

sperm (o) combining word for seed

spermolith (sper'mo-lith) a calculus in the seminal vesicle or spermatic duct

spermoneuralgia (sper'mo-noo-ral'ja) neuralgic pain in the spermatic cord

spermophlebectasia (-fleb'ek-ta'zha) varicosity of spermatic veins

sp gr specific gravity

sphacelate (sfa'se-lat) to become gangrenous

sphacelation (sfas'a-la'shun) the occurrence of gangrene

sphacelism (sfas'a-lizm) necrosis; sloughing

sphaceloderma (sfac'a-lo-der'ma) gangrene of the skin

sphacelous (sfas'e-lus) a slough; a gangrenous mass

sphatika (s) quartz

sphenion (sfe'ne-on) the point at the sphenoid angle of the parietal bone

sphen (o) combining word for sphenoid bone; wedge-shaped

sphenoid (sfe'noid) 1. wedge-shaped 2. sphenoid bone *see* table of bones **sphenoidal** adj

sphenoiditis (sfe'noi-di'tis) inflammation of sphenoid sinus

sphenoidotomy (sfe'noi-dot'a-me) incision of a sphenoid sinus

sphere (sfer) a ball; globed **segmentation s** 1. morula 2. a blastomere

sphere (o) combining word for round; sphere

spherocyte (sfer'o-sit) a small globular, completely haemoglobinated erythrocyte without central pallor seen in hereditary spherocytosis

spherocytosis (sfer'o-si-to'sis) a defect in erythrocyte membrane causing an increase in osmotic fragility and autohaemolysis **hereditary s** an autosomal dominant condition exhibiting anaemia, intermittent jaundice, splenomegaly, gall stones and leg ulcers

spheroid (sfe'roid) a local axonal dilatation filled with degenerated organelles

spheroidal (sfer'oi'd'l) resembling a sphere **s keratitis** excess exposure to sunlight causing opacities in the cornea

spider naevi small red spots consisting of a central arteriole with radiating branches. They get blanched on application of pressure and are found in the face, upper limbs and upper part of the body, are seen in liver cell failure, pregnancy, starvation and intake of oral contraceptives

sphincter (sfingk'ter) a circular muscle constricting an orifice **bladder s** the smooth muscle about the opening of bladder into the urethra **cardiac s** the smooth muscle at the oesophagogastric junction **pyloric s** the smooth muscle around the opening of the stomach into the duodenum **s ani** the sphincter that closes the anus. It consists of sphincter ani externus of striated muscle and sphincter ani internus of smooth muscle **s of Oddi** a circular muscle at the opening of the common bile duct and main pancreatic ducts in the duodenum

sphincteralgia (sfingk'ter-al'jah) pain in a sphincter

sphincterectomy (-ek'to-me) surgical removal of a sphincter

sphincterismus (-iz'mus) spasm of a sphincter

sphincteritis (-i'tis) inflammation of a sphincter

sphincterolysis (-ol'isis) the operative procedure of separating the iris from the cornea in anterior synechia

sphincteroplasty (sfingk'ter-o-plas'te) surgical reconstruction of a sphincter by converting Y incision to V

sphincterotomy (sfingk'ter-ot'a-me) incision of a sphincter

sphingolipid (sfing'go-lip'id) any lipid containing a long chain base like sphingosine, a constituent of nerve tissue

sphingolipidosis (-lip'i-do'sis) a group of inborn errors of sphingolipid metabolism in which lysosphingolipids accumulate which includes Fabry's disease, Gaucher's disease, Krabbe's disease, Niemann-Pick disease and gangliosidosis

sphingolipodystrophy (-lip'o-dis'tra-fe) any of a group of disorders of sphingolipid metabolism

sphingomyelin (-mie'e-lin) ceramide-phosphocholine compound

sphingosine (sfing'go-sen) a long chain, monounsaturated aliphatic amino alcohol found in sphingomyelin

sphygmic (sfig'mik) pertaining to the pulse

sphygm (o) combining word for pulse

sphygmodynamometer (sfig'mo-di'na-mom'e-ter) an instrument for measuring the force of the pulse

sphygmogram (sfig'mo-gram) the tracing of the arterial pulse by a sphygmograph. The curve has a sudden rise followed by a sudden fall, after which there is a gradual descent marked by a number of secondary elevations

sphygmograph (-graf) an instrument to record the movement, form and force of the arterial pulse

sphygmoid (sfig'moid) resembling the pulse

sphygmomanometer (sfig'mo-ma-nom'e-ter) an instrument for measuring the arterial blood pressure

sphygmoscope (sfig'mo-skop) an instrument making the pulse beat visible

sphygmotometer (sfig'mo-to-nom'e-ter) an instrument for measuring the elasticity of the arterial walls

spica (spi'ka) figure of eight bandage or plaster especially as applied to bigger joints

spicule (spik'ul) a sharp, needle-like body

spiculum (spik'u-lum) spicule

spider (spi'der) 1. an arthropod of the class Arachnida, some species are venomous 2. a spider-like naevus **s angioma** a superficial spider-like cluster of capillaries composed of a central 'feeder' vessel and multiple minute tortuous and dilated radiating vessels that blanch on pressure seen in cirrhosis of the liver, pregnancy **s cell** 1. an epithelial cell seen in cervical metaplasia 2. an undifferentiated mesenchymal cell with a small central, acidophilic mass connected by thin striations to the cell periphery, seen in myxoma, rhabdomyomas and rhabdomyosarcomas **s colony** colony of *Actinomyces israelii* **s-leg deformity** deformity seen on pyelogram of renal calyces around hypernephroma **s naevus** spider angioma **s web dot** cob web clot seen in CSF in tuberculous meningitis

spike (spik) 1. a sharp upward deflection in a curve 2. a sharp peak seen in beta or gamma region in semen electrophoresis **s and dome contour** carotid arterial pulse showing an abrupt rise and fall during midsystole (spike) and then showing a second rise at a slower rate during late systole, as in idiopathic hypertrophic subaortic stenosis

spina (spi'na) pl **spinae** a spine; a projection like a thorn **s bifida** failure of closure of the spinal canal due to defective fusion of the vertebral arch in the lumbosacral region and is associated with depression, pigmentation or presence of hair **s cystica** cystic swelling such as meningocoele or meningomyelocoele **s occulta** with no external or visible abnormality

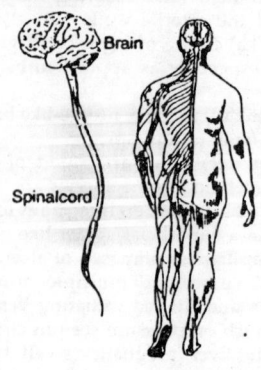

Spinal nerves

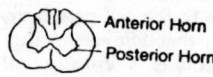

Spinal cord-section

spinal (spi'n'l) pertaining to a spine or to the vertebral column **s cord** an elongated mass of nerve tissue located in the vertebral canal from which 31 pairs of spinal nerves originate **s dysraphism** any congenital split of spine **s muscle atrophy** degeneration of the anterior horn cells with associated muscle weakness and atrophy **s process** 1. a sharp projection from the vertebra; a spine 2. a sharp ridge running diagonally across the posterior surface of the scapula **s shock** a flaccid paralysis below the site of spinal injury **s tap** withdrawal of cerebrospinal fluid from the subarachnoid space in the lumbar region

spinate (spi'nat) having thorns

spina ventosa a fusiform expansile lesion of phalangeal bones with cortical and trabecular destruction and ballooning of the cortex, in tuberculosis and congenital syphilis

spindle (spin'd'l) 1. any fusiform cell or structure 2. a structure consisting of microtubules that helps in the alignment and movement of chromosomes during cell division

spine (spin) 1. spina 2. the spinal column

spinifugal (spi-nif'u-gal) moving or conducting away from the spinal cord

spinipetal (spi-nip'i-t'l) moving or conducting towards the spinal cord

spinnbarkeit (spin'bar-kit) *Ger* the stretchability of cervical mucus or length that strands of cervical mucus reach before breaking. The maximum length coincides with the time of ovulation

spinobulbar (spi'nobul'bar) pertaining to the spinal cord and medulla oblongata

spinocerebellar (-ser'e-bel'ar) pertaining to the spinal cord and cerebellum

spinous (spi'nus) 1. like a spine 2. pertaining to a spine

spiradenoma (spir'ad-e-no'ma) a benign tumour of the sweat glands, particularly of coiled portion

spiral (spi'ral) winding about a centre like coil **Curschmann's s' s** coiled mucous fibrils sometimes found in sputum of patients with bronchial asthma **s computed tomography** helical CT imaging in which a large image volume is obtained by continuous rotation of the detector and scanning images at a speed of 10 mm/sec in a single breath **s organ** the organ of hearing consisting of supporting cells and hair cells that rest on the basilar membrane and extend into the endolymph

spiramycin a macrolide antibiotic used in toxoplasmosis in pregnancy

spireme (spi'rem) the thread-like figure formed during prophase by the chromosome material

spirilla (spi-ril'a) pl. **spirillum,** a flagellated aerobic bacterium with an elongated spiral shape, of the genus Spirillum; *S. minus* a causative agent of rat bite fever

spirillicidal (spi-ril'i-si'dal) destroying spirilla

spirillosis (spi'ri-lo'sis) a disease caused by the presence of spirilla in the blood

Spirillum (spi-ril'um) 1. a spiral-shaped bacterium 2. an organism of the genus *Spirillum*

spir (o) combining word for coil; spiral; breath; breathing

spirit 1. any volatile or distilled liquid 2. a solution of a volatile material in alcohol

Spirochaeta (spi'ro-ke'ta) a genus of slender, spiral organisms belonging to the family Spirochaetaceae, order spirochaetales

spirochete (spi'ro-ket) any member of the order spirochactales. It includes agents responsible for leptospira, borrelia and treponema infections

spirocheticide (spi'ro-ke'ti-sid) an agent which destroys spirochetes **spirocheticidal** adj

spirochetolysis (-ke-tol'i-sis) the destruction of spirochaetes by lysis

spirochetosis (-ke-to'sis) infection with spirochaetes

spirogram (spi'ro-gram) a record made by a spirometer

spirograph (-graf) a device for representing graphically the lung volumes and its subdivisions.

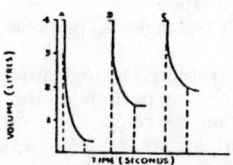

A. Normal;   B. Restrictive ventilatory defect;
C. Obstructive ventilatory defect

Spirogram

spiroid (spi'roid) resembling a spiral

spirolactone (spi'ro-lak'ton) a group of compounds capable of opposing the action of aldosterone on renal transport of sodium and potassium

spirometer (spi'rom'e-ter) a device that measures the volume of air inspired or expired and records the time over which the volume changes. Vital capacity and its subdivisions are obtained. The spirometers may be of closed system—wet type (Bell spirometer with a water seal) or dry type (bellows, piston, wedge spirometer) or open system (using a pneumatachograph with a differential pressure transducer or turbine or vane type volume transducer)

Spirometra (spi'ro-me'tra) a genus of tapeworm and a larval infection (sparganosis) may occur on ingestion of inadequately cooked food

spirometry (spi-rom'e-tre) pulmonary function studies done by a spirometer, that helps to determine FVC, FEV_1, and FEV_1/FVC ratio

spironolactone (spir'o-no-lak'ton) a diuretic that blocks the action of aldosterone on the distal convoluted tubules and collecting tubules of the kidney

spissated (spis'at-ed) inspissated

splanchnectopia (splangk'nek-to'pe-a) displacement of one or more visceral organs

splachnesthesia (splank'nes-the'zhah) visceral sensation

splanchnic (splangk'nik) pertaining to the viscera

splanchnicectomy (splangk'ni-sek'ta-me) excision of a portion of the greater splanchnic nerve

splanchnicotomy (-kot'a-me) splanchinicectomy

splanchn (o) combining word for viscera, viscus, splanchnic nerve

splanchnocoele (splank'no-sel) hernial protrusion of a viscus

splanchnodiastasis (splangk'no-di-as'ta-sis) displacement of a viscus or viscera

splanchnography (splangk'nog'ra-fe) descriptive anatomy of the viscera

splanchnolith (splangk'no-lith) an intestinal calculus

splanchnology (spangk-nol'a-je) the scientific study of the viscera of the body

splanchnomegaly (splangk'no-meg'a-le) visceromegaly; enlargement of viscus

splanchnopathy (splangk'nop'a-the) disease of abdominal viscera

splanchnosclerosis (splangk'no-skelero'sis) hardening of the viscera

splanchnoskeleton (-skel'e-ton) the body structures connected with the viscera

splanchnotomy (splangk-not'o-me) the dissection of the viscera

splanchnotribe (splangk'no-trib) an instrument to crush the intestine

splashback protrusion of tissue from a bullet's entrance wound

splay (spl'a) **Spread out** s **foot** flat foot

spleen (splen) a large mass of lymphatic tissue between the fundus of the stomach and the diaphragm that functions in phagocytosis, production of lymphocytes, and blood storage. It has an outer capsule of dense connective tissue and smooth muscle fibres, from which trabeculae extend into the pulp consisting of lymphocytes and a network of venous sinuses

splen spleen

splenalgia (sple-nal'jah) pain in the spleen

splenectomy (sple-nek'ta-me) excision of the spleen

splenectopia (sple'nek-to'pe-a) displacement of the spleen; floating spleen

splenectopy (sple-nek'to-pe) splenectopia

splenic (splen'ik) pertaining to the spleen s **flexure syndrome** abdominal distension and discomfort by swallowed gas, relieved by defecation or passing of flatus

splenitis (sple-ni'tis) inflammation of the spleen

splenium (sple'ne-um) a band-like structure; a bandage or compress

splenisation (splen'i-za'shun) engorgement of an organ giving the appearance of the tissue of the spleen

srien (o) combining word for spleen

splenocoele (sple'no-sel) hernia of the spleen

splenocolic (sple'no-kol'ik) pertaining to the spleen and colon

splenocyte (sple'no-sit) a splenic monocyte

splenography (sple-nog'ra-fe) radiography of the spleen after an injection of contrast medium

splenohepatomegaly (sple'no-hep'a-tomg'a-le) enlargement of spleen and liver

splenolysis (sple-nol'i-sis) destruction of splenic tissue

splenoma (sple-no'ma) a tumour of the spleen

splenomalacia (sple'no-ma-la'she-ah) softening of the spleen

splenomedullary (-med'u-lar'e) of or pertaining to the spleen and bone marrow

splenomegaly (-meg-ah-le) enlargement of the spleen. Spleen is enlarged in infections (enteric fever, septicemia, infective hepatitis, brucellosis, malaria, kalaazar, subacute infective endocarditis), congestion (portal hypertension, non-cirrhotic portal fibrosis, tropical splenomegaly), anaemias, leukaemias, myelofibrosis, amyloidosis, lipid storage disorders, Felty's syndrome and Still's disease

splenomyelogenous (-mi'e-loj'e-nus) formed in the spleen and bone marrow

splenopancreatic (-pan'kre-at'ik) pertaining to the spleen and pancreas

splenopathy (sple-nop'a-the) any disease of the spleen

splenopexy (sple'no-pak'se) surgical fixation of the spleen

splenoptosis (sple'nop-to'sis) downward displacement of the spleen

splenorrhagia (sple'no-ra'je-ah) bleeding from the spleen

splenorrhaphy (-sple-nor'a-fe) surgical repair of the spleen

splenosis (sple-no'sis) autotransplantation of splenic tissue to unusual sites following open splenic trauma

splenotomy (sple-not'o-me) incision of the spleen

splice junction a segment of DNA involved in RNA splicing

splicing (spli'sing) the cutting and rejoining of strands of linear molecule such as DNA, RNA or protein

splint a rigid device for holding broken bones in place or easing pain

splinter haemorrhage small linear haemorrhages beneath the nails in trauma, psoriasis, subacute infective endocarditis, trichinosis, and rheumatoid arthritis

splinting (splint'ing) 1. application of a splint 2. treatment by use of a splint 3. application of a fixed restoration to join two or more teeth into a single rigid unit 4. rigidity of a muscle

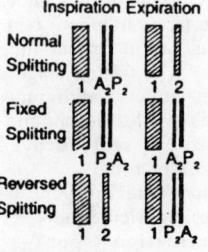

Splitting of second sound

splitting (split'ing) 1. the division of a single object into two or more parts 2. the cleavage of a covalent bond, fragmenting the molecule involved 3. division of a well-defined morbid condition into smaller sub-types **fixed s** the splitting is wide and fixed exhibiting no expiratory variations in ASD **narrow s** splitting becomes narrowed with increased resistance in the pulmonary vascular bed, as in Eisenmenger's complex **paradoxical s** delayed closure of the aortic component may cause splitting to become narrow and pulmonary closure sound precedes the aortic closure sound **s of first heart sound** noted as 'l-lub' over the lower end of the sternum on its left side in right bundle branch block due to delay in the onset of the right ventricular systole **s of second heart sound** the pulmonary valve closes later than the aortic valve and is recognised in the form of split second heart sound in the pulmonary area **wide s** wide splitting when there is delay in the closure of the pulmonary valve, as in RBBB and pulmonary stenosis

spodogenous (spo-doj'e-nus) caused by accumulation of waste products in an organ

spondylalgia (spon'di-lal'jah) pain in a vertebra

spondylarthritis (spon'dil-ar-thri'tis) arthritis of the intervertebral articulations

spondylitic (spon'di-lit'ik) pertaining to spondylitis

spondylitis (spon'di-li'tis) inflammation of vertebra **ankylosing s** a chronic inflammatory arthritis with a predilection for the sacroiliac joints and spine. It manifests by progressive stiffening and fusion of the axial skeleton **s deformans** arthritis and osteitis deformans affecting the spinal column. There is ossification of ligaments and bony ankylosis of the intervertebral articulations to result in kyphosis and rigidity **tuberculous s** Pott's disease.

Tuberculous infection of the spine with a gibbus of spine

spondylizema (spon'dil-i-zema) downward displacement of a vertebra due to destruction of the one below it

spondyl (o) combining word for vertebra; vertebral column; spine

spondylocae (spon'dil-ok'a-se) tuberculosis of the vertebra

spondylodymus (spon'dil-od'i-mus) twin foetuses united by the vertebrae

spondylodynia (spon'di-lo-din'e-a) pain in a vertebra

spondylolisthesis (-lis'the-sis) forward displacement of a vertebra over the one below. It is associated with low back pain aggravated by standing and walking. There can be nerve root compression

spondylolysis (spon'dil-ol'i-sis) a defect in the interarticular part of the vertebra

spondylopathy (spon'dil-op'a-the) any disease of the vertebrae

spondylopyosis (spon'dil-o-pi-o'sis) suppuration of one or more vertebralbodies

spondyloschisis (spon'di-los'ki-sis) congenital fissure of one or more of the vertebral arches

spondylosis (spon'di-lo'sis) 1. ankylosis of a vertebral joint 2. any degenerative lesion of the spine **cervical s** disc degeneration with associated osteophyte formation and osteoarthritis of the joints of cervical spine. It is associated with cervical radiculopathy **lumbar s** degenerative changes in the discs and lumbar spine, associated with low back pain and features of nerve root compression

spondylosyndesis (spon'di-lo-sin-de'sis) spinal fusion

sponge (spunj) 1. a porous absorbent mass 2. the cellular endoskeleton of certain marine animals **s kidney** congenital cyst formation in the renal papillae

spongiform (spon'ji-form) sponge-like **s encephalopathy** neuronal loss, spongiform changes and gliosis with deposition of prion protein

spong (o) combining word for sponge; sponge-like

spongioblast (spun'je-o-blast) a neuroepithelial, filiform ependyma cell

spongioblastoma (spon'je-o-blas-to'ma) a malignant tumour derived from spongioblasts

spongiocyte (spun'je-o-sit) 1. neuroglial cell 2. a vacuolated, lipid-laden cell in the adrenal cortex

spongioid (spun'je-oid) resembling a sponge

spongioplasm (spun'je-o-plazm) a network of fibrils in the cell substance

spongiosa (spon'je-oza) 1. spongy 2. cancellous bone

spongiosaplasty (-plas'te) autoplasty of spongiosa to facilitate new bone formation

spongiosis (spun'je-o'sis) intercelluar oedema of the epidermis

spongiositis (spun'je-o-si'tis) inflammation of corpus spongiosum or corpus cavernosum of the penis

spontaneous involuntary; produced of itself **s bacterial peritonitis** increased susceptibility of patients with cirrhosis to infection of ascitic fluid characterised by sudden onset of abdominal pain, rebound tenderness, absence bowel sounds and fever **s subcortical haematoma** a form of cerebral haemorrhage without hypertension

spoon nails koilonychia

sporadic (spo-rad'ic) occurring singly and is neither epidemic nor endemic

sporangium (spo-ran'je-um) cyst containing spores, as in certain fungi

spore (spor) 1. a resting stage of a cell that resists adverse environmental conditions, as in Clostridium and Bacillus organisms 2. a reproductive element of protozoa or fungi

sporicide (spor'i-sid) an agent which kills the spores, **sporicidal** adj

sporoagglutination (spor'o-a-gloo'tina'shun) specific agglutinins causing clumping of spores of fungi

sporoblast (spor'o-blast) an early stage in the development of a sporocyst prior to the differentiation of sporozoites.

sporocyst (-sist) 1. any cyst containing reproductive cells like spores 2. a stage in the life cycle of a trematode in the first intermediate host where the germinal sac contains germ cells 3. a stage in the life cycle of certain protozoa contained within a oocyst

sporogenic (spor'o-jen'ik) producing spores

sporogony (spo-rog'a-ne) formation of sporozoites in sporozoan protozoa. It is an asexual division within the sporocyte

sporont (spor'ont) the zygote stage within the wall of oocyst, occurring in the life cycle of coccidia

sporoplasm (spor'o-plazm) the protoplasm of the spores

Sporothrix (-thriks) a genus of fungi, including *Sporotrichum schenckii*, the causative agent of sporotrichosis

sporotrichosis (spor'o-tri-ko'sis) infection with *Sporotrichum schenckii* through the wounds presenting with granulomatous lesion, ulcer, and lymphatic spread

sporozoan (-zo'an) 1. sporozoon, an individual organism of sporozoa 2. relating to the sporozoa

sporozoite (-zo'it) spore forms of protozoa

sporozoon (-zo'on) sporozoa; sporozoan

sport 1. to play; to practice field diversions 2. a phenotype trait that appears in an individual spontaneously and is subsequently inherited by his progeny

sporulation (spor'u-la'shun) formation of spores

sporule (spor'ul) a small spore

spot 1. a circumscribed area 2. a macula **Bitot's s** small foamy gray triangular deposits of keratinised epithelium on the conjunctiva associated with vitamin A deficiency **blind s** the optic disc, the site of entrance of the optic nerve and it is not sensitive to light **Cafe au lait s's** sharply defined light brown patches of the skin, seen in neurofibromatosis **cherry red s** red spot on the retina surrounded by oedema as in infantile cerebral sphingolipidosis **cotton wool s's** white opacities in the retina due to retinal ischaemia or infarction in grade 3 hypertensive retinopathy **germinal s** the nucleus of fertilised ovum **Koplick's s's** minute bright red spots with tiny bluish white specks in the centre, found in the buccal mucous membrane during the prodromal stage of measles **liver s** senile lentigo; yellow-brown spots of the face, neck and dorsum of the hands in elderly persons **milk s's** 1. aggregation of macrophages in the omentum 2. white plaques in the epicardium overlying the right ventricle of the heart where it is not covered by lung **mongolian s** smooth mulberry coloured spots in the sacral region found at birth in orientals and dark-skinned races and disappear during childhood **rose s's** rose coloured macules over the abdomen and thighs during first week of typhoid fever **Roth's s's** round white spots in the retina during subacute infective endocarditis **yellow s** macula retinae

spotted fever 1. group of rickettsial infections 2. meningococcal meningitis or septicemia with petechial rash

spp species

sprain (spran) partial tear of joint ligament

sprawn to produce, to bring forth

sprue (sproo) 1. a chronic malabsorption syndrome with steatorrhoea 2. in dentistry, the hole made of wax or metal through which molten metal is allowed to flow into a mold **collagenous s** extensive deposition of collagen in the lamina propria of the colon that does not respond to withdrawal of dietary gluten **non-tropical s** coeliac disease where patients are intolerant to the proteins found in wheat (gluten and gliadin) **tropical s** chronic progressive malabsorption in a patient in or from tropics with partial villous atrophy presenting with diarrhoea, abdominal distension, anorexia, fatigue and weight loss. It responds to tetracyclines

spur a small projection from any structure **s cell** acanthocyte

sputum (spu'tum) spit; expectoration. The material expelled by coughing contains cellular debris, mucus, blood, pus and micro-organisms **bloody s** haemoptysis **nummular s** sputum in discoid masses resembling a coin **rusty s** a reddish brown expectoration in lobar pneumonia

squama (skwah'ma) pl. **squamae** 1. a thin plate of bone 2. an epidermic scale

squame (skwa'me) squama

squamocolumnar junction the zone of transition from squamous epithelium to secretory and glandular epithelium that occur in the nasopharynx, oesophagogastric junction, uterine cervix and anus

squamooccipital (skwa'mo-ok-sip'i-til) pertaining to the squamous portion of the occipital bone

squamoparietal (-pa-ri'i-til) pertaining to the squamous portion of the temporal bone and parietal bone

squamosoparietal (skwa-mo'so-pa-ri'til) squamoparietal

squamous (skwa'mus) 1. scale-like 2. relating to or covered with scales **s bone** upper anterior portion of temporal bone **s cell** a flat scaly epithelial cell **s epithelium** the flat form of epithelial cells **s epithelioma** tumour produced by a squamous epithelium **s pearl** a compact, round cluster of keratinocytes found in well differentiated squamous cell carcinoma

squatting (skwat'ing) a position assumed by a child with cyanotic heart disease, especially Fallot's tetrology in acute hypoxaemia. It relieves the dyspnoea by decreasing right-to-left shunt and increasing the systemic vascular resistance and pulmonary blood flow

squeezing technique prevention of premature ejaculation by pressure below glans penis

squint (skwint) 1. strabismus 2. an abnormality in which the right and left visual axes fail to meet toward an objective point simultaneously **concomitant s** non-paralytic squint. An imbalance in the action of opposing muscles and squint is present at rest in all directions of gaze and it is not associated with diplopia **paralytic s** squint due to weakness of one or more extraocular muscles; the squint is noticeable when the patient attempts to move the eye in the direction of action of paralysed muscle and diplopia occurs in such positions of the eyes which depend upon the contractions of the paralysed muscles

Sr chemical symbol, strontium

SRH somatotropin-releasing hormone

SRS-A slow-reacting substance of anaphylaxis

SSPE subacute sclerosing panencephalitis

ss se'mis; one half

ST ECG segment lying between the end of the QRS complex and the beginning of the T-wave

stabile (sta'bil) stable

stability (sta-bil'i-ti) the condition of being stable or resistant to change

stadium (sta'de-um) a stage or period in the progress of the disease **s decrementi** the period of decrease in severity of a disease **s fluorescentiae** the stage of eruption in an exanthematous disease **s incrementi** the period of increase in the intensity of a disease **s sudoris** the sweating stage of malaria

staff (staff) 1. a specific group of workers **attending s** the physicians and surgeons who are members of the hospital staff and attend their patients at the hospital and supervise and teach students, interns and residents **consulting s** the specialists attached to hospital **house s** physicians and surgeons under training who take care of the patients in the hospital

stage (staj) 1. a period in the course of a disease 2. distribution and extent of spread of a malignancy 3. the part of microscope on which the slide is placed for examination **algid s** period marked by collapse in cholera **amphibolic s** the stage of an infectious disease between the acme and decline at a time when outcome is not certain **anal s** the second stage of psychosexual development in a child when its activities and interests are on the anal zone **cold s** the period of chills or rigor in malaria **defervescent s** the period of decline in fever **eruptive s** 1. the period of appearance of exanthema 2. tooth eruption **exoerythrocytic s** developmental stage of malarial parasite outside of red blood cells, in the liver parenchymal cells **expulsive s of labour** the stage of dilatation of uterine cervix during which child is expelled from uterus; second stage of labour **first s of labour** period when the foetal head is moulded and cervix dilated **fourth s of labour** the post partum period following expulsion of the placenta **hot s** period of pyrexia in malaria **imperfect s** the asexual life cycle phase of a fungus. **intuitive s** a stage of development in child when a child's thought processes are determined by the most prominent aspects of the stimuli **latent s** incubation period **oral s** the earliest stage of psychosexual development when the infant's needs and expressions are centred on the oral zone to be followed by anal stage **phallic s** the third stage of psychosexual development during which period of sexual interest of the child is centred on the penis in boys and clitoris in girls. It is preceded by anal stage **preeruptive s** a stage in infectious disease before appearance of eruptions **predromal s** incubation period **second s of labour** expulsive stage of

labour **sweating s** occurrence of sweating as a terminal stage of malaria **third s of labour** the placental stage of labour

staggers (stag'erz) vertigo and confusion noted in decompression illness

staghorn calculus a renal stone of magnesium ammonium phosphate with broad arborescence filling the renal pelvicaliceal system

stagnant-loop blind loop

staging (staj'ing) 1. the determination of different periods in the course of a disease 2. the classification of neoplasms according to the extent of the tumour **international s** this system describes the size, local extent of tumour, regional lymph node involvement, and presence or absence of metastases beyond the mediastinum **TNM's staging** of tumours according to tumour (T), node (N) and metastases (M).

stain (stan) 1. dye used in histologic and bacteriologic examinations 2. a procedure in which the dye and reagents are used to colour the constituents of cells and tissues **acid s** a stain in which the anion is the coloured component of the dye molecule. Eosin is commonly used to stain the cytoplasm **acid fast s** stain containing carbol fuchsin which is retained by mycobacteria **basic s** a stain in which the cation is the coloured component of the dye molecule. Methylene blue is employed to stain nuclear elements of the cells **contrast s** differential stain that facilitates differentiation of various elements in a specimen **counter s** a contrast stain used after staining of specific elements of a tissue **dental s** discolouration accumulating on the surface of teeth or dentures **differential s** a stain that helps to differentiate among different types of bacteria **double s** a mixture of acid and basic stains **Giemsa s** a stain containing azure II-eosin and azure II used for staining Negri bodies, differential staining of blood smears and chromosomes **Gram's** s a method of differential staining of bacteria which are stained with crystal violet, washed and then flooded with iodine solution. It stains bacteria either dark or purple. Then acetone is added. It decolourises the gram-negative bacteria without affecting gram-positive ones. Then it is counter-stained with safronine or neutral red. Gram-positive organisms appear violet and gram-negative organisms appear red against pink background **haematoxylin-eosin** s a mixture of a hematoxylin in distilled water and aqueous eosin solution to stain tissues. Nuclei are stained a deep blue-black with haematoxylin and cytoplasm is stained pink after counter-staining with eosin **immunofluorescent** s staining resulting from a combination of fluorescent antibody-with antigen-specific for the antibody **intravital** s a stain which is taken up by living cells after parenteral administration **iodine** s stain for amoebae, amyloid, cellulose and starch **metachromatic** s a stain having an ability to produce different colours on staining cells and tissues **Papanicolaou** s *see* Papanicolaou stain **supravital** s stain that colours living cells or tissues that have been removed from the body **vital** s intravital stain **Wright's** s a polychrome stain containing eosin and methylene blue used for demonstration of cells and malarial parasites

staining (stan'ing) a series of dyes used selectively to colour tissues or cells for microscopic examination. Haematoxylin and eosin (H & E) stains nuclei blue and the stroma light pink and is commonly used for tissues removed during surgery. Other stains are acid-fast stain for mycobacteria, gram stain for bacteria, congo red for amyloid, periodic acid Schiff stain for complex carbohydrate and Prussian blue stain for iron

stalagmometer (stal'ag-mom'e-ter) an instrument used to determine the number of drops in a given quantity of liquid

stalk (sta'wk) a narrowed connection with an organ or structure

stammering (stam'er-ing) a speech disorder with hesitation and repetition of sounds

standardisation 1. making a solution of definite strength to be used as a comparison 2. making a drug conform to the standard

standstill (stand'stil) cessation of activity **cardiac** s cardiac arrest

stannosis pneumoconiosis from inhalation of metallic tin dust and it is associated with mottled shadows or nodular opacities in the chest radiogram

stannous (stan'us) containing tin

stannum (stan'um) tin, symbol Sn

stanozolol (stan'o-zo-lol) anabolic steroid

stapedectomy (sta'pe-dek'to-me) excision of stapes

stapedial (sta-pe'de-al) pertaining to the stapes

stapediotenotomy (sta-pe'de-o-te-not'a-me) cutting of the tendon of stapedius muscle

stapediovestibular (-ves-tib'u-lar) pertaining to the stapes and vestibule

stapedius small muscle of middle ear *see* table of muscles s **reflex** contraction of stapedius in response to sudden loud noise

stapedotomy (sta'pe-dot'a-me) a surgical creation of a small opening in the foot plate of the stapes

stapes (sta'pes) *see* table of bones

staphyledema (staf'il-e-de'ma) oedema of the uvula

staphyline (staf'l-lin) 1. pertaining to the uvula 2. shaped like a bunch of grapes

staphylitis (staf'i-li-tis) inflammation of the uvula

staphyl (o) combining word for staphylococci; uvula; resembling a bunch of grapes

staphylococcemia (staf'i-lo-kok-se'mea) staphylococci in the blood

staphylococcus (-kok'us) pl. **staphylococci** a genus of micrococci, order Eubacteriales. They are gram-positive organisms. *S. epidermidis* commonly found on normal skin *S. saprophyticus* an agent that may cause urinary tract infections *S. aureus* an agent responsible for wide variety of suppurative conditions.

staphyloderma (-der'ma) staphylococcal infection of the skin

staphylodialysis (-di-al'i-sis) relaxation of the uvula

staphylolysin (staf'i-lol'i-sin) a haemolysin produced by staphylococci

staphyloma (staf'i-lo-ma) herniation of sclera or cornea with uvea included

staphyloncus (staf'i-long'kus) swelling of the uvula

staphyloplasty (staf'i-lo-plas'te) surgical repair of the soft palate and uvula

staphyloptosia (staf'i-lop-to'se-a) elongation of the uvula

staphylorrhaphy (staf'i-lora'a-fe) suture of a cleft palate

staphyloschisis (staf'i-los'ki-sis) fissure of the uvula and soft palate

staphylotomy (stat'i-lot'a-me) 1. incision of uvula 2. excision of staphyloma

stapler semiautomatic device for gut anastomosis instead of sutures

starch polymers of glucose linked by 1-4 glycoside linkages. Nutrient found in cereals, roots and legumes, providing largest proportion of calories. They are digested promptly by amylase, or slowly digested or escape digestion

Starling's law energy of contraction of heart muscle varies directly with the length of muscle fibres at the end of diastole, named after Ernest Starling British physiologist

Starr-Edwards valve Ball-in-cage aortic valve prosthesis, designed by Albert Starr, US surgeon and M.L. Edwards, US physician

starvation a condition of being without food for a long period of time resulting in undernutrition and loss of weight

stasis (sta'sis) stoppage of flow, growth or activity

stat station; at once

state (stat) condition; situation

state of art relatively new

static combining word for inhibition; maintenance of a constant level **s traction** A steady traction force applied and maintained for an extended time interval

statim (sta'tim) at once

statins lipid lowering agents that inhibit cholesterol biosynthesis in the liver, activate hepatic LD1 receptor and, increase LDL catabolism. Simvastatin and pravastatin are examples

station (sta'shun) 1. a position or location 2. the relationship in centimetres between the leading bony portion of foetal head and the level of ischial spines that is used to determine the level of application of forceps to aid in delivery

stationary resistant to change

statistics (sta-tis'tiks) the science ɩ collection, arrangement, analysis a ɩd interpretation of facts having a bɩ ɩring on the condition of people

statoacoustic (stat'o-a-koo'stiκ) ᵖ rtaining to balance and hearing

statoconia (-ko'ne-a) particles of calcium carbonate and protein adhering to the utricle and saccule; otolith

statolith (stat'o-lith) statoconia

statometer (sta-tem'e-ter) an apparatus for measuring the degree of exophthalmos

stature (stach'ur) body proportion

stavudine aṅ antiretroviral agent

status (sta'tus) standing; condition. **s asthmaticus** acute severe asthma **s epilepticus** a major attack of epilepsy succeeding another without the patient regaining awareness between attacks

status quo (stat-us-kw'au) L the existing situation or state of affairs

staxis (stak'sis) haemorrhage

STD sexually transmitted disease

steady state pertaining to the time period during which a physiologic function remains at a constant value

steal (stel) diversion of blood via alternate routes or reversed flow. A partial blockage of a large artery causing a temporary ischaemia in one segment of its territory by diverting the blood to cater to the excessive demands in another

stearate (ste′a-rat) a salt of stearic acid

stearic (ste-ar′ik) **acid** straight-chain saturated 18-carbon fatty acid, used in ointments, suppositories and soaps

stear (o) combining word for fat

steotitis (ste′a-ti′tis) inflammation of adipose tissue

steat (o) combining word for fat; adipose tissue

steatocystoma (ste′a-to-sis-to′ma) sebaceous cyst

steatogenous (ste′a-toj′e-nus) lipogenic

steatolysis (ste′a-tol′i-sis) emulsion of fat in the digestive process

steatoma (ste′a-to′ma) pl **steotomata** 1. lipoma 2. a fatty mass within a sebacious cyst

steatomatosis (ste′a-to′ma-to′sis) 1. an epithelial cyst 2. lipomatosis

steatonecrosis (-ne-kro′sis) fat necrosis

steatopygia (ste′a-to-pij′e-a) excessive fatness of the buttocks

steatorrhoea (-re′a) excess amount of fat in the feces

steatosis (ste′a-to′sis) fatty degeneration of the liver **macrovascular s** a single fat globule fills the liver cell and pushes the nucleus to the periphery, found in alcoholism, obesity, diabetes mellitus, starvation and malabsorption **microvascular s** small fat vacuoles giving the liver cells foamy appearance found in fatty liver of pregnancy, Reye's syndrome, certain inherited metabolic disorders and drugs

Stein-Leventhal (stin-lev′en-thal) **syndrome** chronic anovulation with hyperandrogenism, described by Irving Stein and Michael Leventhal, US obstetricians.

Steinmann's (stin′-manz) **pin** a metal rod used for internal fixation of a fracture, named after Fritz Steinmann, Swiss surgeon

stellate (stel′at) star-shaped; arranged in rosettes **s cell** any cell having a star shape as astrocytes and Kupffer's cells **s fracture** a fracture with many fissures that radiate from central point of injury **s ganglia** fused lower cervical and first thoracic ganglia of the sympathetic chain

stellectomy (ste-lek′ta-me) excision of a portion of the stellate ganglion

Stellwag's sign infrequent blinking in thyrotoxicosis, named after Carl Stellwag, Austrian ophthalmologist

stem any stalk-like structure **s cell** an undifferentiated cell that can differentiate in more than one direction **s cell factor** growth factor influencing proliferation and differentiation of stem cells

sten(o) combining word for narrow; contracted; constriction

stenochoria (sten′o-kor′e-a) stenosis

stenocoriasis (-ka-ri′a-sis) contraction of the pupil

stenopic (-pe′ik) having a narrow opening; slit

stenosed (ste-nozd) narrowed, constricted

stenosing tenosynovitis fibrous thickening of tendon sheath especially of wrist and palm, affecting their movement

stenosis (ste-no′sis) a stricture or narrowing of any canal, especially of the cardiac valves **aortic s** narrowing of the aortic valve orifice or of the aorta near the valve **cicatrical s** stenosis from any contracted cicatrix **hypertrophic pyloric s** congenital pyloric stenosis due to hypertrophy of the pyloric sphincter presenting with projectile vomiting in second or third week of life **idiopathic hypertrophic subaortic s** left ventricular outflow obstruction due to hypertrophy of the ventricular septum **lumbar s** narrowing of lumbar canal from overgrowth of laminae of vertebrae **mitral s** narrowing of the mitral valve **pulmonary s** narrowing of the opening between pulmonary artery and the right ventricle **pyloric s** hypertrophy of the walls of pyloric orifice causing obstruction **tricuspid s** narrowing of the orifice of the tricuspid valve

stenothermal (sten'o-ther'mal) able to withstand only slight changes in temperature

stenothermic (-ther'mik) developing within a narrow range of temperature, referring to bacteria

stenothorax (-thor'aks) a narrow contracted chest

Stensen's duct parotid duct, named after Niels Stensen, Danish anatomist

stent 1. a device used to maintain a bodily orifice or cavity during skin grafting 2. a slender rod or thread placed within the lumen of a tubular structure to provide support that are anastomosed **coronary s** a piece of coated metallic 'scaffolding' that can be deployed on a balloon to maintain dilatation of a stenosed coronary artery after PTCA **urologic s** a cylindrical device, made of mesh introduced into urethra or ureter during cystoscopy

stephanion (ste-fa'ne-on) intersection of the superior temporal line and the coronal suture

sterc (o) combining word for faeces

stercobilin (ster'ko-bi'lin) brown-orangered pigment, an oxidised product of stercobilinogen, excreted in the stool

stercobilinogen (-bi-lin'o-jen) substance formed by metabolism of conjugated bilirubin by colonic bacteria, excreted in the stool

stercolith (ster'ka-lith) faecalith

stercoroma (ster'ko-ra'ma) accumulation of inspissated faeces in the colon or rectum giving an appearance of abdominal tumour

stercus (ster'kus) faeces; dung **stercoral** adj

stereo combining word for solid; firmly established; three-dimensional

stereoarthrolysis (ster'e-o-ar-throl'i-sis) production of a new joint with mobility in bony ankylosis

stereoauscultation (-aus'kul-ta'shun) auscultation by a stethoscope with two chest pieces that may be placed on different parts of the chest

stereocompimeter (-kam-pim'e-ter) an instrument to measure visual field of both eyes simultaneously

stereocinefluorography (-sin'e-floor-og'rafe) motion picture photography of images providing a three-dimensional visualisation

stereoencephalotome (-en-sedf'a-la-tom) a guiding instrument used in stereotaxic surgery

stereoencephalotomy (-en-sef'a-lot'a-me) destruction of deep-seated brain structures by use of three-dimensional coordinates

stereognosis (ster'e-og-no'sis) recognition of the commonly used object by feeling its size, shape, weight and form when kept in hand while the eyes are closed and it is dependent on the sense of touch, position and movement

stereoisomer (ster'e-o-i'so-mer) a molecule having the same number and type of a groupings as another but in a different arrangement to give different properties

stereoisomerism (-i-som'er-izm) isomerism exhibiting different spatial arrangement of the same groups

stereoscope (ster'e-o-skop) an instrument that produces an impression of solidity or depth of objects by combining images of two similar pictures of an object

stereotactic (-tak'tik) 1. pertaining to stereotactic surgery 2. characterised by precise positioning in space

stereotaxis (-tak'sis) surgical technique depending on accurate three-dimensional localisation within the skull

stereotropism (ster'e-ot'ra-pizm) growth or movement of a part of an organism and may be positive toward or negative away from a solid body

stereotypy (ster'e-o-ti'pe) repetition of meaningless, often bizarre action

steric (ster'ik) pertaining to stereochemistry

sterilant (ster'i-lant) an agent that destroys microorganisms

sterile (ster'il) 1. aseptic, free from living microorganisms 2. barren; not fertile

sterilisation (ster'i-li-za'shun) 1. a process that destroys pathogens by autoclaving pressurised moist heat or by dry heat 2. any procedure like vasectomy or tubectomy making an individual incapable of reproduction

steriliser (ster'i-li'zer) an apparatus for rendering objects aseptic

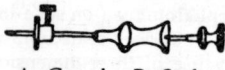

A. Guard;   B. Stylet

Sternal puncture needle

sternal (ster-n'l) of or relating to the sternum s **angle** junction of the manubrium with the body of the sternum and it corresponds with the attachment of the second costal cartilage on either side of the sternum and is recognised as a transverse bony ridge s **puncture** marrow aspiration from the centre of manubrium sterni or body of the sternum by a short bevelled wide bore needle with a stylet fitted with an adjustable guard in front

sternalgia (ster-nal'ja) pain in the sternum

sternebra (ster'ne-bra) any of the segments of the sternum in early life that fuse to form the body of the sternum

stern(o) combining word for sternum

sternoclavicular (ster'no-kla-vik'uler) pertaining to the sternum and clavicle

sternocleidomastoid (-kli'do-mas'toid) pertaining to the sternum, clavicle and mastoid process

sternocostal (-kos't'l) pertaining to the sternum and ribs

sternodymus (ster-nod'i-mus) conjoined twins fused at the anterior chest wall

sternohyoid (ster'no-hi'oid) pertaining to the sternum and hyoid bone

sternoid (ster'noid) resembling the sternum

sternomastoid (ster'no-mas'toid) pertaining to the sternum and mastoid process

sternopagus (ster-nop'a-gus) sternodymus

sternopericardial (ster'no-per'i-kar'de-al) pertaining to the sternum and pericardium

sternoschisis (ster-nos'ki-sis) congenital fissure of the sternum

sternothyroid (ster'no-thi'roid) pertaining to the sternum and thyroid cartilage or gland

sternotomy (ster-not'a-me) operative cutting through the sternum

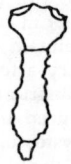

Sternum

sternum (ster'num) see Table of bones

sternutatory (ster-nu'ta-tor'e) causing sneezing

steroid (ster'oid) any of a group of polycyclic compounds containing in its chemical nucleus perhydrocyclopentanophenanthrene ring

steroidogenesis (ster-roi'do-gen'e-sis) production of steroids

sterol (ster'ol) a steroid of 27 or more carbon atoms with one OH group

stertor (ster'tor) the act of snoring

stethalgia (steth-al'jah) pain in the chest,

steth(o) combining word for chest

stethogoniometer (steth'o-go'ne-om'e-ter) an apparatus for the measurement of curvature of the chest

stethometer (steth-om'e-ter) an instrument to measure circular dimension or expansion of the chest

stethoscope (steth'os'ka-pe) an instrument consisting of ear piece, metal frame, rubber or plastic tube and chest piece (bell and diaphragm) used to transmit sounds produced in the body to the examiner's ears

stethoscopy (steth-os'ka-pe) examination with stethoscope

stethospasm (steth'o-spasm) spasm of the chest

sthenia (sthe'ne-a) a condition of activity

sthenic (sthen'ik) a stocky and muscular body configuration

Stevens-Johnson syndrome severe bullous erythema multiforme with involvement of several mucosae including the mouth, eye and genitals accompanied by constitutional disturbance often from drug sensitivity, named after Albert Stevens, and Frank Johnson US paediatricians

stibialism (stib'e-a-lizm) chronic antimonial poisoning

stibium (stib'e-um) antimony symbol Sb

stibocaptate (stib'o-kap'tat) potassium antimony dimercaptosuccinate

stibogluconate a pentavalent antimony compound used intravenously in the treatment of visceral leishmaniasis

stigma (stig'ma) 1. visible evidence of a disease 2. any spot or blemish on the skin 3. mark of disgrace

stilet (sti'let) stylet

stilboestrol synthetic oestrogen used in cancer of prostate and breast

still birth (stil'berth) delivery of a dead foetus **s b ratio** the number of still births per thousand still and live births in the same period

still born born dead

Still's disease juvenile rheumatoid arthritis, named after Sir George Still, British physician

stimulant (stim'u-lant) 1. stimulating 2. an agent that increases activity

stimulate (stim'i-lat) to increase the functional activity of an organ or structure

stimulation (stim'u-la'shun) 1. arousal of the body or its parts to increased functional activity 2. the condition of being stimulated

stimulator (stim'u-la'tor) stimulant

stimulus (stim'u-lus) pl **stimuli** 1. stimulant 2. that which can elicit response in an excitable tissue

sting 1. sharp momentary pain produced by puncture of the skin 2. the venomous apparatus of a stinging organism 3. the organ used to inflict such an injury

stippling (stip'ling) 1. punctate appearance 2. *rad* white granularity in a radiolucent background

stirrup (stir'up) stapes

stitch (stich) 1. suture 2. a momentary sharp pain

Stockholm syndrome a phenomenon where the victim starts to sympathise and identifies with the cause of his or her aggressor, term coined after a 1973 bank robbery in which four Swedes held in a bank vault became attached to their captors

stoichiology (stoi'ke-ol'a'je) the physiology of the cellular elements of tissues

stoke (stok) a unit of viscosity

Stokes-Adams syndrome *see* Adams-Stokes syndrome

stoma (sto'ma) 1. the mouth 2. a minute opening 3. an artificial opening between two cavities or canals

stomach (stom'ak) the J-shaped musculomembranous enlargement of the alimentary canal directly under the diaphragm in the epigastric, umbilical and left hypochondriac regions of the abdomen, between the oesophagus and small intestine. It consists of a cardiac part, a fundus, a body and a pyloric part. Its glands secrete gastric juice which when mixed with food forms chyme making it suitable for further digestion **cascade s** a form of hourglass stomach in which there is constriction between the cardiac and pyloric portions **hourglass s** division of stomach into two parts by scar in chronic duodenal ulcer resembling an hourglass in shape **leather bottle s** a type of stomach with hypertrophy of its walls by infiltration with malignant tissue **watermelon s** gastric antral vascular ectasia where linear angioid streaks converge at the pylorus in the pattern reminiscent of watermelon, which presents with acute gastric bleeding or chronic iron deficiency anaemia

stomachalgia (stum'a-kal'jah) pain in the stomach

stomal ulcer ulcer at the site of gastrojejunostomy

stomatalgia (sto'ma-tal'jah) pain in the mouth

stomatitis (sto'ma-ti-tis) inflammation of the mucous membrane of the mouth

stomat (o) combining word for mouth

stomatocytes cup-shaped erythrocytes

stomatodeum common precursor of nasal cavity and mouth

stomatodynia (sto'ma-to-din'e-a) pain in the mouth

stomatognathic (sto'ma-tog'nath'ik) referring to the mouth and jaws together

stomatology (sto'ma-tol'a-je) branch of medicine concerned with the mouth and its diseases

stomatomalacia (sto'ma-to-ma-la'hah) softening of the structures of the mouth

stomatomenia (-me'ne-a) bleeding from the gums occurring as a form of vicarious menstruation.

stomatomycosis (-mi-ko'sis) any fungal disease of the oral cavity

stomatopathy (sto'ma-top'a-the) any disease of the mouth

stomatorrhagia (sto'ma-to-ra'jah) bleeding from the mouth

stomocephalus (sto'mo-sef'a-lus) a foetus with poorly developed mouth and jaw

stomodeum (-de'um) an ectodermal depression at the cranial end of an embryo that forms front part of the mouth.

-stomy combining word for creation of an opening into or a communication between

stone (ston) a calculus **bile duct s** common bile duct stone may develop from biliary sludge due to dysfunction of sphincter of Oddi many years after cholecystectomy or may migrate from the gall bladder **dental s** a hemihydrate of gypsum used in the preparation of dental models **gall bladder s** gall stones which may be cholesterol or pigment stones **salivary s** a calcified stone present in the ducts of salivary glands **urinary tract s** aggregates of crystals and small amount of protein and glycoprotein found as sand anywhere in the urinary tract or as a round stone in the bladder

stool (stool) 1. faeces 2. evacuation of the bowel **bloody s** blood in the stools as in dysentery **fatty s** stools containing fat as in malabsorpition syndrome and pancreatic disease **lienteric s** stool that contains undigested material **mucous s** stools containing large amount of mucus **pea soup s** liquid stools of enteric fever **pipe stem s** stools resembling a pipe stem in stricture of rectum **rice water s** watery stools in cholera **tarry s** stools appearing like a tar as in upper GI bleed

storiform (stor'i-form) a matted irregularly whorled patterns

storm 1. an exacerbation of symptoms 2. a crisis in the course of a disease

strabismometer (stra-biz-mom'e-ter) an instrument for measuring strabismus

strabismus (stra-biz'mus) failure of eyes to fix at the same point; squint

strabotomy (stra-bot'a-me) division of one or more ocular muscles or their tendons for the correction of squint

straight tubule a duct in a testis leading from a convoluted seminiferous tubule to the rete testis

strain (stran) 1. to exert to the utmost 2. subline of species 3. a hereditary tendency 4. to filter

strait (strat) opening of pelvic canal **inferior s** the lower opening or outlet of pelvic canal **superior s** upper opening or inlet of the pelvic canal s **back syndrome** loss of normal dorsal curvature leading to chest deformity and cardiac abnormalities

strands epithelial cells in single file between collagen bundles

strangle (strang'gl) to suffocate; to choke

strangulated (strang'gu-la-ted) constricted so as to prevent passage of sufficient amount of air, as through the trachea or to cut off venous return as in a hernia

strangulation (strang'gu-la'shun) 1. asphyxiation by neck compression 2. passage of a motile tissue through an orifice, as in hernia, tight enough to stop blood flow

strangury (strang'gu-re) frequent painful passage of urine

strap to apply overlapping strips of adhesive plaster s **cell** an elongated eosinophilic cell with vague cross-striations seen in rhabdomyosarcoma

stratification selection of groups in clinical trials to be equal in terms of a factor such as age that can affect the outcome

stratiform (strat'i-form) occurring in layers

stratigraphy (stra-tig'ra-fe) tomography

stratum (stra'tum) pl **strata** a layer s **basalis** the outer layer of the endometrium next to the myometrium that is maintained during menstruation and gestation s **functionalis** the inner layer of endometrium; the layer next to the uterine cavity that is shed during menstruation and that forms the maternal part of the placenta during gestation s **germinativum** multiplying layer of the epidermis

streak (strek) a line or stria

street virus virus that is in its natural or genetically unmodified form

strephosymbolia (straf'o-sim-bo'le-a) perception of objects reversed as if in a mirror

strept (o) combining word for twisted; curved

Streptobacillus (strep'to-ba-sil'lus) a genus of gram-negative bacteria that are highly pleomorphic; *S. moniliformis* is a causative agent of rat bite fever

Streptococcaceae (-kok-a'se-a) a family of gram-positive cocci that occur in chains or pairs

streptococcaemia (-kok-se'me-a) streptococci in the blood

Streptococcus (-kok'us) a genus of gram-positive cocci dividing in one direction only forming chains. Some of the species are highly pathogenic **alpha haemolytic** s streptococci causing partial haemolysis of blood on blood agar plates **beta haemolytic** s streptococci causing complete haemolysis of the blood in blood agar plates *S. agalactiae* a group of beta haemolytic species found in raw milk responsible for sepsis in new-born and endometritis in post partum women *S. faecalis* an enterococcus found in the alimentary tract that may cause urinary tract infections *S. pneumoniae* an oval or spherical, gram-positive cocci possessing a capsule with more than 80 serological strains and is responsible for lobar pneumonia and other infections in different parts of the body *S. pyogenes* any of the group of beta haemolytic streptococci causing suppuration *S. viridans* a group of alpha haemolytic streptococci found in upper respiratory tract and a common agent causing subacute infective endocarditis

streptodornase (-dor'nas) DNA-splitting enzyme produced by group A streptococci

streptokinase (-ki'nas) a streptococcus produced plasminogen activator that increases plasmin levels to dissolve recently formed clots

streptolysin (strep-tol'i-sin) haemolysin of haemolytic streptococci

streptomyces (strep'to-mi'sez) a group of soil bacteria order Actinomycetales that are a source of various antibiotics

streptomycin (-mi'sin) an aminoglycoside antibiotic obtained from *Streptomyces griseus* effective against mycobacteria, and a variety of aerobic gram-negative bacilli and some gram positive bacteria

streptosepticemia (-sep'ti-se'me-a) septicemia due to streptococcal infection

streptozocin (-zo'sin) an antineoplastic agent from *Streptomyces achromogenes* used in the treatment of islet tumour of pancreas

stereognosis (ster'e-og-no'sis) ability to recognise the common objects by feeling its size, shape, weight and form when kept in the hand while the eyes are closed. It is dependent on the sense of touch, position and movement.

stress (stres) 1. force exerted in any direction or manner between two bodies **s fracture** a fracture resulting from repeated, relatively trivial trauma to the bone **s profile** a description of a patient's neurophysiological responses to various degrees of stress **test** Treadmill exercise test to assess cardiovascular status **s ulcers** acute peptic ulcer from burns, injury or sepsis

stretch to extend; to draw out; to expand **s receptor** receptor in the walls of the bronchi, bronchioles and lung. that send impulses to the respiratory centre that prevent overinflation of the lungs *see* J receptors **s reflex** a lower motor neuron reaction in which stretching of the muscle makes it contract

stretcher (strech'er) a contrivance to carry sick, injured or dead

stretching a therapeutic method designed to elongate pathologically shortened soft tissue stretched and thereby to increase range of motion. cyclic s a repeated passive stretch usually applied by a mechanical device. passive s a type of mobility exercise in which manual, mechanical or positional stretch is applied to soft tissues and in which the force is applied opposite to the direction of shortening. selective s. the

process of stretching some muscle groups which selectively allow others to become light to improve function in a patient with paralysis.

stria pl **striae** a streak-like, linear, atrophic, pink, purple or white line on the skin due to changes in the connective tissue **s gravidarum** curved pink streaks on lower abdomen following pregnancy due to stretch damage to elastic tissue in the skin

striate (stri'at) striated

striated (stri'at-ed) having stripes or striae

striation (stri'a-shun) 1. stria 2. the act of making striae

striatonigral (stri'a-to-ni'gral) referring to the connections of the striation with substantia nigra

striatum (stri-a'tum) corpus striatum **striatal** adj

strictition the reduction of the total volume when mixed due to solute-solvent interaction

stricture (strik'chur) an abnormal narrowing of a duct or passage

stricturisation (strik'thur-i-za'shun) the process of decrease in caliber

strictureplasty (strik'chur-plas'te) surgical enlargement of a stricture of the bowel by longitudinal incision and transverse suturing of the stricture

stridor (stri'dor) a loud, musical sound of constant pitch heard in laryngeal or intratracheal obstruction. The crowing sounds are accompanied by supraclavicular inspiratory retraction

string sign a radiologically visible thin line of contrast in Crohn's disease

striocerebellar (stri'o-ser'e-bel'or) pertaining to the corpus striatum and cerebellum

strip 1. to express the contents from a canal or tube by running the finger along it 2. subcutaneous excision of a vein in its longitudinal axis

strobila segments of a tapeworm

stroke (strok) a rapidly developing clinical symptoms and/or signs of focal (at times global) disturbance of cerebral function, with symptoms lasting for more than 24 hours or leading to death with no apparent cause other than that of vascular origin **heat s** *see* heat stroke **ischaemic s** sudden onset of stroke due to diminished blood supply to the brain **paralytic s** sudden onset of paralysis from an injury to the brain or spinal cord **s in evolution** cerebral ischaemia progressing to hemiplegia over several hours **s volume** amount of blood pumped by either ventricle per beat and it is dependent upon end-diastolic pressure and peripheral vascular resistance (after load) **s work** external work performed by the ventricle with each beat. It maintains perfusion and oxygen delivery to all organs

stroma (stro'ma) pl **stromata** supporting connective tissue of epithelial organ

stromatosis non-malignant infiltration of uterine muscle by endometrial stroma

stromuhar (strom'oor) an instrument for measuring the blood flow

Strongyloides (stron'ji-loi-dez) a very small nematode (2 mm × 0.4 mm) which parasites the mucosa of the upper part of the small intestine. The eggs hatch in the intestine and larvae are passed in the stool. They moult in moist soil and become infective filariform larvae and penetrate human skin and undergo a developmental cycle

strongyloidiasis (stron'ji-loi-di'a-sis) infestation with the namatode *Strongyloides stercoralis* presenting with itchy rash, abdominal pain, steatorrhoea, and weight loss **systemic s** stronglyloides hyperinfestation syndrome occurring in association with immune suppression presenting with diarrhoea, pneumonia and meningoencephalopathies

strongyloidosis (-do'sis) stronglyloidiasis

strongylosis (stron'ji-lo'sis) infestation with Strongylus

Strongylus (stronji-lus) a genus of parasitic nematode

strontium (stron'she-um) chemical element at. no. 38 symbol Sr.

STP standard temperature and pressure **D STP** a d (dry) complete absence of water STP

straight leg raising test in conditions of sciatica, attempts by the patient to raise his extended leg are restricted by pain. The extended leg cannot be elevated passively with the examiner's hand. This is due to the entrapment of spinal roots

strophulus (strof'u-lus) papular urticaria

struma (stroo'ma) *Ger* goitre, name from a Bulgarian river Struma showing high incidence of the condition

strumectomy (stroo-mek'ta-me) excision of a goitre

Strumpell-Marie disease ankylosing spondylitis, named after Adolf Strumpell, German physician and Pierre Marie, French physician

strurite magnesium-ammonium phosphate found in infective urinary stones

stumitis (stroo-mi'tis) thyroiditis

strychnine (strik'nin) a poisonous alkaloid from *Strychnos nux-vomica*. It causes excitation of all parts of central nervous system by blocking neural impulses and is used in experimental pharmacology

STS serological tests for syphilis

Stuart-Power factor coagulation factor X, vitamin K dependent

stump distal end of a limb left after amputation

student's elbow olecranon bursitis

Student's t test *stat* method of testing significance of difference between means of two populations when one or both samples are small

stunning (stun'ing) loss of function **myocardial s** temporary impairment of myocardial function due to a brief episode of myocardial ischaemia

stunting failure to maintain normal growth and weight gain due to prolonged nutritional deficiency or chronic disease

stupe (stoop) a counter-irritant for topical use

stupefacient (stoo'pe-fa'shent) 1. inducing stupor 2. an agent that induces stupor

stupor (stoo'per) a state wherein the patient shows response on vigorous stimuli but sinks back to the original state as soon as the painful stimulus is withdrawn

Sturge-Weber syndrome encephalotrigeminal angiomatosis presenting as cutaneous vascular portwine naevus on the face, contralateral hemiparesis and hemiatrophy, glaucoma and seizures, named after William Sturge and Frederick Weber, British physicians

stuttering (stut'er-ing) 1. a defective speech pattern wherein there is staccate repetition of the first phoneme of a spoken phrase 2. intermittent progression of disease

stye (sti) hordeolum

stylet (sti'lit) 1. a wire running through a catheter or cannula to make it stiff or to clear its passage 2. a slender probe

styl(o) combining word for stake; pole: styloid process of the temporal bone

stylohyoid (sti'lo-hi'oid) pertaining to the styloid process and hyoid bone

styloid (sti'loid) one of several slender bony processes

styloiditis (sti'loi-di'tis) inflammation of a styloid process

stylomastoid (sti'lo-mas'toid) pertaining to the styloid and mastoid processes of the temporal bone

stylomaxillary (-mak'si-lar'e) pertaining to the styloid process of the temporal bone and the maxilla

stylus (sti'lus) 1. stylet 2. a probe or slender wire or needle for stiffening or clearing a canal 3. a pointed medicinal preparation in the form of a stick

stypsis (stip'sis) use of an astringent

styptic (stip'tik) 1. astringent 2. haemostatic

sub combining word for under; near; almost

subabdominal (sub'ab-dom'i-n'l) below the abdomen

subacromial (-a-kro'me-al) below the acromion **s bursitis** painful gout-like attacks of inflammation following rupture of calcific material into the subacromial bursa

subacute (-a-kut) a condition between acute and chronic **s combined degeneration of cord** a combined system disease and funicular myelitis characterised by progressive spastic and ataxic paraparesis and distal neuropathy due to vitamin B_{12} deficiency. There is symmetric demyelination in posterior and lateral columns **s infective endocarditis** a microbial infection of a heart valve, the lining of a cardiac chamber or blood vessel or a congenital abnormality like septal defect presenting with fever, tiredness, night sweats, weight loss, new signs of valve dysfunction or heart failure. There may be features of embolic stroke or peripheral arterial embolism. Other features are purpura, petechial haemorrhages, splinter haemorrhage, Osler's nodes, digital clubbing, splenomegaly and microscopic haematuria **s necrotic myelitis** a progressive ascending motor, sensory and autonomic paralysis due to necrosis and distension of the spinal cord **s sclerosing panencephalitis** (SSPE) a slow form of measles encephalitis affecting children and adolescents, has an insidious onset manifesting with poor performance in studies, incoordination, ataxia, pyramidal and extrapyramidal manifestations, aphasia and optic atrophy

subalimentation (sub-al'i-men-ta'shun) insufficient nutrition

subaortic stenosis subvalvular aortic stenosis

subaponeurotic (-a'p-o-noo-rot'ik) below an aponeurosis

subarachnoid (sub'a-rak'noid) between the arachnoid and pia mater **s haemorrhage** bleeding into the subarachnoid space. It results in blood spilling over into the cerebrospinal flow resulting in bloody CSF. It presents with sudden severe headache, which frequently spreads to the cervical region, nausea, vomiting with loss of consciousness. There is neck stiffness, focal neurologic deficit and/or cranial nerve palsy

subareolar (-a-re′o-lar) beneath the areola

subastragular (-as-trag′a-ler) below the a stragalus

subaural (sub-aw′ral) below the ear

subcapsular (sub-kap′su-ler) below a capsule, referring to the capsule of the cerebrum

subclass (sub′klas) a taxonomic category subordinate to a class and superior to an order

subclavian (sub-kla′ve-an) below the clavicle **s steal syndrome** a cerebrovascular insufficiency caused by stenosing atherosclerosis of left subclavian artery, proximal to the origin of the vertebral artery which reverses the blood flow to the vertebral artery 'stealing' the blood from posterior cerebral circulation —

subclavicular   (sub-kla′vik′u-ler) subclavian

subclinical (sub-kl′in′i-k′l) without obvious clinical manifestations

subclone (sub′klon) the progeny of a mutant cell arising in a clone

subconjunctival (sub′kon-jungk-ti′val) beneath the conjunctiva

subconscious (sub-kon′shus) 1. partially conscious 2. occurrence of mental processes without the individual being aware of their occurrence

subconsciousness (-nes) a state in which the mental processes occur without the conscious perception of the individual

subcoracoid (-kor′a-koid) under the coracoid process

subcortex (-kor′teks) any part of the brain lying below the cerebral cortex

subcostal (-kos′t′l) **subcortical** adj below a rib or ribs

subcranial (-kra′ne-al) below the cranium

subcrepitant (-krep′i-tint) nearly crepitant

subculture (sub′kul-chur) the transfer of a small part of a culture to a new container to continue its growth

subcutaneous (sub′ku-ta′ne-us) beneath the skin

subdiaphragmatic (sub-di′a-frag-mat′ik) below the diaphragm

subdural (-door′al) between the dura mater and arachnoid **s haematoma** venous blood after trauma

subendocardial (sub′en-do-kar′de-al) beneath the endocardium

subendothelial (-en-do-the′le-al) beneath the endothelium

subepicardial (-ep-i-kar′de-al) below the epicardium

subepidermal (-der′mal) beneath the epidermis

subepithelial (-the′le-al) beneath the epithelium

suberosis an extrinsic allergic alveolitis caused by exposure to cork dust and fungus such as Penicillium

subfamily (sub′fam-i-li) a taxonomic division between a family and a tribe

subfascial (sub-fash′ul) beneath a fascia

subfrontal (-frun′tal) situated underneath the frontal lobe

subgenous (sub′je-nus) a taxonomic category between a genus and a species

subglenoid (sub-gle′noid) beneath the glenoid fossa

subglossal (-glos′al) below the tongue

subglottic stenosis narrowing upper end of trachea or lower end of larynx, usually following prolonged endotracheal intubation

subgrondation (sub′gron-da′shun) a type of depressed fracture of the skull with depression of one fragment of bone beneath another

subhepatic (-he-pat′ik) below the liver

subhyoid (sub-hi′oid) below the hyoid bone

subiculum (su-bik′u-lum) an underlying structure.

subiliac (sub-il′e-ak) below the ilium

subinvolution (sub′in-vo-loo′shun) incomplete involution subjacent (sub-ja'sent) situated beneath

subject (sub-jekt) 1. a person or animal subjected to treatment, observation or experiment 2. to cause, to undergo or submit to

subjective global assessment physician's overall judgement on all available evidence, as in giving fitness certificate for operation

subjugal (sub-joo'gal) below the zygomatic bone

sublatioretinae (-la'she-o-ret'i-ne) detachment of the retina

sublethal (-le'thal) insufficient to cause death

sublimation (sub'li-ma'shun) 1. the conversion of a solid directly into a gas 2. diversion of primitive impulse into acceptable activity

sublime (sub-lim) 1. to bring to a state of vapour by heat and condense again by cold 2. awakening feelings of awa

subliminal (-lim'i-n'l) below the threshold of consciousness

sublingual (-ling'gwal) beneath the tongue

sublinguitis (sub'lingwi'tis) inflammation of the sublingual gland

subluxation (-luk-sa'shun) incomplete dislocation, especially when joint surfaces remain in contact but displaced from normal position

submammary (sub-mam'a-re) below the mammary gland

submandibular (sub'man-dib'u-ler) below the mandible

submaxilla (-mak-sil'a) mandibula

submaxillaritis (sub-mak'si-ler-i'tis) inflammation affecting the submandibular salivary gland as in mumps

submaxillary (-mak'si-lar'e) below the maxilla

submental (-men't'l) beneath the chin

submentovertical longest effective diameter of the foetal head as in brow presentation

submersion syndrome a near-drowned condition manifesting with breathlessness, cyanosis and fever

submicroscopic (-mi'kro-skop'ik) too small to be visible with the ordinary light microscope

submucosa (sub'mu-ko'sa) beneath a mucous membrane

submucous (sub-mu'kus) tissue beneath a mucous membrane s fibrosis of mouth severe fibrosis of structures of oral cavity affecting mobility

subnasale (-na-sa'le) the point at which the nasal septum merges with the upper lip in the mid-sagittal plane

subnasion (sub-na'zi-on) subnasale

subneural (sub-noor'al) beneath a nerve

subnormal (-nor'm'l) below normal

subnucleus (-no'kle-us) a secondary nucleus

suboccipital (sub'ok-sip'it'l) below the occiput

suborbital (sub-or'ni-t'l) beneath the orbit

suborder (sub'order) a taxonomic category between an order and a family

subpatellar (sub'pa-tel'er) below the patella

subpericardial (-per-i-kar'de-al) beneath the pericardium

subperiosteal (-per-e-os'te-al) beneath the periosteum

subperitoneal (-per-i-to-ne'al) beneath the peritoneum

subpharyngeal (-fah-rin'je-al) beneath the pharynx

subphrenic (sub-fren'ik) beneath the diaphragm s abscess abscess between the liver and diaphragm s interposition syndrome interposition of the colon between the liver and diaphragm that may cause abdominal distension with air under diaphragm radiologically

subphylum (sub-fi-lum) a taxonomic category between phylum and a class

subplacenta (sub'pla-sen'ta) the decidua basalis

subpleural (sub-ploor'al) beneath the pleura

subpreputial (sub'pre-pu'shal) beneath the prepuce

subpubic (sub-pu'bik) beneath the pubic bone

subpulmonary (-pul'mo-nar'e) beneath the lung

subretinal (-reti'n'l) beneath the retina

subscapular (-skap'u-ler) below the scapula

subscription (-skrip'shun) prescription carrying directions for compounding

subserous (-ser'us) beneath a serous membrane

subspecies (sub'spe-sez) a taxonomic category subordinate to a species

subspinale (sub'spi-na'le) the most posterior midline point between the nasal spine and the crest of maxilla

substance (sub'stans) matter or molecule or group of molecules of plant or animal origin **ground s** amorphous material in which structural elements are embedded **medullary s** 1. the fatty material found in the myelin sheath of nerve fibres 2. the soft marrow-like substance in the interior of an organ or bones **Nissl s** bodies consisting of granular endoplasmic reticulum and ribosomes found in nerve cells and dendrites **reticular s** neural material consisting of closely intermingled gray and white matter extending throughout the length of spinal cord and upward into thalamus **s abuse** the use of illicit, potentially addicting, drugs such as cocaine, misuse of prescribed drugs with stimulatory or depressant effect on CNS such as amphetamines or barbiturates or habitual use of that possess deleterious effects in addition to desired effects such as alcohol and tobacco **s P** a neurotransmitter found in the basal ganglia, posterior horns of spinal cord and sensory nerves of viscera, acts as a strong vasodilator

substantia (sub-stan'she-a) substance **s alba** white matter in the brain and spinal cord largely composed of nerve fibres **s compacta** the compact non-cancellous portion of bone **s gelatinosa** gelatinous substance found in the apical part of the posterior horn of the spinal cord and it is composed of very small nerve cells **s grisea** gray cell bodies and dendrites of nerve cells **s medullaris medulla s nigra** a large cell mass extending from the rostral border of pons to subthalamus, composed of pigmented cells and cells containing dopamine **s perforata** region in the brain through which many small branches of anterior, middle and posterior cerebral arteries pass 1. transparent connective tissue between Bowman's membrane and Descemet's membrane in the cornea 2. dense white fibrous tissue forming the main mass of the sclera **s spongiosa** cancellous bone in which trabeculae form a lattice work with interstices filled with bone marrow

substernal (sub-ster'n'l) below the sternum

substituent (-stich'u-ent) a substitute

substitution (sub'sti-too'shun) 1. replacement of an atom or group in a compound by another 2. *Psy* an unconscious defence mechanism by which an unacceptable thing is replaced by one that is acceptable **s therapy** replacement of substances normally produced by body especially hormones

substrate (sub'strat) specific substance acted on by enzyme

substructure (-struk-chur) a tissue or a structure beneath the surface

subsultus twitch

subtarsal (sub-tar'sal) below the tarsus

subtentorial (sub'ten-to're-al) beneath the tentorium of cerebellum

subtertian occurring more often than every second day

subthalamus (sub-thal'a-mus) that part of the diencephalon interposed between the thalamus, cerebral peduncle, hypothalamus and midbrain tegmentum

subtribe (sub'trib) a taxonomic category between a tribe and a genus

subtrochanteric (sub'tro-kan-ter'ik) below the trochanter

subungual (sub-ung'gwal) beneath a nail **s exostosis** painful bony overgrowth of distal phalanx of great toe under the nail

suburethral (sub'u-re'thral) beneath the urethra

subvaginal (sub-vaji-n'l) 1. under a sheath 2. below the vagina

subvalvular (-val'vu-lar) below the valve **s aortic stenosis** narrowing of left ventricular outflow tract due to a subvalvular membrane or fibromuscular tissue with systolic murmur better audible in third or fourth interspace without a click **s pulmonary stenosis** infundibular pulmonic stenosis, the systolic murmur audible at a lower level in pulmonary area without a click

subvertebral (-ver'te-bral) on the ventral side of the vertebra

subvolution (sub'vo-loo'shun) turning over a flap of mucous membrane to prevent adhesion

succenturiate accessory **s placenta** detached lobule of placenta functioning normally

succimer (suk'si-mer) an oral agent used in the treatment of lead poisoning in children

succinate (suk'si-nat) any salt or ester of succinic acid

succinic (suk-sin'ik) **acid** an intermediate in the tricarboxylic acid cycle

succinylcholine (suk'si-nil-ko'len) a short acting neuromuscular relaxant

succinyl CoA (suk'si-nil-ko-a) succinyl-coenzyme A, an intermediate product of the tricarboxylic acid cycle

succorrhoea (suk'o-re'a) increased flow of a natural secretion

succus (suk'us) juice; any fluid obtained from a living tissue as secretion especially the digestive juices

succussion (su-kush'un) a shaking **s splash** a splashing sound audible over the chest in hydro- or pyo-pneumothorax while the chest is jerked to-and-fro. It is also heard in conditions of severe distension of the stomach, herniation of stomach or of intestine into the thorax and over a large cavity containing fluid and air in the lung

suck 1. draw in with the mouth 2. to draw the breast

sucking wound wound of chest wall comunicating with pleura

sucralfate a basic aluminium salt of sucrose octasulphate. It has no effect on acid secretion but binds to fibroblast growth factor and to ulcer base reducing the access of pepsin and acid in peptic ulcer

sucrase (soo'kras) a hydrolase that catalyses the breakdown of disaccharides to monosaccharides

sucrose (soo'kros) saccharum, a disaccharide made up of glucose and fructose

sucrosemia (su-kro-se'mi-a) presence of sucrose in the blood

sucrosuria (soo'kro-su're-a) presence of sucrose in the urine

suction (suk'shun) the act of drawing, as fluids by exhausting the air **nasogastric s** the suction of fluid, solid or gaseous material from the gastrointestinal tract by use of tube introduced into the stomach or intestine through the nares **post-tussive s** a sucking noise audible immediately after coughing over a cavity in the lung **s abortion** the removal of products of conception from the uterus by a device that sucks **s biopsy** a method to obtain tissues by a device that applies suction

suctorial (suk-tor'e-al) adapted for sucking

sudamen (soo-da'men) minute epidermal vesicles produced by excessive sweating over a prolonged period

Sudan (soo-dan) any of a variety of dyes used to stain for fats

sudanophilia (soo-dan'o-fil'e-a) affinity of tissues for sudan stain

sudation (soo-da'shun) the process of sweating; perspiration

sudden cardiac death an unexpected natural death from cardiac causes within a short period of time,mostly caused by ventricular arrhythmias

sudden death a person previously in apparent good health falls ill and dies within minutes or at most a few hours

sudomotor (soo'do-mo'ter) stimulating the sweat glands

sudoresis (soo'do-re'sis) profuse sweating

sudoriferous (soo'do-rif'er-us) producing sweat

sudorific (soo'do-rif'ik) causing sweat

sudoriparous (soo'do-rip'a-rus) secreting sweat

suffocation (suf'o-ka'shun) asphyxiation

suffodiens undermining

suffusion (su-fu'zhun) 1. extravasation 2. reddening of the surface 3. condition of being wet with a fluid 4. the act of pouring fluid over the body

sugar (shoog'er) a carbohydrate, that is the chief source of energy **extrinsic s** extracted, refined or concentrated sugar such as sucrose **intrinsic s** naturally incorporated sugars in the cellular structure of fruits or milk **s coating** gray-pink plaque like elevations of cerebellar folia seen with medulloblastoma **s intolerance** diarrhoea due to osmotic effect on unabsorbed sugar **s substitutes** a group of carbohydrates such as fructose, sorbital and xylitol used as replacements of usual dietary sugars in diabetics **s tumour** a benign lung tumour with increased vascularity and polygonal glycogen filled clear cells

sugarcane worker's lung bagassosis

suggestion (sug-jes'chun) 1. implanting of an idea in the mind of another by some word or act 2. incitement **post hypnotic s** the act of exercising control over a hypnotised person by communicating some belief or words

suggillation (sug'ji-la'shun) 1. ecchymosis 2. livedo

suicide (soo'i-sid) the act of taking one's own life **attempted s** an attempt that does not inevitably involve fatal intent

suicidology (soo'i-sid-ol'o-je) the study of causes, prediction and prevention of suicides

sukrameha (s) spermatorrhoea

sula (s) colic

Su Jok an acupuncture technique curing diseases using hands and feet which have harmony with all parts of the body

sulbactum (sul-bak'tam) b-lactamase inhibitor that protects penicillin

sulcate (sul'kat) furrowed

sulcus (sul'kus) a groove, furrow, fissure especially of the brain or slight depression **alveololingual s** the space in the floor of the mouth between the base of the tongue and the alveolar ridge **calcarine s** a fissure on the medial surface of the occipital lobe of the brain, separating the cuneus from lingual gyrus **central s** a fissure on the lateral surface of each cerebral hemisphere at the border between the frontal and parietal lobes **cingulate s** a fissure on the medial surface of the cerebral hemisphere binding the gypus cinguli and paracentral lobule **collateral s** a deep sagittal fissure on the undersurface of the temporal lobe between the fusiform and hippocampal gyri **coronary s** atrioventricular groove on the outer surface of the heart **frontal s** fissure on outer surface of each frontal lobe of cerebrum **gingival s** the space between the surface of the tooth and free gingiva **hippocampal s** a shallow groove on the medial side of hippocampal gyrus **intraparietal s** a groove that separates parietal lobe into a superior and inferior parietal lobule **olfactory s** groove on the inferior surface of each frontal lobe of cerebrum **precentral s** a fissure demarcating the anterior border of precentral gyrus **scleral s** a slight groove at the line of union of sclera and cornea **s cuits** the ridges on the skin of the palmar surface of the fingers and toes **s gluteus** furrow between the buttock and thigh **s matricis unguis** the cutaneous furrow in which the lateral border of nail is situated

sulph - combining word for beginning thus

sulpha (sul'fa) sulphonamides

sulphacetamide (sul'fati-set'amid) soluble sulphonamide used in the treatment of ophthalmic infections

sulphadiazine (-di'a-zen) a diazine derivative of sulphanilamide which readily crosses the blood-brain barrier

sulphadimidine (-di'mi-din) a sulpha preparation that is rapidly absorbed and quickly excreted in the urine

sulphamethizole (sul'fa-meth'i-zol) rapidly excreted sulphonamide used in urinary tract infection

sulphamethoxazole (-meth-ok'sa-zol) a sulphonamide preparation used in combination with trimethoprim

sulphanilamide (-nil'a-mid) first sulphonamide preparation to be discovered, used as a potent antibacterial agent

sulphasalazine (-sal'a-zen) sulphonamide possessing no antibacterial activity used in ulcerative colitis. It is a 5-amino salicylic acid bound by an azo bond to sulphapyridine. The colonic bacteria break the azo bond to release aminosalicylate which has an anti-inflammatory effect on colonic mucosa

sulphatase (sul'fah-tas) an enzyme that hydrolyses sulphuric acid esters

sulphate (sul'fat) a salt or ester of sulphuric acid

sulphatide (sul'fah-tid) cerebroside sulphuric ester

sulphaemoglobin (sulf'he'mo-glo'bin) sulphmethaemoglobin, a complex formed by hydrogen sulphide and ferric ion

sulphaemoglobinaemia (-he'mo-glo'bine'me-a) presence of sulphaemoglobin in the blood exhibiting persistent cyanosis

sulphydryl (sulf-hi-dril) the radical, -SH of sulphur and hydrogen

sulphide (sul-fid) a compound of sulphur having a valence of 2

sulphinpyrazone (sul'fin-pi'ra-zon) an uricosuric agent used in gout

sulphisoxazole (sul'fi-sok'sa-zol) a short acting sulphonamide preparation

sulphite (sul'fit) a salt of sulphurous acid

sulphmethaemoglobin (sulf'met-he'mo-glo'bin) sulphaemoglobin

sulphobromophthalein (sul'fo-bro'mothal'e-in) a sulphur and bromine containing compound used in testing hepatic function

sulphonamide (sul-fon'a-mid) para-amino benzene sulphonamide group of antibacterial agents. They have a synergistic action with trimethoprim, dapsone and pyrimethamine

sulphone (sul'fon) an oxidation product of sulphur compound in which two hydrocarbon radicals are attached to -SO_2- group. Dapsone is a preparation of sulphone

sulphonylurea (sul'fo-nil-u-re'a) hypoglycaemic agent whose action is mediated through stimulation of the release of insulin from the pancreatic beta cells, and may also reduce the hepatic release of glucose and diminish insulin resistance. They are used in the treatment of non-obese patients with type 2 diabetes who fail to respond to dietary measures alone **first generation** s chlorpropamide, tolbutamide and tolazamide **second generation** s glipizide, glicazide and glybenclamide

sulphur (sul'fer) a pale yellow crystalline element, at. no. 6 s **granules** yellow aggregates of filamentous branching actinomycotic bacteria s **test** a pinch of flowers of sulphur when sprinkled on urine sample placed in a beaker, sulphur sinks in presence of bile salts due to lowering of surface tension of urine

sulphurated (sul'fu-rat'ed) combined with or impregnated with sulphur

sulphuric (sul-fur'ik) **acid** H_2SO_4, a colourless, corrosive liquid

sulphurous (sul-fur'us) **acid** H_2SO_3, a solution of sulphur dioxide in water

sumatriptan an agonist of serotonin that causes vasoconstriction of cranial vessels and block extravasation of plasma, used in acute migraine

summation (su-ma'shun) an aggregation of a number of similars

sunburn (sun'bern) erythema caused by exposure to critical amounts of ultraviolet light

sunray spiculation radiological appearance in osteogenic sarcoma where the periosteal reaction shows dense filiform spiculations that are perpendicular to the periosteum

sunscreen (-skren) a substance used to protect the skin from ultraviolet radiation **chemical s** absorb specific wavelength of ultraviolet radiation **physical s** reflect ultraviolet radiation and visible light

sunsetting symmetric downward deviation of the eyes

sunstroke (-strok) heat stroke

super a combining word for above; excessive

superacute (soo'per-a-kut) extremely acute with markedly severe manifestations and rapid progress

superalimentation (soo'per-a-li-menta'shun) increased feeding beyond the needs of appetite

superalkalinity (-al'ka-lin'i-te) excessive alkalinity

supercilia (-sil'e-a) eye brow

supercilium (-sil'e-um) pl **supercilia** the line of hairs at the superior edge of the orbit; eyebrow

superclass (soo'per-klas) a taxonomic category between a phylum and a class

super ego (soo'per-e'go) an outgrowth of ego that has identified with some important persons from early life as a personal standard

super excitation (-ek'si-ta'shun) overstimulation

superfamily (soo'per-fam'i-le) a taxonomic category between an order and a family

superfecundation (soo'per-fe'kun-da'shun) fertilisation of a second ovum by a second sperm after one has already been fertilised

superfemale XXX syndrome

superfetation (-fe-ta'shun) fertilisation and subsequent development of a second ovum after the first has already been implanted in the uterus

superficial (-fish'al) 1. situated near the surface of the body 2. cursory

superficialis (-fish'e-a'lis) superficial

superficies (-fish'e-ez) an outer surface

superinduce (-in-doos) to induce or bring on in addition to something already present

superinfection (-in-fek'shun) an infection that occurs when the native flora of the body have been markedly reduced, often by antibiotic therapy, allowing invasion by opportunistic organisms

superinvolution (-in'vo-lu'shun) marked reduction in the size of the uterus following child birth

superior (soo-per'e-or) 1. situated above 2. directed upward 3. situated near the vertex of the head **s mesenteric artery syndrome** condition due to compression of superior mesenteric artery presenting with postprandial epigastric pain, distension, nausea and weight loss **s venacaval obstruction** obstruction of superior vena cava presenting with bilateral engorgement of the jugular veins, and oedema affecting the face, neck and arms

superjacent (soo'per-ja'sent) immediately above

superlactation (-lak-ta'shun) hyperlactation

supermotility (-mo-til'i-te) increased motility

supernatant (-na'tant) 1. floating on the surface 2. the clear liquid remaining on the top after precipitate settles

supernumerary (-nu'mer-ar'e) exceeding the normal number

superolateral (-o-lat'er-al) above and to the side

superovulate production of more than normal number of ova

superoxide (-ok'sid) a strong acid molecule. HO_2 ($H^+ + O_2^-$), where O_2^- is superoxide molecule. It is a highly reactive form of oxygen **s desmutase** an enzyme found in all aerobes that serves to protect against the damage by oxygen-free radicals

supersaturate (-sach'er-at) saturate beyond the normal point

superscription (-skrip'shun) the beginning of a prescription, take or recipe

superstructure (soo'per-struk'chur) a structure above the surface

supervascularisation (soo'per-vas'ku-lar-i-za'shun) a relative increase in vascularity following destruction of tumour cells by radiotherapy

supervoltage (soo'per-vol'tij) a very high voltage

supinate (soo'pi-nat) 1. to turn the forearm or hand so that palm faces upward 2. to rotate the leg and foot outward

supine (soo'pin) lying on the back with the face upward

suppository (su-poz'i-tor'e) a solid cone-shaped medicated pellet made up of inert substance, that is inserted into the rectum or vagina where it melts and release the drug

suppressant (su-pres'ant) 1. inducing suppression 2. an agent that stops secretion, or excretion

suppression (su-presh'un) 1. arrest of secretion of a fluid 2. deliberately excluding from conscious thought 3. stopping an abnormal flow or discharge 4. masking of a phenotypic expression of a mutation.

suppressor cells CD8 + T-lymphocytes that inhibit antigen responses by decreasing the activity of T helper (CD4) cells **s test** a clinical test or assay to determine whether a hormone produced in excess is under the control of regulating or releasing factor

suppurant (sup'u-rant) causing suppuration

suppuration (sup'u-ra'shun) the formation of pus

supra - combining word for above; over

supraacromial (soo'pra-a-kro'me-al) above acromion

supraauricular (-aw-rik'u-lar) above the auricle of the ear

suprabulge (soo'pra-bulj) the portion of the crown of a tooth that converges toward the occlusal surface of the tooth

supracerebellar (soo'pra-se-re-bel'ar) above the upper surface of the cerebellum

suprachoroid (-kor'oid) on the outer side of the choroid of the eye

suprachoroidea (ko-roi'de-a) the outermost layer of the choroid

supraclavicular (-kla-vik'u-ler) above the clavicle

supraclusion (-kloo'zhun) projection of a tooth beyond the normal occlusal plane

supracondylar (-kon'di-ler) above a condyle

supracostal (-kos't'l) above the ribs

supracotyloid (-koti-loid) above the acetabulum

supradiaphragmatic (-di'a-fra-mat'ik) above the diaphragm

supraduction (-duk'shun) moving upward of an eye

supraepicondylar (-epi-kon'di-ler) above an epicondyle

suprahyoid (-hi'oid) above the hyoid bone

supraliminal (-lim'i-n'l) above the threshold for conscious awareness

supralumbar (-lum'ber) above the lumbar region or loin

supramalleolar (-ma-le'o-ler) above a malleolus

supramaxillary (-mak'si-lar'e) above the maxilla

supranuclear (-nu'kle-ar) 1. cranial to the level of the motor neurones of the spinal or cranial nerves 2. part of a cell between the nucleus and distal border

supraocclusion (-o-kloo'zhun) an occlusal relationship in which a tooth extends beyond the occlusal plane

supraorbital (-or'bi-t'l) above the orbit

suprapelvic (-pel'vik) above the pelvis

suprapontine (-pon'tin) above the pons

suprapubic (-pu'bik) above the pubes

suprarenal (-re'nal) 1. above a kidney 2. pertaining to the suprarenal or adrenal gland

suprarenalectomy (-re'nal-ek'ta-me) adrenalectomy.

suprascapular (-sca-p'u-ler) above the scapula

suprascleral (-skle'ral) on the outer side of the sclera

suprasellar (-sel'er) above the sella turcica

supraspinal (-spi'nl) above a spine

suprasternal (-ster'nl) above the sternum

supratrochlear (-trok'le-ar) above a trochlea, especially that of the humerus

supravaginal (-vaj'i-nl) above the vagina or any sheathing membrane

supravalvar (-val'ver) above a valve **s aortic stenosis** narrowing of the left ventricular outflow just above the sinuses of valsalva, often associated with mental deficiency, elfin facies, and asymmetric carotid pulsations **s pulmonic stenosis** obstruction in the main pulmonary artery above the pulmonary valve

supraventricular above the ventricles **s tachycardia** abnormally fast heart rate due to reentry within AV node

supravergence (-ver'jens) upward rotation of the eye, while the other eye remaining stationary

supraversion (-ver'zhun) 1. a turning upward 2. a tooth out of occlusal line 3. binocular conjugate movement upward

sura (soo'ra) calf formed by the bellies of gastrocnemius and soleus muscles

sural relating to the calf of the leg

suramin agent used in the treatment of trypanosomiasis and onchocerciasis

surfactant (sur-fak'tant) a chemically heterogeneous material consisting of phospholipids and proteins that are present in the alveolar epithelium as a surface active lining complex. It provides a film at the interface between the air and liquid and reduces the surface tension in the lungs. It is necessary for the normal expansion of foetal lung when the infant is transferred from fluid to gaseous environment

surge any increase in the flow of a substance above a relatively constant base line

surgeon (ser'jun) a medical practitioner specialised in surgery and treats disease, injury and deformity by operation or manipulation

surgery (ser'jer-e) 1. that branch of medicine which treats diseases, injuries and deformites by operation or manipulation 2. a place in a hospital where surgery is performed 3. performance or procedures of an operation **ablative s** operation in which a part is removed **ambulatory s** undertaking operation on patients who are admitted to and discharged from the hospital on the same day **aseptic s** operation carried out under aseptic conditions **conservative s** surgery in which as much as possible a part or structure is retained **cosmetic s** surgery to improve the appearance **cytoreductive s** debulking operation **dental s** oral and maxillofacial surgery **exploratory s** an operation undertaken to establish diagnosis **general s** that which deals with surgical problems of all kinds. **major s** surgery involving increased risk to the life **manipulative s** use of manipulation in surgery or bone setting **maxillofacial s** the branch of dentistry concerned with diagnosis and surgical and adjunctive treatment of injuries and deformities of the oral and maxillofacial region **minor s** a simple operative procedure not causing risk to life **open heart s** surgery concerned with correction of intracardiac disease under direct vision **oral s** maxillofacial surgery **orthopaedic s** surgical correction of musculoskeletal diseases, injuries and deformities **plastic s** surgery concerned with the restoration, reconstruction and improvement of shape and appearance of body structures **radical s** surgery designed to remove a large area of damaged or neoplastic tissue or adjoining areas of lymphatic drainage **reconstructive s** plastic surgery **second look s** surgery undertaken at a later date after original operation to detect recurrence of the disease **stereotaxic s** operation to produce sharply circumscribed lesions in specific regions of the brain after locating the structure by three-dimensional coordinates **subtotal s** an operation in which only a portion of the organ is removed

surgical pertaining to surgery **s drain** an appliance inserted into a body cavity' or wound to allow drainage of fluid, pus or air **s emphysema** presence of gas in the subcutaneous tissue which gives a peculiar crackling sensation to the examining fingers and it is like palpating a horse hair mattress. It may be due to trauma leading to fractured ribs or nasal bone, or infections such as gas gangrene or following administration of saline by subcutaneous route or intercostal tubal drainage subcutaneous emphysema **s jaundice** obstructive jaundice **s spares** material used to close surgical incisions

surrogate (sur'o-git) substitute **marker** an indirect indicator of something, such as measurement of viral load to assess the therapeutic response of a drug **s pregnancy** bearing child with an intention of handing over to another whatever source of ova or sperm

sursumduction (sur'sum-duk'shun) supraduction

sursumvergence (-ver'jens) an upward turning, as of the eyeballs

sursumversion (-ver'zhun) the act of moving the eyes upwards

surveillance close observation kept over a person or group especially suspect

susceptible (ser-sep'ti-bl) 1. easily affected or acted upon 2. lacking resistance

sushumna (s) the cental nervous column along which the main chakaras lie

suspended heart cardiothoracic separation which radiologically presents as if heart is suspended in the mid-thorax. It is of no clinical significance.

suspension (sus-pen'shun) 1. readily affected or acted upon 2. lacking resistance or immunity 3. easily influenced 4. a technique to free a body part from the resistance of friction by suspending the part in a sling attached to a rope.

suspensoid (sus-pen'soid) a colloid suspension in which the disperse particles are solid and are sharply demarcated from the fluid in which they are suspended

suspensory (sus-pen'sor-e) 1. supporting a part as a ligament, muscle or bone 2. a sling or bandage that serves to hold up a part 3. a supporter applied to uplift a dependent part as of scrotum or a pendulous breast

sustentacular cells cells within the epithelium supporting other specialised cells

sustentaculum (sus'ten-tak'u-lum) a structure that serves as a support to another

sutura (soo-tur'ah) suture; a type of fibrous joint where two bones are found in membrane

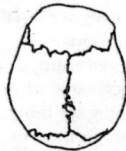

Cravial sutures

suture (soo'cher) 1. surgical stitch used to close an incision of a wound 2. the surgical material so used 3. sutura **absorbable s** a surgical suture material that can be digested by body tissues **apposition s** a suture of the skin only **approximation s** a suture that pulls together the deep tissues **atraumatic s** a suture affixed to the end of an eyeless needle **blanket s** a continuous lock-stitch to approximate the skin of a wound **continuous s** an uninterrupted series of stitches using one suture fastened at each end by a knot **cranial s's** the sutures between the bones of the skull **interrupted s** suture created by passing a needle through both sides of a wound and knotting the ends of the suture material together to one side

SVC 1. slow vital capacity 2. superior vena cava

suxamethonium a short acting depolarising muscle relaxant

svedberg (sfed'berg) (s) a unit of sedimentation co-efficiency equal to 10^{-13} seconds determined by ultra centrifugation, named after Theodor Svedberg, Swedish chemist

swab (swahb) a wad of cotton or gauze attached to one end of a slender stick used for applying medication, removing a substance from a surface or obtaining a piece of tissue or secretion for bacteriological examination

swage (swaj) 1. to shape metal especially around a region to make a close fit. 2. to fuse a suture material to a needle

swallow (swal'o) to pass anything from the mouth through the fauces, pharynx and oesophagus to the stomach; deglutition

swallowing (swal'o-ing) a complicated process initiated voluntarily, then completed reflexly enabling the movement of food from mouth through the pharynx and oesophagus to the stomach

Swan-Ganz catheter a balloon tipped soft, flexible catheter introduced to the right heart through a vein and the balloon guides the catheter to the pulmonary artery. On inflation of the balloon it blocks the flow of blood from the right heart to the lung and enables the recording of the back pressure in the pulmonary artery distal to the balloon, devised by Harold Swan and William Ganz, US physicians

swan-neck a thin curved neck resulting from muscular atrophy, a feature of myotonia dystrophica **s deformity** a deformity of a finger in rheumatoid arthritis, showing marked flexion of the distal interphalangeal joints and hyperextension of the proximal interphalangeal joints

swarming (sworm'ing) the spread of bacteria over a culture medium

swastha (s) health; well-being

swasthvritta (s) regime promoting health

swathya (s) health

sweat (swet) secretion of sweat glands of the skin, a colourless fluid containing sodium chloride, urea and fatty substances. It cools the body by evaporation and also eliminates waste material **s gland** a simple coiled tubular gland found on the body. The coiled secreting part lies in the subcutaneous tissue and the duct passes through dermis and epidermis to its opening, sweat pore. The sweat glands are more numerous in the palms and soles

sweating (swet'ing) 1. the act of perspiration 2. emitting sweat

swedena (s) steam or sweating therapy

sweeny (swe'ne) shoulder slip

sweet 1. pleasing to the taste or senses 2. tasting like sugar 3. beautiful to the eye

Sweet's syndrome a disorder manifesting with fever, raised painful plaques on the face, neck and extremities and polymorphonuclear leucocytosis that responds to corticosteroids, named after Robert Sweet, British physician

swelling (swel'ing) 1. an abnormal enlargement of a part of the body not due to an increase in number of cells 2. an elevation **cloudy s** a degenerative change affecting the protein constituents of the organs presenting a cloudy appearing swelling

Swimmer's itch appearance of papules on the skin of persons who swim in water containing Cercariae of certain schistosomes

swimming pool granuloma a skin granuloma due to *M. marinum* occurring in persons working in marine environment

swoon 1. syncope 2. to faint

Swyer-James lung unilateral transradiant lung or lobe with poor ventilation and perfusion, an acquired condition as an end result of a severe patchy obliterative bronchiolitis occurred in childhood, named after Swyer-James, British physicians

sycoma (si-ko'ma) a large soft wart

sycosiform (si-ko'si-from) resembling sycosis

sycosis (si-ko'sis) deep folliculitis seen in adult males in areas which have coarse hairs. The infection is located in deeper part of hair follicles and lesions consist of painful erythematous papules or pustules **s barbae** sycosis in the beard region **s nuchae** sycosis in the back of the neck

Sydenham's (sid'en-hamz) **chorea** rheumatic chorea, named after Thomas Sydenham, British physician

syllabus (sil'a-bus) an outline of a course of the study

sylvatic plague Bubonic plague that is endemic among wild rodents

sylvian aqueduct a narrow canal from the third to fourth ventricle in the brain, named after Francois Sylvius, Dutch anatomist

symballophone (sim-bal'o-fon) a stethoscope with two chest pieces to lateralise the sounds

symbiont (sim'bi-ont) an organism that lives with another in symbiosis

symbiosis (sim'bi-o'sis) 1. living together of two organisms of different species 2. *Psy* mutually interdependence of two persons

symblepheron (sim-blef'a-run) adhesion of one or both eyelids to the eyeball

symblepharopterygium (-blef'a-ro-fer-ij'e-um) adhesion of the lid to the eyeball through a pterygium-like cicatricial band

symbol something used for or regarded as representing something else

symbolia (sim-bo'le-a) an ability to recognise an object by touch sensation

symbolism (sim'bo-lizm) 1. an abnormal mental state in which everything that happens is considered by the individual as symbolic of his thoughts 2. a process involved in the disguised representation in consciousness of unconscious events

symbolisation (sim'bol-i-za'shun) an unconscious mechanism in which one idea or object comes to represent another because of similarity or association between them.

Syme's operation 1. amputation through the ankle with removal of malleoli 2. excision of the tongue 3. external urethrotomy, named after James Syme, Scottish surgeon

symmelus (sim'e-las) a foetus with fused limbs with or without feet

symmetry (sim'e-tre) equality; correspondence in the shape, size and relative position of parts on opposite sides of the body

sympathectomy (sim'pa-thek'ta-me) excision of a segment of a sympathetic nerve or of one or more sympathetic ganglia

sympathetic (sim-pa-thet'ik) 1. pertaining to the sympathetic nervous system 2. caused by or pertaining to sympathy **s nervous system** one of the two subdivisions of the autonomic nervous system, having cell bodies of preganglionic neurones in the lateral gray columns of the thoracic segment and first two or three lumbar segments of spinal cord (thoracolumbar) **s chain ganglion** a cluster of cell bodies of postganglionic sympathetic neurones lateral to the vertebral column, close to the body of a vertebra. These ganglia extend downward through the neck, thorax and abdomen to the coccyx on both sides of the vertebral column and are connected to one another to form a chain on either side of the vertebral column **s meningitis** mild aseptic meningitis produced by an infective lesion close to meninges. **s ophthalmia** autoimmune uveitis in one eye induced by injury to other

sympathicoblast (sim'path'i-ko-blast) sympathoblast

sympathicoblastoma (sim-pati-ko-blasto'ma) a neuroblastoma arising in one of the sympathetic ganglia

sympathicotonia (-to'ne-a) an increased tonus of the sympathetic nervous system exhibiting a marked tendency for vascular spasm, high blood pressure, tremors of hands, may be seen in thyrotoxicosis

sympathicotripsy (-trip'se) crushing of a sympathetic ganglia

sympathicotropic (-trop'ik) 1. exhibiting an affinity to sympathetic nervous system 2. an agent having an affinity for or exerting its action on sympathetic nervous system

sympathoadrenal (sim'pa-thoa-dre'nl) concerning the sympathetic nervous system and the adrenal medulla

sympathoblast (sim-path'o-blast) a primitive cell from the neural crest glia which forms the adrenal medulla

sympathogonia (sim'op-tho-gone-a) the completely undifferentiated cells of the sympathetic nervous system

sympathogonioma (-go'ne-o'ema) a tumour containing undifferentiated cells of the sympathetic nervous system

sympatholytic (-litik) antagonism to or inhibition of transmission of impulses from the postganglionic fibres to effector organs, inhibiting the smooth muscle contraction and glandular activity

sympathomimetic (-mi'met'ik) 1. producing effects that mimic those caused by the sympathetic nervous system 2. an agent that produces such an effect

sympathy (sim'pa-the) 1. the mutual relation between two organs, systems or parts of the body 2. an emotional concern for and sharing of mental and emotional state of another person

symphalangia (sim'fa-lan'je-a) congenital fusion of contiguous phalanges of a digit

symphyseal (sim-fiz'e-al) relating to symphysis; fused

symphysiorrhapy (sim-fiz'e-or'a-fe) suture of a divided symphysis

symphysiotomy (sim-fiz'e-e-otah-me) division of symphysis pubis to facilitate labour, very rarely performed

symphysis (sim'fi-sis) a line of union; a form of cartilaginous joint without cavity **mental s** the fibrocartilaginousunion of the two halves of the mandible that gets ossified during the first year **pubic s** the firm fibrocartilaginous joint between the two pubic bones

sympodia (sim'po'de-a) fusion of lower extremities

symport (sim'port) process by which two substances move in the same direction across a cell membrane; cotransport

symposium a published collection of opinion or comments on a particular subject; a conference at which a subject is discussed

symptom (sim'ph'tom) an alteration in the body function, appearance or sensation that indicates the presence of a disease or disorder of the body **accessory s** a minor symptom **cardinal s** the primary symptom in the diagnosis of the disease **concomitant s** a symptom accompanying the primary symptom **constitutional s** symptom indicating that the disease has become general **deficiency s** a manifestation of lack of some essential nutrient **delayed s** a symptom appearing sometime after the precipitating cause **equivocal s** a symptom noticed in a variety of diseases **focal s** a symptom at a specific location **general s** constitutional symptom **negative s** absence of symptom expected in a disease **pathognomonic s** a symptom characteristic of a particular disease **presenting s** the symptom for which patient seeks relief **prodromal s** a symptom indicative of beginning of a disease **subjective s** symptom perceptible only to the patient **withdrawal s** symptoms following sudden withdrawal of a substance to which a person has been addicted

symptomatic (simp'to-mat'ik) 1. suggesting presence of underlying condition 2. treatment directed to comfort rather than cure

symptomatology (simp'to-ma-tol'a-je) 1. the branch of medicine dealing with symptoms of various diseases 2. all the manifestations of a given disease

symptomatolytic (simp-to-mat-o-lit'ik) causing the disappearance of symptoms

symptosis (simp-to'sis) gradual wasting of the body or of an organ

sympus (sim'pus) a foetus with fused extremities

syn combining word for union, association; together

synapse (sin'aps) the functional junction between the neurones or between a neuron and an effector such as a muscle or gland. The transmission of impulse occurs by a chemical transmitter or by a direct propagation of the bioelectric potential

synapsis (si-nap'sis) the pairing of homologous chromosomes during prophase I of meiosis

synaptic (si-nap'tik) relating to synapse or synapsis

synaptosome (sin-ap'to-som) synapse isolated from its cell

synarthrodia (sin'ar-thro'de-a) fibrous joint

synarthrophysis (sin-ar'thr'o-phi-sis) the process of ankylosis

synarthrosis (sin-ar-thro'sis) an immobile joint; joint without synovial cavity

syncanthus (sin-kan'thus) adhesion of the eyeball to the structures of the orbit

syncephalus (-sef'a-lus) a conjoined twin having a single head, single face and four ears

synchilia (-ki'le-a) congenital adhesion of lips

synchiria (-ki're-a) a disorder of sensibil-

ity in which a stimulus applied to one side of the body is referred to both sides

synchondrosis (sin'kon-dro'sis) a cartilaginous joint in which the connecting material is a hyaline cartilage or fibrocartilage.

synchondrotomy (-kon-drota-me) division of synchondrosis

synchronism (sin'kro-nizm) simultaneous occurrence of two or more events **synchronous** adj

synchrony (sing'kra-ne) the occurrence of two events simultaneously or with a fixed time interval between them

synchysis (sin'ki-sis) liquefaction of the vitreous body of the eye **s scintillans** appearance of glistening spots in the eye due to cholesterol crystals floating in a fluid vitreous

syncliticism (sin-klit-izm) 1. a condition of parallelism between the planes of the foetal head and of the pelvis 2. normal synchronous maturation of the nucleus and cytoplasm of blood cells

synclitism (sin'kliit-izm) syncliticism

synclonus (-klo-nus) clonic spasm or tremor of several muscles

syncopal (sin'ko-pal) relating to or marked by syncope

syncope a transient loss of consciousness accompanied by loss of postural tone and followed by spontaneous recovery **cardiac s** syncope of cardiac origin due to severe obstruction to cardiac output or disturbances of cardiac rhythm **carotid s** compression of carotid sinus leading syncope that may be cardio-inhibitory manifesting in bradycardia, sinus standstill and AV block that can be prevented by atropine, or vasodepressor manifesting with hypotension prevented by atropine or adrenaline **cough s** markedly raised intrathoracic pressure during paroxysms of prolonged bouts of cough producing syncopal attack**defecation s** sudden rectal emptyingproducing syncope **micturition s** syncope during or immediately after passing urine **multifactorial s** precipitation of syncope in elderly by vascular instability from diseases or physical stresses **neurologic s** syncope due to obstruction of vertebrobasilar artery and is associated with neurologic signs **orthostatic s** occurrence of syncope when a person assumes upright posture and it is due to uncompensated gravitational stress on circulation

syncitial (sin-sish'al) of or relating to a syncytium

syncytioma (-sit'e-oma) a tumour of chorion

syncytiotrophoblast (-sit'e-o-trof'o-blast) the outer syncitial layer of the trophoblast

syncitium (-sish'e-um) a multinucleated mass of protoplasm produced by union of cells

syndactyly (-dak'ti-le) fusion of fingers which may be cutaneous due to bridging of soft tissues or osseous due to bony fusion

syndectomy (-dek'ta-me) excision of a circular strip of conjunctiva around the cornea

syndesis (sin'de-sis) 1. arthrodesis 2. the condition being bound together

syndesmectomy (sin'dez-mek'to-me) the excision of a portion of a ligament

syndesmectopia (-mek-to'pe-a) abnormal position of a ligament

syndesm (o) combining word for connective tissue; ligament

syndesmology (-mol'a-je) study of the ligaments and joints

syndesmoplasty (sin-dez'ma-plas'te) plastic surgery of a ligament

syndesmosis (sin'dez-mo'sis) a joint in which the bones are united by interosseous membrane or ligament

syndesmotomy (-mot'ah-me) surgical division of a ligament

syndrome (sin'drom) a group of signs and symptoms of disease occurring together

syndrome X insulin resistance with central trunkal obesity, impaired glucose tolerance, hypertriglyceridaemia, hypertension and accelerated atherosclerosis

syndromology (sin'drom-ol'a-je) the field concerned with the taxonomy, aetiology and patterns of congenital abnormalities

synechia (si-nek'e-a) pl **synechiae** adhesion especially of iris, cornea and conjunctiva **annular s** an adhesion of iris to the lens throughout its entire pupillary margin **anterior s** an adhesion of the iris to the cornea **posterior s** an adhesion of the iris to the lens **total s** an adhesion of the entire surface of the iris to the lens **s vulvae** a congenital fusion of the labia minora

synechotomy (sin'e-kot'a-me) the division of a synechia or adhesion

synencephalocoele (-en-sef'a-lo-sel) protrusion of brain substance through a defect in the skull and adhesions prevents its reduction

syneresis (si-ner'i-sis) release of part of fluid content of gel

synergism (si-ner'i-jizm) cooperative interaction between two or more components in a system; the combined effect is more than the sum of each individual constituent

synergist (-er-jist) a structure or a drug that aids the action of another

synergy (-er-je) working together, of enzymes and drugs, whose combined effect exceeds their sum

synesthesia (sin'es-the'zhah) inappropriate sensory perception

synesthesialgia (-es-the'ze-al'ja) a painful synesthesia

syngamy (sing'gah-me) conjugation of gametes in fertilisation

syngeneic (sin'je-ne'ik) 1. of same species but not genetically identical 2. immunologically compatible, accepting grafts from each other.

syngenesis (sin-jen'e-sis) sexual reproduction

syngraft (sin'graft) a graft between genetically identical persons, typically between identical twins

synizesis (sin'i-ze'sis) 1. an occlusion or closure 2. a clumping of chromatin at one side of the nucleus during the prophase of mitosis **s pupillae** closure of the pupil of the eye

synkinesis (-ki-ne'sis) involuntary movement of one muscle induced by voluntary movement of another

synecrosis (-ne'kro'sis) association between group or individuals is mutually detrimental

synonym (sin'o-nim) a name or word having the same meaning with another; one of two or more words which have the same meaning

synophthalmus (-of-thal'mus) a congenital defect in which two orbits merge to form a single cavity containing one eye

synorchism (sin'or-kizm) congenital fusion of testes into a single mass

synoscheos (sin-os'ke-us) an adhesion between the penis and the scrotum

synosteotomy (sin'os-te-ot'a-me) dissection of joints

synostosis (-os-to'sis) a joint in which the dense fibrous connective tissue uniting the adjacent bones at a suture has been replaced by bone, resulting in a complete fusion across the suture line

synotia (si-no'she-a) fusion of the lobes of the ear with absence or incomplete development of the mandible

synovectomy (sin'o-vek'ta-me) resection of overgrown synovium in rheumatoid arthritis to prevent destruction of joint cartilage

synovia (si-no've-a) synovial fluid

synovial fluid fluid in the joint cavity which is highly viscous due to presence of hyaluronic acid synthesised by type B cells. It also contains electrolytes, albumin, glucose and water that have their origin from filtration from subsynovial capillaries. The fluid maintains the nutrition of the avascular articular cartilage and lubricates the joint

synovialis (si-no've-a'lis) synovial

synovial membrane the smooth lining of a joint cavity with one or two layers of cells. The cells are of connective tissue origin and are of two types: type A (a phagocytic cell) and type B (fibroblast with well developed endoplasmic reticulum).

synovioma (si-nove-n'o'ma) a highly malignant synovial sarcoma occurring in the knee, ankle, foot or other joints.

synoviorthesis (si-no'ove-or-the'sis) irradiation of synovium to destroy the inflamed synovial tissue

synovitis (sin'o-vi'tis) inflammation of a synovial membrane

synteny (sin'te-ne) the location of two or more genes on the same chromosome

synthase (-thas) synthesis promoting enzyme; synthetase

synthesis (-the-sis) 1. a building up, putting together 2. formation of compounds by the union of elements 3. a period in cell cycle 4. *Psy* the integration of various elements of the personality

synthetic (sin-thet'ik) artificially produced

syntonic (sin-ton'ik) having even tone or temperament

syntrophoblast (sin-trof'o-blast) the outer syncytial layer of the trophoblast

syntropic (-trop'ik) 1. pointing in the same direction 2. denoting correlation of several factors in the development of disease

syntrophy (sin'tra-pe) 1. the tendency of two diseases merging into one 2. a number of similar anatomical structures inclined in one direction as the ribs

syphilid (sif'i-lid) any of the skin lesions of secondary syphilis

syphilis (sif'i-lis) a sexually transmitted disease due to infection with *Treponema pallidum* **acquired s** condition begins as a painless ulcer at the site of infection usually on the genitals and the regional lymph nodes are enlarged (primary s). 6-8 weeks later there is macular or papular rash, mucosal ulcers and lymphadenopathy (secondary s). Later there is development of gumma (syphilitic granuloma) affecting the skin, mucosa and bones (tertiary s). Cardiovascular syphilis and neurosyphilis develop at a quaternary stage **congenital s** foetus developing syphilis by contacting it from the mother. The child may be born dead, or present with vesicles, bullae and mucosal ulcers, hepatosplenomegaly and CNS involvement

syphiloma (sif'i-lo'ma) a gumma of syphilitic origin

syringe (sir'inj) an instrument used for injecting or withdrawing fluids **air s** a small, fine nozzled syringe through which air is forced to blow debris from or to dry a cavity in preparing teeth for restoration **chip s** air syringe **dental s** a small syringe containing an anaesthetic solution used in operative dentistry **hypodermic s** a small syringe, with a calibrated barrel, used to administer drugs into the subcutaneous tissue **Luer-Lok s** a glass syringe with a metal tip and locking device to secure needle, used for intravenous or hypodermic use

syringectomy (sir'in-jek'ta-me) fistulectomy

syringitis (sir'in-ji'tis) inflammation of the eustachian tube

syringo combining word for tube; fistula

syringoadenoma (si-ring'go-ad'e-no'ma) syringocytadenoma

syringobulbia (-bul'be-a) development of fluid filled cavity in the medulla presenting with dysarthria, palatal palsy, Horner's syndrome, nystagmus and sensory loss on the face

syringocarcinoma (-kar'si-no'ma) a carcinoma of a sweat gland

syringocoele (si-ring'go-sel) 1. central canal of the spinal cord 2. a meningomyelocoele in which there is a cavity in the ectopic spinal cord

syringocystadenoma (si-ring'go-sis'ted-e-no'ma) papilloma of sweat gland ducts

syringoma (sir'ing-go'ma) a sweat gland tumour located on the eyelids, neck, upper anterior chest and vulva, most common in pubertal females and it appears as multiple flesh coloured to yellowish papulonodules

syringomyelia (si-ring'go-mi-e'le-a) development of a fluid-filled cavity near the centre of the spinal cord and the expanding cavity disrupts the spinothalamic tract, damage anterior horn cells and compress long fibre tracts. It is characterised by dissociated sensory loss (loss of pain and temperature sensation with preservation of posterior column modalities), trophic lesions, wasting of small muscles of hand, and upper motorneuron lesion signs in the lower limb

syringotomy (sir'ing-got'a-me) fistulotomy

syrinx (sir'inks) 1. Eustachian tube 2. lesion of syringomyelia

syrup (sir'up) 1. the saccharine solution left after refining of sugar 2. a concentrated solution of sugar 3. a liquid preparation of medicinal substances in a concentrated solution of a sugar

systaltic (sis-tal'tik) pulsating

system (sis'tim) the association of organs that have common functions **alimentary s** digestive system **autonomic nervous s** that part of the nervous system which represents motor innervation to smooth muscle of internal organs, cardiac muscle and glands. It consists of two distinct mutually antagonistic divisions as sympathetic and parasympathetic systems, the name has been derived as it was thought to be self-governing or spontaneous **cardiaovascular s** the heart and blood vessels by which blood is pumped and circulated through the body **CD s** Cluster designation, a system for classifying cell surface markers expressed by lymphocytes **centimetre-gram-seconds s** (CGS) metric system expressing fundamental physical units of length, mass and time and those units derived from them, in centimetres, grams and seconds **central nervous** s (CNS) that portion of nervous system consisting of the brain and spinal cord **centroencephalic** s the neurones in the brain stem **chromaffin** s chromaffin cells of the body staining readily with chromium salts, found along sympathetic nerves, in adrenal medulla, and in various other organs **circulatory** s a system concerned with circulation of nutrient fluids that includes cardiovascular and lymphatic systems **conducting** s **of the heart** a system of specialised muscle fibres that generate and transmit electrical discharges and coordinate contractions, comprising the sinus node, atrioventricular node, Bundle of His and bundle branches and their terminal ramifications into Purkinge system **digestive** s alimentary system from the mouth to anus with associated organs and glands concerned with ingestion, digestion and absorption of food stuffs and nutrients, and elimination of undigested material **endocrine** s ductless glands secreting hormones into the blood which includes pituitary, pineal body, thyroid, parathyroid, pancreas and adrenal glands, paraganglia and gonads. **extrapyramidal motor** s basal ganglia (corpus striatum), its associated structures (substantia nigra, subthalamic nucleus) and its descending connections with the midbrain, concerned with maintenance of equilibrium and muscle tone **genitourinary** s urogenital system **haversian** s basic unit of compact bone consisting of a haversian canal and its concentrically arranged lamellae **haematopoietic** s the tissues concerned with the production of blood including the bone marrow and lymph nodes **hypothalamohypophyseal portal** s a system of veins from median eminence of the hypothalamus pass downwards along the stalk and pars tuberalis of the hypophysis and reach

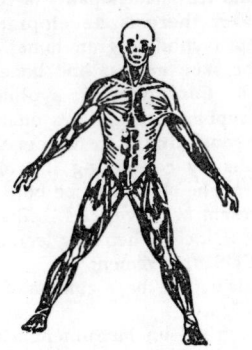

Skeletal muscles

anterior lobe of the pituitary where they arborise into a second capillary bed and convey releasing factors to the anterior lobe **limbic** s a heterogeneous group of brain structures at or near the edge (limbus) of the medial wall of the cerebral hemisphere (hippocampus, amygdala and gyrus funiculatus) **lymphatic** s the lymphatic vessels, lymph nodes and lymphoid tissue **lymphoreticular** s the tissues of the lymphoid and reticuloendothelial systems **masticatory** s the bony and soft structures of the face and mouth involved in mastication; jaws, teeth, temporomandibular articulations, masticatory muscles, tongue, lips, cheeks and oral mucosa **muscular** s voluntary or skeletal muscles of the body **nervous** s spinal cord, ganglia and nerves **neuromuscular** s the muscles of the body collectively and the nerves supplying them **parasympathetic nervous** s one of the two subdivisions of the autonomic nervous system having cell bodies of preganglionic neurones in the nuclei of the brain stem and in the lateral gray matter of the sacral portion of the spinal cord **peripheral nervous** s that part of the nervous system other than the CNS **portal** s an arrangement of vessels in which blood after passing through one capillary bed, enters a second capillary network **properdin s** an alternate pathway for complement consisting of many distinct proteins that react in a serial manner and activate C3 **renal s** urinary system **reproductive s** male or female gonads, associated ducts and external genitalia **respiratory s** the system concerned with the supply of oxygen to and elimination of carbon dioxide from the cells of the body and maintenance of normal acid base balance, consists of gas conducting airways and lungs (alveoli, terminal and respiratory bronchioles and blood vessels surrounding the alveoli) **reticular activating s** (RAS) that part of brain stem reticular formation (an extensive branched nerve cells) that receives collaterals from the ascending sensory pathways and project to the higher centres. When it is activated, a generalised alert or arousal behaviour results **reticuloendothelial s** the cells of different organs concerned with phagocytosis found in connective tissue and lymphatic structures, Kupffer cells, histiocytes, alveolar macrophages, and microglia **skeletal s** the bony framework of the body **somatognathic s** all structures involved in speech and in receiving, mastication and deglutition of food **sympathetic nervous s** one of the two divisions of autonomic nervous system having cell bodies in the preganglionic neurones in the lateral gray columns of the thoracic segments and first two or three lumbar segments of the spinal cord **urinary s** the kidneys, ureters, bladder and urethra **urogenital s** genit-ourinary system, consisting of organs involved in the formation and excretion of urine and in reproduction **vascular s** circulatory system consisting of cardiovascular and lymphatics **vegetative nervous s** autonomic nervous system

systema (sis-te'ma) system
systemic (sis-tem'ik) 1. affecting the whole body: generalised 2. relating to a system **s inflammatory response** (SIR) a part of metabolic response to injury that may be sepsis, trauma, or burns. It is associated with encephalopathy, spiking fever, marked tachycardia, hyperventilation, signs of increased sympathetic tone, bleeding and leucocytosis **s lupus erythematosus** (SLE) an autoimmune disorder of undetermined aetiology with a variety of clinical manifestations. There is non-organ specific autoimmunity with the presence of a group of autoantibodies directed against components of the cell nucleus, such as antinuclear antibody, circulating immune complexes and widespread immunologically determined tissue damage. It is characterised by arthritis, arthralgia, fever, photosensitive erythematous, butter fly rash across the face, livedo reticularis, Raynaud's phenomenon, pericarditis, myocarditis, endocarditis, pleurisy, fibrosing alveolitis, acute lupus pneumonitis, nephrotic syndrome and renal failure **s mycosis** systemic infection by fungi acquired by inhalation **s vasculitis** generalised inflammation of blood vessels that may be a primary disorder or may be part of or secondary to another disease process such as SLE. There is infiltration of one or more layers of the blood vessels with polymorphonuclear cells in acute stage and with lymphocytes in the chronic stage. There may be giant cells, granuloma and fibrinoid necrosis. The vasculitis may affect large vessels (Giant cell arteritis, Takayasu's arteritis) medium sized vessels (Polyarteritis nodasa, Kawasaki's disease) or small vessels (Wegener's granulomatosis, Churg-Strauss syndrome, Henoch-Schonlein purpura)

systole (sis'to-le) the phase of contraction of the heart muscle especially of the ventricles in the cardiac cycle

systolic pertaining to systole **s bladder** excessively contracted bladder following tuberculous fibrosis **s blood pressure** the force exerted by blood on arterial walls during ventricular contraction **s hypertension** marked rise in systolic blood pressure without rise of diastolic

systremma (sis-trem'a) a muscular cramp in the calf of the leg

syzygy (siz'i-ge) binding together of gametes without fusion of cells or nuclei

T

T symbol for temperature; abbreviation for tumour

T translocation

T$_{1-12}$ symbol for thoracic nerve or vertebra

T$_3$ symbol for tri-iodothyronine

T$_4$ symbol for tetraiodothyronine; thyroxine

T-cell T lymphocyte

T-disease thalassaemia

TAA tumour associated antigen

TAB Typhoid paratyphoid A and B vaccine

tabacosis (tab'a-kosis) extrinsic allergic alveolitis from occupational exposure to tobacco dust.

tabacum (ta-ba'kum) tobacco

tabagism (tab'a-jizm) poisonous effects of excessive use of tobacco.

tabanus (ta-na'nus) blood-sucking biting flies which can transmit trypanosomes

tabatiere anatomique (ta-ba'te-ar'a-na'to-mek) anatomical snuff box. The triangular area of the dorsum of the hand at the base of the thumb. When the thumb is extended, the area appears depressed and is bound by the tendons of long and short extensor muscles of the thumb

tabella (ta-bel'a) a medicated tablet

tabes (ta'bez) any chronic condition leading to wasting of the body **t dorsalis** syphilis of the spinal cord and its appendages. There is degeneration of sensory neurons and wasting of dorsal columns and optic atrophy characterised by lightning pains, sensory ataxia, and visual failure **t mesenterica** intestinal tuberculosis, calcified mesenteric lymph nodes

tabetic (ta-bet'ik) pertaining to tabes **t crisis** paroxysms of pain or other acute manifestations in tabes dorsalis **t gait** a high steppage gait associated with tabes **t foot** twisted foot

table (ta'bl) a flat layer or surface; a thin flat plate

tablespoon (ta'bl-spoon) a rough measure using a household spoon

tablet (tab'let) a small piece of solid dosage form of a medication **compressed t** a tablet made by forcibly compressing the powdered substances **enteric-coated t** tablet having an outer layer resisting dissolution by gastric juice **sublingual t** small, flat, oval tablet kept beneath the tongue to permit direct absorption

taboo (ta'boo) something unacceptable or improper

taboparesis (ta'bo-par-e'sis) a combined form of tabes dorsalis and general paralysis of insane

tabular (tab'u-lar) resembling a table **t bone** a flat bone

tache (t'osh) a crescentic discolouration of the skin or mucosa.

tachy- a combining word for, meaning rapid

tachyarrhythmia (tak'e-a-rith'me-a) irregularity of the heart combined with tachycardia

tachycardia (tak-e-kar'de-a) increased heart rate. It occurs during and immediately after exercise, in febrile conditions, thyrotoxicosis, anaemia, anxiety, nervousness, congestive heart failure, after haemorrhage, paroxysmal tachycardia, atrial fibrillation and atrial flutter. Tachycardia acts to increase the amount of oxygen delivered to the cells of the body by increasing the heart rate **atrial t** rapid heart rate arising from an atrial focus with less than 200 beats per month **bidirectional ventricular t** a rare form of ventricular tachycardia with right bundle branch block and alternating polarity of QRS in the frontal axis **nodal t** tachycardia occurring because of an increase in rhythmicity of the AV node over the SA node **paroxysmal atrial t** PAT episodes of atrial tachycardia beginning and ending suddenly. **paroxysmal supraventricular t** rapid ectopic atrial beats originating proximal to bifurcation of bundle or in an accessory pathway. It is sudden in origin and transient in nature **supraventricular t** SVT a regular tachycardia with a rate of between 140 and 220 due to reentry within the AV mode **ventricular t** a rapid succession of beats arising from a ventricular focus at a rate greater than 100 beats per minute

tachylalia (tak'e-la'le-a) rapid speech

tachyphonia (tak'ki-fo'ne-a) hoarseness of voice

tachyphylaxis (tak'e-fi-lak'sis) rapid immunisation against the effects of toxic doses of a substance; repeated administration of some drugs result in a marked decrease in effectiveness

tachypnoea (tak'ip-ne'a) increased respiratory rate. Normal rate of respiration is 16-20 per minute at rest in a normal adult. The rate is increased in pneumonia, pleurisy, hypoxic conditions, cardiac failure, during excitement, exertion and fever

tachysterol (ta-kis'te-rol) one of the isomers of ergosterol formed after ultraviolet irradiation of ergosterol

tactoid pseudocrystalline structure formed when haemoglobin S is deoxygenated and molecules of haemoglobin polymerise

tactile (tak'til) of or pertaining to the sense of touch **t agnosia** an impairment of tactile object recognition caused by unilateral damage to parietotemporal cortices **t anaesthesia** lack of sense of touch in the fingers **t corpuscles** minute elongated bodies enclosing the afferent fibres and serving as receptor for touch or slight pressure. They are located in dermal papillae just beneath the epidermis and are found in large numbers on fingertips, toes, soles, palms,

lips, nipples and tip of tongue **t disc** tiny expanded end of a secondary nerve fibre in the epidermis and in hair roots **t discrimination** ability to localise two points of presssure on the surface of the skin **t hyperaesthesia** an abnormal increase in the sense of touch **t image** a mental concept of an object as perceived through the sense of touch **t localisation** ability to accurately identify the site of tactile stimulation **t sensation** the sensation of touch **t system** part of the nervous system concerned with sense of touch **t vocal fremitus** TVF detection of vibrations transmitted to the palpating hand from the larynx through the bronchi, lungs and chest wall. It is increased in solidified lung or superficial cavity, and diminished in airways obstruction, collapse, fibrosis, pleural effusion, pneumothorax and pleural thickening

taction (tak'shun) the sense of touch; contact

tactometer (tak-to'et-er) an instrument to determine the acuity of touch sensitiveness

tactus (tak'tus) touch

tadpole sign a comma-shaped shadow located directly below a malignancy which is of lesser sonographic density and is related to necrotic tissue

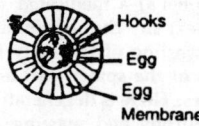

Ova of Taenia solium and T. saginata

taenia (te'ne-a) 1. a tapeworm 2. a flat band or strip of tissue **t coli** one of three large bands of the large intestine into which muscular fibres are collected **t echinococcus** dog is the definitive host of the tiny tapeworm *E. granulosus*. Man acquires the disease by handling a dog or drinking contaminated water with eggs. The embryo through blood reaches liver or lung or brain and gives rise to multiple cysts referred as hydatid cysts. **t saginata** beef tapeworm. It has a scolex of the size of a pinhead and four suckers. The adult worm produces little or no intestinal upset. The segments appear in the stool. Praziquantel is drug of choice. **T solium** pork tapeworm. The scolex has in addition to sucker, two circular rows of hooklets. Adult gets the disease by eating undercooked pork containing cysticerci. The larvae liberated from eggs in the stomach, get distributed to different parts of the body where they develop and cysticercosis in the brain causes epilepsy, personality changes, and staggering gait

taeniacide (ta'ne-a-sid) an agent that destroys tapeworms

taeniafuge (ta'ne-a-fuj') an agent that expels tapeworms

taeniasis (tenia-sis) infestation with tapeworms of the genus *Taenia*

tag a small appendage; label **haemorrhoidal tag** anal skin tag from an old external haemorrhoid **radioactive t** a radioactive isotope incorporated into a chemical or organic materials **skin t** a small outgrowth of skin often noted in the neck, axilla and groin

tagged labelled with radioactive or other easily identifiable material

tail a slender appendage extending from the posterior end of the trunks **t sign** comet tail of bronchogenic carcinoma tapering towards the pleura and may be associated with pleural retraction **t fold** a curved ridge formed at the caudal end of the early developing embryo

taila (s) oil, medicated oil(s)

Takayasu's disease pulseless disease or aortic arch syndrome, named after Japanese ophthalmologist, Michishige Takayasu. It is a chronic inflammatory granulomatous panarteritis of elastic arteries such as aorta and its major branches; common in women and is associated with loss of pulse

take to be effective such as successful grafting, or administration of vaccine

talalgia (tal-al'je-a) pain in the heel or ankle

talantropia nystagmus

talar (ta'lar) pertaining to talus, the ankle

talc (talk) magnesium silicate or malgnesium aluminium silicate used in making lubricants, talcum powder and dusting powder **t granuloma** a foreign body giant cell reaction seen in peritoneum, lungs and subepithelial tissues of external genitalia

talcosis (tal-ko'sis) pneumoconiosis resulting from inhalation of talc

talcum (talk'um) talc; hydrous magnesium polysilicate, an inert powder having a cooling effect on the skin

taliped (tali-pe'd) club-footed

talipes (tal'i-pez) club-foot, a congenital deformity wherein the foot is twisted out of shape and position **t arcuatus** high plantar arch **t calcaneovalgus** dorsiflexed and abducted (evertion) foot and its dorsum lies almost in contact with the skin. There is tightness of the dorso-lateral soft tissue, responds to repeated manual stretching and should be begun immediately after birth **t calcaneus** fixed dorsiflexion and walking on heel **t equinovarus** club-foot; the foot is adducted and inverted and is held equinus (plantar flexion) at the ankle. It requires operative correction in early infancy **t planus** flat-foot **t valgus** outward turning of foot **t varus** inward turning of foot

talipomanus (tal'ip-om'an-us) deformity of hand which is twisted out of shape and position

talo- pertaining to the ankle

talocalcaneal (ta'lo-kal-ka'ne-al) pertaining to the talus and calcaneus

talocrural pertaining to the talus and leg bones

talus (ta'lus) articulation between the upper tarsal bone and the lower ends of tibia and fibula to form ankle joint

tama(s) swelling of the feet and legs

tambour (tam-boor) a shallow, drum-shaped appliance

Tamm-Horsfall protein glycoprotein secreted by renal tubules. It is normal in urine, precipitated as casts in albuminuria, named after Igor Tamm, Russia-born US virologist and Frank Horsfall Jr., US physician.

tamoxifen (ta-moks'i-fen) selective oestrogen receptor modulator without androgen activity, used to treat early oestrogen receptor-positive breast cancer

tampon (tam'pon) a pack of cotton wool or gauze useful to stop haemorrhage, or absorb secretions

tamponade (tam'pon-ad) pathologic compression of a part; insertion of tampon to stop bleeding **balloon t** producing pressure against some object by a catheter surrounded by an elongated balloon, often to arrest oesophageal bleeding from varices **cardiac t** pathologic condition resulting from accumulation of excess fluid in the pericardium

tan brownish discolouration of the skin from exposure to sun

tandem a curved stainless steel tube inserted into uterus during brachytherapy

tandem repeats a sequence of oligonucleotides present in multiple copies and adjacent to each other i.e. in tandem.

tang 1. a strong taste or flavour 2. a long slender projection from a chistle, file or knife

tangent a branching off, divergence

tangentiality a disturbance wherein one exhibits an inability to have goal-directed associations of thought and the patients fail to get the desired goal from desired point

tangential speech the speaker wandering away from the intended point, moving to areas that are less and less relevant and never returning to the original idea

tanned red cells red blood cells treated with tannic acid, which enables them to act as antigen carriers

Tangier (tan-jer) **disease** familial high-density lipoprotein deficiency with reticulo-endothelial storage of cholesterol, first found in Tangier island, Chesapeake Bay Bay, USA

tannic (tan'ik) **acid** polymers of polyhydroxy benzoic acids which render proteins insoluble used as astringent and protein precipitant

tannin (tan'in) tannic acid, found in tea and coffee

tantalum (tan'ta-lum) a noncorrosive and malleable metal used to make prosthetic appliances or plates, at no. 73

tantrum (tan'trum) a violent display of bad temper

tap (tap) a light blow; to withdraw fluid from a cavity

tape (tap) a long narrow strip of linen, cotton, paper or plastic

tapering arch a dental arch that converges from the molars to the central incisors

tapetum (ta-pe'tum) a membranous layer

tapeworm a ribbon-shaped parasitic worm of the genus *Taenia* class Cestoda. It lives in the intestines. It is acquired from eating undercooked meat or fish that is infested with cysts containing larva

tapophobia fear of being buried alive

Tapia's syndrome hemiparalysis of larynx and tongue, described by Spanish otologist, Antonio Tapia

tapioca a starchy food

tapotage (ta-pot'-age) percussion with partly flexed fingers over the chest to dislodge thick secretions

tapotment (ta-pot-mon't) percussion with hand of tissue while massaging

tapping (tap'ing) paracentesis

tar 1. a dark viscid mass of complex chemicals obtained by distillation of coal, shale and organic matter 2. a sticky brown substance that is inhaled in tobacco smoke

tarantula (ta-ran'tu-la) a venomous spider

Tardieu's (tar'dyuz) **spots** petechiae of head and neck from asphyxia, described by French medicolegal expert, Auguste Tardieu

tardive (tar'div) late or slow in appearance **t dyskinesia** choreiform or athetoid movements especially of face noted after long term use of psychotropic drugs

tardy late; behind time

tartar a hard, crust-like deposit that can form on the crowns and roots of teeth and in the gums

target (tar'get) site of action **t cell** helmet cell, an abnormal erythrocyte with a rounded deeply staining area surrounded by lightly staining area which in turn is surrounded by dense cytoplasm at the periphery of the cell **t couple** couple who have one child or even newly married couples to develop acceptance of the idea of family planning from the earliest possible stage **t lesion** a vesicle surrounded by a haemorrhagic maculopapule as in erythema multiforme **t organ** an organ intended to receive a therapeutic dose of irradiation; an organ most affected by a specific hormone **t sign** a smoothly contoured radioopacity with both central and peripheral radiolucency seen in pedunculated colonic polyps in double-contrast barium studies **t symptoms** symptoms of an illness that are most likely to respond to a specific treatment

tarsadenitis (tar'sad-en-i'tis) inflammation of the tarsal borders of the eyelids

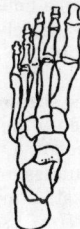

Tarsal and metatarsal bones

tarsal (tar'sal) referring to the edge of an eyelid; instep; any of the bones of the tarsus (back part of the foot) **t bone** any one of seven bones making up the tarsus of foot consisting of the talus, calcaneus, cuboid, navicular and three cuneiforms **t gland** one of numerous modified sebaceous glands on the inner sufaces of eyelids **t tunnel syndrome** compression of posterior tibial nerve following long standing or walking, presents with pain, paraesthesia and cyanosis of foot

tarsalgia (tar-sal'je-a) pain in the ankle or foot

tarsitis (tar-si'tis) inflammation of the tarsus or margin of an eyelid

tarso combining word for flat of foot; eyelid

tarsometatarsal (tar'so-met'a-tar'sal) pertaining to the tarsal and the metatarsal bones

tarsorrhapy (tar-sor'a-fe) suturing of the eyelids to protect the cornea when the person cannot close the eyelids

tarsotomy (tar'sot'o-me) incision of the tarsus of the eyelid

tarsus (tar'sus) 1. articulation between the foot and the leg where talus articulates with tibia and fibula, the cuboid and cuneiform bones with the metatarsals 2. connective tissue framework that provides internal support for the eyelid

tartar (tar'tar) potassium bitartrate; a hard crust-like deposit on teeth

tart cell a segmented neutrophil that has retained some nuclear fragments in its evolution towards becoming a full-fledged LE cell

taste a chemical sense dependent upon sense organs on the surface of the tongue. The nerve impulses are carried to the brain by the lingual and glossopharyngeal nerves from the anterior two-thirds and posterior-third of the tongue respectively **after t** the persistence of a taste sensation after removal of original stimulus **t area** area in the cerebral cortex **t buds** oval sensory end organs located on the surface of tongue also found on soft palate, epiglottis and portions of the pharynx. Each bud contains sensory and gustatory cells and supporting cells. When stimulated by chemical stimuli they produce one or a combination of the four fundamental taste sensations - sweet, bitter, sour and salty **t cells** neuroepithelial cells within a taste bud that act as receptors for the taste sense

tat **gene** 1. a gene present in retroviruses that encodes the *tat* transactivating protein 2. oncogenic inducing mesenchymal tumours experimentally

tattooing (ta-too'ing) practice of marking the skin with permanent patterns of picture design or name by injecting minute amounts of indelible pigments

taurine (taw'rin) a product of taurocholic acid which is present in bile

taurocholate (tow'ro-ko'lat) a salt of taurocholic acid

Taussig-Bing (taw'sig-bing) **heart** a congenital defect with aorta arising from right ventricle, and pulmonary artery from both right ventricle and left ventricle, named after Helen Taussig, US paediatrician and Richard Bing, US surgeon

tautologism repetition of same information in different words

tawny (ta-ni) brownish yellow

taxis (tak'sis) a movement of an organism towards or away from the stimulus; application of force in the manual replacement of a displaced or injured part

taxon a grouping based on similarities without specifying its level of abstraction

taxonomy (taks-on'o-me) a systematic classification of animals and plants

Tay-Sachs' (ta'saks) **disease** an autosomal recessive disorder presenting with mental and physical retardation, blindness, cherry-red spots on the macula, spasticity, enlarged head and convulsions. It is due to an absence of an enzyme, hexosaminidase- A necessary in the metabolism of sphingolipid, described by Warren Tay, British physician and Bernard Sachs, US neurologist

tb tubercle bacillus

TB tuberculosis

T bandage bandage resembling the letter T, used for the head and the perineum

Tbs tablespoon

tc symbol for technetium

T cell a T lymphocyte, thymus derived cell is the most complex cell of the immune system. It mediates cellular immune responses **T cell leukaemia** leukaemia in which the abnormal white blood cells are T-lymphocytes

tds to be taken thrice a day (*ter di'e sumen'dum*)

tea pot stomach markedly short lesser curvature of the stomach

tear (tar) to separate or pull apart by force causing discontinuity in a structure; a drop of lacrimal secretion **t drop cell** a deformed red cell that has squeezed through a reticuloendothelial system bearing increased connective tissue **t duct** a tiny channel that carries tears from the surface of the eye to the back of nose

tears (ters) watery secretion by the lacrimal glands. They lubricate the surfaces between eyeball and eyelids

tease (tez) to pull tissue apart or separate with needles for microscopic examination

teaspoon (te'spoon) a household measure equal to approximately 5 ml

teat (tet) the nipple of the mammary gland

technetium (tek-ne'she-um) a radioactive element obtained in the fission of uranium atomic weight 99 widely used in radio-isotope studies

technical (tek'ni-kal) 1. involving applied sciences 2. of terms used with special senses in technical context

technician (tek-nish'an) a person possessing the knowledge and skill necessary to carry out specific technical procedure

technique (tek′nek) the specialised procedure or method

technologist (tek′nol′o-jist) a person specialised in the application of scientific knowledge to solve the practical or theoretical problems

technology (tek-nol′o-je) scientific study of a technique; applied science **t transfer** the process of providing the private sector access to technological advances developed by the scientists in Government sector

tectorium (tek-to′re-um) an overlying structure; any roof-like structure

tectum (tek′tum) any roof-like structure

teeth (teth) hard bony projections in the jaws **anterior t** teeth located close to the midline of the dental arch on either side of the jaw **deciduous t** 20 teeth making up the first dentition, which are shed and replaced by the permanent teeth **Hutchinson's teeth** upper central permanent incisors are

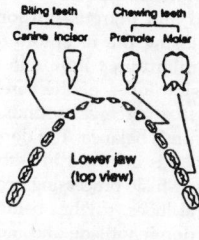

Teeth

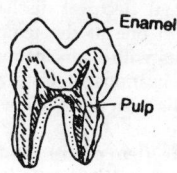

Section of tooth

peg-shaped and notched in congenital syphilis, named after Sir Jonathan Hutchinson, English surgeon **milk t** deciduous teeth **Moon t** the dome-shaped first permanent molars, named after Henry Moon, English surgeon **permanent t** the teeth that develop as second dentition replacing the deciduous teeth. They are 32 in number, 16 in each jaw. They include incisors (central and lateral), canines (cuspids), premolars (bicuspids) and molars

teething (teth′ing) eruption of deciduous teeth

teflon polytetrafluoroethylene, a polymeric molecule that is resistant to organic solvents useful in surgical implants

tegmen (teg-men) a covering

tegmental (teg-men′tal) relating to a tegmentum **t nucleus** one of the several masses of gray matter lying in the tegmentum of the midbrain and upper pons

tegmentum (teg-men′tum) 1. a covering or roof 2. the dorsal portion of cruri cerebri of the midbrain

teichoic acid a major constituent of gram-positive bacterial cell walls

tela (te′la) a thin web-like structure

telalgia (tel-al′je-a) referred pain

telangiectasia (tel-an′je-ek-ta′zea) a vascular abnormality formed by proliferation of a group of small blood vessels in the skin, usually on the nose and cheeks

telangiectasis (tel-an′je-ek-ta-sis) the site on the skin containing dilated small blood vessels

telangiitis (tel-an-je-itis) inflammation of the capillaries

telangion (tel-on′je-on) a terminal arteriole

tele combining word for distant, far

telecardiography (tel′e-kar′de-o-g′ra-fe) the recording of an electrocardiogram by transmitting impulses to a site away from the patients

telediagnosis (tel′e-di′ag-no′sis) identification of a disease by analysing the transmitted data of a patient at a diagnostic centre

telefluoroscopy (tel'e-floo'or-os'ko-pe) television transmission of fluoroscopic images to a distant place

telemedicine the use of telecommunication equipment to transmit the image and information about a patient at a distant site. It provides to obtain medical and surgical consultation

telemetry the technique of transmission of data to a distant point from the individual

telencephalon (tel-en-sefa-lon) end brain

teleneuron (tel'e-nu'ron) a nerve ending

teletherapy (tel-e-ther'-a-pe) treatment wherein the source of the therapeutic agent (radiation) is away from the body; teleradiotherapy

telogen (tel'o-gen) resting phase of hair follicle cycle

telomere (tel'o-mer) the distal extremity of a chromosome arm. They are long in immortalised cells and markedly short in normal cells undergoing senescence

telophase (tel'o-faz) the final stage of mitosis wherein the nucleus is formed from each group of chromosomes produced by anaphase or meiosis following the migration of chromosomes to the poles of the cell

temper the state of an individual's mood, disposition or mind

temperament (tem'per-a-ment) the individual's peculiarity of thinking, feeling and acting

temperature 1. a measure of sensible heat associated with the metabolism of human body normally maintained at a constant level (37°C) 2. a relative measure of sensible heat or cold **subnormal t** body temperature below 36.6°C which can occur suddenly in peripheral circulatory failure, following myocardial infarction, overwhelming infections and after prolonged exposure to cold, or gradually in patients with hypothyroidism and chronic wasting diseases **t**

elevation a raise in body temperature above 37.7°C in a resting individual from the normal range; fever or pyrexia **t recording** performed with a centigrade clinical thermometer which is kept beneath the tongue, in the axilla, fold of groin or rectum. The temperature of the mouth and rectum are half a degree higher than that of axilla or groin **t sense** a superficial sensation tested using test tubes filled with hot and cold water

template (tem'plat) a mold; pattern determining the shape of a substance. It acts as a guide to form a copy of the original

temple (tem'pl) the flattened lateral side of the head above the zygomatic arch

temporal (tem'por-al) relating to the temple; pertaining to time **t arteritis** inflammation of arteries of head referred as giant cell arteritis in elderly persons. It is associated with severe headaches and scalp tenderness. The temporal arteries are thickened and tender. Corticosteroids are useful **t bone** a bone on either side of skull at its base. It is composed of squamous, mastoid and petrous portions, the latter enclosing the receptors for hearing and equilibrium **t lobe** one of the two lower side lobes of the cerebral hemisphere that perceives sounds and smell, and controls balance. The dominant temporal lobe is involved in verbal comprehension. Music processing occurs in both temporal lobes, rhythm being processed on the dominant side and melody/pitch more on the non-dominant side **t lobe epilepsy** a form of epilepsy in which abnormal electrical discharges are confined to one of the temporal lobes. It presents with hallucinations and abnormal sensations of taste and smell

temporalis (tem'po-ra'lis) pertaining to the temple

temporate (tem'per-it) moderate

temporomandibular joint syndrome incordinated function of the jaw joints

and their supporting muscles and ligaments. It is characterised by headache,
facial pain and restriction of jaw movement

temulence intoxication

tenacious (te-na'shus) holding fast; sticky

tenaculum (tem-ak'u-lum) a small, sharp
pointed hook set in a handle to seize
and hold the tissues in operations

tenalgia (ten-al'je-a) pain in a tendon

tenascin X a large extracelular-matrix
protein

tenderness (ten'der-nes) sensation of pain
on touch or pressure **rebound t** inten-
sification of pain when pressure is released

tendinitis (ten'din-i'tis) painful inflammation of a tendon caused by injury,
over-use or prolonged pressure **rotator
cuff t** shoulder pain from pressure on
the tendons of shoulder especially that
of supraspinatus. It follows injury or
overuse during activities involving repeated elevation of the arm as in
cricket

tendinoplasty (ten'din-no-plas-te) the surgical repair of a defect in a tendon

tendocalcaneus Achilles tendon. The large
tendon at the lower end of the gastrocnemius muscle inserted into os calcis

tendon (ten'dun) a dense, inelastic fibrous cord of connective tissue by which
muscle gets attached to a bone or other
structure **t reflex** a reflex act in which
a muscle contracts when its tendon is
percussed **t transfer** a surgical procedure in which a tendon is repositioned
to make a muscle perform a new func-
tion   **t**

tenesmus painful straining to pass stools
and less commonly urine

tennis elbow damage by repeated small
injuries and overuse at the attachment
of forearm extensors to the lateral
epicondyle of humerus and presenting
with pain. There is tenderness on the
lateral epicondyle and in the outer
part of the antecubital fossa. Pronation
of the forearm accentuates the pain

tennis leg acute rupture of soleus that
may occur following any violent exercise in which the rapidly moving body
abruptly changes its directions

tenodesis (ten-od'e-sis) surgical fixation
of a tendon

Tenon's (te'nonz) **capsule** fascial sheath
of eyeball in which it rotates named
after French surgeon, Jacques Tenon

tenonitis (ten'on-itis) inflammation of tendon or sheath

tenoplasty (ten'o-plas'te) the surgical repair of a defect in a tendon

tenorrhaphy (ten-ar'a-fe) suture of a divided tendon

tenositis (ten'o-si'tis) inflammation of a
tendon

tenosynovitis (ten'o'sin'o-vi'tis) inflammation of the thin synovial lining of a
tendon sheath. It is caused by mechanical irritation or by bacterial infection

tenotome (ten'o-tom) a cutting instrument
used in tenotomy

tenotomy (te-not'o-me) surgical division
of a tendon

tenovaginitis (ten'o-vaj'in-a'tis) a mild
chronic inflammation or thickening
of the fibrous wall of the sheath that
surrounds a tendon. The cause is unknown

TENS transcutaneous electrical/electronic
nerve stimulation

tense (tens) tight

tension (ten-shun) the act of stretching;
mental strain **t headache** a headache
associated with emotional strain or
anxiety or spasm of muscles of the
head and neck **t pneumothorax** a
valvular condition allowing entry of
air into pleural cavity raising pleural
pressure

tensor (ten'sor) a muscle that stretches or
tightens some part of the body **t fascia
lata** mucocutaneous flap **t tympani** small
muscle lying in a bony canal above
eustachian tube whose tendon is inserted on malleolus. It helps to
dampen excessive vibrations

tent covering over bed to maintain a controlled atmosphere

tentacle (ten'ta-k'l) a slender whip-like process

tentative (ten'ta-tiv) indecisive **t diagnosis** a diagnosis made on available information that is subject to change

tenth cranial nerve vagus nerve

tenting 1. *ECG* symmetrical peaking of T wave which is associated with lengthening of PR interval, seen in hyperkalaemia 2. severe dehydration is associated with a delay in flattening or tenting on pinching of a patient's skin

tentorial hernia herniation of brain tissue under tentorium pushing midbrain against opposite side of tentorium

tentorium (ten-to're-um) a tent or a membranous covering **t cerebelli** the process of dura mater between the cerebrum and cerebellum supporting the occipital lobes

tentum the penis

tephromalacia (tef'ro-mal-a'she-a) the softening of the gray matter of the brain or spinal cord

tephrosis (tef-ro'sis) incineration

tepid (tep'id) moderately warm; lukewarm

tepor (te'por) lukewarm

teratic (ter-at'ik) relating to severely malformed foetus

teratoblastoma (ter'a-to-blas-to'ma) a neoplasm of embryonic elements without having all the germinal layers

teratogen (ter-at'o-jen) an agent such as a drug, viral infection or radiation responsible for physical defects in a developing embryo

teratogenesis (ter'a-toje-ne-sis) the production of physical defects in the embryo or foetus; production of a monstrous growth

teratogenic (ter-a-toje-nik) causing abnormalities in foetus

teratology (ter-a-tol'o-je) study of foetal malformations

teratoma (ter-a-to'ma) a neoplasm representing all the germinal layers of an embryo usually found in an ovary, testis and mediastinum

teratospermia (ter'a-to-sper'me-a) presence of abnormal sperms

terbutaline a sympathomimetic bronchodilator

teres (te'rez) long and round

terfenadine H_1 receptor blocking antihistamine

tergal (ter'gal) the dorsal surface of the body

ter in die (ter'inde'a) L. tid, three times a day

term word; boundary; specified time of duration

terminal (ter'mi-nal) situated at or forming the end **t bar** the portion of the cell below and perpendicular to the cilia in the ciliated columnar cells **t bronchiole** the airway immediately proximal to the respiratory bronchiole **t cancer** a malignant condition that is expected to cause the patient's death within a short period of time **t disease** seriously disabling disease which is fatal **t duct carcinoma** a low grade malignant salivary gland tumour, common in palate

termination of pregnancy abortion

terminology (ter-mi-nolo'je) scientific vocabulary

terminus (ter'mi-nus) an ending.

terra (ter'a) earth; soil

terror intense fear

terry section rapid frozen section for surgical diagnosis

tertian (ter'shun) recurring every third day **t fever** fever characterised by febrile paroxysms occurring every third day as in malaria that may be benign (*Plasmodium vivax*) or malignant (*P. falciparum*)

tertiary (ter'she-ar-e) third in order; third stage **t health care** health care offered at super-speciality institutions **t hyperparathyroidism** continuous stimulation of parathyroids in secondary hyperparathyroidism may result in adenoma formation and autonomous PTH secretion. Serum calcium level is raised **t syphilis** third and most advanced stage of syphilitic gumma and aortitis occurring 5-10 years after infection **t prevention** measures available to reduce or limit impairments and disabilities, to minimise suffering caused by existing departures from good health and to promote the patient's adjustment to irremediable condition

tesla a unit of measure of magnetic strength, named after Nikola Tesla, US physicist

test a chemical reaction; trial; examination

Tes tape dip-strip enzyme based test for glucose in urine

testes (tes'tes) plural of testis. **t determining factor** a gene on the Y chromosome determines the male sex

testicle (tes'ti-kl) the testis; male sex organs suspended in the scrotum

testicular of or pertaining to the testis **t feminisation** XY individuals exhibiting insensitivity to androgens **t feminisation syndrome** a rare genetic disorder wherein an individual who is genetically male develops female sex characters as the body tissues fail to respond to testosterone

testis (tes'tis) the male gonad situated on either side in the scrotum, produces sperms and testosterone. Each testis contains hundreds of comparments containing tiny tubes called seminiferous tubules in which sperms are produced. Sperms mature in the epididymis at the back of the testis before passing into the vas deferens **t determining factor** a protein encoded by a gene on the short arm of Y chromosome which is responsible for development of primary male organs

test meal a meal of small quantity and composition given to aid chemical analysis of the stomach contents or radiological examination of the stomach

testosterone (tes-tos'ter-on) a sex hormone that stimulates bone and muscle growth

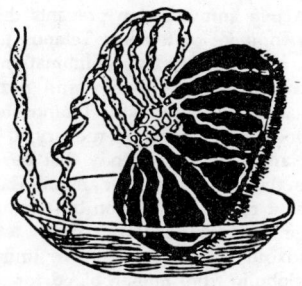

Testis

and the development of male characteristics. It is produced by the testes and in small amounts by the ovaries

test tube baby a full-term gestational product resulting from *in vitro* fertilisation of an egg that was implanted in a uterus and carried to term

tetanolysin (tet'a-nol'i-sin) the haemolytic fraction of the exotoxin formed by *Clostridium tetani*

tetanospasmin (tet'a-no-spas'min) a neurotoxin of *Clostridium tetani*, that is most toxic substance known to man, causing profound muscle spasms due to tetanospasmin, s, blockage of the release of glycine

tetanus (tet'a-nus) an infectious often fatal disease characterised by violent tonic muscle spasms and rigidity caused by toxin of *Clostridium tetani*. It presents initially with trismus, tonic rigidity involving muscles of the face, neck and trunk. The back is slightly arched and there is board-like abdominal wall. Contraction of the frontalis and the muscles of the angles of the mouth gives rise to the risus sardonicus. Violent spasms lasting for a few seconds to 3-4 minutes occur. They are painful, exhausting. They gradually increase in frequency and severity. Death may occur from exhaustion, asphyxia or aspiration pneumonia. The absorbed toxin has to be neutralised and further toxin production has to be prevented. Active immunisation prevents the development of tetanus. Tetanus toxoid is commonly given in combination with the diphtheria toxoid and pertusis vaccine in childhood. Tetanus toxoid booster has to be given every 10 years **t antitoxin** an antibody that develops in the humans or other animals (horses) as a result of infection by tetanus organism or inoculation with tetanus toxoid **t immunoglobulin** immunoglobulin from human blood for use in persons not previously immunised against tetanus **t neonatorum** umbilical infection due to dressing with mud, dung etc. **t toxoid** a highly effective vaccine for *C. tetani* that selectively elicits helper immune response

tetany (tet'a-ne) severe tonic muscle spasm often due to a deficiency of ionised calcium from low blood calcium or respiratory alkalosis

tetracosactrin synthetic corticotropin. Useful to test adrenal cortical function

tetracycline (tet'ra-si'klen) a broad spectrum antibiotic active against most pathogenic bacteria, rickettsias, chlamydias and mycoplasma

tetrad (tet'rad) a group of four similar or related entities

tetradactyly (tet'ra-dak'ti-le) four digits on the hand or foot

tetragonum (tet-rag'on-um) a square

tetralogy a combination of four factors or anomalies **t of Fallot** *See* Fallot's tetralogy

tetraplegia (tet'ra-pleje-a) paralysis of all four limbs

tetraploid (tet'ra-ployd) a cell having chromosomes which are four times the basic or haploid number

tetrasomy (tet-ra-so'me) the presence of two additional chromosomes of one type

T fracture a type of intercondylar fracture of the distal femur that occurs in falls from a height with the feet extended resulting in a violent impact of femur on the tibial plateau

TGF transforming growth factor(s) a group of distinct polypeptides that have been isolated from virus-transformed rodent cells, capable of altering cell phenotype. **TGF a** polypeptide synthesised by transformed cells that is a potent stimulant of cell growth. **TGF b** a regulatory peptide produced by various normal and neoplastic cells bearing TGF b receptors

thalamectomy (thal'amek'to-me) surgical removal of a portion of the thalamus

thalamic syndrome infarction of sensory tracts in or below thalamus presenting with hemianaesthesia and severe pain on minimal stimulus

thalamus (thal-a-mus) an ovoid gray nuclear mass deep within the brain in the lateral wall of lateral ventricle through which sensory impulses pass to reach the cerebral cortex. It may also play a part in long term memory

thalassemia (thal-a-se'me-a) a hereditary haemolytic anaemia having decreased synthesis of haemoglobin polypeptide chains a **thalassemia** defective formation of a chains **t major** homozygous b-chain defect with a reduction of Hb-A and an increase of Hb-F **t minor** heterozygous chain defect with mild hypochromic anaemia without iron deficiency

thalidomide (tha-lid'o-mid) hypnotic and antiemetic, teratogenic. Its use was abandoned as it caused severe foetal malformations, if taken in early pregnancy. Now has found new indications as an immunosuppressive agent

thallium (thal'e-um) a heavy, soft malleable metallic, radioactive element at no. 81 **t scanning** a radionuclide scanning to assess the heart function by determining how well different areas of heart muscle absorb thallium after it has been injected into the blood

thanatology (than'a-to'logi) study of death and dying after Thanatos, Greek figure representing death

thatched roof disease allergic alveolitis seen in New Guinea

thea tea

theaism (the'a-izm) chronic caffeine poisoning from excessive tea drinking

theasaurus dictionary of synonyms or words of similar meanings

thebesian (the-be'ze-an) **veins** venules conveying blood from the myocardium to the atria or ventricles, named after Adam Thebesius, German physician

theca (the'ka) sheath enclosing an organ or structure **t cell tumour** a benign, yellow, solid ovarian tumour

thelarche (the-lar'ke) pubertal development of nipple or breast occurring before other signs of puberty

thelitis (the-li'tis) inflammation of the nipples

thelium (the'le-um) 1. a papilla 2. a nipple 3. a cellular layer

thenar (the'nor) 1. the palm of the hand or sole of the foot 2. fleshy part on the outside of the palm of the hand **t eminence** a prominence at the base of the thumb **t fascia** a thin membrane covering the short muscles of the thumb **t muscle** the abductor or flexor muscle of the thumb

theophylline (the'o-fil'en) xanthine compound inhibiting breakdown of cyclic AMP

theory (the'o-re) the doctrine or the principles of explanation

therapeutic (ther-a-pu'tik) of or relating to the treatment or cure of a disease **t drug monitoring** TDM the regular measurement of the serum levels of those drugs that require close 'titration' of doses in order to ensure that they are in sufficient levels in the blood to be therapeutically effective, while avoiding potentially toxic excess **t index** the ratio of drug's toxic level to therapeutic level **t nihilism** abandonment of all attempts of treatment **t range** the dosage range over which a drug has a beneficial effect without causing side effects **t window** 1. the range of a drug's concentration in which the desired effect occurs, below which there is little desired effect and above which toxic effects appear 2. the gap between the dose needed to provide desired effect and that needed for undesired effect **t vaccine** a vaccine-like product used to improve the immune function of a person who has already an infection

therapeutics (the'r-a-pu'tiks) branch of medicine concerned with the details of treatment of disease

therapist (ther'a-pist) a person skilled in giving therapy

therapy (ther'a-pe) the treatment of a disease **acrion t** use of ionisers to increase the number of negative ions in the air breathed **aroma t** treatment via the sense of smell alone **clay t** burying people to the neck in the earth as a therapy for a variety of illnesses **Gestalt t** *Ger* shape, form, figure or pattern; a psychotherapy born in Berlin which considers the whole determines the parts **maintenance t** administration of medication for a period of time following initial treatment, to stabilize the condition or prevent recurrence or deterioration **music t** use of music for therapy **Reichian t** treatment to unblock body tensions and free breathing patterns to increase the flow of biological energy through the body **urine t** drinking one's own urine for health of life

thermal (ther'mal) pertaining to heat or caused by heat

thermoanalgesia (ther'mo-an'al-je-si-a) a condition in which the application of heat produces pain

thermoanaesthesia (ther'mo-an'es-the'ze-a) loss of ability to feel cold or heat sense

thermocoagulation (ther'mo-ko-ag-u-la'shun) coagulation of tissue by the action of high frequency currents

thermodilution (ther'mo-di-lu'shun) a method of measuring the ventricular blood volume and cardiac output utilising a thermistor

thermogenic (thermo-jen'ik) producing heat.

thermometer (ther-mom'e-ter) an instrument for measuring temperature

thermophile (ther'mo-pil) an organism that grows well at an elevated temperature.

thermoplegia (ther'mo-ple'je-a) heatstroke; sun stroke.

thermoreceptor (ther-mo-re-sep'tor) a sensory receptor stimulated by a rise in body temperature

thermoregulation (ther'mo-reg'u-la'shun) heat regulation

thermoregulatory centre a centre in the hypothalamus that regulates heat production and heat loss so as to maintain a normal body temperature

thermostat (ther'mo-stat) a device present in the heating system to maintain the temperature

thermosterilisation bacterial sterilisation by use of heat

thermotherapy (ther'mo-ther'a-pe) treatment of disease by means of heat

thesis a long essay written as a qualification for higher degree

thiabendazole broad-spectrum antihelminthic, effective against most types of round worms in the gut

thiamine the first component of B complex; aneurin; vitamin B_1 It is essential for energy production, and nerve and muscle function

thiazides sulphonamide-related diuretics that inhibit distal tubular resorption used in hypertension, heart failure and nephrogenic diabetes insipidus

thigh (thi) the part of the lower limb situated between the hip and the knee

thimble bladder grossly contracted and fibrosed bladder

thinking mental activity involving imagination, appraisal, evaluation, forecasting, planning. creation and will **abstract t** the ability to assume a mental set, to keep simultaneously in mind all aspects of a complex situation and to extract common properties **concrete**

t a disturbance in the ability to form abstract concepts and is encountered in organic mental disorder

thioacetazone a synthetic, cheap bacteriostatic antituberculosis drug

thiopentone a short acting barbiturate, used as intravenous anaesthetic for induction and minor surgery

thiotepa alkylating cytotoxic agent

thiouracil antithyroid drug

third cranial nerve oculomotor nerve

third generation cephalosporins a group of broad-spectrum antibiotics (cefatoxime, cefazidine, ceftriaxone) that are structurally related to penicillins and useful against pencillinase-producing bacteria

third heart sound a low pitched gallop sound occurring early in the diastole about 0.15 sec. after the aortic closure sound. It corresponds to the 'v' wave of the jugular vein. It may be produced from either the left or right ventricle.

third intention healing of a wound by filling with granulation tissue

Thomsen's (tom'senz) **disease** myotonia congenita, named after Asmus Thomsen, Danish physician

third ventricle a narrow cavity between the two optic thalami. It communicates anteriorly with the lateral ventricles and posteriorly with the fourth ventricle

thirst a bodily sensation for desire to drink water

Thomas's splint a splint used for fracture of femur. It has padded ring bearing on ischial tuberosity and bars extending beyond feet, for extension, named after Hugh Thomas, UK orthopaedic surgeon

thoracentesis (tho'ra-sen-te'sis) aspiration of fluid from the pleural space

thoracic (tho'-ras'ik) of or pertaining to the thorax. **t duct** the main trunk of lymphatic system opening into venous system. The duct enters the thoracic cavity posteriorly to the oesophagus and to the right of the aorta. In the superior mediastinum the duct arches to the left crossing the midline at approximately the level of T_4 to T_6 vertebrae and merges with the left internal jugular vein **t gas volume** TGV the gas volume in the thorax and it is measured by body plethysmography and it can be measured at different lung volume levels such as TLC, FRC or RV **t inlet injury** traumatic injury to the base of the neck involving superior mediastinal vessels **t outlet syndrome** Scalenus syndrome. A condition caused by compression of brachial plexus and subclavian artery between a cervical rib and the scalenus anticus muscle

thoracoabdominal (tho'rak-o-ab'do-mi-nal) pertaining to the thorax and abdomen

thoracolumbar (tho'rak-o-lum'bar) pertaining to the thoracic and lumbar parts of the spine

thoracolysis (tho'rak-ol'i-sis) the separation of adhesions of the lung from the chest wall

thoracopagus (tho'ra-kop'-a-gus) two malformed foetuses joined at thorax

thoracoplasty (tho'ra-ko-plas'te) surgical removal of the ribs facilitating the chest wall to move in and cause compression of a diseased lung

thoracopneumograph (tho'ra-ko-nu-mo-gra'ph) an instrument to record the respiratory movements of the chest

thoracoscope (tho'ra-ko-skop) an endoscope facilitating the examination of the pleural cavity

thoracoscopy inspection of the pleura using an endoscope inserted through an incision in the side of the chest

thoracotomy (tho'rak-ot'o-me) a surgical procedure in which chest is opened for operation on a diseased lung, heart or other organ lying in the thoracic cavity

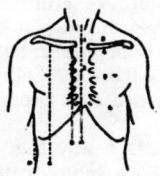

Thorax-anterior view
area: 1) suprasternal 2) sternal
3) supraclavicular 4) infraclavicular
5) mammary and 6) inframammary

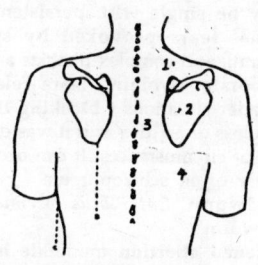

Thorax-pasterior view
area: 1) supraclavicular 2) scapular
3) interscapular 4) scapular

thorax (tho'raks) region of the trunk between the neck and abdomen; the chest. By drawing certain imaginary vertical lines the thorax is divided into various regions such as supraclavicular, suprasternal, clavicular, infraclavicular, mammary between third and sixth costal cartilages, inframammary between the sixth rib and costal arch, sternal, axillary, infraaxillary, suprascapular, scapular (supraspinous and infraspinous), interscapular and infrascapular regions

thorn sign a vaguely-defined spicular radiologic shadow that tapers medially from the lateral chest wall which corresponds to a thickening of the minor fissure, seen in right sided pleural effusion

Thorn test a test of adrenal insufficiency which involves administration of corticotropin. It causes decrease in circulating eosinophils in healthy person but not in those with adrenal insufficiency, named after George Thorn, US physician

thread (thred) 1. any thin filamentous structure 2. a suture material

thought a state of individual experience in cognitive operations and activities **obscessive** t rigid and repetitive thoughts concerning any aspect of mental life **phobic** t irrational fears which may be single with persistent, irrational fears provoked by specific stimuli, and complex phobias are more elaborate involving fears related to broader situations t **blocking** the sudden loss of an idea as if it was dropped out of circumstances. It can occur normally or in schizophrenia

threadworm Enterobius vermicularis; pinworm

threatened abortion moderate haemorrhage without dilatation of cervix

three point suture intradermal suture to hold point of skin flap without distortion

threshold (thresh'old) limit of perception; point above which the substance is eliminated t **dose** the minimum dose that will produce an effect on the patient t **limit value** the concentration of an airborne chemical or potentially toxic or radioactive substance below which persons may work over an eight-hour period without known adverse effect

thrill (thril) a sensation of vibration appreciated on palpation. It is caused by turbulent blood flow through a heart valve or a hole in the septum of the heart

throat (throt) the pharynx and the fauces; gullet, the anterior aspect of the neck t **culture** the study of cultures of flora in the throat t **swab** a sterile swab of cotton wool wrapped around the end of a strong and thin wooden stick is passed towards pharynx or tonsillar region while a tongue depressor facilitates exposure of posterior wall of pharynx and prevents the swab touching oral cavity. The swab is rubbed firmly over mucosal surface, exudates, membrane and withdrawn. A smear is made from the material and stained. The swab is kept in a broth facilitating its culture

throb (throb) a pulsating movement

throbbing (throb'ing) beating or pulsation

thrombasthenia (throm'bas-the-ne-a) defective clot retraction due to a platelet abnormality causing bleeding

thrombectomy (throm-bek'to-me) removal of a thrombus from a blood vessel, to restore blood flow

thrombi (throm'bi) plural of thrombus

thrombin (throm'bin) the enzyme which converts fibrinogen into fibrin

thromboangiitis (throm'bo-an'je-i'tis) inflammation of inner wall of a blood vessel with thrombosis t **obliterans** see Buerger's disease

thromboclasis (throm-bok'la-sis) dissolution of a thrombus; thrombolysis

thrombocyte (throm'bo-sit) a blood platelet which aids coagulation of the blood

thrombocythaemia (throm'bo-si-the'me-a) an increase in the number of circulating blood platelets

thrombocytopaenia (throm'bo-sito-pe'nea) the decrease in the number of circulating blood platelets

thrombocytopaenic purpura a bleeding disorder that results from a deficiency of platelets in the blood. It is characterised by purple or reddish brown discoloured areas on the skin

thrombocytopoiesis (throm'bo-si-to-poye'sis) the production of blood platelets

thrombocytosis (throm'bo-si-to'sis) increased number of platelets in the peripheral blood

thromboembolism (throm'bo-em'bo-lizm)

obstruction of a blood vessel by a fragment that has broken off from a thrombus elsewhere in the circulation

thromboendarterectomy (throm'bo-end'ar-ter-ek'to-me) removal of an obstructing thrombus together with the inner lining of an obstructed artery

thromboendarteritis (throm'bo-end-ar'ter-i'tis) inflammation of the inner lining of an artery with formation of thrombus

thrombogenesis (throm'be-jen'e-sis) the formation of blood clots

thrombokinase a clotting factor that is activated by tissue injury

thrombolysis (throm-bol'i-sis) dissolution of a thrombus

thrombopaenia (throm-bo-pe'ne-a) an abnormal decrease in the number of blood platelets

thrombophilia (throm-bo-fil'e-a) a tendency to the occurrence of thrombosis

thrombophlebitis (throm'bo-fle-bi'tis) inflammation of a vein often with the formation of a thrombus in part of a vein present near the surface of the body **t migrans** thrombosis developing and receding in different parts of the body, often associated with carcinoma of pancreas

thromboplastic (throm'bo-plas'tik) causing clot formation in the blood

thromboplastin (throm'bo-plas'tin) a substance necessary in the coagulation, which facilitates conversion of prothrombin to thrombin in presence of calcium ions

thromboplastinogen (throm'bo-plas-tin'o-jin) blood clotting factor VIII

thrombopoiesis (throm'bo-poy-e'sis) formation of thrombus

thrombopoietin a stimulant of platelet production in the bone marrow

thrombosis (throm'bo'sis) the formation of a fibrinous clot in any part of the circulatatory system **coronary t** thrombosis of a coronary artery, a common cause of myocardial infarction **deep vein thrombosis** DVT thrombosis of deep veins in the legs or pelvis. It is en-

couraged by low cardiac output, sluggish flow, increased coagulability of blood, endothelial damage, post-operative and post partum states and in carcinoma

thrombotic thrombocytopaenic purpura TTP. A rare condition of thrombocytopaenia, and normal coagulation factors presenting with splenomegaly, varying neurologic signs, disseminated intravascular coagulation and fever

thromboxanes substances produced from arachidonic acid by cyclooxygenase which generates prostaglandin G2 that is subsequently converted by thromboxane (Tx) synthetase into Tx A_2. It increases after vascular injury, eliciting a primary haemostatic response, inducing platelet aggregation and vasoconstriction

thrombus (throm'bus) a fibrinous clot consisting of platelets, fibrin and cellular elements which obstructs a blood vessel or is formed in one of the chambers of the heart

thrush white creamy patches on the oral mucosa caused by a fungus, *Candida albicans*; candidiasis

thrust push forcibly or drive with force

thumb (thum) the first digit of the hand with two phalanges which can oppose the other fingers **t sign** protrusion of the thumb across the palm and beyond the clenched fist, seen in Marfan's syndrome **t sucking** the habit of sucking one's thumb

thymectomy (thi-mek'to-me) surgical removal of the thymus gland.

thymic (thi-mik) pertaining to the thymus

thymidine (thi'mi-den) a nucleoside present in deoxyribonucleotide

thymine (thi'min) a pyrimidine base present in DNA where it is paired with adenine

thymocyte (thi'mo-sit) a cell formed in the thymus as the precursor of T (thymus derived) lymphocyte

thymoma (thi-mo'ma) a tumour of thymus

thymoprivous (thi-mo-pri'vus) atrophy of the thymus

thymus (thi'mus) a lymphoid gland situated in the anterior mediastinum playing an important role in the development of immunologic competence. It weighs 10-35 g at birth, increasing to 20-50 g by puberty, involuting to 5 g or less in elderly. It consists of two flat symmetric lobes and contain cortex and medulla. The cortex is a dense lymphoid tissue containing thymocytes in large number. Medulla contains less number of thymocytes and thymic (Hassall's) corpuscles

thyroarytenoid (thi'ro-a-rit'en-oyd) pertaining to the thyroid and arytenoid cartilages of the larynx

thyrocalcitonin (thi'ro-kal'si-to'nin) a polypeptide hormone elaborated by thyroid gland

thyrocardiac (thi'ro-kar'de-ak) pertaining to the thyroid and heart

thyroglobulin (thi'ro-glob'u-lin) an iodine-containing protein

thyroglossal (thi'ro-glos'sal) pertaining to the thyroid gland and the tongue **t cyst** unobliterated part of the thyroglossal duct and is found in the midline of the neck forming a closed space into which secretions accumulate **t duct** a duct that in embryo connects the thyroid diverticulum with the tongue **t fistula** a discharging opening in the neck from persistence of a part or whole of thyroglossal tract **t tract** a tract extending from the tongue to isthmus of thyroid gland, that gets obliterated

thyrohyoid (thi'ro-hi'oyd) pertaining to the thyroid gland or cartilage and the hyoid bone

thyroid (thi'royd) resembling a shield, a bilobed endocrine gland in the neck that is essential for growth and metabolism **t cartilage** largest cartilage of the larynx which projects in men as

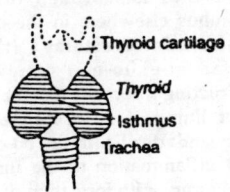

Thyroid gland

'Adam's apple' **t gland** an endocrine gland in the base of the neck on either side of the lower part of larynx and upper part of the trachea. It consists of two lateral lobes connected by an isthmus. It contains a large number of follicles that contain a homogeneous susbtance (colloid). It contains thyroglobulin with active substances like thyroxine and triiodothyronine **t hormone** hormones secreted by the thyroid gland **t thrill** a palpable thrill is often felt in fingers laid lightly over an uniformly enlarged thyroid gland due to increased vascularity **t stimulating hormone** a hormone secreted by the pituitary gland that stimulates the thyroid gland to increase its secretion of hormones **t storm** a hypermetabolic state superimposed on hyperthyroidism, may be triggered by infection, surgery, trauma or withdrawal from thyroid blocking drugs

thyroidectomy (thi'royd-ek'to-me) surgical removal of all or a part of thyroid gland, in situations of hyperthyroidism, goitre or thyroid tumours

thyroidism (thi'royd-izm) condition due to overactivity of the thyroid gland

thyroiditis (thi-royd-i'tis) inflammation of the thyroid gland **Hashimoto's t** a condition of goitrous hypothyroidism presenting with a small or moderately sized diffuse goitre which is firm or rubbery in consistency. Thyroxine therapy is indicated, named after

Hakaru Hashimoto, Japanese surgeon **post partum** t unmasking of previously unrecognised subclinical autoimmune thyroid disease, within 6 months of delivery **Riedel's** t a rare condition in which there is extensive infiltration of the thyroid and surrounding structures with fibrous tissue. It presents with a slow-growing goitre which is irregular and hard, named after Bernhard Riedel, German surgeon **subacute** t a virus (Coxsackie, mumps or adenovirus) induced inflammation of thyroid gland which results in release of colloid and its constituents into the circulation. There is hyperthyroidism characterised by pain in the region of thyroid gland, raised levels of thyroid hormones and systemic abnormalities

thyromegaly (thi'ro-meg'a-le) goitre

thyrotropic hormone, TSH, thyroid-stimulating hormone released by anterior pituitary gland

thyrotropin releasing hormone a hormone released by the hypothalamus that stimulates pituitary gland to release TSH

thyrotoxicosis (thi'ro-tok'i-ko'sis) a toxic condition caused by overactivity of thyroid gland

thyrotropin (thi-rot'ro-pin) a hormone secreted by anterior pituitary that stimulates the thyroid gland

thyroxine (thi'roks'in) a thyroid hormone of the thyroid gland. It helps to control the rate of energy production in the body

TIA abbreviation for transient ischaemic attack

tibia (tib'e-a) the inner, thick bone of the leg extending from the knee to the ankle articulating with the femur above and talus below; the shin -bone **saber** t a deformed tibia that is curved outwards due to gummatous periostitis of syphilis t **valga** a bulging of legs in which the convexity is inward t **vara** a bowing of the legs in which the convexity is outward

tibial (tib'e-al) pertaining to the tibia

tic (tik) twitching; a sudden, repetitive involuntary muscular contraction including eye blinking, facial gestures and shoulder shrugging t **douloureux** trigeminal neuralgia, paroxysmal severe pain over the face.

ticarcillin synthetic penicillin, more active against Pseudomonas

tick (tik) a small, eight-legged blood-sucking creature, some of which spread infectious diseases such as Lymē disease, Kyasanur forest disease and Rocky Mountain Spotted fever t **typhus** Rickettsia infection transmitted by ticks

tid three times a day, ter in die

tidal volume, V_T the volume of air inhaled or exhaled with each breath during resting, quiet respiration

tide an alternate rise and fall

Tietze's syndrome costochondritis; a painful condition resulting from inflammation of the cartilages that attach the ribs to the sternum, named after Alexander Tietze, German surgeon

tikta (s) bitter

tilting disc disc with eccentric hinge, opened by pressure on one side, device used for heart valve prosthesis

timbre (tim'ber) the characteristic quality of a sound independent of pitch and loudness

time (tim) the interval between beginning and ending t **distribution** description of disease by the time of its occurrence t **frame** the limits of time for any event

timolol beta blocker used in hypertension, myocardial ischaemia and glaucoma

tinctorial (tink-to're-al) pertaining to staining

tincture (tink'chur) an alcoholic solution containing medicinal substances t **of iodine** an alcoholic solution of iodine

tine a sharp projecting point t **test** a disposal plastic disc with four tines of 2 mm length dipped into tuberculin is used for tuberculin test

tinea (tin'e-a) superficial fungal infection affecting the skin, hair or nails; ringworm **t barbae** fungal involvement of hairs of beard region presenting as localised boggy swellings **t capitis** fungal infection primarily involving scalp hair, occurs mainly in children **t corporis** tinea infection of the surface of the skin of the trunk, face and extremities and presents as markedly itchy circular or irregular lesions **t cruris** tinea lesions in the groin seen in adult males **t interdigitale** fungal infection of interdigital spaces between adjoining toes or finger **t manum** fungal infection of the palms and it is markedly itchy **t pedis** fungal infection of the soles that appear as circumscribed areas of scaling and fissures in adults **t unguium** fungal infection of nails **t versicolor** fungal infection by *Malassezia furfur* forming discrete hypo- or hyperpigmented macules with overlying fine scaling over the trunk, proximal extremities and face

Tinel's (ti'nelz) **sign** nerve regeneration indicated by occurrence of tingling sensation on percussion over the site of nerve injury, named after Jules Tinel, French neurosurgeon

tingible bodies macrophages that contain fragments of lymphocyte nuclei

tinkle a sound like the ringing of a small bell

tinnitus (tin-i'tus) a persistent ringing sound heard in the ear

tipped uterus inclination of the uterus backward instead of being slightly forward

tipping (tip'ing) angulation of a structure

tire (tir) become exhausted

tissue (tish'u) an aggregation of similar cells united to perform a particular function **t culture** growth of tissue *in vitro* on artificial media **t plasminogen activator** tPA a thrombolytic protease that converts plasminogen into plasmin, activating fibrinolysis, without affecting the circulating plasminogen or fibrinogen **t typing** a series of tests of a donor and recipient before transplant surgery

titre (ti'ter) the quantity of a substance required to produce a reaction with a given volume of another substance **antibody t** a measure of the amount of antibody against a particular antigen present in the blood

titubation (tit'u-ba'shun) shaking of the trunk and head; staggering

tiw abb. Three times a week

TLC 1. total lung capacity 2. total leucocyte count

t lymphocyte a type of thymic lymphoid cell that fights infections and cancer cells directly

toadskin (tod'skin) a condition characterised by excessive dryness, wrinkling and scaling of skin, as in Vitamin A deficiency

tobacco (to-bak'o) dried leaves of *Nicotiana tabacum*. It contains nicotine. It is widely used in the form of cigarettes, *beedies*, cigars, snuff and chewing tobacco

TNM classification tumour, nodes, metastases; an international system for staging cancer by giving numerical values to each of these

Tobey-Ayer test in thrombosis of transverse sinuses, the compression on jugular vein of the affected side does not cause rise in CSF pressure, named after George Tobey Jr, US otolaryngologist and James Ayer, US neurologist

tobramycin an aminoglycoside antibiotic

tocolytic (to'ko-li-tik) an agent that arrests uterine contractions in labour

tocolysin any drug reducing force of uterine contraction

tocometer instrument recording the uterine contractions

tocopherol (to-kof'er-ol) vitamin E

Todd's palsy prolonged episodes of partial seizures may leave paresis of the involved limb lasting for several hours after the seizure ceases, named after Robert Todd, British physician

toe (to) one of the digits of the foot

togaviruses a family of medium-sized viruses with single-strand RNA and lipid envelope. Many arboviruses and rubella are examples

toilet 1. cleaning of a wound following operation or of an obstetrical patient 2. an area for use during defecation and urination

tolbutamide an oral hypoglycaemic agent of sulphonylurea group

tolerance (tol'er-ans) the ability to endure without ill effect; endurance; need to take increasingly higher doses of a drug to obtain the same effect

tolerant (tol'er-ant) forbearing, indulgent

tolnaftate topically used antifungal agent for ringworm

toluene a hydrocarbon derived from coal tar

tomogram (to'mo-gram) a roentgenogram of a selected layer of the body

tomograph (to'mo-graf) an x-ray apparatus to produce a tomogram

tomography (to'mog'ra-fe) body section roentgenography; laminography. A diagnostic imaging technique that produces a cross-sectional image of an organ or part of the body computed t CT, tomography in which transverse planes of tissue are swept by radiographic beam and a computerised analysis of variance in absorption produces a precise reconstructed image of that area computerised axial t CAT, positron emission t PET, reconstruction of brain sections using positron-emitting radionuclides. The coloured images indicate degree of metabolism or blood flow single position emission computed t SPECT an imaging method for reconstructing cross-sectional images of radiotracer distributions

tone (ton) normal degree of tension in muscle; quality or character of sound

tongs an instrument having two arms joined by a hinge

tongue (tung) the movable muscular organ on the floor of mouth functioning in tasting, eating and speaking. It consists of a body and root and is attached by muscles to the hyoid bone below, mandible in front, styloid process behind and the palate above and by the mucous membrane to the floor of the mouth, the lateral walls of pharynx and the epiglottis. The surface of the tongue has numerous papillae (filiform, fungiform and vallate). Taste buds are present on the papillae especially the vallate papillae. The mucous and serous glands open on the surface black hairy t fungal infection associated with a brown fur due to elongated growth of the filiform papillae without desquamation geographic t appearance of a map on the tongue due to localised irregular red areas of desquamation of filiform papillae surrounded by a whitish border megenta t a megenta-coloured tongue in riboflavin deficiency scrotal t a furrowed and fissured tongue resembling the skin of the scrotum smooth t smooth surface tongue due to atrophy of papillae as in anaemia strawberry t red tongue in scarlet fever due to hypertrophy of fungiform papillae t-tie a midline mucosal fold on the under-surface of the tongue, binding it to the floor of the mouth impeding its movements

tonic (ton'ik) continuous tension; a substance that invigorates or strengthens t atrophy wasting of muscles with active reflexes. t clonic fits grand mal seizures t phase early rigid stage of contraction of all muscles as in major fits t pupil delayed reaction to light and accommodation t reflex maintenance of muscle tone

tonicity (to'nis'i-te) 1. tone 2. property of possessing tone 3. a physiological process dependent upon the selectively permeable characteristics of a membrane

tonometer (ton-om'e-ter) an instrument to measure tension of a gas in a liquid or pressure usually intraocular pressure; an instrument to measure frequencies of tones as a tuning fork

tonometry (ton-om'e-tre) the measurement of tension or pressure of the fluid inside the eye as intraocular pressure; the measurement of the frequencies of tones

"T on p" phenomenon *ECG* sinus tachycardia with prolongation of Q-T and a delayed T wave followed or overlapped by the succeeding P wave, as in alkalosis

tonsil (ton'sil) 1. a small oval mass of lymphoid tissue on each side of the fauces 2. rounded projection towards the midline of the posterior end of lower surface of each cerebral hemisphere **faucial t** palatine tonsil **lingual t** mass of lymphoid tissue in the root of the tongue **nasal t** lymphoid tissue on the nasal septum **palatine t** a mass of lymphoid tissue lying in the tonsillar fossa on each side of the oral pharynx between the glossopalatine and pharyngopalatine arches **pharyngeal t** lymphoid tissue on the roof of the posterior wall of the nasopharynx.

tonsillar (ton'si-lar) pertaining to a tonsil **t fossa** a depression located between the glossopalatine and pharyngopalatine arches in which the palatine tonsil is situated

tonsillectomy (ton-sil-ek'to-me) the operative removal of a tonsil or the tonsils. It is performed in those with recurrent severe tonsillitis

tonsillitis (ton-sil-i'tis) inflammation of the tonsils, especially faucial tonsil. It has a sudden onset with fever, chills, head ache, pain in tonsils while swallowing. The tonsils appear enlarged and red

tonus (to'nus) the slight, continuous tension in muscle

tooth (toth) one of a set of small hard bodies attached in a row to each jaw pl. **teeth** They c , grind and process food in the mouth for ingestion. Each tooth consists of a crown which projects above the gum, two to four roots, embedded in the alveolus and a neck between the crown and the root. Each tooth contains a cavity filled with pulp, and it is richly supplied with blood vessels and nerves. The solid portion of the tooth consists of dentin; and the enamel covers the exposed portion of the crown. Two sets of teeth appear at different periods of life; the 20 deciduous teeth appear during infancy and 32 permanent teeth during childhood and early adulthood **impacted t** a tooth that is unable to erupt due to adjacent teeth or malposition of the tooth **t surface** the external aspect of tooth that has labial, lingual, mesial, distal and occlusal surfaces

toothache pain in the tooth or region about a tooth

toothpaste a dentifrice used with a brush to clean the exposed surfaces of the teeth

tophaceous (to'fa'shus) hard or gritty

tophus (to'fus) a chalky deposit of urates in the soft tissue about joint and in the pinna of the ear. pl. **tophi**

topical a particular part of the body; pertaining to matters of current interest

topognosis (to'pog-no'sis) ability to localise tactile sensations

topographic (top'o-graf'ik) pertaining to specific position relative to one another

topology (to-pol'o-je) the relation between the presenting part of the foetus and the birth canal

TORCH agents *Toxoplasma gondi*, other transplacental infections, rubella virus, cytomegalovirus and herpes virus infection of the uterus that may induce major malformations in the foetus and cause prominent neurologic defects

torpor lack of response to normal stimulus; apathy; inactivity

torque (tork) a rotary force

torr (tor) a unit of pressure required to support a column of mercury one mm high at 0°C and standard gravity, named after Italian mathematician Torricelli

Torsade de pointes *ECG* a form of ventricular tachycardia with prolonged QT intervals that are initiated by a premature ventricular depolarisation stricking near the apex of a delayed T-wave. They have irregular rates of 200-250/min, with marked variability in amplitude and direction of a QRS wave that seems to twist around an isoelectric baseline

torsion (tor'shun) the act of twisting **t dystonia** a disorder of basal ganglia exhibiting a prolonged muscular contraction and the part of the body thrown into spasm **t of testicle** twisting of the cord that is attached to a testicle. It interrupts its blood supply and may destroy it

torso (tor'so) the trunk of the human body

torticollis (tor'ti-kol'is) wry neck, a contracted state of the cervical muscles causing twisting of the neck and inclination of the head to one side

tortuous full of turns, twists or bends

torture a deliberate form of cruel, inhuman and degrading punishment. It is an act by which severe pain or suffering whether physical and/or mental, is intentionally inflicted on a person to obtain a confession or information **t medicine** a multi-disciplinary medical specialty providing holistic care to the victims of torture

torulosis (tor-u-lo'sis) cryptococcosis

torulus (tor'u-lus) a small elevation

torus (to'rus) a rounded ridge **t fracture** an incomplete fracture of the diaphysis of long bones with buckling of the cortex on the side opposite the fracture

total hip replacement a procedure that replaces the femoral head and its articular surface with a completely synthetic device

total iron-binding capacity TIBC, a quantitative measurement of transferrin's ability to transport iron

total ischaemic burden the sum total of all episodes of myocardial ischaemia

total knee replacement a procedure that substitutes a painful arthritic knee and its articular surface with a synthetic substitute

total lung capacity the total volume of air contained in the lung after a maximal voluntary inspiration; TLC. It consists of four fractions - tidal volume, inspiratory reserve volume, expiratory reserve volume and residual volume

total parenteral nutrition TPN intravenous hyperalimentation that attempts to provide all body's need for nutrition without using gastrointestinal tract

totipotent (to-tip'o-tent) an ability of a part to develop in any manner; a cell capable of differentiating into any type of cell

touch (tuch) to perceive by the tactile sense to feel with the hands

toucheurism sexual satisfaction from touching opposite sex

tour de maitre (toor'de-ma'tr) *Fr* a method of introducing a catheter or sound into the male bladder or into the uterus

Tourette's syndrome a disorder characterised by recurrent twitching, snorting and sniffing noises and involuntary shouting of obscenities. *see* Gilles de la Tourette's syndrome

tourniquet (toor'ni-ket) an appliance to compress a blood vessel to reduce blood flow **t test** capillary fragility test. Appearance of 10 or more petechiae within a circle of 2.5 cm in diameter on the forearm when the sphygmomanometer cuff is left inflated for 15 minutes on the arm at a pressure midway between the systolic and diastolic pressures. It may occur in thrombocytopaenia, non thrombocytopaenic purpura and scurvy

Touton giant cell a type of multinucleate histiocytic giant cell present in some granulomas in which the lipid content is great, named after Karl Touton, German dermatologist

Town's view fronto-occipital radiography

toxaemia (toks-e'me-a) a general intoxication due to a presence of toxins in the blood stream. **t of pregnancy** pree-clampsia or eclampsia

toxic (toks'ik) pertaining to a poison **t epidermal necrolysis** TEN, a severe mucocutaneous reaction pattern characterised by fever, systemic toxicity, tenderness, erythema and widespread exfoliation **t megacolon** an acute colitis with partial or complete colonic dilatation occurring as a life threatening complication of ulcerative colitis and Crohn's disease **t shock syndrome** TSS, a life threatening condition caused by staphylococci associated most often with the use of some highly absorbable tampons **t state** a condition typically seen in third week of typhoid at which the patient is markedly sick, disoriented and having greatest risk for intestinal perforation and haemorrhage **t vacuolisation** rounded 'empty' cytoplasmic spaces within neutrophils seen in gram-negative bacteraemia and endotoxaemia.

toxicity (toks-isi-te) the quality of being poisonous

toxicology (toks'i-kol'o-je) scientific study of poisons, its effects, manifestations and treatment

toxicosis (toks'i-ko'sis) any disorder produced by the action of a poison

toxin (toks'in) any of a group of poisonous substances produced by microorganisms, or plants or of animal origin

Toxocara a nematode worm, *Toxocara canis* or *T. cati*

toxocariasis infestation with the larvae of round worms of the genus Toxocara that normally live in the intestines of dogs

toxoid (toks'oyd) a modified bacterial exotoxin which has lost its toxicity but retains the property of stimulating the formation of antibodies

toxoplasma (toks'o-plas'ma) an intracellular protozoan parasite of genus Sporozoa

toxoplasmosis a protozoan parasitic disease caused by *Toxoplasma gondii* con-

genital **t** occurs from transmission from mother infected during pregnancy to foetus. The manifestations are cerebral with hydrocephalus or microcephaly associated with convulsions, tremors or paralysis **acquired t** toxoplasma organism invades lymph nodes and spleen. It may be asymptomatic or present with features of pneumonia, or enlarged lymph nodes

tPA abbreviation for tissue plasminogen activator

TPN abbreviation for total parenteral nutrition

TPR abbreviation for temperature, pulse and respiration

trabecula (tra-bek'u-la) 1. a supporting connective tissue strand 2. bony plate of cancellous bone

trace element a mineral required by the body only in minute amounts, such as cobalt, copper, magnesium, manganese, selinium and zinc

tracer readily recognisable element, usually radioactive or radical introduced into a metabolite

trachea (tra'ke-a) windpipe; the cartilaginous tube from the larynx to its bifurcation into the right and left main bronchi; trachea is 12 cm long and consists of a framework of 16 to 20 C-shaped cartilaginous plates with a dense connective tissue

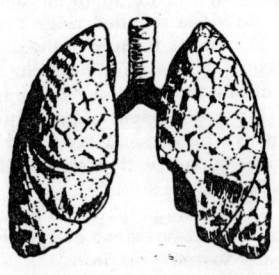

Trachea and lungs

tracheal (tra'ke-al) pertaining to the trachea **t tug** downward pull with each pulsation of the heart seen in aortic aneurysm

tracheitis (tra'ke-i'tis) inflammation of the trachea usually caused by infection

tracheobronchial (tra'ke-o-brong'ke-al) pertaining to the trachea and bronchi

tracheobronchitis (tra'ke-o-brong'ki-tis) inflammation of the trachea and bronchi

tracheooesophageal pertaining to the trachea and oesophagus **t fistula** an abnormal passage between trachea and oesophagus. It may occur as a birth defect or following surgery

tracheomalacia (tra'ke-o-ma'a-she-a) softening of the tracheal cartilages

tracheostenosis (tra'ke-o-sten-o'sis) narrowing of the trachea

tracheostomy (trak'ke-os'to-me) the surgical creation of an opening into the trachea through the neck. It provides an airway during tracheal obstruction

tracheotomy (trak'ke-ot'o-me) incision of the trachea through the skin and muscles of the neck in which a tube is inserted into the trachea to keep the airway open

trachoma (trak-ko'ma) a chronic infection of the conjunctiva and cornea caused by *Chlamydia trachomatis*. Transmission occurs by direct contact responds to tetracyclines, or erythromycin

tract (trakt) bundle of nerve fibres having common origin and termination and subserving similar function; a number of organs arranged in series subserving a common function

traction (trak'shun) a procedure of exerting a pulling force, along the long axis of a structure. To align two adjoining structures or to hold them in place. A traction technique is used to align some types of fracture of the femur

traditional medicine the sum total of all the knowledge and practices, whether explicable or not, used in diagnosis, prevention and elimination of physical, mental or social imbalance and relying exclusively on practical experience and observation handed down from generation to generation whether verbally or in writing

tragi (tra'ji) hair growing on the pinna of external ear

tragus (tra'gus) cartilaginous projection anterior to the external opening of the ear

trailing phenomenon perceptual abnormality associated with hallucinogenic drugs where moving objects appear as a series of discrete and discontinuous images

trait (trat) any genetically determined observable characteristic or condition; a disposition or tendency to act in a certain manner

tram-tracking radiologically when seen longitudinally the thickened airway walls appear as parallel, curved lines in bronchiectasis

trance (trans) a profound degree of sleep from which the person cannot be aroused easily **t state** altered state of consciousness with markedly diminished or selectively focussed responsiveness to environmental stimulus

tranquilizer (tran'kwi-liz'er) an agent which has calming effect without inducing sleep

trans- prefix meaning through; across

transabdominal (trans'ab-dom'i-nal) through the abdominal wall

transaminase (trans-am'in-as) an enzyme that catalyses the reversible transfer of an amino group

transbronchial needle biopsy *see* biopsy

transcend (tran's-end) to rise above, excel

transcervical balloon tuboplasty a procedure attempting to reestablish the patency of fallopian tubes

transcortin cortisol binding globulin

transcript handwritten or typed copy of the original

transcription (tran-skrip'shun) synthesis of a single-stranded RNA molecule from a double standard DNA template in the nucleus, during protein production **t activator** a protein that binds to DNA, activating its transcription machinery **t factors** DNA-binding proteins necessary for gene activity **t unit** a DNA sequence that is transcribed into a coherent peptide

transcutaneous through the skin **t electrical nerve stimulation** TENS a method of relieving pain by application of minute impulses to nerve endings beneath the skin **t oxygen monitor** skin electrode using polarography to measure blood oxygen

transdermal therapy use of topical prolonged release forms of drugs such as nitroglycerine or testosterone

transducer (trans-du'ser) a device that receives energy from one system and retransmits in a different form to another

transduction (trans-duk'shun) transfer of genetic material from one cell to another by viral infection

transection (tran-sek'shun) a cross section cut transversely

transfection (trans-fex'shun) acquisition of new genetic markers by incorporation of added DNA into eukaryotic cells

transferase (trans-fer-as) any of the enzymes that catalyses the transfer of an organic group from one compound to another

transferrin (trans-fer'rin) serum beta globulin that binds and transports iron, throughout the body in the blood stream

transfer RNA a molecule of RNA that picks up a specific amino acid in a cell and joins it with other aminoacids in a correct sequence to make a particular protein

transfix (trans-fiks) to pierce through with a pointed weapon.

transfixion (trans-fik'shun) a weapon cutting through from within outward

transformation (trans'for-me'shun) a change of form from one to another

transfusion (trans-fu'shun) administration of blood or blood components directly into the blood stream **t medicine** a subspecialty involved in patient management through administration of blood cells and blood products **t reaction** any untoward response to nonself blood products which elicit febrile reactions that are either minor from non-specific leucocyte derived pyrogens or major due to a true immune reaction

transgenation mutation

transient of brief duration **t ischaemic attack** TIA, a brief interruption in the blood supply to the brain that results in temporary impaired sensation, movement, vision or speech. The disability is less than 24 hours duration. TIAs often precede cerebral infarctions or strokes

transiliac (trans-il'e-ak) across two ilia

transillumination (trans'il-lu'mi-na'shun) the passage of light through body tissues for purpose of diagnosis

translation (trans'la'shun) the conversion of genetically coded instructions into a sequence of aminoacids to make an essential protein inside a cell

translocation (trans'lo-ka'shun) transfer of a segment of one chromosome to another part of homologous chromosome; rearrangement of genetic information on a chromosome

translucent (trans-lu'sent) diffuse transmission of light so that objects beyond are not clearly visible

transmembrane protein a protein that is fully integrated in the plasma membrane

transmission (trans-mish'un) transfer, as in communicable diseases, transmitted from reservoir or source of infection to susceptible host **airborne t** the spread of infectious agents by aerosal or dust particles **placental t** the transmission of substances in the mother's blood of foetus through placenta **synaptic t** the release of neurotransmitters by a neuron that either initiates or inhibits the passage of an electrical impulse to the next neuron **vertical t** passage of infection from mother's body fluid to the infant either in utero, during delivery or during breast feeding

transmissible capable of being transferred from one person to another

transmural (trans-mu'ral) across the wall of an organ or structure

transplacental (trans'pla-sen'tal) through the placenta

transplant (trans-plant) to transfer an organ or tissue from one person to another or from one part of the body to another or any organ or tissue that is transplanted

transplantation (trans'plan-ta'shun) the grafting of tissues or organ taken from the same body or from another to replace a malfunctioning part **t rejection** host immune responses evoked when an allograft tissue is transplanted into a recipient

transport transfer of substances in a biologic system

transposition (trnaz'po-zishun) displacement of a viscus to opposite side

transposon (tranz-po'zon) vehicle of transfer of genetic material between individual bacteria

transpupillary thermotherapy a technique in which heat is delivered to the choroid and retinal pigment epithelium through the pupil using a modified diode laser, useful in choroidal melanoma

transsexual (trans-seks'u-al) change of external anatomy of a person to that of opposite sex; a person affected by transsexualism

transsexualism a gender identity disorder characterised by a persistent belief on the part of the affected individuals that they belong to the opposite sex **female t** present masculine appearance and behaviour **male t** behaves that he will grow up to be a woman and lose his genitals

transudate (trans'u-dat) a fluid that has

passed through a membrane or extruded from tissue. This fluid has protein less than 3 gm% specific gravity less than 1015 and fewer cellular elements

transudation (trans-u-da'shun) the passage of fluid through a membrane or tissue surface

transurethral (trans-u-re'thral) performed through the urethra **t prostatectomy** removal of prostate with a resectoscope which is passed up through the urethra

transvaginal (trans-vajinal) performed through the vagina

transversalis (trans'ver-sa'lis) transverse

transverse foramen a canal through the transverse processes of the cervical vertebrae for passage of the vertebral arteries

transverse lie a non-cephalic, non-breech position in which the foetus 'long axis is perpendicular to that of the mothers' due to lower uterine obstruction. Such shoulder presentation are managed by caesarian section

transverse myelitis an acute inflammatory, demyelinating disorder affecting the spinal cord over a variable number of segments. It presents with subacute paraparesis with a sensory level

trapped lung a portion of infected lobe of the lung and visceral pleura fixing the affected lung in a partially collapsed state, seen in empyema

trapped nerve nerve compression

transversion (trans-ver'zhun) eruption of a tooth in a position normally occupied by another

transvesical (trans-ves'i-kal) through the bladder

transvestism (trans-vest'izm) a sexual deviation having an excessive desire to wear the dress of the opposite sex

trapezium (tra-pe'ze-um) 1. a quadrilateral plane figure of which no two sides are parallel 2. the first bone on the radial side of the distal row of the bones of the wrist, os trapezium. It articulates with the base of metacarpal bone of the thumb

trapezius (tra-pe'ze-us) a broad flat muscle on either side of upper and back of the neck, shoulders and thorax

trapezoid (trap'e-zoyd) having the shape of a four-sided place with two sides parallel and two diverging

T ratio *stat* used to determine whether the results obtained are due to chance - alone

trauma (traw'ma) a wound or physical injury; a severe emotional shock **t centre** an hospital providing care for critically injured patients **t score** numerical grading system that combines the Glasgow Coma scale and measurement of cardiopulmonary function as a gauge of severity of injury and to predict the outcome.

traumatic (traw-mat'ik) produced by a trauma **t arthritis** arthritis developing after an injury to a joint **t tap** a diagnostic lumbar puncture in which there is incidental haemorrhage from tearing of vessels. It is differentiated from subarachnoid haemorrhage by absence of xanthochromia, rapid coagulation of blood and decreasing erythrocytes in serial tubes

traumatology (traw-ma-tol'oje) the branch of surgery dealing with wounds or injuries

traveller's diarrhoea a diarrhoea that can occur when a person visits a foreign country and ingests contaminated food or water

tray (tra) a flat surface with raised edges *trayi* (s) three fold

treadmill test an exercise test to assess a person's risk of death from cardiovascular events. The score is calculated as the duration of exercise in minutes − (5 × the maximal ST segment deviation in mm during or after exercise) − (4 × the treadmill angina index i.e. 0 = no angina during exercise 1 = non limiting angina, 2 = exercise limiting angina)

treatment (tret'ment) care and management of a patient to combat disease **active t** treatment directed specifically towards cure of the condition **causal t** treatment directed towards the removal of cause of the disease **conservative t** withholding medicine unless indicated; preservation of an organ or part of it during operative procedure **dental t** treatment of the teeth and adjacent tissues **dietetic t** treatment of disease based on regulation of diet **empiric t** treatment based on observation and experience **palliative t** treatment designs to relieve symptoms **preventive t** treatment directed at the prevention of disease **specific t** treatment directed at the cause of disease **supportive t** measures to supplement specific therapy **surgical t** treatment by operative procedure **symptomatic t** treatment of the symptoms than disease

trehalose non-reducing disaccharide found in some mycobacteria and fungi

trematoda (trem'a-to'da) parasitic flukes; platyhelminthes; flat worms

tremble (trem'bl) to shiver, quiver or shake.

tremor (trem'or) regular rhythmic oscillatory movements around a fixed axis due to alternating contraction and relaxation of the muscles **essential t** coarse postural termor noted in upper extremity, head and neck. Noted with muscle contraction, exaggerated by emotional and physical stress **flapping t** movements simulating the beating of wings with rapid flexion and extensions at the wrist and metacarpophalangeal joints seen in hepatic precoma, respiratory and renal failure **hysterical t** variable tremors with a bizarre picture involving a limb or whole body **intention t** appearance of tremors in a limb with a goal directed action due to loss of modulating effect of cerebellum on voluntary movement, seen in brain stem or cerebellar disease **k tremor** intention tremor due to affection of cerebellum and its outflow pathways0 **pill-rolling t** tremors as rotary movements between the index finger and the thumb **postural t** fine tremors at a fast rate in a limb held in an antigravity posture, noted in situations of catecholamine excess such as thyrotoxicosis, anxiety state, hypoglycaemia and in alcoholism **static t** rapid tremors which are rhythmically alternating in flexor and extensor muscles that are marked at rest as in Parkinsonism **toxic t** postural tremors seen in excess smoking and ingestion of drugs such as caffeine, theophylline, amphetamine, beta 2 agonists and tricyclic antidepressants

tremulous (trem'o-lus) shaking, trembling

trench fever infection with *Rickettsia quintana* with typhus-like condition

trench foot cold trauma due to prolonged exposure to cold

trench mouth fusospirochaetal stomatitis

trend general direction, course

Trendelenburg test a test of stability of the hip and particularly of the ability of the hip abductors (gluteus medius and gluteus minimus) to stabilise the pelvis upon the femur. When the patient stands on the affected limb and lifts the sound leg from the ground, the iliac crest falls on the lifted side indicating the abductor muscles are incapable of stabilising the pelvis upon femur. It is noted in poliomyelitis, congenital dislocation of the hip and ununited fracture of the femoral neck.

Trendelenburg operation Sephanous ligation for varix, named after Friedrich Trendelenburg, German surgeon

Trendelenburg position marked head down tilt of whole body especially for pelvic operations

trepanation (tre'pan-a-shun) the drilling of a hole in the skull to relieve distress, one of the earliest known surgical procedures

trephine (tre-fin') a saw for removal of a circular disc of bone; an instrument for removal of a circular area of cornea

trepidation (trep'i-da'shun) trembling

Treponema (trep'o-ne'ma) spiral bacteria. *T. carateum* causative agent of pinta, *T. pallidum* causative agent of syphilis, *T. pertenue* causative agent of yaws

treponemal (trep'o-ne-ma-l) caused by Treponema

treponemiasis (trep'o-ne-mi'a-sis) infection with treponema; syphilis

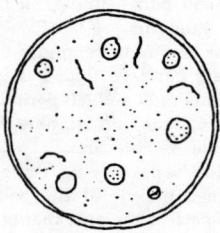

Treponema pallidum

trepopnoea (trep-op'ne-a) a condition in which breathing is most comfortable when the patient is turned to a definite recumbent position

Treves' bloodless fold ileocaecal fold of peritoneum that connects antimesenteric border of end of ileum to mesentery of appendix, named after Frederick Treves, British surgeon

TRF abbreviation for thyrotropin-releasing factor

TRH abbreviation for thyrotropin-releasing hormone

triad (tri'ad) a group of three entities; an association of three clinical or pathologic findings, characteristic of a disease

triage (tre-azh') a system to sort out and categorise casualties to determine priority of need and proper place of treatment

triamcinolone a synthetic glucocorticoid

triamterene mild diuretic causing retention of potassium

triangle (tri'ang-gl) a three-cornered area **t of codman** a wedge-shaped periosteal elevation of bone seen on a plain film of the long bones characteristic of Ewing's sarcoma **t test** a method to investigate the neighbourhood of the shoulder joint for bony injury. The triangle is formed by three bony points, namely the tip of acromion, the tip of the coracoid process and the most prominent part of the great tuberosity of the humerus

triangular having three angles **t bandage** a square bandage folded diagonally **t ligaments** right and left peritoneal folds between liver and diaphragm on either side of bare area

triceps (tri-'seps) having three heads **t muscle** a muscle at the back of the upper part of the arm that straightens the elbow joint **t skin fold thickness** estimation of corporal fat by measuring on the right arm halfway between the olecranon process of the elbow and the acromial process of scapula

trichiasis (trik-i'a-sis) a condition of ingrowing eyelashes that causes them to rub against eyeball

Trichinella (trik'i-nel'la) a nematode parasite *Trichinella spiralis* one of the smallest nematodes causing trichinosis

trichinosis (trik'in-o'sis) disease due to *Trichinella spiralis* which spreads by eating undercooked meat. Symptoms occur from secondary invasion of tissues mainly striated muscle in which larvae encyst. Initially the condition presents with diarrhoea, later by fever, oedema of face, eyelids and conjunctiva, stiffness, pain and tenderness of muscle. There is eosinophilia and albendazole is useful

trichobezoar (trik'o-be'zor) a hair ball formed in the stomach or intestine

trichoglossia (trik'o-glos'e-a) hairy tongue due to thickening of papillae

trichologist (trik'o-logi-st) a person qualified to work in the field of trichology

trichology (trik'o-logi) the study of the hair and scalp in healthy and disease conditions

trichomonas (trik'o-mo'nas) a parasitic flagellate protozoa called *Trichomonas vaginalis* that is sexually transmitted

trichomoniasis (trik'o-mo-ni-a-sis) infection with *T. vaginalis*, common in women, presents with burning, redness and itching of vulvar tissue and profuse vaginal discharge. It may be malodorous. Metronidazole is useful

trichonosis (trik-o-no'sis) any disease of the hair

trichophytobezoar (trik-o-fi'to-be-zor) a bezoar composed of animal hair and vegetable fibres

trichophyton (tri-kof'it-on) a genus of imperfect fungi **t rubrum** dermatophytic infection where fungus remains confined to stratum corneum only

trichotillomania (trik'o-till'o-man-ia) compulsive hair pulling

trichrome stain a stain used in histopathology, that stains collagen green, muscle red-purple and myelin brown. Useful to determine muscle invasion in certain carcinomas

trichthecenis (trik'the-sen-sis) mycotoxin produced by Fusarium and Stachybotrys

trichuriasis (trik'-u-ri'a-sis) infection caused by nematode, Trichuris. Intense infections in children present with persistent diarrhoea or rectal prolapse and stunting. Treatment is with mebendazole

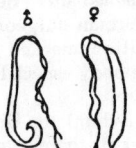 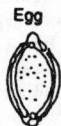

Trichuris trichura

Trichuris (tri-kri'ris) an intestinal nematode, whipworm. *T. trichiura* a species

of *Trichuris* that infects humans when the ova are ingested. The larvae develop into adults which inhabit large intestine, caecum, lower ileum and anal canal

tricuspid (tri-kus'pid) three cusps **t atresia** absent tricuspid orifice, hypoplastic right ventricle with right atrium to left atrium shunt **t insufficiency** incompetence of tricuspid valve leaking the blood backward **t stenosis** narrowing of the opening of tricuspid valve **t valve** the valve that guards the opening between the right atrium and right ventricle, and it has largest circumference

tricyclic antidepressant drug used to treat depression

trident (trident) three-pronged **t hand** short fifth finger seen in mongolism

tridosha (s) three pathogenic factors - *Vata*, *Pitta* and *Kapha*

trigastric (tri-gas'trik) having three bellies, a muscle interrupted by two tendons

trigeminal fifth cranial nerve **t ganglia** ganglia situated lateral to cavernous sinus that receives sensory fibres of all three branches of trigeminal nerve

trigeminy *ECG* a form of arrhythmia in which every third QRS wave is a ventricular premature beat

trigger finger thickening and constriction of the mouth of a fibrous digital sheath interfering with the free gliding of the contracted flexor tendons. It may affect the fingers in middle aged and the thumb in infants. In adults there is tenderness at the base of affected finger and locking of the finger in full flexion. Infants are unable to straighten the thumb which is locked in flexion. The treatment consists of incising the mouth of the fibrous flexor sheath longitudinally

trigger points areas of the body which become unusually tender or sensitivie at the onset of a particular disease

trigger thumb a congenital fixed flexion deformity of the thumb related to a narrow flexor pollicis longus

triglyceride glycerol with all three hydroxyls linked to fatty acids

trigger zone relatively circumscribed regions adjacent to nerves often in the head and neck when stimulated even with light touch may elicit marked neuralgia accompanied by lightning pain

trigonal (trig'o-nal) triangular

trigone (tri'gon) a triangular area **t of bladder** a triangular area at the base of the bladder between the two openings of the ureter and urethra

trika (s) sacrum

trikurccham **(s)** trocar for evacuating abscesses

trilogy (tril'o-je) a combination of three elements or events

trimester (tri-mes'ter) one of the three periods of approximately 3 months each into which pregnancy is divided

trimethoprim TMP, folic acid antagonist **t-sulphamethoxazole** SMX, a combination anti-bacterial agent formulated as a 1:20 ratio of TMP to SMX, effective against genitourinary, gastrointestinal and respiratory tract infections and to treat *Pneumocystis carinii* pneumonia

tripara (trip'a-ra) a woman who has had three pregnancies that have lasted beyond 20 weeks

triphasic pills oral contraceptives in which the progesterone levels vary every seven days during the cycle while the oestrogen levels remain constant

triple A syndrome an inherited familial disorder characterised by primary adrenocortical insufficiency, chalasia of the cardia and alacrimia, see Allgrove syndrome

triple fusion arthrodesis of talus, calcaneum and cuboid bones to stabilise the foot

triplet (trip'let) one of three individuals produced at the same birth after a long period of gestation

triple response a triad of transient skin changes seen in immediate hypersensitivity when the skin is firmly stroked by a pointed object, characterised by an immediate response or stroke due to local release of histamine and prostaglandin, flare as a red halo due to vasodilation and wheal with a swelling and blanching of the stroke due to histamine release from mast cells and oedema of intercellular junctions with protein and fluid accumulation, described by Lewis

triple X syndrome a chromosome abnormality in which a female has an extra X chromosome. It may be associated with mental retardation

triploidy having three sets of otherwise normal chromosomes

tripod (tri'pod) a stand having three supports

triquetral (tri-kew'tral) triangular t bone 1. the third carpal bone in the proximal row, enumerated from the radial side 2. any wormian bone

trismus (tris'mus) spasm of muscles of mastication with difficulty to open the mouth and in mastication; lock jaw

trisomy (tri'so-me) the presence of an additional chromosome of one type in a diploid cell which results in severe genetic disorders t 13 mental defect, microphthalmia, polydactyly and congenital heart disease; Patau's syndrome t 18 mental defect, micrognathia, deformed hands and feet, congenital heart disease; Edward's syndrome t 21 Down's syndrome; mongolism

trituration (tri'tur-a-shun) a controlled grinding and mixing process by which substances are added to a base

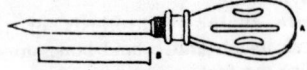

A. Trocar with handle; B. Cannula

Trocar and cannula

trocar (tro'kar) a sharp-pointed obturator contained in a cannula to pierce the wall of a cavity

trochanter (tro-kan'ter) either of the two processes below the neck of the femur greater t a thick process at the upper end of femur projecting upwards externally to the union of the neck and shaft lesser t a conical tuberosity on the inner and posterior surface of the upper end of the femur at the junction of shaft and neck third t an unusually prominent gluteal ridge of the femur

troche (tro'ke) losenze. It releases drug as it dissolves in the mouth

trochlea (trok'le-a) a pulley-shaped structure

trochlear (trok'le-ar) 1. pertaining to a trochlea 2. of the nature of a pulley. t muscle superior oblique muscle of eye t nerve see tables of nerves

troika triad

trombicula (trom-bik'o-la) the chigger mite

trophic (trof'ik) referring to nutrition

trophoblast (trof'o-blast) a layer of extraembryonic ectodermal tissue on the outside of blastocyst. It develops into placenta and aminotic sac

trophoblastic tumour an abnormal growth that arises from the trophoblast

trophozoite (trof'o-zo'it) the active motile feeding stage of a protozoa

Troisier's (trwa-ze-az) sign left supraclavicular node as first sign of carcinoma of stomach, named after Charles Troisier, French physician

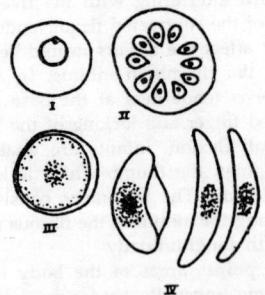

Trophozoite of P. vivax stage I, II, III & IV

trophic ulcer *see* ulcer

trophoblast outer layer of conceptus, responsible for attachment to and chemical exchanges with the host

trophozoite (trof'o-zo':t) stage of simple growth of protozoa.

-trophy referring to nutrition or growth

-tropic of direction 1. movement in response to a stimulus 2. aim of a specific object 3. hormones stimulating specific object

tropical occurring chiefly in hot climate lying between cancer and capricorn t abscess amoebic liver abscess t polymyositis *Staphylococcus aureus* infection causing abscesses in muscle t pulmonary eosinophilia a respiratory disorder occurring as a hypersensitivity response to a filarial origin and presenting with cough, paroxysmal attacks of dyspnoea and eosinophilia t spastic parapesis demyelination of the long motor neurons in the spinal cord due to infection from human T cell lymphotropic virus (HTLV) t splenomegaly gross splenomegaly affecting malnourished children and adults in malaria-endemic regions and occurs as an exaggerated immune response to malaria t sprue a chronic progressive malabsorption in a patient in or from tropics. There is partial villous atrophy, diarrhoea, abdominal distension, anorexia, fatigue and weight loss. Tetracyclines are useful in the management t ulcer ulceration of legs and feet seen in malnoished, bare footed labourers with multiple infections in tropics

tropomyosin protein of voluntary and cardiac muscle, spirally wrapped round actin filament

troponin (tro'po-nin) an inhibitory protein in the muscle fibres

trough (trof) 1. a shallow longitudinal depression 2. being administered over a prolonged period that has potential side-effects

Trousseau's sign a sphygmomanometer cuff is placed around the arm and the pressure is raised to 200 mmHg. If tetany is present, typical contractions of the hand like obstetrician's hand occur within 5 minutes, named after Armand Trousseau, French Physician

true (troo) real; genuine t pelvis the portion of the pelvis below the iliopectineal line t ribs the seven upper ribs on either side of the chest with cartilages articulating directly with the sternum

truncal (trung'kal) pertaining to the trunk t ataxia inability to walk due to midline cerebellar lesion

truncate (trung'kat) to amputate

truncus (trung'kus) a stem; trunk t arteriosus the arterial trunk from the embryonic heart

trunk 1. that portion of the body exclusive of the head and limbs 2. the main stem of a nerve, lymphatic or blood vessel coeliac t the trunk arising from abdominal aorta that supplies blood to the stomach, duodenum, liver, gall bladder, pancreas and spleen pulmonary t the great vessel arising from the right ventricle of the heart that gives the right and left pulmonary arteries to the lungs sympathetic t the two long chains of ganglia connected by sympathetic nerve fibres that extend along the vertebral column.

trusion (troo'zhun) malposition of a tooth

truss (trus) an elastic appliance to retain a reduced hernia within the abdominal cavity

Trypanosoma (tri'pan-o-so'ma) a protozoan parasite with a whiplike flagella. *T. cruzi* causative agent of American trypanosomiasis. *T. gambiense* causative agent of African sleeping sickness *T. rhodesiense* causative agent of sleeping sickness in East Aftrica.

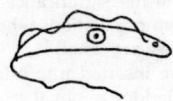

Trypanosoma gambiense

Trypanosomiasis (tr-pan'o-so-mi'a-sis) infection with protozoa of the genus trypanosoma **African t** African sleeping sickness caused by *T. gambiense* conveyed to humans by the bites of infested tsetse flies. It is characterised by irregular bouts of fever, and enlargement of lymph nodes, head ache, changed behaviour, insomnia by night and sleepiness by day and mental confusion. The Rhodesian infections are more acute and severe. It is managed by suramin or pentamidine. Difluoroethyl ornithine is used when nervous system is involved **American t** *see* Chagas disease

trypanosomicidal (tri-pan'o-so-mi-ci-dal) destructive to trypanosomes

trypsin (trip'sin) a proteolytic enzyme formed in the intestine from the action of enterokinase of intestinal juice on trypsinogen secreted by pancreas. It catalyses the hydrolysis of peptide bonds in partly digested proteins

trypsinogen (trip-sin'o-gen) a proenzyme found in pancreatic juice

tryptophan (trip'to-fan) an essential amino acid. It is found in high concentration in animal and fish protein. It is a precursor of serotonin

tsetse (she'she) blood sucking diptera confined to Africa. It is an important transmitter of trypanosomes, the causative agents of African sleeping sickness

TSH abbreviation for thyroid-stimulating hormone

TSH-RF abbreviation for thyroid-stimulating hormone releasing factor

tsutsugamushi (soot-soo-ga-moo'shi) **disease** Scrub typhus

t-test a statistical procedure designed to compare two sets of observations and to determine the significance between means of two populations when one or both samples are small

t-tube a devise inserted into biliary duct after gall bladder removal to facilitate drainage from bile duct

tuba (too'ba) a tube

tubal pertaining to a tube especially fallopian tube **t ligation** a female sterilisation procedure in which the fallopian tubes are surgically tied off and cut **t pregnancy** implantation of a fertilised egg in a fallopian tube. It is associated with severe abdominal pain and light vaginal bleeding **t reanastomosis** a surgical reconstruction procedure when the cut ends of a fallopian tube are joined together

tube (tub) a long hollow cylindrical structure **stomach t** a rubber tube to introduce food or to perform a wash **test t** a glass tube closed at one end **uterine t** fallopian tube

tubectomy (too-bek'to-me) excision of a portion of the uterine tubes

tube feeding providing fluid and food into the stomach through a nasogastric tube

tuber (tu'ber) a swelling, protuberance **t cinereum** a part of the base of hypothalamus that is connected by infundibulum with the posterior pituitary

tubercle (tu'ber-kl) 1. small, rounded nodule produced by infection with *Mycobacterium tuberculosis* 2. a small rounded elevation on a bone 3. a small nodule

tubercular (tu-ber'ku-lar) resembling tubercles **t chancre** extremely rare form of primary cutaneous tuberculosis with painless nodules which breakdown in a week to form an ulcer with enlargement of regional lymph nodes

tuberculid (tu-ber'ku-lid) a papular skin eruption probably due to allergy to tuberculosis

tuberculin (tu-ber'ku-lin) a sterile liquid containing the growth products of or specific substances extracted from the tubercle bacillus **t test** a test to determine the presence of tuberculosis infection based on positive reaction to tuberculin. It is useful in epidemiological survey to get a picture of prevalence of tuberculosis in a community and to select a group requiring BCG vaccination. The test is performed by either old tuberculin or tuberculin purified protein derivative. Mantoux test, Heaf's test or tine test are useful.

tuberculoid (tu-ber'ku-loyd) resembling tubercle.

tuberculoma (tu-ber'ku-lo'ma) a tumour-like mass from an enlarged caseous tubercle

tuberculosis (tu-ber'ku-lo'sis) an infectious disease caused by *Mycobacterium tuberculosis*. Lungs form the common site of the disease. Other sites are gastrointestinal and genitourinary systems, CNS, bones, joints, lymph nodes and skin **avian t** tuberculosis of birds caused by *Mycobacterium avium* **bovine t** tuberculosis of cattle caused by *Mycobacterium bovis* **endogenous t** tuberculosis originating from a primary lesion **exogenous t** tuberculosis acquired from an exogenous source **miliary t** presence of widespread lesions of tuberculosis occurring after a haematogenous dissemination of tubercle bacilli. It occurs in individuals who have inadequate cell-mediated immunity **multidrug resistant t** MDR-TB *Mycobacterium tuberculosis* that is resistant to therapy with a variety of antituberculosis agents that had been effective in treatment **open t** tuberculosis in which the tubercle bacilli are present in the sputum **post primary t** the pathological changes are as a result of interaction between tubercle bacilli and the host immunological responses. Tubercle is the primary lesion of tuberculosis, which undergoes caseous necrosis and forms a cavity. It can undergo fibrosis or get disseminated. Clinically it presents with fever, cough, loss of weight and haemoptysis. The condition is diagnosed by chest radiograph and sputum examination for presence of acid fast bacteria. It is treated with short course chemotherapy using rifampicin

INH, pyrazinamide, ethambutol and/or streptomycin **primary t** lesion due to an infection with *M. tuberculosis* in individuals who have never had previous experience with tubercle bacilli. The spread of the disease is by inhalation of airborne droplet nuclei containing tubercle bacilli. It is characterised by formation of tubercles and caseation, fibrosis and calcification

tuberosis (tu'ber-o'sis) a condition associated with the development of nodules

tuberosity (tu-ber-osi-te) an elevation or protuberance

tuberous sclerosis an autosomal dominant condition with hamartomas affecting many systems. Classically it is characterised by mental retardation, epilepsy and skin lesions like small white oval (ash leaf) macules or pink or yellowish papules on the centre of the face (adenoma sabaceum)

tuboplasty (tu'bo-plas'te) a surgical procedure to repair a narrowed or blocked fallopian tube

tubo-ovarian (tu'bo-o-va're-an) pertaining to a uterine tube and ovary

tubular (tu'bu-lar) shaped like a tube **t breathing** high pitched bronchial breathing heard over an area of consolidation of the lung as in lobar pneumonia

tubule (tu'bul) a small tube **renal t** the part of a nephron through which renal filtrate from the renal corpuscle flows and is changed to urine by absorption and secretion

tuft a cluster; a coil

tularemia (tu-lar-e'me-a) a bacterial infection by *Fancisella tularensis*. It is transmitted by ticks or acquired while skinning infected wild rabbits. It presents as a skin ulcer and painful regional lymphadenopathy. Streptomycin, gentamycin and tetracyclines are useful. It is named after Tulare in California where disease was first discovered

tulle gras a close-meshed net cut into squares and impregnated with soft paraffin, Peruvian balsam and vegetable oil to treat raw surfaces

tumefacient (tu-me-fa'shent) tending to cause swelling

tumefaction (tu'me-fak'shun) a swelling

tumescence (tu-mes'ens) swollen

tumid swollen

tumour (tu'mor) swelling, one of the cardinal signs of inflammation; a neoplastic growth with an uncontrolled, multiplication of cells **t associated antigens** molecules such as CA 19-9, CA 125 and CA 195 that may be associated with specific tumours **t doubling time** *see* doubling time **t markers** non-specific substances, which under certain circumstances can be used to detect recurrence. The tumour markers include carcino embryonic antigen - CEA, oncofetal antigens (- fetoprotein), and tumour associated antigens (CA125, CA 19-9) **t necrosis factor** TNF, a molecule that mediates shock and tumour related cachexia divided into TNF-α and TNF-β **t promoter** cocarcinogen. A substance that has no intrinsic carcinogenic potential, but which when applied repeatedly, is capable of amplifying the cancer-inducing effects of other substances **t seeding** the spillage of tumour cells and then subsequent growth into tumour colonies. The spillage can occur from an operative field and along needle biopsy tracts **t specific antigen** a substance secreted by some tumours and in some conditions **t suppressor gene** a growth regulatory gene that encodes a protein capable of suppressing malignant transformation

tunic (tu'nik) a covering

tunica (tu'ni-ka) a covering or coat **t albuginea** white fibrous capsule of testis **t vaginalis** serous cavity surrounding testis and epididymis

tuning fork a two-pronged fork-like instrument whose prongs when struck give off a musical note

tunnel vision a visual defect in which only objects that are straight ahead can

be seen. There is concentric constriction of the visual fields

turbid (tur'bid) cloudy

turbidity (tur-bid'i-te) cloudiness

turbinate (tur'bi-nat) shaped like a top **nasal t** three conchae of lateral nasal wall

Turcot's (tur'kotz) **disease** autosomal recessive condition described by Jacques Turcot, Canadian physician. Colonic adenomatous polyps and glioblastomas of the central nervous system

turgescence (tur-jes'ens) swelling of a part

turgid (tur'jid) congested

turgor 1. normal consistency of living tissue 2. distension

turista (too-ris'ta) a severe type of gastroenteritis, afflicting many people from west who travel to tropical or subtropical regions

Turner's syndrome a genetic disorder affecting females who have only one X chromosome, described by Henry Turner, US physician. There is failure of the ovaries to respond to pituitary hormone stimulation. It is characterised by amenorrhoea, failure of sexual maturation, short stature, webbing of neck and cubital valgus

TURP abbreviation for transurethral resection of prostate

turpentine (tur'pen-tin) a volatile oil used in liniments

tus cough

tussive (tus'iv) pertaining to cough **t ulcer** ulcer in the tongue by contact with lower incisors in prolonged coughing

TWAR agent a fastidious strain of *Chalamydia psittaci* that causes upper and lower respiratory tract infections and pneumonia. The name derives from first two isolates, which had been designated TW-183 and AR-39

T wave the portion of the electrocardiogram that is due to ventricular repolarisation.

Tweedledee and Tweedledum syndrome *Psy* a variety of paranoid schizophrenia in which two closely related persons shares a delusional system

Tween (t-wen) a non-ionic detergent consisting of fatty acid esters of polyoxyethylene sorbitan

twelfth cranial nerve *see* hypoglossal nerve

twilight state disturbed consciousness with hallucinations **t sleep** a dream-like state of conscious sedation

twin one of two offsprings born at one birth **fraternal t** twin comes from two separate fertilised ova and the two individuals growing from them are like ordinary siblings except that they are born together **identical t** twin coming from the same fertilised ova which instead of growing into one individual, becomes split into two. The nuclei of the two cells contain exactly the same hereditary determinants. Such twins resemble each other, in almost complete detail

twitch (twich) a brief contraction of a skeletal muscle

two glass test the patient is instructed to pass some urine into the test glass no. 1 and the remaining in the test glass no. 2. If the first glass contains pus and second does not contain, it suggests anterior urethritis. On the other hand, the first is clear and the second is turbid with pus and/or prostatic threads, it suggests posterior urethritis

two point discrimination ability to distinguish two touches close together

tyloma (ti-lo′ma) callosity

tylosis (ti-lo′sis) formation of a callus; palmo-plantar hyperkeratosis

tympanectomy (tim′pan-ek′to-me) excision of tympanic membrane

tympanic (tim-pan′ik) pertaining to the tympanum **t membrane** ear drum **resonance** a sound produced by percussion over an air fitted cavity or gas-filled cavity

tympanites (tim-pan-i′tez) distension of the abdomen due to presence of gas or air in the intestine or in the peritoneal cavity.

tympanitis (tim-pan-i′tis) otitis media

tympanoplasty (tim′pan-o-plas′te) surgical procedure to repair the hearing mechanism of the middle ear. It consists of repair of the ear drum and/or repositioning of the tiny bones of the middle ear to treat hearing loss

tympanum (tim′pan-um) the cavity of middle ear

tympany (tim′pa-ne) a bell-like percussion note

type a category to classify people who share similar traits

type A personality a personality behaviour associated with competitive drive, restlessness and a sense of urgency or impatience, are more coronary prone

type B personality individuals who are more calm and more relaxed and philosophical

typhlitis (tif-li′tis) inflammation of the caecum

typhlon (tif′lo-n) the caecum

typhoid (ti′foyd) an infectious disease caused by *Salmonella typhi* **t fever** caused by *S. typhi* which are transmitted by the faecal-oral route. The bacilli localise mainly in the lymphoid tissue of the small intestine in the Peyer's patches where they ulcerate. It presents with fever, headache, myalgia, bradycardia, constipation, splenomegaly, abdominal distension, diarrhoea and delirium. It may be associated with complications such as haemorrhage, perforation and septicemia. Ciprofloxacin, amoxycillin, cotrimoxazole and chloramphenicol are effective. Injectable or oral vaccines are available for prevention

typhus (ti′fus) arthropod-borne infectious disease caused by rickettsia. Rickettsiae multiply in vascular endothelial cells and produce lesions in different parts of the body. The common clinical features are fever, severe prostration, mental disturbance and often rash **endemic t fever** flea-borne typhus caused by *R. mooseri*; the clinical features resemble those of a mild louse-borne typhus **epidemic t fever** louse-borne typhus caused by *R. prowazeki*. It has sudden onset with malaise, headache, fever, pain in the back and limbs and rash. There is splenomegaly, dry tongue, condition responds to tetracycline or chloramphenicol

typing (ti'ping) classification according to type

tyramine (ti'ra-men) a decarboxylation product of tyrosine and it is a sympathomimetic amine

tyrosine (ti'ro-sin) an amino acid present in most proteins

tyrosinaemia (ti'ro-si-ne-mi-a) increased levels of tyrosine in blood associated with increased urinary excretion of tyrosine and tyrosyl compounds. The condition arises as an autosomal recessive condition with hepatosplenomegaly, cirrhosis of the liver, renal tubular dysfunction and vitamin D-resistant rickets

tyrosinosis (ti'ro-sin-o'sis) a rare disorder of tyrosine metabolism, wherein there is an increased urinary excretion of tyrosyl metabolites following ingestion of tyrosine

tyrosinuria (ti'ro-si-nu'ri-a) excretion of tyrosine in the urine

Tzanck (tsank) **cell** a degenerated cell from the keratin layer of the skin and is seen in pemphigus, named after Arnault Tzanck, Russian dermatologist in Paris

U

U unit; chemical symbol for uranium; international unit of enzyme activity

uberous (u'ber-us) fertile; prolific

uberty (u'ber-te) fertility

ubiquinone (u-bek'-wi-non) coenzyme Q, a protein that acts as a hydrogen carrier which is linked to intramitochondrial electron transport cascade

ubiquitous (u-bik'wi-tus) present everywhere, omnipresent

ubiquity (u-bik'wi-te) state or capacity of being everywhere

Uchlinger disease hyperostosis generalisata with pachydermia

udharana (s) example

udaka (s) water, *u. meha* diabetes insipidus

udana (s) upward moving

udara (s) abdomen, belly

udasina (ṡ) indifferent

udder (ud'er) mammary gland of animals.

uddesa (s) enumeration

uhya(s) imagining, a function of mind

ugly aggressive or malignant condition

UIP usual interstitial pneumonia.

ulalgia (u-lal'je-a) pain in the gums

ulatrophy (u-lat'ro-fe) recession of gums.

ulcer (ul'ser) a circumscribed depressed lesion on the skin or mucous membrane of any internal organ following sloughing of necrotic inflammation **anastomotic u** ulcer at the anastomotic site as in gastrojejunostomy **annular u** ring-like ulcer **aphthous u** painful ulcer affecting oral mucous membrane with necrosis of subepithelial blood vessels **Barrett's u** peptic ulcer of the oesophagus in heterotropic gastric mucosa **Buruli u** necrotising ulcer of skin and subcutaneous tissue of the extremities from *My. ulcerans*, named after Buruli in Uganda **corneal u** ulcer in the cornea **carcinomatous u** hard and indurated ulcer with everted raised edges **Curling's u** an ulcer of the duodenum following severe burns **decubitus u** an ulceration caused by prolonged pressure in a patient who is bedridden for a prolonged period of time, pressure sore **dendritic u** ulcer of the cornea branching in different directions as in herpes simplex infection **dental u** ulcer on the oral mucosa from trauma inflicted by the teeth **duodenal u** peptic ulcer situated in the duodenum **flask u** flask-shaped ulcer in the intestine in amoebic dysentery **gastric u** an ulcer of gastric mucosa **girdle u** a tuberculous ulcer spreading along the wall of the intestine in an encircling manner **gravitational u** occurrence of ulcer over the medial or lateral malleolus from varicosity of long or short saphenous vein respectively **Gwalior u** cutaneous leishmaniasis **Hunner's u** chronic interstitial cystitis with ulcers involving all layers of the bladder **jejunal u** ulcer developing in jejunum following gastrojejunostomy **kissing u** ulcers developing on directly opposing surfaces of the stomach in lesser curvature **marginal u** a gastric ulcer in the jejunal mucosa near the site of gastrojejunal anastomosis **meatal u** ulcer at the external urinary meatus often after circumcision in small boys **peptic u** a group of ulcerating lesions affecting the upper gastrointestinal tract **perforating u** an ulcer involving the entire thickness of an organ **phagedenic u** ulcer that spreads rapidly causing disintegration of tissues with slough and discharge. **plantar u** a deep neurotrophic ulcer of the sole of the foot as in diabetes mellitus, leprosy **preauricular u** ulcer at the root of helix with a preauricular sinus **prosthetic u** ulcer over the gums due to an ill-fitting denture **rodent u** ulcerating basal cell carcinoma of the skin **serpiginous u** a creeping ulcer that heals in one part and extends to another **stomal u** marginal ulcer **stress u** peptic ulcer developing from stress such as burns, surgery, prolonged corticosteroid therapy, acute infections or cerebral trauma **traumatic u** an ulcer due to a local injury **trophic u** an ulcer due to imperfect nutrition of the part **tropical u** lesion of cutaneous leishmaniasis; chronic painful phagedenic ulcer occurring in lower extremities in malnourished children in tropics **varicose u** ulcer in the leg associated with varicose veins **venereal u** ulcer caused by a venereal disease

ulcerate (ul'ser-at) to form an ulcer

ulceration (ul'ser-a'shun) the formation of an ulcer

ulcerative (ul'ser-a'tiv) causing ulceration **u colitis** a non-specific inflammation of large bowel especially rectum characterised by diarrhoea with blood and mucus. It occurs in young and middle aged adults of either sex. It runs a chronic course with remissions and relapses. Corticosteroids and sulphasalazine are used in treatment **u jejuno-ileitis** complication of coeliac disease which responds poorly to a gluten-free diet, and exhibits multiple ulcers in jejunum **u stomatitis** ulcers with ragged necrotic margins on the gums, palate, lips and inner aspects of the cheeks. Occur in adults with malnutrition and poor dental hygiene

ulcerogangrenous (ul'ser-o-gang'gre-nus) an ulcer that contains gangrenous tissue

ulcerogenic (ul'ser-o-jen'k) causing ulceration

ulceromembranous (ul'ser-o-mem'brah-nus) ulceration and a membranous exudation **u gingivitis** fusospirochaetal destructive inflammation of gums

ulcerous (ul'ser-us) affected with ulceration

ulcus (ul'kus) ulcer

ulectomy (u-lek'to-me) excision of scar tissue to relieve tension

ulemorrhagia (u'lem-o-ra'je-a) bleeding from the gums

ulerythema (u'ler-i-the'ma) an erythematous disease of skin with formation of cicatrices and atrophy

uletic (u-let'ik) pertaining to the gums

ulitis (u-li'tis) inflammation of the gums; gingivitis

Ullmann's (ul'manz) **line** a line from the anterior edge of the first sacral vertebra when extended upward at a right angle to the superior surface of the sacrum will pass through the last lumbar vertebra in spondylolisthesis, named after Emerich Ullmann, Hungarian surgeon

ulna (ul'na) the larger of the two bones of the forearm lying parallel with the radius. It extends from the elbow to the wrist on the side of the little finger. It articulates with the humerus and with the head of the radius above and with the radius and bones of the carpus below pl. **ulnae**

ulnad (ul'nad) in the direction of the ulna

ulnar (ul'nar) pertaining to the ulna, or to ulnar (medial) aspect of the arm **u artery** one of the terminal branches of the brachial artery. Originating in cubital fossa, supplies muscles of forearm and palm, contributes in anatomosis around elbow joint and terminates in palm by joining superficial palmar arch **u bursa** tendon sheath of finger flexors in the palm extending into the little finger **u deviation** pull of flexor tendons on unstable proximal interphalangeal joints as in rheumatoid arthritis **u drift** a change of metacarpophalangeal joints in chronic rheumatoid arthritis wherein the long axis of the fingers makes an angle with the long axis of the wrist **u nerve** *see* Table of nerves **u neuritis** interference of ulnar nerve function by constriction or recurrent friction causing numbness or tingling in the ulnar distribution and often of clumsiness in performing fine finger movements **u refill time** appearance of palmar blush by filling *via* ulnar artery within 5 seconds on releasing pressure when both the ulnar and radial arteries are occluded by pressure at the wrist

ulnaris (ul-na'ris) ulnar

ulnocarpal (ul'no-karpal) pertaining to the ulna and carpus

ulnoradial (ul'no-ra'de-al) pertaining to the ulna and radius

ul(o) combining word for scar ; gingiva

ulocarcinoma (u'lo-kahr'sino'ma) carcinoma of the gums

ulodermatitis (u'lo-der-ma-ti-'tis) inflammation of the skin resulting in destruction of tissue and the formation of scars

uloglossitis (u'lo-glos-si'tis) inflammation of the gums and the tongue

uloid (u'loyd) resembling a scar

ulorrhagia (u'lo-ra'jah) bleeding from gums

ulorrhoea (u'lor-re'a) slow bleeding from the gums

ulotomy (u-lot'o-me) l. incision of scar 2. incision of gums

ulotripsis (u'lo-trip'sis) massage of gums

ultimate (ul'tim-it) final; last

ultimobranchial (ul'ti-mo-brang'ke-al) body embryonic pharyngeal pouches getting separated from the pharynx and incorporated into substance of thyroid gland, and secrete calcitonin

ultimum moriens (ul'ti-mum mo're-enz) L. last to die such as right atrium, upper part of the trapezius muscle

ultra going beyond what is usual or ordinary

ultracentrifugation (ul'trah-sen-trif'uga' shun) subjection of material to an exceedingly high speeds with high gravitational force which enables separation and sedimentation of the molecules of a substance

ultracentrifuge (ul'trah-sen'-tri-fuj) a high speed centrifuge for subjecting solutions to forces many times that of gravity and producing concentration differences depending on the weight of the molecule

ultradian (ul-tra'de-an) refers to a period of less than 24 hours **u rhythm** rhythmic repetition of certain phenomenon in living organisms occurring in cycles of less than a day

ultrafilter (ul'tra-fil'-ter) a filter for purifying solutions having a membrane with pores sufficiently small to prevent the passage of the suspended particles

ultrafiltrate (ul'tra-fi'trat) a liquid that has been passed through an ultrafilter

ultrafiltration (ul'tra-fil-tra'shun) filtration through an ultrafilter capable of removing very minute particles

ultralente (ul'tra-len'te) longer than lente, of insulin active for 24 hours

ultramicroscope (ul'tra-mi'kro-skop) an instrument using scattering phenomenon to detect the position of objects too small to be seen by an ordinary microscope. **ultramicrosopic,** adj

ultramicroscopy (ul'tra-mi-kros'ko-pe) the use of the ultramicroscope

ultrasonic (ul'tra-sonik) a frequency above the audiofrequency and range of sound waves having a frequency greater than 20000 Hz, which is beyond the range of normal human audibility **u cleaning** use of ultrasonic energy to clean medical and surgical instruments

ultrasonication (ul'tra-son'ika-shun) use of ultrasound to disintegrate solids including microorganisms

ultrasonics (ul'tra-son'iks) the branch of science that deals with ultrasonic phenomenon

ultrasonogram (ul'tra-son'o-gram) an image made by ultrasonography

ultrasonograph (ul'tra-son'o-gra-f) an apparatus that sends sound impulses towards an organ which in turn echoes the sounds, which are graphically displayed on a fluorescent screen

ultrasonography (ul'tra-son'o-gra-fe) a process of imaging deep structures of the body based on the differences in the acoustic impedance of different tissues, electricity applied to a piezoelectric crystal in the transducer causes a high frequency mechanical vibration. The transducer generates the ultrasound beam and detect the returning echo **A mode u** a modality providing simple displays that are plotted as a series of peaks whose height represents the depth of echoing structure from the transducer **B mode u** ultrasonography modality having a wide range applications, often used to perform real-time two-dimensional evaluation of the foetus presenting images in rapid succession **Doppler u** measurement of velocities of moving fluid such as blood based on principles of the Doppler effect, there is shift in frequency between emitted ultrasonic waves and their echoes **Duplex u** an ultrasonographic modality combining B mode display with pulsed Doppler signals and it reflects motions within a tissue such as blood flow **M-mode u** a modality wherein the echo signal is recorded on a continuously moving strip of paper with the transducer held in a fixed position over mitral or aortic valves adj. **ultrasonographic**

ultrasound (ultra-sownd) sound waves having frequency higher than the range audible to the human ear (over 20000 vibrations per second) **A mode u** sonography presented as a single line representing the time taken for the ultrasound wave to reach the interface of a structure and reflect back to the transducer **real time u** a sonographic procedure providing rapid, multiple images of an anatomical structure in the form of motion **u scanning** a diagnostic imaging procedure wherein high frequency sound waves are passed into the body and reflected back, on which a computer

builds up an image of internal structures **u therapy** ultrasonic waves when projected as a beam from a transducer penetrate and strike the tissues and the energy is converted into heat which is used for relief of pain

ultrastructure (ul'tra-struk'tur) the fine structure of tissues such as membranes, microtubules and microfilaments visible on electromicroscopic study

ultraviolet (ul'tra-vi'o-let) beyond the visible violet portion of the spectrum **u light** invisible rays of sunlight producing burning effects, antirachitic effect by producing vitamin D **u radiation** the segment of the electromagnetic spectrum lying between 200 and 400 nm **u therapy** treatment with ultraviolet radiation

ultravirus (ul'tra-vi'rus) an ultramicroscopic virus capable of passing through the finest bacterial filters

Ultzmann's (ooltz'mahnz) **test** appearance of emerald-green colour in presence of bile pigments on addition of potassium hydroxide and hydrochloric acid to urine, named after Robert Ultzmann, German urologist

ululation (ul'u-la'shun) loud crying of hysterical patients

Ulysses syndrome a complication of false positive tests which leads to prolonged search to elucidate the nature of a non-existent disease, named after Ulysses who fought in Trojan war, needed 20 years to return home due to unnecessary *detours*

umbilical (umbil'ikal) pertaining to umbilicus or umbilical cord **u adenoma** a pedunculated, raspberry-like mass in the umbilicus **u carcinoma** a secondary carcinomatous nodule at the umbilicus, often referred as Sister Joseph's (of Mayo clinic) nodule **cord** structure connecting the umbilicus of the foetus with the placenta in the gravid uterus and carrying two umbilical arteries and a vein **u fissure** that part of hepatic longitudinal fissure in which the umbilical vein is located **u fistula** a fistulous tract in the umbilicus may discharge urine (urachal fistula), faeces (patent omphalomesenteric duct) or mucus **u hernia** a hernia of the umbilicus. It may be congenital seen in infants or acquired where a scar gives way. In adults the hernia, is paraumbilical where umbilicus is either above, or more commonly just below the hernial protrusion **u sepsis** infection of umbilicus by careless handling or cutting of the cord without antiseptic measures **u souffle** a hissing sound from the umbilical cord **u vesicle** that part of the embryonic yolk sac leading from the umbilicus

umbilicate (um-bil'i-kat) resembling the umbilicus

umbilication (um-bil'i-ka'shun) a depression or a pit resembling the navel

umbilicus (um-bil'I-kus) the depressed area of scar in the middle of the abdominal wall where the umbilical cord was attached to the foetus; navel

umbilectomy (um'bi-lek'to-me) excision of the umbilicus

umbo (um'bo) 1. a rounded elevation 2. the slight projection at the centre of the inner surface of the tympanic membrane

umbonate (um'bo-nat) knob-like; button-like raised centre

umbra (um'bra) shade, shadow

umbrella cells multinucleated superficial cells of the bladder epithelium covering multiple underlying transitional cells

umbrella filter a stainless steel filter placed in the inferior vena cava to prevent emboli from passing that point

un a prefix meaning 'not'

Unani-tibbi a mixture of Ayurveda and traditional medicine of Persia and Arabia

unborn not yet born

uncal (un'kal) pertaining to the uncus of the brain

uncertain doubtful

unciform (un'siform) hook-shaped, hamate **u bone** hamate bone on ulnar side of distal row of the carpus **u fasciculus** bundle of fibres connecting frontal cerebral lobes with the temporosphenoid lobes **u process** a hook-like process of hamate; anterior end of hippocampal gyrus; long thin portion of bone from orbital plate of the ethmoid articulating with the inferior turbinate

uncinaria (un'sin-a-ri'a) nematodes having a hook-like structure

uncinariasis (un'sin-a-ri'a-sis) infestation by uncinaria in the intestine, ankylostomiasis; hookworm disease

uncinate (un-sin-at) 1. hooked or hook-shaped 2. unciform **u convolution** uncinate gyrus **u epilepsy** form of epilepsy characterised by olfactory and gustatory hallucinations **u fasciculus** curved bundle of fibres connecting orbital gyri of frontal lobe with rostral part of temporal lobe **u gyrus** recurved rostral portion of the hippocampal gyrus in the temporal lobe of the brain **u process** a curved bony process

uncipressure (un'si-presh'ur) pressure applied with a hook to stop bleeding

unconditioned natural **u reflex** an inborn reflex that is not dependent upon previous experience

unconjugated not united to another compound, such as bilirubin, not united with glucuronide

unconscious (un-kon'shus) inability to respond to any sensory stimuli or being unaware of the surroundings; insensible **u system** mental contents and processes at a given moment outside the sphere of consciousness by a censoring or repressing counterforce

unconsciousness (un-kon'shus-ns) a state of loss of awareness from which a person can't be aroused

uncontrolled trials trials with no comparison group

uncoupling 1.separation of a metabolic process 2. separation of activities in receptor-ligand interactions

uncovertebral (ung'ko-ver'tah-bral) pertaining to the uncinate process of a vertebra

unction (ungk'shun) application of an ointment

unctuous (ungk'tus) nature or characteristic of an ointment, oily or greasy

uncus (ung'kus) hook-shaped structure; hooked anterior portion of hippocampal gyrus, one of the convolutions on the inferior surface of the temporal lobe.

undecylenic (un-des'i-len'ik) **acid** an unsaturated fatty acid used as a tropical antifungal agent

underbite underdevelopment of mandible

undercoverage inadequate coverage, refers to case left out in surveys

underexposure to expose a film for too short a period

underfed (un'derfed) to feed insufficiently

under-five clinic a clinic taking care in illness, preventive care and growth monitoring of children below five years

under general surgical procedure performed under general anaesthesia

under local a surgical procedure performed under local anaesthesia

undermine to make a hollow or tunnel underneath

undernourished not provided with sufficient food for normal growth

undernutrition (un'der-nu-tri'sh'un) nutritional deficiency arising from lack of food or from an inability to absorb it

understain (un'der-stan) to stain less deeply than usual

undertoe (un'der-to) great toe being displaced under other toes

underweight (un'der-wat) a condition in which the body weight is 10% less than that of a normal

Underwood's (un'der-woodz) sclerema neonatorum, named after Michael Underwood, British paediatrician

undeveloped (un'deve'lop-ed) not developed

undifferentiated (un-dif'er-en'she-at-ed) without identifiable pattern, a term applied to the cellular arrangement of neoplastic tissue

undine (un'din) a small glass flask used in irrigation of the eyes

undoing a compulsive act that is performed in an attempt to prevent or undo the consequences that the patient irrationally anticipates from a frightening obsessional thought or impulse

undulant (un-du-lant) undulating; wave like pattern or motion **u fever** brucellosis

undulation (un'du-la'shun) a wave-like movement

undulate (un-du-lat) to fluctuate in wave-like pattern

unfit not fit, unsuitable.

ungual (ung'gwal) pertaining to the nails **u phalanx** terminal phalanx of each finger and toe **u tuberosity** spatula-shaped extremity of terminal phalanx that gives support to the nails

unguentum (un-gwen'tum) an ointment

unguent (ung'gwent) an ointment

unguis (ung'gwis) 1. a finger nail or toe nail 2. the lacrimal bone 3. white prominence on floor of the posterior horn of the lateral ventricle pl. **ungues**

ungula (un'gu-la) instrument for removal of dead foetus from the uterus; hoof of an animal.

ungulate (ung'gu'lat) a hoofed mammal

unhappy gut dysfunctional gastrointestinal smooth muscle leading to functional colitis

unhealthy sick; unwell

uni- (L) combining word for one

uniarticular (u'ne-ar-tik'u-lar) pertaining to a single joint

uniaxial (u'ne-ak'se-al) 1. having one axis only 2. development in axial direction

unicameral (u'ni-kam'er-al) having only one cavity

UNICEF United Nations International Children's Emergency Fund

unicellular (u'ni-sel'u-ler) having one cell such as protozoa or bacteria

uniceps (u'ni-seps) having a single head or origin

unicornous (u'ni-kor'nus) having one horn or cornu

unicuspid (u'ni-kus'pid) having a single pattern, one cusp

unidirectional (u'ni-di-rek'shun-al) flowing in only one direction

unifactorial (u'ni-fa-k-to-real) having a single causative factor

unifocal (u'ni-fo'kal) arising from single focus

uniform identical shape or form

unigravida (u'ni-grav'i-da) primigravida; woman pregnant for the first time

unilaminar (u'ni-lam'i-nar) having a single layer

unilateral (uni-lat'er-al) affecting only one side **u hyperlucent lung syndrome** a small unilateral transradiant lung or a lobe with poor ventilation and perfusion, named after MacLeod, and Swyer and James

unilobar (u'ni-lo'bar) having one lobe only

unilocular (u'ni-lok'u-lar) having only one cavity

uninucleated (-noo'kle-at'ed) mononuclear

uniocular (u'ne-ok'u-lar) having only one eye

unio mystica an oceanic feeling, one of mystic unit with an infinitive power

unhealthy sick; unwell

union (un'yun) the process of healing; establishment of continuity between the edges of the broken ends of a bone

uniovular (u'ne-ov'u-lar) arising from one ovum

unipara (u-nip'a-ra) a woman having one pregnancy over 20 weeks

uniparental (u-nipa-ran-tal) **disomy** the inheritance of two copies of a chromosome from one parent

uniparous (u-nip'a-rus) giving birth to one offspring at a time

unipolar (u'ni-po'lar) having one pole **u disorder** a mood disorder with recurrent depression

unipotential (u'ni-po-ten'shul) possessing only one power, such as producing cells of one type only

unisex lack of sex distinction by external appearance

uniseptate (u'ni-sep'tat) having only one seputm

unisexual (u'ni-seks'u-al) having sexual organs of one sex only

unit (unit) 1. single thing 2. an element in a group 3. a standard measurement of a quantity symbol U **Bodansky u** the quantity of alkaline phosphatase that liberates 1 mg of phosphate ion from glycerol 2-phosphate in 1 hour under standared conditions **coronary care u** a specially designed and equipped hospital section providing constant observation and treatment of patients with severe heart disease; CCU **intensive care u** a section in the hospital with special equipments and skilled staff concerned with the care of seriously ill patients who require immediate and continuous attention; ICU **international u** a unit of biological substances such as enzymes, hormones, vitamins etc. established by the International Conference for the unification of formulas **King-Armstrong u** unit to describe amount of alkaline phosphatase **motor u** producing motor activity **S.I. u** any of the units of the Systeme International d'Unites (International System of Units) *see* table 10 and 11 **somogyi u** amount of amylase which will liberate reducing equivalents equals to 1 mg of glucose per 30 minutes under defined conditions **terminal respiratory u** gas exchanging unit of the lung which consists of a respiratory bronchiole, alveolar ducts, alveolar sacs and alveoli **Todd u** the reciprocal of the highest unit that inhibits haemolysis by enzymes such as antistreptolysin 'O' **tuberculin u** 0.00002 mg of purified protein derivative in 0.1 ml corresponds in potency to 1:10,000 solution of old tuberculin

unitarian (u-ni-tar'e-an) composed of a single unit

Tabel 11: SI units (Systeme International d'Unites) or International System of Units

Quantity	Name of the unit	Symbol
Base units		
length	metre (me'tre)	m
mass	kilogram (kil'o-gram)	kg
time	second (sek'und)	s
electric current	ampere (am'per)	A
temperature	kelvin (kel'vin)	K
luminous intensity	candela (kan-del'ah)	cd
amount of a substance	mole (mol)	mol
Derived units		
area	square metre	m^2
acceleration	metre per second squared	m/s^2
concentration of a substance	mole per cubic metre	mol/m^3
luminescence	candela per square metre	cd/m^2
mass density	kilogram per cubic metre	kg/m^3
specific volume	cubic metre per kilogram	m^3/kg
speed velocity	metre per second	m/s
volume	cubic metre	m^3

Table 12: SI derived units with special name

Quantity	Name of derived unit	Symbol	Expression in other units
Electric			
capacitance	farad (far'ad)	F	C/V
charge	coulomb (koo'lom)	C	$A \cdot s$
conductance	siemens (se'menz)	S	Ω-1
potential	volt (vol)	V	J/C
resistance	ohm (orn)	Ω	V/A
energy, work	joule (jool)	J	$N \cdot m$
force	newton (noo'ton)	N	$Kg \cdot m/s^2$
frequency	hertz (hertz)	Hz	S^{-1}
inductance	henry (hen're)	H	Wb/A
illumination	lux (luks)	lx	lm/m^2
luminous flux	lumen (loo'men)	lm	$cd \cdot sr$
magnetic			
flux	weber (we'ber)	Wb	V.s
flux density	tesla (tes'la)	T	Wb/m^2
power	watt (waht)	W	J/S
pressure	pascal (pas'kal)	Pa	N/m^2
radiation			
absorbed dose	gray (gra)	Gy	J/Kg
absorbed dose equivalent	sievert (se'vert)	SV	J/Kg
activity	becquerel (bek-rel)	Bq	S^{-1}
temperature	degree celsius (sel'se-us)	°C	K-273.15

unitary (u'ni-tar'e) related to a single unit

United Nations International Children's Emergency Fund UNICEF, one of the specialised agencies of the United Nations with activities covering programmes of assistance in child survival, protection and development and has undertaken a campaign for a "child health revolution"

univalence (uni-va'lens) having a valence of one.

universal (u'ni-ver'sal) applicable to all conditions **u antidote** antidote used in poisoning where specific antidote is not available such as activated charcoal **u donor** a person whose blood group is O Rh negative can be transfused into persons belonging to any of the other ABO blood groups without any untoward reactions **u dressing** a large flat bandage that can be folded in such a way as to make a large or small bandage **u immunisation programme** global immunisation programme to protect all children of the world against six vaccine-preventable diseases, namely diphtheria, whooping cough, tetanus, polio, tuberculosis and measles. The programme was launched in India in 1985 **u recipient** a person with AB blood group Rh positive whose serum will not agglutinate the cells of the other ABO blood

University of Wisconsin preservation solution 1 litre of solution at 4°C is perfused through the donor portal vein and 2-3 litres through the aorta to perfuse the liver and kidneys. This enables extension of organ storage such as liver after retrieval

unload to remove a load

unmada (s) insanity; mental aberration

unmask expose

unmedullated (un-med'u-lat'ed) a nerve that does not contain a myelin sheath

unmyelinated (un-mie-li-nat'ed) a nerve fibre without a myelin sheath

Unna's (oo'naz) **dermatosis** seborrhoeic dermatitis, named after Paul Unna, German dermatologist

unpaired student t test determination of statistical significance while studying 2 groups of different people

unphysiologic (un-fiz-e-olog'ik) not physiologic

unrest irregularity, instability, or turbulence

unsaturated (un-sach'ur-at'ed) 1. not holding all of a solute which can be held in solution by the solvent **u fats** fats which have a lower content of hydrogen than saturated fats **u fatty acid** an alkyl chain fatty acid that contains one or more double bonds between carbon, and are liquid at room temperature

unstable angina patients exhibiting rapidly worsening angina, severe angina at rest or prolonged and severe ischaemic chest pain. ST-T depression in ECG is common. Coronary spasm is responsible in many, also called preinfarction angina

unstriated (un-stri'at-ed) without striations, as smooth muscle fibre

Unverricht disease a genetic disorder associated with myoclonic epilepsy, named after Heinrich Unverricht, German physician

Unverricht-Lundborg syndrome an autosomal recessive progressive myoclonic epilepsy named after Heinrich unverricht, German Physician and Herman Bernhard, Swedish physician. The defective gene encodes cystatin B, inhibitor of cysteine protease

unwell sick, ill or indisposed

upa-dhatu (s) secondary constituents produced as a result of the action of fire in each of the body constituents

upadrava (s) secondary disease

upakrama (s) introduction; beginning of treatment of a patient

upamana (s) analytical reasoning involving comparison

upanga (s) appendage, auxiliary branch

upasamhara (s) conclusion

upasaya (s) amelioration relief from the distressing symptoms

upavasa (s) fasting

upayantra (s) minor or accessory instrument

upamana (s) analogical reasoning, involving comparison.

update to bring up to date

upper airway obstruction obstruction in upper airway may occur from inhalation of foreign bodies, acute oedema or infections. The condition may also develop slowly from tumours, tracheal stenosis and laryngeal abnormalities enabling examination of the oesophagus, stomach and duodenum.

upper GI term for radiocontrast studies of the upper gastrointestinal tract **upper GI bleeding** bleeding in the upper GI occurs from peptic ulcer, oesophageal varices, gastric erosions, gastric carcinoma commonly

upper motor neuron UMN a descending fibre (corticospinal or pyramidal) system with cells of origin in the precentral gyrus of cerebral cortex, that descends and after decussation to the opposite side innervates cranial nerve nuclei and the anterior horn cells **UMN lesion** a neurological condition caused by damage to the pyramidal tract. It causes paralysis of movement, increased tone with spasticity hyperreflexia and extensor plantar response

upper respiratory tract URT consists of nose, nasopharynx and larynx lined by vascular mucous membranes with ciliated epithelium. It participates in air conditioning, swallowing **URT infection** bacterial or viral infections affecting the upper respiratory tract

upside-down stomach a rare variety of para oesophageal hiatus hernia wherein the entire stomach is in the thoracic cavity

upsiloid (up'si-loyd) shaped like the letter U or V

uptake (up'tak) absorption and incorporation of a substance by living tissues

urachal (u'ra-kal) fistula connection of bladder to exterior at umbilicus and the discharge may be urine

uracil (ur'-ah-sil) a pyrimidine base

urachus (u'ra-kus) remnant of allantois a canal present in the foetus between the umbilicus and the apex of the bladder, which changes as a fibrous cord after birth **urachal** adj

uracrasia (u'ra-kra'zhah) inability to retain urine

uraemia (u-re'me-a) a toxic condition caused by retention in the blood of waste substances especially products of protein metabolism normally excreted in the urine

uraemic (u-re'mik) related to uraemia **u frost** cutaneous precipitation of urea in severe renal failure **u polyneuropathy** sensory-motor neuropathy noted in patients on chronic dialysis

uragogue (u'rah-gog) agent increasing production of urine, diuretic

uraniscoplasty (u'ran-is'ko-plas'te) repair of cleft palate

uraniscorrhaphy (u'ran-is-kor'ra-fe) suturing of cleft palate

uraniscus (u'rah-nis'kus) the palate

uranism (u'rah-nizm) homosexuality

uranium (u-ra'ne-um) a hard white naturally occurring radioactive metallic element. Symbol U, at no. 92

uranochisis (u'ran-oa'ki-sis) cleft palate

uranoplasty (u'ran-o-plas'te) repair of the palate

uranoplegia (u'ra-no-ple'je-a) paralysis of muscles of soft palate

uranorrhaphy (u-ran-or-ra-fe) suturing of a cleft palate

uranoschisis (u-ran-os'kis-is) cleft palate

uranostaphyloschisis (u'ran-o-staf 'ilos'ki-sis) fissure of the soft and hard palate

uranostaphyloplasty (u'ran-o-staf'il-o-plas'te) operative correction of a defect of the soft and hard palates

urataemia (u'ra-te'me-a) presence of urates in the blood

urate (u'rat) a salt of uric acid, a normal constituent of urine

urathritis (ura-thritis) gouty arthritis

uratoma (u'ra-to'mah) a concretion of urates

uratosis (u'ra-to-sis) deposition of crystalline urates in the tissues

uraturia (u'rah-tu're-ah) urates in the urine

Urbach-Oppenheim (ur'bak-ope'en-him) **disease**. necrobiosis lipoidius diabeticorum, described by Erich Urbach and Maurice Oppenheim, US dermatologists

urban (ur'ban) pertaining to a city area **u factor** atmospheric pollution of urban air from exhaust fumes of automobiles, dust and smoke from factories **u plague** plague associated with domestic rodents **u rabies** rabies in dogs **u typhus** endemic typhus

urbanisation migration of people to cities because of employment opportunities, attraction of better living conditions and availability of social services

ur-defenses (ur'de-fens'es) humans defend against psychologic disorganisation and traumatisation by belief in their physical invulnerability, the fantasy that others are potential friends and faith in a celestial order

urdhava (s) upward

urdhvagah (s) ascending

urea (u-re'a) the chief nitrogenous end product of protein metabolism **u breath test** test to determine the amount of urease in Helicobacter pylori infection **u frost** minute white flaky deposits of urea on the skin of the face in patients with advanced uraemia **u clearance** measurement of renal function, which is dependent on glomerular filtration rate and tubular reabsorption

urease (u're-as) an enzyme that promotes the breakdown of urea into ammonia and carbon dioxide, first enzyme to be prepared in the crystalline state

urecchysis (u'rek'i-sis) the extravasation of urine into the tissue

ureoedema (u-re-de'ma) subcutaneous swelling from extravasated urine

uremia (u-re'me-a) accumulation of excess amount of nitrogenous end products of protein metabolism due to renal insufficiency **uremic** adj. **post-renal u** conditions preventing urine al-

ready formed from being excreted out of the body from obstructions in the urinary tract **renal u** disorders of kidney with deranged or destroyed parenchyma **prerenal u** poor renal blood flow resulting in renal failure **u serositis** a syndrome of pericarditis, pleural effusion and sometimes ascites **u syndrome** condition noted when BUN exceeds 100 mg/dl

uremic (u-re'mik) pertaining to uraemia

uredo urticaria

ureodeoxycholic acid UDCA useful in treatment of gall stones. It suppresses absorption of dietary cholesterol from the intestine and prevents compensatory increase in hepatic biosynthesis of cholesterol

ureogenesis (ur'e-o-jen'e-sis) formation of urea

ureolysis (u're-ol'i-sis) decomposition of urea to carbon dioxide and ammonia

ureometer (u're-om'et-er) instrument to measure the amout of urea in urine

ureometry (u-re-om'et-re) estimation of amount of urea in urine

ureopoiesis (u-re'o-poi-e'sis) formation of urea

uresiesthesis (ure'se-es-the'sis) the normal impulse to pass the urine

uresis (u-re'sis) urination, the passage of urine; urination

ureter (u-re'ter) one of a pair of long slender muscular tubes that convey urine from the pelvis of the kidney to the base of the bladder. Each kidney has one ureter which measures 28-34 cm in length and a diameter of 1 mm to 1 cm, and its wall consists of mucosal, muscular and fibrous layers. **ureteric** adj. **ureteric colic** excruciating pain passing from the loin to the groin

ureterectasis (u-re'ter-ek'ta-sis) distension of a ureter

ureterectomy (u-re'ter-ek'tah-me) surgical removal of a ureter or a segment of it

ureteritis (u-re'ter-i'tis) an inflammation of a ureter

ureterocoele (u-re'ter-o-sel) cystic dilatation of the lower portion of the ureter near its opening into the bladder

ureterocolostomy (u-re'ter-o-ko-los'to-me) surgical anastomosis of a ureter to the colon

ureterocystoscope (u-re'ter-sis'to-skop) a cystoscope combined with a urethral catheter

ureterodialysis (u-re'ter-o-di-al'isis) rupture of a ureter

ureteroenterostomy (u-re'ter-o'en'ter-os'to-me) the surgically created anastomosis between a ureter and the intestine

ureterogram (u-re'ter-og-ram) a roentgenogram of a ureter taken after injection of a radio-opaque substance.

ureterography(ure'ter-og'ra-fe) radiography of the ureter following injection of a contrast medium

ureterohydronephrosis (u-re'ter-o-hi'drone-fro'sis) dilatation of ureter and pelvis of the kidney. This may occur from a mechanical or inflammatory obstruction in the urinary tract

ureteroileostomy(uer'ker-o-il'e-os'tome) anastomosis of a ureter to a loop of the ileum which is drained through a stoma on abdominal wall

ureterolith (u-re'ter-o-lith) a stone in the ureter

ureterolithiasis (u-re'ter-o-li-th'-i'as-sis) formation of a stone in the ureter

ureterolithotomy (u-re'ter'o-li-th-ot'o-me) surgical removal of a stone from a ureter

ureterolysis (u-re'ter-ol'i-sis) 1. rupture of the ureter 2. surgical procedure of separating the ureter from adhesions 3. paralysis of the ureter

ureteroneocystostomy (u-re'ter-o-ne'o-sistos'to-me) transplantation of a ureter to a different site in the bladder

ureteropathy (u-re'ter-op-ah-the) any disease of the ureter

ureteronephrectomy (u-re'ter-o-nef-rek'to-me) excision of a kidney and its ureter

ureteropelvioplasty (ure'ter-o-pel've- o-plas'te) surgical reconstruction of the junction of the ureter and renal pelvis

ureteroplasty (u-re'ter-o-plas'te) surgical reconstruction of the ureter

ureteropyelitis (u-re'ter-o-pi'e-li'tis) inflammation of a ureter and renal pelvis

ureteropyeloneostomy(u-re'ter-o-pi'el-o-ne-os'to-me) surgical creation of a new communication between a ureter and the renal pelvis.

ureteropyelonephritis (u-re'ter-o-pi'el-o-nef-ri'tis) inflammation of the ureter, renal pelvis and kidney

ureteropyosis (u-re'ter-o-pi-o'sis) suppurative inflammation of a ureter

ureterorenoscope (u-re'ter-o-ren'o-sco-pe) a fiberoptic endoscope used to visualise the ureter and the kidney

ureterorenoscopy (u-re'ter-o-ren'osco-pi) visualisation of the interior of the ureter and kidney by ureterorenoscope and performing biopsy or removal or crushing of stones

ureterorrhagia (u-re'ter-or-ra'je-a) a discharge of blood from a ureter

ureterorrhaphy (u-re'ter-or'ra-fe) suture of the ureter

ureteroscope (u-re'ter-o-skope) fibreoptic endoscope to visualise the ureter

ureteroscopy (u-reter-o-sko'pe) examination of the ureter by ureteroscope

ureterosigmoidostomy (u-re'ter-o-sigmoyd-os-to-me) anastomosis of a ureter to the sigmoid colon

ureterostenosis (u-re'ter-o-sten-o'sis) stricture of the ureter

ureterostoma (u're'ter-os'to-ma) the orifice through which the ureter enters the urinary bladder

ureterostomy (u-re'ter-os'to-me) attachment of the divided distal end of a ureter to the skin of the lower abdomen

ureterotomy (u-re'ter-ot'o-me) incision of a ureter

ureterotrigonoenterostomy (u-re'ter-o-trig'ono-en'ter-os'to-me) surgical removal of the trigone of the bladder with the openings of the ureters and implanting it into the intestine

ureterouterine (u-re'ter-o-u'ter-in) relating to a ureter and uterus

ureterovaginal (u-re'ter-o-vaj'i-nal) relating to a ureter and vagina

ureterovesical (u're'ter-o-ves'i-kal) relating to a ureter and the bladder

urethra (u-re'thra) a membranous canal for the external discharge of urine from the bladder. Male urethra is 18-20 cm long, having S-shaped curves, extends from bladder neck to top of the penis. During its course it passes through the prostate, sphincter urethrae and corpus spongiosum of penis. It also discharges seminal fluid. Female urethra is 4 cm. long, extending from bladder neck, runs downward and forward, embedded in anterior wall of vagina, ending by external urethral orifice in the vestibule between the vagina and clitoris

urethral (u-re'thral) relating to the urethra u caruncle a pouting granulomatous- like tissue from the urethral meatus; raspberry tumour u catheterisation passage of a latex or silicone catheter through urethra into the urinary bladder to drain bladder as a temporary measure or to retain it for a few days to measure urine output following major surgery, or in comatose patients u crest vertical ridge on posterior wall of prostatic part of urethra u glands small mucous glands in the cavernous part of the urethra, known as Littre's glands u stricture narrowing in the urethral passage causing obstruction u syndrome symptoms of urethritis and cystitis usually in female without any bacteria on culture of the urine

urethralgia (u're-thral'jah) pain in the urethra

urethrectomy (u-re-threk'to-me) surgical removal of the urethra

urethritis (u're-thri'tis) inflammation of the urethra gonococcal u infection of urethra by Neisseria gonorrhoeae causing dysuria and purulent discharge non-gonococcal u NGU, urethritis of nongonococcal origin, milder than gonococcal urethritis

urethro- combining word for, in relation to urethra

urethrocoele (u-re'thro-sel) prolapse of the female urethra into the vagina caused by a weakness in the muscles of the front wall of the vagina

urethrocystitis (u-re'thro-sis-ti'tis) inflammation of the urethra and the bladder, usually resulting from infection

urethrocystogram (u-re'thro-sis'to-gram) a roentgenogram of the urethra and bladder

urethrodynia (u-re'thro-din'e-a) pain in the urethra

urethrography (u-re-throg'ra-fe) the roentgenographic study of the urethra

urethromet-y (u're-throm-i'tre) measuring resistance in urethra for a retrograde flow of fluid

urethroperineal (u-re'thro-per'i-ne'al) pertaining to the urethra and perineum

urethropexy (u're'thro-pek'se) surgical fixation of urethra to the symphysis pubis and fascia of rectus abdominis muscle, performed in stress incontinence in the female

urethroplasty (u-re'thro-plas'te) surgical repair of a wound or a defect of the urethra

urethroprostatic (u-re'tho-pros-tat'ik) pertaining to the urethra and prostate

urethrorrhagia (u-re'thro-ra'je-a) bleeding from the urethra

urethroscope (u-re'thro-skop) a lighted instrument to examine the interior of the urethra

urethroscopy (u-re'thros'ko-pe) visual examination of the urethra with a urethroscope

urethrostenosis (u-re'thro-ste-no'sis) stricture of the urethra

urethrostomy (u're-thros'ta-me) surgical formation of a opening of urethra at the perineal surface

urethrotome (u-re'thro-tom) an instrument for cutting a urethral stricture

urethrotomy (u-re'throt'o-me) incision of a urethral stricture

urethrovaginal (u-re-thro-vaj'i-nal) relating to the urethra and vagina

urethrovesical (u-re'thro-ves'i-k'l) pertaining to the urethra and bladder

urge to drive or force onwards

urge incontinence urinary incontinence in elderly due to to detrusor instability

urhidrosis (u-ri-dro'sis) presence of urea or uric acid in the sweat

URI upper respiratory infection

URT upper respiratory tract

uric (u'rik) **acid** an acid occurring as an end product of purine metabolism

uricaemia (u-ri-se'me-a) excess uric acid in the blood

uricometer (u'rik-om'e-ter) instrument for quantitative estimation of uric acid in the urine

uricosuria (u'ri-ko-su're-a) excess excretion of uric acid in the urine

uricosuric (u'ri-ko-su'rik) an agent causing increased excretion of uric acid in the urine and useful in the management of gout; probenecid, sulphinpyrazone and colchicine are examples

uridine (u'ri-den) a nucleoside from nucleic acid, which on hydrolysis yields uracil and ribose

uridine diphosphate epimerase deficiency condition with excretion of galactose in the urine due to an inability to metabolise galactose

urinal (u'ri-n'l) a receptacle for urine

urinalysis (u-ri-nal'i-sis) physical, chemical and microscopic examination of urine for diagnostic purpose.

urinary (u'ri-nar'e) relating to urine. **u antiseptic** an antibiotic used in the treatment of recurrent infections of the urinary tract **u bladder** receptacle for urine excreted by the kidneys **u calculi** stones formed in the urinary passages that may contain urates, calcium, oxalate, phosphate and cystine **u casts** casts formed from the glycoprotein synthe-

sised and secreted in the ascending limb of the loop of Henle and distal convoluted tubules, along with cellular elements in an acid medium. The coagulated protein appears cylindrical in shape as they are casted according to lumen of renal tubules **u catheter** the catheter used to drain the bladder, may be non-retaining (Gibbon's catheter used temporarily) or self-retaining (Foley's catheter to retain catheter for few days). They are made of latex or silicone. Their size is mentioned by Charriere gauze or French gauge **u crystals** in acid urine, crystals of uric acid (reddish brown rhombic prisms), urates (granular particles) or calcium oxalate (envelope-shaped) may be seen. Calcium phosphate crystals (colourless prisms) and ammonium magnesium phosphates (triangular prisms) may be seen in alkaline urine **u diversion** a surgical procedure to allow urine to pass through a channel other than the urethra **u incontinence** involuntary emptying of bladder from neurologic disease, prostatic enlargement or weakness of pelvic floor muscles **u infection** infection of the urinary tract **u pigment** urochrome, urobilin, uroerythrin and haematoporphyrin **u retention** inability to empty the bladder completely **u system** kidneys, ureters, bladder and urethra **u tract** the structures involved in the formation, storage and excretion of urine-kidneys, ureters, bladder and urethra **u tract infection** UTI, infection of urinary tract **u tract obstruction** obstruction above the bladder or in the bladder outflow tract. In the former there is bilateral hydronephrosis and in the latter frequency, slowing of the stream, over-flow incontinence or complete retention

urinate (u'ri-nat) to discharge urine

urination (u'ri-na'shun) the act of passing urine, micturition.

urine (u'rin) the fluid formed by the kidneys, transported by the ureters,

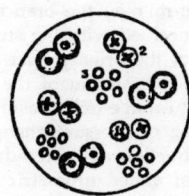

Cells: 1. Epithelial cells; 2. Pus cells; 3. RBC's

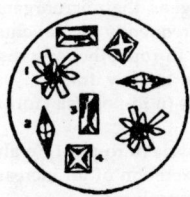

Crystals: 1. Uric acid; 2,4. Calcium oxalate; 3. Ammonium magnesium phosphate (triple phosphate)

stored in the bladder and eliminated through urethra during micturition **urinary** adj. **febrile u** passage of high coloured, concentrated urine **cloudy u** urine with cloudy appearance which may be due to presence of phosphates, urates or pus **chylous u** milky urine from presence of chyle or fat **midstream u** a specimen of urine collected while voiding urine. It eliminates organisms in urethra to a great extent as many of them come out at the beginning or at the end of urinary stream **residual u** urine remaining in the bladder after urination **u analysis** examination of the urine for presence of protein, sugar, bile pigments, bile salts, urobilinogen, ketone bodies, specific gravity and microscopy for casts, erythrocytes, leucocytes, crystals **u eggs** *Schistoma haematobium*

urinoglucosometer (u'ri-no-gloo'k-o-som'e-ter) an instrument for measurement of glucose in the urine

urinoma (u'ri-noma) a tumour-like urine filled cyst in the renal capsule secondary to congenital urethral obstruction

urinometer (u'ri-nome'ter) an instrument to determine the specific gravity of urine or other fluids; hydrometer. It has calibrations from 1000 to 1060 for a temperature of 15°C. Urine or other fluids (pleural or ascitic fluid) are collected in a jar and allowed to cool to room temperature. Urinometer is allowed to float by spinning it in the fluid. It should not touch the sides. Reading of the miniscus is recorded. Specific gravity of urine varies fom 1015 to 1025 and it is influenced by the amount of urea and sodium in the urine. The specific gravity is high in diabetes mellitus and in conditions of proteinuria. It is low in diabetes insipidus. The specific gravity becomes fixed at 1010 in renal failure with loss of concentrating power of kidney. An exudative fluid has a specific gravity of 1015 or more and a transudative fluid less than 1015

urinometry (u'ri-nom'e-tre) determination of specific gravity of the urine

urinothorax (ur'in-o-tho-raks) pleural fluid with pleural fluid/serum creatinine ratio > 1

urinous (u'ri-nus) pertaining to the urine

urobilin (u'ro-bi'lin) a brownish pigment formed by oxidation of urobilinogen

urobilinaemia (u'ro-bi'lin-e'me-a) the presence of urobilin in the blood

urobilinogen (u'ro-bi-lin'o-jen) product obtained following reduction of bilirubin. A red colour appears when Ehrlich's aldehyde reagent is added to urine

urobilinogenaemia (u'ro-bi'lin-o-jan-e'me-a) the presence of the urobilinogen in the blood

urobilinuria (u'ro-bi'lin-u're-a) excess amount of urobilin in the urine

urochrome (u'ro-kroom) the pigment that gives urine its yellow colour

urocoele (u'ro-sel) distension of the scrotum with extravasated urine

urocrisia (u'ro-kriz'e-a) diagnosis by examining the urine

urocystitis (u'ro-sis-ti'tis) inflammation of the urinary bladder

urodynamics (u'ro-di-nam'iks) the dynamics of the propulsion and flow of urine in the urinary tract. **urodynamic** adj

urodynia (u'ro-din'e-a) pain accompanying urination

urogastrone (u'ro-gas'tron) a polypeptide inhibits the secretion of gastric acid, a fluorescent pigment extracted from urine

urogenital (u'ro-jen'i-tal) pertaining to urinary system and genitalia **u sinus** outpouching of hindgut from which bladder and urethra develop

urogenous (u-roj'e-nus) producing urine

urogram (u'ro-gram) a roentgenogram of any part of the urinary tract

urography (u-ro-g'ra-fe) roentgenography of any portion of the urinary tract **intravenous u** urography after intravenous injection of an opaque medium which is rapidly excreted in the urine **retrograde u** urography after injection of a contrast medium into the bladder through urethra

urokinase (u-ro-ki'nas) a proteolytic enzyme activating the fibrinolytic system by converting the plasminogen to plasmin. It is used as a thrombolytic agent

uroporphyrin (u'ro-por'fi-rin) degradation product of haem, which is excreted in the urine along coproporphyrin and urine may turn reddish-brown on standing

urolith (u'ro-lith) a stone in the urinary tract

urolithiasis (u'ro-li-thi'a-sis) the formation of urinary stone and the resultant disorder

urologic (u-ro-loj'ik) pertaining to urology

urologist (u-rol'o-jist) a specialist in urology

urology (u-rol'o-je) the branch of medicine concerned with the study of disorders of the urinary tract and of the reproductive system of the male

urometry (u-rom'e-tre) measurement and recording of pressure changes caused by contraction of ureter during peristalsis of ureter. **urometric** adj

uromodulin (u-ro-mo'du-lin) an acid glycoprotein secreted by epithelial cells in ascending loop of Henle and distal convoluted tubules

uropathogens the microorganisms found most frequently in patients with UTI

uropathy (u-rop'a-the) any disease affecting the urinary tract

uropoiesis (u'ro-poi-e'sis) formation of the urine

uroporphyria (u'ro-por-fir'e-ah) porphyria with excretion of an increased amount of uroporphyrin

uroporphyrin (u'ro-por'fi-rin) porphyrins produced by oxidation of uroporphyrinogen, which are excreted in urine in excess amount

uroporphyrinogen (u'ro-por'fi-rin'o-jen) a porphyrinogen formed from porphobilinogen

uroradiology (u'ro-ra-de-ol'ah-je) radiology of the urinary tract

urorrhagia (u'ro-ra'je-a) an excess flow of urine

uroscopy (u'ros'kah-pe) diagnostic examination of the urine, **uroscopic** adj

urosepsis (u'ro-sep'sis) septic poisoning from retained and absorbed urinary substances

urticant (ur'ti-kant) producing urticaria

urticaria (ur-ti-ka're-a) sudden eruption of transitory, itchy wheals of variable size and shape due to a particular food or food additive, a drug and rarely an underlying systemic disease; hive. **urticarial** adj. **allergic u** urticaria from type I hypersensitivity reaction to a foreign protein resulting in release of histamine and other vasodilator substances **bullous u** superimposition of bullae on the wheals **cholinergic u** urticaria occurring on exposure to heat from sunlight or other sources **chronic u** urticaria persisting for more than 6 weeks **cold u** urticaria due to cold **dermographic u** development of urticarial wheals on light stroking of the skin **giant u.** angioneurotic oedema **papular u** appearance of small papules and wheals as a hypersensitivity reaction **pressure u** urticarial wheals developing on prolonged pressure **solar u** unusual susceptibility to sun rays **u medicamentosa** urticaria following ingestion of certain drugs **u pigmentosa** abnormal accumulation of mast cells in the skin presenting with multiple, irregular hypopigmented macules, noted in infancy

urticarial (ur-ti-ka're-al) pertaining to urticaria

urtication (ur'ti-ka'shunt) the development of urticaria

urustambha (s) paraplegia

ushah-pana drinking water soon after getting up early in the morning is regarded as hygienic

Usher's syndrome a genetic disorder characterised by congenital deafness, and retinitis pigmentosa, named after Charles Usher, British ophthalmologist

ushna (s) hot in potency

USMLE United States Medical Licencing Examination

Usual Interstitial Pneumonia UIP a disease with prominent fibrotic component, dense interstitial inflammation with destruction of the alveolar architecture characterised by insidious deterioration of respiratory function

uteralgia (u'ter-al'jah) pain in the uterus

uterectomy (u'ter-ok'to-me) removal of uterus through the abdomen or vagina

uterotonic (u'ter-o-toni'ik) increasing the tone of uterine muscle

uteropexy (u'ter-o-pek-si) hysteropexy

uterovaginal (u'ter-o-vaj'i-n'l) pertaining

to the uterus and bladder

uterine (u'ter-in) relating to the uterus **u apoplexy** a uterus in which myometrial vessels have been stripped of a protective endometrium and are actively bleeding **u bleeding** bleeding from uterus either physiologically (menstruation) or pathologically (menorrhagia, polymenorrhoea). It can occur as a nonmenstrual bleeding (metrorrhagia), withdrawal bleeding (following oestrogen therapy) or breakthrough bleeding from progestational agents) **u inertia** inability of the uterus to produce sufficiently strong contractions during labour to move the foetus through the birth canal **u prolapse** descent of the uterus from its normal position **u souffle** a vascular sound audible in a pregnant uterus **u subinvolution** failure of the uterus to return to normal size after child birth **u tube** one of the two small fallopian tubes attached to either side of the uterus

uteroabdominal (u'ter-o-ab-dom'i-n'l) pertaining to the uterus and abdomen

uterocervical (u'ter-o-ser'vi-k'l) pertaining to the uterus and cervix uteri

uterofixation (u'ter-o-fiks-a'shun) fixation of a displaced uterus

uterogestation (u'ter-o-jes-ta'shun) uterine pregnancy which is normal

utero-ovarian (u'ter-o-o-va're-un) pertaining to uterus and ovary

uteroplacental (u'ter-o-plah-sen'tal) pertaining to the placenta and uterus

uterorectal (u'ter-o-rek't'l) pertaining to or communicating with uterus and rectum

uterosalpingography (u'ter-o-sal-ping-og'ra-fe) radiography of the uterus and fallopian tubes after the introduction of a contrast medium

uterovaginal (u'ter-o-'vaj'i-nal) pertaining to the uterus and vagina

uterovesical (u'ter-o-ves'i-kal) relating to the uterus and the bladder

uterus (u'ter-us) a hollow pear-shaped muscular organ of female reproductive system situated in the pelvis which allows the fertilised ovum to implant and provide nourishment to the developing foetus. It consists of a main part (corpus) with an elongated lower part (cervix) with an opening at the end (os). The upper rounded part of the uterus is the fundus at each end of which is the cornua where the uterine tubes join it **bicornuate u** uterus having two lateral horns due to imperfect fusion of the para mesonephric ducts **double u** uterus bicorpus **gravid u** the pregnant uterus **inversion u** a turning inside out of the uterus, one of the rarest complications of labour **involution u** uterus diminishing in its size following delivery **prolapse u** downward displacement of uterus which may be of first degree with cervix being within the vaginal orifice; second degree with cervix outside the vaginal orifice or third degree with whole uterus remaining outside the vaginal orifice **rudimentary u** hypoplastic uterus measuring 1 to 3 cm in length **parturient u** uterine contractions of labour **u rupture** rupture of uterus may be spontaneous due to weakening of the uterine wall of previous caesarean section scar or trauma during pregnancy **septate u** uterus divided into two cavities by a septum **unicorn u** a one-horned uterus where one half is developed and the other undeveloped or absent

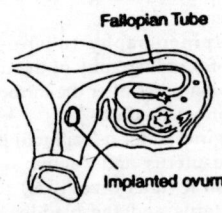

Uterus with implanted ovum

UTI urinary tract infection showing presence in an appropriately collected midstream specimen of urine of more than 10^5 colony forming units per ml. of urine.

utility the value placed by the individual on a particular health state

utpanna (s) arise

utpala-patram (s) knife shaped phlebotome

utpatti (s) origin

utricle (ut'ri-kal) the larger of the two sacs of the membranous labyrinth in the vestibule of the ear **prostatic u** a minute pouch in the prostatic opening on the summit of the seminal colliculus

utsarga (s) strength

uttara vasti (s) urethral syringe

utter to speak

uvea (u've-a) the pigmented vascular layer of the eye consisting of the choroid, ciliary body and the iris

uveitis (u-ve-i'tis) inflammation of the uvea

uveoparotid (u've-o-pa-rotid) pertaining to the uvea and the parotid gland

uveoparotitis (u've-o-par-o-ti'tis) inflammation of the uvea and the parotid gland

uveoscleritis (u've-o-sk'e-ri'tis) scleritis due to extension of uveitis

uviform (u'vi-form) grape-like

uvula (u'vu-la) 1. the conical fleshy mass of tissue projecting down from the posterior border of the soft palate **bifid u** split uvula 2. part of inferior vermis of cerebellum belonging to Palaeocerebellum. 3. uvula vesicae; elevation on the trigone immediately posterior to the urethral orifice produced by the median lobe of prostate

uvulatome (u'vu-lo-tom) an instrument for cutting the uvula

uvulectomy (u'vu-lek'to-me) surgical removal of the uvula

uvulotomy (u-vu-lot'me) incision of the uvula

uvulitis (u'vu-li'tis) inflammation of the uvula

uvulopalatopharyngoplasty extensive surgical resection of the soft palate in the oropharynx. It may be of help in removal of pharyngeal obstruction in a selected subgroup of patients exhibiting severe obstructive sleep apnoea. The procedure is to increase the size of the airway by removal of the uvula, part of the soft palate and other redundant pharyngeal tissue

U-wave a small rounded deflection following the T wave in the electrocardiogram. Its significance is undetermined

V

V symbol for pulmonary ventilation

Va volume of alveolar gas

V_1-V_6 *ECG* unipolar ECG chest leads placed on a horizontal line from V_1 at the right edge of the sternum at fifth intercostal space to V_6 at left mid-axillary line

V-genes codes for variable parts of immunoglobulin light and heavy chains

V-squint eyes are widely separated while looking upwards and are close while looking down

v- prefix for viral genes

V_a-Q ventilation-perfusion ratio

vaccinal (vak'sin-al) pertaining to vaccine or vaccination

vaccinate (vak'sin-at) to inoculate vaccine to produce immunity.

vaccination (vak'si-na'shun) the inoculation of vaccine to produce immunity; immunisation

vaccinator (vak'si-na'tor) a person who vaccinates.

vaccine (vak'sen) a suspension of live, live-attenuated, killed, complete or incomplete micro-organisms or products obtained therefrom which contains antigens, administered to induce active immunity against a specific infectious disease **inactivated v** killed vaccine. Organisms killed by heat or chemicals when injected into the body stimulate active immunity (pertusis, cholera, typhoid, rabies, salk vaccine) **live v** vaccines prepared from live attenuated organisms (BCG, oral polio, measles) **v lymph** material obtained from cowpox **sabin v** live poliovaccine **salk v** killed polio vaccine administered parenterally

vaccinia (vak-sin'e-a) cowpox

vacuity emptiness

vacuolar (vak'u-o-lar) pertaining to a vacuole

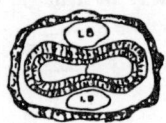

Vaccinia virus

vacuolation (vak'u-o-la'shun) the formation of vacuoles

vacuole (vak'u-ol) small cavity formed within the protoplasm of a cell

vacuum (vak'u-um) a space devoid of air **v aspiration** a method of removal of foetus and placenta using a suction device and can be carried out in early pregnancy upto 14th week **v extraction** a procedure that helps easy delivery by a suction **v extractor** device to assist labour wherein the cup adheres to scalp by vacuum to which traction is applied **v phenomenon** a linear or oval radiolucency corresponding to gas in the inter-vertebral space, seen in degenerative disc disease **v sign** a normal radiologic finding noted when traction is applied to a joint causing coalescence of gas within a joint. It disappears in effusion

Vade Mecum (wa'de-me'kum) a book for ready reference

Vagabond's disease pediculosis corporis seen among beggars and uncared adolescents belonging to the lower socio-economic groups

vagal (va'gal) pertaining to a vagus nerve

vagina (va-ji'na) a muscular canal, in the female extending from the vulva to the uterine cervix; a sheath

vaginal (vaj'in-al) pertaining to the vagina; resembling a sheath **v adenosis** hyperplasia of mucous glands in vagina due to high oestrogen therapy during pregnancy **v hydrocoele** hydrocele limited to tunica vaginalis in male **v ring** a flexible silicone ring that is inserted into the vagina to give support to the uterus following its prolapse

vaginalitis (vaj-in-al-i'tis) inflammation of tunica vaginalis testis

vaginate (vaj'in-at) sheathed

vaginismus (vaj'in-iz'mus) an involuntary spasm and tightening of the opening of the vagina and perineal muscles preventing intercourse

vaginitis (vaj-in-i'tis) inflammation of the vagina and it can be caused by infection, allergic reaction or oestrogen deficiency **atrophic v** soreness, itch and pale atrophic appearance of vagina due to oestrogen deficiency

vaginoscope (vaj'in-o-skop) a vaginal speculum

vaginosis a vaginal infection noted in women of reproductive age, without leucocyte infiltration **bacterial v** infection from *Gardenerella vaginalis* and anaerobes causing smell and white discharge

vaginotomy (vaj'i-not'o-me) colpotomy

vagitus (va-ji't-us) first cry of a newly born infant

vagolysis (va-gol'i-sis) surgical destruction of the vagus nerve

vagotomy (va-got'o-me) interruption of the impulses transmitted by vagus nerve by its surgical division

vagotonia (va'go-to'ne-a) hyperexcitability

vague not clearly stated

vagus (va'gus) wandering **v nerve** either of the tenth cranial nerves that regulate various functions such as swallowing, talking, heart rate and digestion. This mixed cranial nerve takes its origin in an elongated nucleus in the floor of the fourth ventricle and emerge along the internal aspect of the medulla and leave the skull through the jugular

foramen along with 9th and 11th cranial nerves. It carries sensation from the pharynx, larynx, oesophagus, heart, respiratory passages and abdominal viscera. The motor fibres innervate the muscles of the soft palate, pharynx and larynx

vaidya (s) physician

vairagya (s) detachment, dispassion

vajikarana a process or a drug which makes a man sexually as strong as a horse

valciclovir antiviral agent when given early shortens the disease like chickenpox

valgus (val'gus) bent outward.

validate to confirm

validity (va-lid'i-te) *stat* extent to which figure derived from the test actually measures intended object in statistics

valine (val'en) an essential amino acid

vallecula (val-lek'u-la) a depression or furrow on any surface

Valley fever pneumonic form of coccidioidomycosis

vallum (val'um) a wall

valproate anticonvulsant useful in primary and secondary generalised tonic clonic seizures and myoclonus

Valsalva's (val-salvaz) **manoeuver** increase of intrathoracic pressure by forcible exhalation effort against closed glottis, named after Italian anatomist, Antonio Valsalva **V's aneurysm** dilatation of aortic wall from a congenital defect which can rupture into the right ventricle or right atrium **V's sinus** slight bulge of aortic wall behind each aortic valve cusp

valsartan angiotensin II receptor antagonist having similar effects to ACE inhibitors. It does not influence bradykinin metabolism and does not cause cough

values qualities that a person has learned to believe are important or worthwhile

valva (val'va) a valve

valve (valv) a membranous fold in a

canal or passage to allow flow in one direction and to retard or to prevent regurgitation of the contents passing through it

valvotomy (val-vot'o-me) a surgical procedure of opening or slitting of a narrowed heart valve

valvula (val'vu-la) a small valve

valvulae conniventes mucosal folds of jejunum

valvular (val'vu-lar) having the form or function of a valve **v heart disease** a defect in one or more heart valves which may be congenital or acquired **v pneumothorax** tension pneumothorax. **v vegetations** variably sized excrescences that are present on the heart valves

valvulitis (val'vu-li'tis) inflammation of valve leaflets of the heart

valvulo- of valves

valvuloplasty (val'vu-lo-plas'te) reconstructive operation to repair a defective heart valve

vamana (s) emesis

vanaspati (s) substances obtained from medicinal plants and herbs

vampire blood sucking bat; a clinician who requests excessive blood tests, potentially causing iatrogenic anaemia

vancomycin glycopeptide bactericidal antibiotic and is indicated in serious infections such as endocarditis or septicemia

Van Gogh syndrome *Psy* self mutilation which may be associated with dysmorphic delusions, distrubances of body image

vanillylmandelic acid VMA main urinary metabolite of adrenaline and noradrenaline. It is raised in urine in pheochromocytoma and neuroblastoma

vanishing disappearing **v diabetes mellitus syndrome** a marked reduction in the requirement of exogenous insulin that occurs secondary to complete destruction of the pituitary gland especially the anterior lobe; Houssay phenomenon **v lung** giant bullous emphysema especially in the apices of the lungs. Radiologically there is disappearance of lung markings. There is absence of concomitant emphysema **v twin** a spontaneous regression of a second gestational product in twin pregnancies

vanjanya (s) substances from plant kingdom.

vanti (s) vomiting

Van den Bergh reaction test to distinguish unconjugated from conjugated bilirubin, named after Dutch physician, Van den Bergh

Vaquez's disease *see* polycythaemia rubra vera named after Louis Vaquez, French physician

var variant, variety.

variable (va're-a-b'l) *stat* changing from time to time; a value subject to change; not constant; characteristics of individual groups that can be expressed as numerical value in statistics **v expressivity** variable expression of autosomal dominant trait in affected individuals

variance *stat* an estimate of variability. The sum of the square deviation around the mean, divided by the number of cases

variant (var'e-ant) tendency to differ in some characteristic from the class to which it belongs **v angina** Prinzmetal's angina. Vasospasm of coronory arteries causing chest pain at rest with elevated ST segment

variation (va're-a'shun) deviation in characters in an individual from those typical of the group to which it belongs

variceal (var'i-se'al) pertaining to or caused by a varix **v banding** application of a band through endoscope for control of bleeding **v bleeding** occurs from oesophageal varices located within 3-5 cm of the oesophago-gastric junction or from gastric varices

varicella (var'i-sel'a) chickenpox

varicella–zoster virus herpes virus that can cause chickenpox and herpes zoster

varices (var'i-sez) plural of varix

varicocoele (var'i-ko-sel) varicose condition of the veins of the spermatic cord surrounding a testicle in the scrotum giving a sensation like a bag of worms

varicography (var'i-kog'ra-fe) roentgenologic visualisation of varicose veins following injection of a radiopaque medium

varicose (var'i-kos) unnatural and permanent dilatation of a vein **v aneurysm** dilatation of anastomotic channel in AV shunt **v veins** enlarged and twisted veins just below the skin, usually in the legs **v ulcer** venous ulcer

varicosity (var'i-kos'i-te) a varicose condition

variola (va-ri'o-la) smallpox **v minor** mild form of smallpox (alastrim)

varix (va'riks) an enlarged and tortuous vein, artery or lymphatic vessel

varna (s) appearance

varsha (s) rainy season

varus (va'rus) bent inward; bending with outward convexity

vas (vas) any canal to carry a fluid pl. **vasa**

vasana (s) past impressions

vasanta (s) spring

vascular (vas'ku-lar) relating to blood vessels **v headache** a headache caused by spasm of blood vessels in the brain and scalp **v sling** a congenital malformation in which the left pulmonary artery arises from the right pulmonary artery, crossing to the left between the trachea and oesophagus forming a sling around the trachea. It is associated with tracheal stenosis with stridor, wheeze and choking

vascularization (vas'ku-lar-i-za'shun) formation of new blood vessels

vasculature (vas'ku-la-tur) the vascular network of the body

vasculitis (vas'ku-li'tis) inflammation of blood vessels, leading to end-organ or tissue damage **large vessel v** temporal arteritis, pulseless disease **medium size v** polyarteritis nodosa, Kawasaki disease **small vessel v** microscopic polyangiitis, Wegener's granulomatosis, Churg-Strauss syndrome, Leucocytoclastic vasculitis, Hanoch-Schonlein purpura and essential mixed cryoglobulinaemia

vas deferens one of a pair of narrow elongated tubes of 47 cm length that store and carry sperms from the testicles to ejaculatory duct which empties into the prostatic urethra

vasectomize to perform a vasectomy

vasectomy (vas-ek'to-me) surgical interruption of the vas deferens by excision of a portion of it to prevent sperm reaching the urethra; a male sterilising procedure following which the man is capable of ejaculation normally but semen is devoid of sperms

vaso- relation to a vessel or to a duct

vasoactive (vas'o-ak'tiv) exerting influence upon the calibre of blood vessels **v intestinal polypeptide**, VIP, a neuropeptide present in the nerve fibres of smooth muscle, blood vessels and in the glands of the upper respiratory tract. It stimulates adenylate cyclase causing potent vasodilation, pancreatic and intestinal secretion, inhibition of gastric acid secretion, increased cardiac output, glycogenolysis, bronchodilation and inhibition of macromolecule release from mucous glands **v substances** a group of circulating substances that regulate vascular tone causing either vasodilation (atrial natriuretic peptide, kinins and VIP) or vasoconstriction (angiotensin II, adrenaline and noradrenaline and vasopressin)

vasoconstriction (vaso-kon-strik'shun) the diminution of the calibre of blood vessels

vasoconstrictor (vas'o-kon-strik'tor) an agent causing constriction of the blood vessels

vasodepressor (vas'o-de-pres'or) an agent causing lowering of blood pressure by reducing peripheral resistance

vasodilatation (vas'o-dil-a-ta'shun) increase in the calibre of blood vessels; vasodilation

vasodilator (vas'o-di-la'tor) an agent causing dilatation or relaxation of the blood vessels

vasography (vas-og'ra-fe) roentgenography of blood vessels or vas deferens following injection of contrast medium into the lumen

vasomotor (vas'o-mo'tor) an agent regulating the diameter of the blood vessels **v rhinitis** rhinorrhoea, and sneezing without any evidence of infection or allergy

vaso-occlusive crisis occlusion of small vessels by sickled red cells and ischaemia in sickle-cell anaemia

vasopressin (vas'o-pres'in) one of the hormones formed by the hypothalamic nuclei and stored in the posterior lobe of the pituitary gland; antidiuretic hormone (ADH); used in the management of diabetes insipidus

vasopressor (vas'o-pres'or) an agent causing contraction of the muscular tissue of the capillaries and arteries and raising the blood pressure

vasospasm (vas'o-spazm) spasm of the blood vessels causing a decrease in their calibre

vasovagal (vas'o-va'gal) relating to the action of vagus nerve on the blood vessels **v attacks** a sudden slowing of the heart causing temporary loss of consciousness; fainting

vasovasostomy (vas'o-va-sos'to-me) surgical reanastomosis of vasa deferentia in a vasectomised person

vasti (s) enema

vastus (vas'tus) vast, great, extensive

vata (s) wind; one of the *doshas*; joint pain

vataka (s) small pill

VATS abbreviation for video-assisted thoracic surgery

vault (vaw'lt) a dome-like structure

vayu (s) air

VC vital capacity

VCG vector cardiogram

VD venereal disease

VDRL Venereal Disease Research Laboratories **v test** a reaginic screening test for syphilis. Heat inactivated serum is added to the VDRL antigen and agglutination is viewed by light microscopy at 4 minutes

vection (vek'shun) the carrying of causative agent of a disease from an infected person to a healthy person

vector (vek'tor) an invertebrate animal acting as a carrier transmitting an infective agent from one host to another; *mol* a cloning vehicle such as plasmid, phage, cosmid, yeast, artificial chromosome into which DNA to be cloned can be inserted

vectorcardiogram (vek'tor-kar'de-o-gram) the graphic record produced by vectorcardiography

vectorcardiograph (vek'tor-kar'de-o-gra-f) the instrument used in vectorcardiography

vectorcardiography (vek'tor-kar'de-o-gra-fe) a method to determine the direction and magnitude of electromotive forces of the heart as represented by vector loops

vedana (s) pain *vsthapana* analgesic

vegetable (vej'e-ta-bl) **cell** a large cell with clear, lipid and glycogen-laden cytoplasm, angulated borders and a small hyperchromatic nucleolus arranged in bundles, encountered in renal cell carcinomas

vegetation (vej-e-ta'shun) a morbid growth; variably sized excrescences found on the heart valves **bacterial v** friable, necrotic lesions on the valves **lupus erythematous v** lesions consisting of mucoid substance, fibrinoid degeneration and collagenous fibrosis on tricuspid and mitral valve **non-bacterial thrombolic v** small foci of organising thrombi along the line of the valve leaflet's closure or on either side of the ventricle

vegetative (vej'e-ta'tiv) to exist in an inactive and passive way devoid of

mental activities **v state** a deeply comatose state in which only the basic body
functions are maintained

vehicle (ve'i-kl) a substance having no
therapeutic action used as a medium
for active remedies *mol* a self-replicating DNA molecule such as virus,
plasmid or phage that serves as a vector
for insertion of a segment of DNA into
a host.

veil (val) a covering structure

veiled appearance myositis ossificans exhibiting punctate linear radiodensity
parallel to the shaft and cortex of long
bones

veiled cell *imm* an antigen presenting
cell of the mononuclear phagocytic
system that is present in the marginal
sinus of afferent lymphatics.

vein (ven) one of the systems of branching vessels carrying deoxygenated
blood from various parts of the body
to the heart (*see* Table 13)

Table 13: Veins

Axillary v.	present in axilla accompanying axillary artery. Continues as subclavian vein at the outer border of the 1st rib
Azygos v.	on the right side in front of vertebra, begins as lumbar azygos vein ends into superior vena cava
Basilic v.	begins on the ulnar side on the dorsum of hand, ascends up, joins cubital veins, becomes deep in the upper arm and continues as axillary vein
Basivertebral v's	emerge from foramina on posterior surface of vertebral bodies, communicate with external vertebral plexes, opens into anterior internal vertebral plexus
Brachiocephalic v's	two large trunks at the root of the neck formed by union of internal jugular and subclavian vein. They unite to form superior vena cava
Cardiac v great	begins at the apex of the heart, lies in anterior interventricular groove, enters the beginning of coronary sinus
Cardiac v middle	begins at the apex of the heart, lies in posterior interventricular groove and ends in the coronary sinus near its termination
Cardiac v small	runs in the coronary sulcus posteriorly, opens into the end of coronary sinus, drains back of right atrium and ventricle
Cephalic v	begins from the dorsal venous network on radial side of hands, ascends on the forearm, gives median cubital vein, ends in the axillary vein just below the clavicle
Cerebellar v's inferior	placed on the inferior surface of cerebellum, includes median and lateral vessels, drains into straight sinus, sigmoid sinus or petrosal sinuses
Cerebral v's anterior	small vein accompanying anterior cerebral artery. Joins to form basal vein which ends into great cerebral vein.
Cerebral v's great	formed by union of internal cerebral veins, opens into straight sinus

Cerebral v's inferior	drains inferior surface of cerebral hemispheres. Communicate with superior sagittal, cavernous, superior petrosal and transverse sinus through superior, basal and middle cerebral veins
Cerebral v's internal	right and left vein, drains internal deep parts of cerebral hemispheres unite to form great cerebral vein
Cerebral v's middle, deep	runs in the floor of lateral cerebral sulcus, drains insula and neighbouring gyri, joins basal vein
Cerebral v's middle, superficial	begins on the lateral surface of hemisphere, ends in the cavernous sinus
Cerebral v's superior	8-12 in number, drains superolateral and medial surfaces of hemisphere, open into superior sagittal sinus against the current of blood in it
Cubital v. median	present in front of elbow region. Communicates with cephalic vein and deep veins. Joins basilic vein
Cystic v	runs between gall bladder and liver, vary considerably, drains gall bladder and cystic duct, joins hepatic veins
Diploic v.	occupy diploe of the cranial bones, develops after 2 years of age. They are devoid of valves and communicate with meningeal veins and sinuses of dura mater frontal, temporal, parietal, and occipital bones
Dorsal v's of penis, deep	drains glans penis and corpora cavernosa, enters prostatic plexus, communicates with internal pudendal veins
Dorsal v's of penis – superficial	drains prepuce and skin of the penis, ends in external pudendal vein
Emissary v.	passes through openings in skull bones. Communicates scalp veins with cranial venous sinuses, e.g. mastoid, parietal and condylar
Facial v	formed by union of supraorbital and supratrochlear vein, ends in internal jugular vein. It has no valves and communicates with cavernous sinus through ophthalmic and pterygoid venous plexus
Femoral v	begins as continuation of popliteal vein, receives many tributaries, communicates with great saphenous vein, becomes external iliac vein at the margin of inguinal ligament
Hemiazygos v	starts on the left in front of vertebral column, ends in azygos vein, communicates with left renal vein, drains lower intercostal spaces
Hemiazygos v accessory	ascends in front of thoracic vertebra on the left, drains 4 to 6 intercostal spaces, joins azygos vein
Hepatic v's	commence in the liver as intralobular veins, opens into sublobular veins, which unite to form hepatic veins, ends into inferior vena cava

Iliac v common	result from the union of external and internal iliac veins, lies in front of sacroiliac joint. Veins of two sides unite to form inferior vena cava
Iliac v external	upward continuation of femoral vein, begins behind inguinal ligament, joins internal iliac vein to form common iliac vein
Iliac v internal	formed by confluence of the veins, draining pelvis corresponding to the branches of the internal iliac artery. Joins external iliac vein to form common iliac vein
Intercostal v's posterior	eleven on each side run with branches of posterior intercostal arteries, first intercostal ends in brachiocephalic vein. Other veins open into azygos vein
Intervertebral v	drains veins from spinal cord, communicates with vertebral venous plexus, ends in vertebral, intercostal, lumbar and sacrial veins
Jugular v anterior	starts at the level of hyoid bone, communicates with internal jugular vein, ends into external jugular vein
Jugular v external	drains mostly scalp and face, formed by union of retro-mandibular vein and posterior auricular vein, ends into subclavian vein
Jugular v internal	collects blood from brain, face and neck. Begins at the jugular foramen as continuation of sigmoid sinus. It joins subclavian vein to form brachiocephalic vein
Meningeal v's middle	communicates with superior sagittal sinus, diploic veins and middle cerebral veins, drains meninges, ends in cavernous sinus or pterygoid venous plexus
Paraumbilical v's	establishes anastomosis between the veins of anterior abdominal wall and portal vein, runs along *ligamentum teres*, ends in left branch of portal vein
Popliteal v	formed by union of tibial veins, runs in popliteal fossa, becomes femoral vein
Portal v	formed by union of superior mesenteric and splenic vein at the level of second lumbar vertebra, enters *porta hepatis*, divides into right and left branch to enter substance of liver
Pulmonary v	commence in the capillary network in the walls of alvéoli of lungs, joining together, ultimately two veins emerge from each lung, opens separately in the upper posterior part of the left atrium
Rectal v's inferior	formed by external rectal venous plexus in the lower part, drains into internal pudendal vein.
Rectal v's middle	begins in the rectal venous plexus, receives tributaries from bladder, prostate, seminal vesicle, ends in internal iliac vein
Rectal v superior	starts from the rectal venous plexus, continues as inferior mesenteric vein

Retromandibular v	descends in the parotid glands, divides into anterior and posterior branches. Anterior branch joins posterior auricular to form external jugular vein
Saphenous v great	longest in the body, begins on the medial margin of foot, ends in femoral vein, has 10-15 valves and communicates with deep veins of the leg
Saphenous v small	begins as continuation of lateral marginal vein of foot ends in popliteal vein, has 10-12 valves and communicates with deep veins of leg and great saphenous vein
Splenic v	starts from union of splenic tributaries, ends behind the neck of the pancreas by uniting with superior mesenteric vein to form portal vein
Subclavian v	continuation of axillary vein, unites with the internal jugular to form the brachiocephalic vein
Testicular v	formed by tributaries of veins of epididymis, emerge at the back of testis, ascends as pampiniform plexus, coalesce into two veins, becomes single vein which opens into inferior vena cava (right) and left renal vein (left)
Thyroid v's middle	drains lower part of thyroid gland, larynx and trachea joins internal jugular vein
Thyroid v superior	formed by superficial tributaries, drains thyroid gland, ends by joining internal jugular or facial vein
Vena cava, inferior	formed by junction of two common iliac veins, in front of lumbar 5th vertebra, ascends up, perforates the diaphragm, passing through pericardium, opens in the lower part of right atrium
Vena cava, superior	collects blood from upper half of body, formed by junction of right and left brachiocephalic veins, opens in the upper part of right atrium

velamentous (vel'a-men'tus) veil-like

velocardiofacial syndrome a malformation with dominant microdeletion characterised by broad nose, wide eye spacing, cleft palate, mental retardation, cardiac abnormality such as Fallot's tetrology, right aortic arch, and VSD

vellus (vel'us) fine body hair which appears after fall of the lanugo hair and present before puberty

velum (ve'lum) a covering

vena (ve'na) a vein. pl. **venae**

vena cava either of two large veins that drain deoxygenated blood from the body into the right atrium of the heart

venacavography (ve'na-ka-vog'ra-fe) radiography of a vena cava

venereal (ve-ne're-al) due to sexual contact **v disease** any sexually transmitted disease which include syphilis, gonorrhoea, AIDS, nonspecific urethritis, chalmydiosis and chancroid **v sore** chancroid **v wart** reddish elevation on the genitals and anus

venereologist (ve-ner'e-ol-jist) a specialist in venereology.

Venereology (ve-ner'e-ol'a-je) the branch of medicine dealing with the study and treatment of venereal diseases

venesection (ven'e-sek'shun) phlebotomy

venin (ven'in) any of the several poisonous substances found in snake venom

venipuncture (ven'i-punk'chur) puncture of a vein with a needle to withdraw blood or to inject fluid or drugs

Venkataraman and Ramakrishnan fluid a medium for transporting vomitus or stools for culture of cholera vibrio

veno- pertaining to or of veins

venoclysis (ve'nok'li-sis) intravenous infusion

venodilator agent causing dilatation of veins and reduce preload such as organic nitrate

venogram (ve'no-gram) phlebogram

venography (ve-nog'ra-fe) a diagnostic imaging procedure to examine veins following injection of a contrast medium

venom (ven'om) a poison which certain snakes or insects secrete and introduce into the victims by biting or stinging

venomous (ven'o-mus) having gland or glands secreting venom

veno-occlusive (ve'no-o-kloo'siv) obstruction to the veins **v disease** centrilobular liver damage leading to the thrombosis of central veins and later cirrhosis caused by drinking bush tea in Jamaica

venoscan study for deep vein thrombosis by injection of technetium-labelled fibrinogen

venostasis (ve'no-sta'sis) retardation of venous outflow from a part.

venous (ve'nus) pertaining to or of the nature of a vein or veins; pertaining to the blood in the pulmonary artery **v hum** a continuous murmur due to increased blood flow in jugular veins **v nipping** compression of retinal veins by thickened arterioles in hypertension **v thrombosis** a condition characterised by a clot in a vein **v ulcer** ulcer in leg from varicose veins or deep vein thrombosis

vent an opening serving as an outlet; expression

venter (ven'ter) the abdomen; any hollowed cavity

ventilate fleshy part

ventilation (ven'ti-la'shun) process of exchange of gas between the lungs and ambient air; replacement of vitiated air by a supply of fresh outdoor air, and control of the quality of incoming air with regard to its temperature, provide an environment that is comfortable and free from risk of infection **alveolar v** ventilation of alveoli where gas exchange takes place **controlled mandatory v** CMV, it is done by intermittent positive pressure ventilation through an endotracheal tube **deadspace v** ventilation occurring in alveoli which are not perfused with blood and ventilation becomes ineffective **intermittent mandatory v** IMV, used for weaning the patients from controlled ventilation. It maintains respiratory muscle function and prevents asynchronous breathing **intermittent positive-pressure v** IPPV, it assists in delivery of bronchodilator aerosols and humidification of the bronchial passages. The inspiratory process is done by the machines with a peak inspiratory pressure of 15 to 25 cm of water. It increases the tidal volume and enables better distribution of inhaled gas to poorly ventilated areas of the lung **mechanical v** artificial ventilation from exhaust, fans and air conditioning; the partial or complete replacement of a patient's own respiratory muscle function by external mechanical support to improve gas exchange and reduce the work of breathing **natural v** simple system of ventilating small houses, school and offices. **non-invasive intermittent positive pressure v** NIPPV, provides pressure support of 25 cm H_2O at the onset of inspiration which ceases at the onset of expiration. It may be applied *via* a face or nasal mask **non-invasive negative pressure v** NINPV, it operates by producing negative pressures within an internal tank or iron lung that increases all or part of the thorax. It has been replaced by NIPPV. **pressure support v** PSV, breaths initiated by the patient are assisted by a preset positive pressure supplement. It may help weaning from CMV or SIMV **synchronised intermittent mandatory v** SIMV, the ventilator is programmed to deliver a predetermined number of mechanical breaths of specified tidal volume after a suitable pause in the patient's spontaneous ventilatory efforts. It may help weaning from CMV **v scan** an image produced by radionuclide scanning of the lungs following inhalation of a radioactive gas

ventilation-perfusion imaging useful in the detection of pulmonary thromboemboli, which appear as 'filling defect'. ^{131}Xe gas is inhaled in ventilation scan and 99 m Tc-labelled macroaggregates of albumin microspheres are injected intravenously, the particles becoming transiently trapped in pulmonary microvessels providing the 'perfusion' scan

ventilation-perfusion ratio measure of efficiency of gas transfer in the lung. Perfusion defect is indicated by a ratio above 1; and a ratio below 1 indicates ventilation defect

ventilator a machine that takes over the breathing of a person who is unable to breath on his or her own **pressure-cycled v** allow the flow of gas (oxygen, compressed air) into the lungs till a preset gauge pressure (40 cm H_2O) is reached. Then the machine shuts off allowing exhalation to occur as a passive event **time-cycled v** tank respirator which sucks air into the lungs by creation of a negative pressure while the body is confined within an airtight tank **volume-cycled v** allow the flow of gas into the lungs till a preset tidal volume is reached. They are able to deliver the desired concentration of

oxygen at a pressure upto 80 to 100 cm H_2O

ventilatory failure the failure of the lungs to oxygenate the blood to a normal level and to maintain the arterial CO_2 pressure at or below the normal level when breathing air at normal PO_2

ventrad (ven'trad) towards the ventral side

ventral (ven'tral) towards the belly surface **v hernia** a hernia through the abdominal wall especially in the epigastrium

ventricle (ven'trik-l) a small cavity referring to either of the two lower thick-walled chambers on each side of the heart or one of a series of intercommunicating cavities of the brain filled with cerebrospinal fluid

ventricose protruding belly

ventricular (ven'trik'u-lar) pertaining to ventricle **v aneurysm** full thickness myocardial infarction followed by thinning and stretching of the infarcted segment **v assist device** a portable, battery-powered device that assists the blood flow while a patient is awaiting heart transplantation **v asystole** ventricular stand still when there is cessation of the stimuli reaching the ventricles. It may occur in myocardial infarction necessitating cardiac massages **v ectopic beats** VEB, extrasystoles; premature beats. It is characterised by irregular pulse with weak or missed beats. They produce a low stroke volume as left ventricular contraction is premature and ineffective. Patients are asymptomatic but may complain an irregular heart beat and its significance depends on underlying heart disease such as acute myocardial infarction, heart failure or digoxin toxicity. They may occur in normal people **v fibrillation** rapid, ineffective, uncoordinated contractions of the ventricles of the heart, which is rapidly fatal if untreated **v gallop** triple rhythm with extra sound in systole **v septal defect** VSD, a congenital heart disease having a hole in the septum between the ventricles of the heart **v standstill** *see* v asystole **v stroke work** VSW, the external work performed by the ventricle with each beat. It is calculated from stroke volume (SV) and the pre- and after load pressures. VSW = SV (afterload-preload) ml/mmHg. **v tachycardia** an abnormally fast heart beat at a rate of 140 to 220 beats per minute that are initiated in the ventricles and it does not show any response to pressure on carotids

ventriculocaval shunt communication through a tube from lateral ventricle *via* jugular vein to superior vena cava in hydrocephalus

ventriculoperitoneal shunt communication through a tube subcutaneously from lateral ventricle to subphrenic space in hydrocephalus

ventriculogram (ven-trik'u-lo-gram) a roentgenogram of the cerebral ventricle following injection of air or gas as a contrast medium

ventriculography (ven-trik'u-lo'gra-fe) roentgenography of the cerebral ventricle or ventricle of the heart following injection of a contrast medium

ventriculopuncture (ven-trik'u-lo-pun-k'tur) the puncture of a ventricle of the brain with a needle

ventriculostomy (ven-trik'u-los'to-me) the formation of a drain for cerebrospinal fluid from the ventricles of the brain

ventriculus (ven-trik'u-lus) the stomach; a small cavity; a ventricle of the brain or heart

ventro- abdomen, towards front surface

ventrolateral nucleus major division of thalamus. It relays proprioceptive pathway from cerebellum to prefrontal cortex

ventrosuspension operation to correct retroversion of uterus

Venturi effect pressure falls in narrow segment of tube through which fluid passes, named after Venturi, Italian physicist **v mask** holes in the mask to draw in constant proportion of air to join oxygen flow

venula (ven'u-la) venule; a minute, vein tributary

venus (ve'nus) Roman goddess of love and beauty **mount of v** the mons pubis **necklace of v** eruption around the neck in secondary syphilis

verapamil calcium channel blocking agent, useful in treatment of supraventricular tachycardia and control of atrial fibrillation

verbatim (ver-ba'ti-m) word for word

verbigeration (ver-bij'er-a'shun) *Psy* meaningless repetitions of specific words or phrases

vermi- combining word for worm

vermian (vermi-an) pertaining to the vermis of the cerebellum

vermicidal (ver'mi-si'dal) destructive to worms

vermicide (ver'mi-sid) an anthelmintic drug

vermicular (ver-mik'u-lar) worm-like appearance

vermiform (ver'mi-form) resembling a worm in shape **v appendix** a long narrow worm-shaped tube connected to caecum. Its distal end is closed and is lined with mucosa similar to that of large intestine

vermifuge (ver'mi-fuj) an agent that expels worms

vermin (ver'min) parasitic insects such as lice and bed bugs

vermis (ver'mis) worm-like structure, the median lobe of the cerebellum

vermix (ver'mi-ks) vermiform appendix

vernix (ver'niks) the fatty material consisting of sebum and desquamated epithelial cells covering the skin of a newborn

vernal (ver'nal) pertaining to or appearing in spring **v conjuctivitis** recurrent allergic conjuctivitis.

Verner-Morrison syndrome pancreatic adenoma secreting VIP presenting with severe watery diarrhoea, hypokalaemia and achlorhydria, described by Verner-Morrison, US physician

Vernet's (ver-naz') **syndrome** paralysis of palate, pharynx and larynx due to damage to XIth, Xth and XIth cranial nerves in jugular foramen, inside the skull, named after Maurice Vernet, French neurologist

verruca (ver-roo'ka) wart; or wart-like lesion, an epidermal tumour caused by a papillomavirus. The virus grows only over the skin commonly seen in children. Often it is asymptomatic with an irregular verrucous surface and grow at a very slow rate **v filiform** finger-like projection of wart on the neck or face **v plantaris** skin coloured flat-topped papules on the dorsal aspects of the hands and the face **v vulgaris** skin coloured or brownish papules with irregular surface on the dorsal aspects of the hands, the forearm and the face

verrucose (ver'roo-kos) wart-like excrescences or elevations

Verrey's needle needle with guarded point for introduction of gas into peritoneum before laparoscopy

versicolor (ver'si-kol'or) variegated; changeable in colour

version (ver'zhun) an abnormal direction of the axis; turning; manipulation of a foetus in the uterus to change its position, to facilitate delivery; the procedure by which an unfavourable presentation of foetus *in utero* is changed **bipolar v** turning of the foetus with the aid of fingers introduced into the cervix during the first stage of labour **cephalic v** the version in which head is made to present **external v** the foetus can be turned by abdominal manipulation if there is sufficient amount of amniotic fluid, if the uterus is not contracting, if the presenting part is not engaged and if the abdominal muscles are relaxed **internal v** a very old obstetric procedure and consists of introduction of the hand into the uterine cavity, grasping a foot and with the help of abdominal manipulation, turning the foetus so as to bring down the

half breech **podalic v** the version in which the breech is made to present

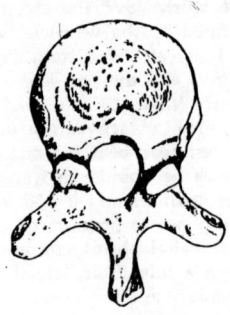

Vertebra

vertebra (ver'te-bra) any of the 33 bones that form the vertebral column pl. **vertebrae**. There are 7 cervical, 12 thoracic, 5 lumbar, 5 sacral and 4 coccygeal vertebrae. In adults the sacral vertebrae are fused to form a single bone, the sacrum and 4 rudimentary coccygeal vertebrae fuse to form the coccyx. A vertebra consists of a ventral body and a dorsal or neural arch. The bodies of successive vertebrae articulate with one another and are separated by intervertebral discs. The discs consist of fibrocartilage enclosing a central mass, *nucleus pulposus*. The movements such as flexion, extension, lateral flexion and rotation are possible

vertebral (ver'te-bral) pertaining to a vertebra **v artery** one of the pair of arteries passing up the neck to supply blood to the brain. **v canal** spinal canal **v column** spinal column **v foramen** the hollow space enclosed by a vertebral arch **v groove** the groove lying on either side of the spinous processes of the vertebrae **v percussion** the spinous processes of vertebrae are percussed from above downwards with the percussing finger or a small percussion hammer. Tenderness over a par-

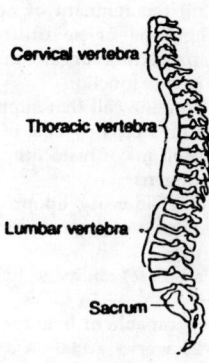

Vertebral column

ticular vertebra is indicative of disease and it is of particular value in the dorsal region **v scalloping** an exaggerated concavity of either the anterior or posterior cortex of a vertebral body, resembling the edge of a scallop shell

vertebrate (ver'te-bra't) animal having a vertebral column or backbone

vertebrobasilar insufficiency the branches of vertebrobasilar artery supply the entire brain stem, cerebellum and the vestibular apparatus. An impairment in blood supply results in episodes of vertigo, dizziness, diplopia, dysarthria, dysphasia, incoordination of gait and bilateral signs of sensory-motor deficit

vertex (ver'teks) a summit or top; the highest point; the crown of the head **v presentation** head-down position of a foetus at the time of delivery

vertical (ver'ti-kal) perpendicular to the plane or horizontal; upright **v transmission** appearance in successive generations characteristic of dominant inheritance; maternal transmission of infection to the foetus, through placenta as in TORCH (toxoplasmosis, rubella, cytomegalovirus, herpes) infections, syphilis and HIV

vertigo (ver'ti-go) dizziness; or a condition in which a person, or his surroundings seem to be turning round

verumontanum (ver'u-mon'ta'num) mountain ridge

very high density lipoprotein VHDL, a plasma protein with density greater than 1210 kg/l. It consists of 57% protein (predominantly apolipoprotein AI and AII), 21% phospholipid, 17% cholesterol and 5% triglycerides. It transports cholesterol from the intestine to the liver.

very low density lipoprotein VLDL, a plasma lipoprotein that has a density of 0.95 to 1.0 kg/l. It consists 6-10% protein (apolipoprotein B-100 and apolipoprotein C), 15-20% phospholipid, 20-30% cholesterol and 45-65% triglycerides. It is essentially endogeneous triglyceride of hepatic origin

vesica (ve-si'ka) a bladder

vesical (ves'i-kal) of or pertaining to a bladder

vesicant (ves'i-kant) causing a blister or blisters

vesication (ves'i-ka-shun) formation of blister or vesicle in the skin

vesicle (ves'i-kl) a circumscribed elevation of skin, less than 0.5 cm in diameter and containing clear fluid

vesicocoele (ves'i-ko-sel) a hernial protrusion of the bladder

vesicosigmoidostomy (ves'i-ko-sig'moy-dos'to-me) the operation to establish a permanent communication between the urinary bladder and sigmoid colon

vesicostomy (ves'i-kos'to-me) the formation of an opening into the bladder

vesicotomy (ves'i-kot'o-me) incision of the urinary bladder

vesicoureteral (ves'i-ko-u-re'ter-al) pertaining to the urinary bladder and the ureter

vesicoureteric reflux backward flow during the process of micturition, of urine from urinary bladder to ureter which results in recurrent ascending urinary infection

vesicourethral (ves'i-ko-u-reth'ral) pertaining to the urinary bladder and the urethra.

vesicovaginal (ves'i-ko-vaj'i-nal) communication between the urinary bladder and vagina

vesicula (ve-sik'u-la) a vesicle; a small bladder

vesicular (ve-sik'u-lar) of or pertaining to a vesicle or vesicles **v emphysema** alveolar emphysema **v mole** hydatidiform mole

vesiculitis (ve-sik'u-li'tis) inflammation of the seminal vesicle. Seminal vesicle may be enlarged and fibrous as a result of chronic inflammation, usually of gonococcal origin

vesiculography (ve-sik'u-log'ra-fe) radiography of seminal vesicles

vessel (ves'el) a tube or duct, as an artery or vein or the like for carrying blood or other body fluid to another

vestibular (ves-tib'u-ler) pertaining to noncochlear part of the inner ear **v ganglion** eighth cranial nerve ganglion **v neuronitis** lesion of vestibular division of eighth cranial nerve resulting in attacks of vertigo and nystagmus without any loss of hearing **v nucleus** a large nucleus in the floor of fourth ventricle receiving vestibular sensations **v nystagmus** inner ear lesions causing nystagmus of short duration

vestibular (ves-tib'u-lar) **glands** two small glands situated on either side of the opening of the vagina that secrete a clear lubricating mucus during sexual stimulation

vestibulocochlear (ves-tib'u-lo-kok-lear) eighth cranial nerve or acoustic nerve

vestibule (ves'ti-bul) a space or cavity at the entrance to another space or cavity

vestibulo-ocular reflex a reflex in which a movement of the eyes is produced that is equal and opposite to the movement of the head. Vestibular disease may be associated with loss of the reflex

vestibulum (ves-ti-b'u-lum) vestibule

vestige (ves'tij) the remnant of a structure having little or no utility, but which in preceding organisms performed a useful function

veto cell an immune cell that suppresses the activity of T cells capable of reacting against self major histocomptibility complex antigens

VHDL very high density lipoprotein

VF vocal fremitus; ventricular fibrillation

via by way of

viability (vi'a-bil'i-te) ability to live after birth

viable (vi'a-bl) capable of living **v foetus** foetus of 22 weeks gestation and 500 gm weight

vial (vi'al) a small bottle

Vi-antigen the capsular antigen of *Salmonella typhi* which is specifically associated with its virulence

vibration (vi-bra'shun) a rapid to and fro movement **v sense** appreciation of vibrations when a foot of a vibrating tuning fork is kept on bone prominences of the body. It is lost in lesions of the posterior column and earliest sensation to be lost in diabetes mellitus and old age.

vibrio (vib'reo) short, actively motile gram-negative rods of the genus Vibrio which cause acute gastroenteritis *V. cholera* bacteria responsible for cholera. It is classified into *Inaba, Ogawa* and *Hikojima* based on lipopolysaccharide antigen. *El tor* biotype is responsible for majority of outbreaks in India *V. parahaemolyticus* cause of food poisoning

vibriocardiogram (vib'reo-kar'de-o-gram) VCG; the graphic record by vibriocardiography

vibriocardiography (vib'reo-kar'de-o-grafe) the graphic recording of mechanical vibrations produced by the heart

vibrissa (vi-bris'a) one of the stiff, brisk hairs growing about the mouth of certain animals

vicarious (vi-ka're-us) pertaining to the performance of one organ of part of the functions normally performed by another **v menstruation** non-genital bleeding at the time of menstruation **v movements** movements by other muscles after paralysis of those normally involved

vice versa in reverse order

vicia broad bean

viction a person who suffers from an injurious action

Victor Horsley's sign in advanced cases of middle meningeal haemorrhage the temperature taken in the axilla on either side in fracture of posterior cranial fossa, the temperature is higher on the paralysed side, named after Sir Victor Horsley, British surgeon

video-game epilepsy a light-sensitive epilepsy

videognosis (vid'e-og-no'sis) diagnosis using the data and radiographic images transmitted by the use of television

viderabine (vi-dar'a-ben) an antiviral agent effective against herpes simplex and herpes zoster-varicella virus

Vidian (vid'e-an) **nerve** vasomotor supply to nasal mucosa, named after Grido Vidius, French neurologist

vidradhi (s) abscess

view box a box with a uniform light source used to view a radiograph

vigabatrin (vi-ga-ba-tren) an anticonvulsant agent useful in partial secondary generalised tonic-clonic seizures and infantile spasms

vigilance the conscious and semiconscious focusing and sustained attention to subtle sensory signals within a determined modality such as auditory or visual, while eliminating or distracting internal and external stimuli

village health guide a person with an aptitude for social service and is not a full time government functionary

vihar entertainment and activities

vikalpa (s) doubt

vikriti (s) transformation

viksipta (s) restless state of mind

villaret (ve-lar-az) **syndrome** metastases, meningioma, carotid dissection and carotid body tumour at the posterior retropharyngeal space near carotid artery may result in lower cranial nerve (9, 10, 11and 12) paralysis with Horner's syndrome

villus one of the millions of small hairlike vascular protrusions on certain mucous membranes such as small intestine which absorb digested nutrients pl. **villi**.

vinblastine (vin-blas'ten) a chemotherapeutic alkaloid that interferes with the microtubules of the mitotic spindle causing the lysis of rapidly dividing cells. Used in the treatment of Hodgkin's disease, leukaemia and other lymphoproliferative disorders.

vinca (vin'ka) **alkaloids** anti-tumour alkaloids from *Vinca rosea*. They act on mitotic spindles

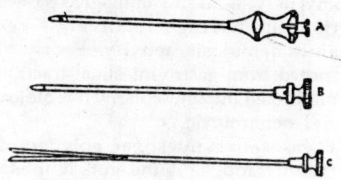

A. Cannula; B. Trocar; C. Split needle

Vim Silverman needle

Vim Silverman needle cutting type liver-biopsy needle. It consists of three parts—an outer cannula, trocar and split needle. The cannula with trocar in position is introduced through the skin and intercostal muscles. The patient is asked to hold his breath at the end-expiratory phase. The trocar is advanced quickly forwards to about three-fourths of its length. Then the trocar is removed and the split needle is introduced through the cannula while the patient has held his breath. The blades of the needle is longer than the cannula, the outer cannula is advanced by 2.5 cm so as to bring to the level of the split needle. Then the needle with the cannula is withdrawn quickly and the patient is asked to breathe normally. The liver tissue of 0.5-2.0 cm length will be seen adhering to the prongs of the needle.

Vincent's angina (vin'sents an-ji'na) necrotising ulcerative gingivitis usually associated with poor oral hygiene, named after French physician, Henri Vincent

vincristine (vin-kris'ten) a chemotherapeutic alkaloid that interrupts the mitotic spindles causing lysis of proliferating cells. Used to treat leukaemia and other malignancies

Vincent's organism *Borrelia vincenti*

vindesine a plant alkaloid that inhibits cell division by binding to tubulin and disrupting the mitotic spindle

violaceous (vi'e-la-shus) of a violet colour

viomycin (vi-o-mi'sin) aminoglycoside antibiotic having relatively weak antituberculosis activity. Poorly absorbed from gastro-intestinal tract; administered intramuscularly. It is ototoxic and nephrotoxic

VIP vasoactive intestinal polypeptide, found throughout the gut. It inhibits gastric secretion but increases pancreatic and intestinal secretions, increases cardiac output, glycogenolysis and bronchodilation

vipaka (s) systemic changes

viparita – bhavana (s) contrary thought

viparyasa (s) distorted conception

viparyaya (s) illusion, misconception.

viper (vi'fer) a venomous snake of the family Viperidae

VIPoma an endocrine tumour in the gut or pancreas producing vasoactive intestinal polypeptide

V/Q ventilation/perfusion

V/Q scan a radioisotope evaluation of the ratio of pulmonary ventilation (v) to pulmonary perfusion (q) useful in detection of pulmonary embolism

viral of or pertaining to or caused by a virus **v gastroenteritis** gastroenteritis in infants usually from rotavirus **v hepatitis** parenchymal liver disease caused by specific hepatitis viruses (A-E) and rarely by cytomagalovirus, Epstein-Barr virus, herpes simplex virus and yellow fever virus **v load** measurement of the amount of virus in a sample undetectable v load a level of viral load that is too low to be detected **v meningitis** aseptic meningitis commonly mild without any sequelae

viraemia (vi'rem'e-a) the presence of viruses in the blood

Virchow's (veer-sho-vz) **triad** endothelial injury, alterations in normal blood flow and hypercoagulability leading to haemostasis, named after German pathologist

Virchow's law (ver-koz) every cell is derived from another cell, enunciated by Rudolf Virchow, German pathologist

Virchow's sign enlargement of left supraclavicular lymph nodes in gastric carcinoma

Virchow's triad causes of venous thrombosis are damage to the wall, slowing of blood flow and hypercoagulability

virechana (s) purgation; purgative

virgin (ver'jin) **lymphocyte** prior to any kind of antigen stimulation

virile (vir'il) masculine

virilism (vir'il-izm) masculinity; a female disorder in which there is development of secondary male sexual characteristics

virilization (vir'i-li-za'shun) the development of male secondary sex characters in female due to overproduction of androgens. The features include hirsutism, temporal balding, deepened voice, acne, enlarged clitoris.

virion (vi're-on) an elementary viral protein particle

virocyte (vi'ro-site) atypical enlarged lymphocytes with foamy cytoplasm and coarse nuclear chromatin that react to viral infections; Turk cells

viroid a small circular segment of single stranded RNA that causes disease in higher plants

virologist (vi-rol'o-jist) a specialist in virology

virology (vi-rol'o-je) a branch of microbiology concerned with viruses and viral diseases

virtual reality a computer-based simulated environment in which users interact with a high-performance computer, graphics, specialized software, and devices providing visual, tactile and auditory feedback, thereby simulating a true-life environment

virucide (vir-u-sid) agent destroying a virus

virulence (vir'u-lens) the relative ability of a micro-organism to cause disease by overcoming body defences; being extremely poisonous

virulent (vir'u-lent) pertaining to virulence

virus (vi'rus) 1. any of a group of ultramicroscopic infectious agents that reproduce only in living cells. They contain either RNA or DNA, but not both. The virus genome is enclosed in a protein shell and in some cases by a lipid envelope. They are intracellular diverting host cell's metabolites to its own reproduction. Glycoproteins on the virus surface recognise specific cellular receptors which determines the cells the virus infects and hence the type of disease produced. 2. a programme designed to damage a computer system

virya (s) potency, semen *v pradana* potency oriented

visarpa (s) erysipelas

visarpi (s) erysipelas

vis-à-vis face to face; opposite

viscera (vis'er-a) organs in the cavities of the body

visceral (vis'er-al) of or pertaining to the viscera **v larva migrans** migration of

Table 14 Vitamins: Action

Name	Alternative name	Action	Daily requirement	Effects of deficiency	Effects from excess intake
Fat soluble					
Vitamin A	retinol	night vision	1 mg	night blindness,	raised intracranial pressure, liver damage, skin changes
		epithelial function antioxidant		xerophthalmia perifollicular hyperkeratosis	
Vitamin D	Vitamin D$_2$ Vitamin D$_3$	calcium metabolism	3 mcg	ricketts, osteomalacia	hypercalcaemia
Vitamin E	tocopherols	red cell function antioxidant	10 mg	mild haemolytic neuropathy in children	
Vitamin K		synthesis of clotting factors (II VII, IX, X)	100 mcg	bleeding	

Water soluble

Thiamine	Vitamin B_1	carbohydrate metabolism	1 mg	beri-beri peripheral neuropathy Wernicke-Korsakoff syndrome	
Riboflavin	Vitamin B_2	cellular oxidation	1.5 mg	angular stomatitis, cheilosis	
Niacin	nicotinic acid nicotinamide	cellular oxidation	15-20 mg	pellegra	flushing
Vitamin B_6	Pyridoxine	transamination decarboxylation	3 mg	peripheral neuropathy	
Folate	folic acid	haemopoiesis	200 mcg	megaloblastic anaemia	
Vitamin B_{12}	cobalamin	haemopoiesis	3 mcg	megaloblastic anaemia subacute combined degeneration of the spinal cord	
Vitamin C	ascorbic acid	collagen synthesis antioxidant	30-60 mg	scurvy, impaired healing, bleeding into tissues and joints	raised urinary oxalate and urate

Table 15: Vitamins: Sources

A	animal foods - liver, fish, egg yolk, milk, ghee, cheese, butter and as carotene in dark green leafy vegetables, carrot, pumpkin, papaya, mangoes, Red palm oil	Thiamine	cereals, sprouting green leafy vegetables, liver, pork, legumes
		Riboflavin	liver, meat, eggs, kidney, milk and other dairy products, green leafy vegetables, sprouted cereals and pulses
D	exposure to ultraviolet irradiation of sun light, milk, butter, cheese, egg yolk, fish liver oils	Niacin	liver, pulses, whole cereals, fish, meat, milk, eggs, groundnut, coffee
E	all vegetable oils, wheat-germ, egg yolk, butter, peas	Pyridoxine	yeast, liver, meat, whole grain cereals, groundnuts, banana, legumes
K	green leafy vegetables, liver, pulses, also synthesised by colonic bacteria	Folic acid	yeast, liver, nuts, green vegetables, chocolate
		Vitamin B_{12}	meat, liver, egg, dairy products, yeast
		Vitamin C	fresh fruits, green leafy vegetables, germinating pulses

helminthic larva in the viscera of the body **v leishmaniasis** *see* kala azar

viscero – of organs of body especially larger organs within serous cavities of the trunk

visceromegaly (vis'er-o-meg'a-le) organomegaly

visceroptosis (vis'er-op-to'sis) descent of an organ from its normal position

viscid (vis'id) sticky

viscosity (vis'kos'i-te) resistance of fluid to deforming forces

viscus (vis'kus) internal organ

visha (s) poison *v guna* poisonous properties

vision (vizh'un) sight; power of sensing with the eyes

visual (vizh'u-al) pertaining to vision **v acuity** sharpness of vision **v aphasia** word blindness **v agnosia** inability to recognise objects or persons **v hallucination** false perception involving sight consisting of both formed images (people) and unformed images (flashes of light) **v pigment** combination of retinal pigment with opsin

vital (vi'tal) of or necessary to life **v capacity** maximum volume of air that can be exhaled or inhaled following a maximum expiratory or inspiratory effort respectively **v sign** indications of life such as pulse, heart beat, chest movements, constriction of pupil when exposed to light **v statistics** statistics concerned to human life or the conditions affecting human life and maintenance of population.

vitalometer instrument to measure vital capacity

vitamins (vi'ta-minz) a group of organic substances present in foods essential in small quantities for normal functioning of the body (*see* tables 13 and 14) **lipid soluble v** vitamin A, B, D, E and K. **water soluble v** vitamin B complex and vitamin C.

vitarka (s) examination

viveka (s) discrimination

vitellin (vi-tel'in) a phosphoprotein found in the yolk of eggs.

vitellointestinal (vi'tel-o-in-tes'tin-al) **duct** communication between the midgut and yolk sac

vitiligo (vit-il-i'go) depigmented macule of variable size and shape in the skin or any part of the body including the mucous membranes of the lips and genitalia. There is no other change in the skin and it is due to lack of melanin formation by the melanocytes

vitium (vish'e-um) defect

vitrectomy (vi-trek'to-me) removal of vitreous

vitrellum small glass capsule releasing volatile drug when broken

vitreous (vit're-us) glass-like; hyaline; transparent gel **v haemorrhage** bleeding into the vitreous humour, usually encountered in diabetic retinopathy **v humour** the transparent, gelatinous substance filling the posterior chamber of the eye

vivax malaria tertian malaria, caused by *Plasmodium vivax*

vivi- combining word for alive

viviparous (viv-ip'ar-us) bearing living young

vivisection (viv'i-sek'shun) the performance of surgical procedures upon living animals for the experimental purpose

VLDL very low-density lipoprotein. It transports triglycerides to tissues to be used as energy or stored as fat. High level in the blood is associated with ischaemic heart disease

VMA vanillyl mandelic acid

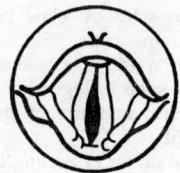

Vocal cord

vocal (vo'kal) pertaining to the voice or the organs of speech **v cords** either of the two pairs of folds of mucous membranes projecting into the cavity of the larynx that vibrate as air is breathed out and are responsible for voice production **v ligament** ligament stretched between thyroid cartilage in front and arytenoids behind

vocal cord dysfunction syndrome VCDS Throat tightness and loss of voice from incomplete adduction of the vocal cord. The attacks are rapid to develop and also to dissolve

Vogt-Koyanagi syndrome uveitis, retinal detachment, vitiligo, alopacia and deafness, described by Vogt-Koyanagi, German ophthalmologist

vola (vo'la) a concave surface; palm of the hand or sole of the foot

volar (vo'lar) pertaining to flexor surface

volitional (vo-lish'un-al) voluntary **v collapse** loss of the 'will to live' ·

Volkmann's (volk'manz) **ischaemia** impairment of arterial blood supply from an injury of the extremity by direct pressure from a tight plaster cast or oedema. Early signs are pain, pallor, puffiness (oedema), pulselessness and paralysis, named after Richard von Volkmann, Professor of surgery, Halle

Volkmann's ischaemic contracture ischaemic contracture is liable to follow an injury of the extremity when the arterial blood supply to the part is impaired. It is a late stage characterised by flexion of fingers in case of the forearm. The fingers can be partially extended by flexing the wrist implying that the contracture is in the flexor group of muscles. A 'claw hand' occurs in extreme cases

volubility (vol'u-bil'i-te) copious, coherent, logical speech; logorrhoea

volume (vol'um) measure of the quantity; amount

voluntary (vol'un-ter'e) accomplished at one's own accord **v health agency** an organisation that is administered by autonomous agency which collects funds for its support and spends money to conduct programmes directed to furthering the public health by providing health services or health education.

volvulus (vol'vu-lus) twisting or knotting **v of intestine** twisting of a loop of intestine that causes intestinal obstruction

vomer (vo'mer) the unpaired flat bone of the nasal septum

vomeronasal organ an olfactory structure that is anatomically and physiologically distinct from the main nasal system. It has a duct like opening within the nose. And the duct terminates in an ovoid-shaped cul-de-sac lined with pseudostratified columnar epithelium

vomit (vom'it) to eject contents of the stomach through the mouth

vomiting (vom'it-ing) expulsion of the contents of the stomach through the mouth.

vomitoxin (vom'it-ok-sin) a mycotoxin, deoxynivalenol, a contaminant of wheat and corn

von Gierke's (ger'kez) **disease** a glycogen storage disorder due to glucose–6 phosphatase deficiency characterised by retarded growth, accumulation of glycogen in the liver and kidney. It requires frequent carbohydrate feeds and liver transplant, named after Edgar von Gierke, German pathologist

von Hippel Lindau (hip'el-lin'dow) **disease** haemangioblastoma of the cerebellum associated with angioma of the retina and cysts of the pancreas and kidneys. There may be polycythaemia, named after Eugen von Hippel, German ophthalmologist and Arvid Lindau, Swedish pathologist

von Recklinghausen's (rek'ling-how'zenz) **disease** 1. generalised neurofibromatosis, a hereditary disorder characterised by multiple nodules all over the body and it may be associated with 'café au lait' spots 2. primary hyperparathyroidism exhibiting osteitis fibrosa cystica, named after Friedrich von Recklinghausen, German pathologist

Voorhees' (voor'ez) **bag** an inflatable rubber bag for dilating the cervix to induce and facilitate labour, named after James Voorhees, American obstetrician

voracious greedy in eating, immoderate, insatiable

von Willebrand's disease a congenital bleeding disorder due to the deficiency of factor VIII presenting with bleeding tendency at an early age usually as epistaxis and easy bruising. There is prolonged bleeding time, named after Erik von Willebrand, Finnish physician

von Graefe's (von gra'fez) **sign** failure of the upper eyelid to move downward with the eye ball in exophthalmic goitre, named after Albrecht von Graefe, German ophthalmologist

vortex (vor'teks) a whorled arrangement. pl. **vortices**

vorticose (vor'tik-os) one of the four veins that receive blood from all parts of the choroid of the eyes

vox (voks) voice

voyeurism (voy'yer-izm) sexual gratification derived from looking at sexual objects or acts

VR vocal resonance

vrana (s) ulcer

vriddhi (s) enlargement

vrshana (s) testes

VSD ventricular septal defect

vulnerable (vul'ner-a-bl) susceptible

vulsella (vul-sel'a) a forceps with claw-like hooks at the end of each blade

vulva (vul'va) external visible part of female genitalia consisting of the clitoris and the labia, vestibule of the vagina and the opening of the urethra and of the vagina; pudendum

vulvar relating to vulva

vulvitis (vul-vi'tis) inflammation of the vulva, caused by infection, allergic reaction and ageing

vulvovaginitis (vul'vo-vaji-ni'tis) inflammation of the vulva and vagina by an infection

v wave the wave in the normal jugular venous pulsations corresponding to the atrial diastole

V-Y advance a surgical incision in plastic surgery that allows lengthening of a contracted scar, where a 'Y' shape is sewn into a V-shaped incision

vyadhiksamtva (s) natural resistance and immunity of the body

vyadi (s) disease *vyadhikshamatva* increase in immunity

vyana (s) moving alround

vyavasaya (s) objective knowledge

vyayama (s) physical exercise

W

W 1. chemical symbol for the element tungsten 2. a unit of hardness of x-rays

w watt, a unit of electric energy

Waardenburg (vah'r-den-boorg) **syndrome** a genetic disorder characterised by wide-bridge of nose, frontal white blaze of hair, growing together of the two eyebrows, white eyelashes, lateral displacement of the inner canthi, cutaneous hypopigmentation and deafness, described by Petrus Waardenburg, Dutch ophthalmologist

Wada test test to determine cerebral dominance by injecting barbiturate into the carotid artery in left handed individual, before undergoing surgery near language area, devised by Juhn Wada, Japanese-born Canadian neurosurgeon

waddling to walk with short steps, swaying from side to side and hip elevation like a duck noted in osteomalacia, pseudohypertrophic muscular dystrophy, bilateral dislocation of hip and advanced pregnancy

wafer (wa'fer) a thin sheet of flour paste to enclose a medicine in powder form; a flat vaginal suppository

Wagner-Jauregg (vahg'ner-yow'reg) **treatment** treatment of dementia paralytica by infecting the patient with malaria, described by Julius Wagner von Jauregg, Austrian neuropsychiatrist

Wagner-Meissner (vahg'ner mis'ner) **corpuscle** a small, special pressure sensitive sensory end-organ attached to a single nerve fibre, named after Rudolph Wagner, German physiologist and Georg Meissner, German anatomist

Wagstaffe's (wag'stafs) **fracture** fracture with separation of the internal malleolus of the ankle, named after William Wagstaffe, a British surgeon

waist (wast) the part of the body between the thorax and the hips

waist-to-hip girth ratio measurement of waist and hip circumference with a measuring tape helps in estimation of body fat distribution. There is an increased risk of ischaemic heart disease, stroke and death when the waist/hip ratio is more than 1.0 in male or more than 0.8 in female

wakefulness the ability to be aroused, mediated by ascending reticular activating system

Walcher's (Vol'kerz) **position** assumption of dorsal recumbent posture with hips at the edge of the bed and legs hanging down, described by Gustav Walcher, a German gynaecologist

Waldenstrom's (val'den-stremz) **disease** osteochondritis deformans juvenilis, described by Johann Waldenstrom, a Swedish orthopaedic surgeon

Waldenstrom's macroglobulinaemia a malignant disease of B-cells that appear to be a hybrid of lymphocytes and plasma cells which secrete characteristically an IgM paraprotein, and may present with hyperviscosity syndrome and is treated with plasmapheresis

Waldeyer's (vahl'di-erz) **gland** sweat glands of the eyelids especially prominent in lower eyelid margin, described by Wilhelm Waldeyer, a German anatomist

Waldeyer's ring lymphoid tissue formed by the lingual, pharyngeal and faucial tonsils arranged in the form of a ring at the level of the nasopharynx and oropharynx

walk (wok) to move on foot with alternate steps; the particular way a person moves

walker (wok'er) a mobile device that assists a person in walking. It consists of a stable platform made of light weight metal tubing that can be grasped by the hands and used as a support while taking a step

walking (wok'ing) act of moving on foot **heel w** walking on heels as in peripheral neuropathy **sleep w** somnambulism **w cast** a cast that allows the patient to be ambulatory. **w pneumonia** Mycoplasma pneumonia

wall (wawl) the limiting structure of a space such as a cell, vessel or cavity; boundaries of a cavity

Wallenberg's (vol'en-bergz) **syndrome** occlusion of the posterior inferior cerebellar artery or one of its branches supplying the lower portion of the brain stem resulting in ipsilateral loss of temperature and pain sensations of face and contralateral loss of these sensations in the extremities and trunk, ipsilateral ataxia, dysphagia, dysarthria and nystagmus, named after Adolf Wallenberg, a German physician

Wallerian (wol-e're-an) **degeneration** the degeneration of a nerve fibre that has been severed from its cell body, in which there is axonal and myelin sheath disintegration and digestion by Schwann cells distal to the interruption while proximal to transection the nerve degenerates to the nearest node of Ranvier, described by Augustus Waller, English physician

wall eye (wahl'i) 1. the eye jumps when uncovered; 2. crossed eyes 3. strabismus 4. absence of colour in the iris. 5. dense opacity of cornea

Walter Reed staging a system for clinical staging of AIDS

Walthard's islets microscopic inclusions of the germinal epithelium of the ovary found in or near its serosal covering, described by Max Walthard, Swiss gynaecologist

Walther's (vahl'terz) **ducts** minor ducts draining the sublingual gland, named after August Walther, German anatomist

wambles (wahm'b'lz) milk sickness

wan looking ill, sad, tired, anxious

wandering (wan'der-ing) moving about; not fixed **w abscess** abscess appearing on a site distant from its origin **w kidney** floating kidney **w mind** day dream **w spleen** floating spleen **w pacemaker** dual rhythm wherein both SA and AV nodes discharge spontaneously with variable asynchronicity

Wangensteen (wan'gen-sten) **tube** a double-lumen tube passed through the nose into the stomach and connected to a special suction apparatus to maintain decompression of the stomach and duodenum in post-operative conditions, introduced by Owen Wangensteen, American surgeon

Warburg (war'boorg) **apparatus** a capillary manometer for determination of oxygen consumption and carbon dioxide production in small bits of tissue, introduced by Otto Warburg, German biochemist

ward (word) a large hall in a hospital to accommodate for the care of several patients

Wardrop's (war'dropz) **operation** ligation of an artery for aneurysm at a distance beyond the sac, named after James Wardrop, British surgeon

warfarin (war'fah-rin) **poisoning** a toxic condition due to ingestion of warfarin accidentally in the form of a rodenticide or by overdose of anticoagulation.

warfarin sodium coumarin anticoagulant, named after Wisconsin Alumni Research Foundation

war gas any chemical agents used to produce poisonous or irritant effects. Organophosphates which bring about irreversible inhibition of acetylcholinesterase are the important examples

warm antibody haemolysis an autoimmune haemolytic anaemia (AIHA) with presence of warm anti-red cell antibody. These antibodies react with red cells at 37°C and destroy red cells by means of opsonization. The condition may be idiopathic or secondary to chronic lymphatic leukaemia, lymphoma, SLE or certain drugs

warm blooded having a relatively high and constant body temperature encountered in humans, other mammals and birds

warm shock septic shock febrile patient with hypotension, who in early stages may be warm

warm-up physical and mental preparation for exercise

wart (wort) a circumscribed cutaneous elevation due to hypertrophy of the papillae and hyperplasia of all layers of the epidermis **common w** firm papules with a rough horny surface **filiform w** fragile small filiform projections commonly seen in males on the face and neck **genital w** a wart of the genitalia caused by human papilloma virus (HPV) **plane w** smooth, round, polygonal, flat or slightly raised lesion noted on the face and dorsum of the hands **plantar w** small shiny rounded flat painful lesion beneath pressure points **seborrhoeic w** benign epidermal tumour showing raised and stuck-on appearance, unrelated to sebaceous glands **venereal w** vegetating growth upon skin especially on the mucocutaneous junctions of the genitals **viral w** wart due to infection from human papilloma virus **water w** molluscum contagiosa , shiny white, hemispherical lesions with an umbilacated look

Wartenberg's (wor'ten-bergz) **sign** when the flexed fingers locked with examiner's flexed fingers are pulled away, the thumb of the patient normally extends. In pyramidal lesion, the thumb adducts and flexes, described by Robert Wartenberg, American neurologist

Warthin Frinkeldey cells reticuloendothelial giant cells in hyperplastic lymphoid tissue in measles Aldred Worthin, US Pathologist and Wilhelm Frinkeldey, German Pathologist

Warthin's tumour adenolymphoma of parotid gland that contains both epithelial and lymphoid tissues which produces a slowly growing painless swelling in the lower part of parotid gland

wash (wosh) act of cleaning a part or all of the body; a solution used for cleansing or bathing a part, such as an eye or mouth

washed red cells red blood cells that have been washed in sterile saline prior to transfusion, which removes most leucocytes, useful in IgA-deficient patients

washerwoman's fingers cold white slightly wrinkled skin noted after prolonged immersion in cold water and in dehydration

washerwoman's itch eczema of the hands of laundry workers exposed to soaps and detergents

wasp (wosp) hymenopterous insect **w sting** injection of wasp venom into the skin resulting in a painful wound

Wasserhelle (vos'er-hel'le) *Ger* waterclear referred to parathyroid chief cells

Wassermann (wos'er-man) **reaction** a complement fixation test to diagnose syphilis, named after August Wasserman, a German bacteriologist

waste (wast) decay, useless material; wasting; emaciation **w products** products of metabolism or wear and tear of tissues that are removed from the body by elimination

wasted ventilation the volume of air that ventilates the physiologic dead space in the respiratory system

wasting (wast'ing) emaciating; to shrink in physical bulk or strength

water (wah'ter) a colourless, odourless clear liquid formed by a combination of hydrogen and oxygen, H_2O. It forms the principal constituent of all body fluids, secretions and urine **potable w** water suitable for drinking **w balance** maintenance of balance between intake of water and losses through urine, insensible perspiration, expired air and faeces **w bath** a water filled vessel to hold racks of test tubes whose temperature is controlled by a thermostat at 37°C **w bed** a rubber mattress partially filled with warm water **w bottle cardia** a globose cardiac shadow due to pericardial effusion **w brash** reflex salivary hypersecretion in response to peptic oesophagitis, heart burn **water cure** hydrotherapy **w care** water treatment of a condition **w depletion** loss of water from the body resulting in hypertonic extracellular fluid volume and rise in plasma sodium **w excess** an excess of total body water occurs when water intake exceeds renal and cutaneous losses. It is unlikely in presence of normal renal function. It occurs in renal impairment, cirrhosis of the liver, heart failure, nephrotic syndrome, and inappropriate ADH secretion **w for injection** distilled and sterilised water for parenteral use **w intoxication** overhydration of the cells leading to inflation of cell volume and impaired cerebral function. There is profound hyponatraemia **w on brain** abnormal increase in cerebrospinal fluid, hydrocephalus **w reactive** a substance that produces hazardous vapours or that release energy when it comes into contact with water or humid air **w retention** retention of sodium being accompanied by retention of an approximately iso-osmotic amount of water **w syringe** a syringe to deliver water spray to a localised area in dentistry **w trap** under water seal

water-bite (wah'ter-bit') trench foot.

water-borne (wah'ter-born) spread by contaminated drinking water

water carriage system sewerage system concerned with collection and transportation of human excreta and waste water from residential, commercial and industrial areas by a network of underground pipes to the place of ultimate disposal

water-cell a glycogen rich parathyroid chief cell, that is clear and large

water deprivation test after estimation of serum sodium concentration and osmolality, water is not allowed for 8

hours from 8 a.m. Timed hourly urine collections, serum osmolality measurements and body weight are recorded. The test is discontinued if there is loss of 3% of body weight. At the end of 8 hours the urine osmolality should exceed 800 osmol/kg. It occurs in normal persons and patients with primary polydipsia. If the urine concentration does not occur 1 microgram desmopressin is given intravenously and further samples are taken. In ADH-deficient diabetes insipidus there is prompt urine concentration. The osmolality remains low in nephrogenic diabetes insipidus

water hammer a hermetically sealed tube containing a vacuum partly filled with water. When the tube is inverted quickly the water drops abruptly and imparts a palpable shock to that end of the container **w pulse** combination of an abrupt percussion wave, ill-sustained crest and rapid collapse of the pulse seen in peripheral vasodilation and hyperkinetic circulatory states

Waterhouse-Friderichsen (wah'ter-hous frid'er-iksen) **syndrome** fatal vasomotor collapse and shock in meningococcal infection due to haemorrhage into the adrenal gland, named after Rupert Waterhouse, an English physician and Carl Friderichsen, a Danish physician

Water-lily sign rupture of hydatid cyst giving a radiological shadow of an air and water-filled cavity with a floating membrane

Water-pot perineum trauma to the urethra, in which multiple fistulas associated with inflammatory strictures and diverticuli develop, forming draining sinuses

waters (wah'terz) amniotic fluid surrounding the foetus

Waters' view occipitomental view for x-ray of paranasal sinuses, named after Charles Waters, US radiologist

watershed (wat'ter-shed) **lesions** lesions between areas of distribution of arteries as in ischaemic lesions of brain

water soluble capable of being dissolved in water

Watkins' (wot'kinz) operation an operation for prolapse and procedentia of uterus wherein the bladder is separated from the uterus, named after Thomas Watkins', an American gynaecologist

Watson-Crick (wat'son-krik) helix a double helix with each chain containing chemical compounds arranged in a specific sequence. It is the structure of DNA carrying genetic information, discovered by James Watson, American biochemist and Francis Crick, British biochemist.

Watson-Jones pin three-flanged pin for femoral neck fractures, named after Watson-Jones, English orthopaedic surgeon

watt (wot) a unit of electric power, being the work done at the rate of 1 joule per second, named after James Watt, a Scottish engineer

wave (wav) 1. a double oscillation shown by the moving parts 2. vibrating motion 3. oscillation noted in graphic records of physiologic activities

wavelength (wav'length) the distance between the top of one wave and the identical phase of the succeeding one

wax (waks) esters of various fatty acids deposited in the form of a plastic substance by insects or obtained from plants or petroleum; a mixture of secretions of the ceruminous and sebaceous glands present in cartilaginous part of the ear canal and it may form a tight ring, in the ear causing deafness, tinnitus, ear ache and ear wax

waxy (waks'e) resembling wax **w cast** a dense highly refractile urinary cast seen in chronic renal diseases **w exudates** hard yellow-white macular aggregates of fatty and proteinaceous material that leaks into the retina, seen in diabetes mellitus

W B C white blood cell; white blood count

weak (wek) loss of physical strength or vigour

weakness subjective feeling of lack of strength

weal mark on the skin made by a blow of stick or whip

wean (wen) to discontinue the breast feeding of an infant with substitution of other foods; the slow discontinuation of ventilatory support

weaning (wen'ing) 1. infant changed from breast to other feeding 2. the process of gradually withdrawing mechanical support

weanling a child which has recently been weaned

weasand (we'zand) *Ger* the trachea

weaver's bottom ileogluteal bursitis with pain and tenderness over ischial tuberosities aggravated by sitting and lying; tailor's bottom

web 1. a membrane or a tissue extending across a space 2. world wide web, www. The graphical, multimedia portion of the Internet. It comprises millions of web pages. 3. a membrane or a tissue extending across a space oesophageal w web in upper oesophagus causing dysphagia for solids **w browsing** software. Software that is used to explore www. Internet explorer is the web browsing software included with Windows 98. **w site** a group of related Web pages. **w style** a desktop display options

webbed (webd) having a membrane or tissue connecting adjacent structures **w toes** an abnormality in which the toes are connected by webs of skin

Weber-Christian (web'er-kris'chan) disease relapsing febrile non-suppurative nodules in subcutaneous tissue with central depression, noted in a generalised disorder of fat metabolism, named after Frederick Weber, English physician and Henry Christian, American physician

Weber's (web'erz) disease localised epidermolysis bullosa, described by Frederick Weber, English physician

Weber's (va'berz) **glands** mucous glands on the lateral borders of the tongue, described by Moritz Weber, a German anatomist

Weber's syndrome ipsilateral oculomotor paralysis and contralateral paralysis of the face, arm and leg due to a damage to pyramidal tract in the brain stem, named after Hermann Weber, an English physician

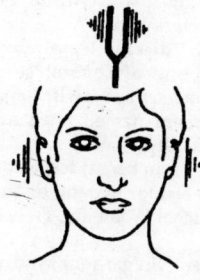

Weber's text

Weber's test test performed by placing the stem of vibrating tuning fork on the head in the midline and asking the patient whether the tune is heard in both the ears or better in one ear than in the other. In unilateral conduction deafness, the tune is appreciated in the affected ear and in unilateral nerve deafness the tune is appreciated in unaffected ear, named after Friedrich Weber, a German otologist

Weber-Christian (ve'bur-kris'chi-an) **disease** a skin disorder characterised by recurring inflammation in the fat layer of the skin, with features of relapsing fibroid nodular nonsuppurative panniculitis, named after Frederik Weber, English Physician and Henry Christian, US Physician

Webster's (web'sterz) **operation** an operation to fix the retrodisplaced uterus by passing round ligaments through the perforated broad ligaments, named after John Webster, an American gynaecologist

Wechsler (wek'sler) **adult intelligence scale** American psychologist Alfred Wechsler defined intelligence as the aggregate or global capacity of the individual to act purposefully, to think rationally and to deal effectively with his environment and it forms the basis in widely used intelligence scale in adults

wedge (wej) **fracture** a vertebral fracture with anterior compression

wedge pressure pulmonary artery wedge pressure measured by introducing cardiac catheter into a branch of pulmonary artery which is approximately equal to left atrial pressure

wedge resection the surgical excision of a part of an organ

WEE western equine encephalitis

Weech's formula formula to predict adult height at maturity from that of a children aged 2-12 years

Weeks' (weks) **bacillus** *Haemophilus aegyptius*, named after John Weeks, American ophthalmologist

weeping shedding tears **w eczema** dermatitis with vesicles exuding serous fluid **w sinew** a circumscribed cystic swelling of a tendon sheath

Wegener's (veg'nerz) **granulomatosis** a triad of necrotising angiitis and aseptic necrosis of the upper respiratory tract and paranasal sinuses, granulomatous pulmonary vasculitis, and a non-specific segmental necrotising glomerulonephritis, named after Friedrich Wegener, a German pathologist. The level of antineutrophil cytoplasmic autoantibodies reflects the activity of the disease and is treated with immunosuppressive agents

weight (wa't) 1. the gravitational force exerted on an object, usually by the earth 2. heaviness *see* table of weights 15, 16 **apothecaries' w** a system of weightsused in compounding prescriptions based on the grain (equivalent 64.8 mg) **atomic w** the sum of the masses of the constituents of an atom, expressed in atomic mass units or SI units **avoirdupois w** the system of weight commonly used for ordinary communities and its units consist of dram, ounce and pound **equivalent w** weight of a chemical element that is equivalent to and will replace a hydrogen atom in a chemical reaction **metric w** a system of weights founded on the French metre-dividing or multiplying by ten **molecular w** the sum of all the atomic weights of all the elements in one molecule of a compound **w gain** an increase in weight due to an imbalance between energy intake and energy expenditure **w traction** traction applied to a limb or part of a limb by means of a suspended weight

Table 16. Measures of weight (metric system)

The gram or gramme, the unit of weight, is the weight of a cubic centimetre of distilled water at 4°C

Scale	Table	Grams
Pico	1 Picogram	10^{-12}
Nano	1 Nanogram	10^{-9}
Micro	1 Microgram	10^{-6}
Milli	1 Milligram	0.001
Centi	1 Centigram	0.01
Deci	1 Decigram	0.1
Unit	1 Gram	1.0
Deca	1 Decagram	10.0
Hecto	1 Hectogram	100.0
Kilo	1 Kilogram	1000.0

Table 17 Metric and British Weights

Metric	British
1 Decigram	1.543 grain
1 Gram	15.432 grains
1 Decagram	0.353 ounce
1 Hectogram	3.527 ounces
1 Kilogram	2.2046 pounds
1 ton (1000 kilo)	2204.6 pounds

weightlessness the condition of not being acted on by the force of gravity as seen in astronauts flying in areas where the force of gravity is totally absent

Weigert's (vi'gerts) **stain** staining for gram-positive bacteria and fibrin devised by Karl Weigert, German pathologist

Weil-Felix (vil-fa'liks) **reaction** serological test to diagnose rickettsial disease, named after Edmund Weil, Austrian bacteriologist and Arthur Felix, German bacteriologist

Weil's (vilz) **disease** leptospirosis caused by any one of several serotypes of *Leptospira interrogans* with hepatocellular involvement named after Adolf Weil, German physician

Weinberg's (vin'bergz) **test** a complement fixation test for hydatid disease, named after Michel Weinberg, French pathologist

Weingarten (vin'gar-ten) **syndrome** tropical pulmonary eosinophilia with chronic cough, nocturnal bronchospasm and miliary pulmonary infiltrates, described by German physician R.J. Weingarten at Madanapalle, India

Weir's (werz) **operation** appendicostomy, named after Robert Weir, American surgeon

Weismannism (wis'man-izm) theory propounded by August Weismann, a German biologist, which states that acquired charateristics are not inherited

Weiss (vis') **test** test for presence of urochromogen in urine, named after Moriz Weiss, an Austrian physician

Welch's (welsh'ez) **bacillus** *Clostridium perfringens* the causative organism of gas gangrene, named after William Welch, American pathologist

well baby clinic a clinic that supervises and offers services for healthy infants

well differentiated resembling the original histologic characteristics

Wellen's (wel'lenz) **syndrome** occlusion of the left anterior descending coronary artery presenting with symmetrically inverted T waves without any change in ST segment or R wave

wellness a state of fitness

welt wheal

wen 1. sebaceous cyst of the scalp 2. epidermal cyst.

Wenckebach's (ven'ke-baks) **phenomenon** second degree AV block with dropped beats wherein conduction through the bundle of His fails altogether from time to time so that ventricular beats are dropped, which is characterised in ECG by shortened PR interval after drop of the beat, but subsequently lengthens progressively from cycle to cycle until conduction again fails. It is named after Karel Wenckebach, a Dutch physician. It is detected by noting a changing a-c intervals in the neck and variation in the intensity of first heart sound

Werdnig-Hoffmann (verd'nig-hof'man) **paralysis** a hereditary, progressive infantile muscular atrophy due to degeneration of anterior horn cells of the spinal cord, named after Guido Werdnig, an Austrian neurologist and Ernst Hoffman, a German neurologist

Werlhof's (verl'hofs) **disease** idiopathic thrombocytopaenic purpura, named after Paul Werlhof, German physician

Wermer's (ver'merz) **syndrome** multiple endocrine neoplasia, first described by Paul Wermer, American physician

Werner's (ver'nerz) **progeria** familial premature senility, hypogonadism, cataracts and atropic changes in skin, named after Werner, German gynaecologist

Wernicke's (ver'ni-kez) **aphasia** inability to comprehend the spoken or written word due to injury to Wernicke's area

Wernicke's area area in the superior temporal lobe and adjoining parietal lobe of dominant cerebral hemisphere of the brain. It recalls, recognises and interprets words and sounds in understanding language, described by Karl Wernicke, German neurologist

Wernicke-Korsakoff (ver'ni-ke-kor-sak'of) **syndrome** ophthalmoplegia (horizontal nystagmus and paresis of lateral gaze), ataxia and disturbed mentation, confabulation commonly accompanies deficits in memory and cognitive function. Alcohol related deficiency syndrome dramatically resolves following administration of thiamine, named after Karl Wernicke German neurologist and Sergéi Korsakoff, Russian neurologist

Wernicke's (ver'ni-kez) **disease** haemorrhagic polioencephalitis

Wernicke's encephalopathy cerebral form of thiamine deficiency often presenting acutely, usually in an alcoholic where the patient is confused and shows ophthalmoplegia

Wertheim's (ver'timz) **operation** radical hysterectomy for cancer of the cervix, named after Ernst Wertheim, Austrian gynaecologist

Wertheim-Schauta (ver'tim-show'tah) **operation** an operation for cystocoele wherein the uterus is interposed between bladder and vagina, named after Ernst Wertheim and Friedrich Schauta, Austrian physicians

Westergren's (west'er-grenz) **method** method to determine erythrocyte sedimentation rate, named after Alf Westergren, Swedish physician. About 0.02 ml of 3.8% sodium citrate is taken in a syringe and 1 ml of blood is drawn into it from a vein. It is introduced into a bottle and shaken. Then it is sucked into the graduated pipette 2.5 mm in diameter upto zero mark. It has markings from 0 to 200 mm. The tube is allowed to stay vertically in the stand. After one hour it is read and the distance to which the blood has settled is noted in mm. It is referred to as sedimentation rate. The normal value is 3-7 mm in first hour. It is high in infections, carcinoma, lymphoma, collagen diseases, rheumatic fever, pregnancy and anaemia. It is low in polycythaemia, haemoglobinopathies and congestive heart failure

Westermark's sign vascular oligaemia distal to the thromboembolism, seen in chest roentgenogram, named after Neil Westermark, German radiologist

Western blot test a precise immunoblot test to confirm the presence of antibodies to HIV, It also detects presence of anti HIV antibodies

Western blotting a technique to analyse protein antigens by transferring from gel to nitrocellulose

West Nile fever Arbovirus infection characterised by fever, rash and encephalitis seen in Egypt and Northern Uganda

Westphal's (ves'fahlz) **sign** loss of knee jerk in tabes dorsalis, named after Karl Westphal, a German neurologist

Westphal Strumpell (vest'fal-strim'p'l) **disease** hepatolenticular degeneration, named after Karl Westphal and Ernst Strumpell, German physicians

West's (ves'tez) **syndrome** infantile spasms

wet soaked with water **w beri beri** high output circulatory state with cardiac failure noted in thiamine deficiency **w brain** increase in amount of cerebrospinal fluid **w cough** productive cough **w dream** nocturnal seminal emission **w dressing** a moist dressing applied to relieve symptoms of certain skin disorders **w lung** non-cardiogenic pulmonary oedema **wet-nurse** a woman who breast feeds the child of another **w pack** application of cold pack to reduce fever **w pleurisy** pleurisy in which the inflammation has progressed to an effusion

Wetzel's (wet'selz) **grid** a graph used in evaluation of growth and development of children aged 5 and 15 years, devised by Norman Wetzel, US paediatrician

Wetzel's (wet'selz) **test** examination of blood for carbon monoxide, named after George Wetzel, German anatomist

Wharton's (hwar'tonz) **duct** duct of the submandibular salivary gland opening into the mouth by the side of the *frenum linguae*, named after Thomas Wharton, British anatomist

Wharton's jelly substance of the umbilical cord consisting of a special form of embryonic connective tissue consisting of small stellate cells with long processes, which anastomose with each other, the meshes of which are filled with a gelatinous material

wheal (hwel) urticarial lesion presenting on the skin as a smooth, slightly elevated area which is redder or paler than the surrounding skin accompanied by itching **w and flare reaction** a test for immediate hypersensitivity to an antigen, presenting with erythema and swelling

wheat (hwet) edible cereal grain, wheat preparations include *Chapati, upma, vermicelli* and *noodles*

wheel a disc attached through its middle to a rotating axle **wheelchair** a special chair having two large and two small wheels for transportation of patients

wheeze (hwez) 1. a continuous high pitched whistling sound heard in patients with generalised airways obstruction 2. rhonchi

whey (hwa) watery fluid remaining after separation of the curd and cream from milk

whiff slight puff or breath

whiplash (hwip'lash) **injury** an injury to the spine at the junction of the fourth and fifth cervical vertebrae occurring from a rapid acceleration or deceleration of the body where upper four cervical vertebrae act as the lash and lower three act as the handle of the whip. Such injuries are common in rear-end auto collisions, and sometimes in football players

Whipple's (hwip'elz) **disease** intestinal lipodystrophy, named after George Whipple, American pathologist. It presents with malabsorption, weight loss, enlarged lymph nodes, fever, pigmentation, anaemia and joint pains

Whipple's operation radical pancreato-duodenectomy, named after Allen Whipple, American surgeon.

Whipple's triad insulin secreting pancreatic islet cell tumour presenting with spontaneous hypoglycaemia, central nervous or vasomotor symptoms and improvement of symptoms following administration of glucose

whip worm a round worm *Trichuris trichiura* often parasitic in human intestines. The adult worms are found in the large intestine with their anterior ends deeply embedded in the mucosa and measure 30 to 50 mm in length. Female worm produces 5000 eggs each day. The eggs appear like grenades

whirl (hwurl) to revolve rapidly; to feel giddy **w bone** 1. the patella 2. the head of the femur

whisky (hwis'ke) a distilled alcoholic liquor made from grain and it consists of ethyl alcohol

whisper (hwis'per) speech without using vocal cords. The gentle hiss of exhaled breath is shaped as in normal speech, by the teeth, tongue, lips and palate. The vocal cords are held rigid without vibration

whispering pectoriloquy increased transmission of whispered sounds clearly to the chest wall, heard in consolidation of the lung

whistle (hwis'el) a sound produced by pursing lips and blowing

white (hwit) achromatic colour of maximum lightness that reflects all rays of the spectrum **white blood cells** leucocytes; white cells **w coat hypertension** border-line or variable elevation of blood pressure in apprehensive patients when faced with the white coat of the physician **w gangrene** gangrene by local loss of blood supply **w hairy tongue** enlarged papillae on the dorsal surface of the tongue. It requires frequent brushing **w head** milium; tiny, hard painless blemish occurring in clusters on the cheeks, nose and around

the eyes **w leg** *Phlegmasia alba dolens* occurs during puerperium from deep vein thrombosis **w line** 1. white attachment of oblique and transverse muscle of abdomen also called as *linea alba.* 2. dense zones of provisional calcification seen in x-ray of long bones in scurvy **w matter** nervous system composed by white medullated nerve fibres **w nails** leuconychia; nails appearing white due to opacity of nail bed as in cirrhosis of the liver **w of egg** albumin of an egg. **w of eye** sclera **w pox** variola minor **w sponge** naevus; a hereditary condition showing diffuse white thickening of the oral mucosa. There may be involvement of other mucosal surfaces such as vagina and rectum **w transverse line** seen in nails in arsenical poisoning

White's (hwitz) **operation** removal of testes for prostatic hypertrophy, named after William White, American surgeon

Whitehead's (hwit'hedz) **operation** haemorrhoidectomy, named after Walter Whitehead, an English surgeon

Whitfield's (hwit'feldz) **ointment** ointment containing 3% salicylic acid and 6% benzoic acid in petroleum base, named after Arthur Whitfield, British dermatologist

Whitlow (hwit'lo) an inflammation of deeper tissues of a finger or toe especially of the terminal phalanx usually terminating in suppuration

Whitman's (hwit'mahnz) **operation** hip joint arthroplasty, named after Royal Whitman, American orthopaedic surgeon

Whitmore's (hwit'morz) **bacillus** *Pseudomonas pseudomallei* responsible for infective melioidosis, named after Alfred Whitmore, who was in Indian Army Medical Service.

Whitmore's disease melioidosis

WHO World Health Organisation with headquarters at Geneva.

whole (hol) **blood** blood that is unmodified except for the presence of an anticoagulant, and is used for transfusion

whole body counter an instrument that detects the radiation present in the entire body

whole bowel irrigation administration of electrolyte-balanced, inert solutions to flush mechanically the gut material. In poisoned patients large volumes of a mixture of polyethylene glycol and salts are administered to flush toxic substances out of the body before they can be absorbed

whoop (hoop) the sonorous and compulsive inspiration of whooping cough

whooping cough (hoop'ing kawf) infection from *Bordetella pertusis* characterised by catarrh of respiratory tract and paroxysms of cough ending with a whooping inspiration. The organism spreads by droplets from infected untreated patients. The incubation period varies from 7 to 14 days. Pertusis is noted in children below five years and it passes through three stages – catarrhal, paroxysmal and convalescent – each lasting upto 2 weeks. There can be complications such as otitis media, pneumonia, bronchiectasis, pneumothorax, seizures and encephalopathy. The condition is treated by erythromycin. It is prevented by active immunisation

whorl (hwerl) circular arrangement of like parts around a point on an axis as in skin ridges giving a spiral pattern of finger prints; a turn of the cochlea or of a nasal concha; spiral arrangement of cardiac muscle fibres

Whichmann's (vik'mahnz) **asthma** laryngeal stridor, named after Johann Whichmann, a German physician

Wickham's (vik'hamz) **striae** fine white network on the surface of the papules in lichen planus

Widal (ve'dahl) **test** test for diagnosis of typhoid fever, named after Georges Widal, French physician. It detects and measures the H and O agglutinins of typhoid and paratyphoid bacilli in the patient's serum. The antibody titres increase steadily after the first week till the fourth week and then decline

wide complex arrhythmia ECG blockage of sodium channels in cardiac cells results in widening of QRS complex. It may respond to intravenous administration of sodium bicarbonate bolus. Tricyclic antidepressant overdose is associated with sinus tachycardia with markedly prolonged QRS duration

widow's hump dorsal kyphosis with exaggerated cervical lordosis from vertebral compression due to osteoporosis

Wilder's (wil'derz) **sign** an early sign of Grave's disease demonstrating a slight twitch of the eyeball when it adducts or abducts, named after William Wilder, an American ophthalmologist

wild type the form of the gene normally present in nature **w virus** virus that has not been exposed to the drugs before

will mental faculty enabling one to decide on a course of action; process of exercising the power of choice

William's (wil'yamz) **sign** a dull tympanitic resonance over second intercostal space in massive pleural effusion, named after Charles William, English physician

Williamson's (wil'yam-sunz) **sign** markedly decreased blood pressure in the leg compared to the arm on the side of pleural effusion or pneumothorax, named after Oliver Williamson, English physician

William's syndrome supraclavicular aortic stenosis, peripheral pulmonic stenosis, associated with mental deficiency, 'elfin' facies, hoarse voice and loquacious personality

Williams-Campbell syndrome congenital bronchial cartilage deficiency with bronchiectasis, named after Howard Williams, and Peter Campbell, Australian Physicians

Willis' (wil'is) **circle** anastomosis of the internal carotid, the anterior and posterior cerebral arteries, the anterior and posterior communicating arteries in the base of the brain encircling the optic chiasma and hypophysis, named after Thomas Willis, English anatomist

Willis' nerve accessory nerve

Willis' phenomenon an accelerated reaction with rapid tuberculin conversion in individuals after revaccination of BCG

willow bark an astringent bark containing salicin, the glycoside of salicylic acid

Wilms (vilmz) **tumour** nephroblastoma, named after Marx Wilms, German surgeon occurs in children of 1-7 years of age, arises from the entrapped embryonic nephrogenic tissue and presents with enlargement of kidney. There can be pain, fever and hypertension. Kidney is of enormous size, and soft in consistency and the shape is lost

Wilson's (wil-sunz) **disease** hepatolenticular degeneration, named after Samuel Wilson, British neurologist. A genetic disorder in which copper accumulates in the liver, brain, cornea and kidneys. The plasma concentration of ceruloplasmin is low and it presents with cirrhosis of the liver, Kayser-Fleisher ring and movement disorders. D-penicillamine is used to chelate copper

Wimberger's (wim'bar'gerz) **sign** radiologic abnormality giving ring-like appearance of epiphysis due to a thin ring of bone around empty or poorly formed centre of epiphysis as in scurvy, described by Heinrich Wimberger, German radiologist

Wilson-Mikity (wil'sun-mik'ite) **syndrome** a pulmonary dysmaturity syndrome seen in premature infants, described by Mirlam Wilson, US paediatrician and Victor Mikity, US radiologist

windborne carried by the wind, as pollen

windburn exfoliation of skin from excessive exposure to wind

window (win'do) 1. a circumscribed opening in a plane surface; an aperture **aortic w** a lateral view of chest radiograph showing a clear area bounded by the aortic arch, the bifurcation of the trachea and the pericardial border **cochlear w** *fenestra cochleae* **oval w** *fenestra vestibuli* **round w** cochlear window **w period** an interval between the time of inoculation or exposure to a microorganism and the ability to demonstrate its presence by serologic assays 2 the rectangular portion of the screen that displays an open program or the contents of a folder or disk

windpipe (wind'pip) trachea

wind wane an instrument to observe the wind direction

wine (win) fermented beverage of any form usually made from grapes. It contains 10% to 15% alcohol **w glass** a fluid measure of 60 ml

wing either of the anterior appendages of birds which are modified for flight

winging of scapula raised medial border of scapula due to paralysis of serratus anterior muscle

Winiwarter's (vin'i-var'terz) **operation** cholecystoenterostomy, named after Alexander Winiwarter, German surgeon

wink quick closing and opening of the eyelids

Winslow's (winz'loz) **foramen** opening between greater and lesser peritoneal sacs above first part of duodenum, named after Jacob Winslow, French anatomist

Winterbottom's (win'ter-bot'ums) **sign** prominent lymph nodes in the posterior cervical triangle in trypanosomiasis, named after Thomas Winterbottom, British physician

Wintergreen (win'ter-gren) **oil** methyl salicylate, a flavouring substance and a counter-irritant

Wintrich's (vin'triks) **sign** change of pitch of the percussion note occurring over a cavity when the mouth is opened and closed, named after Anton

Wintrich, a German physician

Wintrobe's (win'tro-bz) **method** method to determine erythrocyte sedimentation rate. The haematocrit tube is filled to the 100 mm mark with oxalated blood and it is kept vertically for one hour before the reading is taken. The same tube can be used to estimate packed cell volume (PCV). The ESR varies from 0 to 9 mm in men and 0 to 2 mm in women, named after Maxwell Wintrove, American haematologist

wire (wir) a long slender, flexible metallic structure of variable thickness

wiring the fixing into position by wire in surgery and dentistry

Wirsung's (ver'soongz) **duct** pancreatic duct, named after Johann Wirsung, German physician

wisdom (wiz'dom) **tooth** last molar tooth on either side of jaw usually erupting between 18 and 25 years

Wiskott-Aldrich (wis'kot-awl'drich) **syndrome** a sex-linked recessive disorder with a defect in both T and B cell function, described by Alfred Wiskott, German paediatrician and Robert Aldrich, American paediatrician. It is characterised by eczema, thrombocytopaenia with bleeding tendency, and infections

witch doctor a man in some primitive societies who attempts to cure sickness and to exorcise evil spirits by the use of magic

witches' milk milk of newborns under the influence of hormones in the mother's blood, colostrum

withdrawal stopping of administration of a drug especially a narcotic or alcohol to which the individual has become addict either physiologically or pathologically **w behaviour** the physical or psychologic removal of oneself from a stressor **w bleeding** occurrence of vaginal bleeding following discontinuation of hormonal medication, noted at the end of each cycle of oral contraceptive pill **w method** a contraceptive technique where male withdraws his penis before occurrence of ejaculation **w syndrome** physical and psychological disturbances expressed by a narcotic addict when deprived of the required drug dosage

withdrawn behaviour a condition in which there is a blunting of the emotion and a lack of social responsiveness

Witkop disease diffuse white thickening of the oral mucosa with gelatinous plaques on the bulbar conjunctiva, a name derived from a South African term for favus

witness a person who was actually present at a particular event

Witzel's (vit'selz) **operation** gastro stomy, named after Friedrich Witzel, a German surgeon

wobble (wob'ble) move unsteadily from side-to-side **worm w** overdoses of piperazine or its accumulation in patients with renal failure causes neurological abnormalities such as visual disturbances, seizures, cerebellar ataxia and electroencephalographic abnormalities

Wolff-Chaikoff (vol'f-che'y-kaf) **phenomenon** an inhibitory effect on thyroid hormone secretion following administration of approximately 2 mg of iodide in normal men named after J. Wolff, US physiologist and Israel Chaikoff, British born US physiologist

Wolffian (wool'fean) **body** mesonephros, described by Kaspar Wolff, German anatomist

Wolffian duct mesonephric duct in the embryo extending from the mesonephros to the cloaca

Wolff-Parkinson-White syndrome WPW syndrome ventricular pre-excitation that is associated with AV bypass tracts which conduct in an antegrade direction and produce a typical ECG pattern of a short PR interval (<0.12 sec), a slurred upstroke of the delta wave and a wide QRS complex, named after Louis Wolff, American cardiologist, John Parkinson, British physician and

Paul White, American cardiologist

Wolff's (volfs) **law** development of structure by bone that is suited to resist the forces acting upon it, described by Juslins Wolff, German anatomist

Wolfram's (wool'framz) **syndrome** a rare autosomal condition with a deficiency of vasopressin exhibiting diabetes insipidus, diabetes mellitus, optic atrophy and deafness. DIDMOAD it is named after D.J. Wolfram, US physician

Wolman's disease an inherited metabolic disorder in which infants show hepatosplenomegaly, adrenal calcification and foam cells in the bone marrow, named after Moshe Wolman, an Israeli physician

woman an adult human female **w year 1** year in the reproductive life of a sexually active woman

womb (woom) uterus which protects and nourishes the foetus **w leasing** surrogate motherhood **w stone** calcified hydatidiform mole or fibroid

wonder drug a drug usually recently discovered and noted for its startling curative effect; miracle drug

wood alcohol methyl alcohol

Wood's light (woodz) long wavelength ultraviolet light used in the diagnosis of fungal infections of the scalp, named after Robert Wood, American physicist

Woolsorter's disease anthrax; fatal disseminated anthrax probably from inhalation of the spores of *Bacillus anthracis* presenting with cyanosis, dyspnoea, mediastinitis and haemoptysis

Woodman's disease extrinsic allergic alveolitis developing from inhalation of penicillium species from oak and maple trees

wood tick *Haemophysalis spinigera*, a soft wood tick, whose nymphal forms spread Kyasanur forest disease

Wood trimmer's disease extrinsic allergic alveolitis from rhizopus and mucor species inhaled from contaminated wood trimmings

Woodworker's lung extrinsic allergic alveolitis developing from inhalation of oak, cedar and mohogany wood dust

woody legs occurrence of haemorrhage into deep tissues of the thighs and legs causing tense induration in adults due to vitamin C deficiency

Wool-sorter's disease haemorrhagic bronchopneumonia due to inhalational anthrax

word blindness infarction in the distribution of posterior cerebral artery, tumour or haemorrhage resulting in an inability to comprehend written words; visual aphasia; alexia

word deafness lesion in superior temporal gyrus from infarction, tumour, or abscess resulting in impaired auditory comprehension, inability to repeat a sentence or write a dictation; auditory aphasia

word salad use of incoherent mixture of words and phrases as in schizophrenia

work a force moving a resistance; occupation

workman's compensation a type of insurance which provides medical care and wage compensation for workers or their dependents for economic losses caused by industrial diseases or injuries

work-up the process of obtaining all the relevant data to diagnose and treat a patient

World Health Organisation, WHO an international agency of United Nations with headquarters at Geneva with an objective of the attainment by all people of the world the highest level of health. It has defined health as a state of complete physical, mental and social wellbeing and not merely the absence of disease or infirmity

worm (wurm) an elongated, flat, round or segmented invertebrate; helminth

wormian (wur'me-an) **bones** small, irregular bones in the course of the cranial sutures, described by Olaus Worm, Danish anatomist

wort herb **St John's w** perinnial aromatic herb which flowers on June 24, St. Johns' day, used as an antidepressant

worthlessness (wurth'les-nes) a component of low self-esteem, characterised by feelings of uselessness

wound (wund) injury caused by physical means wherein there is disruption of the normal continuity of structures **bullet w** a puncture from a bullet **incised w** any sharp cut in which the tissues are not severed **lacerated w** a torn wound with ragged edges **nonpenetrating w** wound in which surface of the skin remains intact **open w** contusion in which skin is broken **penetrating w** wound in which the causative weapon or bullet entered the body and emerged **puncture w** wound by a sharp pointed instrument **w irrigation** the rinsing of a wound by a medicated solution, water or antibiotic liquid preparation **w repair** restoration of the normal structure following an injury

wreath (reth) an encircling structure resembling a circle of flowers

Wright's stain stain containing eosin and methylene blue used in the study of blood cells and malarial parasites, introduced by James Wright, US pathologist

wrinkle (ring'kl) ridge or furrow on the surface due to contracture, folding, especially of the kind produced by age

W-plasty plastic surgery to repair straight scars requiring the redistribution of tension

Wrisberg's (ris'burgz) **cartilages** the cuneiform cartilages of the larynx, named after Heinrich Wrisberg, German anatomist

Wrisberg's ganglion a ganglion of the superficial cardiac plexus between the aortic arch and the pulmonary artery

wrist (rist) region of the articulation between the forearm and hands; carpus **w drop** paralysis of the extensors of the hand and fingers from radial nerve lesions due to injury, compression or lead palsy; drop hand

writer's cramp spasmodic contraction of the muscles of the thumb and forefinger after prolonged writing, sometimes accompanied by pain

writhe to twist the body as in pain.

wry (ri) twisted

wry neck (ri'neck) torticollis; a contracted state of one or more muscles of the neck resulting in a characteristic attitude of the head. There is lateral inclination of the head towards the shoulder on the affected side.

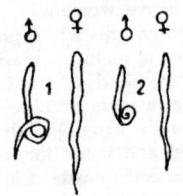

1. Wuchereria bancrofti
2. Wuchereria malayi

Wuchereria (voo'ker-e're-a) filarial nematodes, named after Otto Wocherer, German physician **W bancrofti** white threadlike nematode which causes lymphangitic filariasis **W malayi** Brugia malayi

wuchereriasis (voo-ker-e-ri'a-sis) *see* filariasis, elephantiasis

w/v weight per volume. It indicates the amount by weight of a solid substance dissolved in a measured quantity of liquid

X

X symbol for any unknown quantity

x symbol for abscissa (horizontal axis); *stat* mean

xanth (o) - yellow or yellowish

xanthelasma (zan-thah-laz'ma) subcutaneous cholesterol deposits at the inner margins of the eyelids, that are most common in normocholesterolaemic elderly or hypercholesterolaemic younger subjects

xanthemia (zan-the'mi-a) 1. presence of yellow colouring matter in the blood 2. carotenaemia

xanthic (zan'thik) yellow or yellowish in colour

xanthine (zan'thin) 1. sympathomimetic agent affecting cyclic 3' 5' AMP system of the bronchial smooth muscle and cause bronchodilatation 2. a purine base found in body tissues and fluids 3. oxidation product of guanine and hypoxanthine x oxidase an enzyme facilitating breakdown of purines

xanthinuria (zan'thin-ur'i-a) 1. excretion of large amounts of xanthine in the urine 2. a hereditary disorder of purine metabolism due to a deficiency of the enzyme, xanthine oxidase, causing excess elimination of xanthine in urine, and may be associated with xanthine stones in the urinary tract; xanthuria

xanthochromatic (zan'tho-kro-mati'k) yellow coloured

xanthochromia (zan'tho-kro'mi-a) an yellowish discolouration, as of the skin or cerebrospinal fluid

xanthochromic (zan'tho-kro'mik) having a yellow discolouration, as applied to cerebrospinal fluid

xanthocyanopsia (zan'tho-si-an-op'se-a) a form of colour blindness in which yellow and blue are distinguishable, but not red and green

xanthocyte (zan'tho-sit) a cell containing yellow pigment

xanthoderma (zan'tho-der'ma) yellow colouration of the skin

xanthodontous (zan-tho-dont-ous) yellowish teeth

xanthoerythrodermia (zan'tho-e-rith'roder'me-a) a yellowish red coloured skin

xanthogranuloma (zan'tho-granu-lo'ma) an infiltration of retroperitoneal tissue by lipid macrophages, exhibiting histologic features of both granuloma and xanthoma, occurring mostly in women

xanthoma (zan-tho'-ma) xanthomata, raised yellow papule, nodule or plaque-like lesions in the skin on tendons from deposition of lipid-laden histiocytes found in hypercholesterolaemia, hypertriglyceridaemia, lipoprotein lipase deficiency or b lipoproteinaemia. **eruptive x**, wax yellow lesions especially over extensors of the elbows and knees, and on the back and buttocks, in patients exhibiting severe hyperlipidaemia. **x disseminatum** presence of xanthoma throughout the body especially on the face, in the tendon sheaths and mucous membranes **x multiplex**, xanthomatosis. **x palpebrarum** small yellow-grey plaques around the eyes, **x planum** yellowish macules or plaques. **x tendinosum**, subcutaneous nodules on the dorsal aspect of fingers and the Achilles tendon **x tuberosum**, nodules over the elbows and knees

xanthomatosis (zan'tho-ma-to'sis) 1. an accumulation of an excess of lipids in the internal organs due to an altered metabolism of lipids with hypercholesterolaemia. 2. x-disseminatum or multiplex

xanthomatous (zan'tho-ma-tus) pertaining to xanthoma

xanthophyll (zan'tho-fil) a yellow pigment derived from carotene

xanthopsia (zan-thop'si-a) abnormal vision in which all objects appear yellow

xanthopsin (zan-thop'sin) the visual purple produced by light acting on rhodopsin

xanthopsis (zan-thop'sis) a yellowish discolouration of degenerating tissues especially in malignancy

xanthorrhoea (zan'tho-rea) yellowish discharge from the vagina

xanthosarcoma (zan'tho-sar-ko'ma) a giant cell tumour of tendon sheath

xanthosis (zan-tho'sis) yellowish colouration of the skin seen in carotenaemia

xanthous (zan-th'us) yellowish

xanthurenic (zanth'u-ren'ik) **acid** a minor catabolite of tryptophan which is found in increased amounts in urine in pyridoxine deficiency

xanthuria (zan-thu're-a) excretion of excess of xanthine in the urine; xanthinuria

X axis axis of abscissa, usually horizontal, along which the abscissa and ordinate are measured

X body cytoplasmic inclusions in macrophages in Langerhans' cell granulomatosis

X cells ganglion cells of the retina, chiefly central and are necessary for recognition of large objects

X chromatin nuclear material forming sex chromosomes during cell division

X chromosome a chromosome that determines female sex characteristics. In the normal female there are two X chromosomes, and in the male one X chromosome and one Y chromosome

X chromosome inactivation random inactivation of one of the two female X chromosomes during early embryonic development

X disease aflatoxicosis occurring after consumption of groundnuts contaminated by *Aspergillus flavus* that produce aflatoxin

Xe chemical symbol for xenon

xeno strange or relation to foreign material

xenobiotic (zen'o-bi-ot'ik) an active chemical substance foreign to a living system

xenodiagnosis (zen'o-dia'g-no'-sis) a biologic diagnosis of some diseases caused by insects, ticks or vectors by feeding uninfected vectors on patient and later examining them for infection.

xenogeneic (zen'o-jen-e'ik) 1. xenogenic 2. tissues from individuals of different species utilised in transplantation

xenogenesis (zen'o-jen-e-sis) 1. generation of offspring different from the parent 2. heterogenesis

xenogenic (zen-o-jenik) 1. xenogeneic 2. originating outside of the organism, or from a foreign substance introduced into the organism

xenogenous (zenoj'e-nus) caused by a foreign body

xenograft (zen'o-graft) 1. a graft of tissue transplanted between animals of different species, that are closely (concordant) or distantly (discordant) related 2 heterograft

xenology (zen-cl-o-je) the study of parasites and their hosts

xenomania (zen-o-mah-ne-a) an inordinate attachment to things foreign

xenomenia (zen-o-me-ne-a) vicarious menstruation.

xenon (ze'-non) a heavy, colourless, chemically inactive gaseous element, with symbol Xe, at. no. 54

Xenon 133 (^{133}xe) a radio-isotope with gamma emission utilised to determine the distribution of gas and perfusion of various areas in the lungs

xenoparasite (zen'o-par'a-sit) an organism that becomes a parasite only in debilitated individuals

xenophobia (zen'o-fo'bi-a) an irrational fear of strangers, and strange customs

xenophonia (zen'o-fo'ne-a) change in the quality of the voice

xenophthalmia (zen'of-thal'-mi-a) inflammation caused by the presence of a foreign body in the eye

Xenopsylla (zen'op-sil'a) a genus of fleas, common example being *Xenopsylla cheopis* the rat flea, which carries plague bacillus from rodents to man

xenorexia (zen'o-rek-se-a) perverted appetite leading to frequent swallowing of foreign bodies

xenotropic (zen'o-trop'ik) a virus found in cells of an animal species, undergoes replication only when it infects cells of a different animal species

xerantic (se-ran'tik) causing dryness

xerasia (ze-ra'se-a) disease of the hair characterised by abnormally dry and brittle hair

xero- (zir'o) a combining word for pertaining to dryness

xerochelia (zer-o-kile-ah) dry lips

xerocyte (zer-o-sit) an erythrocyte with a defect in the membrane which allows loss of potassium and water, causing dehydration of cells, which appear half dark and half light

xeroderma (zer'o-der'ma) dry, rough discoloured skin **x pigmentosum** an autosomal recessive disorder presenting with photodermatosis. There is defective repair of the damaged DNA induced by sunlight due to an enzymatic deficiency

xerogram (zir'o-gram) image produced by xerography

xerography (zerog'ra-fe) 1. a method of radiography to obtain image on paper 2. xeroradiography

xeroma (ze'ro'ma) 1. abnormally dry conjunctiva 2. xerophthalmia

xeromammogram (zer'o-ma-mo-gram) a breast radiograph image

xeromammography (zer'o-ma-mog'rah-fe) an alternative x-ray technique using photoconductor which produces a final image of soft tissue architecture of the breast on paper rather than film

xeromenia (ze'r-o-meni-a) a condition in which menstruation occurs without any blood flow

xeromycteria (ze'ro-mik-te're-a) dry nasal mucosa

xerophagia (ze'ro-faje-a) eating dry food

xerophobia (ze'ro-fa-bea) inhalation of saliva due to fear

xerophthalmia (zer'of-thal'me-a) 1. abnormal dryness of conjunctiva and cornea due to keratinisation from vitamin A deficiency and it may also occur in Sjogren's syndrome 2. xeroma.

xeroradiography (zer'o-ra'di-og rah-fi) 1. recording of x-ray images by a dry photoelectric process wherein the metal plates are coated with a semiconductor such as selenium, and a dry powder is used instead of liquid chemicals to develop 2. xerography

xerosialography (zer'o-si'ah-log'rah-fi) radiography of salivary ducts where images are recorded by xeroradiography

xerosis (ze-ro'sis) dryness of the conjunctiva, cornea, skin or mucous membranes **x conjunctivae** a dry, thickened and pigmented bulbar conjuctiva **x corneae** a dull, hazy lustreless cornea

xerostomia (zer'o-sto'me-a) 1. dryness of oropharyngeal mucosa due to decreased or arrested salivary secretion, and is characteristic of Sjogren's syndrome and it may also occur in HIV-1 and candida infection, malignancy and systemic sclerosis 2. xerostoma

xerotic (ze-rot'ik) dry; dryness **x keratitis** an inflammation of the cornea developing from dry conjunctiva

xerotocia (ze'ro-to-se-a) dry labour due to decreased amount of amniotic fluid

xerotomography (zer'o-to-mog'rah-fe) tomography wherein the images are recorded by xeroradiography

xerotripsis (ze'ro-trip-sis) dry friction

xiphisternal (zif-i-ster'nal) relating to the xiphisternum

xiphisternum (zif'i-ster'num) xiphoid process, lowest part of the three segments of the sternum. **xiphisternal**, adj

xiphocostal (zif'o-kos'tal) refers to the xiphoid process and ribs

xiphodynia (zif'o-din'e-a) pain in the xiphisternum

xiphoid (zif'oid) 1. sword-shaped 2. ensiform **x process** the lowest portion of the sternum; a sword-shaped cartilaginous process to which no ribs are attached

xiphoidalgia (zif'oi-d-al'gea) pain in the xiphoid process

xiphoiditis (zif'oi-di'tis) inflammation of the xiphoid process

xiphopagotomy (zi-fop'a-got'o-me) surgical separation of twins joined at the xiphoid process

xiphopagus (zi-fop'ah-gus) symmetrical conjoined twins fused at the xiphisternum

XLD agar xylose-lysine-deoxycholate agar, a highly selective bacterial growth medium used to isolate gastroenteric pathogens

X linkage sex linkage; disorders determined by mutant genes carried on the X chromosomes

X-linked (eks'linkt) sex-linked transmission by the genes on the X-chromosome and the individuals affected are males **x disorder** a disease caused by genes located on the X chromosome **x dominant** transmission of a dominant gene on X chromosome. All of the daughters of an affected male are affected but none of the sons. Hypophosphataemic vitamin D-resistant rickets is an example **x inheritance** a pattern of inheritance wherein the transmission of traits varies according to the sex of the individual. The genes on X chromosome have no counterparts on the Y chromosome. The pattern of inheritance may be dominant or recessive. The characteristic determined by a gene on the X-chromosome is always expressed in males **x recessive** condition caused by a gene carried on the X-chromosome. It affects males and is transmitted by healthy female carriers.

45 XO chromosome constitution symbol

to depict the presence of only one sex chromosome wherein the other X or Y chromosome is missing. Turner's syndrome

XO/XY mosaicism a normal chromosome complement with part of an X chromosome missing, as in some patients with a classic Turner's phenotype

X radiation exposure to x-rays or treatment with x-rays

X-ray (eks' rae) 1. roentgen ray named after discoverer, Wilhelm Rontgen, German physicist 2. electromagnetic radiation similar to light but of shorter wavelength and capable of penetrating solids 3. a radiogram made by x-rays **x-r film** a radiograph made by projecting x-rays through organs or structures of the body onto a photographic film **x-r fluoroscopy** real time imaging using an x-ray source that projects through the patient onto a fluorescent screen or image intensifier **x-r pelvimetry** a radiographic examination used to determine the dimensions of the bony pelvis of a pregnant woman

X wave x descent in jugular venous pressure wave due to atrial relaxation and downward displacement of the tricuspid valve in ventricular systole

XTE syndrome a rare autosomal dominant condition characterised by xeroderma, talipes and enamel defect

46 XX syndrome homologous sex chromosomes representing female

47 XXX syndrome triple X syndrome. Females with such chromosomal constitution may exhibit amenorrhoea and mental retardation without any bodily abnormalities

48 XXXX syndrome rare disorder of sex chromosomes characterised by menstrual irregularity, infertility and mental retardation

49 XXXXX syndrome rare disorder of sex chromosomes characterised by infertility, mental and growth retardation

47 XXY syndrome Klinefelter's syndrome

48 XXXY syndrome sex chromosome abnormality characterised by multiple X chromosomes accompanied by one Y chromosome, with mental and growth retardation and testicular atrophy

49 XXXXY syndrome sex chromosome abnormality characterised by multiple X chromosomes accompanied by one Y chromosome, with mental and growth retardation, small undescended testes, muscle hypotonicity, and hypoplastic external genitalia

xylene (zi' len) dimethylbenzene 1. useful as a solvent in microscopy 2. aromatic hydrocarbon, which is depressant of central nervous system

xylo- a combining word for, pertaining to wood

xylocaine a trade name for a local anaesthetic, lidocaine

xylose (zi'los) an aldopentose, wood sugar, used to test intestinal absorptive capacity

xylosuria (zilo-su're-a) presence of xylose in the urine

xylotherapy (zi'lo-ther'ah-pe) treatment by application of certain woods to the body

xylulose (zilu-los) a pentose sugar

xyrospasm (zi'ro-spazm) an occupational spasm involving the fingers and arms, seen in barbers

xysma (ziz'ma) membranous shreds in the faecal material

xyster (zis'ter) a surgeon's file to scrape the bones

47 XYY syndrome presence of an extra Y-chromosome in male, largely asymptomatic. Often tall. There may be behavioural problems in later life

Y

Y symbol for yttrium, pyrimidine, tyrosine

YAG yttrium aluminium garnet laser

yakrt (s) liver

yakshma (s) consumption *raja y* pulmonary tuberculosis

yam a starchy tuberous root used as a food.

yamika (s) very short duration.

yana (s) vehicle

yang Chinese philosophy characterising the positive, bright and masculine principles in nature that influence the destiny

Yankauer's speculum a speculum used to examine the nasopharynx

yapya (s) diseases which are incurable, but may be relieved from discomfort and distress

yaw an individual lesion of yaws **mother yaw** the initial skin lesion of yaws occurring at site of inoculation

yawn opening the mouth involuntarily with a prolonged, deep inspiration of air often accompanied by stretching of the body and is considered a sign of fatigue

yawning (yawn'ing) taking deep inspiration with mouth wide open

yaws (yawz) a chronic nonvenereal infectious disease caused by *Treponema pertenue* which spreads by direct contact usually in children, and is characterised by an initial granulomatous lesion usually in the lower limb which gets crusted leaving behind a scar. It is followed by a secondary stage with multiple granulomatous papules and later periostitis. It is treated with penicillin **crab y**, yaws characterised by hyperkeratosis with fissuring and ulceration of the soles

Y-axis axis of ordinance, a vertical axis along which ordinate is measured or from which the abscissa is measured

Yb chemical symbol of a rare metal

Y body a rounded mass corresponding to the Y chromosome found in fluorescently ‹ stained metaphase and interphase nuclei of genotype male cells - buccal mucosa, fibroblasts, spermatozoa and amniotic cells

Y cartilage most elastic cartilage consisting of elastic fibres in a flexible fibrous matrix. It is yellow and found in the external ear, auditory tube, epiglottis and the larynx

Y cell ganglion cell of retina found in its periphery

Y chromosome a sex chromosome carrying genes which produce male characteristics in man

yeast (yest) 1. single celled rounded fungus of the family Saccharomycetaceae, that multiplies by budding and it can transform to a mycelial stage or remain single celled 2. frothy yellow fungus capable of fermenting carbohydrates **brewer's y** yeast obtained during the brewing of beer **y chromosomes** yeast chromsomes used in recombinant DNA procedures, and they carry large segments of foreign DNA in the sequencing of nucleic aids

yellow (yel'o) a primary colour resembling a ripe lemon

yellow artificial chromosome YAC, a cloning vector allowing cloning of large segments of DNA

yellow atrophy shrinkage of liver often seen in last months of pregnancy, having grave prognosis

yellow beeswax the purified wax from the honey comb of the honeybee

yellow blood a unit of packed red blood cells giving a milky-yellow white discolouration. It implies bacterial contamination and it should not be used

yellow body the corpus luteum

yellow fever an acute, often fatal viral infection seen in Africa and South America between latitudes of 15° north and 15° south of the equator, transmitted by mosquito, *Aedes aegypti* and characterised by high fever, vomiting, jaundice and bleeding. **Yellow fever vaccine** a vaccine produced from live, attenuated yellow fever virus grown in chick embryo and used for immunisation against yellow fever

Y descent negative wave in jugular venous pulsation corresponding to right ventricular filling with atrial emptying and it follows second heart sound

Y fork a Y-shaped region in a replicating DNA molecule

yellow marrow material in the central hollow of the shaft of bones

yellow nail syndrome a clinical complex characterised by thickened yellow nail plate in association with chronic lymphoedema of hands, feet, ankles, and face. It may be associated with pleural effusions, chronic pulmonary infections and bronchiectasis

yellow ointment an ointment containing yellow wax and petrolatum

yellow spot Y.S. 1. a small circular yellow area on the retina opposite the pupil which is the point of clearest vision 2. yellow nodule on anterior end of vocal cords

yellow vision xanthopsia, a condition in which objects appear yellow in colour

Yentl (yen'tl) **syndrome** a phenomenon wherein a woman receives equal medical treatment when she exhibits herself to be equal to a man in terms of risk factors for coronary artery disease, named after Yentl, heroine of Bashevis story, who had disguised herself as a man

Yersinia (yer-sin'i-a) a genus of nonmotile, nonencapsulated ovoid or rod-shaped, bi-polar staining gram-negative bacteria belonging to the family Enterobacteriaceae, named after Alexandre Yersin, French bacteriologist *Y.*

enterocolitica an enteric pathogen that spreads through raw pork and causes febrile enterocolitis or yersiniosis *Y. pestis* plague bacteria, causing plague in humans and rodents, transmitted to humans by rat flea, *Xenopsylla cheopis. Y. pseudotuberculosis* a bacterial illness causing acute mesenteric lymphadenitis

Yersiniosis (yer-sini-o'sis) an infection caused by *Yersinia enterocolitica* and is characterised by fever, diarrhoea and abdominal pain

Yersin's serum antiplague serum, named after Swiss bacteriologist, Alexandre Yersin

Y fracture a y-shaped intercondylar fracture

yin Chinese philosophy characterising the negative, dark and feminine principles in nature that influence the destiny

Y ligament a y-shaped band-like structure covering the upper and anterior part of the hip joint

Y-linked (wi'linkt) referring to genes carried on the Y chromosome or to the characteristics or conditions they transmit

yoga Hindu philosophy advocating union of physical and mental disciplines to attain union of the self with the supreme *hatha y* one of the six traditional forms of yoga that unites two opposites

yogurt (yog'hurt) a curdled milk produced by fermentation with *Lactobacillus bulgaricus*

yohimbine (yo-him'ben) an alkaloid from the bark of the tree *Corynanthe yohimbi* known to possess aphrodisiac properties

yoke (yok) jugum, 1. a connecting structure 2. a depression or ridge connecting two structures

Yokohama asthma a smog induced asthmatic condition, described in Yokohama, Tokyo's port city

yolk (yok) 1. yellow of the egg 2. stored nutrient in the ovum entering into the formation of the embryo **Y sac** membranous sac surrounding yolk in the embryo **y stalk** the umbilical duct connecting yolk sac with the embryo **y sac carcinoma,** a non-seminomatous germ cell lesion

yoni (s) vagina *y-vronekshanom* instrument used in vaginal examination

Yonyavekshnana yantra (s) instrument used in vaginal examination

Young-Helmboltz theory (Yung-helm'bolts) theory of vision suggesting that coloured light stimulates the three types of cones corresponding to the colours red, green and violet in various proportions. It was proposed by British physician, Thomas Young and German physician, Helmholtz

Yoon's rings rings to occlude fallopian tubes in laparoscopic sterilisation

Yorkes-Bridges test a modified and improved form of the Binet test for intelligence

Young's (Yungz) **operation** partial prostatectomy, described by Baltimore urologist, Hugh Young

Young's rule rule enunciated by English physician, Thomas Young, to calculate the dose of a drug prescribed to a child. It is obtained by multiplying the adult dose by the age in years and dividing the result by the sum of the child's age plus 12

Young's syndrome a disorder of men characterised by dilated bronchioles associated with less number of sperms due to obstruction to their flow in the epididymis from inspissated secretions. The condition manifests with recurrent sinopulmonary infections and azoospermia. The ciliary functions are normal

youth (yooth) period between childhood and mature adult

Yo-yo effect a disturbed peristalsis in an obstructed megaureter where a bolus of contrast material that has reached the bottom of the dilated segment cyclically regurgitates it into the upper ureter while a small amount passes into the bladder

Yo-yo liver a carnitine deficiency state exhibiting an abrupt increase and decrease in the size of the liver from an intermittent storage of a metabolic product

Yo-yo syndrome the repeated weight loss, followed by weight gain, experienced by many dieters

Y-plasty (wi'plaste) use of a y-shaped incision to reduce scar contractures

Y-protein a hepatic protein that binds unconjugated bilirubin in the hepatic cytosol; ligandin

ypsiliform (ip-sili-form) y-shaped

Y-set a plastic device used to administer intravenous fluids through a primary intravenous line connected to a combination drip chamber from which two separate plastic tubes lead to fluid sources and the set includes three clamps

ytterbium (i-tur-be-um) a metal, symbol Yb, at. no. 70

yttrium (it-re-um) a metallic element, symbol Y, at. no. 39

yttrium 90 a radioactive trivalent metallic element used in the treatment of pituitary tumours.

yugma-sanku (s) instrument with twin hooks

Yuppie flu debilitating stress-related viral condition

Z

Z symbol for atomic number

z zero; zone

zafirlukast a short-acting oral leukotriene antagonist useful in the management of mild to moderate asthma

Zahn infarct a subcapsular, wedge-shaped lesion in the liver characterised by sinusoidal dilatation from obstructed intrahepatic portal veins, named after Friedrich Zahn, German-born Swiss Pathologist

zalcitabine dideoxycytidine, a nucleoside inhibitor to bind the reverse transcriptase of human immuno-deficiency virus

zanamivir a sialic acid analogue inhibitor of neuraminidases of influenza A and B

zangal copper subacetate formed by action of vegetable acids on copper cooking vessels which are not properly lined

zaphyr (ja-fire) soft breeze, after Zephyrus, Greek God of the west wind

Zang's (zangz) **space** space between the two lower tendons of the sternomastoid muscle in the supraclavicular fossa, described by German surgeon, Christoph Zang

zaranthan (zah-ran'than) hardening of the breast

Zaufal's (tsow'fahlz) **sign** saddle nose, named after Prague rhinologist, Emanuel Zaufal

Z-axis the axis along which values of Z are measured and at which both X and Y are equal to zero

z band a thin, dark band passing through transversely across the striated muscle fibre

Z-deformity radial deviation at the wrist with ulnar deviation of the digits in rheumatoid arthritis; hitch hiker's thumb. Often there is palmar subluxation of the proximal phalanges

z disk *see* **z band**

zea corn or maize

zebra body a lysosome that contains broad transversely-stacked myelinoid membranes, seen in certain lysosomal storage diseases **z myopathy** a congenital, non-progressive myopathy with presence of striped and rod-shaped bodies in muscle fibres, visible on electron microscopy

zebra pattern alternating light and dark bands of the hair shaft seen by polarizing light microscopy in trichoschisis due to decreased sulphur content of hair shaft. Other features are growth and mental retardation, ichthyosis and ectodermal dysplasia

ZEEP abbreviation for zero-end expiratory pressure

zein (ze'in) corn protein

zeiosis (ze'o-sis) a form of lymphocyte mediated cytolysis demonstrating nuclear disintegration and mitochondrial swelling

Zeis (ze'is) **glands** sebaceous glands in the lid margin, described by German ophthalmologist, Eduard Zeis

zeism (ze'izm) condition developing from excessive intake of maize, refers to pellegra

Zeitgeber *Ger* time-keeper, any factor in the environment with periodicity, capable of synchronising the endogenous circadian rhythm into a 24-hour cycle

Zellballen *Ger* nest-like clusters of uniform round-to-polygonal chief cells that are surrounded by delicate richly vascular tissue, seen in paraganglioma

Zellweger's syndrome cerebrohepatorenal syndrome, described by Hans Zellweger, US paediatrician

zenana eunuch

zenith (zen'ith) climax, apex, summit, highest point

Zenker's (zeng'kerz) **degeneration** degeneration of skeletal muscles especially in typhoid, described by Freidrich Zenker, German pathologist; zenkerism

Zenker's diverticulum outpouching of the wall of the oesophagus in its upper or lower third, named after German pathologist, Freidrich Zenker. It causes bad breath, regurgitation of saliva and food particles consumed several days earlier. The diagnosis is made with a barium swallow and treatment is surgical

Zenker's fluid a tissue fixative consisting of mercuric chloride, potassium dichromate, glacial acetic acid, and water useful in the study of nuclei, named after Konrad Zenker, German histologist

zeolite naturally occurring fibrous silicate mineral. Its exposure leads to development of pleural mesothelioma

zero (zir'o) nought, symbol O, neutral fixed point on the graph from which all divisions of a scale is measured; the point on a scale at which the graduations begin. Numeral is a significant contribution from India

zero fluid balance a state in which the amount of fluid intake is equal to the amount of fluid output

zero order kinetics the rate of drug elimination is linear with time and proportional to the concentration of the enzyme responsible for catabolism and independent of substrate concentration

zero-end expiratory pressure ZEEP, pressure that has returned to atmospheric level at the end of exhalation

zest great interest keen enjoyment, a lively and enthusiastic relish for life, and it is an aspect of personality that fluctuates with health and state of mind

zero population growth the population neither increases nor decreases at a given period of time, where the number of births is equal to the number of deaths

zestocautery appliance used for therapeutic application of superheated steam

zetacrit (za'ta-krit) a method for determining erythrocyte sedimentation rate which is not affected by haemotocrit. Zeta sedimentation rate is linear with respect to fibrinogen and gamma globulin. It has no male : female differences

zeugmatography (zoog'metog'rafe) magnetic resonance imaging

zidovudin (zi-do-vu-den) a thymidine analogue which inhibits the human immunodeficiency virus reverse transcriptase thereby impairing viral replication; ZDV

Ziegler's (zeg'lerz) **operation** V-shaped iridectomy to create an artificial pupil, described by US ophthalmologist, Samuel Ziegler

Ziehen-Oppenheim (ze'hen-op'en-him) **disease** dystonic muscular deformity, described by German neurologists, Georg Ziehen and Herman Oppenheim.

Ziehen's (ze'henz) **test** test for mental functions requiring description of difference between contrasting objects, such as cat and dog, described by German neurologist, Gerog Ziehen.

Ziehl-Neelsen (zel-nel'sen) **method** smear staining technique to demonstrate acidfast bacteria, described by German bacteriologists, Franz Ziehl and Friedrich Neelsen. A sputum smear prepared on a slide is heat-fixed and dried. It is covered with a small piece of filter paper which is moistened with 5 to 7 drops of carbolfuchsin. The slide is gently heated from below to steaming. After 5 minutes the filter paper is removed and the slide is washed in water. It is then decolourised with acid alcohol for 2 minutes and then washed in water till no stain appears in washing. It is then counterstained with 0.1% methylene blue for one minute. Then it is washed and dried and examined with 100X oil immersion objective. The bacilli appear red under the light blue background

Ziemann's (ze'menz) **dots** small pink dots in the red cell membrane sometimes noted in *P. malariae*

Zieve's (ze'eve) **syndrome** excess alcohol intake in patients with chronic liver disease produces frank haemolysis associated with abdominal pain, jaundice and hyperlipidaemia, described by US physician, Leslie Zieve

ZIFT zygote intrafallopian transfer, a method to treat infertility by artificially placing a fertilised egg into a woman's fallopian tube

zig-zag progression of a line showing sharp turns first to one side and then to the other **z QRS Waves** *ECG* sinusoidal QRS complex in ventricular flutter

zileuton a 5-lipo-oxygenase inhibitor, useful in mild to moderate chronic asthma

z line *see* z band

zinc (zingk) hard bluish white metal, a micronutrient present in many enzymes. Daily requirement is 15 mg, found in shell fish, meat, poultry and whole grain. Its malabsorption leads to growth retardation, severe diarrhoea and hair loss **z carbonate** a mild astringent found in dusting powders **z chills** metal fume fever **z chloride** white granular powder used as antiseptic **z deficiency** a condition developing from insufficient amounts of zinc in the diet, characterised by fatigue, decreased taste and odour sensitivity, poor appetite, delayed healing of wounds and susceptibility to infection **z exposure** an intense exposure to fumes of zinc generated from smelting, welding or foundry work cause a flu-like illness (*metal fume fever*) Zinc is a major ingredient of smoke bombs, which obscures vision and causes tracheobronchitis **z finger** a tertiary protein structure motif of higher organisms consisting of a protein loop held together at both ends by a zinc ion which is present in transcription factors **z insulin** Lente insulin produced

by crystallisation in the presence of an excess of zinc. It can be crystalline zinc (ultralente) or amorphous zinc (semilente) **z ointment** an ointment containing 20% zinc oxide mixed with petrolatum and white ointment used topically to treat skin diseases **z oxide** white odourless, water insoluble powder used as antiseptic and astringent in the treatment of some skin disorders and also acts as a reflector of sunlight **z phosphate** dental cement for luting of dental inlays, crowns, bridges and orthodontic appliances **z pyrithione** a shampoo useful for scalp involvement in seborrhoeic eczema **z sandwich** a hormone receptor complex in which a hormone binds to another forming a bridge between histidine and glycine residues and zinc **z sulphate** colourless crystalline powder used as an astringent and as an emetic

zincalism (zingk'al-izm) chronic zinc poisoning

zingiber ginger **Z officinalis** *sunthi* plant root used for cooking. Important ingredient in ayurvedic medicine

Zinn's (zinz) **ligament** connective tissue attached to the recti muscles of the eye, named after Johann Zinn, German anatomist

zipper proglottid presence of 15-20 lateral zipper-like branches in the proglottid of *Taenia saginata* demonstrable on injection of safronin and India ink

zirconium (zir-ko'ne-um) symbol Zr, rare metallic element, at. no. 40.

z-lines transverse lines giving striated appearance to myocardial fibrils

Zn chemical symbol for the element zinc, at. no. 30

zoacanthosis (zo'ak-an-tho'sis) any dermatitis caused by animal structures, such as bristles, sting or hairs

zoanthropy (zo-an'thro-pe) a mental disorder in which a patient believes himself to be an animal

zoetic (zo-et'ik) pertaining to life

Zolmitriptan a second-generation sumatriptan-like drug used in the treatment of migraine headache

Zollinger-Ellison (zol'lin-jer-el'li-son) **syndrome** 1. gastrinoma syndrome 2. tumours or hyperplasia of the D cells of the islets of the pancreas secreting large amounts of gastrin, stimulate the parietal cells of the stomach to secrete maximal amount of gastric acid resulting in severe peptic ulceration, diarrhoea, occasionally with malabsorption, described by Robert Zollinger, US surgeon and Edwin Ellison, US physician. The ulcers are often multiple and severe in duodenum and may be found in unusual sites like jejunum or oesophagus and recur. There can be bleeding, perforation and pyloric stenosis. It is treated with large doses of omeprazole or H_2-receptor antagonist

zombie effect personality changes due to extrapyramidal effects of haloperidol with features identical to idiopathic Parkinsonism

zona (zo'na) 1. a band or girdle 2. herpes zoster, pl. **zonae** **zonal** adj. **z arcuata** the inner third of the basilar membrane of the cochlear duct **z glomerulosa** outer layer of the adrenal cortex secreting aldosterone (mineralocorticoid) **z haemorrhoidalis** the part of anal canal between anus and anal valves containing the rectal venous plexus **z fasciculata** thick middle layer of adrenal cortex secreting cortisol (glucocorticoid) **z orbicularis** circular fibres in the capsule of hip joint forming ring around neck of femur **z pellucida** a transparent membranous envelope of the ovum **z reticularis** innermost zone of the adrenal cortex concerned with production of androgens **z vasculosa** entry of a number of capillaries from the mastoid bone to the external acoustic meatus

zonal (zo'nal) pertaining to a zone or zones

zone (zon) an encircling area or division distinguished for some purpose **epileptogenic z** a cortical region whose stimulation causes seizure **erogenous z** a part of the body, whose stimulation excites sexual feelings **trigger z** the area on stimulation by touch or pressure causes pain **z electrophoresis** electrophoretic technique in which components are separated into zones or bands in a buffer and stabilised in solid medium **z of equivalence** a region in an antigen-antibody reacting system where the ratio of antigen to antibody is equivalent **z of interaction** *psy* refers to areas or channels through which the tension of needs and the way of relief are sensed in conjunction with the outside **z therapy** the treatment of a disorder by mechanical stimulation and counter-irritation of a body area in the same longitudinal zone as the affected area **z of uncertainty** intellectual function with IQ of 70

Zondek-Aschheim (zon'dek-ash'him) **test** biological test of pregnancy which demonstrates chorionic gonadotropin in the urine in large quantities, described by German gynaecologists, Bernhard Zondek and Selmar Aschheim

Zondek's syndrome post-partum metrorrhagia, galactorrhoea and hyperthyroidism, described by German born Israeli obstetrician, Bernhardt Zondek.

zonesthesia (zo'nes-the'zi-ah) painful sensation of constriction experienced around the waist or abdomen

zonifugal (zo-nif'u-gal) moving outward from any zone or region

zoning phenomenon layering of atypical platelets in the bone marrow in myelofibrosis; three microscopic zones of osteochondroma-like growth in myositis ossificans

zonipetal (zo-nip'et-al) moving toward a zone or region

zonisamide (zo-ni's-mide) a benzisoxazole

sulphonamide, an antiepileptic agent

zonked highly intoxicated from drugs or alcohol

zonoskeleton (zon'o-skel'e-ton) the proximal bones to which limbs attach, such as the hip bone, scapula and clavicle

zonula (zo'nu-la) little zone or area pl. **zonulae, z ciliaris** suspensory ligament of the lens **z occludens** intracellular tight junctions that regulate the intestinal epithelial barrier, and its permeability

zonular (zon'u-lar) pertaining to a zonula **z cataract** a cataract with opacity limited to certain layers of the lens **z occludens toxin** Zot. toxin elaborated by *Vibrio cholera* that acts as a morphogenetic phage peptide for the *Vibrio cholerae* phage and as an enterotoxin that modulates intestinal tight junctions **z space** a space between the fibres of the ligaments of the lens

zonulin system system regulating paracellular pathways in intestinal epithelium responsible for the movement of fluid, macromolecules and leucocytes between the blood stream and the intestinal lumen and vice versa

zonulitis (zon'u-li'tis) inflammation of the ciliary zonule

zonulolysis (zo-nu-lol'i-sis) disintegration of the ciliary zonule by enzymes instilled into the anterior chamber

zonulotomy (zon'u-lot'o-me) incision of the ciliary zonule

zoo a combining word for pertaining to an animal

zoo blot a method to detect conservation of DNA sequence during evolution among different species

zoodermic (zo'o-der'mik) performed with animal skin as in skin grafting

zoogenous (zo-oje-nus) 1. acquired from animals 2. viviparous

zooglea (zo'o-gle'a) a colony of bacteria embedded in a gelatinous matrix. pl. **zoogleae**

zoogony (zo'og'o-ne) the production of living young from within the body. **zoogonous**, adj.

zoograft (zo'o-graft) a graft of tissue from that of a lower animal to a human

zooid (zo'oyd) animal-like; an individual in a colony of animals

zoolagnia (zo'o-lag'ne-a) sexual attraction towards animals

zoolite a hydrated double silicate

zoological (zo-ol'oj-i'kal) pertaining to zoology

zoology (zo-ol'ah-je) branch of biological science dealing with animals

zoomania (zo'o-ma'ne-ah) a morbid affection for animals

zoomastigophora (zo'o-mas'ti-go-for'a) a class of unicellular organisms which includes flagellates having a vesicular nucleus and lacking chromatophores (unicellular organisms with flagella includes *Giardia lamblia*

zoonosis (zo-o-no'sis) any infectious or parasitic disease transmissible to man from animals. pl. **zoonoses zoonotic** adj.

zoonotic (zo'o-not'ik) **helminths** helminths transmitted to man from animals such as *Trichinella spiralis, Toxocara canis, Ankylostoma braziliensis, Gnathostoma spinigerum*

zooparasite (zo'o-par'a-sit) any parasitic animal or species, **zooparasitic** adj.

zoopathology (zo'o-path-ol'o-je) the science of the diseases of animals

zoophagous (zo-of'ah-gus) carnivorous

zoophilia (zo'o-fil'e-a) 1. abnormal love of animals 2. a paraphilia in which intercourse or sexual activity is preferred method to achieve sexual excitement

zoophilic transmission to man from animals

zoopharmacology (zo'o-fahr'mah-kol'o-je) veterinary pharmacology

zoophobia (zo'o-fo'be-a) abnormal fear of animals

zooplasty (zo'o-plast'ti) the transplantation of living tissue from a lower animal to the human body; zoografting

zoopsia (zo-op'se-ah) a hallucination in which the patient thinks he sees animals

zoosis (zo-o'sis) any disease due to animal agents

zoospore (zo'o-spor) a motile spore produced by certain protozoa, fungi and algae

zootomy (zo-ot'ah-me) the dissection or anatomy of animals

zoosperm presence of live spermatozoa in the ejaculated semen

zootoxin (zo'o-tok'sin) a toxic substance of animal origin such as venom of snakes, spiders and scorpions or serum produced by means of such toxin

zoster (zos'ter) herpes zoster, a belt, encircling structure, girdle or shingles **z ophthalmicus** a herpes infection of the eye

zosteriform (zos-ter'i-form) any band-like unilateral skin lesion located along the cutaneous distribution of a spinal or a branch of trigeminal nerves, usually seen in the recrudescence of herpes zoster

z-plasty (ze'plas-te) a plastic operation for relaxation of scar contractures by Z-shaped incision, and transposition of two triangular flaps in such a way so that their apices cross the line of contracture

z protein a protein that is normally present in the Z band of striated muscle

z QRS waves *ECG* sinusoidal QRS complexes seen by electrocardiography in ventricular flutter

Zr chemical symbol, zirconium

z score the deviation of a score referring to the difference between the score and the mean divided by the standard deviation

z test use of Z score to determine significance

z-track a method of giving injection in such a way as to prevent backward flow of the injected solution

Zuckerkandl's (tsook'er-kon'd'lz) **bodies** paraganglia near the bifurcation of aorta, described by German anatomist, Emil Zuckerkandl

Zulu dancer's hip occupational arthritis developing in Zulu people

z value a statistical test for the hypothesis that a population's mean does not differ from the target value

z wave fall of atrial pressure between atrial and ventricular contractions

zwitterion (tsvit'er-i'on) *Ger* an ion having both positive and negative regions of charge

zyg (o) - a combined word for joined or a junction or yoked

zygal (zi'g'l) yoke-shaped; H-shaped

zygapophysis (zi'gah-pof'i-sis) paired articular processes on superior and inferior surfaces of the neural arch of a vertebra to interlock each vertebra with the ones above and below. pl. **zygopophyses**

zygion (zij'e-on) the most lateral point on the zygomatic arch. pl. **zygia**

zygodactyly (zi'go-dak'ti-le) union of digits by skin and soft tissues without bony fusion of the phalanges unlike syndactyly

zygogene cells cells of the stomach that secrete pepsin

zygogenesis (zi'gojen'esis) the formation of a zygote

zygoma (zi-go'ma) the zygomatic process of the temporal bone fused with zygomatic bone, forming an arch. **zygomatic** adj.

zygomatic (zi'go-matik) pertaining to zygoma **z arch** the bony arch below the orbit of the skull formed by the union of the processes of temporal and zygomatic bone; forming the prominence of the cheek and part of the orbit. **z nerve** sensory branch of maxillary division of trigeminal nerve supplying the skin of temple and cheek bone

zygomaticofacial (zigo-mat'iko-fa'shul) pertaining to zygoma and face

zygomaticotemporal (zigo-mat'iko-tem'pah-rul) pertaining to zygoma and temporal bone

zygomaticus (zi'go-mat'ik-us) a facial muscle that draws the upper lip upward and outward. There is a major and a minor zygomaticus muscle on either side of the face

zygomycetes (zi'go-mi-se'tez) a group of fungi such as Absidin, Mucor, Rhizopus which grow in compromised hosts

zygomycosis (zi'go-mi'ko'sis) an infection from fungi of the family Mucoraceae occurring in ill patients. It may be confined to subcutaneous tissue or invade the blood vessels

zygopodium (zi-go-po-de-um) the intermediate-distal portion of the limb such as ulna and radius, and the tibia and fibula

zygosis (zi go-sis) union of a male and a female gamete (an egg and a sperm) resulting into a fertilised ovum.

zygosity (zi-gos'i-ti) to determine whether a certain twin pair is monozygotic (from one zygote) or dizygotic (two zygotes) the condition relating to conjugation or to the zygote as 1 or 2; to determine specific character being identical (homozygosity) or different (heterozygosity)

zygote (zi'got) the cell produced by zygosis. **zygotic** adj.

zygotene (zi'go-ten) stage during prophase of cell division

zym(o)- a combining word for enzyme; fermentation

zymase (zi'mas) 1. enzyme 2. intracellular enzyme of yeast

zymogen (zi-mo-jen) any substance that may change into an enzyme due to some internal alteration; proenzyme

zymogenesis (zi-mo-jen'e-sis) transformation of zymogen into an active enzyme

zymolysis (zi-mo-lie'sis) digestive and fermentative action of enzymes

zymose (zi-mos) invertin, an enzyme that converts a disaccharide into a monosaccharide

zymosis (zi-mo'sis) 1. fermentation 2. an infectious disease

zymotic (zi-mot'ik) **disease** an infectious disease caused by germs introduced into the body from outside which act in a manner similar to fermentation

ZZ homozygous phenotype as in a_1-antitrypsin deficiency

New Words

A

ABC *abb* abacavir, absolute basophil count, absolute bone conduction, acalculous biliary colic, acid balance control, airway, breathing and circulation, aneurismal bone cyst, antigen-binding capacity, antigen-binding cell, aspiration biopsy cytology, assessment of basic competency

abdominal cocoon mass of palpable bowel loops in abdomen causing small bowel obstruction

abdominoplasty (ab'domino-pla'sti) a type of cosmetic surgery in which excess fat and skin are removed from the abdominal area; tummy tuck

Abernathy malformation a congenital anomaly of the splanchnic vasculature in which the portal venous blood is diverted into the inferior vena cava

abortus (ab'ar-tus) number of pregnancy losses before 20 weeks regardless of cause

abuse a maladaptive pattern of substance use

abusive head injuries brain, skull and spinal injuries associated with shaking abuse inflicted on infants see shaken baby syndrome

abutment tooth *dent* a crowned tooth that stablises a bridge or partial denture

ACC *abb* American College of Cardiology

access (ak'ses) the point where a needle or catheter is inserted for dialysis

access site the vein tapped for vascular access in haemodialysis treatment

accreditation(ak'kre-di-ta'shun) the process of certifying, usually by a national body, that an institution meets the procedural standards

aceruloplasminaemia (a'ceru-lo'plas-min'emea) an autosomal recessive disorder of iron overload exhibiting a loss of function, mutation in ceruloplasmin and accumulation of iron in neural and glial cells of brain, hepatocytes and pancreatic islet cells

acinar *add* **a pattern** *radiol* a collection of round or elliptic, ill-defined discrete or partly confluent opacities in the lung **a shadow** *radiol* a round or slightly elliptic pulmonary opacity that is considered to represent an anatomic acinus rendered opaque by consolidation

ACPO abbreviation for acute colonic pseudo-obstruction a variant of ileus, characterised by massive colonic dilatation resulting from either increased sympathetic stimulation or decreased parasympathetic activity

actin filament a protein filament formed by the polymerization of globular actin molecule

acute motor axonal neuropathy an axonopathy without demyelination, noted in northern China, often called Chinese paralytic syndrome; AMAN

adherin's junction a cell junction in which the cytoplasm face of the membrane is attached to actin filaments

adiponectin (adi-po-nek-tin) an adipocyte-derived hormone having an important role in maintenance of glucose homeostasis and insulin sensitivity

adjustment disorder *psy* a debilitating reaction usually lasting less than six months, to be a stressful event or situation

ADL *abb* activities of daily living

ADR *abb* adverse drug reaction

advance care planning process of discussing the type of treatment and care that a patient would or would not wish to receive in the event that they lose capacity to decide or unable to express a preference

advance decision a statement of a patient's wish to refuse a particular type of medical treatment or care if they become unable to make or communicate decisions for themselves

advance directive a legal document designated to help to ensure that care decisions made on a person's behalf are consistent with his or her preference

advanced sleep phase disorder converse of the delayed sleep phase disorder, occurs in older people

aerid (a'rid) a sharp, bitter or unpleasantly pungent taste or smell

affective disorder *psy* an emotional disorder involving abnormal highs and/or lows in mood

affective flattening *psy* a loss or lack of emotional expressiveness

afterload the load against which the cardiac muscle exerts its contractile force

age-related macular degeneration degeneration of the macula that leads to loss of central vision in elderly persons

age spots brown spots on the skin that resemble freckles and that are caused by long-term exposure to sun

aggrephagy (ag're-faji) a selective pathway in which denatured and polyubiquitinated proteins are assembled into organized structures called aggresomes and then targeted to autophagosomes for degradation by autophagy

agni (s) ayu digestive fire or digestive capacity

agnosia (ag'no-sis) inability to recognize familiar faces, locations or objects

AHA American Heart Association

air inspired atmospheric gas **a bronchiologram** *radiol* the radiologic shadow of an air-containing bronchiole **a bronchogram** *radiol* the radiographic shadow of an air-containing bronchus surrounded by airless lung **a fluid level** *radiol* a local collection of gas and liquid creating a radiologic shadow characterised by a sharp horizontal interface between gas density above and liquid density below **a space** the gas containing part of the lung parenchyma

a trapping retention of excess gas in the lung during expiration

akash (s) sky, space

Alberti's regimen use of small doses of either intramuscular or intravenous insulin for the treatment of diabetes ketoacidosis

Alexander method a somatic method for improving the physical and mental functioning, named after the originator, Frederick Alexander from Australia

algor mortis (al'gor-mor'tis) *for* cooling of the body used to assess time since death

Alice in wonderland syndrome bizarre disturbances of body image, macropsia/ micropsia, feeling of levitation, alteration of sense of passage of time, depersonalization, and doubting personality

allodynia (all'o-dy'nea) perception of pain in response to stimuli that are not normally painful

Alogia (al'o-jia) *psy* an impoverishment in thinking that is inferred from observing speech and language behavior

ALS advanced life support, an emergency care that may include airway management, defibrillator and use of drugs and medication

alterative (al'ter-at'iv) a substance that promotes a gradual change in nutrition or in the body without creating a particular effect of its own

altergoism (awl'ter-e'go-izm) identified with people of similar personality to one's own

alternate splicing use of different exons in the formation of messenger RNA from initially identical transcripts, which can result in generation of related proteins

altostasis (al'to-sta-sis) ability to maintain stable functions in the face of a change in the environment

alveolarisation *radiol* the opacification of groups of alveoli by a contrast medium

alveoplasty (al've-o'plasti) *den* surgical reshaping of the bone structures in the mouth being fitted for dentures

alymphia (ah-lim'fe-ah) deficiency or absence of lymph

amalgam dent a mixture of silver and several other metals used to make fillings for cavities

AMBU acronym for air mask bag unit

AMC abbreviation for army medical corps

amelogenesis *den* imperfect den insufficient enamel in the outer layer at the teeth

amok *psy* a dissociative episode characterized by a period of brooding followed by an outburst of violent, aggressive or homicidal behavior directed at people and objects

amphipathic having both hydrophobic regions, as in a phospholipid

amplification an increase in the copy number of a particular gene which can be either inherited or somatic

amusia (a-mu'sia) acquired brain defects of music processing

Amyand's hernia presence of vermiform appendix in inguinal hernia sack, named after Cladius Amyand, who performed a successful appendectomy in 1735 in England

amylin (a'my-lin) a polypeptide hormone secreted along with insulin from pancreatic beta cells

analytical validity of a test ability to measure accurately and reliably the component of interest

anaphrodisiac (an' afro-de'sik) a substance that reduces sexual desire and/ or potency

anchoring junction a cell junction that attaches cells to each other

Angelman syndrome a rare neurogenetic disorder in which children exhibit an unusual, happy demeanour, jerky movements and flapping of hands, named after Harry Angelman, an English paediatrician, see Happy puppet syndrome

angioid streaks grey, orange or red wavy branching lines in Bruch's membrane

angiomyolipoma (an'ji-o-lip'oma) a neoplasm composed of varying admixture of blood vessels, smooth muscle cells, adipose tissue, typically occurs within lung

angiospasm (an'ji'o'spa'sm) spasmodic contractions of a blood vessel with increase in blood pressure

anhedonia (an'hid-o'nea) psy a loss of interest in things that are normally pleasurable

anicteric (an'ic-teric) not jaundiced

ANM abbreviation for auxiliary nurse midwife

annotation (an'not-a-shun) identification of the location and coding regions of genes in a genome and the prediction of functions for these regions

annotation catalogue a map denoting the function of specific genomic regions

anorgasmia (an'or-ga-s'mea) inability to achieve sexual satisfaction despite normal desire and excitement

antegrade trafficking trafficking across the secretory stations from the endoplasmic reticulum toward the plasma membrane or the lysosomes

anthropomorphic (an'th-ro-po-:nor'fic) having human characteristics

anti-aging factors factors that delay or stop aging

anticonvulsant hypersensitivity syndrome a rare and potentially fatal complicated condition from use of anticonvulsants with features of fever, rash and internal organ involvement, *see* DRESS syndrome

antigen presentation a process by which immune cells capture foreign antigens to facilitate their recognition by T-cells

antigen presenting cell a cell of the immune system, such as a monocyte, that presents pieces of an invading microbe or antigen to lymphocytes

antilithic (an'ti-lith'ik)l preventing calculus formation 2 an agent that prevents calculus formation

antiperiodic a substance that counteracts intermittent diseases

antiporter a membrane carrier protein that transports two different molecules across a membrane in opposite directions

antisocial personality disorder a long-standing pattern of behavior noted in adults which interferes with functioning; ASPD

aortopulmonary window a mediastinal space bounded anteriorly by the posterior surface of the ascending aorta, posteriorly by the anterior surface of the aortic arch, inferiorly by the superior surface of the left pulmonary artery, medially by the left side of the trachea, left main bronchus and oesophagus, and laterally by the left lung, and contains fat, the ductus ligament, the left recurrent laryngeal nerve, and lymph nodes

ap (s) water

apart (s) life sustaining energy centred in the large intestine in expulsion activity

apatarpana ayu catabolic

APC gene adenomatous polyposis coli gene

apical ballooning syndrome an acute, reversible cardiac dysfunction that is noted in post-menopausal females

apiocetomy *dent* root resection

apoB abbreviation for apolipoprotein B, a component of LDL cholesterol

apperception (aper'sep-shun) process of understanding through linkage with previous experience

aprotinin (ap'ro-tin'in) a haemostatic agent that inhibits the fibrinolytic enzyme plasmin

aromatherapy (aa'roma-ther-a'pe) the use of essential oils from plants for massage or inhalation

arrhythmogenic right ventricular cardiomyopathy a disorder characterised clinically by ventricular arrhythmia, heart failure and sudden death, and histologically by cardiomyocyte loss and replacement with fibrosis or fibrous-fatty tissue

ART abbreviation for 1. anti-retrovirus therapy 2. assisted reproductive technology

arthrodiastasis (ar-thro'di-ast'asis) distraction of the joint with an articulated external fixator

arthropneumoradiography (ar'thro-nu'mo-ra-de-og/ra-fe) radiographic examination of a joint after injection with air

artificial sphincter an inflatable cuff implanted around the upper urethra to squeeze the urethra shut and provide urinary control

ascending reticular activating system a complex pathway from pons to midbrain to intraluminar thalamic nuclei of basal forebrain with different cortical communications that are concerned with arousal; ARAS

ASCUS abbreviation for atypical squamous cells of undetermined significance

Asherman's syndrome cessation of menstruation and /or infertility caused by intrauterine adhesions

Asherman's disease cessation of menstruation and/or infertility caused by intrauterine adhesions, named after Israeli Gynaecologist Joseph Asherman

Asperger syndrome *psy* children who have autistic behavior without problems with language

assay analysis of the chemical composition or strength of substance

aster (a'ster) the star-shaped arrangement of microtubules that is characteristic of a mitotic or meiotic spindle own tissue

Aston-patterning an integrated system of movement eduction, body work, ergonomic adjustments, and fitness training to establish the relationship between the body and mind

asymptomatic without signs or symptoms of disease

atherectomy (a'ther-ec'tamy) an invasive surgical procedure designed to clear clogged arteries by ablating the obstruction

Atkins diet a low-carbohydrate diet used to promote weight loss, and was promoted by Robert Atkin

atransferrinaemia (a'trans-fer'in-emea) a rare autosomal recessive hereditary disorder having iron overload and hypochromic anaemia exhibiting reduced delivery of iron to bone marrow and reduced haemoglobin synthesis

ATS abbreviation for American Thoracic Society

audit *add* **clinical a** process used by clinicians who seek to improve patient care, involves comparing aspects of care (structure, process and outcome) against explicit criteria **comparative a** audit studies that compare the occurrence of certain outcomes between surgeries, between departments, between hospitals or between countries

autogenic transplant a patient receiving a transplant of his or her own tissue

autoimmune polyendocrinopathy-candidiasis-ectodermal dystrophy a rare inherited autosomal recessive disorder caused by mutations in the autoimmune regulator gene presenting with autoimmune polyendocrine syndrome type 1 with manifestations of Addison's syndrome, hypoparathyroidism, type 1 diabetes, primary hypothyroidism, chronic mucocutaneous candidiasis, nail dystrophy and dental enamel hypoplasia; APECED

autologous blood donation donation of a person's own blood before scheduled surgery to make the blood available in case a transfusion is necessary during or after surgery

automatic thoughts *psy* thoughts that automatically come to mind when a particular situation occurs

autophagic flux autophagic activity as represented by completion of the entire autophagy pathway from the fusion of cargo-laden autophagosomes to lysosomes to cargo degradation within the lysosome

autophagocytosis (auto'fag-o'sy-tosis) a catabolic process causing degradation of a cell's own components through lysosomes that has significant influence in cell growth, development and homeostasis; autophagy

autophagosome double-membrane cytosolic vesicle that sequesters cytoplasmic contents and delivers them to the lysosome for subsequent degradation

autophagy (auto'fa-ji) a catabolic pathway involving the degradation of cellular components through the lysosomal machinery. **a proteins** a family of proteins originally identified in yeast as being crucial for the regulation of autophagy

auxiliary liver transplantation a technique in which all or part of the graft is placed in the abdomen and the native liver being left in situ

avatar (s) incarnation in human form, embodiment, as a concept

aVF, aVL, aVR abbreviation for augmented electrocardiographic leads from the left foot, left arm and right arm respectively

avolition (a'vol-i-shun) *psy* a condition in which a person lacks energy, spontaneity and initiave, noted in schizophrenia

axonal polyneuropathy occurrence of sensory and motor dysfunction in a progressive, symmetric, length-dependent manner

AYUSH abbreviation for ayurveda, yoga and naturopathy, unani, siddha and homoeopathy

B

B Pharma abbreviation for Bachelor of Pharmacy

BAC abbreviation for bacterial artificial chromosome

bacterial artificial chromosome a chromosome-like structure constructed by genetic engineering that carries genomic DNA to be cloned; BAC

bacterial artificial chromosome a cloning vector whose accommodation DNA inserts of up to 1 million base pairs

bahramdipity (ba'hram-di'piti) derived from Bahram Gur, the Persian dictator, an irresponsible publication of a publicity seeking article by a journal editor where discoveries are suppressed or not even allowed to be completed or verified

balavridhi (s) ascending energy level

balpains CA2+ -dependent cysteine proteases that modulate cellular function

balsum (bal'sam) a resinous substance from trees that has soothing or healing action

BAMS abbreviation for Bachelor of Ayurvedic Medicine and Surgery

Bare lymphocyte syndrome a rare recessive condition with major histocompatibility complexes are not exposed and manifest with severe immune defects

bare lymphocyte syndrome a rare recessive disorder without any expression of major histocompatibility complexes and present with severe combined immune deficiency

BAROS bariatric analysis and reporting outcome system to standardise and compare outcomes of bariatric surgical services which defines five outcome groups as failure, fair, good, very good and excellent based on a scoring system that is used to evaluate 3 main areas such as percentage of excess weight loss, changes in co-morbid medical conditions and quality of life

base 1 A substance that can accept a proton in solution 2. Purine and pyrimidines in DNA and RNA are organic bases referred to simply as base

base line a return to an original state

base pair two nucleotides (always a pyrimidine with a purine) that are paired and held together by a hydrogen bond

baseline a condition against which later changes are compared

basiphobia (bas'i-fo'be-a) morbid fear of walking

basii (s) a method of an enema

basti ayu administration of medicated enema

bath *add* **bed b** the cleaning of a patient in bed **b blanket** a flannel covering that can be used to prevent chilling **colloid b** a medicated bath prepared by adding soothing agents **contrast b** alternate immersion of a patient in hot water and cold water **emollient b** a bath in a soothing and softening **liquid paraffin b** the dipping of an extremity into a warm solution of paraffin to provide pain relief and increased mobility **sitz b** immersion of only the hip and buttocks to relieve pain and discomfort following rectal surgery, cystoscopy or vaginal surgery **sponge b** one in which the patient's body is not immersed but wiped with a wet cloth or sponge **tepid b** one

in water 30° to 35°C **warm b** one in water 32° to 40°C **whirlpool b** one in which the water is kept in constant motion by mechanical means for massaging action

bathy (ba'th-i) combining word for deep

battered child syndrome unexplained or inappropriately explained physical trauma and other manifestations of severe repeated physical abuse of children, usually by parents

bayonet apposition side-to-side alignment of the fracture fragments

BDS abbreviation for Bachelor of dental surgery

Beckwith-Wiedeman syndrome an epigenetic overgrowth syndrome, caused by mutations in growth regulating genes on chromosome 11, characterised by omphalocele, macroglossia and macrosomia

behavior modification a form of therapy that uses rewards to reinforce desired behavior

behavioural therapy *psy* psychotherapy that helps a person to change the way he or she responds to certain circumstances

behaviourism (be'havi-ur'izm) a system of psychology in which all behaviour, normal and abnormal, is seen as a set of conditioned reflexes separate from individual's will

bench marking a process defining a level of care set as a goal to be obtained

Bender-Gestatt test *psy* a psychological assessment used to evaluate visual-motor functioning, visual-perceptual skills, neurologic impairment and emotional disturbances

Berkow (ber'ko) **formula a** method for determining the percentage of the total body surface affected by burn and it is calculated from the rule of nines

Bernheim (ber'n-heme) **effect** normally there is a slight displacement of the inter ventricular septum into the right ventricular cavity due to higher pressures on the left side of the heart **reverse B e** displacement of the interventricular septum into the left ventricular cavity when there is right ventricular overload

Bethesda system a system for reporting cervical or vaginal cytologic findings and diagnoses, named after Bethesda, Maryland, USA, headquarters of National Institute of Health

BHAT beta blocker heart attack trial showing therapy with a nonselective adrenergic blocking agent improves survival

Bhattacharyya-Connor syndrome a rare defect of sitosterolemia-xanthomatosis due to an increased absorption of sitosterol and defective turnover with accumulation in tissues, described in 1974 by AK Bhattacharyya and WE Connor

BHMS abbreviation for Bachelor of Homoeopathic Medicine and Surgery

Bhore committee a committee appointed by Government of India in 1946 under the chairmanship of Sir Joseph Bhore, to survey the then existing position regarding the health in the country and health organization and to make recommendations for the future development

bibliotherapy (bib'li-o-the-rapi) use of books to improve one's understanding of personal problems and/or to heal painful feelings

bifid bacteria a group of bacteria normally present in the intestine

binge eating disorder a loss of control over eating behaviours

biobank a bank of biological specimens for biomedical research

biocitizenship individual and collective welfare claims made by biologically damaged population; biological citizenship

biodynamics (bi'o-dyna'miks) a therapy that works on the idea that the digestive system reacts to the moods and emotions of the individual

bioenergetics (bi'o-ener-je'tiks) a therapy that aims to unblock the flow of life energy relieving tension and bringing emotional release

bioenergetics (bi'o-ener'je-tiks) system of therapy that combines breathing and body exercises, psychological therapy and the free expression of emotions to release blocked

biogerontology (bi'o-ger-o'n-toloji) study of biological basis of ageing

biohazard (bi'o-ha-jar'd)an organism or substance derived from an organism, that poses a threat to human health

bioidentical hormones compounds that have exactly the same chemical and molecular st ture as hormones that are produced in the human body

bioinformatics (bi-o-infor'mat-iks) the study of genetic and other biologic information using computer and statistical techniques

biological age age according to metabolic function as opposed to chronological age

biological imaging in vitro characterisation and measurement of biological processes at the cellular and molecular level, and the images include those in the metabolic, biochemical, physiological and functional categories

biological target volume a specific volume of target depending upon its biological property, such as high tumour burden; BTV

biomarker (bi-o-mar'ker) the measurement of any molecule or material such as cells or tissue, that reflects the disease process

biomarker a biochemical substance that can be detected in blood samples that indicates the presence of a cancerous growth

biomechanics (bi-o-mek'ani-ks) study of the physical limits of the human body, forms the basic science underlying sports medicine

biomedical waste any waste, which is generated during the diagnosis, treatment or immunization of human beings or animals or in research activities pertaining thereto or in the production or testing of biologicals

biopharmaceutics (bi'o-farma'su-tiks) a study of the relevant factors influencing the rate and amount of drug that reaches systemic circulation

biorhythm (bi'o-ry'dam) dependence of the health and performance of the individual on three fixed length cycles that include a physical cycle lasting 23 days that affects vitality, confidence and sex drive, an emotional cycle lasting 28 days that affects creativity and an intellectual cycle of 33 days affecting mental function

biosafety (bi'o-saf-ti) the application of knowledge, techniques and equipment to prevent personal, laboratory and environmental exposure to potentially infectious agents of biohazards

biosamples samples of biological specimens for biomedical research

biosphere (bi'o-spi-ar) the world of living organisms

bioterrorism (bi-o'ter'ori-zm) use of biological or chemical weapons for terroristic activity

biotype a variant strain of a bacterial species with distinctive physiological characteristics

BIP trial Benzafibrate infarction prevention trial showing reduction in cardiovascular events and cardiovascular mortality in patients with diabetes treated with beta blocker

Birquet's syndrome a somatisation disorder running a chronic and fluctuating course with pain, vomiting, nausea, headache, dizziness, menstrual irregularities and sexual dysfunction seen in women

birth weight the weight of a neonate determined immediately after delivery

bite *den* occlusion contact between opposing upper and lower teeth **b guard** a plastic dental appliance that fits over the biting surface of the upper or lower teeth

bivalirudin (bi'va-li-ru'din) a direct thrombin inhibitor

bivent.icular pacing electrical pacing in both ventricles see cardiac resynchronization therapy

bizarre *psy* a delusion that involves a phenomena that the person's culture would regard as totally implausible

Bjornstad syndrome an autosomal recessive disorder associated with sensorineural hearing loss and twisted hairs

bladder training a behavioural modification programme used to treat stress incontinence

blank a negative control specimen required for certain assays and quality assurance in laboratory tests

blepharoptosis (ble'pah-rop-to'sis) drooping of an upper eyelid

blooming (bloom'ing) in radiology, a change in size of the focal spot, usually an increase

blotting a technique for transferring DNA (Southern blotting), RNA (Northern blotting), or proteins (Western blotting) from an agarose or polyacrylamide jel to a nylon membrane

Blount's disease breaking and fragmentation of the medial tibial epiphysis, named after Waler Blount, US orthopaedic surgeon; tibia vara

blur lack of sharpness in an x-ray image, usually due to patient motion

BMI abbreviation for body mass index

body contour surgery surgical procedures performed to improve body shape by removing fat and skin

body dysmorphic syndrome *psy* a psychiatric disorder characterized by preoccupation with an imagined physical defect

Bolan principle a doctor is not guilty of negligence if he or she has acted in accordance with a practice that is accepted as proper by a responsible body of medical personnel skilled in that particular act

bonding 1. development of an emotional attachment between parents and newborn 2. den application of synthetic material o teeth

bone spur an overgrowth of bone; osteophyte

Bordet-Biedl syndrome a rare autosomal recessive genetic disorder with clinical features of retinitis pigmentosa,

Polydactyly, obesity, learning disabilities, hypogonadism and renal abnormalities

botox (bo'toks) trade name for a preparation of botulinum toxin type A

Bouchard' nodes swelling of the middle joint of the finger

BPT abbreviation for Bachelor of Physiotherapy

bracer *den* an orthodontic appliance consisting of brackets cemented to the surface of each tooth and wires of stainless shall or nickel titanium alloy, used to treat malocclusion by changing the position of the teeth

bramhana ayu treatment which increases the size of the body making it stronger

Braxton Hicks contraction tightening of the uterus or abdomen throughout pregnancy. These contractions do not cause changes in the cervix; false labour

BRCA abbreviation for breast cancer gene

breakthrough (brak'throo) 1. a significant step forward in theory development or research 2. in psychotherapy, a change in attitude or behaviour following a period of little or no change in sight

breast crawl human babies when kept in skin-to-skin contact between their mother's breasts can initiate breast feeding on their own

breast implant a soft pouch, filled with saline or silicone that is surgically implanted beneath the skin and muscle of the chest wall to form a reconstructed breast after mastectomy

breast reconstruction any surgical method used to create a new breast after mastectomy

breast reduction a surgical procedure performed in order to decrease the size of breast

breast self examination a monthly routine in which a woman follows several steps to detect any changes or suspicious lumps in her breast; BSE

bridge *den* a permanent or removable substitute for a missing tooth or teeth

bridge *dent* an appliance of one or more artificial teeth anchored by crowns on the adjacent teeth

broncho-oto-renal syndrome a rare autosomal dominant disorder charactrised by bronchial cysts of fistulae, external ear malformations and/or preauricular sinus, hearing loss and renal anomalies, Melnick-Fraser syndrome, BOR syndrome

Bronz baby syndrome a condition in which the skin, serum and urine develop a dark, grayish-brown discolouration following phototherapy in infants with cholestasis

Bruch's membrane a membrane in the eye between the choroid membrane of the retina

Brugada (bru'ga-da) **syndrome** an inherited arrhythmogenic disease with polymorphic ventricular tachycardia characterised by typical electrocardiographic pattern of ST-segment elevation >2 mm in precordial leads V1 through V3, incomplete bundle branch block in the right precordial leads and an increased risk of sudden cardiac death as a result of ventricular fibrillation

BT abbreviation for bleeding time

bubonulus (bu'bo-nu'lus) primary stage of LGV with large tender lymphangial nodule and lymphangitis of distal penis

buck teeth *den* varying degrees of abnormality protruding upper teeth

Bucks' fascia deep connective tissue of the penis

buddhi (s) intellect

buddhi (s) judgement

BUMS abbreviation for Bachelor of Unani Medicine and Surgery

burn out a form of mental distress manifested in normal individuals who experience decreased work performance resulting from negative attitudes and behaviours

Bx abbreviation for biopsy

C

CABG *abb* coronary artery bypass grafting

Caffey disease a rare disorder of unknown aetiology characterised by cortical hyperostosis with inflammation of the contiguous fascia and muscle; infantile cortical hyperostosis

calciphylaxis (kal'ci-fy-lak'sis) a small-vessel vasculopathy characterised by mural calcification, intimal proliferation, and microthrombosis seen in patients with renal disease; calcific uraemic arteriopathy

calmative (ca'ma-tiv) a substance used as a tranquillizer or sedative

CAM complementary and alternative medicine; a group of diverse medical and health care systems, practices and products that are not presently considered to be part of conventional medicine

canaliculodacryosystorhinostomy (kan-a-;ol'lo-dak're-o-sis'to-ri-nos'tomi) a surgical procedure to relieve a stricture found at the junction of lacrimal canaliculus and conjunctiva

cancer genome entire set of unique DNA that makes up a specific cancer

cancer stemlike cells cancer cells found within tumours or haematologic cancers that possesses characteristics associated with normal stem cells

candidate gene a gene that has been selected on the basis of a perceived match between the known or presumed function of the gene and the biologic characteristics of the disease in question

Canker sore a painful sore inside the mouth

CAP abbreviation for community acquired pneumonia

capase a protease involved in the initiation of apoptosis

CAPD abbreviation for continuous ambulatory peritoneal dialysis

capnogram (kap'no-gram) a continuous record of the carbon dioxide content of expired air

CAPRICON trial Carvedilol post-infarct survival control to evaluate the role of beta-adrenergic blocking drugs in patients with significant post-myocardial infarction ventricular dysfunction

cardiac arrest catastrophic event in which the heart stops beating, resulting in lss of consciousness and death

cardiac resynchoronisation therapy a procedure to improve the left ventricular ejection fraction and functional status by minimising regional left ventricular delay caused by prolonged ventricular conduction, reducing mitral regurgitation and left ventricular reverse remodeling and normalizing neurohormonal factors, CRT

cardiac resynchronization therapy treatment using a pacemaker that stimulates both ventricles simultaneously; see biventricular pacing, CRT

cardiotoxic triad cardiac dysfunction resulting from hypertension, coronary artery disease and a specific diabetic cardiomyopathy in a diabetic patient

care, *add* **c giver** a lay person who assumes responsibility for the physical and emotional needs of another who is incapable of self-care **managed c** a system of health care in which a person's use of resources is 'managed' to cut costs

carinal angle the angle formed by the right and left main bronchi at the tracheal bifurcation

cartilage-hair hypoplasia a condition noted during second year because of growth deficiency affecting the limbs, accompanied by flaring of the lower rib cage, a prominent sternum, bowing of the legs, short hands and feet and very short fingers with extreme ligamentous laxity; metaphyseal chondrodysplasia

catacholaminergic polymorphic ventricular tachycardia a syndrome of exercise or emotion-mediated polymorphic ventricular tachycardia or ventricular fibrillation in children or young adults occurring in a structurally normal heart; CPVT

cataractogenesis (kat'a-rak-to-jen'e-sis) the process of cataract formation

CBHI abbreviation for central bureau of health intelligence

CCU abbreviation for coronary care unit; critical care unit

celibacy (sel'i-besi) abstinence from sex

cell adhesion molecule a cell surface protein that is used to connect to each other; CAM

cell block a paraffin-embedded specimen derived from dried mucus, sputum or debris present in clear fluids

cell cycle control system a term of regulatory proteins that governs progression through the cell cycle

cell division cycle gene a gene that controls a specific step in the cell cycle; CDS gene

cell fate the final differentiated state that a pleuripotent embryonic cell is expected to attain

cell mediated immune response activation of specific cells to launch an immediate response against an invading microbe

cella (sel'a) a cell or room

centriole a cylindrical array of microtubules that is found at the centre of a centrosome in antimal cells

cetuximab an IgGl chimeric monoclonal antibody against epidermal growth factor receptor

CF abbreviation for cystic fibrosis

CFC abbreviation for chlorofluorocarbon

CFTR abbreviation for cystic fibrosis transmembrane regulator

CFTR gene cystic fibrosis transmembrane conductance regulator gene

CGHS abbreviation for Central Government Health Services

chala (s) mobile

Chandra-Khetarpal syndrome a congenital malformation consisting of levocardia, bronchiectasis, and sinus abnormalities described by RK Chandra and SK Khetarpal in 1963

chaperone (cha'per-on'e) **complex** an oligomeric protein that assists in the folding, unfolding, assembly, or disassembly of other macromolecular structures without being permanently incorporated into the assisted structures

character *psy* set of attitudes and behavior patterns that the individual acquires or learns over time

Charles Bonnet syndrome a condition characterised by visual hallucinations alongside deteriorating vision, usually in elderly people, named after Swiss Naturalist Charles Bonnet

CHC abbreviation for community health centre

cheiloscopy (ke'li-o-sko-pi) *for* lip print used as a tool for identification in forensic sciences

cheirospam spasm of the muscles of the hand as in writer's cramp

chelation (ke'la-shun) the act of drawing substances out of the body through urination or defecation

chemical peel a cosmetic surgery procedure that uses chemicals to remove damaged outer layers of the skin, improving the skin's appearance and texture

Chernobyl nuclear accident high incidence of cancer of thyroid gland due to release of large doses of radioactive iodine in 1986 at the site of nuclear reactor at Chernobyl, Russia

chi chi an internal life force, energy *c kung* (qui-gong) an internal energy exercise

chintan (s) thinking

chintana (s) thinking

chondroclast (kond'ro-kla'st) a cell concerned in the absorption of cartilage

chordoid (kar-do'id) **glioma** a rare, low-grade circumscribed, fusiform-shaped glioma arising in the viscinity of lamina terminalis in the region of third ventricle

chromoblastomycosis a chronic soft tissue fungal infection commonly caused by Fonsecacea pedrosoi

chromosome *add* **bacterial artificial c** a chromosome-like structure, constructed by genetic-engineering, that is used as a vector to clone DNA fragments of genome in cells of the bacterium Escherichia coli **c replacement therapy** a cytosurgical procedure that extracts existing chromosomes from a particular diseased cell and insert new ones in their place in that same cell

chromosome banding the treatment of chromosomes to reveal characterstic patterns of horizontal bands

chromosome condensation compaction of entire chromosomes in preparation for cell division

chronic prostatitis-chronic pelvic pain syndrome a type of prostatits characterized by chronic genitourinary pain that may be associated with urinary and sexual dysfuncntion

chronological age age in calendar years

chronopharmacology (kron'o-far'ma-kol'oje) a branch of chronobiology concerned with effect of drugs on times of biologic rhythm

CHUK conserved helix-loop-helix ubiquitous kinase gene that has essential role in the proliferation and differentiation of skin epidermis and its derivatives

cilia microtubule-based structures found on cells

ciliopathy diseases characterized by dysfunction of cilium

cilium a hair-like cellular organelle

cinching (sin'ch-ing) surgical shortening of an ocular muscle by placating

circumscribed (cir'kum-skr'i-bd) having a complete or nearly complete visible border

circumstantial conversation *psy* a disturbance in speech in which a person goes into unnecessary details, some of which may be inappropriate

cistron (sis'tron) the smallest unit of genetic material that must be intact to function as a transmitter of genetic information; gene

claw toe a deformity involving hyperextension at the metatarsophalangeal joint and flexion at both the proximal and distal interphalangeal joints

clean catch specimen a urine specimen that is collected from the middle of the urine stream after the first part of the flow has been voided

cleidocranial dysplasia a condition recognised in infants because of drooping shoulders, open fontenellaes, prominent forehead, mild short stature and dental abnormalities

clinical *add* **c governance** a framework through which health organisations are accountable for continuously improving the quality of their services an safeguarding high standards of care b creating an environment in whic excellence in clinical care will flourish

guidelines systematically develope statements to assist practitioner an patient decisions about appropriat health care for specific circumstances

clinical target volume a tissue volume tha contains as demonstrable gross tumou volume and/ or subclinical microscopi malignant disease which is to b eliminated; CTV

clinical utility of a test likelihood that th test will lead to an important outcome

clinical validity of a test ability to detec or predict the presence or absence o clinical disease or predisposition to disease

clinician a health professional involved in clinical practice

cloning the process of generating multiple exact copies of a particular piece of DNA to allow it to be sequenced or studied in some other way

club drugs generic term for psychoactive drugs, usually illegal, that are used by participants of the rave and dance clubs and recreational drug subculture

CMO abbreviation for Chief Medical Officer, Casualty Medical Officer

Cobb's angle a measure of curvature of scoliosis, determined by measurements made on vertebrae

cocoon syndrome a lethal inherited condition due to deficiencies in CHUK characterized by multiple foetal malformations such as defective face and seemingly absent limbs, which are bound to the trunk and encased in a tight. abnormally thick and adhesive skin and the foetuses are spontaneously aborted

coding region portion of a gene's DNA or RNA that codes for its corresponding gene product

codon (cod'on) a three nucleotide sequence of DNA or RNA that specifies a single amino acid

cofactor a substance that works in combination with something else to bring about a certain effect

Cogan's syndrome interstitial corneal keratitis associated with sudden onset of deafness and vestibular symptoms, named after David Cogan who described the condition in 1945

cognitive as an ability to think, learn and memorize **c restructuring** the process of replacing maladaptive thought patterns with constructive thoughts and beliefs

cognitive behavioural therapy a psychotherapy with an aim to find the patterns of thinking that underlie a disorder and the ways to reinforce those thoughts

coinfection invasion of the body by two microorganisms at about the same time

coinosite (koi'no-sit) a free commensal organism; conasite

cold chain a system of storage and transport of vaccines at low termperature from the manufacturer to the actual vaccination site.

collateral blood vessels tiny, latent vessels that may spontaneously enlarge and become functional

collodion baby syndrome an extremely rare, fatal disorder where the babies are born covered by a tight yellow shiny membrane. As the membrane dries it leaves cracks on the skin which could result in infection, dehydration, and bleeding

coloclysis (ko'lo-kli'sis) irrigation of the colon

colony formation a phenotypically recognizable characterstic of cell transformation and a measure of malignant tumour-cell behaviour

colpocephaly (kol'po-si'fali) an isolated dilatation of the occipital horn presenting with mental retardation, spastic diplegia and visual impairment

colposuspension (kol'po-sus'pen-shun) suspension of the anterior vaginal wall at the level of the bladder neck in women with stress incontinence

columella (col'u-me-II-ah)the strip of skin running from the tip of the nose to the upper lip, which separates the nostrils

combination therapy the combination of various treatment methods

COMET Carvedilol or metaprolol European trial confirming the superiority of carvediolol over metaprolol in patients with heart failure

compages (kem-pa'jez) a joining together or that which is joined together

compartmental (kum-pahrt-men'tal) syndrome a condition in which increased tissue pressures in a confined anatomical space cause decreased blood flow leading to ischaemia and dysfunction of contained myoneural elements

compassion satisfactory pleasure derived from the work of helping of other **c fatigue** cost of caring for others in emotional pain that has led helping professionals to abandon than work with traumatised persons

complementary DNA a DNA molecule synthisised by an RNA dependent DNA polymerase from an RNA template

complex condition a condition caused by the interaction of multiple genes and environmental factors

complex regional pain syndrome reflex sympathetic dystrophy and casualgia

compression fatigue cost of caring for others in emotional pain that has led helping professionals to abandon that work with traumatized persons

compression satisfaction pleasure derived from the work of helping others

comptocormia (com'to-kor-miya) postural abnormality characterized by involuntary truncal flexion induced by standing or sitting, often associated with other neurologic disorders

comptomelic dysplasia a condition noted in newborn infants characterised by bowing of long bones especially in lower legs, short bones, respiratory distress and other anomalies that include defects of the cervical spine, central nervous system, heart and kidneys

compulsory gambling disorder an impulse control disorder in which an individual cannot resist gambling despite repeated losses

computed tomographic angiography a diagnostic study in which a contrast substance is injected into the circulation and its movement is the tracked by a tomographic X-ray device

computed tomographic calcium scoring a diagnostic study that allows visualization of calcium deposits in the blood vessels, especially the coronary arteries

conduct disorder *psy* a repetitive and persistent pattern of behavior in which the basic rights of others are violated or major age-appropriate rules of society are broken

confidence interval *stat* a range of values for a random sample within lies, with reasonable probability the true value of something being studied in a given population

conflict *psy* an emotional struggle that arises from opposing issues

confocal fluorescence microendoscopy in vivo microscopic observation of the airways and alveoli with a device using a blue laser which has been adapted within a small probe that can be advanced through the working channel of the bronchoscope into the distal airways and alveoli to induce fluorescence; alveolscopy

conisation (ko'ni-ze'shun) removal of a cone-shaped section of tissue from the cervix for diagnosis or treatment; cone biopsy

connectome (con'ec-tom) major neural connections in the brain

Contarini's (kon'tar'i-ni) **condition** bilateral pleural effusion with pus on one side and clear fluid on other secondary to cardiac decompensation, named after 95th doge of Venice

contextual therapy the study and treatment of a phobia in the actual setting in which the phobia reactions occur

contig (kon-tig) the result of joining an overlapping collection of sequences or clones **fingerprint clone c** contigs produced by joining clones inferred to overlap on the basis of their restriction digest fingerprints **initial sequence c** contigs produced by merging overlapping sequence reads obtained from a single clone in a process called sequence assembly **merged sequence c** contigs produced by taking the initial sequence contigs contained in overlapping clones and merging those found to overlap **sequence c** merged sequence contigs **sequenced-clone c** contigs produced by merging overlapping sequenced clones

contrast a substance injected into the body that illuminates certain structures that would otherwise be hard to see on the radiograph

contrast solution any material used in imaging tests to help outline the body parts being examined

conventional therapy treatments that are widely accepted and practiced

cooling treatment a treatment modality to lower body temperature in order to relieve pain, swelling, constriction of blood vessels and to decrease the likelihood of cellular damage by slowing the metabolism

coping *psy* a person's patterns of response to stress

coplanar(co'pla-nur) within the same plane

COPP a cancer chemotherapy regimen consisting of cyclophosphamide, oncovin (vincristine), procarbazine and prednisone

copy number variation variation from one person to next in the number of copies of a particular gene or DNA sequence

copy-number aberration an increase or decrease in the number of copies of DNA segments oftens to hundreds of base pairs in size

cord colitis syndrome a persistent diarrhoeal illness in a patient undergoing cord blood haematopoietic stem cell transplantation

cordocentesis (car'do-sen-te'sis) a procedure for delivering a blood transfusion to a foetus that involves threading a fine needle through a pregnant woman's abdomen and into the umbilical cord with the aid of ultrasound imaging

corpulent (cor'pu-lent) bulky

corpus diictii *for* body of evidence which denotes homicide

corset (cor'set) support device for the back

cosmeceutical (cos'me-su'ti-cal) agents that are active topically

costa *add* **c cervicalis** cervical rib **c fluctuantis** floating ribs, the lower two ribs on either side which ordinarily have no ventral attachment **c spruriae** false ribs, the lower five ribs on either side **c varae** true ribs, upper seven ribs on either side

counterpulsation (kown'ter-pul-sa'shun) a technique for assisting the circulation and decreasing the work of the heart by synchronising the force of an external pumping device with cardiac systole and diastole

COX 2 abbreviation for cyclooxygenase-2

CPD courses continuing professional developmental courses

CPPB abbreviation for continuous positive pressure breathing

Cri du chat syndrome a chromosomal disorder wherein a piece of chromosomal material is missing from a particular region of chromosome 5 and presents .with unusual facial features, hypotonia, microcephaly, mental retardation and cat-like cry; chromosome-5 deletion syndrome, cat cry syndrome

Cronkite Canada syndrome marked epithelial disturbances in the gastrointestinal tract and epidermis characterised by a triad of epidermal changes including alopaecia, onychodystrophy and generalised hyperpigmentation, described by Cronkite and Canada in 1955

cross match a test to determine if patient and donor tissue are compatible

crud an ill defined bodily ailment

cruor (kroo'or) a blood clot

crush syndrome failure of the kidneys resulting from violent compression of muscle tissue

cryonics (kri'o-niks) practice of freezing dead persons in hopes of later restoring life

cryopreservation (kri'o-pre-ser'va-shun) preservation of tissue, sperm, fluid, blood or plasma at extremely low temperatures

C-section caesarean section

CSF1 abbreviation for colony stimulating factor 1

CTGF abbreviation for connective tissue growth factor

cud (kud) the bolus of partially digested food

cudding (kud'ing) rumination

cue (q) a pattern of stimuli to which a person has learnt to respond

cuffing (kuf'ing) the formation of a cuff-like surrounding border

curly toe a condition caused by contracture of the flexor digitorum longus, presenting with flexion at the metatarsophalangeal and interphalangeal joints and medial deviation of the toes

cushingoid (koosh'in-goid) resembling the features of Cushing syndrome

CUSP abbreviation for clinical ultrasonography in practice, enables doctors to keep track of advances in the field of ultrasonography and its application

cut off a critical value for an analyte above or below which the value is considered abnormal

cutdown surgical incision of the skin to expose a vein and permit the insertion of a catheter or needle for administration of medication, withdrawal of blood or diagnostic or therapeutic catheterization

cyanphobia (si'no-fo-be-a) irrational fear of dogs

cyber knife an image-guided frameless stereotactic radiosurgery delivery system, consisting of a light-weight linear accelerator mounted on a robotic arm and uses real-time X-rays to establish the position of lesion during treatment and then brings the radiation beam into alignment with the observed position of treatment target

cyclic vomiting syndrome a rare idiopathic disorder characterized by recurring periods of vomiting in an otherwise normal child or adult

cyclothymic disorder *psy* disorder a mood disorder characterized by mild mood swings

cystography (sis'to-gra-fi) a detailed x-ray examination of urethra and bladder that uses contrast dye to enhance the images

cystometrography (sis'to-met'ro-gra-fi) a procedure that measures varying pressure levels as bladder fills with, and then releases, urine

cytochrom P450 a heterogenous group of enzymes that catalyses various oxidative reactions in the human liver, intestine, kidney, lung and central nervous system

cyton (si'ton) perikaryon

cytonecrosis (si'to-ne-kro'sis) death of individual cells

cytopaenia (si'to-pe'ne-a) deficiency in number of any of the cellular elements of the blood

D

D and E abbreviation for dilatation and evacuation

D Ch abbreviation for Diploma in child health

D F M abbreviation for Diploma in Forensic Medicine

D G O abbreviation for Diploma in Obstetrics and Gynaecology

d/c abbreviation for discontinue

DA abbreviation for Diploma in Anaesthesia, developmental age

DALYs abbreviation for disability adjusted life years

Damocles syndrome a person with cancer is so preoccupied with their uncertain future that they find it difficult to get on with their day-to-day life

Dance's sign detection of an elongated mass in the right upper quadrant or epigastrium with an absence of bowel in the right lower quadrant in intussusception

DASH Dietary approaches to Stop Hypertension, a low-fat, low-cholesterol diet plan with a low sodium-content, that lowers blood pressure

day surgery planned operative procedure on patients who are admitted and discharged home on the same day of the surgery

de novo mutation any DNA sequence change that occurs during replication

de novo mutation any DNA sequence change that occurs during replication in a family for the first time

death *add* **neonatal d** the death of a live-born infant during the period that commences at birth and ends 28 completed days after birth **perinatal d** the death of a foetus weighing at least 500 gm or the death of an infant during the first week of life

death trance *for* obvious absence of apparent signs of life which cannot be determined by ordinary clinical tests due to suspended state of activity of heart, lungs, brain etc associated with a state of insensibility or loss of voluntary power; suspended animation

debulking surgical procedure in which subcutaneous tissue is removed by lymphoedematous limb

decubitus ulcer a pressure sore resulting from ulceration of the skin occurring in persons confined to bed for a long period of time

deep bite *den* a deep or excessive overbite in which the lower incisors bite too loosely to or into the gum tissue, or palate behind the upper teeth

deep sequencing genetic sequencing at sufficiently high coverage to identify low-frequency mutations

deficiency disease any disease caused by a lack of an essential nutrient

defloration (di'flo-ra'shun) for loss of virginity

defloration *for* loss of virginity

deformation (di'for-ma'shun) temporary or permanent damage in a dimension of a body under external loading

delayed sleep phase disorder a condition characterized by reported sleep onset and wake times are intractably later than desired, though actual sleep times are nearly the same

deletion removal of a piece of a genetic material

delle (del'lay) a central, lighter coloured portion of the erythrocyte as observed in a stained blood film

demagogue (de'mo-gog) one who leads using emotional appeals

dendromer (den'dro-mer) tree-shaped synthetic molecules formed with a regular branching structure

denial *psy* a defense mechanism whereby one refuses to acknowledge what is present and often obvious to others

Denver classification the classification of human chromosomes on the basis of size and centromere position; the 23 pairs of chromosomes are classified in 7 groups in order of decreasing length

Denys-Drash syndrome a constellation of nephropathy with ambiguous genitals and bilateral Wilm's tumour

depersonalisation *psy* a dissociative symptom in which the patient feels that his or her body is unreal, is changing or is dissolving

depot dosage a form of medication that can be stored in the patient's body tissues for several days or weeks, thus minimizing the risk of the patient forgetting daily doses

depot injection a medicating technique in which a drug is released over a period of two to four weeks

deprivation a condition of having too little of something

derailment (de'rale-me'nt) *psy* a pattern of speech in which a person's ideas slip off one track onto another that is completely unrelated or only obliquely related

derealisation *psy* a dissociative symptom in which the external environment is perceived as unreal

dermabrasion a technique for removing the upper layers of skin with plain wheals powered by compressed air

developmental delay the failure to meet certain developmental milestones such as sitting, standing, walking and talking at the average age

DEXA dual energy X-ray absorpiometry; use of low dose radiation of two different energies to mesure bone mineral content at different anatomical sites

dharana (s) to fix one's mind

dhat ayu psy severe anxiety and hypochondriacal concerns associated with the discharge of semen, whitish discolouration of the urine and the feelings of weakness and exhaustion

dhatu ayu body tissues

dhee(s) reception

dhi ayu power of discrimination between right and wrong, good and bad, useful and harmful

dhriti (s) retention

dhriti ayu ability to retain experiences as memory

dhyana (s) meditation

diabesity (di-a'be-siti) obesity and diabetes developing together

DIAPPERS acronym representing causes of urinary incompetence, Delirium, Infection, Atrophic urethritis, Pharmacological (drugs), Psychological, Excess urine output as in diabetes, congestive heart failure, Restricted mobility, Stool impaction

diastrophic dysplasia a characteristic disorder recognised at birth by the presence of very short extremities, club foot and short hands with proximal displacement of the thumb producing a hitchhiker appearance

dicer an RNase III enzyme involved in cleaving hairpin-shaped double-stranded RNA precursor structures

dichroism (dy'kro'izm) the property of seeming to be differently coloured when seen from different directions

DIDMOAD syndrome hereditary association of diabetes insipides, diabetes mellitus, optic atrophy and deafness; Wolfram's syndrome

diopterics (di'of-ter'iks) the branch of optics concerned with the refraction of light

dioxin (di'oxi-n) a highly toxic organic compound coming as an unwanted by-product of industrial and combustion activity

discombobulate (dis'kom-bu'lat) to upset, confuse

disease marker specific molecular signature of disease, physiological measurements, genotype structural or functional characteristics, metabolic changes or other determinants that may simply the diagnostic process

disease toxonomy the science of disease classification

disfluency an interruption in speech flow

disorder *add* **adjustment d** the development of emotional or behavioural symptoms in response to an identifiable stressor(s) occurring within 3 months of the onset of the stressor(s) **Asperger's d** qualitative impairment in social interaction **body conduct d** a repetitive and persistent pattern of behaviour in which the basic requests of others or major age-appropriate societal norms or values are violated **depersonalisation d** persistent or recurrent experiences of feeling detached from, and as if one is an outside observer of, one's mental process or body developmental coordination **d performance** in daily activities that require motor coordination is substantially below that expected given the person's chronological age and measured intelligence **dysmorphic d** preoccupation with an imagined defect in appearance **factitious d** intentional production or freigning of physical or psychological signs or symptoms **female orgasmic d** persistent or recurrent delay in, or absence of, orgasm following a normal sexual excitement phase **female sexual arousal d** persistent or recurrent inability to attain, or to maintain until completion of the sexual activity, an adequate lubrication-swelling response of sexual excitement **gender identity d** a strong and persistent cross-gender identification **hypoactive sexual desire d** persistently or recurrently deficient or absent sexual fantasies and desire for sexual activity **intermittent explosive d** several discrete episodes of failure to resist aggressive impulses that result in serious assault acts or destruction of property **male erective d** persistent or recurrent inability to attain, or to maintain until completion of the sexual activity, an adequate erection **male orgasmic d** persistent or recurrent delay in, or absence of, orgasm following a normal sexual excitement phase **nightmare d** repeated awakenings from the major sleep period or naps with detailed recall of extended or extremely frightening dreams, usually involving threats to survival, security, or self esteem **oppositional defiant d** a pattern of negativistic, hostile and defiant behaviour **gender identity d** a strong and persistent cross-gender identification **hypoactive sexual desire d** persistently or recurrently deficient or absent sexual fantasies and desire for sexual activity **intermittent explosive d** several discrete episodes of failure to resist aggressive impulses that result in serious assault acts or destruction of property **male erective d** persistent or recurrent inability to attain, or to maintain exection until completion of the sexual activity, an adequate erection **male orgasmic d** persistent or recurrent delay in, or absence of, orgasm following a normal sexual excitement phase **nightmare d** repeated awakenings from the major sleep period or naps with detailed recall of extended or extremely frightening dreams, usually involving threats to survival, security, or self esteem **oppositional defiant d** a pattern of negativistic, hostile and defiant behaviour lasting at least 6 months **rumination d** repeated regurgitation and re-chewing of food for a period of at least 1 month following a period of normal functioning **schizotypal personality d** a pervasive pattern of social and interpersonal deficits marked by acute discomfort with, and reduced capacity for, close relationships as well as by cognitive or perpetual distortions and eccentricities of behaviour, beginning by early adulthood **separation anxiety d** development of inappropriate and excessive anxiety concerning separation from home or from those to whom the individual is attached **sexual aversion d** persistent or recurrent extreme aversion to, and avoidance of all genital sexual contact with a sexual partner **shared psychotic d** development of delusion in an individual in the context of a close relationship with another person(s), who has an already established delusion **sleep walking d** repeated episodes of rising from bed during sleep and walking about, usually occurring during the first third of the major sleep episode **stereotypic movement d repetitive** seemingly driven, and non-functional motor behaviour

dissociative *psy* identity disorder condition in which two or more distinctive identities or personality states alternate in controlling a person's consciousness and behaviour

DM abbreviation for diabetes mellitus, Doctor of Medicine, diastolic murmur, dopamine

DME abbreviation for Director of Medical Education

DMER abbreviation for Director of Medical Education and Research

DMLT abbreviation for Diploma in Medical Laboratory Technology

DMRD abbreviation for Diploma in Medical Radiodiagnosis

DMRT abbreviation for Diploma in Medical Radiotherapy

DNA adducts chemical changes in DNA molecule that have not been specified by the four bases

DNA helicase an enzyme that separates and unwinds the two DNA strands in preparation for replication or transcription

DNA library a collection of DNA fragments that are cloned into plasmids or viral genomes

DNA ligase an enzyme that joins two DNA strands together to make a continuous DNA molecule

DNA methylation the addition of a methyl group to DNA at the 5-carbon of the cytosine pyrimidine ring that precedes a guanine

DNA methyltransferases family of enzymes that catalyze the transfer of a methyl group to DNA using S-adenosyl methionine as the methyl donor

DNA microarray a technology that is used to study many genes or other sequences at once

DNA primate an enzyme that synthesizes a short strant of RNA that serves as a primer for DNA replication

DNA repair capacity ability of natural cellular processes to repair mistakes that occur in DNA

DNB abbreviation for Diplomat of National Board

DNR *abb* do not resuscitate

DO abbreviation for Diploma in Ophthalmology

DOA abbreviation for date of admission

DOB abbreviation for date of birth

DOD abbreviation for date of discharge

DOE abbreviation for dyspnoea on exertion

DON abbreviation for Director of Nursing

double cortex syndrome a genetic defect with presence of a band of grey matter within the subcortical white matter presenting with mental retardation and epilepsy

double outlet ventricle a complex congenital defect in which both the aorta and pulmonary artery arise from one rather than two ventricles

DPB abbreviation for Diploma in Pathology and Bacteriology

DPH abbreviation for Diploma in Public Health

DPI abbreviation for dry powder inhaler

DPM abbreviation for Diploma in Psychological Medicine

Dr abbreviation for Doctor

drainage angle the tiny channel through which fluid leaves the eyeball

DRESS syndrome drug rash with eosinophilia and systemic symptoms; a severe form of cutaneous drug reaction characterised by fever, skin rash, lymphadenopathy, haematological abnormalities, and internal organ involvement

drip rate rate in which the fluid drips from the intravenous bag into the intravenous line

drooling (dru'ling) slow seepage of saliva from the mouth

drop attack sudden loss of tone

drosha RNase III enzyme involved in cutting the endogenous double-stranded RNA segments into short, hairpin-shaped double stranded RNA precursor structures

drusen tiny yellow dots on retina that can be soft or hard and that usually do not interfere with vision

dry socket *Dent* a painful condition following tooth extraction in which a blood clot does not properly fill the empty socket, leaving the bone underneath exposed to air and food

DS abbreviation for double strength

Duke criteria clinical criteria described at Duke University, North Carolina for the diagnosis of infective endocarditis that includes two major criteria such as positive blood culture and evidence of valvular heart disease

Duke's criteria clinical criteria described by Duke University, North Carolina, US for

the diagnosis of infective endocarditis that include the major criteria of a positive blood culture, and evidence of valvular disease, and minor criteria of fever and evidence of embolism

dying declaration *for* a statement-written or oral-made by a dying person since then dead, as to the cause or circumstances bearing material facts relating to his/her impending death

dysaesthesia unpleasant parasthesia

dysbiosis (dis'bi-o-sis) the condition that results when the natural flora of the gut are thrown out of balance such as when antibiotics are taken

dysbiosis (dis'bi-o-sis) an immune response to the newly established microbiota in the ileal pouch

dyskeratosis congenita a rare form of ectodermal dysplasia characterised by reticulated hyperpigmentation of the face, neck and shoulders, dystrophic nails and mucous membrane leukoplakia

dysmelodia (dis'mel-o-de'a) selective impairment of cortical module that perceives melody of the music

dystimbria (dis'tim-bri'a) selective impairment of cortical module that perceives timbre of the music

E

e health record a system capable of providing health information and data, result management, order entry and support and decision support; EHR

early detection of health impairment the detection of disturbances of homoeostatic and compensatory mechanisms while biochemical, morphological and functional changes are still reversible

early neonatal death death of a live born neonate during the first 7 days after birth

echopraxia (ek'o-pra'ksia) psy repetition by imitation of the movements of another

ectrodactyly (ek'tro-dac'tili) malformation consisting split hands and feet

Edward's syndrome disorder characterized by multiple physical abnormalities and severe mental retardation caused by an extra copy of chromosome 18; trisomy 18 syndrome

effector protein a protein that is secreted by microbes directly into a host cell to alter physiological processes in the host

efferocytosis (ef'er-o'sito-sis) a process by which apoptotic or necrotic cells are removed by phagocytosis

effusive-constrictive pericarditis a clinical condition consisting of both pericardial effusion and constrictive pericarditis

EGFR abbreviation for epidermal growth factor receptor

egg on side sign a radiologic appearance of Ebstein's malformation exhibiting pulmonary oligaemia, severe right atrial dilatation and an inapparent aorta

ego alien *psy* thoughts that are repugnant, recurrent, unwanted, undesired and not consistent with a person's usual thinking

egomania (eg'o-ma'nea) extreme self appreciation

ejaculation *add* **premature e** persistent or recurrent ejaculation with minimal sexual stimulation before, on, or shortly after penetration and before the person wishes it

ejection fraction the fraction of all blood in the ventricle that is ejected at each heart beat

Ekbom syndrome a rare psychiatric disorder manifesting as a delusion, or hallucination of parasitic infestation, named after Karl Ekbom, a Swedish neurologist who described the condition in 1938; delusions of infestation, parasitophobia, neurodermatitis

El Nino effect a shift of a warm equatorial water from the Western to Eastern Pacific ocean, occurring every 2 to 7 years leading to extremely dry conditions, drought, devastating fires in many regions of the World and torrential rains and flooding in other regions

electrical alternans alternating amplitude of the QRS complexes with every other beat in ECG

electrocautery (e'lek-tro-kat-eri) application of direct current flowing in one direction

electrochemical gradient a differential concentration of an ion or molecule across the cell membrane that serves as a source of potential energy and may polarize the cell electrically

electromagnetic navigation bronchoscopy ENB; a bronchoscopic procedure that allows biopsy instruments directly reaching the mediastinal lymph nodes or peripheral nodules

electrophysiological testing a diagnostic study done in a catheterization laboratory in which a catheter is guided to the heart and electrodes are used to make detailed recordings of the heart's electrical system and activity

elimination zero disease in a defined geographic area as a result of deliberate efforts, and control measures needed to prevent reestablishment of transmission

eltrombopag (el'trom-bo'paj) orally active thrombopoietin-receptor agonist that stimulates thrombopoiesis

elution (e-loo'shun) separation of material by washing

emmenagogue (em'me-na-gog) a substance that encourages menstrual flow

emotional exhaustion feelings or being overextended and depleted of one's emotional and physical resources

empirical based on experience

EMR abbreviation for electronic medical record

EMS abbreviation for emergency medical service

encatarrhaphy (en'cat-a'ra-fi) the artificial implantation of an organ or tissue in a part where it does not naturally occur

encode process of giving exact genetic instructions for building protein

encopresis (en'ko-pres'is) repeated passage of faeces into inappropriate places

end of life care multi-dimensional and multi-disciplinary physical, emotional and social care of patients with terminal illness

end stage the final period in the course of a progressive disease leading to a patient's death

end-diastolic volume the volume of blood in the ventricle at the end of diastole

endoscopy *add* **endoluminal e** introduction of flexible or rigid endoscopes into hollow organs or systems **perivascular e** access into the body planes in the absence of a natural cavity such as mediastinoscopy, retroperitoneoscopy

engagement descent of the foetus head into the mother's pelvis

enhanced external counterpulsation a treatment for angina in which pressure cuffs compress blood vessels to increase the return of blood to the heart during the diastolic phase

enhancer a DNA regulatory sequence that provides a binding site for transcription factors capable of increasing the rate of transcription for a specific gene

Enterobacter sakazakii a gram-negative non-spore forming bacteria belonging to the Enterobacteriacease family, whose infection leads to sepsis, meningitis, encephalitis and necrotizing enterocolitis

entrainment the patterning of body processes and movements to the rhythm of music

entrapment neuropathy sensory and motor symptoms in the distribution of individually entrapped peripheral nerves

eosinophilic pustular folliculitis a chronic and relapsing dermatosis seen in East Asian population. The condition begins as small papules which enlarge and coalesce into a large plaque, usually on the face; Ofuji's diseae

EPI abbreviation for expanded program of immunisation

epialleles (epi'al-lels) genes along with their respective epigenetic factors stable through a few transgnerations in a cellular population

epidermolytic (ep'i-derm-mo-ly'tik) damaging the top layer of the skin

epigenesis (epi'jene-sis) a fundamental regulatory system beyond nucleotide sequence information of DNA

epigenetic inheritance inheriting traits transmitted by mechanisms not directly involving gene's nucleotide sequence

epigenetic related to heritable phenotypes or modifications not based in the DNA sequence add before epigenetic inheritance

epigenetics (epi'gen-e'tiks) study of heritable changes in gene expression that do not involve changes in DNA sequence

epigenome (epi'ji-nom) the overall epigenetic state of a cell

epileptologist a physician specialized in the treatment of epilepsy

epimutations (epi'mut-a-shuns) heritable defects in gene expression that do not involve changes in DNA sequence

epiphenomenon (epi'fena-me'non) an additional condition or symptom in the course of a disease, not necessarily connected with the disease

Epley manoeuvre a gentle but specific manipulation of rotation of the patient's head to shift the loose otoliths from the semicircular canal as a treatment of benign paroxysmal positional vertigo

equator imaginary line encircling the eye ball and dividing the eye into a front and back hall

eradication (e'radi-ka-shun) zero disease globally as a result of deliberate efforts and control measures no longer needed

Erdheim-Chester disease a relentlessly progressive non-Langerhans' cell systemic histiocytosis presenting with pain and sclerotic lesions in the long bones, extraskeletal involvement including the orbit, the hypothalamic-pituitary-sella area, the retroperitoneum and periaortic tissues, the lungs and the heart

erotographomania (er'o-to-fo'ma-nea) sexual gratification obtained by obscene writing

erotographomania sexual gratification obtained by obscene writing

errhine (er'rin) a substance that induces sneezing and nasal discharge

ERV abbreviation for expiratory reserve volume

EST expressed sequence tag a short sequence from a coding region of a gene that identifies the gene

et al and other people

ethical analysis a process of thinking through ethical problems and reaching a conclusion; moral reasoning

ethical matters involving 1 moral principles or practices, 2 matters of social policy involving issues of morality in the practice of medicine

Evan's syndrome a clinical condition characterised by immune thrombocytopaenia and autoimmune haemolytic anaemia with no known underlying cause, described by Evans and colleagues in 1951

evidence-based medicine conscientious explicit, and judicious use of current best evidence in making decisions about the case of individual patients. It integrates individual clinical expertise with the best available external clinical evidence from systematic research; EBM

evisceration (eve'ser-a'shun) removal of eye contents

executive profile a battery of laboratory parameters that may be measured annually in executives in order to detect any disease

exercise stress test an electrocardiogram that is done while a person exercises on a treadmill or stationary bicycle

exhumation (ex'hu-ma-shun) for lawful disinternment or taking out of an already buried body from the grave for medicolegal purpose when autopsy examination is imperative

EXIT procedure ex-utero intrapartum treatment procedure adapted in circumstances in which an airway obstruction is predicted at the time of delivery due to the presence of a large neck mass

exome (ek-some) all the expressed messenger RNA-sequences in any tissue

exome the portion of the genome which includes all the coding DNA

expiration date the last date in which a medicine should be used

exposome characteristics of both exogenous and endogenous exposures that can have differential effects at various stages during person's life time

external beam radiation therapy radiation that is focused on the area affected by cancer from a source outside the body; EBRT

extractable nuclear antigen nuclear components that are solutes in saline; ENB

extramedullary haematopoiesis development and growth of haematopoieic tissue outside of the bone marrow; EMH

extremely low birth weight a newborn whose weight is less than 1000 gms

extrophy (ecs'tro-fi) being turned inside out combined with being outside the body

ezetinibe (eze-ti'nib) a selective cholesterol and related phytosterols absorption inhibitor from small intestine

F

face association *psy* a technique used in psychoanalysis in which the patient allows thoughts and feelings to emerge without trying to organise or censor them

face lift surgery a cosmetic procedure that involves redirecting some of the skin and muscle tissue of the face and neck to counter signs of aging produced by gravity

failed back syndrome a condition experienced by patients who undergo a surgical procedure with unsatisfactory results

failure to thrive an infant or child does not gain weight or grow in height at a normal rate

falling out a sudden collapse which sometimes occurs without warning but sometimes preceded by feelings of dizziness

false negative test results showing no problem when one exists

false positive test results showing a problem when one does not exist

FAMS abbreviation for Fellow of Academy of Medical Sciences (India)

FAST scan focussed abdominal sonar for trauma

fate mapping method used to determine the cellular derivatives of a cell or population of cells

FDA abbreviation for federal drug administration

Feldenkrais method a therapy based on creating a good self image by correction and improvements of body movements, named after Moshe Feldenkrais

female athletic triad a combination of disorders frequently found in female athletes that includes disordered eating, osteoporosis and oligo- or amenorrhoea

fervescence (fer-ve'sens) increase of fever or body temperature

festoon (fes-toon) a carving in the base material of a denture that simulates the contours of the natural tissues it is replacing

FGFR abbreviation for fibroblast growth factor receptor

FICA abbreviation for Fellow of Indian College of Physicians

FICS abbreviation for Fellow of International College of Surgeons

fiducials (phi'du-se-yals) markers that help to precisely identify the targeted tumour location

fight-or-flight response reaction to stress produced by the adrenal glands and autonomic nervous system

filling *dent* dental material that occupies the space remaining within a tooth after the decayed portion has been removed

filopodia (fil'o-pod'ea) *dent* cytoplasmal extension

fine mapping an experimental approach to narrowing a genome-wide association signal by typing all known SNPs in the haplotype lock containing the tap SNP

finger stick a technique for collecting a very small amount of blood from the finger tip region

Fitz-Hugh-Curtis syndrome inflammation of the liver capsule associated with genital tract infection

five (5)-year survival rate the percentage of people with a given cancer who are expected to survive 5 years or longer with the disease

fixative a chemical that is used to preserve cells and tissues

flap a section of tissue moved from one area of the body to another **tissue f** section of tissue detached from its blood supply, moved to another part of the body and reattached by microsurgery to new blood supply **pedicle f** a section of tissue with its blood supply intact, which is maneuvered to another part of the body

flashback *psy* a recurrence of a memory, feeling or perceptual experience from the past

flat affect an absence of facial expression

flat *psy* absence or near-absence of any signs of affective expression remove existing and add this

floccillation (fla-ci-la-shun) an aimless plucking at the bed clothes; corphologia

flossing (fla'sing) *den* preventive dental procedure involving soft nylon or silk thread

fluid sign a focal, linear or triangular area of strong hyperintensity, which is isointense relative to CSF or T2 weighted sagittal images

fluorescein (flu're-sin) a fluorescent chemical used to examine the cornea

fluorescence in situ hybridization a laboratory technique for detecting and locating a specific DNA sequence on a chromosome; FISH

FNAB abbreviation for fine needle aspiration biopsy

FNAC abbreviation for fine needle aspiration cytology

FNB abbreviation for Fellow of National Board

FOB abbreviation for fiberoptic bronchoscopy

foetal alcohol syndrome a cluster of birth defects that includes abnormal facial features and mental retardation caused by the mother's consumption of alcoholic beverages during pregnancy

FOGSI abbreviation for Federation of Obstetric and Gynaecologic Societies of India

fondaparnux a synthetic pentasaccharide causing rapid and predictable inhibition of factor Xa

Fontan procedure a surgical procedure for advanced and complex congenital heart disease that redirects blood from the venous system directly to the pulmonary arteries without passing through the usually deformed or obstructed ventricle, first described by Francois Marie Fontan of France

foot progression angle angle between long axis of foot and direction of gait

foot thigh angle angle between line of foot and thigh

forensic medicine branch of medical discipline which deals with the application of medical knowledge to the administration of law

Forestier (for'es-tear) **disease** diffuse, idiopathic skeletal hyperostosis characterised by a tendency toward ossification of ligaments, especially spine giving an appearance of candle wax dripping down the spine

forward and reverse strands two strands of a double stranded DNA molecule

four-dimentional coformal radiation therapy measurement of the natural tumour motion that occurs during treatment, that is included in the treatment plan to ensure that the tumour is targeted throughout the treatment cours

FP abbreviation for family planning

fracture *add* **avulsion f** two fragments of bone are pulled apart **burst f** fracture caused by hyperflexion of the spine usually accompanied by axial compression, and fragments of bone are pushed circumferentially **butterfly f** if a bone is struck a direct blow when two break lines spread out obliquely from the point of contact of the blow producing a free-floating butterfly fragments between the two fractures **commuted f** occurrence of fracture when a large amount of energy is dissipated into bone. The bone breaks into fragments which may impact into each other or separate and become displaced **compression f** if load applied along the length of a bone exceeds that of its strength then it may collapse into itself **distraction f** avulsion fracture **Galeazzi f** a distal radius fracture with separation of the distal ulnar epiphysis rather than a true joint disruption **green stick f** occurrence of fracture in young people where bones are very flexible. They bend and then may buckle or partially break when over loaded **Hangman's f** a fracture of the pedicle of C2 vertebra caused by hyperextension of the spine **Jefferson f** fracture of the ring of C1 vertebra, usually caused by axial loading, named after Jefferson, English neurosurgeon **Manteggia f** injury characterised by a dislocation of the radial head at the elbow together with a ulna fracture **partial f** green stick fracture **pathological f** occurrence of fracture when the strength of bone is reduced by disease **stress f** occurrence of fracture when bones are subjected to a very large number of loads, none of which alone would be enough to break the bone but which means that the mechanical structure of the bone can gradually fatigue **tear-drop f** fracture-dislocation where part of the injury goes through the lower part of the vertebra and part of the injury is ligamentous **traumatic f** occurrence of fracture when an excessive load is applied to normal bone **wedge f** most common lower cervical spine fracture caused by hyperflexion of the spine where bone is compressed

frailty (fra'l-ti) a collection of biomedical factors which influence on individual's physiological state in a way that reduces his or her capacity to withstand

Framingham risk score a multivariable statistical model that uses age, sex, smoking history, blood pressure, cholesterol, high-density lipoprotein cholesterol, and blood glucose levels or history of diabetes to estimate coronary event risk among individuals without previously diagnosed coronary heart disease. FRS

FRCOG abbreviation for Fellow of Royal College of Obstetricians and Gynaecologists

FRCP abbreviation for Fellow of Royal College of Physicians

FRCS abbreviation for Fellow of Royal College of Surgeons

free radical an unstable molecule that causes oxidative damage by stealing electrons from surrounding molecules, thereby disrupting activity in the body's cells

free water a concept describing the movement of water independent of sodium

frotheurism (fro'th-ur'izm) recurrent, intense sexually arousing fantasies, sexual urges, or behaviour involving touching and rubbing against a non-consenting person, over a period of at least 6 months

frottage (fro'ta-j) pervert way of obtaining sexual pleasure by rubbing sexual organs against someone

frozen shoulder a shoulder that becomes scarred and cannot move

functional MRI a technique to map the functioning of human brain that is dependent on regional blood perfusion, blood volume and blood oxygenation that accompany the neuronal activity, fMRI

fundoplication (fun'du-pli-ka-shun) a surgical procedure that increases presence on the lower oesophageal sphincter by stretching and wrapping the upper part of the stomach around the sphincter

FW abbreviation for family welfare

G

gadolinium a very rare metallic element useful for its sensitivity to electromagnetic resonance

gambler's fallacy the erroneous belief that the outcomes of recent random events have some bearing on future random events: the Monte Carlo fallacy

gamma knife a non-invasive surgical procedure that uses computer-guided gamma rays produced by radioactive material, cobalt-60. The blades of the knife act as the beams of gamma radiation programmed to target lesion at the point where they interact

gandha (s) smell sensation, aroma

Ganser's syndrome an unusual factitious disorder characterized by dissociative symptoms and absurd answers to direct questions

gap junction a communication channel in the membranes of adjacent cells that allows free passage of ions and small molecules

gastroparesis (gas'tr-o-par-e'sis) a syndrome characterised by delayed gastric emptying with features of postprandial fullness, nausea, vomiting and bloating in the absence of mechanical obstruction of the stomach

gender dysphoria *psy* persistent aversion toward some or all of those physical characters or social roles that cannot one's own biological sex

gender identity disorder a male or female that feels a strong identification with the opposite sex and experiences considerable disturbances because of their actual sex

gene deserts large intergenic regions

gene dosage the copy number for a specific gene as determined in analytic approaches that do not assess single cells but describe the average copy number profile of a complex tumour in which some cell populations may harbor copy number alterations of the gene and some may not

gene knock-down techniques by which the expression of one or more of an organism's genes are reduced by treatment with a specific sequence of RNA that targets a specific gene

gene regulatory protein any protein that binds to DNA and thereby affects the expression of a specific gene

gene repressor protein any protein that binds to DNA and blocks transcription of a specific gene

general intelligence factor a dominant, underlying factor determining intelligence; g factor

generic drugs non-proprietory drugs

generic name non-proprietary name of a medication

genetic anticipation a process in which successive generations of patients with some genetic disorders present earlier and with progressively worse symptoms. It is due to expression of the trinucleotide repeat within the disease gene with each generation

genetic association a relationship that is defined by the nonrandom occurrence of a genetic marker with a trait, which suggests an association between the genetic marker and disease pathogenesis

genetic linkage a relationship that is defined by the coinheritance of a genetic marker with disease in a family with multiple disease affected members

genetic medicine use of knowledge about single genes to improve the diagnosis and treatment of single-gene disorders

genetic test laboratory studies of blood or other tissue to identify genetic disorders

genogram (je'no-gram) a family assessment tool consisting of a family tree diagram depicting family dispersals, losses, roles of organisational patterns over three or more generations

genome reduction a decrease in the genome size during evolution of an organism

genomewide association study an approach used in genetics research to look for associations between many specific genetic variations and particular diseases

genomewide scan an assay that measures hundreds of thousands to millions of points of genetic variations across a person's genome simultaneously

genomic islands regions of a genome with distinct nucleotide composition or with clusters of genes that encode specialized functions

genomic library a collection of DNA fragments, obtained by digesting genomic DNA with a restriction enzyme, that are cloned into plasmid or viral vectors

genomic medicine use of knowledge about interactions between the genome and non-genomic factors from which new diagnostic and therapeutic approaches are emerging

genotype a person's complete collection of genes

Gertie Marx needle needle used for epidural anaesthesia for women in labour, named to honour Gertie, a US anaesthesiologist

Gestalt therapy *Ger* a humanistic therapeutic technique that focuses on gaining an awareness of emotions and behaviour in the present rather than in the past

gestogenic (ges'to-gen'ik) inducing progestational effects in the uterus

ghrelin (gre'lin) a secretion by endocrine cells of oxyntic glands in the fundus of the stomach that regulate appetite

Gitelman syndrome a rare autosomal recessive condition of hypokalaemic metabolic alkalosis with distinct features of hypocalciuria and hypomagnesaemia, noted in later childhood or early adulthood

Gleason grading system a method of predicting the tendency of a tumour in the prostate to metastasise

Gleason system a system that grades prostate cancer using numbers from 1 to 5 based on how much the cells in the cancerous tissue look like normal prostate tissue, named after Donald Gleason, an US Pathologist remove existing and add this

Global action plans proposals that outline specific steps or activities for a strategy to suceed

Global strategies proposals that offer a strategic vision of how to tackle health challenges, listing specific objectives and guidance to stakeholders

glossopharyngeal neuralgia sharp, recurrent pain deep in the throat that extends to the area around the tonsils and even the ear

glucagon-like peptide-1 a incretin hormone released from gastrointestinal tract capable of stimulating insulin secretion, GLP-1

Gnathostomiasis (nath'o-sto'mi-asis) a foodborne zoonosis by infection with larvae of Gnathosoma species. Humans may become accidental hosts after ingesting third-stage larvae, where they are unable to mature

GOBI abbreviation for growth and development, oral rehydration, breastfeeding and immunisation

Goldenhar's syndrome a developmental malformation of the first 2 bronchial arches that presents a combination of several anomalies such as dermal epibulbar tumours, peri-auricular apprendices and malformation of the ears; oculo-auriculo-vertebral dysplasia

Good Samaritan law a law that provides protection against claims of malpractice for medical practitioners who render emergency care at the scene of an accident except when gross negligence or wilful misconduct can be proved

GP abbreviation for general practitioner

gravel debris which is formed from a fragmented kidney stone

gravidity (gra'vi-di-ti) number of confirmed pregnancies

green tobacco sickness symptoms such as headache, giddiness, nausea and general ill health from nicotine absorbed through skin, by a person while handling green leaves of tobacco during cultivation, curing and manufacture

gross tumour volume gross palpable or visible/demonstrable extent and location of malignant growth; GTV

ground-glass pattern *radiol* finely granular pattern of pulmonary opacity within which normal anatomic details are partly obscured, and it resembles etched or abraded glass

group therapy *Psy* a form of psychosocial treatment where a small group of patients meet regularly to talk, interact and discuss problems with each other and the therapist

growth plate the place in. long bones where growth occurs during childhood

guided imagery use of relaxation and mental visualization to improve mood and /or physical wellbeing

guidelines policies or methods of professional practice that are approved by the Review Committee and designed to promote evidence-based health policies or clinical interventions

Gunther's disease a rare inherited autosomal recessive condition exhibiting a deficiency of uroporphyrinogen III synthetase and presenting as congenital erythropoietic porphyria with marked sun sensitivity

gurney (ger'ne) a wheeled cot used in hospitals

guru (s) 1. heavy 2. teacher, guide

gutta percha *dent* an inert latex-like substance used for filling root canals

H

H and E haematoxylin and eosin stain

h structure the general underlying segmentation of the genome

haematocolpometra (he'mat-o-kal'po-metra) accumulation of menstrual blood in the vagina and uterus

haematophobia (he'mat-o-fo'bea) fear of blood

haemodiafiltration (he'mo-di'a-fil'tra-shun) a technique for extracorporeal blood treatment for urea at end stage renal disease

haemoglobin H disease a condition arising from heterozygocity for alpha thalassemia, noted in parts of Asia and around the Mediterranean

haemophagocytic lymphohisticytosis a rare, potentially life-threatening condition characterised by uncontrolled activation of macrophages and lymphocytes

HAFF abbreviation for hypoglycaemia-associated autonomic failure

hair bulb root of a strand of hair from which the colour develops

hair cells sensory receptors in the inner ear that transform sound vibrations into messages that travel to the brain

half time the time required for one half of a quantity of a substance to be eliminated from a system

half-and-half nail azotemic onychopathy showing finger nail bands with red, pink, brown transverse distal bands occurring at least in 20-60% of nail length and with the remaining nail showing a dull whitish aspect

halo sign an earliest radiologic sign of invasive aspergillosis exhibiting a micronodule surrounded by perimeter of ground glass opacity corresponding to alveolar haemorrhage

hammer toe a joint involvement with flexion at the proximal interphalangeal joint with or without the distal interphalangeal joint and the metatarsophalangeal joint may be hyperextended

haplotype (hap'lo-type) a series of polymorphisms that are close together in the genome

haplotype (ha'pl-o-typ)a combination of related genes on the same chromosome, which are usually inherited together

hapMap a catalogue of common genetic-variation in humans compiled by an international partnership of scientists and funding agencies with a goal to determine the identity and length of haplotypes across the genome in different human populations

happy puppet syndrome a puppet-like gait, fits of laughter and characteristic facial characteristics see Angleman syndrome

haptics study pertaining to the way how people use touch

HAV hepatitis A virus

HBV hepatitis B virus

HCV hepatitis C virus

head lag backward flop of an infant's head when placed in a sitting position

healing crisis when the body begins to eliminate toxins at an accelerated rate unpleasant sensations may be experienced

health promotion the process of enabling people to increase control over, and to improve health

health protection the provision of conditions for normal mental and physical functioning of the human being individually and in the group and it includes the promotion of health, the prevention of sickness and curative and restorative medicine in all its aspects

health systems a system composed of all organisations, institutions and research that are concerned with efforts to improve people's physical and mental well being

helical CT method allowing continuous 360 degree radiologic image; spiral CT

hellerwork a therapy to realign the body following stress, illness and bad posture

Henderson's equation equation formulated by Lawrence Henderson, describes the dynamic equilibrium that occurs when weak acids are in solution

Hendra virus an enveloped RNA virus closely related to Nipah virus causing respiratory infection, noted in Queensland, Australia

HER2 abbreviation for human epidermal growth factor receptor type 2

herbalism (her'b-a-li-zm) the use of plant to prevent and treat illness

heritability the proportion of inter-individual differences in a trait that is the result of genetic factors

Hermansky-Pudlok syndrome a rare inherited disorder bearing the names of two doctors in Czechoslovakia who in 1959 recognised similar abnormalities in two unrelated adults, who presented with albinism, tendency to bleed easily, and pulmonary fibrosis, and the condition is most commonly noted in Peurto Rico

heteroplasmy (het'er-o-pla'smi) individuals with mitochondrial DNA disease harbouring both mutant and wild type mitochondrial DNA

Heubner's (hu'b-nerz) **artery** a medial lenticulostriate artery that arises from the proximal segment of the anterior communicating artery, that supplies the anterior medial part of the head of the caudate nucleus and the anterior internal capsule

Hib disease an infection caused by Haemophilus influenza type B in children

hibernian fever *see* TNR receptor-associated periodic syndrome

hibernoma (hi'ber-noma) uncommon, benign soft-tissue tumours that histologically mimic brown fat, and may be noted in the neck, axillae, mediastinum, and periaortic and perirenal zones.

hidradenitis suppurativa a chronic recurrent inflammatory disease affecting skin that bears apocrine glands

HIF hypoxia-inducible factor that induces expression of genes involved in angiogenesis, erythropoiesis and cell metabolism, proliferation and survival

high spot *dent* an area of a tooth or restoration that feels abnormal or uncomfortable because it hits its opposing tooth before other teeth meet

hippocampal sclerosis a disorder characterized by hippocampal neuronal loss that causes medical temporal lobe epilepsy

Hirayama's disease a form of juvenile muscle atrophy characterized by an imbalance in growth between the vertebral column and the spinal canal contents, which causes abutment of the anterior spinal cord against the vertebral column and detachment of the posterior dura, leading to microcirculatory disturbances and ischaemic changes in the cord

hirsute (hir'su-t)hairy

histrionic personality disorder psy personality disorder characterized by feelings of emptiness, coupled with an intense need to be liked and to be the centre of attention

HMG-CoA beta-hydroxy beta-methyl glutaryl CoA, a key intermediate in the synthesis of ketone bodies, of sterols, and of fenesyl geranyl derivatives

holiday heart syndrome occurrence of supraventricular arrhythmia usually atrial fibrillation and atrial flutter following an acute alcoholic binge in chronic alcoholics

holistic pertains to the entire person, including the mind, body and spirit **h medicine** therapy that attempts to treat the patient as a whole person

holmgren (holm'gren) **test** test to detect imperfect perception of colour, based on matching various trends of yarn

holoendemic (ho'lo-ende-mik) parasitaemic rate in adults greater than 75%

holoprosencephaly (ho'lo-pro'cen-si'fali) a condition where two cerebral hemispheres . instead of being separated by a cleavage remain united having a centrally placed single ventricle

Holt-Oram syndrome a congenital cardiac defect and skeletal abnormalities of upper limb first reported by Mary-Clayaton Holt and Samuel Oram

homogeneous (ho'mo-gen-e'us) uniform opacity or texture throughout

homolog one of two or more genes that have a similar sequence and are descended from a common ancestor gene

homunculus (hom'an-cu-lus) little person

HOPE the heart outcomes prevention evaluation study demonstrating significant benefits of ACE inhibitors in patients with documented coronary, cerebral or peripheral vascular disease

horizontal gene transfer exchange of genetic material between contemporaneous, extant organisms

hospitalism (hos′pi-tal′izm) a general morbid condition of the building or of its atmosphere, productive of disease

hot flushes a perimenopausal manifestation exhibiting a wave of heat triggered by the hypothalamic response to oestrogen withdrawal

hot spot a region of DNA whose mutation and recombination occur at much higher than normal rate

hot tub folliculitis a skin infection caused by P aeruginosa that often follows bathing in a hot tub or public swimming pool

house keeping gene a gene that codes for a protein that is needed by all cells, regardless of the cell's specialization

HSV herpes simplex virus

Hubris (hub′ris) **syndrome** a condition linked with power where a person exercises power for a long period with pride and self confidence treats others with insolence and contempt

human development index a composite index combining indicators representing three dimension-longevity, knowledge and income

Hutchinson-Gilford progeria syndrome a rare, sporadic autosomal dominant syndrome that involves premature ageing, generally leading to death within approximately 13 years of age due to myocardial infarction or stroke

hydrogenated fats vegetable oils that have been converted into a solid form

hydrogenation process of adding hydrogen to a compound

hydrotherapy (hi-dr-o-ther′api) the use of water as a therapy as in taking health giving baths and drinking spa water

hydrotherapy (hi′dr-o-tir′a-pi) use of water, ice, steam of hot and cold temperatures to maintain and restore health

hyperendemic (hy′per-en′de-mik) parasitaemic rate in adults in the range of 51-75%

hyper-IgD syndrome an autosomal recessive disorder with persistently raised serum IgD levels causing recurrent attacks of fever, abdominal pain, diarrhoea, lymphadenopathy, arthralgia, skin lesions and aphthous ulceration due to a mutation in the gene for mevalonate kinase involved in the metabolism of cholesterol; HIS hyperphagia over eating

hyphema collection of blood in the eye

hypoendemic (hy′po-ende-mik) parasitaemic rate in adults less than 10%

hypoplastic left heart syndrome a congenital defect involving a rudimentary mitral valve and left ventricle, and with a hypoplastic aortic valve and ascending aorta

I

IAP abbreviation for Indian Academy of Paediatrics

ICAM-1 abbreviation for intercellular adhesion molecule-1

ICD add abbreviation for 2. implantable-cardioverter-defibrillator 3. intercostal drainage

ICMR abbreviation for Indian Council of Medical Research

ID1 abbreviation for inhibitor of differentiation 1

idealization psy a defense mechanism for dealing with internal conflicts and insecurities by overtly valuing the qualities of another individual

identification (i′den-ti′fi-kashun) *for* determination or establishment of individuality of a person-living or dead

idiopathic CD4 lymphocytopaenic syndrome a syndrome characterised by a low CD4 cell count that is unexplained by HIV infection or other medical conditions; ICL

IFN abbreviation for interferon

IG immunoglobulin

IGF-1 insulin-like growth factor-1

image analysis a computerized method for extracting information from digitized microscopic images of cells or cell organelles

image-guided biopsy a technique in which computer images are used to guide a biopsy needle to a lump that cannot be felt but has shown up on a mammogram; stereotactic biopsy

image-guided radiation therapy use of imaging methods to assist in targeting a lesion during radiation treatment

imagery *psy* a technique in behaviour therapy in which the patient is conditioned to substitute pleasant fantasies to counter the unpleasant feelings associated with anxiety

immune reconstitution inflammatory syndrome a manifestation of increased immune activity usually in response to anti-retroviral therapy; IRIS

immunoisolation (imm'yun-i'so-la'shun) encapsulated cells hiding from the effect of immune system

impacted tooth *Dent* tooth that is growing against another tooth, bone or soft tissue

impaired fasting glucose a metabolic state referring to a range of fasting plasma glucose levels between 'normal' and that diagnostic for diabetes. The value ranges from 110 mg/dl to 125 mg/dl. IFG

impaired fasting glucose a plasma glucose level of 110-126 mg/dl

impaired glucose tolerance blood glucose of 140-199 mg/dl 2 hours following a 75g glucose lading dose, or fasting blood glucose of 100-125 mg/dl after a 8 hour fast

impar (im'par) not even, unequal, unpaired

implantable cardioverter defibrillator a small device, like a pacemaker, that is implanted in the chest in order to automatically detect ventricular fibrillation or ventricular tachycardia; if it happens, it administers an electrical shock to restore a normal heartbeat; ICD

impression (im'pre-shun) den a mold of the teeth, and the gums

impression *dent* an imprint of the upper

and lower teeth made in a pliable material that sets

impulsivity (im'pul-si-ti-vi-ti) psy a tendency to act according to a sudden urge or impulse without planning ahead

in extremis (in-eks-tre'mis) at the point of death

in tela a tissue, relating especially to stained histologic preparations

inactivating mutation a change in the DNA sequence of a specific gene that results in loss of biologic function

incidental finding a mass or other lesion detected by CT, MRI or other modality performed for an unrelated reason; incidentaloma

incretin (in'cret-in) a hormone released from the gastrointestinal tract in response to ingestion of food that stimulates secretion of insulin

India ink test a dye added to a sample of CSF to detect Cryptococcus neoformans

infanticide (in'fen-ti-side) for murder of an infant within one year of its birth

inferior liver margin sign a supine radiograph in pneumoperitoneum revealing collection of free gas under the inferior surface of the liver

infibulation (in'fi-bu-le'shun) a procedure where the tissue around the vagina is sewn leaving only a small opening for the passage of urine and menstrual blood

infliximab a chimeric monoclonal antibody to tumor necrosis factor-alpha and is a potent immunosuppressive agent

infraclusion *dent* the state wherein a tooth has failed, to erupt to the maxillo-mandibular plane of interdigitation

iniencephaly (ini'en-ke'fali) a developmental error occurring in early pregnancy with arrest and imperfect development of base of the skull mainly in the vicinity of foramen magnum

inlay dent a filling that is made outside of the tooth and then cemented into place

inotropic agent a drug that increases the contraction strength of the heart muscle

INR abbreviation for International normalised ratio

insertion mutation a type of mutation involving the addition of genetic material

insight psychotherapy psy psychotherapy that aims to relieve emotional conflict by helping the patient understand the cause of a conflict

instant needle burner a portable, compact, destroyer into which the contaminated syringe with needle when inserted, it generates a high temperature above 1600° C thereby completely burning the needle and reducing it to ashes in a few seconds

instep the dorsal part of the arch of the foot

institutional review board a group of physicians, scientists, ethicists, lawyers and community members that review human subjects research to ensure that the research will be performed ethically and that will benefit patients

insulin ball hard, more discrete amyloid lumps of insulirt

insulin resistance tissues targeted by insulin fail to respond leading to increased production of pancreatic insulin

intake (in'tak)that which is taken into the body

intellectualisation psy a defense mechanism whereby one deals with internal conflicts and insecurities by the excessive persuit of knowledge along with the excessive use of cleaver words to defend against emotions

intemperance (in-tem'per-ans) lack of proper self control, applied to use of alcoholic beverages

intensity modulated radiation therapy an advanced method of conformal radiation therapy in which the beams are aimed from several directions and the intensity of the beams is controlled by computers; IMRT

intercadent (in'ter-ka'den't) irregular in rhythm

intercurrent occurring during the course

interface radiol common boundary between the shadows of two juxtaposed structures

intergenic regions segments of DNA that do not contain or overlap genes

intermediate density lipoprotein a plasma lipoprotein composed of protein, phospholipid, cholesterol and triglyceride which transports cholesterol from the intestine to the liver; IDL

intermediate syndrome cranial nerve and brain stem lesions with a proximal neuropathy that starts 1-4 days after acute intoxication and lasts for 2-3 weeks

intermittent explosive disorder Psy a mental disturbance characterized by specific episodes of violent and aggressive behavior that may involve harm to others or destruction of property

internal radiation therapy treatment involving implantation of a radioactive substance into the body

interstitial radiation therapy a type of treatment in which a radioactive implant is placed directly into the tissue

intersystole the period intervening between the systole of the atrium and that of the ventricle of the heart

intestinal capillariasis an infection caused by C phillippinensis, acquired by ingestion of raw freshwater fish and presenting with abdominal pain, borborygmus and intermittent diarrhoea, may cause death from cardiomyopathy from irreversible electrolyte losses

intracytoplasic sperm injection process to inject a single sperm into each egg before the fertilized eggs are put back into the uterus: ICSI

intraoperative radiation therapy delivery of a single, high dose of external beam radiation to the tumour site; IORT

intrarenal resistive index a noninvasive ultrasound-based method to assess vascular resistance and elasticity used to assess the renal allograft function and the prediction of allograft and patient survival

intravenous line a method of supplying fluids and medication by using a needle or a thin tube inserted to a vein

introjection psy a defense mechanism whereby one deals with emotional conflicts by accepting blame beyond what is realistic

introns the portions of a gene that are removed before translation to a protein

invasive (in'va-siv) penetrating

inversion a chromosomal segment that has been broken off and reinserted in the same place, but with the genetic sequence in reverse order

involuntary smoking breathing in the smoke from others or from burning cigarettes, especially by a nonsmoker; passive smoking

irrigation the practice of washing out or flushing a wound or body opening irrigation with a stream of water or another fluid

isocentre the centre of the treatment area in relation to the paths of the radiation beams

isotretinoin a drug that decreases sebum production and dries up acne

J

J point QRS-ST junction in ECG

J wave notched or slurred QRS in ECG

JaK STAT signaling pathway one of several cell-signaling pathways that activates gene expression. The pathway is activated through cell-surface receptors and cytoplasmic Janus .kinases (JaKs), and signal transducers and activators of transcription (STAT)

JAMA abbreviation for Journal of the Amercian Medical Association

Jaw wiring surgical procedure where metal pins and wires are anchored into the jaw bones and surrounding tissue to keep the jaw from moving; maxillomandibular fixation

Jensen metaphyseal chondrodysplasia a rare dominantly inherited chondrodysplasia characterised by severe shortening of limbs associated with an unusual facial appearance

Jervell and Lange-Nielsen syndrome a rare form of long QT syndrome presenting with prolonged QT interval, and congenital deafness. The condition was reported by authors in 1957

Jesuits' bark an archaic term for cinchona bark

Jeun's syndrome autosomal recessive disorder that results in a constricted and narrow rib cage with generalised chondodystrophy and pelvic, phalangeal and neurologic anomalies with renal and hepatic disorders; thoracic-pelvic-phalangeal dystrophy; asphyxiating thoracic dystrophy

JIPMER Jawaharlal Nehru Institute of Postgraduate Medical Education and Research, located at Puducheri

JNC-7 seventh report of the Joint National Committee on Prevention, Detection, Evaluation and Treatment of high blood pressure

JIMA abbreviation for Journal of Indian Medical Association

Jorcha-Levin syndrome a spectrum of short neck, skeletal dysplasia with variable involvement of the vertebrae and ribs, described by Jorcho and Levin in 1938

Joubert's syndrome nephronopathisis associated with mental retardation and ataxia

K

keratoacanthoma (ker'ato-akan'thoma) a benign crateriform neoplasm that often involutes spontaneously after a few months of rapid growth

keratomileusis surgical alteration of refractive errors by changing the shape of a deep layer of the cornea

keratonosis (ker'a-to-no'sis) any abnormal non-inflammatory affection of the horny layer of the skin

kerion celsi an inflammatory form of tinea capitis caused by a T-cell mediated hypersensitivity reaction to the causative dermatophyte

Kesaree-Wooley syndrome a phenotypic female with 49 chromosomes: penta-X

keyhole surgery surgery performed via an endoscope through small incision see minimally invasive surgery

key-way (ke'we) *Dentistry*, the female portion of a precision attachment

khara (s) granular

kick (kik) a brisk mechanical **stimulus** kidney *add* **cement k** calcified kidney from tuberculosis replacement of kidney by caseous material from tuberculosis

Kikuchi-Fujimoto's disease a rare, self-limiting inflammatory process of cervical lymphadenopathy seen in children and young adults of Asian heritage, described independently in 1972 by Kikuchi and Fujimoto and others in Japan; histiocytic necrotizing lymphadenitis

kilobase unit of length of DNA fragments equal to 10000 nucleotides; kb

Kimura disease a rare condition seen in Far-East, characterized by cervical lymphadenopathy, eosinophilia and hyperimmunoglobulinaemia (IgG) and subcutaneous masses especially in head and neck, named after Kimura from Japan who gave a detailed description of the condition in 1948

kinase (ki'nase) an enxyme that transfers a phosphate group to a substrate

kindling *psy* phenomenon by which a psychiatric condition becomes more Lesch-Nyhan syndrome resistant longer it is left untreated

kindred (kin'dred) an aggregate of genetically related people

kinematics (kin'e-mat'iks) the science concerned with movements of the parts of the body

kinesin a motor protein that uses energy obtained from the hydrolysis of ATP to move along a microtubule

Kleine-Levin syndrome a disorder occurring primarily in young males 3 or 4 times in a year marked by episodes of hypersomnia, hypersexual behaviour and excessive eating

Knock pouch a type of ileostomy in which the surgeon forms an artificial rectum from a section of the ileum

knock-in (nak'in) **technique** an innovative genetic procedure to alter the function of a gene

knock-out (nak'out) **technique** a mechanism to shut down or turn off a particular gene from producing a specific protein in a test organism

kopophobia (kop'o-fo'ne-a) morbid fear of fatigue

Kuttner's tumour a tumour-like inflammatory condition of the salivary glands usually submandibular glands, described by Kuttner in 1896; chronic sclerosing sialadenitis

KVO line keep vein open, refers to intravenous drip rate that runs as a rate sufficient to keep a line open for medication administration

L

La Nina a positive cold event of Southern oscillation having far reaching effect on public health

labialism (la'be-al-izm) a form of stammering with confusion in the use of the labial consonants

labiaplasty (lae'bea-pla'sti) surgical procedure in which labia minora are cut down to achieve reduction in size or better symmetry

labitome (lab'i-tom) a forceps with sharp-blades

langhana ayu treatment which causes lightness or reduces the size of the body

lck of personal accomplishment feelings of incompetence and under achievement at work

lcunes small ischaemic infarcts in the deep regions of the brain or brain stem

landau-Kleffner syndrome a rare condition of unknown cause presenting with a loss of language function characterised by loss of language skills in a previously normal child; LKS

Laron syndrome a genetic disorder with dwarfism due to lack of receptors necessary for body growth though growth hormone levels are normal and presents with deep set eyes, small hands and feet, high-pitched voice and obesity

larvate (lar'vat) a concealed, masked or undeveloped

lase (laz) to cut, divide or dissolve a substance

LASEK acronym for laser-assisted epithelial keratoplasty

laser skin resurfacing a cosmetic surgery in which a laser is used to treat wrinkles, scars and various skin lesions

late neonatal death death of a neonate after 7 days but before 29 days

latency of similars horn a principle of homoeopathic treatment according to which substances that cause specific symptoms in healthy people are given to sick people with similar symptoms

latency the period of inactivity between the time of a stimulus and the time of a response

lathology (lath'o-loji) study of errors

Lazarus sign a reflex movement in brain dead or brain-stem failure patients

Lazarus syndrome a spontaneous return of circulation after failed attempts of resuscitation, named after the biblical figure Lazarus of Bethany

lazy leukocyte syndrome impaired neutrophil motility to chemotactic stimulation

LBW abbreviation for low birth weight

left shift an increase in the peripheral blood smear of immature granulocytes with decreased nuclear segmentation due to increased production of myeloid series in the marrow

left shift appearance of immature white cells in the peripheral blood

Leigh's syndrome a disorder caused by abnormalities in mitochondrial energy metabolism that affect vascular endothelium, and exhibiting haemorrhagic necrosis in the deep grey matter structures of the brain, brain stem and spinal cord, named after Denis Leigh who originally described the condition; mitochondrial encephalopathy

Lemierre's syndrome an acute oropharyngeal infection with secondary thrombophlebitis of its internal jugular vein, named after Andre Lemierre who charcterised the condition; postanginal septicemia

leprechaunism (lep're-cha'vu-nizm) a syndrome characterised by intrauterine growth retardation, fasting 1 hypoglycaemia and postprandial hypoglycaemia in association with profound resistance to insulin

leptin (lep'tin) a protein hormone that affects feeding behaviour and hunger in humans

Lesch-Nyhan syndrome a rare genetic disorder that affects male children, and is due to total absence of enzyme hypoxanthine guanine phosphoribosyl transferase that affects the level of uric acid in the body presenting with physical handicaps, mental retardation and kidney problems, described by Michael Lesch and William Nyhan in 1964

leukaphresis (luk'a-fe-re'sis) a procedure to remove leucocytes from withdrawn blood and reintroduction of reminder of the blood into the donor

LFT abbreviation for liver function tests, lung function tests

LHF abbreviation for left heart failure

LHV abbreviation for lady health visitor

life span (lif'span) duration of life of an individual

life support process in which a person is kept alive artificially with a ventilator, to maintain breathing, and/or a pacemaker, to sustain the heart beat

ligator (li'ga-tur) an instrument used in the ligation of vessels

LIGHT a platelet-derived ligand of the tumor necrosis factor, that is lymphotoxin-like inducible super-family protein that competes with glycoprotein D for herpes virus entry mediated on T lymphocytes that promotes vascular influences

linear accelerator radiotherapy machine that emits photon- or electron radiation megavolts redirected in many arcs for treating benign or malignant tumours throughout the body; linac

lingua villosa nigra black discolouration of the tongue characterised by hypertrophy and elongation of filiform papillae and lack of normal desquamation, often attributed to poor oral hygiene. It is secondary to infection with porphyria-producing chromogenic bacteria or yeast

linkage analysis an approach to the discovery of the genetic basis of a disease that correlates the patterns of disease inheritance within families with specific alleles of genetic markers of known location

linkage disequilibrium the nonrandom association of genetic markers

lipid profile an abbreviated battery of tests performed on an automated chemical analyser that includes total cholesterol, LDL cholesterol, HDL cholesterol and triglycerides

lipidome (li'pi-dom) the totality of lipids in the cells

lipoblastoma rare soft tissue neoplasm derived from foetal adipose tissue, occurs in infants and young children

lipophage (li'po-faj) the selective targeting of lipids to autophagosomes for degradation through the autophagy pathway

liposhaving removal of fat that lies close to the skin surface by using a needlelike instrument that contains a sharp edged shaving device

lithotresis (li'tho-tre'sis) the boring of holes in a calculus to facilitate its crushing

littoral (lit'o-ral) relating to or growing on or near a shore especially of the sea

Liver X receptor master regulators of whole body cholesterol homeostasis; LXR

living cell a written advanced directive made by competent persons prior to incapacitation when they would be unable to express their wishes for treatment, resuscitation and terminal care

living will an advance directive prepared by a competent person that indicates his or her wishes regarding life-sustaining medical treatments

livor mortis *for* purplish or reddish purple areas of discolouration in the dependent parts of the body due to gravitation of accumulated fluid, blood in the vessels after death, showing up through the skin

LMWH abbreviation for low molecular weight heparin; substance derived by cleavage of unfractionated heparin to yield smaller chains of unfractionated heparin

load forces acting on a body

long QT syndrome abnormal QT interval prolongation in the surface ECG and an increased risk of sudden death usually due to ventricular fibrillation

longitudinal study a research study that collects repeated observations of the same items over a long period of time

loss of function mutation a mutation that reduces or eliminates the function of the protein encoded by the gene in which the mutation lies

loss-of-function mutation a mutation that decreases the production or function of a protein

low birth weight a newborn whose weight is less than 2500 g

Lowe's syndrome a rare inherited disorder that is characterized by congenital cataracts, glaucoma and severe mental retardation

LP abbreviation for lumbar puncture

LTBI latent tuberculosis infection, an individual infected but has no symptoms or signs of active disease

lucency (lu'sen-si) *radiol* any circumscribed area appearing dark than the surrounding

lues maligna a skin disorder of secondary syphilis in which areas of ulcerated and dying tissue are found

lux a standard unit of measurement for illumination

luxate (lu'x-at) dent to loosen or dislocate tooth from the socket

Lynch syndrome hereditary colorectal cancer presenting at younger age

M

M cyclin a eukaryote enzyme that regulates mitosis

M phase the period of the cell cycle-mitosis or meiosis-which the chromosomes separate and migrate to the opposite poles of the spindle

MAC technique abbreviation for monitored anaesthesia care, technique

macroautophagy (ma'kro-auto-fa'ji) a cellular process that involves the sequestration of cytoplasmic components into double-membrane autophagosomes that fuse with lysosomes where their cargoes are delivered for degradation and recycling

macrobiotics (ma'kro-bio-tiks) group of vegetarian-based diets with varying restrictions

macrodont *dent* a tooth abnormality large and frequently distorted proportion

macromastia (mak'ro-mas'tia) excessive size of the breasts

macronutrients (mak'ro-nu'tre-ents) nutritional substances such as carbohydrates, proteins, and fats required in large amount

macropathology (mak'ro-pa-thol'o-je) pathology that pertains to the gross anatomical changes in disease

macroprolactin (mak'ro-pro'lak-tin) a hormonally inert large molecular weight prolactin-immunoglobulin G complex

macropsia (ma'kro-p-sia) *psy* the visual perception that objects are larger than they actually are

Madelung's disease a rare disease of unknown aetiology characterized by multiple symmetric lipomatosis, predominantly seen in men, often in alcoholics

make-a-picture story *psy* a psychological test in which a person creates a story with fictional characters using cut-out figures, animals and objects to illustrate the story

mala ayu waste product of the body

malaplakia (mal'a-pla'kiya)an acquired granulomatous disorder

malar (ma'lar) relating to the cheek or cheek bones

malingering (mal'in-ger'ing) the act of intentionally feigning or exaggerating physical or physiological symptoms for personal gain

Mallampati classification classification based on the structures visualized with mouth opening and tongue protrusion in sitting position that correlates with the difficulty of intubation preoperatively, named after Seshagiri Mallampati

malocclusion *dent* misalignment of opposing teeth in the upper and lower jaws

malpraxis (mal'pra-k-sis) want or lack of reasonable care and skill or willful negligence on the part of the medical practitioner in course of professional attendance on his patient leading to his bodily injury, sufferance or even loss of life

mammotome (ma'mo-to'm) a biopsy that uses suction and a large tube to withdraw breast tissue

managed care a contractual arrangement whereby an agency or insurance company mediates between physician and patients, negotiating the payment for service and overseeing the treatment given

manda (s) slow

mantie (man'tei) a covering layer

Marchiafava-Bignami disease a symmetrical demyelination and necrosis of the middle part of corpus callosum noted in people with chronic alcoholism

marma ayu extremely sensitive nerve points which should be guarded from injury

MARS molecular adsorbent recirculating system; a specific type of extracorporeal blood treatment which combines the removal of water and albumin-bound toxins from patient's blood

marsupialisation (mar'su-pea-li'sha-shun) cutting out a wedge of the cyst wall and putting in stitches so the cyst cannot recur

maschalyperidrosis (mas'kali-per'i-dro-sis) excessive sweating in the axilla

mastocytosis an abnormal growth and accumulation of neoplastic mast cells in various organs

mastopexy (mas-to-pek'si) surgical procedure to lift up a breast

maternal mortality number of women dying per 100,000 live births while pregnant or within 42 days of termination of the pregnancy, irrespective of the duration and the site of pregnancy, from any cause related to or aggravated by the pregnancy or its management but not from accidental or incidental causes.

mati (s) intelligence

maze procedure a surgical method to create a maze of permanent new electrical pathways through heart muscle to treat chronic atrial fibrillation

McCune-Albright syndrome a genetic syndrome characteristically seen in girls and is characterized by development of ovarian cysts and puberty before the age of 8, together with abnormalities of bone structure and skin pigmentation

McKittrick-Wheelock syndrome a rare complication of villous adenoma usually of rectosigmoid region presenting with large volume secretory diarrhoea, prerenal acute renal failure, and severe electrolyte dysfunction, described in 1954

MDI abbreviation for metered-dose inhaler

MDR-TB multi-drug resistant tuberculosis that is resistant to rifampicin and isoniazid

MDS abbreviation for Master of Dental Surgery

Meckel's syndrome an autosomal recessive disease with dysplasia and malformation of multiple organs characterised by occipital meningoencephalocoele, microphelomia, lung hypoplasia, polycystic kidneys or renal hypodysplasia or dysplasia, bile duct dilatation, postaxial Polydactyly and situs inversus

meda ayu fatty tissue

medical device any instrument, apparatus, appliance, material or health care product, excluding pharmacological drugs, used in a patient for diagnosis, prevention, monitoring, replacement and treatment

medical error science that deals with what can go wrong in medicine

medical humanities a sustained interdisciplinary enquiry into aspects of medical practice, education and research expressly concerned with the human side of medicine

medical jurisprudence science dealing with the legal aspects of medical practice

medical transcription (med'i-kal tran-skrip'shun) machine transcription of physician dictated medical reports concerning a patient's health care

medicalisation (med'i-kal'i-shun) definition and treatment of condition that were not previously construed as medical problems

medication label a label that contains important information to help the healthcare professional deliver the required medication to the patient

medicolegal autopsy examination for a special type of examination of a dead body as per laws of the land towards administration of justice and prosecution of the guilty

megabase unit of length for DNA fragments equal to 1 million nucleotides; Mb

MELAS abbreviation for mitochondrial enceph'aiomyopathy with lactic acidosis and stroke-like episodes

MELD score model for end-stage liver disease determined by using the total serum bilirubin concentration, the international normalized ratio for the prothrombin time, and the serum creatinine concentration

Melnick-Fraser syndrome *see* broncho-oto-renal syndrome

membrane channel a protein complex that forms a pore or channel through the membrane for the free passage of iqns and small molecule

Menkes disease a fatal neurodegenerative disorder of infancy from diverse mutations in a copper transport gene

mentastics (men'tas-tiks) a form of movement reeducation in which 'person learns to reexperience movement as pleasurable and positive

meridian *chi* the traditional Chinese medicine describing the channels which run beneath the skin through which the body's energy flows

mesoendemic (me'so-en'de-mik) parasitaemic rate in adults in the range of 11-50%

meta analysis a method to estimate the relative risk as a composite number through all trials in the aggregate

metabolic profiling identifying the types and amounts of known metabolic intermediates present in a biological specimen

metabolic syndrome presence of 3 of the following: abdominal obesity, elevated triglyceridaemia, low high density lipoprotein cholesterol, elevated blood pressure and elevated fasting glucose occurring in the same patient

metabolome (met'a-bo'lom) (1) all the metabolites produced by a person (2) low molecular weight chemicals in a biological system

metabolomics a systematic study of metabolomes

metagenomic analysis genomic analysis that is performed directly on a mixture of heterogeneous organisms, genomes, or genes

metastatic quotient a prognostic framework measuring how adept the cells are with respect to metastatic functions

metatarsus adductus a condition noted in newborns presenting with adduction of the forefoot relative to the hind foot

miasm *Horn* a general weakness or predisposition to chronic disease transmitted down the generational chain

MIC minimal inhibitory concentration; the lowest concentration of antibiotic sufficient to inhibit growth of bacteria in vitro

MICRO HOPE a sub-study of the HOPE trial, the microalbuminuria, cardiovascular and renal outcomes prevention, evaluation study showing ramipril lowering the risks of cardiovascular disease and renal disease in patients with diabetes

microarray a technology used to study many genes at once **m based profiling** the use of gene expression signatures fro mcancer samples to define some aspect of outcome

microbivore (mi'kro-bi-vor) an artificial mechanical white blood cell of microscopic size

microchemarism (mic'ro-kemer-izm) the intermingling of some cells from one person inside the body of another

microdeletion syndrome a syndrome caused by a chromosomal deletion spanning several genes that is too small to be detected under the microscope with the use of conventional cytogenetic methods

micrograph photograph taken through a light or electron microscope

micronychia (mi'kro-nik'e-a) abnormal smallness of nails

Micropsia (mi'kro-p-se'a) psy the visual perception that objects are smaller than they actually are

microRNA a small, regulatory non-coding RNA in plants and animals that inhibits gene expression by binding to imperfect complementary sites within the 3' untranslated regions of their target-messenger RNA transcripts; miENA

microsatellites short sequences of codomly repeated segments of DNA, two to five nucleotides in length. These regions are inherently unstable and susceptible to mutation

microscintigraphy (mi'kro-sin-tig'ra-fi) imaging of small anatomic structures by use of radionuclide in conjunction with special collimator which magnify the image

MIDCAB minimally invasive coronary artery bypass while the heart is still beating through small incisions in the chest wall, without use of heart-lung machine

Middle East Respiratory Syndrome a flu-like respiratory infection that progresses to pneumonia caused by a corona virus with strong tropism for non-ciliated bronchial epithelial cells; MERS

mid-life crisis crisis of confidence about a person's life choices, usually occurring in middle age

Miller-Fisher syndrome a variant of Guillain-Barre syndrome characterised by the acute onset of oculomotor dysfunction, ataxia, and loss of deep tendon reflexes with relative sparing of strength in the extensors and trunk, named after Charles Miller-Fisher, a Canadian Neurologist MFS

Mini CEX a method for assessing clinical evaluation exercise

minimal access surgery a combination of modern technology and surgical innovation that aim to accomplish surgical therapeutic goals with minimal somatic and psychological trauma; MAS

Mirizzi's syndrome obstructive jaundice caused by compression of common hepatic duct by a stone in the cystic duct or the neck of gall bladder

miRNA micro RNA involved in regulation of gene expression through RNA interference

misdiagnosis incorrect diagnosis of a morbid condition

misopedia (mis'o-pedea) hatred of children

mis-sense mutation the alteration of a single DNA nucleotide so that the resulting codon specifies a different amino acid

mitochondrial DNA small circular chromosome found inside mitochondria mitotic chromosome highly condensed duplicated chromosome held together by the centromere

mitophagy (mi'to-fa-ji) the selective targeting of damaged or dysfunctional mitochondria to autophagosomes for degradation through the autophagy pathway

mitotic chromosome highly condensed duplicated chromosome held together by the centromere

mittelschonerz Ger midcycle pain

mixoscopia (mi-kso-sko'pia) psy obtaining sexual satisfaction by observing a couple during the act of sexual intercourse

mm Hg an abbreviation for millimeters of mercury, to measure blood pressure

MMP abbreviation for matrix metalloproteinase MODS multiple organ dysfunction syndrome

MODS multiple organ dysfunction syndrome

Mondor's (man'dorz) **disease** a benign, self-limited thrombophlebitis of the subcutaneous veins of the anterolateral thoracoabdominal wall, may be associated with breast cancer

MONICA project acronym for MONItoring trends and determinants in CArdiovascular disease morbidity and mortality, risk factors and medical care of cardiovascular diseases from its numerous populations

monogenic disease a disorder caused by a mutation in a single gene

Monteggia's fracture fracture of proximal third of ulna with dislocation of the head of the radius, named after Giovanni Battista Monteggia

Morgellous disease a mysterious, most bizarre disease that mimics scabies or lice causes burning or itching sensation on the skin and the feeling of bugs crawling over under or on top of it, characterized by open sores on the face or body and sting like fibres emerge from their wounds, and the name has origin from a description of an illness in the medical case-history essay

morning after pill high doses of oral contraceptives taken to prevent pregnancy after a single act of unprotected sex

morphogenomics a combination of morphology and genomics

morphometrics (mor'fo-met-ri'ks) a technique using computer-modeling software to identify craniofacial characteristics

morphoproteomics a combination of morphology and proteomics

mortality *add* **early neonatal m** number of child deaths less than 7 days of life expressed as per 1,000 live births in the reference year **infant m** probability of dying between birth and exactly one year of age expressed per 1,000 live births **late neonatal m** number of child deaths of 7 days to 28 completed days of life expressed as per 1,000 live births in the reference year **perinatal m** number of deaths of foetuses weighing at least 500 g plus the number of early neonatal deaths, per 1,000 total births **post neonatal m** number of child deaths of 29 days to less than 1 year of age expressed as per 1,000 live births in the reference year **under-5 m** probability of dying between birth and exactly five years of age expressed per 1,000 live births

mosaicism (mos'ay-sis'm) a genetic condition resulting from a mutation crossing over, or non disjunction of chromosomes during cell division causing a variation in the number of chromosomes in the cells

mother tincture How the first stage in the preparation of a homoeopathic remedy consisting of soaking a plant, animal or mineral or mineral product in a solution of alcohol

motif an element of structure or pattern that may be a recurring domain in a variety of proteins

MOTT abbreviation for mycobacteria other than M tuberculosis; and M bovis; atypical mycobacteria

MP abbreviation for malarial parasite

MRS abbreviation for magnetic resonance spectroscopy, a non-invasive technique in which magnetic resonance is used to determine the molecular structure of a compound or to detect the presence of a compound and it detects characteristic signals produced by atomic nuclei with an odd number of protons and neutrons, to obtain in situ concentration of chemicals in normal and diseased tissues

MTP abbreviation for medical termination of pregnancy

MU abbreviation for million units

mucilaginous (mu'si-la'ji-nus) gummy or having the consistency of gelatin

mucociliary escalator the coordinated action of cilia on the surface of cells lining the respiratory tract which moves mucus up and out of the respiratory tract

Mudaliar committee A committee appointed by Government of India under the chairmanship of Dr A L Mudaliar in 1962 to have a fresh look at the health needs and resources in the country

multifocal motor neuropathy a rare but treatable acquired motor neuropathy that may simulate motor neuron disease

multileaf collimator multiple metal 'leaves' that can be adjusted individually to shape the radiation beam to the contour of the tumour and to variably modulate the dose and found in the linear particle accelerator

multipass transmembrane protein a membrane protein that passes back and forth across the lipid layer

multiple systems atrophy features of Parkinsonism, often without tremor with varying degrees of autonomic features, cerebellar involvement and pyramidal tract dysfunction seen sporadically in middle-aged and elderly patients; MSA

musicotherapy an adjunctive treatment of medical disorders by music

myelipoma a benig 1 tumour composed of fat and interspe >ed haematopoietic elements that resemble bone marrow

myelokanthexis (my'lo-kyan-tek-sis) discordance between hypercellular bone marrow and neutropaenia in the peripheral blood

N

NAD abbreviation for 1. no appreciable disease, 2. nothing abnormal detected

NAME acronym for naevi, atrial myxoma, myxoid neurofibromatosis, and ephelides

nanomedicine (nan'o-med'i-sin) the medical diagnosis, monitoring and treatment at the level of single molecule or molecular assemblies providing structure, control, signalling, homeostasis and motility in the cells at the nanoscale

nanopore (nan'o-por) surface perforated with holes of nanoscale

nanoshell (nan'o-shel) a platform for nanoscale drug delivery

nanotechnology (nan'o-tek-no'logi) study of structure one to one hundred nanometers in scale

narrative medicine practice of medicine with narrative competence such as to hear, discern, absorb and interpret stories that may enhance clinical expertise and offer doctors important evidence relating to the feelings and emotions surrounding the illness experiences

National Cancer Registry Programme programme offering a comprehensive picture of the magnitude and pattern of cancer in the country, that includes database of cancer cases both at the level of population and hospital; NCRP

natural history the progression of a disease if it is left untreated

naturotherapy (na'tu-ro'the-ra-pi) treatment of disease by utilizing the body's inherent ability to heal

Naxos disease arrhythmogenic right ventricular cardiomyopathy

nd abbreviation for notifiable disease

necrolytic migratory erythema a rare inflammatory dermatosis developing more frequently in glucagonoma syndrome and present with polymorphic mucocutaneous manifestations encompassing multiple annular erythematous scaling and crusting patches with hypopigmentation

necrophobia (nek'ro-fo'bea) fear of death

NEDD9 abbreviation for neural precursor cell expressed developmentally down regulated 9

Nelson's disease bilateral diffuse adrenal cortical hyperplasia due to corticotroph adenoma, enlarging after adrenalectomy, absence of the negative feedback by glucocorticoids may lead to stimulation of an undetected small pituitary tumour and uncontrolled corticotrophin secretion, named after American endocrinologist Don Nelson who described the condition in 1960

neonatal mortality rate the number of neonatal deaths per 1000 live births

nephronophthisis renal cysts that are restricted mostly to corticomedullary junction and forming most frequent genetic cause of end stage renal disease during the first three decades of life

neural therapy a treatment that uses injections of anaesthesia to remove short circuits in the body's electrical network

neuroid (nu'royd) resembling a nerve

neuroplasticity (nu'ro-pla-sti-citi) ability of the brain throughout life to recognize neural pathways based on new experiences

neuropraxia (nu'ro-prak'sia) a local block to conduction of nerve impulses at a discrete area along the course of a nerve

neurotmesis (nu'rot-me'ses) a state in which the nerve has been completely severed or so seriously disorganised that spontaneous recovery is not possible

next generation sequencing DNA sequencing that harnesses advances in miniaturization technology to simultaneously sequence multiple areas of the genome rapidly and at low cost

NICU abbreviation for neonatal intensive care unit

nidovirus positive-strand RNA virus named for its strategy of replication wherein there is formation of a nested set of messenger RNAs in the 3' position. The examples include coronavirus and torovirus

night guard a removable, custom-fitted plastic appliance that fits between the upper and lower teeth to prevent them from grinding against each other

night terror sleep disorder, occurring mainly in children, in which an individual awakens suddenly in an agitated, almost terrified state

NIH *abb* National Institute of Health

niyama (s) practice of rules laid down for the proper conduct

NNF abbreviation for National Neonatology Forum

nocebo (no'se-bo) experiencing worsening of symptoms from an inert substance

nomogram (no'mo-gra-m) a graphic image in which a straight line connects known values to find an unknown value

nomophobia (nom'o-fob'ea) fear of being out of mobile phone contact

non palpable cannot be felt by hand

nonadjuvant chemotherapy treatment of tumour with drugs before surgery to reduce the size of the tumour

non-alcoholic steatohepatitis a small group of patients with non-alcoholic fatty liver who have inflammation as well as fat on liver histology: NASH

noncoding RNAs segments of RNA that are not translated into amino acid sequences but may be involved in the regulation of gene expression

noncoplanar (non'co-plan'ar) within different planes

noninvasive (non'in-va-siv)medical technique or procedure that does not require incision or the introduction of a foreign object or needle into the body

noninvasive procedure that does not penetrate the body

nonsense mutation the alteration of a single DNA nucleotide so that the resulting codon signals a termination of translation

nonsynonymous single-nucleotide polymorphism a polymorphism that results in a change in the amino acid sequence of a protein

normal flora mixture of bacteria normally found at specific body sites

norms a fixed or ideal standard mean score for a particular age group

NRHM abbreviation for National Rural Health Mission

NRUM abbreviation for National Urban Health Mission

ns abbreviation for not significant

NSAIDs abbreviation for non-steroidal anti-inflammatory drugs

nude mouse a researcher's tool for transplant research, specially created by mutation. It does not possess a thymus gland and lacks immune system and body hair

nulltiple (nul'ti-ple) a scientific discovery published zero times

nutraceutical (nu-tre-su'ti-kal) a chemical substance considered a nutrient and used for prevention or treatment of disease

nutritive (nu'tri-tiv) pertaining to nutrition

nyasa (s) nasal therapy

O

O blood type in the ABO blood group; eye (oculus)

OA abbreviation for osteoarthritis, occipitoanterior position

object relation *psy* emotional bond between an individual and another person

objective structured clinical examination an examination based on planned clinical encounters in which the candidate interacts with a standard pattern; OSCE

occipital neuralgia pain on one side of the back of the head caused by entrapment of one or more nerves

occult blood presence of blood that can't be seen with the naked eye

occult primary malignancy a histologically proven metastatic malignant tumour with no identifiable primary on routine investigations

ombrophobia (om'bro-fo'be-a) morbid fear of rain

onomatopoeic (on'o-ma-to-poik) related to the use of words whose sound suggest their sense

onychogryphosis (ony'ko-gri-fo-sis) thickened, curved discoloured, toe-nails penetrating adjacent toes; Ram's horn nails

OP abbreviation for out-patient, osmotic pressure, occipitoposterior position

open bite *den* a malocclusion in which some teeth do not meet the opposite teeth

operational care a sustained complete response for a prolonged period

operon two or more prokaryote genes that are transcribed into a single mRNA

oppositional defiant disorder *psy* a recurring patten of negative, hostile, disobedient and defiant behaviour in a child or adolescent lasting for at least six months without serious violation of the basic rights of others

opsoclonus (op'so-clo-nus) a paraneoplastic syndrome describing rapid, chaotic conjugate spontaneous eye movements that disturb ocular fixation, associated with ataxia and other brain-stem disturbances

opsoclonus (op'so-klo'nus) rapid, chaotic, conjugate spontaneous eye movements that distort ocular fixation

optical coherence tomography an imaging technology using an infrared light to obtain cross-sectional images of tissues; OCT

optokinetic (op'to-kine-tik) a reflex that causes person's eyes to move when their field of vision moves

oral rehydration therapy the administration of fluid by mouth to prevent and correct the dehydration that is a consequence of diarrhoea; ORT

organelle (or'gan-el'ae) specialized structures within a cell which is separated from the rest of the cells by a membrane composed of lipids and proteins, where chemical and metabolic functions take place

organic food food grown with addition of only animal or vegetable fertilizers to the soil and without the use of artificial pesticides and chemical fertilizers

orgasmic disorder impairment of the ability to attain sexual climax

orlistat (or'li-stat) an agent that inhibits pancreatic and gastric lipases thereby reducing the hydrolysis of ingested triglycerides to free fatty acids in intestine

orphan drug drug that treats a rare disease

orthodeoxia (or'tho-de'oc-sia) a reduction of partial pressure of oxygen in arterial blood by 4 mm Hg or more when the patient moves from a supine to an upright position

orthognothic (or'tho-no'thik) having a face without projecting jaw

orthotic (or'th-o-tik) a device or brace to control, correct or compensate for a bone deformity

orthotropia (or'th-o-tro'pea) straight eyes without any ocular deviation

Osborn waves hypothermic (J) waves seen on the electrocardiogram in hypothermia, are rounded waves that occur immediately after the QRS complex

osmotic demyelinating syndrome severe electrolyte disturbances leading to seizures or encephalopathy

osteogen (os'te-o-jen) a bone matrix producing tissue or layer

osteopathy (os'te-o-pati) a form of manipulation of the spinal and other joints based on realignment

osteopoikilosis (os'te'o-po'i-ki-lo-sis) an autosomal dominant condition characterized by multiple, discrete round or ovoid radiodensities in cancellous bones in an asymptomatic individual; spotted bone disease

OTC abbreviation for over-the-counter

outcome research the systemic study of the effects of different therapeutic interventions on health outcomes add to outcome

outcome result of an intervention

output liquid that is excreted from the body

over bite *den* protrusion of the upper teeth over the lower teeth

overactive bladder the leakage of large amounts of urine at unexpected times, including during sleep

overlap syndrome combination of chronic obstructive pulmonary disease and sleep apnoea-hypopnoea syndrome

over-the-counter drug a drug sold lawfully without a prescription in a pharmacy or drug store; OTC

oxymoron (oxi'mo-ran) combination of contradictory or incongruous words

oxysteroid a metabolite of cholesterol

Oz abbreviation for ounce

outcome result of an intervention

ozomator (ozo-na'tur) an apparatus for generating ozone and diffusing it in the atmosphere of a room

P

P a per anum, through the anus; yearly; pulmonary arterial

PM abbreviation for post-mortem, post-meridian

pack years number of packets of cigarettes (20 in each packet) smoked per day multiplied by the years of smoking

pagophagia (fa'go-fa-zea) a common form of pica with compulsive ingestion of large amount of ice, a symptoms of iron deficiency anaemia

painful arc syndrome a disorder in which the arm can't be raised between 45 and 160 degrees laterally

Paget-Schroetter syndrome a spontaneous primary upper-extremity deep vein thrombosis noted in young healthy adult men, described, independently by von Schroetter in 1884 in Vienna and by Paget in 1875 in London

pallesthesia (pa'li-es-the'sea) loss of vibrating sensation

palliative care the holistic care of patients with advanced progressive, incurable illness, focused on the management of a patient's pain and other distressing symptoms and the provision of psychological, social and spiritual support to patients and their family

palmar fasciitis and polyarthritis syndrome a rare paraneoplastic syndrome reported mainly for ovarian cancers, presenting with polyarthritis, rapid flexor contractures of hands with palmar nodules due to palmar fasciitis

Panayiotopoulos (pan-a'yio-to-polus) syndrome benign childhood epileptic syndrome characterised by episodic symptoms comprising of ictal vomiting, eye deviation, fever, and unconsciousness.

panchakarma ayu five purification therapies consisting of emesis, purgation, enema, medication through nostril and blood letting

PANDAS disorders a group of childhood disorders associated with streptococcal infections and acronym stands for Paediatric Autoimmune Neuropsychiatric Disorders Associated with Streptococcal infections

panidrosis (pan'i-dro'sis) sweating of the entire surface of the body

pantoscopic (pan'to-skop'iik) designed to observe objects at all distances denoting bifocal lenses

parachute valve malformation of an atrio-ventricular valve in which tension apparatus springs from a single papillary muscle or muscle group

paraphenylene diamine a common ingredient in hair dye preparation, that accelerates dyeing and may be associated with local or systemic toxic effects; PPD

paraplanitis (para-pla-ni;tis) an inflammation of the peripheral part of retina and/or para plana

paraspinal line *radiol* a vertically oriented interface in a frontal chest radiograph commonly to the left of the thoracic vertebral column, extending from the aortic arch to the diaphragm

paratendinitis (para-ten'di'-ni'tis) inflammation of the investing para tendon, diagnosed by eliciting tenderness around the full circumference of the tendon

parthenophobia (par'the-r.ɔ-fo;be-a) morbid fear of girls

partial agonist a drug that does not produce maximal effects

partial pressure the pressure exerted by one of the gases in a mixture of gases

paruresis (par'yu-re'sis) inhibited urination, especially in the presence of strangers

passive smoking *see* involuntary smoking

Patau syndrome a congenital disorder associated with the presence of an extra copy of chromosome 13, named after Kalu Patau; trisomy 13

PBC practice-based commissioning; engaging practices and other primary care professionals in the commissioning of service

PDGF-1 platelet-derived growth factor-1

pedigree (pi'di-gri) lineage

peglylation (pig'ly-ka-sh'un) the process by which a polyethylene glycol moiety is attached to protein or a drug to decrease renal clearance and increase bioavailability and efficacy

pelvic floor exercises exercises to strengthen the pelvic floor

pendiculation (pen'di-ku-la'shun) stretching

penetrance the likelihood that a person carrying a particular genetic variant will have a detectably altered phenotype

penile implant an artificial device placed in the penis during surgery to restore erection

pentology of Cantrell a midline closure defect from an interference in the embryological development of the abdominal wall, presenting with lower sternal defect, abdominal wall defect, anterior diaphragm defect, pericardial defect and intracardiac defect, described by Cantrell and colleagues in 1958

percussion myotonia a persistent dimpling after a sharp blow on a muscle

perfusion imaging diagnostic study using radionuclide scanning to visualize the pattern of blood flow in the heart

pericoronitis *Dent* irritation or inflammation of the gum produced by the crown of an incompletely erupted tooth

perilipin an adipocyte-specific protein that coats lipid droplets, required for optimal lipid incorporation and release from the droplets

perimenopause (peri' men-o'pas) 5 to 10 year transitional state before menopause

perinatal mortality rate the number of still births plus neonatal deaths per 1000 total births

peripartum cardiomyopathy a type of heart muscle disease that develops during or immediately after pregnancy

persecutory delusions psy a fixed, and inflexible belief that others are persecutory delusions engaging in a plot or plan to harm an individual

persistent vegetative state a condition of life without consciousness or will as a result of brain damage.

personalised medicine tailoring of medical treatment to the individual characteristics of each patient; precision medicine

personality *psy* enduring pattern of perceiving, relating to, and thinking about one's environment and one's self

personality disorders *psy* persistent and pervasive patterns of inner experience and behavior that deviate markedly from the expectations of the individual's culture and cause significant distress or impaired functioning **antisocial p d** a pervasive pattern of disregard for-and violation of-the rights of others **avoidant p d** a pervasive pattern of social inhibition, feelings of inadequacy, and hypersensitivity to negative evaluation by others **borderline p d** a pervasive pattern of instability of interpersonal **dependent p d** a pervasive pattern of excessive need to be taken care of leading to submission and clinging behavior and fears of separation **histrionic p d** a pervasive pattern of excessive emotionality and attention seeking **narcissistic p d** a pervasive pattern of grandiosity, need for admiration, and lack of empathy for other people **obsessive-compulsive p d** a pervasive pattern of preoccupation with orderliness, perfection, and control of oneself and others at the expense of flexibility, openness, and efficiency **paranoid p d** a pervasive pattern of distrust and suspicion of others, so that their motives are seen as malevolent **schizoid p d** a pervasive pattern of detachment from social relationships, combined with a restricted range of emotional expression in interactions with other people **shizotyal p d** a pervasive pattern of social and interpersonal deficits, including acute discomfort and reduced capacity for close relationships, cognitive or perceptual distortions, and eccentricities of behavior

personalized medicine therapy customized for the individual patient

PGI Postgraduate Institute of Medical Education and Research located at Chandigarh

phacomatosis (fa'ko-ma-to'sis) the coexistence of an extensive vascular naevus and various melanocytic lesions

phaeohyphomycosis (fi'o-hif'o-mi'cosis) fungal infections by pigmented moulds or yeasts

phalilali'a (fa'li-la-liya) involuntary echoing of the last word, phrase, sentence or sound vocalized by oneself

phantom breast sensation that a surgically removed breast is still present

phlegmasia alba dolens extensive swelling of the entire leg with no tissue ischaemia

phlegmasia cerules dolens extensive deep venous thrombosis with signs of arterial insufficiency

phonics (fo'ni-ks)a system to treat the reading by treating the speech sounds associated with single letters, letter combinations and syllables

phoria (fo-rea) a latent tendency to deviate, held in control by fusion

phosphoinositides a group of membrane lipids that undergo cycles of phosphorylation and dephosphorylation through organelle-specific phosphoinositide kinases and phosphoinositide phosphatases, which leads to distinct subcellular distributions of the individual phosphoinositide species

photodynamic therapy a novel mode of treatment that uses a combination of special rays and drugs to destroy the cancerous cells

photopsin (fo'to-p'sin) colour detector inside cone cells consisting of a highly sensitivie chemical, retinol

phototherapy light therapy; the administration of bright light in order to normalize the body's internal clock or relieve deression

phronesis (fro'ne-sis)the art of knowing what to do when you don't know what to do

physician finger the finger next to the little finger; ring finger

physis (fy'sis) growing part of a bone

phytonutrient biologically active substances that give fruits and vegetables their colour, flavour, smell and natural disease resistance

Pierre-Robin syndrome micrognathia usually accompanied by a high arched palate and fore-shortened floor of mouth

piggyback a medication infusion that is attached to an already existing intravenous line

Pilates (pi'lat-es) a physical-mind method consisting of a series of non-important exercises designed by Joseph Pilates to develop strength, flexibility, balance and inner awareness

pithiatism (ti'a-ti'zum) a disorder created by suggestion and curable by persuation; hysteria

placenta accreta placenta adhering to myometrium with no intervening deciduas

placenta increta presence of placenta within the myometrium

placenta percreta presence of placental tissue in extrauterine region or on uterine serosa

planning target volume selection of appropriate beam sizes and beam arrangements, taking consideration all the possible geometrical variations to ensure the prescribed dose is actually absorbed in the clinical target volume; PTV

plasmid (pla's-mid) an extrachromosomal, self-replicating piece of DNA

plastinate (plas'ti-na't) creation of an anatomic specimen through plastination

plastination (plas'ti-na'shun) preparation of an anatomic specimen by injection of polymers into the vessels, cavities and other spaces

platypnoea-orthodeoxia syndrome a rare disorder characterized by dyspnoea and hypoxaemia when the patient is in the upright, but not the supine position

pleonaemia (ple-o-ne'mea)ncreased blood flow to the lungs that shows an increased width of pulmonary vessels radiologically

ploidy 1. total number of chromosomes that a cell has 2. amount of DNA in a given cell relative to a haploid nucleus of the same organism

pneumocephalus (nu'mo-ce'fa-lus) presence of air in the ventricles of the brain

podobromhidrosis (podo'brom-hid-ro'sis) smelly feet

polarity therapy a holistic energy-based system that includes body work, diet, exercise and life-style to flow to restore and maintain proper energy throughout the body

pollakidipsia (po'Ua-ki'dip-siya) unduly frequent thirst

pollex (po'leks) thumb

polotherapy (po'lo-the-ra'pi) a proliferative therapy that rejuvenates the body by injection of natural substances to stimulate the growth of collagen in order to strengthen weak or damaged joints, ligaments or muscles

Pomeray technique removal of part of the fallopian tubes as a sterilizing method of birth contro

Pompe disease an autosomal recessive disorder affecting glycogen storage with lysosomal accumulation of glycogen in numerous tissues manifesting in a progressive neuromuscular disorder, named after D.C. Pompe who described the condition in 1932

pontic (pon'tik) Dent an artificial tooth

population attributable risk the difference in the rate of disease between a population that is exposed to a given factor and one that is not

pornographomania (por'no-gr'a-fo'ma-nea) a form of sexual deviation where there is abnormal interest in collection or in intractable perusal of pornographic material

portCAB port-access coronary artery bypass, a surgical procedure to perform coronary artery bypass through small incisions (ports) in the chest wall; see MIDCAB

portogram (por't-o'gram) a single sheet of paper on which there is a graphic representation of progress in labour

positional cloning an approach for determining the position of a gene that when mutated causes monogenic disease

postpolio syndrome a functional deterioration after a prolonged period of stability in an individual who had acute poliomyelitis at a young age, characterised by fatigue, weakness, joint and muscle pain and worsening functional abilities

post-term neonate a neonate born any time after completion of the 42nd week, beginning with day 295

potentiation *Horn* process of increasing the power of homoeopathic preparation by successive dilutions and succession of a mother tincture

pouchitis (pow'chi-tis) nonspecific inflammation of ileal pouch developing as an immune response to the newly established microbiota

prakara (s) intense condition

prakruti ayu physical nature or constitution

pramlintide (pra'ml-in'tide) a soluble non-aggregating injectable synthetic analogue of amylin that improves glycaemic control

Prasad syndrome presence of geophagia, retarded growth, pallor, severe hypochromic anaemia, hypogonadism, chronic hepatosplenomegaly noted in males in Iran and Turkey, described by AS Prasad and colleagues in 1961

pratyaksha (s) direct perception

prebiotic living microorganisms providing health benefits beyond general nutrition following ingestion in adequate amounts

pre-embryo a human embryo or fertilized ovum in the first fourteen days after fertilization before implantation in the uterus has occurred

prehypertension a condition in which blood pressure is higher than normal (above 120/80 mm Hg but below 140/90 mm Hg), putting a person at higher risk of developing high blood pressure

premature rupture of membranes an event that occurs during pregnancy when the sac containing foetus and the amniotic fluid bursts or develops a hole prior to the start of the labour; PROM

presbycusis (pre's-bi-ku-sis) hearing loss of the higher frequencies brought on by age

presbyoesophagus (pre's-bi-eso'fa-gus) an age-related oesophageal motility dysfunction

preterm neonate a neonate born before 37 completed weeks

preventive dentistry branch of dentistry concerned with avoiding tooth decay ad gum diseases

primal scene the occasion in which a child becomes aware of its parents' sexual intercourse

primal therapy *psy* psychotherapy which focuses on a patient's earlier emotional experiences and encourages verbal expression of childhood suffering

primary care an integral part of the whole health system that ensures greater community participation, and acts as the first point of contact for health and social needs

primary end point main result measured at the end of the study to see if the treatment has worked

primary gain *psy* immediate relief from guilt, anxiety or other unpleasant feelings that a patient derives from a symptom

primary graft failure injury to the graft in lung transplantation manifesting in hypoxaemia and diffuse radiographic infiltrates associated with capillary leak into the graft; PGD

prithvi (s) earth, world

proarrhythmia increased occurrence of existing arrhythmias, a serious reaction to anti-arrhythmic medications in some people

probiotic non-digestible substances providing beneficial physiological effect on host by selectively stimulating growth or activity of a limited number of indigenous favourable bacteria

Proder-Willi syndrome a genetic defect characterized by a failure to thrive in infancy, mild learning difficulties and abnormal satiety response to food intake

prodrome (pro'dro-m) running ahead of a symptom or group of symptoms that appears shortly before an acute attack of illness

professional competence the habitual and judicious use of communication, knowledge, technical skills, clinical reasoning, emotions, values and reflection in daily practice for the benefit of the individual and the community being served

profusion radiot number of small opacities per unit area or zone of lung

projective test *psy* a type of psychological test that assesses a person's thinking patterns, observational ability, feelings and attitudes

prolabium the exposed carmine margin of lip

prolotherapy (pro'lo-ther'a-pe) use of inflammation inducing injections in periarterial soft tissue to strengthen ligaments and tendons

promoter methylation an epigenetic mechanism to regulate the expression of a gene

promoter-inactivation mutation a genetic variation in the promoter of an otherwise normal gene that results in a dramatic reduction in gene expression

propensity a greater risk for developing a disease

prostate specific antigen a protein made by the cells of the prostate that is increased by both benign prostate hypertrophy and prostate carcinoma

prostate-specific antigen a protein made by the prostate gland; PSA

prosthetist a health care rofessional who is skilled in making and fitting artificial parts for the human body

protein-activated receptor a thrombin receptor on platelets; PAR-1

proteome (pro'te-yom) locations and features of all the proteins in the body

proteome the complete set of proteins encoded by the genome

proteus syndrome a somatic mosaicism characterized by patchy or segmental overgrowth and hyperplasia of skin, connective tissue, and other tissues along with susceptibility to the development of tumours

PSA abbreviation for prostate-specific antigen

P-selectin an adhesion molecule on activated platelets and endotheli.il cells
P-s glycoprotein ligand-1 an adhesion molecule on leucocytes that o binds to P-selection; PSGL-1

pseudocavity (sud'o-cav-iti) a pulmonary nodule or mass having a central portion that is more lucent than its periphery due to presence of necrotic tissue with an increased amount of lipid with no true cavity

pseudogene (su'do-gen) a mutated form of a gene that is no longer functional, either because parts of the coding regions are missing or altered or because it is no longer transcribed

pseudogenes (sud'o-gen'us) molecular remains of broken genes, which are unable to function because of leth.il injury to their structures

pseudohypoglycemia a common artifact of measurement caused by the continued consumption of glucose by cells in the collection tube

psyche (sy'k) the human soul, mind or spirit

psychedelic (sy'ke-de'lik) relating to or denoting drugs that produce hallucinations

psychodelic (syko'del'ik) hallucinogenic LSD whose effect on the mind is to 'fathom hell or soar angelic'

psychosocial ability of the mind to adjust and relate the body to its social environment

pulp den soft innermost layer of a tooth containing blood vesels and nerves **p chamber** area within the natural crown of the tooth occupied by dental pulp

purpura fulminans (per'pu-ra-ful'mi-nans) a life threatening cutaneous haemorrhage and necrosis caused by disseminated intravascular coagulation and 4eyr\al vascular thrombosis

pus cell a neutrophil

pygmalionism (pig'ma-li'o-ni'sum) psy sexual interest in viewing or handling nude statues

pyknodysostosis (pik'no-dis'osto-sis) an autosomal recessive bone dysplasia presenting in early childhood as short limbs, characteristic facies, an open anterior fontenella, a large skull with frontal and occipital bossing and dental abnormalities

pyromania (pi'ro-ma-nea)deliberate and purposeful fire setting on more than one occasion

Q

Qi chin chi basic life energy

qigong (chee-gong) chi any practice which is concerned with exercise to get energy

qod abbreviation for every other day

quadranectomy (kwa'dran-tek'tomi) a partial mastectomy involving removal of the quadrant of the breast in which the tumour is located

quiddity (kwi'ddi-ti) the inherent nature; a distinctive feature

quietus death or something that causes death

quodque (kwod'kwe) each, every

quot op sit abbreviation for as often as necessary

R

R/O abbreviation for rule out

RAAS abbreviation for renin-angiotensinogen-angiotensin system

radiesthesia (ra'de-es'the-sea) the use of dowsing with a pendulum to diagnose and treat illness

radiofrequency ablation a technique for removing a tumour by heating it with a radiofrequency current passed through a needle electrode

radiogenics (ra'de-o-jen'iks) science of radiation

radionuclide scanning to produce a three-dimensional image by a camera that rotates around the person being examined; SPECT

rakta ayu blood *r* moksha blood letting

raktamokshna (s) method of blood letting

randomised clinical trial a study in which the participants are assigned by chance to separate groups that compare different treatments

range of movement the arc of measurable movement through which the joint moves in a single plane

RANK-1 the ligand for the receptor activator of nuclear factor

rare variant a genetic variant with a minor allele frequency of less than 1%

rasa (s) taste sensation

rasa ayu taste

rasayana (s) a substance that retains all its qualities in different ailments, seasons and acts as a tonic

reactogenicity (re-ak-to-je-ni-si'te) state of being able to produce adverse reaction

rearrangement a structural alteration in a chromosome, usually involving breakage and reattachment of a segment of chromosomal material, resulting in an abnormal configuration

recombinant DNA DNA that has been artificially engineered to include segments that were not originally part of the sequence

recreational drugs drugs taken on an occasional basis for enjoyment

redman syndrome range of orange-red discolouration of the skin, facial and periorbital oedema as a toxic reaction among children inadvertently given excess doses of rifampicin

reduce to restore a part of the body to its normal position or place as in treating a fracture or a dislocation

reefing (ref'ing) reducing the extent of a tissue by folding it and securing with sutures

refection (re-fek'shun) recovery; repair

refeeding syndrome condition occurring after feeding has restored in severely malnourished patient

reference range a set of values for an analysate being measured in a patient which is regarded as encompassing the usual maximum or minimum for the given analysate

referred pain pain felt at a site different from the location of the injured or diseased part of the body

reflexology a therapeutic method of relieving pain by stimulating predefined pressure points on the feet and hands

reiki (ree'ki) jap an ancient Japanese form of energy healing, based on premise that our physical body is alive because of the 'life force energy' that is flowing through

rejection *add* **acute** *r* occurrence during the first six months of transplantation mediated by T cell-dependent immune response **chronic allograft r** occurrence after first six months, most common cause of graft failure and non-immune factors may contribute to pathogenesis **hyperacute r** immediate graft destruction due to ABO or pre-formed anti-HLA antibodies

reparatory horn a reference book consisting of description of symptoms

replication bubble local dissociation of the DNA double helix in preparation for replication

replication fork the Y-shaped region of a replicating chromosome

replication origin the location at which DNA replication begins

representative sample a random sample of people that adequately represent the test taking population in age, gender, race and socioeconomic study

repression *psy* unconscious psychological mechanism in which painful or unacceptable ideas, memories or feelings are removed from conscious awareness or recall

respiratory arrest sudden, life-threatening stoppage of breathing

respiratory gating tracking patient's normal respiratory cycle with an infrared camera and a marker placed on the chest or abdomen

respirocyte (res'pir-o-site) artificial mechanical red blood cell

rest, rice, compression and elevation standard self-treatment routine for most strains sprains and muscle pains; RICE

restorative (res'to-ra'tiv) a substance capable of reviving consciousness or normal bodily functions

restriction enzyme an enzyme that cuts DNA at specific sites

restriction map the size and number of DNA fragments obtained after digesting with one or more restriction enzymes

retainer *den* an orthodontic appliance that is worn to stablise teeth in a new position

retainer *dent* an orthodontic appliance that is worn to stabilize teeth in a new position

reticulon proteins conserved proteins residing mainly in the endoplasmic reticulum and influencing trafficking between the endoplasmic reticulum and the Golgi complex, vesicle formation, and membrane morphogenesis

retinal-renal syndrome nephronophthisis associated with retinal degeneration

retinoic acid syndrome a complication of therapy with all-trans retinoic acid in patients with acute promyelocytic leukaemia and present with fever and respiratory distress

retreatment process of removing diseased or damaged pulp from a tooth and then filling and scaling the pulp chamber and root canals

retrograde trafficking trafficking in the direction opposite to that of anterograde trafficking

retrospective study a study that looks back in time to determine the cause of a present condition

Rett disorder *psy* the development of multiple specific defects following a period of normal functions after birth, named after Austrian Paediatrician Andreas Rett who described the condition in 1966

RHF abbreviation for right heart failure

ribosomal RNA noncoding ribonucleic acid that binds proteins to form the two subunits of the ribosome

Richter's (ri-ch-ers) **syndrome** development of aggressive large cell lymphoma during the course of chronic lymphatic leukaemia, usually associated with worsening of systemic symptoms

Rigler's sign a radiograph of pneumoperitoneum revealing both sid"s of the bowel wall

rigor mortis (ri'gor-mor'tis) cadaveric rigidity

riluzole (ri'lu-jol) a glutamate antagonist tried in motor neuron disease

rimonabant (re'mon'a-blan-t) a cannabinoid receptor antagonist leading to increased levels of serotonin and dopamine, causing decreased appetite

risk assessment a process used to determine the potential hazards of a substance

risk ratio rate of the event occurring in the treatment group: RR

RMP abbreviation for registered medical practitioner

RNA interference the inhibition of gene expression by noncoding RNA molecules

RNTCP abbreviate n for revised National tuberculosis control programme

robotic surgery use of a computerized robot to assist in surgery; may be utilized by the on-site operating team or manipulated from a distant location

rolfing (rol'fing) a treatment procedure to improve the structural alignment of the body especially in those with poor posture and low vitality

root canal *dent* the space within a tooth that runs from the pulp chamber to the tip of the root

root canal treatment *den* dental procedure that saves the outer teeth when he inside is irreparably diseased add to root canal

Rosai Dorfoman disease benign, self limited disease of unknown aetiology on a worldwide distribution seen in children and adolescents with massive symmetric painless cervical lymphadenopathy, fever, leucocytosis, raised ESR and polyclonal elevation of IgG

Rose river virus Australia's most common and widespread mosquito-borne pathogen causing debilitating polyarthritis, rash, and constitutional symptoms

rotator cuff a synthesis of the capsule of the glenohumeral joint with the tendons of the subscapular, supraspinatus, infraspinatus and teres minor muscles

ruksha (s) dry

rukshana ayu treatment producing dryness, and roughness

Rumack-Matthew nomogram to estimate the likelihood of hepatic injury due to acetominophen toxicity for patient with a single ingestion at a known time

running amok for homicidal mania developed under the influence of long continued use of cannabis where the person will kill or go on killing persons without any rhyme or reason

rupa (s) visual sensation

S

salvage therapy treatment measures taken late in the course of disease after other therapies had failure; rescue therapy

samadhi (s) final stage of bliss

samana (s) life-sustaining energy centred in the small intestine caused by side-to-side motion

samyavastha (s) normal condition

sandra (s) viscous, solid

sankalp (s) intention

sankalpa (s) determination

santarpana ayu anabolic

SAPS 2 Simplified acute physiology score, a scoring system used in critical care management to measure severity of illness

sarcopaenia (sar'ko-pe'nea) age-related loss of muscle

scaffold *add* 2. the result of connecting contigs by linking information from paired end reads from plasmids, paired-end reads from BACs, known messenger RNAs or other sources **draft genome s** the sequence produced by combining the information from the individual sequenced clones (by creating merged sequence contigs and then employing linking information to create scaffolds) and positioning the sequence along the physical map of the chromosomes **sequence-contig s** scaffolds produced by connecting sequence contigs on the basis of linking information **sequenced-clone-contig s** scaffolds produced by joining sequenced-clone contigs on the basis of linking information

schistocystis (sis'to-sis-tis) fissure of the bladder

schizencephaly (se'zen-se'fali) a rare, developmental disorder of neuronal migration in which there are clefts spanning the cerebral hemisphere which are characterized by an infolding of the grey matter along the cleft from the cortex into the ventricles epilepsy, mental retardation and presence of CSF between the clefts

schizoaffective disorder psy a mental illness that shows the psychotic symptoms of schizophrenia and the mood disturbances of depression or bipolar disorder

Schmidt's syndrome autoimmune polyendocrine syndrome type 2 with occurrence in the same individual of two or more autoimmune endocrine disorders such as Addison's disease, primary hypothyroidism, Grave's disease, pernicious anaemia, primary hypogonadism, type 1 diabetes, vitiligo, coeliac disease and myasthenia gravis

scoliometer (scko'li-o-met'er) an instrument to measure trunk asymmetry

screening practice of assessing people for the presence of a disease before the disease has a chance to develop

sealants (see'lan-ts) den protective synthetic material applied t the grinding surfaces of the teeth

seasonal affective disorder psy a mood disorder characterized by depression during the winter months

secondary end point study of other variables at the end of the study, such as side effects in the treatment group

secondary gain psy the social, occupational or interpersonal advantages that a patient derives from symptoms

secondhand smoke smoke breathed in from someone else's smoking; passive smoking, environmental tobacco smoke

self-mutilation deliberate attempt to cause injury to oneself without the conscious intent to commit suicide

senescence (se'ne-sens) the phenomenon by which normal diploid cells lose the ability to divide

sensate focus technique a therapy technique designed to treat sexual disorders

sensors (sen'sors) devices capable of detecting and measuring chemical, biological, electrical or other physical signals

sensory integration disorder a neurological disorder that results from the brain's inability to integrate certain information received from body's five basic sensory systems

sentinent (sen'ti-nent) 1. having sense perception, conscious 2. Experiencing sensation feeling

sepsis management bundle consists of administration of low-dose steroids, and recombinant human activated protein C, maximum tight glycaemic control and lung protective strategy to prevent excessive inspiratory plateau pressure, to be implemented as early as possible in patients with severe sepsis and should not be delayed for more than 24 hours after hospitalization

sepsis resuscitation bundle consists of serum lactate measurement, blood culture obtained prior to antibiotic therapy, improve time to broad-spectrum antibiotic and treatment of hypotension and/or elevated lactate, to be implemented within first six hours of hospitalization of patient with severe sepsis

sequence *add* **conserved s** a sequence of DNA or an amino acid sequence in a protein) that has remained essentially unchanged throughout evolution **draft s** DNA sequence in which the order of bases is sequenced at least four to five times, which enables reassembling of DNA fragments in their original order **finished s** complete sequence of a clone or genome, with an accuracy of at least 99.99% and no gaps **Raw s** individual unassembled sequence reads, produced by sequencing of clones containing DNA inserts

sequence motif DNA sequences whose functions can be inferred as they are similar to sequences whose function has been biologically determined

serendipity (ser'en-di'piti) making discoveries by accident and sagacity of things not sought, derived from Serendip

(Sri Lanka)

serotonin syndrome a clinical triad of mental status changes, autonomic hyperactivity and neuromuscular abnormalities, often encountered following over dose of proserotonergic agents

severe acute respiratory syndrome a highly contagious pneumonia caused by a SARS associated coronavirus (CoA), SARS

sexual assault nonconsensual sexual penetration including but not linked to sexual intercourse-achieved with physical force or the threat of physical force

sexual harassment any unwanted sexual attention in a situation where there is difference in power between the harasser and the person being harassed

shabda (s) sound

shaken baby syndrome a form of physical non-accidental injury to infants, characterised by acute encephalopathy with subdural and retinal haemorrhages, occurring in a context of inappropriate or inconsistent history and commonly accompanied by other apparently inflicted injuries

shared psychotic disorder *psy* an uncommon disorder in which the same delusion is shown by two or more individuals: folie a deux

Sharif (s) body

sharps any sharp object such as syringe needles, scalpel blades, broken test tubes, glass that my contain human blood, fluids and tissues with pathogenic organisms

sheeta (s) cold

shelterin protective protein associated with telomere DNA

shiatsu jap a manipulative therapy developed in Japan that incorporates the techniques of Japanese traditional massage, acupressure, stretching and Western massage

Shiatsu jap manipulative therapy developed in Japan consisting of traditional massage, acupressure, stretching and Western massage

short bowel syndrome a condition in which bowel is not as long as normal, either because of surgical removal or congenital defect, and bowel has less surface area to absorb nutrients to result in malabsorption syndrome

short interfering RNA a short, double-stranded regulatory RNA molecule that binds to and induces the degradation of target RNA molecules; siRNA

short-rib Polydactyly syndrome a lethal condition noted in newborn with respiratory distress, an extremely small thorax, very short extemities, Polydactyly and a variety of non-skeletal defects

shotgun sequencing an approach in which thousands or millions of short, random fragments of a DNA sample are sequenced simultaneously and then reassembled with the use of computer algorithms on the basis of matching overlapping ends

shronita (s) ovum

shukra ayu semen

Shwachman-Diamond syndrome an inherited autosomal recessive condition with exocrine pancreatic insufficiency, and variable haematologic cytopaenia due to marrow failure

sibutramine (si'bu-tra-m-in) an agent that causes reduction of weight by reducing the food intake through beta-1 adrenoceptor and 5-HT receptor agonists activity

sick building syndrome an illness related to multiple chemical sensitivity in which a person develops symptoms in response to chronic exposure to airborne environmental elements founding a tightly sealed building

signal transduction a process by which a signal is relayed to the interior of a cell where it elicits a response at the cytoplasmic or nuclear level

signaling lymphocyte activation molecule an adhesion molecule found on platelets

silhouette sign *radiol* effacement of an anatomic soft tissue border by either a normal anatomic structure or a pathologic condition

singer's nodes lumps on the vocal cords due to overuse

single nucleotide polymorphism a single nucleotide variation in a genetic sequence: SNP

single photon emission computed tomography a diagnostic test that uses

SiRNA small interfering RNA

SIRS systemic inflammatory response syndrome

sister (sis'ter) nurse in charge of a hospital ward

sitagliptin (sit-a-glip'tin) orally administered dipeptidyl peptidase-IV inhibitor

Sitz bath a warm bath in which just the buttocks and genital areas soak in water

Sjogren-Larsson syndrome a rare inborn error of metabolism caused by deficiency of enzyme fatty aldehyde dehydrogenase, characterized by triad of ichthyosis, spastic paresis, and mental retardation, described in 1957 by Sjogren and Larsson of Sweden

Sken's glands glands of the female urethra

skip lesion any lesion in which normal tissue is interspersed with tissue affected by a pathologc condition

slakshna (s) amorphous

slimsy (sli'm-si) frail

small cuff syndrome occurrence of gross error in auscultatory systolic and diastolic values when a small cuff is used to determine arterial pressures; non-hypertension

small interfering RNA a short, double-stranded regulatory RNA molecule that binds to and induces the degradation of target RNA molecules

small-for-gestational age newborns who are berrirrd the 10th percentile in height or weight for their estimated gestational age

smoking index an average number of cigarettes/bidis smoked per day multiplied by the number of years of use

SMR standardised mortality ratio; observed mortality/predicted mortality

smriti (s) memory

snap gauge a device used to diagnose erectile dysfunction by measuring erections that occur during sleep; strain gauge

snehana ayu treatment increasing viscosity, softness, moisture, fluidity of the body

snigdha (s) unctuous

SNP single nucleotide polymorphism; a single nucleotide position in the genome for which two or more alternative alleles are present at appreciable frequency in the human population

social phobia *psy* fear of being judged or ridiculed by others, fear of being embarrassed in public

somatic mutation a deleterious genetic variation occurring in any cell of the body except sperm and egg cells

somniloquist (som'ni-lo'kist) sleep talker

sos si opus sit, if needed

sounding of the uterus a procedure to measure the depth and position of the uterus

space maintainer *dent* an orthodontic appliance that is worn to prevent adjacent teeth from moving into the space left by an unerupted or prematurely lost teeth

splitting *psy* a psychological defense mechanism in which the individual deals with emotional conflict by compartmentalizing positive and negative qualities into separate parts

spnrsha (s) touch sensation

spontaneous resolution the act of a disease resolving or going away without treatment

splice-site mutation a sequence variation at or near an intron-exon boundary that perturbs normal splicing of the adjacent intron

split liver generation of two grafts from one donor liver

spurious (spu're-us) simulated, not genuine, false

ss abbreviation for single strength

stana (s) breast

standardization the process of determining

established norms and procedures for a test to act as a standard reference point for future test results

stanya (s) breast milk

stat a specimen often from the critical care unit or emergency room that is given priority in the clinical laboratory in order to measure various analytes with immediate potential impact on patient management

stella (stel'ah) star

STEMI ST elevation myocardial infarction, a severe heart attack demonstrated by a rise in ST portion of wave on an electrocardiogram

stent an expandable, 'scaffold-like' device usually of stainless steel that is inserted into an artery to expand the inner passage and improve blood flow

stereotactic radiosurgery a non-invasive surgery wherein specialised equipments can deliver a dose of high energy radiation from many directions to treat small and previously inaccessible tumours in the brain and spinal cord, or lesions deep in the body without any surgical incision; SRS

stereopsis (ste-re'op-sis) visual blending of two similar images, one following on each retina into one with visual perception of depth

stereotaxy (sti'ri-o'ta-ksi) three-dimensional target localisation

Stewrt-Treves syndrome angiosarcoma arising within chronic post-mastectomy lymphoedema described by Stewart and Treves in 1948

sthambhana ayu treatment which blocks, stops or stabilizes the flow within the body

sthira (s) steady

sthula (s) gross

Stickler's syndrome progressive near-sightedness and degenerative arthritis beginning in childhood, and inherited as an autosomal condition, described by Gunnar Stickler in 1960

stiff-person syndrome a rare neurological disorder characterised by stiffness of skeletal muscle with superimposed spans

STK1 abbreviation for serine-threonine kinase 11

stopcock (stop'kok) a valve that regulates the flow of fluid through a tube

STPD standard temperature and pressure dry, denoting a volume of dry gas at 0°C and a pressure of 760 mm Hg

stress fracture a crack in a bone" usually the result of overuse

string of pearls sign an abdominal radiograph showing small bowel obstruction that has resulted in markedly dilated small bowel revealing a line of gas bubbles trapped between the valvular conniventes

stripe *radiol* a longitudinal composite opacity with a width of 2 to 5 mm

structural gene a gene that codes for a protein or an RNA

structural genomic variation variation within the genome that results from deletion or duplication or from inversion of genomic segments

structural variant a genetic variant involving the insertion, deletion, duplication, translocation, or inversion of segments of DNA up to million of bases in length

subgroup analysis *stat* 1. evaluation of treatment effects for a specific end point in subgroups of patients defined by baseline characteristics 2. investigation of consistency of the trial conclusions among different subpopulations defined by each of multiple baseline characteristics of the patients

subsegment a unit of lung tissue supplied by a bronchus of lesser order than a segmental bronchus

subunit vaccine a vaccine containing only part of an antigen or a sequence from the viral coat instead of the whole microorganism

sudden cardiac death abrupt death from heart disese

sudor (soo'dor) sweat, perspiration

sugar daddy an adult male who exchanges

large amounts of money or gifts for sexual favours from a much younger woman

sukshma (s) subtle

sundowning the onset or exacerbation of delirium during the evening or night with improvement or disappearance during the day, often seen in Alzheimer's disease

sunrise-sunset syndrome displacement of intraocular lens as rising or setting sun

superfecundation (su'per-fe-cun'da-shun) fertilization through separate acts of intercourse of two or more ova

superfetation (su'per-fe-ta'shun) fertilization and implantation of an ovum when anther foetus is already present in the uterus

superimposition (su'per-im'posi-shun) for a technique applied to ascertain whether the photograph of a missing person could correspond and corroborate with the skull of the dead body

supernumerary marker chromosome a small chromosome containing a centromere occasionally seen in tissue culture, often in a mosaic state

surgical diathermy application of a high frequency alternating current through the body tissue and the concentration of current to produce an area of high current density liberating heat

surgical ventricular restoration surgical procedure to remodel a ventricle damaged by a heart attack or heart failure

survivin (sur'vy-vin) a unique member of the inhibitor of apoptosis protein family

Susac's syndrome retinocochleocerebral vasculopathy affecting brain, vision and hearing in adults, named after John Susac of US who described the condition in 1979

svanigraha (s) self-control

SVT abbreviation for supraventricular tachycardia

swedana ayu treatment causing perspiration

synaesthesia (sin'es-thi'sia) a sensory phenomenon of a fusion of the senses

synbiotic (syn'bi'o'tik) a combination of pre- and probiotics

synchronise (sin'kr-o-nize) make happen or exist at precisely the same time

synesthesia (sin'ees-the-sea) psy a condition in which a sensory experience associated with one modality occurs when another modality is stimulate

systemic inflammatory response syndrome a systemic inflammatory response to the invasion of microorganisms and their breakdown products; SIRS

systems biology research that takes a holistic approach to understanding organism functions

T

TAAA abbreviation for thoracoabdominal aortic aneurysm

tabloid a combination of two words tablet and ovoid

TAI abbreviation for Tuberculosis Association of India

tai chi chaun chi a Chinese soft martial art performed as a series of graceful postures one flowing into another. It provides exercise to the body and concentration to the mind

Tako-Tsubo (t'a-ko-su'ba) cardiomyopathy a rare, dreadful cardiomyopathy that is a type of non-ischaemic cardiomyopathy due to a temporary weakening of the myocardium from a weakening of myocardial vascularisation from an emotional stress, a Japanese term meaning an octopus trapping the fisherman catching octopus

tampering (tam'per-ing) to change or alter in an illicit or illegal way

tank a device made to receive and/or hold liquids

tanycyte (tan-i'site) specialised glial cell near the ependymal lining in the developing and adult nervous system

tapering gradually reducing the amount of a drug

target cells red blood cells with central staining surrounded by a ring of pallor and an outer ring of staining, noted in thalassaemia, sickle cell disease and liver disease; Mexican hat cells

target heart rate a heart rate at approximately 50 to 75 percent of a person's maximum heart rate

tarsal coalition a painful rigid flat foot deformity due to a congenital fusion or failure of segmentation between 2 or more tarsal bones and peroneal muscle spasm but without true spasticity

tau (ta-vu) a microtubule associated protein that accumulates in neurons in neurofibrillary degeneration

tautomeric (taw-tom'er-ik) relating to the same part

TDI abbreviation for total daily intake

techtodendrimer (tek't-o-den'dri-mer) multi-component nanodevices having a single core dendrimer to which additional dendrimer modules of different types are affixed

tectiform (tek'ti-form) roof shaped

tectorium (tek-to're-um) an overlying structure

tejas (s) solar power

tele doctor a software comprising a comprehensive electronic medical record to include the patient's clinical information along with personal and family history. It supports acquisition of patient's medical data in the form of image, video, audio, binary format and report

telemicroscopy (tel'e-mi-kros'ko-pe) transmission of digitized microscopic images over telecommunication network for study at a far-off place

telepathology (tel'e-pa-thol'o-je) transmission of digitized images of pathology specimens over telecommunication network for study at a far off place

teleradiology (tel'a-ra'de-ol'o-je) interpretation of digitized radiographic images transmitted by telecommunication network

telerobotic surgery a technique where robots are manipulated by telemetric method by a surgeon at a distance

telomerase (tel-o'-me'ras) a reverse transcriptase on RNA template which acts as a die and a catalytic protein

template (tem'pla-t) a single strand of DNA or RNA whose sequence serves as a guide for the synthesis of a complementary or daughter strand

tendinosis (ten'din-o-sis) sudden unexpected rupture caused by the tendon losing much of its strength

terminologia anatomica a system of anatomic nomenclature approved by the International Federation of Associations of Anatomists

terraform (te'ra-fo'rum) alteration of an environment so as to support life

TERT abbreviation for telomerase reverse transcriptase

TGF abbreviation for transforming growth factor

Th abbreviation for T-helper cell

thanatology (than'at-o-loji) scientific study of death

thenad (the'nad) toward the thenar, toward the palm

theotherapy (the'o-ther'a-pe) treatment of disease by prayer

therapeutic cloning cloning of a human embryo for the purpose of harvesting the inner cell mass

therapy _add_ **adjuvant t** use of radiation or chemotherapy to improve survival after a tumour has been treated surgically **neoadjuvant t** use of non-surgical therapy as initial treatment, such as chemotherapy or radiotherapy for cases in which surgery is a suboptimal initial approach **radiation t** use of ionising radiation to destroy cancerous cells while damaging healthy tissue as little as possible

thermic (ther'mik) pertaining to heat

thermolabile (ther'm-o-la'bil) subject to alteration or destruction by heat

thermometry (ther-mom'e-tre) measurement of temperature

thinker's sign hyperpigmented, dry, nonpruritic, hyperkeratotic plaques located on the front lower thirds of both thighs in severely deconditioned patients with chronic lung disease. The lesions arise from irritation of the skin caused by pressure from the elbows of patients who spend long period of time in the tripod position

third hand smoke inhalation of smoke that sticks around for many days or weeks after a cigarette smoked, a residue of toxins that clings to virtually all surfaces in an enclosed space long after the smoke is gone

three-dimensional conformal radiation therapy A 3- dimensional placing system to deliver radiation to the tumour; 3-D CRT

thumb sign a radiographic sign in a lateral soft-tissue radiograph of the neck, due to an enlarged and oedematous epiglottis from an acute infection

tibolone (t'bo-lo'n) a synthetic selective tissue oestrogenic activity regulator with oestogenic, progestogenic and androgenic effects

tikshna (s) fast acting, powerful

tilt slope

TIMI acronym for thrombolysis in myocardial infarction

tip a point

tissue factor a cytokine receptor analogue on the surface of cells that initiates blood coagulation and is engaged in cell signaling events **t f pathway inhibitor** a protein that when bound to factor Xa blocks the activity of the tissue factor Vila complex

tiw three times per week

TNAI abbreviation for Trained Nurses Association of India

TNF receptor-associated periodic syndrome an autosomal dominant disorder causing recurrent periodic fever, arthralgia, serositis and skin rashes with lowered serum levels of the soluble type 1 TNF receptor; TRAP, Hibernian fever

tocography (to'ko-gra'fi) an obstetric procedure to record uterine muscle contractions during childbirth

toll-like receptor transmembrane protein on the surface of immune cells that detects conserved molecular motifs known as 'microbe-associated molecular patterns' from a variety of organisms and react with several adapter proteins to activate transcription factors leading to the production of inflammatory cytokines and the activation of adaptive immunity

Toloso-Hunt syndrome unilateral eye pain, irritation or damage to the third, fourth and sixth cranial nerves due to cavernous sinus inflammation

tomography (to'mo-gra'fi) imaging procedure that shows a tissue plane

toponarcosis (top'o-nahr-ko'sis) local anaesthesia

toponymous disease disease that is named after a place

torus palatinus bony outgrowths from hard palate

traffic light system a referral system to the acute medical service. The patients in the red category are to be seen within 24 hours, those in amber category within 72 hours and those in green category are referred to the general practitioner

tragerwork (tra'ger-work) a form of therapy offering gentle manipulation to cause relaxation

trans fat fat containing fatty acids with at least one double bond in the trans configuration, found chiefly in partially hydrogenated vegetable oils used for frying and baking that has unhealthy effects on blood lipids

transcription factor a protein that binds to specific DNA sequences and thereby controls the transfer of genetic information from DNA to mRNA

transcriptome (trans'kri'p-tom) the complete set of RNAs transcribed from a genome in a particular tissue at a particular time

transference *psy* the process that develops during psychoanalysis in which the patient redirects feelings about early life figures towards analyst

transfusion-related acute lung injury non-cardiogenic pulmonary oedema complicating transfusion therapy; TRALI

transgenic organism a plant or animal that has been transfected with a foreign gene

transient amnestic syndrome an acute inability to retain new information

translation a ribosome-catalysed process whereby the nucleotide sequence of an mRNA is used as a template to direct synthesis of a protein

translational medicine work that connects laboratory-based basic sciences work and patient-related clinical practice

translocation (tra'ns-lo'ka'shun) a chromosomal segment that has been broken off and reinserted in a different place in the genome

transmyocardial laser revascularization use of a laser during heart surgery to create small channels within the muscle wall to improve the blood flow

transposons (tra'ns-po'sans) sequences of DNA that can move around within the genome of a single cell

transrectal ultrasound an imaging test in which a probe inserted into the rectum gives off sound waves to create a picture of the prostate on a screen: TRUS

transurethral microwave therapy heat therapy that uses microwave energy to destroy internal tissue; TUMT

transurethral needle ablation destruction by heat energy that directs radio waves through needles that are inserted into the prostate gland; TUNA

transurethral resection of the prostate an operation that involves removing a part of the prostate gland that surrounds the urethra: TURP

transurethral vaporization of prostate heat therapy involving a metal instrument that emits a high-frequency electrical current used to remove excess tissue from the prostate; TUVP

transverse rectus abdominis myocutaneous flap a section of muscle, skin and fat moved up for reconstruction of breast from lower abdomen to the chest area; TRAM flap

trentinoin (tre'ti-no'in) a drug that works by increasing the turnover of skin cells

treponation (tri'p-o-na-shun) drilling of a hole in the skull to relieve distress

trepopnea (tre'p-op-nia) occurrence of dyspnoea when the patient is lying on one side, but not the other. It usually occurs when there is an abnormality in only one lung resulting in a lateralized ventilation-perfusion mismatch or shunt, and atrial defects including patent foramen ovale

trinucleotide (tri'nu-kle-o'tide) a polymer consisting of three nucleotides

triolism (tri'o-li-sum) psy a form of sexual deviation where sexual pleasure is obtained when a man either shares his wife or girl friend with another man

triple screen a blood test offered to a pregnant woman by 16th and 18th weeks of pregnancy to help to identify if the unborn baby is at risk for defects

triplet repeat sequences of three nucleotides that are repeated in tandem on the same chromosome a number of times

triploidy (tri-p'loi-di) condition in which an individual has three entire sets of chromosomes instead of the usual two

trisomy condition of having three identical chromosomes instead of the normal two in a cell

trituration Horn process of diluting an insoluble substance by grinding it to make a powder and mixing it with lactose powder

tRNA abbreviation for transfer RNA

tropia a constant ocular malalignment

tsunami (tso'nah-mea) a monster sea wave triggered by seismic activity which temporarily rearranges the coastline triggered by seismic activity which temporarily rearranges the coastline

TT abbreviation for tetanus toxoid

tube feedings delivery of nutrients either a special liquid formula or pureed food through tube directly into the gastrointestinal tract

tui na chi Chinese therapeutic massage

tumefactive demyelination presence of demyelioaiing plaques >2 cm in diameter with atypical features of multiple sclerosis

tumour lysis syndrome metabolic consequences resulting from the sudden release of potassium, phosphates and purine metabolites from tumour cells undergoing sell death and is classically associated with acute lymphocytic lymphoma or Burkitt's lymphoma

turn over time time needed for a metabolite, nutrient, therapeutic agent, toxin or other substances to be either completely removed from the system or replaced by more of the same substance

Twiddler syndrome displacement of pacemaker leads due to twisting of the pacemaker box

twin-twin reverse arterial perfusion sequence a condition in which one foetus lacks a heart and the other foetus pumps the blood for both

twin-twin transfusion syndrome a condition in monochorionic twins in which there is a connection between the two circulating systems so that the donor twin pumps the blood to the recipient twin without a return of blood to the donor: TTls

typing classification according to type

tzanck preparation procedure in which skin cells from a blister are stained and examined under microscope

U

udana (s) life-sustaining energy centres in the diaphragm causing upward motion

UDPG abbreviation for uridine diphosphoglucose

UFH abbreviation for unfractionated heparin substance accelerating the ability of antithrombin III to inactive fraction Ha, Xa and IX

uha (s) speculation

UKPDS the United Kingdom Prospective Diabetes Study demonstrating treatment with either an ACE inhibitor or a beta blocker in patients with type 2 diabetes improve clinical outcomes and reduced risk of myocardial infarction

ulegyria (yu'le-giy're-a) a defect of the cerebral cortex showing narrow and distorted gyri

ULN abbreviation for upper limit of normal

underbite an abnormal protrusion of the lower jaw beyond the upper

undinism *psy* sexual pleasure by witnessing the act of urination of some one else on the same or opposite person

unethical (un'ethi-kul) professional conduct which fails to conform to the moral standards or polices

unfolded protein response a response in the endoplasmic reticulm to the accumulation of unfolded proteins in its lumen through the activation of an adaptive response, which is aimed at coping with the increased lead in the endoplasmic reticulum and activates intracellular signal transduction pathways

Universal precaution a set of procedural directions and guidelines on universal blood and body fluid precautions published by US Centers for Disease Control and Prevention

Uranism (ur'a-ni-sum) *psy* a form of sexual perversion where is sexual gratification is obtained by fingering, fondling, even sucking of the genitalia of the opposite sex

Urbach-Wiethe disease a rare autosomal recessive disease with lipoid proteinosis, described by Urbach et Wiethe, characterised by deposition of an amorphous hyaline substance in the skin, mucosa and several internal organs

ureteral stenting threading of thin catheter into segments of the ureter

urinoma (u'ri-n'oma) perinephric swelling caused by leaks in the renal collecting system

uroflowmetry (uro'flo-met-ri) measurement of force of urine flow

urolagnia (uro'lag-nea) *psy* sexual arousal through the sight and odour of urine

urorrhoea (u'ro-re'ah) involuntary flow of urine

V

vajikarana ayu virilification therapy

valid (val'id) effective; producing the desired result

vallate (val'at) bordered with an elevation

valviform (val'vi-form) valve-shaped

vamana ayu vomiting

van Creveld syndrome a rare short limbed disproportionate dwarfism characterized by postaxial polydactyly, severe skeletal, oral, mucosal and dental anomalies, nail dysplasia and presence of congenital cardiac defects, described in 1940 by Richard Ellis and Simon Van Creveld; chondroectodermal dysplasia

variables (var'i-aba-ls) individual characteristics that must be considered in designing an appropriate treatment plan

varicosis (var'i-ko'sis) a dilated state of a vein

variegated (var'i-gae'ted) patchy variation in colour

variegation (var'e-e'ge'shun) alteration of a phenotype produced by a change in the genotype during somatic development

Varivax a vaccine for the prevention of chickenpox

vasana (s) passion

vascular endothelial growth factor a chemical substance that can stimulate growth of new blood vessels; VGEF

vasolabile (va'so-la'bil) active vasomotion of blood vessels

vasotomy (va-sot-o-me) incision into the vas deferens

vasotoria (va'so-to're-a) the tone of blood vessels, particularly arterioles

vayu ayu air

VBAC *abb* vaginal birth after cesarean

vector the ability to acquire, maintain and transmit an infectious agent v **competence** the ability to acquire, maintain and transmit an infectious agent

veerya ayu potency

vegetative stage a coma-like state characterized by open eyes and the appearance of wakefulness

VEGF abbreviation for vascular endothelial growth factor

venation (ve-na'chun) arrangement and distribution of veins

veneer (ve-ner) 1. a thin surface laid over a base of common material 2. *Dentistry* a layer of tooth-coloured material such as porcelain or composite resin attached to and covering the surface of a natural tooth or a metal crown

venenation (ven'a-na'shun) poisoning, as from a sting or bite

Venn diagram pictorial representation of the extent to which two or more constituent quantities or concepts are mutually inclusive or exclusive

venous access introduction of a needle into a vein for purpose of withdrawing blood or administering medication

ventricular assist device a mechanical device that bolsters the heart's ability to pump blood into circulation

vermilion border the line between the lip and the skin

very low birth weight a newborn whose weight is less than 1500 gm

vesica pudica inability to initiate urine flow when other person is watching or waiting in public toilets; shy bladder

vibex (vi'beks) 1. a line or streak 2. a linear subcutaneous effusion of blood

vidagliptin (vid-a'glip-tin) a dipeptidyl peptidase-IV inhibitor

videoconsultation a facet of telemedicine in which video images are transmitted to an expert located at a distance from the patient

vipaka ayu end product of food

virago woman of strength

virechana ayu purgation therapy

virogenetic (vi'ro-je-net'ik) having a viral origin; caused by a virus

virosis (vi'ro-sis) a disease caused by a virus

virtue ethics (var'tu e'thi-ks) a habitual training of physician in compassion, discernment, trustworthiness, integrity and conscientiousness

virucidal capable of destroying a virus

virucide an agent that destroys a virus

viruliferous (vir'yu-lif'er-us) conveying virus

virustatic (vi'ro-stat'ik) 1. inhibiting the replication of viruses 2. an agent that inhibits the replication of viruses

visage (vi'saj) face

visile (v'si-le) relating to vision specifically denoting the type of mental imagery in which the person recalls most readily that which he has seen

vitality (vi-tal'i-te) vital force, energy

vitiolage (vi'ti-o-laj) for throwing of strong sulphuric acid or any concentrated mineral acids, corrosives over the face or body of the victim for the purpose of disfiguring the face, destroying vision or causing injury on the body; acid attack

VL *abb* viral load

vulnerary (vul'ner-a-ri) a substance that promotes cell growth and repair in the case of wounds

vulvodynia chronic burning and/or pain in the vulva without objective physical findings

vyan(s) life-sustaining energy centred in the heart and lung in life force governing circular motion

W

w reduction purposeful weight loss in order to improve health or appearance

Wadia-Swami syndrome rapidly progressive spinocerebellar degeneration associated with abnormal — eye movements and progressive mental deterioration, described by NH Wadia and RK Swami

WAGR syndrome acronym for Wilms' tumour, aniridia, genitourinary anomalies and mental retardation syndrome

waist-to-hip ratio a formula for determining potential health risks based on measurements of abdominal fat using a ratio of waist size over hip size

Walker-Warberg syndrome a condition of lissencephaly with retinal coloboma, non-attachment of retina, micro-ophthalmia

and cataract; WWS

walking (va'king) movement in one direction, as propelled by the legs and feet w aids any device that helps a person walk, either temporarily or permanently

wallet neuropathy neuropathy due to sitting on a fat wallet for long periods that causes compression of nerves in gluteal region

watchful waiting a form of management in which the disease is closely monitored

water testing any test performed on drinking water, usually to detect microorganisms, particularly those originating from improperly processed sewage

waterbrash flow of saliva and gastric acid backup the oesophagus and into the throat or lungs

Water's position a position used to visualize the maxillofacial bones and maxillary sinuses and determine the patency of the maxillary sinuses in which the patient is placed at a 37 degree angle with the orbitomental line perpendicular to the mid-sagittal plane

WDHA syndrome a syndrome presenting with watery diarrhoea, hypochloraemia and achlorhydria

webbing (wen'ing) a congenital condition wherein adjoining structures are joined by a broad band of tissue

Wechsler intelligence test a series of standard tests used to evaluate cognitive abilities and intellectual abilities in children and adults

weight the measurable heaviness of a person or object w loss loss of body weight

well baby care periodic health supervision for infants and children to promote optimal physical, emotional, and intellectual growth and development

wellness (wel'nes) fitness with physical and mental wellbeing

Western blotting the transfer of protein from a polyacrylamide gel to a piece of nylon filter paper

wheal and flare reaction a rapid response to a skin allergy characterized by the development of a red itchy spot in the area where the allergen is injected

WHIM syndrome an autosomal dominant disorder characterized by warts, hypogammaglobulinaemia, infections and myelokanthexis

white coat hypertension a temporary increase in blood pressure during a medical checkup

Whitmore-Jewett staging system a classification system for prostate cancer using the categories A, B, C, or D

whonamedit biographical dictionary of medical eponyms

wildcrafting (vild'kraf-ting) gathering of herbs or other natural materials

wilderness medicine prevention, diagnosis and treatment of injuries and medical conditions that may develop during activities in remote territories

Williams syndrome a rare neurodevelopmental disorder exhibiting 'eflin' facies, a low nasal brige, an unusual cheerful demeanor, neurodevelopmental delay, supravalvular aortic stenosis, and narrowing of the pulmonary artery, described by New Zealander J Williams and colleagues in 1961

Williams-Beuren syndrome a gene deletion disorder presenting with mental retardation, growth retardation, facial abnormalities such as flat nasal bridge, short upturned nose, periorbital puffiness, long fultrum, and delicate chin, friendly personality, hypertension and supravalvular aortic stenosis

window operation cutting out a large oval shaped piece of the cyst wall and putting in stitches to create a window so that cyst cannot recur

witch milk galactorrhoea in new born

WMA abbreviation for World Medical Association

woman who fall syndrome stumbling and falling without apparent reason noted only in females beginning in late childhood

work up 1. the constellation of procedures including obtaining the patient's medical history, performing a physical examination, and ordering and evaluating laboratory tests and imaging procedures upon which diagnosis and therapy are based 2. to evaluate a patient

workaholic (werk-a-hol'ic) person showing a compulsive need to work

working diagnosis a diagnosis based on experience, clinical epidemiology and confirmatory evidence provided by ancillary studies

wrapping (rap'ing) the process of putting a cover around a thing

wrist band an identifying label attached to a patient's wrist at the time of admission to a hospital

X

x abbreviation for times

XDR extremely drug resistant, applied to tuberculosis

XDR-TB extensively drug resistant tuberculosis; MDR-TB that is also resistant to any fluoroquinolone, and to at least one of three injectable second line anti-tuberculosis drugs (capreomycin, kanamycin, amikacin) *remove the one already present

xeromycteria (zer'o-mik-ter'e-a) dryness of the nasal mucus membrane

ximalagatran (si'mal'a-ga'tran) a orally active direct thrombin inhibitor

X-knife system a high-tech radiation treatment for brain tumours and the knife performs a method of zapping brain tumours with highly focussed, high-dose beams of radiation generated by a linear accelerator

XL abbreviation for extended release

Y

yama (s) rules for self conduct

ygiagam acronym for your guess is as good as mine

Yuzpe regimen a form of emergency contraception in which two oral contraceptive pills that contain oestrogen and progestin hormones are taken to prevent pregnancy

Z

zar *psy* experiences of spirits possessing an individual

zemblanity (gem'bla-niti) opposite of serendipity, from the name of Russian Arctic island, Nova Zembla, a cold barren land, making unhappy, unlucky and expected discoveries occurring by design

zetocrit (jet-o-krit) a method to determine erythrocyte sedimentation rate, that is not affected by haematocrit, fibrinogen or immunoglobulin, and there is no male and female difference; zeta sedimentation rate

Zika virus a flavivirus causing human infection, named after Zika forest, Uganda where virus was isolated in 1947

zin zhuang chi a powerful and popular form of Chinese system of exercise

zinc finger a structural motif found on many DNA-binding proteins that requires a zinc atom for activation

zoacanthosis (jo'kan-tho-sis) a cutaneous eruption due to introduction into the human skin of hair, bristles, stinger of animals

zombies a soulless corpse that is raised from the grave and given a half life

zonary (zo'ne-re) zonal

zone of equivalence a region in an antigen-antibody reacting system where the ratio of antigen to antibody is equivalent value

zoning (zon'ing) the occurrence of a stronger fixation of complement in a lesser amount of suspected serum

Tables & Appendices

TABLE A : ABO Blood Groups

Blood group	antigens in red blood cells	antibodies in serum
A	A	anti B
B	B	anti A
AS	A and B	none
O	neither A nor B	anti A and anti B

TABLE B : Apgar Score (after 60 seconds)

points	parameters
1	pale skin, limp, absent respiratory effort, absent heart rate, no reaction to nasal catheter
2	rosy trunk with blue extremities, good motor tone in limbs, slow, irregular respiratory effort, heart rate <100, makes grimaces to the nasal catheter
3	rosy skin, active movement, good respiratory effort, heart rate >100, coughing or sneezing to nasal catheter

Normal range 8-10 points

TABLE C : Cerebrospinal Fluid (CSF)

colour	clear. colourless
volume	130 ml
specific gravity	1005
reaction	alkaline
pressure	60-180 mm of fluid (lying)
	200-250 mm of fluid (sitting)
rate of flow	3 drops/sec
proteins	40 mg/dL
sugar	60 mg/dL
chlorides	720 mg/dL
cells	2-5 cells/cmm, mostly lymphocytes

TABLE D : Cranial Nerves

I	olfacatory		sensory
II	optic		sensory
III	oculomotor		motor
IV	trochlear		motor
V	trigeminal		
		ophthalmic	sensory
		maxillary	sensory
		mandibular	mixed
VI	abducens		motor
VII	facial		mixed
VIII	vestibulocochlear		sensory
IX	glossopharyngeal		mixed
X	vagus		mixed
XI	accessory		motor
XII	hypoglossal		motor

TABLE E : Development of Foetus

gestation age (in weeks)	weight (in grams)	development
12	45	full formation of limbs, sex distinguishable externally
16	200	full formation of body, closed eyelids
20	400	passage of meconium, vernix on brow and chin
24	820	development of epidermis on palms and soles lanugo over the body
28	1000	slight opening of eyelids, maturation of lungs
32	1800	pink smooth skin, increase of vernix, growth of finger nails
36	2500	descent of testes, shedding of lanugo, well formed subcutaneous tissue
40	3000	full development

TABLE F : WHO Performance Scale

Grade	Description
0	fully active, can carry out all functions without restriction
1	restricted in sternuous activity, ambulatory, can carry out light work
2	ambulatory and capable of self care but unable to carry out work activities up and about for more than 50% of working hours
3	capable of limited self-care; confined to bed/chair for more than 50% of working hours
4	completely disabled; confined to bed/chair

TABLE G : Signs and Symbols

±	positive or negative	Mx	molar, mole/litre)
>	greater than	m	metre, meta
<	less than	mg	milligram
°C	degree Celsius	mg/dl	mg/100 ml
Ci	curie	min	minute(s)
cm	centimetre	ml	millilitre
cm²	square centimetre	mM	millimolar, mmole/litre
cm³	cubic centimetre	mm	millimetre
Cx	complaints	N	normal
dL	decilitre	n	nano, nanometre
Dr	doctor	NA	not applicable
g	gram, gravity	o	ortho
h	hour(s)	P	para
H & E	Haematoxylin and eosin (stain)	po	per oral
1M	intramuscular	R	Roentgen
IU	international unit	rpm	resolution per minute
IV	intravenous	SC	subcutaneous
kg	kilogram	sec	second(s)
L	litre	wk	week(s)
M	mega	yr	year(s)

TABLE H : Classification of Blood Pressure Levels
(according to British Hypertension Society)

category	systolic blood pressure (mm Hg)	diastolic blood pressure (mm Hg)
Blood Pressure		
optimal	<120	<80
normal	<130	<85
high normal	130-139	85-89
Hypertension		
Grade 1 (mild)	140-159	80-90
Grade 2 (moderate)	160-179	100-109
Grade 3 (severe)	>180	>110
Isolated systolic hypertension		
Grade 1	140-149	<90
Grade 2	>160	<90

TABLE I : International Classification of Diseases (ICD)
10th revision arranged in 21 major chapters

I	Certain infectious and parasitic diseases (A00-B99)
II	Neoplasms (C00-D48)
III	Diseases of the blood and blood forming organs and certain disorders involving the immune mechanisms (D50-D89)
IV	Endocrine, Nutritional and Metabolic diseases (E00-E90)
V	Mental and behavioural disorders (F00-F99)
VI	Diseases of the nervous system (G00-G99)
VII	Diseases of eye and adnexa (H00-H59)
VIII	Diseases of the ear and mastoid process (H60-H95)
IX	Diseases of the circulatory system (F00-I99)
X	Diseases of the respiratory system (J00-J99)
XI	Diseases of the digestive system (K00-K99)
XII	Diseases of the skin and subcutaneous system (L00-L99)
XIII	Disease of the musculoskeletal system and connective system (M00-M99)
XIV	Diseases of the genitourinary system (N00-N99)
XV	Pregnancy, childbirth and puerperium (000-099)
XVI	Certain conditions originating in perinatal periods (P00-P96)
XVII	Congenital malformations, deformities and chromosomal abnormality (Q00-Q99)
XVIII	Symptoms, signs and abnormal clinical laboratory findings not elsewhere classified (R00-R95)
XIX	Injury, poisbning and certain other consequences of external causes (S00-T98)
XX	External causes of morbidity and mortality (V01-V98)
XXI	Factors influencing health status and contact with health services (Z00-Z99)

In the coding system, the first character of the ICD-10 code a letter and each letter is associated with a particular chapter except for the letter D.

TABLE J : Motor Weakness-grading

0	total paralysis (no movement)
1	presence of a slight flicker of the contraction of muscle without any associate movement at a joint
2	a normal range of power when the opposing force of gravity is removed by appropriate position
3	a normal range of power against gravity but not against resistance 4-movement against a mild degree of resistance
4	a normal range of power against moderate resistance 4+ movement against strong resistance
5	normal or full power

TABLE K : Primary Skin Lesions

lesion	description
macule	circumscribed area of altered color without any elevation
papule	circumscribed eruptions of < 0.5 cm
vesicle	fluid-filled small blister < 0.5 cm
bulla	vesicle > 0.5 cm
pustule	vesicle containing pus
plaque	confluence of papules with flat top
nodule	large, solid, deep-seated round mass > 1 cm
wheal	elevated lesion with central pallor and red margin
scale	desicated thin plate of cornified epidermal cell

TABLE L : TNM Staging of Lung Cancer

T (primary tumour)

TX	primary tumour cannot be determined
TO	no evidence of primary tumour
Tis	carcinoma in situ
T1-T4	increasing size and/or extent of primary tumour

N (regional lymph nodes)

NX	regional lymph nodes cannot be determined
NO	absence of involvement of regional lymph nodes
N1-N3	increasing firmness, fixation of lymph nodes

M (metastasis)

MX	presence of metastasis cannot be determined
MO	absence of metastasis
M1	existence of metastasis to lung (PUL), bone (OSS), liver (HEP), brain (BRA), lymph nodes (LYM), bone marrow (MAR), rib (PLE), peritoneum (PER), skin (SKI), other organs (OTH)

TABLE M : Coagulation Factors

I	fibrinogen
II	prothrombin
III	thromboplastin
IV	calcium (obsolete term)
V	proaccelerin (obsolete term)
VI	accelerin (obsolete term)
VII	proconvertin (obstolete term)
VIII	a composite three separate proteins
VIII-C	low weight component with coagulant activity
VIII-Ag	antigenic portion molecule
VIII-R; RC	supports risttocetin-initiated platelet aggregation
VIII-v WF	von Willebrand factor, platelet adhesion
IX	Christman factor, plasma thromboplastin
X	Stewart-Prowel factor
XI	plasma thromboplastin antecedent
XII	Hageman factor
XIII	Laki-Lorand factor, fibrinoligane

National Immunization Schedule (NIS)

Vaccine	When to Give	Dose	Route	Site	Disease Protected
Pregnant Women					
TT-1	Early in Pregnancy	0.5 ml	Intra-muscular	Upper-arm	Tetanus
TT-2	4 weeks after TT-1	0.5 ml	Intra-muscular	Upper-arm	Tetanus
TT- Booster	if received 2 TT doses in a pregnancy within the last 3 year*	0.5 ml	Intra-muscular	Upper-arm	Tetanus
Infants					
BCG	At birth or as early as possible till one year of age	0.1 ml (0.05ml until 1 month)	Intra-dermal	Left Upper-arm	Tuberculosis
Hepatitis B	At birth or as early as possible within 24 Hours.	0.5 ml	Intra-muscular	Antero-lateral aspect of mid- thigh	Hepatitis B (Jaundice)
OPV 0	At birth or as early as possible within the first 15 days	2 Drops	Oral	Oral	Poliomyelitis
OPV 1,2,&3	At 6 weeks, 10 weeks, & 14 weeks.	2 Drops	Oral	Oral	Poliomyelitis
DTP 1,2,& 3	At 6 weeks, 10 weeks, & 14 weeks.	0.5 ml	Intra-muscular	Antero-lateral aspect of mid-thigh	Diphtheria,Tetanus,Pertussis (Whooping Cough)
Hepatitis B 1,2,&3****	At 6 weeks, 10 weeks, & 14 weeks.	0.5 ml	Intra-muscular	Antero-lateral aspect of mid-thigh	Hepatitis B (Jaundice)
Measles	9 completed months-12 months. (give up to 5 years in not received at 9-12 months age), 2 dose at 16-18 months.	0.5 ml	Sub-cutaneous	Right Upper-arm	Measles
Vitamin A 1st Dose	At 9 months with measles	1 ml (1 Lakh IU)	Oral		Vitamin A deficiency

Source: IAP Guidelines on Immunization, 2013-14 (modified)

994

995

Children

DPT Booster	16-24 Months	0.5 ml	Intra - Muscular	Antero-lateral aspect of mid-thigh	Diphtheria, Tetanus, Pertussis (Whooping Cough)
OPV Booster	16-24 Months	2 drops	Oral	Oral	Poliomyelitis
Japanese Encephalitis **	16-24 Months with DPT/OPV booster	05 ml	Sub-cutaneous	Left Upper-arm	Japanese Encephalitis
Vitamin A *** (2nd to 9th dose)	16 months with DPT/OPV booster Then, one dose every 6 months up to the age of 5 years	2 ml "(2 Lakh IU)	Oral	Oral	Vitamin A deficiency
DT Booster	5-6 Year & 16 Years	0.5 ml	Intra-muscular	Upper-arm	Tetanus
Pentavalent 1,2,&3	6,10,14 Weeks	0.5 ML	Intra-muscular thigh	Antero-lateral aspect of	Diphtheria, Tetanus, Pertussis, Haemophilus influenza Type B, Hepatitis B infactions.

* Give TT-2 or Booster doses before 36 weeks of pregnancy. However, give these even if more than 36 weeks have passed. Give TT to a woman in labour, if she has not previosly received TT

** SA 14-14-2 Vaccine, in select endemic districts after the campaign.

*** The 2 nd to 9th doses of Vitamin A can be administred to children 1-5 Years old during biannual rounds, in collaboration with ICDS.

**** in select states, districts and cities.

***** Pentavalent Vaccine introduced in place of DPT and Hepatitis B 1,2 and 3 in salected States.